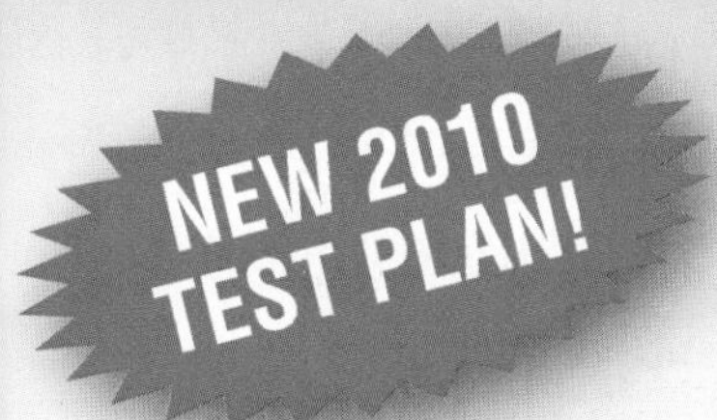
NEW 2010
TEST PLAN!

A guide to...

DAVIS'S Q & A FOR THE NCLEX-RN® EXAMINATION

KATHLEEN A. OHMAN,
EdD, MS, RN, CCRN

Your complete roadmap to NCLEX-RN® success!

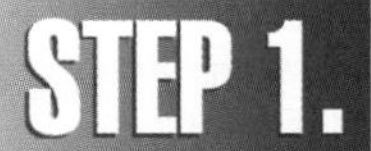
STEP 1.

DEVELOP YOUR PERSONAL COURSE OF ACTION.

- Read the Preface as well as Chapters 1 and 2 to familiarize yourself with the exam and the 2010 Test Plan.
- Review the test-taking strategies in Chapter 3 to build your confidence.
- Check out the tips in Chapter 4 for international and repeat test takers.
- Listen to the five exam-prep audio podcasts online at Davis*Plus*. (See next page for details.)

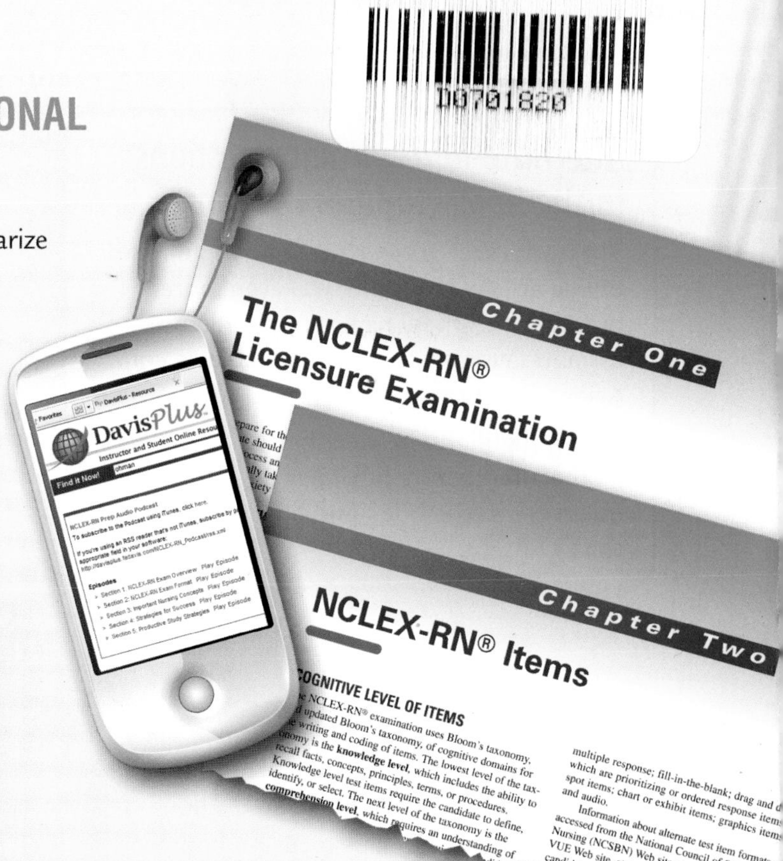
Davis*Plus*
Chapter One
The NCLEX-RN® Licensure Examination
Chapter Two
NCLEX-RN® Items
COGNITIVE LEVEL OF ITEMS

OVER 5,000 QUESTIONS IN ALL!

More alternate-item-format questions than any other NCLEX-RN® review product. **How many? 1,370!**

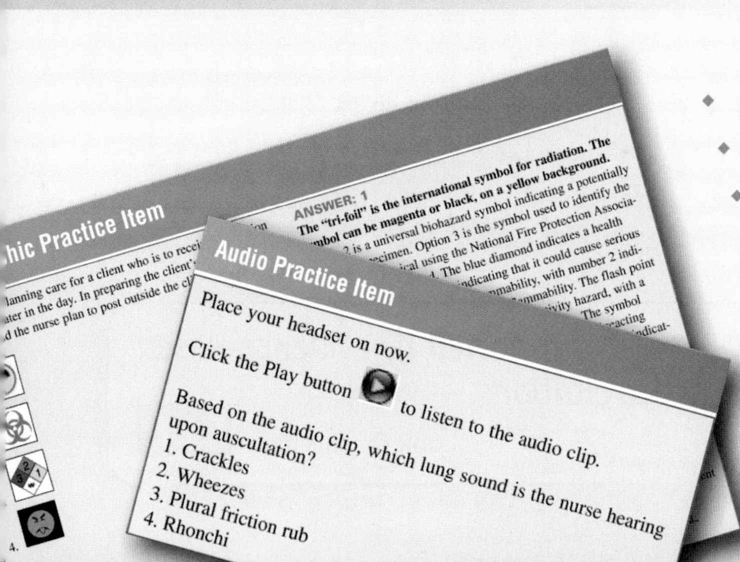
Audio Practice Item
Place your headset on now.
Click the Play button to listen to the audio clip.
Based on the audio clip, which lung sound is the nurse hearing upon auscultation?
1. Crackles
2. Wheezes
3. Plural friction rub
4. Rhonchi

- Multiple Choice
- Multiple Response
- Fill in the Blank
- Drag and Drop (Prioritized or Ordered Response)
- Chart/Exhibit
- Hot Spot
- **New Alternate Format!** Graphic
- **New Alternate Format!** Audio

STEP 2. HONE YOUR SKILLS AND BUILD YOUR KNOWLEDGE BASE.

- Cover the answer column with the bookmark.
- Compare your response to the correct answer.
- Study the rationale for the answer.
- Review the test-taking tip to help you select an option when you are unsure of the response.
- Check out how the question corresponds to the categories on the Test Plan.
- Use the references to find more in-depth explanations of the topic.
- Refer to the citations that support evidence-based practice.

Question categories mirror the 2010 Test Plan

Each question is identified by its Content Area, Category of Health Alternation, Integrated Processes, Client Need category and subcategory, and Cognitive Level.

812 SECTION II Practice Tests

3. Two patient care assistants (PCAs) are helping a client with left-sided weakness to get up from a chair and return to bed. Based on the illustration provided, which action by a nurse observing this transfer is *best*?

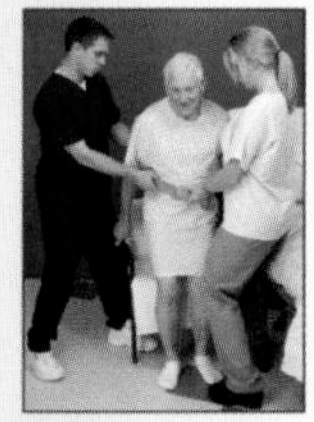

1. Intervene because the chair is incorrectly placed for transferring the client back to bed
2. Compliment the female PCA because she is supporting the client's weak side
3. Compliment the male PCA because he is using a wide base of support
4. Praise the client for using his hand for support on the chair to help prevent a fall

ANSWER: 1

To transfer a client with left-sided weakness back to bed, the client's strong side (not the weak side) should be toward the bed. Though the female PCA is supporting the client's weak side, the male PCA is using a wide base of support, and the client is using the strong side to push from the chair, complimenting and praising are not the best actions to protect the client from injury.

▸ *Test-taking Tip: Select the option that uses ergonomic principles in transferring a client safely. Note three options are similar (complimentary) and one is different.*

Content Area: Fundamentals; *Client Need:* Safe and Effective Care Environment/Safety and Infection Control; *Integrated Processes:* Nursing Process Implementation; *Client Need:* Safe and Effective Care Environment/Safety and Infection Control/Ergonomic Principles; *Cognitive Level:* Analysis

Monahan, F., Sands, J., Neighbors, M., Marek, J., & Green, C. (2007). *Phipps' Medical-Surgical Nursing: Health and Illness Perspectives* (8th ed., pp. 1433–1434). St. Louis, MO: Mosby.

Alternate-item-format questions in the book…and in real time

The audio and graphic questions you'll find online at Davis*Plus* offer you even more practice with these new, alternate-item-formats. Visit http://davisplus.fadavis.com. Keyword: Ohman.

Yellow highlighting identifies all the alternate-item-format questions in the book and on the CD-ROM.

Multiple-Response Practice Item

Which actions should be taken by a nurse when caring for a client who is experiencing dyspnea due to heart failure and chronic obstructive pulmonary disease (COPD)? SELECT ALL THAT APPLY.

1. Apply oxygen 6 liters per nasal cannula
2. Elevate the head of the bed 30 to 40 degrees
3. Weigh the client daily in the morning
4. Teach the client pursed-lip breathing techniques
5. Turn and reposition the client every 1 to 2 hours

ANSWER: 2, 3, 4

Elevating the head of the bed will promote lung expansion. Daily weights will assess fluid retention. Fluid volume excess can increase dyspnea and cause pulmonary edema. Pursed-lip breathing techniques allow the client to conserve energy and slow the breathing rate. Options 1 and 5 are incorrect actions. Applying greater than 4 liters of oxygen per nasal cannula is contraindicated for COPD. High flow rates can depress the hypoxic drive. Because the client with COPD suffers from chronically high CO_2 levels, the stimulus to breathe is the low O_2 level (a hypoxic drive). The situation does not warrant turning the client every 1 to 2 hours. This activity could increase

▸ ***Test-taking Tip:** A multiple-response item requires selecting all of the options that relate to the information provided in the question. Focus on the client's dyspnea and the interventions applicable to both heart failure and COPD.*

Respiratory Management; *Integrated Processes:* Nursing Process Implementation; *Client Need:* Physiological Integrity/Physiological Adaptation/; *Cognitive Level:* Analysis

Reference: ...s, S., Heitkemper, M., Dirksen, S., O'Brien, P., & Bucher, L. (2007). ...*d Nursing: Assessment and Management of Clinical Problems* (7th ed., pp. 640–649, 829). St. Louis, MO: Mosby.

EBP **Evidence-Based Practice (EBP) Reference:** ...ociation of ... *in Individuals with Chronic Obstructive Pulmonary Disease (COPD)*. Toronto, ON: Author. Available at: www.guideline.gov/summary/summary.aspx?doc_id=7008&nbr=004217&string=copd

More than just test-taking tips

Detailed test-taking tips focus on how to read the question for clues to the action required for specific question types and what information is relevant.

Nursing-specific references

Quickly locate sources for in-depth explanations of the content being tested.

Questions supported by evidence-based practice citations.

Look for this icon 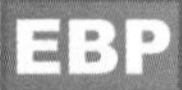

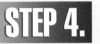

STEP 3. EVALUATE YOUR PROGRESS

- Take the two, 75-question, comprehensive exams that cover all of the content in the book.
- Analyze your performance to identify areas for additional study.

STEP 4. ASSESS YOUR STRENGTHS AND WEAKNESSES.

- 5,000 + questions on the BONUS CD-ROM test your nursing knowledge and skills.
    - Take a comprehensive, 275-question exam, or...
    - Design your own exams.
    - Use the diagnostic program on the CD-ROM to evaluate your performance.

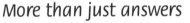

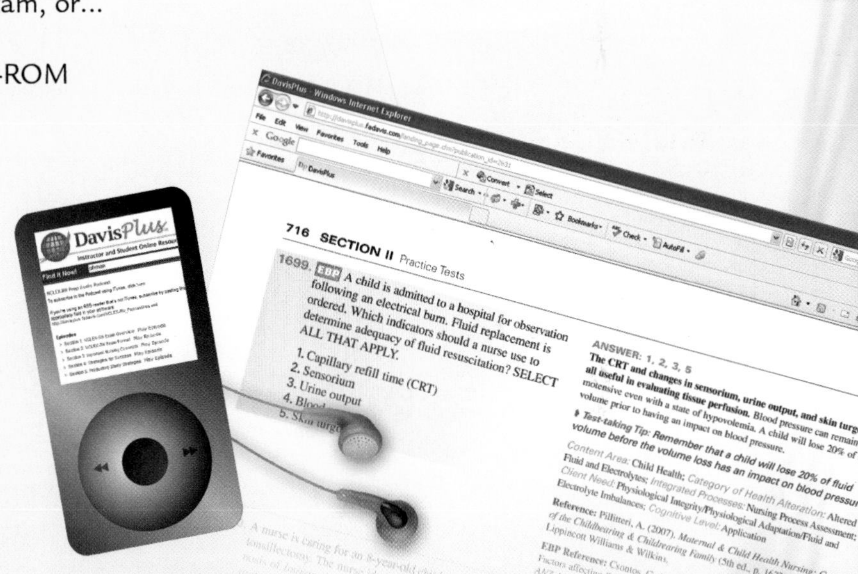
DavisPlus
716 SECTION II Practice Tests
1699. EBP A child is admitted to a hospital for observation following an electrical burn. Fluid replacement is ordered. Which indicators should a nurse use to determine adequacy of fluid resuscitation? SELECT ALL THAT APPLY.
1. Capillary refill time (CRT)
2. Sensorium
3. Urine output
ANSWER: 1, 2, 3, 5

More than just answers

Rationales explain why an answer is correct...and why the incorrect responses are wrong. They walk you step by step through the critical-thinking processes required to arrive at the correct response.

The right level of difficulty

All of the questions are written at the application and analysis levels to reflect the difficulty of the questions you'll encounter on the actual exam.

STEP 5. REDUCE YOUR ANXIETIES

Five exam-prep audio podcasts help you develop an effective plan. Each one addresses an essential step in the process.

1. Exam Overview
2. Review of the Exam Format
3. Important Nursing Concepts
4. Strategies for Success
5. Productive Study Strategies

Download them to your iPod or MP3 player...or listen from your laptop or desktop. You'll find them online at Davis*Plus*, in the Student Resources section for Davis's Q & A for the NCLEX-RN® Examination.

Visit http://davisplus.fadavis.com. Keyword: Ohman.

Davis's Q&A for the NCLEX-RN® Examination

Kathleen A. Ohman, EdD, MS, RN, CCRN
Professor of Nursing
College of St. Benedict/
St. John's University
St. Joseph, Minnesota

F.A. Davis Company • Philadelphia

F. A. Davis Company
1915 Arch Street
Philadelphia, PA 19103
www.fadavis.com

Printed in the United States of America

Last digit indicates print number: 10 9 8 7

Publisher, Nursing: Robert G. Martone
Director of Content Development: Darlene D. Pedersen
Sr. Project Editor: Padraic J. Maroney
Design and Illustrations Manager: Carolyn O'Brien
Developmental Editor: Allison Hale

As new scientific information becomes available through basic and clinical research, recommended treatments and drug therapies undergo changes. The author(s) and publisher have done everything possible to make this book accurate, up to date, and in accord with accepted standards at the time of publication. The author(s), editors, and publisher are not responsible for errors or omissions or for consequences from application of the book, and make no warranty, expressed or implied, in regard to the contents of the book. Any practice described in this book should be applied by the reader in accordance with professional standards of care used in regard to the unique circumstances that may apply in each situation. The reader is advised always to check product information (package inserts) for changes and new information regarding dose and contraindications before administering any drug. Caution is especially urged when using new or infrequently ordered drugs.

Library of Congress Cataloging-in-Publication Data

Ohman, Kathleen A.
Davis's Q&A for the NCLEX-RN(r) examination / Kathleen A. Ohman.
p. ; cm.
Other tittle: Q&A for the NCLEX-RN(r) examination
Includes bibliographical references and index.
ISBN-13: 978-0-8036-2187-9
ISBN-10: 0-8036-2187-6
1. Nursing–Examinations, questions, etc. I. Title. II. Title: Q&A for the NCLEX-RN(r) examination.
[DNLM: 1. Nursing Care–Examination Questions. WY 18.2 O38d 2010]
RT55.O35 2010
610.73076–dc22 2010005467

To Mike and Kris Ohman, Shelly Bass, Garret Ohman, and Donna Walberg for being there especially when I needed love, hugs, and encouragement.

To Garret, my grandson, who is the light of my life, for being such a happy toddler, sharing every weekend with us, and providing a wonderful distraction at just the right times.

To the loving memory of my father, Dean Domino, who helped me through the struggles of writing my first college essay and my mother, Loretta Domino, for her love of my family of 12 brothers and sisters and the many prayers for her children's success.

To the students who have inspired me to write this book.

"To every thing there is a season, and a time to every purpose under the heaven..."
Ecclesiastes 3:1

Foreword

I never expected to be a professor of nursing. My career objective was to be a proficient nurse, meeting the needs of patients and families. The opportunity to teach came to me rather than me seeking the opportunity. My teaching career began when I was approached to temporally relieve a faculty member who was pursuing her master's degree in nursing. Once I became engrossed in teaching, I never left. I am passionate about student learning, facilitating students to reach beyond their expectations to become the best nurses possible.

This temporary teaching position was a turning point in my career. For the next 11 years I taught in a diploma nursing program. When the program closed, I taught at a technical college, then an associate degree nursing program, and then I began teaching at the baccalaureate level. This year will be my 35th year teaching.

Although my primary position is a professor of nursing, I continue to practice as a staff nurse in a hospital setting in the medical-surgical and critical care areas where I also supervise nursing students. I truly love both worlds: working as a nurse and teaching students. My teaching and practice experiences over the years have included teaching in medical-surgical nursing, critical care, fundamentals, leadership and management, gerontology, pharmacology, pathophysiology, women's health issues, South African health care, and nutrition. I have supervised students clinically in the hospital areas including medical-surgical, critical care, the operating room, pediatrics, and maternity and in a nursing home and other community settings. A highlight of my teaching was taking a group of 13 nursing students to Port Elizabeth, South Africa for 4½ months in the fall of 2006. While in South Africa, students completed their medical-surgical and critical care nursing experiences in public and private hospitals and township clinics in Port Elizabeth and the surrounding townships.

Through my teaching career, I have observed the struggles of students taking NCLEX-RN®-type examination questions and assisted many students to overcome their test-taking anxiety. In classes I teach, I address successful test-taking strategies, provide many test items for students to practice, and encourage students to take as many practice items as possible prior to taking the licensure examination.

My interest in helping students with test-taking methods began early in my teaching career. To hone my own item-writing abilities and to refine my methods, I pursued experiences so that I could further help students be successful. My experiences include serving twice as an item-writer for the NCLEX-RN® examination, contributing as an item and chapter writer for multiple products pertaining to the licensure examination, and teaching review courses for the NCLEX-RN® examination. My experiences teaching students the strategies to achieve success and overcoming the obstacles associated with preparing for the NCLEX-RN® Examination led me to dream of writing this book.

My path to writing this book, however, follows a similar path as my career in teaching. This book was a dream that has now become reality. As with the start of my teaching career, the timing was right and the opportunity came to me, rather than me pursuing the opportunity. For this reason, I heartily thank Robert Martone, Publisher, F. A. Davis, for contacting me and making this dream come to fruition.

I also thank you and am pleased that you will be using this book to make your dream of a registered nurse a reality. This book is an opportunity for your success. I like to believe that you were led to this book as I was led to write it for you and your success. I congratulate you on your accomplishments thus far and wish you success and a bright future in nursing. You have selected an awesome profession!

Kathleen Ann Ohman, RN, CCRN, MS, EdD

Preface

THE STUDY PACKAGE

Davis's Q&A for the NCLEX-RN® Examination is a study package reflective of the latest **2010 NCLEX-RN® Detailed Test Plan** and incorporates the latest changes in the NCLEX-RN® Examination! This package provides you with a question and answer (Q&A) review book, an accompanying CD-ROM, and access to the *DavisPlus* Web site (http://davisplus.fadavis.com). Up-to-date information is provided to promote your success on the National Council Licensing Examination for Registered Nurses (NCLEX-RN®). As you embark on this study package, you will find numerous pedagogical features to facilitate your learning whether preparing for course tests or for the NCLEX-RN® Examination.

KEY FEATURES

To ensure your success on the NCLEX-RN® examination and to meet your own study and preparation style, *key features* are incorporated in this study package.

- **More than 5000 questions similar to those on the actual NCLEX-RN® examination.**
  - The book contains **2007** questions, including all item formats found on the actual NCLEX-RN® examination.
  - The accompanying CD-ROM includes all items from the book and an additional **3005** questions.
  - Access to DavisPlus Web site (http://davisplus.fadavis.com) provides audio format questions (a new item format implemented with the NCLEX-RN® Examination (effective April 2010) and other resources to enhance your study.
- **Questions are written at the higher levels of cognitive domain. Effective April 2010, the NCLEX-RN® Examination passing standard is 0.05 logits higher than the previous standard.** Although candidates writing the examination will have a minimum of 75 questions or a maximum of 265 questions, this means that candidates will need to get more items or more of the difficult items correct to pass the examination. Practice with more difficult items is essential!
- ***NEW audio and graphic* format questions are included. These alternate item types are a part of the NCLEX-RN® examination effective April 2010.**
- **All item formats on the examination are included in this study package:**
  - Multiple choice
  - Multiple response
  - Fill in the blank
  - Hot-spot
  - Ordered response (prioritization; drag and drop items)
  - Chart or exhibit
  - Graphic
  - Audio (via the DavisPlus Web site: http://davisplus.fadavis.com)
- **Over 1370 alternate item format questions are included throughout the study package.** There are more alternate item format questions in this package than in any other NCLEX-RN® Q&A package. Each test contains multiple choice questions and alternate format items reflective of the NCLEX-RN® examination.
- **Review tests are organized by content areas.** Organization by content areas facilitates your review for course-specific tests as well as a means of systematic review in preparation for the NCLEX-RN® examination.
- **All *Client Need* categories and subcategories identified in the 2010 NCLEX-RN® Detailed Test Plan are represented in this study package.** Questions target every component of the test plan including the *Client Need* categories, subcategories, and outcome statements to ensure a comprehensive coverage of the behaviors expected of an entry-level registered nurse. Each question identifies the *Client Need* category and subcategory.
- **An answer and rationale section is included with each question in the practice tests.** These provide immediate feedback when answering questions and help refresh or build your knowledge base when progressing to the comprehensive tests. The answer and rationale section for the comprehensive tests is after the questions. This mimics an actual exam and allows you to evaluate your progress in studying for the NCLEX-RN® exam.
- **Evidence-based citations (research studies, summaries of research, or evidence-based resources) support the correct option for 1190 questions.** Currently, no other NCLEX-RN® Q&A or content review books emphasize the evidence-base even though it is being stressed in nursing education and practice.

- **All questions are supported by current nursing references.** References are included so that you can feel confident that every question reflects current nursing practice. Page numbers are also included for your ease in finding the information for additional study on a topic.
- **All questions include the categories used by the 2010 NCLEX-RN® Detailed Test Plan.** The *Client Need* category and subcategory, integrated processes category (i.e., the nursing process, caring, teaching/learning, and communication and documentation), content area and subarea, and cognitive domain level are all included with each question to assist you in focusing on areas that you may need to review. You can feel secure that the expectations in the **2010 NCLEX-RN® Detailed Test Plan** are comprehensively covered in this Q&A package.
- **Test-taking tips are noted in the answer and rationale section.** Strategies for selecting the correct option are included to assist you when you are unsure of the answer and must guess on a question. Tips for remembering key points are addressed with multiple questions to enhance recalling the information in future questions.
- **Comprehensive examinations are uniquely designed to parallel the percentage of test questions assigned to each client needs category and subcategory of the NCLEX-RN® Detailed Test Plan.** The Q&A book contains two 75-item comprehensive exams that parallel the NCLEX-RN® categories of client need and the respective percentages. The CD-ROM contains one 275-item comprehensive exam which reflects a 265-item NCLEX-RN® exam with 10 additional trial questions.
- **Stand-alone pharmacology practice tests and integrated pharmacology questions are included in this study package.** More than **900 questions** are included in this study package on pharmacology and parenteral therapies. Because 13-19% of questions on the NCLEX-RN® Exam pertain to pharmacological and parenteral therapies, taking practice tests that focuses on just pharmacology should boost your confidence in this area.

BOOK ORGANIZATION

This question and answer book is divided into two distinct sections. **Section I** consists of four chapters and provides background and orientation to the NCLEX-RN® examination, as well as chapters on test-taking strategies and guidance for international and repeat test-takers. **Section I** also highlights changes in the examination based on the **2010 NCLEX-RN® Detailed Test Plan.**

Section II consists of seven chapters comprising 48 practice tests and two comprehensive tests. The practice tests in these chapters address subject areas within nursing and are organized around the major themes in the 2010 NCLEX-RN® Detailed Test Plan. Content areas within section II include *Management of care* (such as ethical, legal, and safety issues in nursing, leadership and management, prioritization and delegation, teaching and learning, communication, and cultural diversity), *Safety and infection control: Fundamental concepts of nursing* (such as basic care and comfort, medication administration, disaster preparedness, and infection control) and the more traditional content areas of nursing including medical-surgical, gerontological, obstetric/newborn, pediatric, and mental health nursing. Pharmacology is emphasized in four specialized, stand-alone practice tests which are organized by subject area. Additional questions pertaining to pharmacology are integrated in the medication administration tests, other content tests, and the comprehensive tests. Over 900 pharmacology questions are included within the book and CD.

Finally, **Section II** includes two comprehensive exams reflecting all the subject areas covered in the book and on the NCLEX-RN® Exam. Both of these tests are at a higher level of difficulty and include 75 questions, the minimum number included on the NCLEX-RN® exam itself. A student who performs well on these comprehensive exams should finish the book feeling well prepared for the NCLEX-RN® Examination.

THE CD-ROM

The CD-ROM accompanying this book contains **more than 5000 questions**—all of the questions from the book plus an additional 3000 questions. You can take a 275-item comprehensive test or choose various options to select questions. Questions are categorized by content areas, client need, client need subcategories, integrated processes including nursing process, cognitive level, and alternate item formats. These features allow you to customize your review and to determine your areas of strength and weakness. The extent of categorization is particularly useful when studying for exams within your nursing courses or preparing for a standardized test. The CD-ROM also has a diagnostic feature to allow you to assess your knowledge and to evaluate your study. These diagnostic capabilities will enhance your ability to focus your study on your targeted needs.

HOW TO USE THIS STUDY PACKAGE

It is important that you read the introductory book chapters so you become familiar with the NCLEX-RN® Examination and the Test Plan. Little attention may have been directed at the Test Plan within your nursing program. It is best to know what is being tested before embarking on a study path. Focus on the test-taking strategies and tips included in the introductory chapters and how to apply them when answering the questions. The test-taking tips will help you to remember key information.

Once you have read the introductory chapters, you are ready to develop a plan and begin your practice with the test questions. Use the **PQRST APPROACH** presented in Chapter 3. Remember, success begins with a positive mindset. Focus on your goal, use positive self-talk and self-reassurance as you complete the practice questions, and keep consistent with your study plan.

After you answer the questions, be sure to read the rationales for the correct and incorrect options and the test-taking tips. These provide you with significant information that will help you to understand the basis for the correct option and why the other options are incorrect. The test-taking tip provides a method for selecting an option when you are unsure of the answer or a cue for remembering the information.

As you study, use the CD-ROM to select additional questions in a content area especially if you did poorly on a practice test. Each of the 48 practice tests has approximately 100 questions between the book and the CD-ROM and the CD-ROM features will allow customizing the questions to meet your needs. Using the CD-ROM intermittently throughout your review will also enhance your proficiency in reading and answering questions from the computer screen and prepare you to take the NCLEX-RN® Exam on the computer.

Use the other features of the CD-ROM to take practice tests of 265 questions. This number reflects the maximum number of questions that a student can take on the NCLEX-RN®. Allow yourself 5 hours to complete 265 questions, which is the maximum amount of time allowed on the actual exam, and then evaluate your ability. Once you are consistently answering 75-80% of the questions correctly, you can feel confident that you are well prepared.

Contributors

Nadine M. Aktan, MS, RN, APN-C, Doctoral Candidate
Instructor
William Paterson University
Wayne, New Jersey

Roberta Basol, MA, RN, CNA, BC
CareCenter Director
Intensive Care/Surgical Care and Clinical Practice
St. Cloud Hospital
St. Cloud, Minnesota

Adrienne Beatty, BA, MS, LPC
Placement Specialist
Easter Seals UCP of North Carolina, Inc.
Wilmington, North Carolina

Jodi Lisbeth Berndt, RN, BSN, CCRN, PCCN
Adjunct Instructor
College of St. Benedict/St. John's University
St. Joseph, Minnesota
Staff RN, ICU
St. Cloud Hospital
St. Cloud, Minnesota

Matthew D. Byrne, MS, RN, CPAN, PhD-C
Instructor
College of St. Benedict/St. John's University
St. Joseph, Minnesota

Darlene M. Copley, RN, MS, PMHCNS-BC
Assistant Professor
St. Cloud State University
St. Cloud, Minnesota

Michele McPhee Davidson, PhD, CNM, CFN, RN
Associate Professor
George Mason University
Fairfax, Virginia
Staff Midwife
Women's Healthcare Associates
Lansdowne, Virginia

Katherine H. Dimmock, JD, EdD, MSN, RN
Dean
Chamberlain College of Nursing
Jacksonville, Florida

Constance Domino, BS Child Psychology
Retired
Minneapolis, Minnesota

Dorcas C. Fitzgerald, PhD, RN, CNS
Professor and RN-BSN Completion Program Coordinator
Youngstown State University
Youngstown, Ohio

Augusta Garbarich, RN, BSN
Lake Lillian, Minnesota

Melissa Garno, EdD, RN
Associate Professor
Georgia Southern University
Statesboro, Georgia

Kay Knox Greenlee, MSN, RN, APRN-BC
Director
Clinical Utilization/Quality Resource
St. Cloud Hospital
St. Cloud, Minnesota
Clinical Faculty
North Hennepin Community College
Anoka, Minnesota

Joyce M. Hammer, RN, MSN
Clinical Instructor
Wayne State University
Detroit, Michigan

Sigrid Hedman-Dennis, RN, MSN, CNS
Nursing Faculty
College of St. Benedict/St. John's University
St. Joseph, Minnesota

Debra K. Hoag, RN, MSN, NCSN
Assistant Professor
Fairmont State University
Grafton, West Virginia

Suzanne M. Leson, MS, RD, LD
Instructor and Director of the Coordinated Program in Dietetics
Youngstown State University
Youngstown, Ohio

Margaret M. Mahon, PhD, RN, FAAN
Associate Professor
George Mason University
Fairfax, Virginia

Maria A. Marconi, RN, MS
Assistant Professor
University of Rochester School of Nursing
Rochester, New York

Terri D. McCaffrey, MAN, RN, CNS
Pediatric Clinical Nurse Specialist
Cleft and Craniofacial Center
St. Cloud Hospital
St. Cloud, Minnesota

P. Lea Monahan, BSN, MSN, PhD
Director
Western Illinois University
Macomb, Illinois

Janet Marie Neuwirth, RN, MS
Associate Professor
College of St. Benedict/St. John's University
St. Joseph, Minnesota

Emily Rayman, RN, BSN
Registered Nurse
St. Cloud Hospital
St. Cloud, Minnesota

Rita M. Sarao, MSN, RN, CEN
Instructor
Holy Family University
Philadelphia, Pennsylvania

Darlene Sredl, PhD, RN
Associate Professor
University of Missouri
St. Louis, Missouri

Renotta Stainbrook, BSN, MSN, APRN-BC
Clinical Nurse Specialist
Veterans Administration Medical Center
St. Cloud, Minnesota

Sharon A. Takiguchi, RN, MS, APRN, ABD
Assistant Professor
Hawaii Pacific University
Kaneohe, Hawaii

Linda Turchin, RN, MSN, CNE
Assistant Professor
Fairmont State University
Fairmont, West Virginia

Vanessa V. Uithaler, RN, CCRN
Critical Care Clinical Facilitator
Greenacres Netcare Hospital
Port Elizabeth, South Africa

Karen Helm Vollen, MA, APRN-BC
Clinical Nurse Specialist
Veterans Administration Medical Center
St. Cloud, Minnesota

Bridgette Worlie, RN-BC, BSN
Educator
St. Cloud Hospital/CentraCare Health System
St. Cloud, Minnesota

Reviewers

Marianne Adam, MSN, RN, CRNP
Assistant Professor
Moravian College
Bethlehem, Pennsylvania

Valerie Allen, RN, MSN
Professor of Nursing
Somerset Community College
Somerset, Kentucky

Patrice Balkcom, MSN, RN
Director of Nursing Program
Central Georgia Technical College
Milledgeville, Georgia

Adrienne Beatty, BA, MS, LPC
Placement Specialist
Easter Seals UCP of North Carolina, Inc.
Wilmington, North Carolina

Mary Ellen Bonczek, RN, MPA, CNAA, BC
Senior Vice President/Chief Nurse Executive
New Hanover Regional Medical Center
Wilmington, North Carolina

Wanda L. Brown, MSN, RN
Nursing Instructor
Connors State College
Muskogee, Oklahoma

Lindsey L. Carlson, MSN, RN
Adjunct Instructor of Nursing
William Jewell College
Liberty, Missouri

Michelle D'Arcy-Evans, CNM, PhD
Professor of Nursing
Lewis-Clark State College
Lewiston, Idaho

Carmela Theresa De Leon, PhD, MA, BA
Faculty Member
PIMA Medical Institute
Dobson, Arizona

Valerie Edwards, RN, MSN
Associate Professor
Passaic County Community College
Paterson, New Jersey

Flora Flood, DNP, RNC, WHNP
Associate Professor of Nursing
Oakwood College
Huntsville, Alabama

Jacqueline Galbiati, MSN, RN
Assistant Professor of Nursing and Project Director
Healthcare Careers Grant
Cumberland County College
Vineland, New Jersey

Denise L. Garee, MSN, RN, CEN
Owner
4N6 Nurse Consulting, LLC
Wilmington, North Carolina

Arlene H. Gurganus, RN, BHA
Retired Nurse Manager
Cape Fear Hospital
Wilmington, North Carolina

Janet L. Hartig, MSN, RN
Assistant Professor
Bryan LGH College of Health Sciences
Lincoln, Nebraska

Alice Hildenbrand, MSN, RN, CNE
Assistant Professor
Vincennes University Jasper Campus
Jasper, Indiana

Mary Joanne Hovey, MSN, RN
Nursing A.D. Instructor
Cape Fear Community College
Wilmington, North Carolina

Karen W. Jefferson, MSN, BSN, RN
RN/Clinical Education Specialist
New Hanover Regional Medical Center
Wilmington, North Carolina

Karla Jones, MSN, RN
Faculty, School of Nursing
Treasure Valley Community College
Ontario, Oregon

Mary Beth Koehler, BSN, RNC
Pediatric Clinical Coordinator
New Hanover Regional Medical Center
Wilmington, North Carolina

Wendy Meares, MSN, RN
Associate
Professional Nurse Writers Inc.
Wilmington, North Carolina

Judith P. Moore, MS, RN, BC
Clinical Education Specialist II
New Hanover Regional Medical Center
Wilmington, North Carolina

Janet Marie Neuwirth, RN, MS
Associate Professor of Nursing
College of St. Benedict/St. John's University
St. Joseph, Minnesota

Carla Nye, DNP, RN, CNE
Assistant Professor
University of North Carolina Wilmington School of Nursing
Wilmington, North Carolina

Martha Olson, RN, BSN, MS
Assistant Professor of Nursing
Iowa Lakes College
Emmetsburg, Iowa

Nancy G. Owens, MSN
Professor of Associate Degree Nursing
Somerset Community College
Somerset, Kentucky

Brenda Pavill, RN, PhD
Nursing Faculty, Junior Level Coordinator
College Misericordia
Dallas, Pennsylvania

Sayra Sue Pingleton, MS, RN
Affiliate Professor
William Jewel College, Graceland University, and Johnson County Community College
Shawnee Mission, Kansas

Devon Plumer, MSN, BSN
Pediatric Acute Care Nurse Practitioner
New Hanover Regional Medical Center
Wilmington, North Carolina

Lu Ann Reif, PhD, MPH, RN
Associate Professor of Nursing
College of St. Benedict/St. John's University
St. Joseph, Minnesota

Mary Renquist, MSN, BSN, RN, CDE, CMSRN
Nursing Faculty
Normandale Community College
Bloomington, Minnesota

Shirley Retzlaff, MSN, BSN, RN
Associate Professor
Bryan LGH College of Health Sciences
Lincoln, Nebraska

Elaine M. Rissel-Muscarella, RN, BSN
Lead Instructor
Erie 2 Chautauqua Cattaraugus BOCES
North Warren, Pennsylvania

Shielda Rodgers, PhD, RN
Clinical Associate Professor
School of Nursing at the University of North Carolina at Chapel Hill
Chapel Hill, North Carolina

Karen Moore Schaefer, PhD, RN
Associate Clinical Professor/Associate Chair
Temple University Department of Nursing
Philadelphia, Pennsylvania

Marie E. Seneque, RN, MHA, CCRN, PhD Candidate
CEO and Director of Education
EdComp, Inc.
Leland, North Carolina

Cynthia Small, RN, MSN, APRN-BC
Nursing Instructor
Lake Michigan College
Benton Harbor, Michigan

Ardith Sudduth, PhD, MSN, APRN-BC
Assistant Professor, Hamilton Medical Group Endowed Professorship in Nursing
College of Nursing and Allied Health Professions, University of Louisiana at Lafayette
Lafayette, Louisiana

Julie Smith Taylor, PhD, RNC, WHNP
Assistant Professor and Graduate Coordinator
University of North Carolina Wilmington School of Nursing
Wilmington, North Carolina

Sharon J. Thompson, PhD, RN, MPH
Assistant Professor and Graduate Nursing Director
Gannon University Villa Maria School of Nursing
Erie, Pennsylvania

Lynn Tier, MSN, RN, LNC
Associate Professor
Florida Hospital College of Health Sciences

Marjorie A. Vogt, PhD, CNP
Associate Professor
Otterbein College Department of Nursing
Westerville, Ohio

Barbara Voshall, MSN, BSN
Associate Professor of Nursing
Graceland University
Independence, Missouri

Patricia H. White, RNC, BSN, MSN Candidate
Community Transition Coordinator, RTS Bereavement Coordinator, and NICU Staff Nurse
New Hanover Regional Medical Center
Wilmington, North Carolina

Anita Williams, RPh, PharmD, BCPS
Pharmacist
New Hanover Regional Medical Center
Wilmington, North Carolina

Acknowledgments

My special thanks to:

Robert G. Martone, Publisher, Nursing, F. A. Davis, for considering me for this project, your faith in me, your enthusiasm, and your encouragement.

Padraic J. Maroney, Senior Project Editor, Nursing, F. A. Davis, for your endurance, all that you have done, and all you have been through with managing this project.

Janet Neuwirth and Sigrid Hedman-Dennis, faculty colleagues, Nursing Department, College of St. Benedict/St. John's University, for your item-writing expertise, humor, and keeping me sane.

Allison Hale, RN, MS, Developmental Editor, for joining in this project mid-stream, your editorial competence and attention to detail, and the wonderful working relationship.

Deb Baloun, Office Manager, Nursing Department, College of St. Benedict/St. John's University, for your unwavering support, warm smile, and assistance as able during the project.

Emily Rayman, RN, St. Cloud Hospital for your attentiveness in reviewing and reformatting contributor questions and for the opportunity to work with you.

Those who contributed and reviewed items for your expertise, ideas, and suggestions for enhancement.

Table of Contents

Section

I

Preparing for the NCLEX-RN®

Chapter One

The NCLEX-RN® Licensure Examination

To prepare for the NCLEX-RN® licensure examination a candidate should become familiar with the licensing examination process and the test plan in order to avoid surprises when actually taking the examination. Adequate preparation will ease anxiety and instill confidence!

INFORMATION ABOUT THE LICENSING EXAMINATION

Information about the examination and registration materials is available from the National Council of State Boards of Nursing (NCSBN) Web site at www.ncsbn.org. If Web access is not available, request information by writing to the National Council of State Boards of Nursing at 111 E. Wacker Drive, Suite 2900, Chicago, Illinois 60601.

An application to take the licensure examination should be submitted to the board of nursing in the state in which the candidate wishes to be licensed. The candidate must meet all of the state's board of nursing's eligibility requirements to take the NCLEX-RN® examination. Once eligibility has been verified, the candidate will receive an authorization to test (ATT) and may schedule an appointment at one of the Pearson Professional Center's computer testing sites. Centers are located across and outside the United States, including American Samoa, Guam, Northern Mariana Islands, and the Virgin Islands. A computerized testing site is also planned for the Philippines.

COMPUTER ADAPTIVE TESTING

The NCLEX-RN® examination is administered exclusively as a computerized test. The computerized testing of the NCLEX-RN® began in April 1994. Basic computer skills are necessary for taking the examination. However, a tutorial is provided with the examination that includes instructions on using the mouse and recording answers. Candidates may also request assistance with computer operation during the examination. An on-screen calculator is provided. The tutorial for the NCLEX-RN® examination may be viewed anytime before taking the examination at www.pearsonvue.com/nclex. Completing the tutorial and taking practice examinations on the computer will ease the anxiety that may accompany the use of new technology. These methods also provide the candidate with an opportunity to practice the alternate test item formats that are included in the examination.

Examination Length

Computerized adaptive testing (CAT) is a testing strategy that allows individualized administration of questions based on the ability and competency demonstrated by the candidate on previous questions. Each candidate will be given a varying number of questions ranging from 75 to 265 test items. Of these, 25 are pretest items that are not scored. It is advisable to spend only 1 to 2 minutes per item. Each item must be answered before proceeding to the next item. The answer can be changed until the **option** and the <NEXT> button is selected. Once an item has been answered and the <NEXT> button selected, the computer will not allow a return to previously answered items. Thus candidates cannot skip test items and return to those items later.

Testing Time

The maximum time limit for the examination, including the tutorial, sample items, and breaks, is 6 hours. However, once the minimum number of test items has been answered correctly, the candidate will have demonstrated competency with 95% certainty and the examination will stop. Likewise, if a candidate incorrectly answers a maximum number of test items, the examination will also stop, and the candidate will have failed to demonstrate competency. If neither scenario occurs, then the examination will end when either the maximum number of test items (265) has been taken or the time limit has expired. The length of the examination should not be interpreted as indicating passing or failing.

Examination Results

Results of the examination are not released in the testing center. Rather, the computer scores the examination and then transmits the score to Pearson Professional Centers where it is scored again. The results are then released to the National Council of State Boards of Nursing (NCSBN). The NCSBN Web site address, www.ncsbn.org, provides links to the various state boards of nursing for application purposes and for checking examination results.

The board of nursing (BON) in the state to which the candidate applied to take the examination will provide test results to the candidate approximately 10 days to 1 month after the examination. Some state boards of nursing provide Web access so that applicants can track the progress of their applications. Web services often include viewing examination results and determining the date a nursing license was issued. If a state's BON has a Web site, results may be viewed within 48 hours of taking the examination. It may take longer for results to be available on the Web if taking the examination at peak testing times such as June and July. Accessing the results from the state's BON Web site is usually free.

If a state's BON does not provide access to examination results via their Web site, the candidate may use the *verification of license* option at the Web site to determine if a license has been issued by searching for his or her name. If sufficient time has elapsed since the examination and the candidate has passed the examination, his or her name and license will be displayed. If the candidate did not pass the examination, or if a license has not yet been issued, the candidate's name will not be found. Examination results are not provided when verifying a license.

If a state's BON does not have Web access for examination results, results may be obtained from Pearson Vue's Web site at www.pearsonvue.com/nclex. Results also may be obtained by telephoning Pearson Vue at the number provided with the ATT. There is a fee for obtaining results by using either Pearson Vue's online or phone service.

NCLEX-RN® EXAMINATION STRUCTURE

The content of the examination is based on the knowledge and skills necessary for a newly licensed, entry-level registered nurse to provide safe and effective nursing care. The required knowledge and skill levels are determined by the legal scope of practice as defined by individual state laws and regulations. Required knowledge and skill levels are also determined by a NCSBN study of the practice and job analysis of newly licensed registered nurses in a variety of settings and from varying registered nurse education programs. This study is conducted every 3 years, and the test plan is developed based on these results. The results of the most recent study, published in 2009, provide the structure for the NCLEX-RN® examination test plan effective April 2010. Copies of the test plan are free and available from www.ncsbn.org. A detailed test plan for the NCLEX-RN® examination may also be obtained from the same Web site or by mailing a request to the National Council of State Boards of Nursing at 111 E. Wacker Drive, Suite 2900, Chicago, Illinois 60601.

THE 2010 NCLEX-RN® TEST PLAN

Client Needs Categories and Subcategories

The NCLEX-RN® Test Plan is based on a *Client Needs* framework. The test plan provides a universal structure for defining nursing actions and competencies and focuses on clients in all settings. Four major Client Needs categories and six subcategories are identified in the test plan. Table 1.1 identifies the Client Needs categories and the percentage of test items assigned to each category. Table 1.2 describes the Client Needs categories and subcategories. Examples of examination items that address the Client Needs categories and subcategories are provided in Chapter 2.

Integrated Processes

Integrated throughout the Client Needs categories and subcategories are concepts and processes fundamental to the practice of nursing. These include the nursing process, caring, communication and documentation, and teaching and learning.

- **The Nursing Process.** The nursing process has five phases: (1) assessment, (2) analysis, (3) planning, (4) implementation, and (5) evaluation. An equal number of items on each phase are integrated through the NCLEX-RN® examination.
  - ***Assessment.*** In the assessment phase the nurse gathers information. The nurse collects subjective and objective information about a client, verifies it, gathers additional information if needed, and then communicates relevant assessment findings to other members of the health-care team.

TABLE 1.1
Client Needs Categories and Percentage of Items

Client Needs	Percentage of Items
• Management of Care	16%–22%
• Safety and Infection Control	8%–14%
• Health Promotion and Maintenance	6%–12%
• Psychosocial Integrity	6%–12%
Physiological Integrity	
• Basic Care and Comfort	6%–12%
• Pharmacological and Parenteral Therapies	13%–19%
• Reduction of Risk Potential	10%–16%
• Physiological Adaption	11%–17%

The National Council of State Boards of Nursing. (2009). *2010 NCLEX-RN® Detailed Test Plan.* The National Council of State Boards of Nursing, Inc., Chicago, IL, with permission. Available at: www.ncsbn.org/2010_NCLEX_RN_Detailed_Test_Plan_Educator.pdf

TABLE 1.2

Client Needs Categories and Subcategories

A. Safe Effective Care Environment: The nurse promotes achievement of client outcomes by providing and directing nursing care that enhances the care delivery setting in order to protect clients, family/significant others, and other health-care personnel.

1. Management of Care. Providing and directing nursing care that enhances the care delivery setting in order to protect clients, family/significant others, and health-care personnel.

- Advance Directives
- Advocacy
- Case Management
- Client Rights
- Collaboration with Interdisciplinary Team
- Concepts of Management
- Confidentiality/Information Security
- Consultation
- Continuity of Care
- Delegation
- Establishing Priorities
- Ethical Practice
- Informed Consent
- Information Technology
- Legal Rights and Responsibilities
- Performance Improvement (Quality Improvement)
- Referrals
- Supervision

2. Safety & Infection Control. Protecting clients, family/significant others, and health-care personnel from health and environment hazards.

- Accident/Injury Prevention
- Emergency Response Plan
- Ergonomic Principles
- Error Prevention
- Handling Hazardous and Infectious Materials
- Home Safety
- Reporting of Incident/Event/Irregular Occurrence/Variance
- Safe Use of Equipment
- Security Plan
- Standard/Transmission-based Precautions/Surgical Asepsis
- Use of Restraints/Safety Devices

B. Health Promotion & Maintenance: The nurse provides care and directs nursing care of the client and family/significant others that incorporates the knowledge of expected growth and development principles, prevention and/or early detection of health problems, and strategies to achieve optimal health.

- Aging Process
- Antepartum/Intrapartum/Postpartum and Newborn Care
- Developmental Stages and Transitions
- Health and Wellness
- Health Promotion/Disease Prevention
- Health Screening
- High-risk Behaviors
- Lifestyle Choices
- Principles of Teaching/Learning
- Self-care
- Techniques of Physical Assessment

C. Psychosocial Integrity: The nurse provides and directs nursing care that promotes and supports the emotional, mental, and social well-being of the client and family/significant others experiencing stressful events, as well as clients with acute or chronic mental illness.

- Abuse/Neglect
- Behavioral Interventions
- Chemical and Other Dependencies
- Coping Mechanisms
- Crisis Interventions
- Cultural Diversity
- End-of-Life Care
- Family Dynamics
- Grief and Loss
- Mental Health Concepts
- Religious and Spiritual Influences on Health
- Sensory/Perceptual Alterations
- Stress Management
- Support Systems
- Therapeutic Communications
- Therapeutic Environment

TABLE 1.2
Client Needs Categories and Subcategories (continued)

D. Physiological Integrity: The nurse promotes physical health and wellness by providing care and comfort, reducing client risk potential and managing health alterations.

1. Basic Care & Comfort. Providing comfort and assistance in the performance of activities of daily living.

- Assistive Devices
- Elimination
- Mobility/Immobility
- Nonpharmacological Comfort Interventions
- Nutrition and Oral Hydration
- Personal Hygiene
- Rest and Sleep

2. Pharmacological & Parenteral Therapies. Providing care related to the administration of medications and parenteral therapies.

- Adverse Effects/Contradictions/Side Effects/Interactions
- Blood and Blood Products
- Central Venous Access Devices
- Dosage Calculation
- Expected Actions/Outcomes
- Medication Administration
- Parenteral/Intravenous Therapies
- Pharmacological Pain Management
- Total Parenteral Nutrition

3. Reduction of Risk Potential. Reducing the likelihood that clients will develop complications or health problems related to existing conditions, treatments, or procedures.

- Changes/Abnormalities in Vital Signs
- Diagnostic Tests
- Laboratory Values
- Potential for Alterations in Body Systems
- Potential for Complications of Diagnostic Tests/Treatments/Procedures
- Potential for Complications from Surgical Procedures and Health Alterations
- System-specific Assessments
- Therapeutic Procedures

4. Physiological Adaptation. Managing and providing care for clients with acute, chronic, life-threatening physical health conditions

- Alterations in Body Systems
- Fluid and Electrolyte Imbalances
- Hemodynamics
- Illness Management
- Medical Emergencies
- Pathophysiology
- Unexpected Response to Therapies

The National Council of State Boards of Nursing (2009). *2010 NCLEX-RN® Detailed Test Plan.* The National Council of State Boards of Nursing, Inc., Chicago, IL, with permission. Available at: www.ncsbn.org/2010_NCLEX_RN_Detailed_Test_Plan_Educator.pdf

- ***Analysis.*** Information is interpreted in the analysis phase. The nurse identifies actual or potential client health-care needs and/or problems, collects additional facts if needed, establishes nursing diagnoses, and communicates the analysis findings and nursing diagnoses to relevant members of the health-care team.
- ***Planning.*** In the planning phase, the nurse establishes goals and means to meet client needs. The nurse formulates outcome criteria, develops strategies to achieve the expected client outcomes, modifies the plan of care, and collaborates with and communicates the plan to relevant members of the health-care team.
- ***Implementation.*** In the implementation phase, the nurse initiates or completes nursing actions to accomplish the defined goals of care. The nurse organizes, manages, and provides care, including teaching and counseling, to accomplish the expected client outcomes. The nurse advocates and collaborates on the client's behalf; supervises, coordinates, and evaluates the delivery of care provided by the nursing staff; and records and communicates information to relevant members of the health-care team.
- ***Evaluation.*** In the evaluation phase, the nurse compares the actual client outcomes with expected outcomes of care to determine whether or not outcomes have been achieved and to evaluate the success or lack of success of the interventions in achieving these expected outcomes. The nurse evaluates client adherence to prescribed therapies, documents evaluation information, modifies the plan if indicated, and communicates the

nursing evaluation and client responses to relevant members of the health-care team.

- **Caring.** The interaction between the nurse, client, and family in an atmosphere of mutual respect and trust constitutes caring. Within a collaborative environment, the nurse encourages and offers hope, support, and compassion to the client and family when providing care and facilitating the achievement of desired outcomes.
- **Communication and Documentation.** The verbal and nonverbal interactions between the nurse and the client, the client's significant others, and health-care team members are part of communication and documentation. Observations, events, and activities related to client care are documented in the client's electronic and/or paper record, according to standards of nursing practice and accountability.
- **Teaching and Learning.** Teaching and learning facilitates knowledge acquisition, including skills and attitudes, and disseminates information to others to promote a change in behavior.

CONTENT DIMENSIONS

Various conceptual models are used to organize content in nursing education programs, including the traditional framework of maternal-child, medical-surgical, or psychiatric/mental health nursing. Other frameworks include functional health patterns, head-to-toe formats, stages of maturity, or body systems classification. Regardless of the framework used, the NCLEX-RN® examination integrates components from these frameworks to ensure that all clients' physical and behavioral dimensions across the life span are included. These content dimensions are represented in the Client Needs framework represented in the NCLEX-RN® Test Plan.

The selection of test items in a candidate's examination is controlled by the NCLEX-RN® Test Plan percentages. A candidate will not have a designated percentage of test items from other content frameworks such as the specialty framework of maternal-child, medical-surgical, or psychiatric/mental health nursing. These other content frameworks are not controlled within the candidate's NCLEX-RN® examination. Many test items themselves, however, will focus on clinical situations that entry-level registered nurses are likely to experience. These may involve a neonate, child, adult, or an older adult client or group of clients experiencing a specific health alteration or in need of health promotion, maintenance, or restoration.

Although the percentage of items in the other content frameworks are not controlled within the candidate's NCLEX-RN® examination, combined results on six other content frameworks are provided in the NCLEX-RN® Program Report, a report available to individual nursing programs from the National Council of State Boards of Nursing. These other six content dimensions are (1) nursing process; (2) categories of human functioning; (3) categories of health alterations; (4) wellness/illness continuum; (5) stages of maturity; and (6) stress, adaptation, and coping.

A description of these frameworks is included so that the candidate is able to identify with a particular framework that may have been used in the candidate's nursing program. The candidate should be reassured that there are many approaches used to determine the competence of the entry-level registered nurse and that the content on the examination has likely been addressed within a particular nursing program.

- **Categories of Human Functioning.** This framework describes major disturbances to the wellness continuum. These include (1) protective (safety); (2) sensory-perceptual (cognitive perceptual); (3) comfort, rest, activity, and mobility (activity, sleep, and rest); (4) nutrition (nutritional-metabolic); (5) growth and development; (6) fluid-gas transport; (7) psychosocial-cultural function (psychosocial dimensions); and (8) elimination.
- **Categories of Health Alterations.** This framework describes the body systems that may be impacted from changes in the wellness continuum. These include (1) cardiovascular, (2) endocrine/metabolic, (3) gastrointestinal, (4) reproductive, (5) integumentary/musculoskeletal, (6) immune, (7) nervous/sensory, (8) psychosocial behaviors, (9) renal/urinary, and (10) respiratory systems.
- **Wellness/Illness Continuum.** This framework describes the delivery of services to clients for the purposes of (1) health promotion, (2) health maintenance, (3) health restoration–acute/simple, and (4) health restoration–acute/ complex.
- **State of Maturity.** This framework describes human growth and development and its influences on health and illness for six age categories: (1) natal (prenatal to 1 year), (2) childhood (1 to 10 years), (3) adolescence (11 to 19 years), (4) adulthood (20 to 65 years), (5) older adulthood (66 years and older), and (6) life span. Items that pertain to providing care to clients whose needs are the same, regardless of age or developmental level, are included in the category of life span.
- **Stress, Adaptation, and Coping.** This framework is one in which the nurse promotes adaptive responses in four modes during a client's health and illness. The four modes are (1) physiological needs, (2) self-concept, (3) role function, and (4) interdependence.

The NCLEX-RN® Program Reports also provide a basis for evaluating the strengths and weaknesses in educational programs, to compare graduates from various programs, and to ensure that content essential to entry-level registered nurse practice is included within the nursing program. Examination results for the Client Needs framework, the integrated processes, and the six previously noted dimensions are combined for graduates from a specified nursing program for a 6-month time period and included in the report. The report also compares aggregated examination results for the program's graduates with graduates within the jurisdiction, graduates from the same type of nursing programs (BSN, ADN, or diploma), and with all NCLEX-RN® examination candidates nationally for that particular year.

CHANGES IN THE NCLEX-RN® TEST PLAN

The National Council of State Boards of Nursing made recent changes to the 2010 NCLEX-RN® Test Plan effective April 2010. The *Client Needs* framework, including the eight categories and subcategories of the 2007 NCLEX-RN® Test Plan, was retained for the 2010 NCLEX-RN® Test Plan. However, twenty-two **bulleted concepts** from the 2007 NCLEX-RN® Test Plan were eliminated as stand-alone concepts and either subsumed under another bulleted concept, subsumed under a category, or integrated throughout the test plan (Table 1.3). The terms *changes or abnormalities* were added to the bulleted concept of vital signs for clarification. These changes were based on the practice analysis of the *Report of Findings from the 2008 Practice Analysis: Linking the NCLEX-RN® Examination to Practice* (2008), expert judgment, and feedback from stakeholders.

The **percentage of items** on the NCLEX-RN® Examination was also changed in two client need categories for the 2010 NCLEX-RN® Test Plan. The two client need categories that were changed are illustrated in Table 1.4.

A final change to the 2010 NCLEX-RN® Test Plan was the inclusion of two **additional alternate item types:** Audio item format where the candidate is presented an audio clip and uses headphones to listen and select the option that applies and graphic options in which graphics instead of text are used for the answer options. These are further illustrated in Chapter 2.

CHANGES IN THE NCLEX-RN® PASSING STANDARD

Another recent change to the NCLEX-RN® examination is an increase in the passing standard effective April 1, 2010. Candidates must correctly answer more questions or more of the higher difficulty questions than previously to pass the examination. The increase in the passing standard is in response to U.S. health-care delivery and nursing practice changes. Because entry-level RNs are seeing clients of greater acuity, a higher level of knowledge, skills, and abilities is required to provide safe and effective entry-level RN practice.

TABLE 1.3
2007 NCLEX-RN® Test Plan Bulleted Concepts Eliminated as Stand-Alone Concepts

1 Resource Management
2 Staff Education
3 Disaster Planning
4 Medical Asepsis
5 Disease Prevention
6 Expected Body Image Changes
7 Family Planning
8 Family Systems
9 Growth and Development
10 Human Sexuality
11 Immunizations
12 Psychopathology
13 Situational Role Changes
14 Unexpected Body Image Changes
15 Complementary and Alternative Therapies
16 Palliative and Comfort Care
17 Pharmacological Agents/Actions
18 Pharmacological Interactions
19 Monitoring Conscious Sedation
20 Infectious Diseases
21 Radiation Therapy
22 Accident Prevention and Injury Prevention – combined into single concept

TABLE 1.4
NCLEX-RN® Test Plan Category Changes

2007 NCLEX-RN® Test Plan		2010 NCLEX-RN® Test Plan	
Client Needs Categories/Subcategories	Percentage of Items	Client Needs Categories/Subcategories	Percentage of Items
Safe Effective Care Environment Management of Care	13%–19%	**Safe Effective Care Environment** Management of Care	16%–22%
Physiological Integrity Reduction of Risk Potential	13%–19%	**Physiological Integrity** Reduction of Risk Potential	10%–16%

NCLEX-RN® STRUCTURE IMPLEMENTATION WITHIN THIS STUDY PACKAGE

To ensure success on the NCLEX-RN® examination, all Client Needs categories and subcategories are extensively represented in this book and the accompanying CD and can be found at the end of each item. As you begin your adventure into this book, pay attention to the Client Needs presented. You will have the opportunity to respond to items that test your nursing knowledge and ability for every subcategory in the NCLEX-RN® Test Plan. Focusing on the Client Needs categories and subcategories may assist you in confirming your knowledge or identifying areas for further study.

You will also have the opportunity to respond to items that incorporate the integrated processes, including all five phases of the nursing process, caring, teaching and learning, and communication and documentation. These processes are used in a variety of care situations, integrating concepts from fundamentals, childbearing and family nursing, child health nursing, medical-surgical (adult health) nursing, psychiatric/mental health nursing, pharmacology, and nutrition. As you review questions, you will note that the *Content Area, Category of Health Alteration,* and *Integrated Processes* are included with each item. Again, this information is useful because it can either confirm knowledge or identify areas for further study.

References

Lewis, S., Heitkemper, M., Dirksen, S., O'Brien, P., & Bucher, L. (2007). *Medical-Surgical Nursing: Assessment and Management of Clinical Problems* (7th ed.). St. Louis, MO: Mosby.

National Council of State Boards of Nursing. (2009). *Candidates.* Available at: www.ncsbn.org/1254.htm

National Council of State Boards of Nursing. (2009). *NCLEX-RN® Examination Candidate Bulletin.* Chicago: Author.

National Council of State Boards of Nursing. (2009). *NCLEX-RN® Examination: Test Plan for the National Council Licensure Examination for Registered Nurses, Effective April 2010.* Chicago: Author.

National Council of State Boards of Nursing. (2009). *Frequently Asked Questions.* Chicago: Author. Available at: www.ncsbn.org/1201.htm

National Council of State Boards of Nursing. (2009). *NCLEX-RN® Detailed Test Plan Effective April 2010. Candidate Version.* Chicago: Author. Available at: www.ncsbn.org/2010_NCLEX_RN_Detailed_Test_Plan_Candidate.pdf

National Council of State Boards of Nursing. (2009). *Frequently Asked Questions About the 2010 NCLEX-RN© Test Plan.* Chicago: Author. Available at: www.ncsbn.org/2010_NCLEX_RN_TestPlan_FAQ.pdf

National Council of State Boards of Nursing. (2009). *NCLEX-RN® Examination Program Reports.* Chicago: Author.

Nugent, P. M., & Vitale, B. A. (2008). *Test Success: Test-taking Techniques for Beginning Nursing Students* (5th ed.). Philadelphia: F. A. Davis.

Pearson Vue. (2009). *Online Tutorial for NCLEX Examinations.* Available at: http://www.pearsonvue.com/nclex/

Chapter Two

NCLEX-RN® Items

COGNITIVE LEVEL OF ITEMS

The NCLEX-RN® examination uses Bloom's taxonomy, and updated Bloom's taxonomy, of cognitive domains for the writing and coding of items. The lowest level of the taxonomy is the **knowledge level**, which includes the ability to recall facts, concepts, principles, terms, or procedures. Knowledge level test items require the candidate to define, identify, or select. The next level of the taxonomy is the **comprehension level**, which requires an understanding of data. Comprehension level test items require the candidate to recall, explain, distinguish, or predict. The third level of the taxonomy is the **application level**. At this level, candidates are required to demonstrate, act, intervene, apply, solve, or modify. The **analysis level** involves examining relationships between parts. At this level, candidates are required to analyze, evaluate, select, differentiate, interpret, judge, or prioritize. The **synthesis level** is the highest level of the cognitive domain. During synthesis, information is combined in new and meaningful ways. At the synthesis level, candidates are required to develop, organize, create, or generate.

Because nursing practice requires application of knowledge, skills, and ability, the majority of items on the NCLEX-RN® examination are written at the **application** and **analysis** levels of cognitive ability. These higher levels of cognitive ability require more complex thought processes. For example, rather than posing a question that pertains just to a client experiencing surgery, the item may also include the fact that the client has a diagnosis of chronic obstructive pulmonary disease. The candidate must apply knowledge from both problems and analyze the client's status to answer the question. Boxes 2.1 and 2.2 illustrate questions at the application and analysis levels of cognitive ability.

TYPES OF ITEM FORMATS: MULTIPLE-CHOICE AND ALTERNATE ITEMS

A variety of test item formats are included in the NCLEX-RN® examination. The majority of items will be in the multiple-choice item format. However, alternate test item formats are also included in the examination: multiple response; fill-in-the-blank; drag and drop, which are prioritizing or ordered response items; hot spot items; chart or exhibit items; graphic items; and audio.

Information about alternate test item formats can be accessed from the National Council of State Boards of Nursing (NCSBN) Web site at www.ncsbn.org. The Pearson VUE Web site, at www.pearsonvue.com/nclex, provides a candidate tutorial for practice with the alternate test item formats.

Multiple-choice items present a situation or stem. The candidate selects one response from a list of four answer options to complete the stem or answer the question. Boxes 2.1 and 2.2 provide examples of multiple-choice questions.

Multiple-response items contain a situation or a stem, a list of possible answers, and instructions to select all of the answers that apply. The candidate selects more than one response from a list of possible answer options. Box 2.3 provides a screen shot of a sample multiple-response item from the NCLEX-RN® examination. Box 2.4 exemplifies a multiple-response test item for practice within this book.

Fill-in-the-blank items require typing in a **numerical** answer that is based on the information presented in the item stem. This type of format is used to assess the candidate's ability to perform a calculation, such as a medication dose for an adult or child or an intake and output calculation on a client. It can also be used to respond to situations or questions that require a numerical response, such as the size of a client's pupils. Box 2.5 provides an example of a fill-in-the-blank item.

Drag-and-drop (prioritization or ordered response) test items require the candidate to place items in the correct order (ordered response) or in the order of priority. Based on the situation and the data presented, the candidate will need to determine what is first, second, third, and so forth. When presented with this type of test item on the NCLEX-RN® examination, the candidate uses the computer mouse to click on an item and drag it from one box on the left-hand side of the page to another box on the right-hand side of the page; placing items in the correct order or the order of priority. The specified order could include numerical, alphabetical, or chronological information. To complete

BOX 2.1

Application Level of Cognitive Ability

A client is transferred from a recovery room to a surgical unit after undergoing a pyelolithotomy with placement of a nephrostomy tube. Which nursing action is *least likely* to benefit the client at this time?

1. Calling the physician after noting the urine output is 20 mL per hour
2. Turning the client from side to side to check for bleeding under the client
3. Teaching the client about dietary changes to prevent further stone formation
4. Straining the client's urine from both the nephrostomy tube and the urinary catheter

ANSWER: 3

The immediate postoperative period is an inappropriate time for teaching on dietary changes for stone prevention. Options 1, 2, and 4 are incorrect because these are actions the nurse should perform. The nurse should call the physician for a urine output of 30 mL or less per hour. Turning the client is appropriate after pyelolithotomy. There should be no turning restrictions. Blood can seep under the dressing, through skin folds, and under the client. A nephrostomy tube, placed in the affected kidney to allow stone fragments to pass, also drains urine from that kidney. The nurse should strain urine from both tubes.

Test-taking Tip: An application-type question requires an action. In this question, focus on the key words "least likely." This is a false-response item indicating that the action that should not be performed at this time is the answer. Knowledge of a pyelolithotomy and placement of a nephrostomy tube are needed to decide the appropriate nurse actions and to select the action that would be "least likely."

Content Area: Adult Health; *Category of Health Alteration:* Perioperative Management; *Integrated Processes:* Nursing Process Implementation; *Client Need:* Physiological Integrity/ Reduction of Risk Potential/Potential for Complications from Surgical Procedures and Health Alterations; *Cognitive Level:* Application

Reference: Ignatavicius, D., & Workman, M. (2006). *Medical-Surgical Nursing: Critical Thinking for Collaborative Care* (5th ed., p. 1700). St. Louis, MO: Elsevier/Saunders.

this type of question, all items must be moved from the left-hand side of the page to the right-hand side of the page. Box 2.6 provides a screen shot of a sample ordered response test item from the NCLEX-RN® examination. Box 2.7 provides an example of an ordered response test item for practice within this book.

Hot spot items are used to demonstrate competence in clinical skills that are applied in professional nursing practice. An illustration, graph, or diagram is used as part of the stem or question. The candidate places the cursor over the desired area and clicks the left mouse button to mark an area in the illustration, graph, or diagram. The area can also be deselected with the left mouse button if the candidate wishes to change the location. Box 2.8 provides an example of a hot spot item.

Chart/exhibit items require the candidate to examine and analyze a chart or exhibit to answer the question. For example, after analyzing a list of laboratory values in a client's medical record, the candidate is asked to identify the laboratory value that indicates that the client is experiencing thrombocytopenia. Up to three exhibits may be presented in this type of question. Illustrations may also be provided, requiring the candidate to answer a question related to the illustration provided. Box 2.9 provides a sample NCLEX-RN® screen shot of a chart/exhibit item. Box 2.10 provides a chart/exhibit item for practice within this book.

Graphic items are new alternate format items on the NCLEX-RN® examination effective April 2010. The candidate is presented with a question and options that are graphics rather than text. An example of a graphic item is presented in Box 2-11.

Audio items are also new alternate format items on the NCLEX-RN® examination effective April 2010. The candidate is presented with a play button to listen to an audio clip and then selects an option based on the audio clip presented. The format of an audio item is presented in Box 2-12 and items provided on DavisPlus web site (http://davisplus.fadavis.com).

CONTENT OF ITEMS: THE CLIENT NEEDS FRAMEWORK

Nursing practice requires knowledge of the health needs of the client and the integrated processes fundamental to meeting these needs. The Client Needs is the framework used in developing items for the NCLEX-RN® examination. Details of the scope and content of the NCLEX-RN® examination are described in the 2010 NCLEX-RN® Test Plans available from the NCSBN Web site at www.ncsbn.org.

BOX 2.2
Analysis Level of Cognitive Ability

A client with a diagnosis of acute myocardial infarction has new orders for aspirin 75 mg PO daily, lisinopril (Zestril®) 10 mg PO daily, furosemide (Lasix®) 10 mg PO daily, and potassium chloride (K-Dur®) 20 mEq PO bid. The nurse reviewing the serum laboratory report for the client notes a potassium level of 4.2 mEq/L, creatinine level of 2.3 mg/dL, and platelets of 250 K/µL. Based on the results of the laboratory values, the nurse should plan to consult the physician before administering the:
1. aspirin.
2. lisinopril (Zestril®).
3. furosemide (Lasix®).
4. potassium chloride (K-Dur®).

ANSWER: 2

Lisinopril (Zestril®) should be used cautiously in a client with renal impairment. The serum creatinine level of 2.3 mg/dL is elevated (normal is 0.4–1.4 mg/dL) and indicates renal impairment. The physician should be consulted before administering the lisinopril. Options 1, 3, and 4 are incorrect because these medications are safe to administer. Aspirin will affect platelet aggregation. The platelets are normal. Furosemide results in the loss of potassium; thus, a potassium chloride supplement is given to maintain normal potassium levels. The serum potassium level is normal.

➧ ***Test-taking Tip:*** *An analysis-type question requires critical thinking about the information presented. Recall that angiotensin-converting enzyme (ACE) inhibitors should be used cautiously in clients with renal impairment. Knowledge of the medications and the normal laboratory values is needed to analyze this situation and complete the stem. Recall the medication actions, side effects, and precautions and apply this knowledge when analyzing the laboratory values to accurately interpret which medication requires consulting the physician before administration.*

Content Area: Adult Health; *Category of Health Alteration:* Cardiac Management; *Integrated Processes:* Nursing Process Planning; *Client Need:* Physiological Integrity/Reduction of Risk Potential/Laboratory Values; *Cognitive Level:* Analysis

References: Deglin, J., & Vallerand, A. (2009). *Davis's Drug Guide for Nurses* (11th ed., pp. 171–176, 587–590, 996–1000, 1087–1090). Philadelphia: F. A. Davis; Smeltzer, S., Bare, B., Hinkle, J., & Cheever, K. (2008). *Brunner & Suddarth's Textbook of Medical-Surgical Nursing* (11th ed., p. 877). Philadelphia: Lippincott Williams & Wilkins.

BOX 2.3
Multiple-Response NCLEX-RN®Screen Shot Item

Candidate P Pearson [NCLEX-RN]

Time Remaining 5:58:14

The nurse is caring for a client who has a wound infected with methicilin-resistant *Staphylococcus aureus* (MRSA). Which of the following infection control precautions should the nurse implement? **Select all that apply.**

☑ 1. Wear a protective gown when entering the client's room

☐ 2. Put on a particulate respirator mask when administering medications to the client

☑ 3. Wear gloves when delivering the client's meal tray.

☐ 4. Ask the client's visitors to wear a surgical mask when in the client's room.

☐ 5. Wear sterile gloves when removing the client's wound dressing.

☑ 6. Put on a face shield before irrigating the client's wound.

Select all that apply. Item 2
Click the Next (N) button or the Enter Key to confirm answer and proceed.

Next (N) Calculate (0)

From National Council of State Boards of Nursing. (2005, March). *Fast Facts About Alternate Item Formats and the NCLEX® Examination.* Chicago: Author.

The Client Needs Framework identifies four major categories of needs and six subcategories (see Chapter 1). Examination and practice test items that are reflective of each category and subcategory are presented in Boxes 2.13 through 2.20. Practice items provide an answer section, categorization, and references. The answer section for each practice item provides the correct answer, rationale, and test-taking tip. Categorization of the content, health alteration, client need, integrated processes, and the cognitive level of the test item follows. References, including some evidence-based citations, are included for reviewing the information. This detail is also included in the practice tests in the remaining chapters and on the accompanying CD.

BOX 2.4
Multiple-Response Practice Item

EBP Which actions should be taken by a nurse when caring for a client who is experiencing dyspnea due to heart failure and chronic obstructive pulmonary disease (COPD)? SELECT ALL THAT APPLY.

1. Apply oxygen 6 liters per nasal cannula
2. Elevate the head of the bed 30 to 40 degrees
3. Weigh the client daily in the morning
4. Teach the client pursed-lip breathing techniques
5. Turn and reposition the client every 1 to 2 hours

ANSWER: 2, 3, 4

Elevating the head of the bed will promote lung expansion. Daily weights will assess fluid retention. Fluid volume excess can increase dyspnea and cause pulmonary edema. Pursed-lip breathing techniques allow the client to conserve energy and slow the breathing rate. Options 1 and 5 are incorrect actions. Applying greater than 4 liters of oxygen per nasal cannula is contraindicated for COPD. High flow rates can depress the hypoxic drive. Because the client with COPD suffers from chronically high CO_2 levels, the stimulus to breathe is the low O_2 level (a hypoxic drive). The situation does not warrant turning the client every 1 to 2 hours. This activity could increase the client's energy expenditure and dyspnea.

▶ ***Test-taking Tip:*** *A multiple-response item requires selecting all of the options that relate to the information provided in the question. Focus on the client's dyspnea and the interventions applicable to both heart failure and COPD.*

Content Area: Adult Health; *Category of Health Alteration:* Respiratory Management; *Integrated Processes:* Nursing Process Implementation; *Client Need:* Physiological Integrity/ Physiological Adaptation/Alterations in Body Systems; *Cognitive Level:* Analysis

Reference: Lewis, S., Heitkemper, M., Dirksen, S., O'Brien, P., & Bucher, L. (2007). *Medical-Surgical Nursing: Assessment and Management of Clinical Problems* (7th ed., pp. 640–649, 829). St. Louis, MO: Mosby.
EBP Reference: Registered Nurses Association of Ontario (RNAO). (2005). *Nursing Care of Dyspnea: The 6th Vital Sign in Individuals with Chronic Obstructive Pulmonary Disease (COPD).* Toronto, ON: Author. Available at: www.guideline.gov/summary/summary.aspx?doc_id=7008&nbr= 004217&string=copd

BOX 2.5
Fill-in-the-Blank Item

A physician orders a glucose tolerance test for a client with a suspected diagnosis of diabetes mellitus. The order reads, "Administer glucose 1.0 g/kg for the glucose tolerance test." The client weights 154 pounds. To give the correct dosage, the nurse should administer ______ grams of glucose.

ANSWER: 70

To fill in the blank, first understand what the question is asking. Note that pounds should be converted to kilograms before determining the amount of glucose in grams. Remember, 1 kilogram equals 2.2 pounds. Use the on-screen calculator provided. If the answer seems usually large, recheck the calculations.

Calculation:

1 kg : 2.2 pounds :: X kg : 154 pounds

Multiple the inside, then the outside values.

2.2X = 154

X = 70 kg

Now solve for the amount of grams of glucose to administer

1 g : 1 kg :: X g : 70 kg

X = 70 g

The nurse should administer 70 grams of glucose.

Test-taking Tip: *Recall that 2.2 pounds is equivalent to 1 kilogram. Be sure to double-check calculations if the number seems unusually large.*

Content Area: Adult Health; *Category of Health Alteration:* Endocrine Management; *Integrated Processes:* Nursing Process Implementation; *Client Need:* Physiological Integrity/Pharmacological and Parenteral Therapies/Dosage Calculation; *Cognitive Level:* Analysis

References: Lewis, S., Heitkemper, M., Dirksen, S., O'Brien, P., & Bucher, L. (2007). *Medical-Surgical Nursing: Assessment and Management of Clinical Problems* (7th ed., p. 1258). St. Louis, MO: Mosby/Elsevier; Pickar, G. D. (2007). *Dosage Calculations: A Ratio-Proportion Approach* (2nd ed., p. 46). Clifton Park, NY: Thomson Delmar Learning.

BOX 2.6
Prioritization Item (Ordered Response) NCLEX-RN® Screen Shot

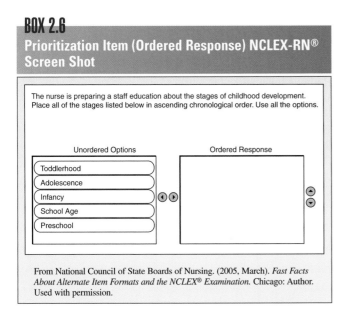

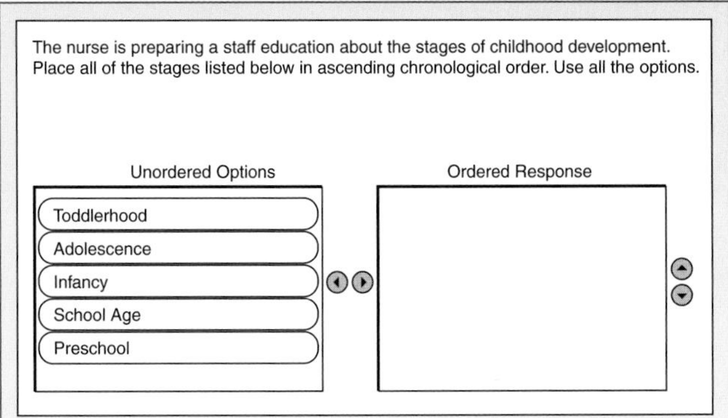

The nurse is preparing a staff education about the stages of childhood development.
Place all of the stages listed below in ascending chronological order. Use all the options.
Unordered Options
Ordered Response
Toddlerhood
Adolescence
Infancy
School Age
Preschool

From National Council of State Boards of Nursing. (2005, March). *Fast Facts About Alternate Item Formats and the NCLEX® Examination.* Chicago: Author. Used with permission.

BOX 2.7
Prioritization (Ordered Response) Practice Item

After receiving an order from a health-care provider to complete a tracheostomy cleaning, a nurse explains the procedure to a client, washes hands, prepares the equipment, opens and sets up the supplies, and performs tracheostomy suctioning. After the suctioning, the nurse uses the gloved hand, which has been kept sterile, to unlock the inner cannula, places the inner cannula in the hydrogen peroxide solution, removes the gloves, and rewashes. Which actions should be taken by the nurse to safely complete the tracheostomy cleaning? Prioritize the nurse's actions by placing the remaining steps in the correct sequence.

______ Rinse the inner cannula in sterile normal saline
______ Clean the inner cannula
______ Put on sterile gloves
______ Replace the inner cannula securely
______ Gently tap the inner cannula to remove excess liquid
______ Remove the inner cannula from the hydrogen peroxide

ANSWER: 4, 3, 1, 6, 5, 2

The nurse should first put on sterile gloves. The next step should be to remove the inner cannula from the hydrogen peroxide. Then, the inner cannula should be cleansed and rinsed in sterile normal saline. The nurse should then gently tap the inner cannula to remove excess liquid. Finally, the nurse should replace the inner cannula securely. This is the correct action sequence of actions to safely clean the tracheostomy tube.

Test-taking Tip: Prioritizing is placing items in the correct sequence. Use visualization to focus on the information in the question and then visualize the remaining steps of the procedure. During the actual NCLEX-RN® examination, the candidate will drag items from one column to another to place them in correct sequence.

Content Area: Fundamentals; *Category of Health Alteration:* Basic Care and Comfort; *Integrated Processes:* Nursing Process Implementation; *Client Need:* Safe and Effective Care Environment/Management of Care/Establishing Priorities; *Cognitive Level:* Analysis

Reference: Potter, P., & Perry, A. (2009). *Fundamentals of Nursing* (7th ed., pp. 947–848). St. Louis, MO: Mosby/Elsevier.

After the scenario, there is a blank line in front of the options to place a number for ordering the options. The answer to the option sequence is 4, 3, 1, 6, 5, 2. This answer sequence is illustrated below:

4___ Rinse the inner cannula in sterile normal saline
3___ Clean the inner cannula
1___ Put on sterile gloves
6___ Replace the inner cannula securely
5___ Gently tap the inner cannula to remove excess liquid
2___ Remove the inner cannula from the hydrogen peroxide

The priority sequence—

Put on sterile gloves
Remove inner cannula
Clean the inner cannula
Rinse the inner cannula in sterile normal saline
Gently tap the inner cannula to remove excess liquid
Replace the inner cannula securely

BOX 2.8
Hot Spot Item

A nurse is assessing an elderly client admitted with a diagnosis of left-sided heart failure and mitral regurgitation. Where should the nurse place the stethoscope to best auscultate the murmur associated with mitral regurgitation? Identify the area by placing an X in the correct location.

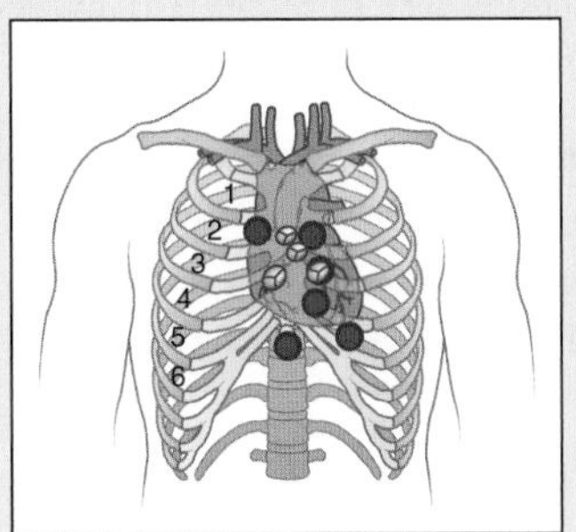

ANSWER:

The mitral valve is best heard with the bell of the stethoscope at the fifth intercostal space in the left midclavicular line.

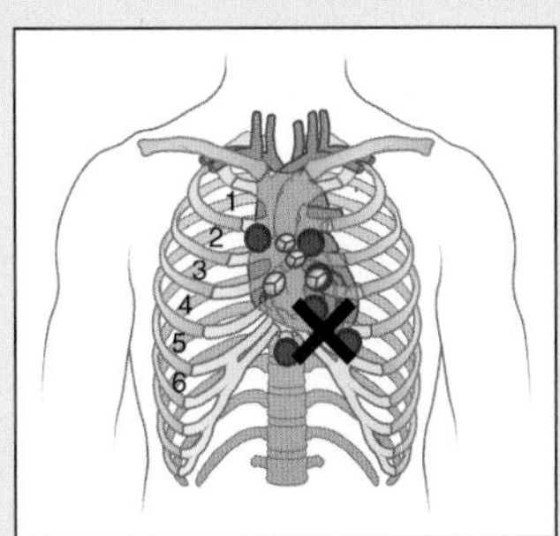

➧ ***Test-taking Tip:*** *Focus on the illustration. Use the mnemonic "All points essential to memorize" to remember the heart valves and auscultation points: aortic valve, pulmonic valve, Erb's point, tricuspid valve, and mitral valve. During the NCLEX-RN® examination, the candidate should position the cursor over the appropriate area on the figure and click the left mouse button to place an X in the selected location. Clicking on the X also deselects the choice and the mouse can be moved to select a different area.*

Content Area: Adult Health; *Category of Health Alteration:* Cardiac Management; *Integrated Processes:* Nursing Process Implementation; *Client Need:* Health Promotion and Maintenance/Techniques of Physical Assessment; *Cognitive Level:* Application

Reference: Black, J., & Hokanson Hawks, J. (2009). *Medical-Surgical Nursing: Clinical Management for Positive Outcomes* (8th ed., pp. 1372–1374). St. Louis, MO: Saunders/Elsevier.

BOX 2.9
Chart/Exhibit Item NCLEX-RN® Screen Shot

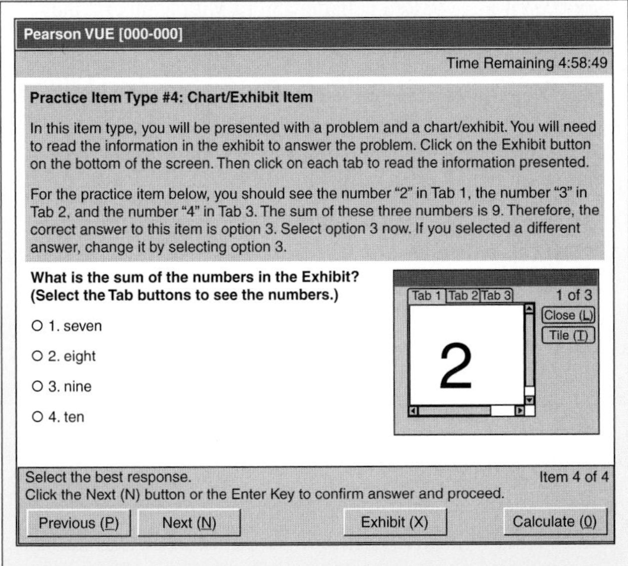

Pearson VUE [000-000]
Time Remaining 4:58:49
Practice Item Type #4: Chart/Exhibit Item
In this item type, you will be presented with a problem and a chart/exhibit. You will need to read the information in the exhibit to answer the problem. Click on the Exhibit button on the bottom of the screen. Then click on each tab to read the information presented.
For the practice item below, you should see the number "2" in Tab 1, the number "3" in Tab 2, and the number "4" in Tab 3. The sum of these three numbers is 9. Therefore, the correct answer to this item is option 3. Select option 3 now. If you selected a different answer, change it by selecting option 3.
What is the sum of the numbers in the Exhibit?
(Select the Tab buttons to see the numbers.)
O 1. seven
O 2. eight
O 3. nine
O 4. ten
Tab 1
Tab 2
Tab 3
1 of 3
Close (L)
Tile (T)
2
Select the best response.
Item 4 of 4
Click the Next (N) button or the Enter Key to confirm answer and proceed.
Previous (P)
Next (N)
Exhibit (X)
Calculate (0)

From The National Council of State Boards of Nursing, Inc. (2006). *Fast Facts About Alternate Item Formats and the NCLEX-RN® Examination.* Chicago: Author, with permission.

BOX 2.10
Chart/Exhibit Practice Item

While performing a physical assessment on a client with a long-term history of tobacco use, a nurse notes changes in the client's fingers (see illustration).

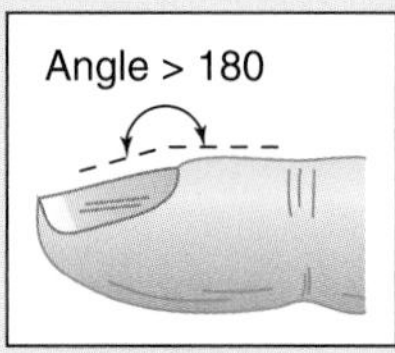

The nurse should best document this assessment finding as:

1. vitiligo.
2. clubbing.
3. keratinized.
4. poor capillary refill.

ANSWER: 2

In this question, the nurse should document the finding as clubbing. The picture shows swelling at the distal end of the finger and loss of the normal 160-degree angle between the base of the nail and the skin. Clubbing results from oxygen deficiency and is often seen in clients with congenital heart defects and long-term use of tobacco. Options 1, 3, and 4 are incorrect findings. Vitiligo is patchy loss of skin pigmentation. Keratinized tissues would be hard or horny. There is no indication that capillary refill has been tested.

▶ ***Test-taking Tip:*** *To answer items in the chart/exhibit format, identify key words in the stem, such as "history of tobacco use" and "best document." Next, focus on the illustration or display and review the accompanying data carefully. Determine what the question is asking.*

Content Area: Fundamentals; *Category of Health Alteration:* Basic Care and Comfort; *Integrated Processes:* Communication and Documentation; *Client Need:* Health Promotion and Maintenance/Techniques of Physical Assessment; *Cognitive Level:* Application

Reference: Berman, A., Snyder, S., Kozier, B., & Erb, G. (2008). *Kozier & Erb's Fundamentals of Nursing: Concepts, Process, and Practice* (8th ed., pp. 582–583). Upper Saddle River, NJ: Pearson Education.

BOX 2.11
Graphic Practice Item

A nurse is planning care for a client who is to receive a radiation treatment later in the day. In preparing the client's room, which sign should the nurse plan to post outside the client's room?

1. 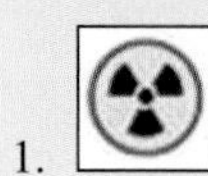
2. 
3. 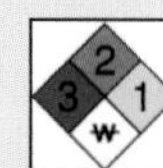

4. 

ANSWER: 1

The "tri-foil" is the international symbol for radiation. The symbol can be magenta or black, on a yellow background. Option 2 is a universal biohazard symbol indicating a potentially infectious specimen. Option 3 is the symbol used to identify the hazard of a chemical using the National Fire Protection Association's (NFPA) diamond. The blue diamond indicates a health hazard; with the number 3 indicating that it could cause serious injury even if treated. Red is flammability, with number 2 indicating that it must be preheated for flammability. The flash point is above 200°F. Yellow is the level of reactivity hazard, with a number 1 indicating that it may cause irritation. The symbol "W" indicates the substance has a special hazard of reacting when mixed with water. Option 4 is the Mr. Yuk symbol indicating that a substance is a poison.

▶ ***Test-taking Tip:*** *To answer items in the graphic format, identify key words in the stem, such as "radiation." Next, focus on the various graphics provided and eliminate options by deciphering the meaning of each graphic.*

Content Area: Fundamentals; *Category of Health Alteration:* Safety, Disaster Preparedness, and Infection Control; *Integrated Processes:* Nursing Process Planning; *Client Need:* Safe and Effective Care Environment/Safety and Infection Control/Accident Prevention; *Cognitive Level:* Application

Reference: Potter, P., & Perry, A. (2009). *Fundamentals of Nursing* (7th ed., p. 845). St. Louis, MO: Mosby/Elsevier.

BOX 2.12
Audio Practice Item

Place your headset on now.

Click the Play button  to listen to the audio clip.

Based on the audio clip, which lung sound is the nurse hearing upon auscultation?
1. Crackles
2. Wheezes
3. Plural friction rub
4. Rhonchi

BOX 2.13
Safe and Effective Care Environment

Management of Care: Providing and directing nursing care that enhances the care delivery setting to protect clients, family/significant others, and health-care personnel.

An unresponsive client is admitted to an emergency room. The client's cardiac rhythm is extremely irregular with no measurable heart rate, no P waves, and no QRS complexes. A nurse leading the resuscitation team should direct the team to perform which action *first*?
1. Defibrillate
2. Administer epinephrine
3. Perform synchronized cardioversion
4. Prepare for pacemaker insertion

ANSWER: 1

The client's signs are characteristic of ventricular fibrillation. Immediate defibrillation is the best intervention for terminating the life-threatening arrhythmia. Epinephrine should be administered according to advanced cardiac life support protocols after defibrillation. Synchronized cardioversion should be performed on a client with atrial fibrillation or atrial flutter. A QRS complex must be present to synchronize the shock. A pacemaker insertion at this time is inappropriate.

▶ ***Test-taking Tip:*** *Note the key word "first." Since the client's heart rate is absent and the rhythm irregular, eliminate options 2, 3, and 4.*

Content Area: Adult Health; *Category of Health Alteration:* Cardiac Management; *Integrated Processes:* Nursing Process Implementation; *Client Need:* Safe and Effective Care Environment/Management of Care/Delegation; *Cognitive Level:* Analysis

Reference: Lewis, S., Heitkemper, M., Dirksen, S., O'Brien, P., & Bucher, L. (2007). *Medical-Surgical Nursing: Assessment and Management of Clinical Problems* (7th ed., p. 855). St. Louis, MO: Mosby.

BOX 2.14
Safe and Effective Care Environment

Safety and Infection Control: Protecting clients, family, significant others and health-care personnel from health and environmental hazards.

EBP A nurse reports to employee health services for an injury to the hand from a needle stick. The needle was used on a client who is known to be HIV positive. Which interventions should be taken by the occupational health nurse in employee health services? SELECT ALL THAT APPLY.

1. Wash the exposed site with soap and water
2. Test for HIV antigens now, in 6 weeks, and then again in 3 months
3. Administer postexposure prophylaxis medications within 1 to 2 hours
4. Counsel on safe sexual practices until follow-up testing is complete
5. Place the employee on leave until testing indicates the employee's HIV status is negative

ANSWER: 1, 3, 4

Occupational blood exposure is an urgent medical concern and care should be sought immediately. Washing can reduce the amount of virus present and may prevent transmission. After an HIV exposure, infection may have occurred even though tests for HIV are negative; it may take up to 1 year for the development of a positive antibody test. Prophylactic treatment is started as soon as possible (preferably within 1 to 2 hours) and lasts for 4 weeks. If results of HIV-antibody testing return positive, treatment continues. HIV-antibody (not antigen) testing is completed at baseline, 6 weeks, 3 months, and 6 months after exposure. Initially, the employee may be sent home on sick leave. However, an employee who is HIV positive can continue to work, but must cover open skin areas and avoid client contact when open skin lesions are present.

➧ ***Test-taking Tip:*** *Apply disease prevention principles. The options that will prevent developing the disease are options 1 and 3. Option 4 prevents the transmission of HIV.*

Content Area: Adult Health; *Category of Health Alteration:* Infectious Disease and Autoimmune Responses; *Integrated Processes:* Nursing Process Implementation; *Client Need:* Safe Effective Care Environment/Safety & Infection Control/Reporting of Incident/Event/Irregular Occurrence/Variance; *Cognitive Level:* Analysis

References: Smeltzer, S., Bare, B., Hinkle, J., & Cheever, K. (2008). *Brunner & Suddarth's Textbook of Medical-Surgical Nursing* (11th ed., pp. 1819–1821). Philadelphia: Lippincott Williams & Wilkins; Berman, A., Snyder, S., Kozier, B., & Erb, G. (2008). *Kozier & Erb's Fundamentals of Nursing: Concepts, Process, and Practice* (8th ed., pp. 859–860). Upper Saddle River, NJ: Pearson Education.
EBP Reference: Panlilio, A.L., Cardo, D., Grohskopf, L., Heneine, W., & Ross, C. (2005, September 30). Updated U.S. public health service guidelines for the management of occupational exposures to HIV and recommendations for post-exposure prophylaxis. *MMWR,* 54(RR09),1–17. Available at: www.cdc.gov/mmwr/preview/mmwrhtml/rr5409a1.htm

BOX 2.15
Health Promotion and Maintenance

The nurse provides care and directs nursing care of the client, family/significant others, that incorporates the knowledge of expected growth and development principles, prevention and/or early detection of health problems, and strategies to achieve optimal health.

When communicating with a normally developed 2-year-old about to undergo a diagnostic test, the nurse would expect the child to communicate:

1. by pointing and imitating.
2. using at least 6 words.
3. in two-word sentences.
4. using complete sentences.

ANSWER: 3

The language development at 24 months includes two-word sentences (a noun-pronoun and verb), such as "Daddy go" and a vocabulary of around 50 words. A child with a hearing impairment who has not acquired language skills would communicate by pointing or imitating. At 15 months, 4 to 6 words are used and at 18 months, 7 to 20. Using full sentences would be the communication skills of a 4 to 5 year old.

▶ ***Test-taking Tip:*** *Visualize a 2-year-old and the language skills before reading each option.*

Content Area: Child Health; *Category of Health Alteration:* Growth and Development; *Integrated Processes:* Communication and Documentation; *Client Need:* Health Promotion & Maintenance/Growth and Development; *Cognitive Level:* Application

Reference: Pillitteri, A. (2007). *Maternal & Child Health Nursing: Care of the Childbearing & Childrearing Family* (5th ed., p. 865). Philadelphia: Lippincott Williams & Wilkins.

BOX 2.16
Psychosocial Integrity

The nurse provides and directs nursing care that promotes and supports the emotional, mental, and social well-being of the client and family/significant others experiencing stressful events, as well as clients with acute or chronic mental illness.

A registered nurse is orienting a new nurse. Together, they are caring for a group of clients diagnosed with enlarged prostates and each is scheduled for a radical prostatectomy. The registered nurse tells the new nurse that one client is likely to need additional support due to the client's high risk for prostate cancer. To which client is the registered nurse most likely referring?

1. 50-year-old Korean man
2. 50-year-old Hispanic man
3. 50-year-old Caucasian man
4. 50-year-old African American man

ANSWER: 4

African American men develop cancer twice as often as white men and at an earlier age. Cancer of the prostate is rare before age 39, but increases with each decade. Asian and Hispanic men have a lower incidence and mortality from prostate cancer than Caucasian men. Caucasian men develop prostate cancer less commonly than African American men, but more commonly than Korean and Hispanic men.

▶ ***Test-taking Tip:*** *Focus on the key words "high risk." Knowledge of cultural differences in the development of prostate cancer is needed to answer this question.*

Content Area: Adult Health; *Category of Health Alteration:* Reproductive Management; *Integrated Processes:* Caring; Teaching/Learning; *Client Need:* Psychosocial Integrity/Cultural Diversity; *Cognitive Level:* Application

Reference: Ignatavicius, D., & Workman, M. (2006). *Medical-Surgical Nursing: Critical Thinking for Collaborative Care* (5th ed., p. 1865). St. Louis, MO: Elsevier/Saunders.

BOX 2.17
Physiological Integrity

Basic Care and Comfort: Providing comfort and assistance in the performance of activities of daily living.

A nurse is calculating the amount of urine output at the end of an 8-hour shift for a client who has a continuous bladder irrigation after a transurethral resection of the prostate (TURP). The nurse emptied the urinary drainage bag twice during the shift. The first time there was 900 mL and the second time there was 1,000 mL. The amount of irrigation hung at the beginning of the shift was 3,000 mL, and there is 1,600 mL left at the end of the shift. The nurse should record that the client had _____ mL of urine output over the 8-hour period. Fill in the blank.

ANSWER: 500

Determine the amount of irrigation solution used: 3,000 – 1,600 = 1,400. Next, subtract the 1,400 mL of irrigation used from the combined amounts in the urinary drainage bag: 1,900 – 1,400 = 500. The client had 500 mL of urine output during the past 8 hours.

➧ ***Test-taking Tip:*** *Read the question carefully to understand what the question is asking. Use the calculator provided on the NCLEX-RN® examination and double-check calculations that seem unusually large.*

Content Area: Adult Health; *Category of Health Alteration:* Renal and Urinary Management; *Integrated Processes:* Communication and Documentation; *Client Need:* Physiological Integrity/Basic Care and Comfort/Elimination; *Cognitive Level:* Analysis

Reference: Ignatavicius, D., & Workman, M. (2006). *Medical-Surgical Nursing: Critical Thinking for Collaborative Care* (5th ed., p. 1860). St. Louis, MO: Elsevier/Saunders.

BOX 2.18
Physiological Integrity

Pharmacological and Parenteral Therapies: Providing care related to the administration of medications and parenteral therapies.

A nurse is administering promethazine (Phenergan®) to a postoperative client. In evaluating the effectiveness of the medication, which finding should the nurse anticipate?

1. Absence of pain
2. Decrease in heart rate
3. Increase in urine output
4. Absence of nausea and vomiting

ANSWER: 4

Promethazine (Phenergan®) has inhibitory effects on the chemoreceptor trigger zone in the medulla with resultant antiemetic properties. It does not have analgesic properties or affect urinary elimination. Bradycardia is a side effect of promethazine.

➧ ***Test-taking Tip:*** *Note the key word "evaluating." Look for the desired action of the medication.*

Content Area: Adult Health; *Category of Health Alteration:* Perioperative Management; *Integrated Processes:* Nursing Process Evaluation; *Client Need:* Physiological Integrity/Pharmacological & Parenteral Therapies/Expected Effects/Outcomes; *Cognitive Level:* Application

Reference: Deglin, J., & Vallerand, A. (2009). *Davis's Drug Guide for Nurses* (11th ed., pp. 1017–1020). Philadelphia: F. A. Davis.

BOX 2.19
Physiological Integrity

Reduction of Risk Potential: Reducing the likelihood that clients will develop complications or health problems related to existing conditions, treatments, or procedures.

The spouse of a client discharged following a transurethral prostatectomy (TURP) calls a clinic because the client continues to have pink-tinged urine 2 days after the procedure. Which response by the nurse is most appropriate?

1. "Bring him right into the clinic so that we can evaluate why his urine is pink-tinged."
2. "This is normal. His urine will be pink-tinged for several days after the procedure."
3. "Is he eating more leafy green vegetables or taking any over-the-counter medications?"
4. "His urine should be clear amber by now so there might be bleeding. Increase his fluids."

ANSWER: 2

The client may continue to pass small clots and tissue debris and have pink-tinged urine for several days after surgery. It is unnecessary to bring the client to the clinic immediately unless the urine is dark red or burgundy, indicating arterial or venous bleeding, respectively. Leafy green vegetables and over-the-counter medications may enhance the effects of anticoagulants. However, this is irrelevant to the situation since the client should not be taking anticoagulants. Having the client's spouse increase his fluid intake will flush the urinary system. However, pink-tinged urine, at this time, is normal.

Test-taking Tip: *Focus on the issue in the stem: pink-tinged urine 2 days after TURP. Eliminate responses 1, 3, and 4 because these imply that the client is bleeding.*

Content Area: Adult Health; *Category of Health Alteration:* Renal and Urinary Management; *Integrated Processes:* Communication and Documentation; *Client Need:* Physiological Integrity/Reduction of Risk Potential/Potential Complications; *Cognitive Level:* Application

Reference: Black, J., & Hokanson Hawks, J. (2009). *Medical-Surgical Nursing: Clinical Management for Positive Outcomes.* (8th ed., pp. 882–884). St. Louis, MO: Saunders/Elsevier.

BOX 2.20
Physiological Integrity

Physiological Adaptation: Managing and providing care for clients with acute, chronic, life-threatening physical health conditions.

Which nursing diagnosis is the highest priority for the client experiencing heart failure?

1. Excess fluid volume
2. Disturbed sleep pattern
3. Activity intolerance
4. Impaired gas exchange

ANSWER: 4

Impaired gas exchange is a basic physiological need according to Maslow's Hierarchy of Needs theory and is the priority nursing diagnosis. Although excess fluid volume is experienced in heart failure, impaired gas exchange would be a higher priority. Disturbed sleep patterns and activity intolerance also may occur in heart failure, but these would be a second-level need for safety and security.

Test-taking Tip: *Note the key word "priority." Use Maslow's Hierarchy of Needs theory to select the basic physiological need for air as the first priority.*

Content Area: Adult Health; *Category of Health Alteration:* Cardiac Management; *Integrated Processes:* Nursing Process Analysis; *Client Need:* Physiological Integrity/Physiological Adaptation/Illness Management; *Cognitive Level:* Analysis

Reference: Lewis, S., Heitkemper, M., Dirksen, S., O'Brien, P., & Bucher, L. (2007). *Medical-Surgical Nursing: Assessment and Management of Clinical Problems* (7th ed., pp. 836–837). St. Louis: MO: Mosby.

References

Anderson, L. W., & Krathwohl, D. R. (Eds.). (2001). *A Taxonomy for Learning, Teaching, and Assessing. A Revision of Bloom's Taxonomy of Educational Objectives.* New York: Addison Wesley Longman.

Berman, A., Snyder, S., Kozier, B., & Erb, G. (2008). *Kozier & Erb's Fundamentals of Nursing: Concepts, Process, and Practice* (8th ed., pp. 582–583). Upper Saddle River, NJ: Pearson Education.

Black, J., & Hokanson Hawks, J. (2009). *Medical-Surgical Nursing: Clinical Management for Positive Outcomes* (8th ed.). St. Louis, MO: Saunders/Elsevier.

Bloom, B. S. (Ed). (1956). *Taxonomy of Educational Objectives: The Classification of Educational Goals, Handbook.* New York: David McKay.

Deglin, J., & Vallerand, A. (2010). *Davis's Drug Guide for Nurses* (12th ed.). Philadelphia: F. A. Davis.

Ignatavicius, D., & Workman, M. (2006). *Medical-Surgical Nursing: Critical Thinking for Collaborative Care* (5th ed.). St. Louis, MO: Elsevier/Saunders.

Lewis, S., Heitkemper, M., Dirksen, S., O'Brien, P., & Bucher, L. (2007). *Medical-Surgical Nursing: Assessment and Management of Clinical Problems* (7th ed.). St. Louis, MO: Mosby.

National Council of State Boards of Nursing. (2009). *NCLEX-RN® Examination Candidate Bulletin.* Chicago: Author.

National Council of State Boards of Nursing. (2009). *NCLEX-RN® Examination: Test Plan for the National Council Licensure Examination for Registered Nurses, Effective April 2010.* Chicago: Author.

National Council of State Boards of Nursing. (2009). *Frequently Asked Questions about the 2010 NCLEX-RN® Test Plan.* Chicago: Author.

National Council of State Boards of Nursing. (2009). *NCLEX-RN® Program Reports.* Chicago: Author.

National Council State Board of Nursing. (2009). *Alternate Format Items.* Chicago: Author.

Nugent, P. M., & Vitale, B. A. (2008). *Test Success: Test-taking Techniques for Beginning Nursing Students* (5th ed.). Philadelphia: F. A. Davis.

Panlilio, A. L., Cardo, D., Grohskopf, L., Heneine, W., & Ross, C. (2005, September 30). Updated U.S. public health service guidelines for the management of occupational exposures to HIV and recommendations for postexposure prophylaxis. *MMWR* 54(RR09), 1–17. Available at: www.cdc.gov/mmwr/preview/mmwrhtml/rr5409a1.htm

Pickar, G. D. (2007). *Dosage Calculations: A Ratio-Proportion Approach* (2nd ed.). Clifton Park, NY: Thomson Delmar Learning.

Registered Nurses Association of Ontario (RNAO). (2005). *Nursing Care of Dyspnea: The 6th Vital Sign in Individuals with Chronic Obstructive Pulmonary Disease (COPD).* Toronto, ON: Author. Available at: www.guideline.gov/summary/summary.aspx?doc_id=7008&nbr=004217&string=copd

Silvestri, L. A. (2006). *Saunders Q&A Review for the NCLEX-RN® Examination* (3rd ed.). St. Louis, MO: Saunders/Elsevier.

Smeltzer, S., Bare, B., Hinkle, J., & Cheever, K. (2008). *Brunner & Suddarth's Textbook of Medical-Surgical Nursing* (11th ed.). Philadelphia: Lippincott Williams & Wilkins.

Wilkinson, J., & Van Leuven, K. (2007). *Fundamentals of Nursing: Thinking & Doing* (Vol. 2). Philadelphia: F. A. Davis.

Williams, L., & Hopper, P. (2007). *Understanding Medical-Surgical Nursing* (3rd ed.). Philadelphia: F. A. Davis.

Chapter Three

Test-Taking Tips and Strategies

Taking the NCLEX-RN® examination can be a stressful experience. Thus, this chapter is designed to help you find ways to read NCLEX-type questions and answer them correctly. Understanding how to take a test and to use strategies to answer test items is just as important as knowing the content. Some test-taking tips are presented in this chapter to help you improve your testing abilities and to pass the NCLEX-RN® examination. Use these strategies and tips to identify the best option to answer a question or complete an item. You can also use these strategies to select an answer for unfamiliar content or for items for which you are uncertain of the answer.

CAREFULLY READ THE NCLEX-RN® ITEMS AND FOCUS ON THE SUBJECT

NCLEX-RN® examination questions are often long and contain more information than what is specifically needed to answer the question. Most questions consist of a case scenario, the question or item stem, and the answer options. Therefore, make sure to read the entire question thoroughly and focus on what the question is asking.

As you read the question, try to answer the question before looking at the options to see if you understand what the question is asking. If you do not know the answer, then rephrase the question in your own words. This may make it easier to understand what the question is asking.

Be sure to read the entire question before reading the options. Decide what information is relevant and what can be omitted. Ask yourself, "What is the question asking?" Focus on the last line of the question. This is the stem of the question and will state what the question is asking or looking for in an answer. In the stem of the question, look for **key words** such as *priority, first,* or *best*. Note the age of the client. If the age is not specified, then assume the client is an adult and answer the question based on principles of adult growth and development or physiological or psychological problems related to adults.

In a multiple-choice question, there will be four answer options and you must select one. Read all of the options thoroughly before selecting an answer. A multiple-response question has many options and you must select all that apply. In a prioritization question, you must list items in order, usually from the highest priority to the lowest priority. These prioritization items can be diverse and include such items as priority of assessments, interventions, nursing skills, pathophysiological concepts, or a variety of other situations that can be sequenced.

THE NURSING PROCESS

After carefully reading the question and options, consider if the nursing process is applied in the question versus the other integrated processes of caring, teaching and learning, or communication and documentation. If the nursing process is being applied, decide which step in the process is the focus of the question. The five steps of the nursing process include (1) assessment, (2) analysis or diagnosis, (3) planning, (4) implementation, and (5) evaluation. A complete description of each step in the process is included in Chapter 1, The NCLEX-RN® Licensure Examination.

Because the nursing process incorporates critical thinking, the licensure examination is designed to test your use of this process within the nursing role and scope of practice. When a step of the nursing process is applied in a question, examine each option to be sure that the option corresponds to that step of the nursing process. For example, if the focus of the question is on assessment but options include implementation, eliminate any options pertaining to implementation as an answer choice. Table 3.1 identifies each step of the nursing process and key words used for that step in test items.

The nursing process can also be used to prioritize actions. Assessment is the first action and thus is the priority in most situations. In a life-threatening situation, if an observation suggests an immediate intervention is needed, only then is an intervention the priority. Boxes 3.1 through 3.5 illustrate using the steps in the nursing process as a test-taking strategy. If after reviewing the examples further explanation is needed, a detailed process for analyzing questions using the nursing process and more specific examples can be found in *Test Success* by Nugent and Vitale (2008).

TABLE 3.1

Steps of the Nursing Process and Key Words in Test Items

Nursing Process Step	Key Words	Key Words	Key Words
Assessment	adaptations ascertain assess check collect communicate determine find out	gather identify inform inspect monitor nonverbal notify observe	obtain information perceptions question signs and symptoms sources stressors verbal verify
Analysis	analysis categorize cluster contribute decision deduction	formulate interpret nursing diagnosis organize problem reflect	relate relevant reexamine significant statement valid
Planning	achieve anticipate arrange collaborate consult coordinate design desired	desired results determine develop effective establish expect formulate goal	modify outcome plan prevent priority select strategy
Implementation	action assist change counsel delegate dependent facilitate give	implement independent inform instruct interdependent method motivate perform	procedure provide refer strategy supervise teach technique treatment
Evaluation	achieved compared desired effective evaluate	expected failed ineffective met	modified reassess response succeeded

THE ABCs

The ABCs—*airway, breathing,* and *circulation*—can be very helpful in answering NCLEX-RN® questions. They can be used when determining the order of priority. Priority-type questions can be identified with words such as *first, priority, initial, main concern,* and *primary*. When choosing the correct answer option, if an option pertains to a client's airway and is pertinent to the situation, then this option should be the nurse's first priority. If no option pertains to airway, then look for an option that pertains to breathing, and so on. Box 3.6 provides an example of this type of item.

MASLOW'S HIERARCHY OF NEEDS

Maslow's Hierarchy of Needs theory states that physiological needs are the most basic human needs (Fig. 3.1); use it as another guide to help prioritize the options to assist in selecting the correct option. Physiological needs are the priority; therefore, physiological needs should be met before psychosocial needs. When a physiological need is not presented in the question or included as one of the answer options, continue using Maslow's Hierarchy of Needs theory and look for the answer option that addresses safety. Continue to move up the hierarchy ladder to identify the priority if needs at the lower levels are not addressed within the

BOX 3.1
Nursing Process Assessment Practice Item

A nurse is caring for a hospitalized 10-year-old client who has chest contusions from a motor vehicle accident. The client is on room air and is being monitored by a pulse oximeter. When the nurse enters the room, the pulse oximeter monitor is alarming and is showing an oxygen saturation of 84%. The nurse should immediately:

1. call the physician for an order for arterial blood gases (ABGs).
2. assess the client's level of consciousness and skin color.
3. replace the machine and probe.
4. administer oxygen through a nasal cannula or by mask.

ANSWER: 2

By immediately evaluating the client's mental status and skin color, the nurse can quickly determine whether or not the signal tracing constitutes an emergency or if it is an artifact. An artifact in the pulse oximeter monitoring system can be caused by altered skin temperature, movement of the client's finger, or probe disconnection. Equipment malfunction can also occur. Calling the physician is necessary only if the reading is accurate. Replacing the machine is only necessary if the machine is malfunctioning. Applying oxygen may be necessary if the nurse is unable to determine the client's pulse oximeter reading within a few seconds.

▶ ***Test-taking Tip:*** *Because assessment is the first step in the nursing process and the situation requires additional information before an intervention can be determined, assessment should be the first action in this situation. Options pertaining to interventions should be eliminated.*

Content Area: Child Health; *Category of Health Alteration:* Respiratory Management; *Integrated Processes:* Nursing Process Assessment; *Client Need:* Physiological Integrity/Physiological Adaptation/Medical Emergencies; *Cognitive Level:* Analysis

References: Ball, J., & Bindler, R. (2008). *Pediatric Nursing: Caring for Children* (4th ed., pp. 685–687). Upper Saddle River, NJ: Pearson Education; Clark, A., Giuliano, K., & Chen, H. (2006). Legal and ethical: Pulse oximetry revisited: "but his O_2 sat was normal!" *Clinical Nurse Specialist: The Journal for Advanced Nursing Practice,* 20, 268–272; Potter, P., & Perry, A. (2009). *Fundamentals of Nursing* (7th ed., pp. 534–535). St. Louis, MO: Mosby Elsevier.

BOX 3.2
Nursing Process Analysis Practice Item

A client is admitted with a tentative diagnosis of hepatitis. A nurse determines which client statement would be consistent with the diagnosis?

1. "I have not been sleeping well because I have so much heartburn at night that it wakes me up."
2. "Whenever I eat dairy products I have diarrhea for a few days."
3. "Lately I have been short of breath during my walk from the bus stop to work."
4. "I am a smoker but lately I can't tolerate the taste of cigarettes."

ANSWER: 4

Anorexia can be severe in the acute phase of hepatitis. Distaste for cigarettes in smokers is characteristic of early profound anorexia. Heartburn at night is a symptom of gastroesophageal reflux disease (GERD). Diarrhea after eating dairy products can be a symptom of lactose intolerance. Increasing shortness of breath can be related to circulatory or respiratory concerns.

▶ ***Test-taking Tip:*** *Analysis questions require understanding of the physiological processes and interpretation of information. In this question, thinking about the signs and symptoms associated with hepatitis is necessary to analyze the client's statements and eliminate options that are inconsistent with the diagnosis. The process of elimination can also be used to eliminate option 3 because it is a sign of activity intolerance often associated with cardiopulmonary problems.*

Content Area: Adult Health; *Category of Health Alteration:* Infectious Disease; *Integrated Processes:* Nursing Process Analysis; *Client Need:* Physiological Integrity Reduction of Risk Potential/Potential for Alterations in Body Systems; *Cognitive Level:* Application

Reference: Lewis, S., Heitkemper, M., Dirksen, S., O'Brien, P., & Bucher, L. (2007). *Medical-Surgical Nursing: Assessment and Management of Clinical Problems* (7th ed., pp. 825; 1004, 1081, 1091). St. Louis, MO: Mosby.

BOX 3.3
Nursing Process Planning Practice Item

A client is admitted with vancomycin-resistant enterococci (VRE) in a leg wound. The wound is draining although dressings are covering the wound. To prevent the spread of the VRE, which is a nurse's best plan of action?

1. Assign the client to a private room
2. Assign only one caregiver to the client
3. Do not allow pregnant staff to enter the room
4. Place the client in a negative-airflow room

ANSWER: 1

Single-client rooms are preferred when there is a concern about transmission of an infectious agent. It is not practical to assign only one caregiver, as the client will likely require multiple caregivers throughout hospitalization. VRE is not spread to pregnant staff at higher rates than to nonpregnant staff. A negative-airflow room is required for airborne diseases. VRE is not an airborne disease.

➧ ***Test-taking Tip:*** *This question is a nursing process planning item that includes planning care for a client. First determine if all options should be included in the nurse's plan. The key words are "best plan of action." Recall that VRE can be transmitted to others, but is not airborne. Eliminate option 4. Of the remaining options, determine which is best.*

Content Area: Fundamentals; *Category of Health Alteration:* Safety, Disaster Preparedness, and Infection Control; *Integrated Processes:* Nursing Process Planning; *Client Need:* Safe Effective Care Environment/Safety and Infection Control/Standard Precautions/Transmission-based Precautions; *Cognitive Level:* Analysis

Reference: Craven, R., & Hirnle, C. (2009). *Fundamentals of Nursing: Human Health and Function* (6th ed., pp. 462–465). Philadelphia: Lippincott Williams & Wilkins.
EBP Reference: Siegel, J., Rhinehart, E., Jackson, M., Chiarello, L., & the Healthcare Infection Control Practices Advisory Committee. (2007). *Guideline for Isolation Precautions: Preventing Transmission of Infectious Agents in Healthcare Settings.* Atlanta, GA. Available at: www.apic.org/AM/Template.cfm?Section=Guidelines&TEMPLATE=/CM/ContentDisplay.cfm&CONTENTID=1174

BOX 3.4
Nursing Process Implementation Practice Item

A postpartum client who delivered an infant vaginally has an outcome written in the plan of care, "To be free of perineal and uterine infection during the postpartum period." Which interventions should a nurse include in the client's care to promote meeting this outcome? SELECT ALL THAT APPLY.

1. Instruct the client on wiping the anal area first after voiding and bowel movements
2. Apply the perineal pad from front to back when changing pads
3. Teach the client to use a "peri" bottle to apply warm water over her perineum after elimination
4. Teach the client to avoid changing the perineal pads more than once a day
5. Prepare a Sitz bath at least once during the shift
6. Assess the level of the fundus every shift

ANSWER: 2, 3, 5

The perineal pads should be applied from front (area under the symphysis pubis) and proceed toward the back (area around the anus) to prevent carrying contamination from the anal area to the perineum and vagina. Squirting the perineum with water after elimination cleanses the area and promotes comfort. Sitz baths increase circulation to tissues, which promotes healing and thus reduces the risk of infection. The client should be taught to wipe the perineum after elimination from front (area under the symphysis pubis) and proceed toward the back (area around the anus) to prevent carrying contamination from the anal area to the perineum and vagina. Perineal pads should be changed at least four times a day to decrease the risk of promoting bacteria growth in the lochia on the pad and transferring that bacteria to the perineum or vagina. Assessing the level of the fundus is not an intervention; it is an assessment.

▶ ***Test-taking Tip:*** *Implementation questions include providing care and teaching. Option 6 pertains to assessment and should be eliminated. Next, eliminate interventions in options 1 and 4 because these would promote bacterial growth rather than prevent an infection.*

Content Area: Childbearing; *Category of Health Alteration:* Postpartal Management; *Integrated Processes:* Nursing Process Implementation; *Client Need:* Physiological Integrity Reduction of Risk Potential/Therapeutic Procedures; *Cognitive Level:* Application

References: Davidson, M., London, M., & Ladewig, P. (2008). *Olds' Maternal-Newborn Nursing & Women's Health Across the Lifespan* (8th ed., pp. 1078–1080). Upper Saddle River, NJ: Prentice Hall Health; Wong, D., Hockenberry, M., Wilson, D., Perry, S., & Lowdermilk, D. (2006). *Maternal Child Nursing Care* (3rd ed., pp. 610–611). Philadelphia: Lippincott Williams & Wilkins.

BOX 3.5
Nursing Process Evaluation Practice Item

A nurse is evaluating teaching for a client who has diabetes and is beginning insulin therapy using an insulin pen. Which behavior should best indicate to a nurse that teaching about the insulin therapy was effective?

1. The nurse showing the client a video that explains how to use the insulin pen
2. The client reading a handout that describes the different types of insulin and insulin pens
3. The nurse demonstrating the correct procedure for preparing the insulin pen for administration
4. The client preparing the insulin pen and self-injecting correctly on the first attempt

ANSWER: 4

The client correctly demonstrating preparing the insulin pen and administering the insulin suggests that the teaching about insulin therapy was effective. Options 1 and 3 are nursing interventions using various teaching strategies. Option 2 is a client action but it does not demonstrate that learning has occurred.

▶ ***Test-taking Tip:*** *Focus on what the question is asking, "indicates teaching . . . was effective" and the nursing process step of evaluation. Options that include nursing interventions should be eliminated as well as any options with client behaviors that do not demonstrate that learning has occurred.*

Content Area: Fundamentals; *Category of Health Alteration:* Medication Administration; *Integrated Processes:* Nursing Process Evaluation; *Client Need:* Health Promotion and Maintenance/Principles of Teaching and Learning; *Cognitive Level:* Application

Reference: Harkreader, H., Hogan, M., & Thobaben, M. (2007). *Fundamentals of Nursing* (3rd ed., p. 284). St. Louis, MO: Saunders/Elsevier.

BOX 3.6
The ABCs Practice Item

A 5-year-old child who is brought to an emergency room is experiencing dyspnea and swelling of the lips and tongue. Audible wheezes, rhinitis, and stridor are also present, and the child is very anxious. Based on these assessment findings, a nurse should *first*:

1. administer oxygen.
2. assess the child's vital signs.
3. administer subcutaneous epinephrine per physician's order.
4. place an intravenous (IV) line to administer antianxiety and other emergency medications.

ANSWER: 1

Securing the airway and administering oxygen is an initial intervention. The child is most likely presenting with symptoms directly related to anaphylactic shock, a potentially life-threatening systemic reaction to an allergen. All of the other interventions are needed to reverse anaphylaxis. The child's vital signs should be known before administering any medications, but that is not the first assessment priority because the information already suggests a life-threatening situation and an intervention is required. Although all of the other interventions are important, they are not the first action. Adrenalin (epinephrine) is an adrenergic (sympathomimetic) agent and cardiac stimulant used to treat anaphylactic shock. An IV line is needed for medications that can act quickly. Agitation increases oxygen demands.

➧ ***Test-taking Tip:*** *Use the ABCs (airway, breathing, circulation) to identify the initial action. Airway is the priority in this situation. In a life-threatening situation, further assessment is not the priority when an observation provides sufficient information to act. Physiological needs are also priority over psychosocial needs; thus the psychosocial option can be eliminated as the priority action.*

Content Area: Child Health; *Category of Health Alteration:* Medical Emergencies; *Integrated Processes:* Nursing Process Implementation; *Client Need:* Physiological Integrity/Physiological Adaptation/Medical Emergency; *Cognitive Level:* Analysis

Reference: Ball, J., & Bindler, R. (2008). *Pediatric Nursing: Caring for Children* (4th ed., pp. 685–687). Upper Saddle River, NJ: Pearson Education.

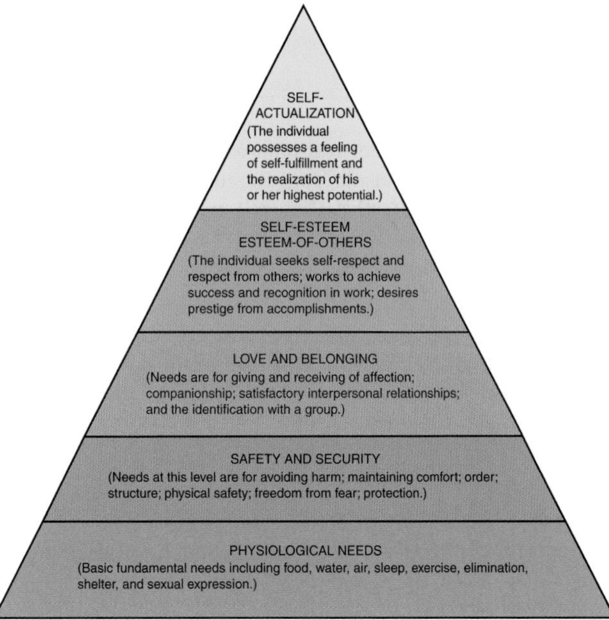

Figure 3-1 Applying Maslow's Hierarchy of Needs to establish priorities. (Adapted from Williams, L. & Hopper, P. (2007). *Understanding Medical-Surgical Nursing* (3rd ed., Fig. 1-3). Philadelphia: F. A. Davis.)

question or options. Box 3.7 provides an example of applying Maslow's Hierarchy of Needs in a practice item.

SAFETY

Safety is a high priority in NCLEX-RN® questions. Carefully read each question and answer options. If an option pertains to safety, which describes a situation that could be life-threatening and affects a physiological need, then safety may be the answer rather than a physiological need that would not be life-threatening. For example, the nursing diagnosis *Risk for injury related to use of restraints* takes priority over the nursing diagnosis *Disturbed sleep pattern related to unfamiliar surroundings*. Although sleep is a basic physiological need, an injury could be life-threatening. Box 3.8 provides an example of applying the principles of safety to practice items.

THERAPEUTIC COMMUNICATION

Some questions relate to therapeutic communication and the nurse's ability to communicate with a client. Therapeutic communication includes both verbal and nonverbal

BOX 3.7
Maslow's Hierarchy of Needs Practice Item

A client hospitalized with a history of vomiting and diarrhea for 2 days has weakness, lethargy, serum CO_2 of 18 mEq/L, and abdominal cramping. The client reports an inability to eat due to nausea. Which should be the nurse's priority nursing diagnosis when caring for the client?

1. Altered nutrition less than body requirements related to diarrhea as manifested by inability to eat
2. Deficient fluid volume related to vomiting as manifested by weakness and low serum CO_2
3. Risk for injury related to weakness and lethargy
4. Acute pain related to increased peristalsis as manifested by abdominal cramping

ANSWER: 2

The client is exhibiting signs of fluid volume deficit (dizziness, weakness, and lethargy). The normal CO_2 is 20 to 30 mEq/L. The decreased serum CO_2 indicates metabolic acidosis, which can be caused by diarrhea. Nutrition, potential for injury, and pain are also concerns, but not the priority, because altered fluid volume can affect perfusion.

▶ ***Test-taking Tip:*** *Note the key word "priority." Focus on the client's symptoms and the low serum CO_2 level. Use Maslow's Hierarchy of Needs theory. Basic physiological needs have priority over safety and security needs. The ABCs (airway, breathing, circulation) can also be used because deficient fluid volume can affect circulation.*

Content Area: Adult Health; *Category of Health Alteration:* Gastrointestinal Management; *Integrated Processes:* Nursing Process Analysis; *Client Need:* Safe and Effective Care Environment/Management of Care/Establishing Priorities; *Cognitive Level:* Analysis

Reference: Lewis, S., Heitkemper, M., Dirksen, S., O'Brien, P., & Bucher, L. (2007). *Medical-Surgical Nursing: Assessment and Management of Clinical Problems* (7th ed., pp. 322; 1036, 1855). St. Louis: MO: Mosby.

BOX 3.8
Safety Practice Item

A nurse is assessing an elderly postoperative client who is exhibiting signs of delirium. The nurse observes that the client is convinced that it is 1954 and is complaining about "the bugs in this hotel." The nurse's priority intervention should be to:

1. obtain a prn order for haloperidol (Haldol®).
2. transfer the client to a room near the nurse's station.
3. call the client's family to come and stay with the client.
4. arrange for a patient care assistant (PCA) to stay with the client.

ANSWER: 4

The nurse's priority intervention should be to arrange for a PCA to stay with the client. The client's immediate safety is the primary concern, and constant observation is the best means of providing a safe environment for this client. Although medication may become appropriate, it should not be the first response to manage a client's behavior. It does not address the issue of observing the client for safety. Transferring the client closer to the nurse's station does not provide the constant observation that is most appropriate for the client at this time. Asking the client's family to stay may not be a realistic expectation.

▶ ***Test-taking Tip:*** *Use Maslow's Hierarchy of Needs theory to determine the priority action. Client safety is always a high priority. Determine which option provides for the most thorough, reasonable, and speedy means of addressing the client's safety needs.*

Content Area: Mental Health; *Category of Health Alteration:* Cognitive, Schizophrenic, and Psychotic Disorders; *Integrated Process:* Nursing Process Implementation; *Client Needs:* Psychosocial Integrity/Behaviorial Interventions; *Cognitive Level:* Analysis

Reference: Mohr, W. (2006). *Psychiatric-Mental Health Nursing* (6th ed., pp. 726–734). Philadelphia: Lippincott Williams & Wilkins.

communication. Normally, communication questions are multiple-choice–type items and incorrect options can be eliminated so that just one answer option remains. The nurse should use communication techniques that focus on the client's concerns and facilitate communication. Therefore, first eliminate the options that are obviously not therapeutic and then look for responses that use barriers to therapeutic communication.

Therapeutic communication includes using techniques such as silence, broad opening statements, focusing, restating, clarifying, validating messages, interpreting body language, sharing observations, exploring issues, and reflecting. Barriers to therapeutic communication include responses such as changing the subject, inattentive listening, giving false reassurance, and giving advice. Tables 3.2 and 3.3 provide a description of common therapeutic communication techniques and barriers to therapeutic communication that you may encounter in the practice items provided or on the NCLEX-RN® examination. Box 3.9 provides an example of applying therapeutic communication in a practice item.

KEY WORDS

Pay attention to key words. There will be questions for which there are more than one correct option; however, based on key words there is only one option that answers the question correctly. Questions may contain key words such as *most appropriate, least appropriate, best, first, last, next,* and *most helpful.* These key words bring your attention to a specific

TABLE 3.2
Therapeutic Communication Techniques

Acknowledging	Indicating an awareness of a change in a client's behavior
Focusing	Collecting additional information to help gain further knowledge on a topic the client addressed after he or she finishes speaking
Giving information	Providing accurate information that a client did or did not request
Offering general leads	Using statements or questions that encourage verbalization, allowing a client to choose the topic of conversation, and facilitating further communication
Offering self	Simply being present or asking if the client needs anything without expecting a client to give the nurse anything
Reflecting	Directing the topic to an idea or feeling that a client stated, which allows for further exploration on that feeling or idea
Seeking clarification	Either stating that what a client said was misunderstood or asking the client to repeat the conversation or basic idea of the message
Sharing observations	Verbalizing what is observed or perceived, which allows client recognition of specific behaviors to compare perceptions with the nurse
Summarizing and planning	Restating the main ideas of a conversation to clarify the important points; often done at the end of an interview
Using silence	Allowing pauses or silences without interjecting a verbal response and allowing a client an opportunity to collect and organize thoughts.

Adapted from Berman, A., Snyder, S., Kozier, B., & Erb, G. (2008). *Kozier & Erb's Fundamentals of Nursing: Concepts, Process, and Practice* (8th ed., pp. 469–471). Upper Saddle River, NJ: Pearson Education.

TABLE 3.3
Barriers to Therapeutic Communication

Asking "why"	Asking why suggests criticism to some and may result in a defensive response from a client.
Belittling the feelings expressed	Conveying a lack of empathy and understanding. This may result in a client feeling insignificant or unimportant.
Changing the subject	Directing the topic into areas of self-interest. This usually indicates that a nurse is unable to handle the topic that is being discussed and avoids listening to what a client is saying and feeling.
Giving nonexpert advice	Telling a client what should be done or how to think. Giving advice focuses on a nurse's opinions and ideas and not on the client's views. This may negate the client's opportunity to participate as a mutual partner in decision making.

TABLE 3.3
Barriers to Therapeutic Communication (continued)

Providing false reassurance	Using clichés or encouraging statements when the situation's outcome is not positive or is unknown. These statements ignore the fears, feelings, and other responses of a client.
Interpreting	Telling a client the meaning of his or her experience.
Passing judgment	Giving opinions or approving or disapproving a client's values. This may result in the client feeling that he or she must think as the nurse thinks and not have his or her own ideas and opinions.
Probing	Asking unnecessary questions; these questions violate a client's rights.
Rejecting	Refusing to discuss certain concerns or topics. This may lead a client to believing that the nurse is rejecting not only the client's concerns but also the client.
Stereotyping	Generalizing groups of people based on experiences that a nurse has previously experienced; categorizes the client and does not look at each client as an individual.

Adapted from Berman, A., Snyder, S., Kozier, B., & Erb, G. (2008). *Kozier & Erb's Fundamentals of Nursing: Concepts, Process, and Practice* (8th ed., pp. 469–471). Upper Saddle River, NJ: Pearson Education.

BOX 3.9
Therapeutic Communication Practice Item

In a written record of a conversation between a nurse and client, which statement by the nurse best encourages therapeutic communication?

Client: "I just learned I might have cancer and I am having surgery tomorrow morning."

1. Nurse: "I see. Why are you afraid? Do you think surgery will reveal that you have cancer?"
   Client: "I am afraid because I don't want to have cancer."
2. Nurse: "Are you afraid that it might be cancer?"
   Client: "I guess."
3. Nurse: "Having a possible diagnosis of cancer is frightening. Tell me more about how you are feeling about this."
   Client: "I'm afraid I will die. My mother died of cancer when I was 10, and I have a 10 year old."
4. Nurse: "This really hits close to you."
   Client: "Yes. I don't want my 10 year old to grow up alone."

1. Response 1
2. Response 2
3. Response 3
4. Response 4

ANSWER: 3

The statements in option 3 use therapeutic communication techniques of sharing observations and using an open-ended statement. The statement allows the client to elaborate further about the client's feelings and fears, while building a trusting nurse–client relationship. Asking the client "why" questions belittles the client's feelings and may cause the client to withdraw from the interaction. Response 2 is an example of restating and clarifying the client's response but it does not stimulate further conversation. Asking the client a "yes"/"no" question, as in response 2, ends the conversation and does not allow for further opportunity to build a relationship. Response 4 is an example of restatement. Although the statement allows the client to further elaborate and is therapeutic, response 3 is the best statement because it uses two therapeutic communication techniques, whereas response 4 uses one.

▸ ***Test-taking Tip:*** *Read through the written conversation carefully. Choose the option that uses more than one therapeutic communication technique and encourages further communication.*

Content Area: Adult Health; *Category of Health Alteration:* Oncological Management; *Integrated Processes:* Communication and Documentation; *Client Need:* Psychosocial Integrity/Therapeutic Communications; *Cognitive Level:* Analysis

Reference: Harkreader, H., Hogan, M., & Thobaben, M. (2007). *Fundamentals of Nursing* (3rd ed., pp. 266–269). St. Louis, MO: Saunders/Elsevier.

point that you need to consider when answering the question. The key words can indicate a priority or negative polarity. Tables 3.4 and 3.5 provide examples of key words.

For priority items, all or most of the options are correct, but you must determine the best option that fits with the key word or phrase to correctly answer the question. Looking for a key word in each of the options that may be a synonym for a key word in the question is also a technique for selecting the correct option. The previously discussed strategies (ABCs, Maslow's Hierarchy of Needs theory, Nursing Process, and Safety) can be used to determine the best option for items that set a priority with a key word.

TABLE 3.4
Key Words That Set a Priority

Best	Last	Most likely
Early	Least appropriate	Most suitable
Essential	Least helpful	Next
First	Least likely	Priority
Highest priority	Most appropriate	Primary
Immediate	Most important	Safest
Initial	Most helpful	Vital

TABLE 3.5
Key Words Indicating Positive and Negative Polarity

Positive Polarity	Negative Polarity
Acceptable	Avoid
Correct	Contraindicated
Effective	Incorrect
Indicate	Ineffective
Most appropriate	Least appropriate, helpful, or likely
Most helpful	Unacceptable
Most likely	Unlikely
Most suitable	Unrelated
Safest	Unsafe
	Violate

Negative polarity items, sometimes called false-response items, are those in which you would select the option that is incorrect. The stem of the item is negatively worded and asks you to identify an exception, detect an error, or identify unacceptable nursing actions or contraindicated actions by the nurse or client. Negative polarity items may or may not appear on your NCLEX-RN® examination.

ABSOLUTE WORD OPTIONS

Absolute words used in options tend to make those options incorrect. Some absolute words include *must, always, never, all, none, every,* and *only*. Eliminating options containing absolute words can make it easier to answer the question.

SIMILAR OPTIONS

At times there may be two or more options that appear to be similar. When you are answering questions, look for these similar options because they can usually be eliminated in multiple-choice items. For these types of items, there is only one correct option to each question and *usually* the option of choice is different from those that are similar. Be careful as you read the stem of the question, however, because the option that may be different may not fit with the question or situation presented. Box 3.10 provides an example of a practice item containing similar options.

In multiple-response items, look for similar options that can include similar assessment findings, actions, or concepts. Similar options are most likely the correct options in multiple-response types of questions.

BOX 3.10
Similar Options Practice Item

A 2-year-old client is hospitalized with lymphoma. Which nursing observation, after a parent has left the room, poses the most immediate and serious safety threat to the child and should be removed or changed?

1. Coloring book and crayons left in the crib
2. Placing a doll with movable eyes in the crib
3. Hanging a mobile over the crib
4. Leaving the crib rail halfway down

ANSWER: 4

The greatest threat to the child is a fall. Crib rails should be raised and secured unless an adult is in attendance. Although all options pose a safety threat, the most immediate and serious of these is the crib rails in a halfway position. A 2-year-old child's developmental stage focuses on mobility and exploring the environment. Crayons can pose a choking hazard if the child should chew on these. Movable eyes in a doll can pose a choking hazard if the eyes can be removed. A mobile could pose a safety risk if the child were to attempt to use this to climb out of bed.

► *Test-taking Tip: Note the similarities in the risk posed in options 1 and 2, that option 3 may or may not pose a risk, and that option 4 presents a different risk. Often, the option that is different is the answer in a multiple-choice type question.*

Content Area: Child Health; *Category of Health Alteration:* Hematological and Oncological Management; *Integrated Processes:* Nursing Process Evaluation; *Client Need:* Safe and Effective Care Environment/Safety and Infection Control/Accident Prevention; *Cognitive Level:* Analysis

Reference: Ball, J., & Bindler, R. (2008). *Pediatric Nursing: Caring for Children* (4th ed., pp. 320–323, 416). Upper Saddle River, NJ: Pearson Education.

OPTIONS THAT ARE OPPOSITES

In both multiple-choice and multiple-response items, look for options that are opposites, such as tachycardia and bradycardia. Either one or both of these options may be incorrect. Focus on eliminating one or both of these options before focusing on the other options. Box 3.11 provides an example of a practice item with options that are opposites.

GLOBAL OPTIONS

A global or umbrella option is one that will be more comprehensive than the other options and frequently includes information or concepts from one or more of the other options. The three distracter options are usually more specific than the global option. Therefore, the global option will be the correct option. Box 3.12 provides an example of a practice item with a global option.

BOX 3.11
Opposite Options Practice Item

Two hours after initiating total parenteral nutrition (TPN), a nurse assesses a client and notes diuresis and decreased blood pressure. The nurse recognizes that these signs may indicate that the:

1. glucose content of the TPN solution is too high.
2. TPN solution is infusing too slowly.
3. TPN solution is infusing too rapidly.
4. protein content of the TPN solution is too low.

ANSWER: 3

If the TPN solution is infusing too rapidly, hyperosmolar diuresis occurs from rapid infusion of glucose, which results in a rapid increase in blood glucose and rapid metabolism. It is the rapid infusion of the glucose, rather than the amount of glucose, causing the symptoms. Protein content will not cause diuresis.

▶ ***Test-taking Tip:*** *Note that options 2 and 3 are opposites. Examine these options first to determine if one or both can be eliminated. Focus on the time frames of 2 hours and the information that this is the initial infusion of the TPN. Think about the nutrient content of TPN solution and which of those nutrients is metabolized quickly.*

Content Area: Adult Health; *Category of Health Alteration:* Gastrointestinal Management; *Integrated Processes:* Nursing Process Analysis; *Client Need:* Physiological Integrity/Pharmacological and Parenteral Therapies/Total Parenteral Nutrition; *Cognitive Level:* Analysis

References: Smeltzer, S., Bare, B., Hinkle, J., & Cheever, K. (2008). *Brunner and Suddarth's Textbook of Medical-Surgical Nursing* (11th ed., p. 1198). Philadelphia: Lippincott Williams & Wilkins; Wilkinson, J., & Van Leuven, K. (2007). *Fundamentals of Nursing: Theory, Concepts and Applications.* (Vol. 1, p. 617). Philadelphia, F. A. Davis.

BOX 3.12
Global Options Practice Item

A nurse is teaching day-care providers caring for young children about infectious disease transmission. About which most common sources for disease transmission should the nurse teach the day-care providers?

1. Fecal, oral, and respiratory routes
2. Contact with toys that are shared
3. Urinary, oral, and respiratory secretions
4. Sneezing, coughing, and rubbing a runny nose and then touching others

ANSWER: 1

Because young children have not fully developed good hygiene behaviors, transmission of infectious diseases is facilitated by fecal, oral, and respiratory routes among other children in their play or school group. Although toys are a source of disease transmission, this option is not as inclusive as option 1. The urinary route is less contagious than the fecal route, which transmits *Escherichia coli.* Option 3 is concerned with disease transmission only from the respiratory route.

▶ ***Test-taking Tip:*** *Note the plural "sources" of infectious disease in the stem and select the option that is most inclusive. Option 1 is the broadest option addressing the various "routes of transmission."*

Content Area: Child Health; *Category of Health Alteration:* Infectious Disease; *Integrated Processes:* Teaching/Learning; *Client Need:* Physiological Integrity/Physiological Adaptation/Infectious Diseases; *Cognitive Level:* Application

Reference: Ball, J., & Bindler, R. (2006). *Child Health Nursing: Partnering with Children and Families.* (p. 597). Upper Saddle River, NJ: Pearson Education.

DUPLICATE INFORMATION AMONG OPTION ITEMS

Some test items are designed so that more than one point or fact is included within each option. For these types of questions, first look for the options with duplicate information and determine if that information is correct or incorrect. If it is incorrect, then you can eliminate all items with the duplicate information. Box 3.13 provides an example of a practice item with duplicate information among answer options.

DELEGATION AND ASSIGNMENT ITEMS

Most likely, there will be questions that ask you to delegate or assign certain clients or tasks to other health-care personnel. Read the question thoroughly so that you understand the task or to whom the task is being delegated or assigned. Carefully look at what is being asked and match the skill with the scope of practice of the appropriate caregiver. Use the five rights of delegation: the right task, under the right circumstances, to the right person, with the right direction and communication, and the right supervision and evaluation. Remember that registered nurses (RNs) are responsible for assessing, evaluating, teaching, and making decisions about client care and that these tasks cannot be delegated. Note that observations, but not assessments, can be delegated. Because the scope of practice varies by state, you should encounter only the universal tasks that can be delegated. Table 3.6 illustrates examples of tasks that may and may not be delegated to unlicensed assistive personnel.

NCLEX-RN® questions may also ask you to decide when to notify a physician or other health-care provider. On the NCLEX-RN® examination, the option of notifying the physician may or may not be the correct option. NCLEX-RN® is testing the RN's ability to work safely. Sometimes choosing the option of notifying the physician or other health-care personnel, such as the charge nurse, is relegating your responsibility to someone else when further assessment or an immediate intervention is needed. If you are unable to determine if you must call the physician or if another action is indicated, make sure that client safety has been addressed first and that all information necessary to notify the physician has been obtained. Remember, a person's safety is the priority, especially if an unsafe situation can be life-threatening. Box 3.14 provides an example of a delegation practice item.

LABORATORY VALUES

Laboratory values are included in the NCLEX-RN® examination. The 2010 NCLEX-RN® Detailed Test Plan (2009) identifies essential laboratory values that you need to know. These include arterial blood gases [ABGs (pH, Po_2, Pco_2,

BOX 3.13
Duplicate Information Among Options Practice Item

A client is newly admitted with a diagnosis of left-sided heart failure. On assessment of the client, which findings should a nurse expect?

1. Chest tightness and ascites
2. Dyspnea on exertion and ascites
3. Dyspnea on exertion and crackles
4. Neck vein distention and crackles

ANSWER: 3

Dyspnea and crackles are signs of pulmonary congestion. This occurs in left ventricular failure from back pressure into the left atrium and pulmonary venous system. Neck vein distention and ascites result from right-sided heart failure. Chest tightness could occur from either right-sided or left-sided heart failure from inadequate tissue oxygenation. Clients with left heart failure can develop right-sided failure.

➧ *Test-taking Tip: This item is testing your knowledge of the difference between right and left heart failure. Duplicate information is presented in the options. If you know one of the facts, such as dyspnea on exertion, you then can eliminate the other options (1 and 4). Now, just examine options 2 and 3. Note that option 3 pertains to just the lungs, whereas option 2 pertains to two different body areas.*

Content Area: Adult Health; *Category of Health Alteration:* Cardiac Management; *Integrated Processes:* Nursing Process Assessment; *Client Need:* Physiological Integrity/Reduction of Risk Potential/System Specific Assessments; *Cognitive Level:* Analysis

Reference: Smeltzer, S., Bare, B., Hinkle, J., & Cheever, K. (2008). *Brunner & Suddarth's Textbook of Medical-Surgical Nursing* (11th ed., p. 950). Philadelphia: Lippincott Williams & Wilkins.

TABLE 3.6

Tasks That May and May Not Be Delegated to Unlicensed Assistive Personnel

Tasks That *May* Be Delegated to Unlicensed Personnel	Tasks That *May Not* Be Delegated to Unlicensed Personnel
Bathing	Administering parenteral medications
Feeding	Assessment
Gastrostomy feedings in established systems	Care of invasive lines
Maintaining safety	Client education
Measuring and recording intake and output (I&O)	Creating a nursing care plan
Performing basic life support (CPR)	Evaluation of care effectiveness
Performing simple dressing changes	Giving telephone advice
Postmortem care	Insertion of nasogastric tubes
Suctioning of chronic tracheostomies	Interpretation of information and data
Taking vital signs	Making a nursing diagnosis
Transferring and ambulating clients	Performing triage
Weighing clients	

Adapted from Berman, A., Snyder, S., Kozier, B., & Erb, G. (2008). *Kozier & Erb's Fundamentals of Nursing: Concepts, Process, and Practice* (8th ed., p. 518). Upper Saddle River, NJ: Pearson Education.

BOX 3.14

Delegation Practice Item

A nurse is assigned to six clients, along with a licensed practical nurse (LPN) and an unlicensed assistive personnel (UAP). One client is scheduled for surgery in 15 minutes, another is having pain, one is complaining of a sudden onset of itching after receiving a new medication, and another has family who wants to talk to the physician right away. Which action should the nurse take to best manage and delegate client care?

1. Ask the LPN to give the client in pain an analgesic and the UAP to get the client ready for surgery
2. Assess the client with itching and ask the UAP to get a cart for the client needing to go to surgery
3. Ask the LPN to talk to the family and the UAP to notify the client with pain that an analgesic will be administered soon
4. Assess the client with pain and ask the LPN to let the family know the doctor is coming

ANSWER: 2

The client with itching should be assessed immediately as this may be the first sign of an anaphylactic reaction to a new medication. Delegation of retrieving a cart is appropriate for a UAP. It is appropriate for the LPN to give medication, but it is not appropriate for the UAP to prepare the client for surgery. In preparation for surgery, the client may require additional preoperative teaching, medication administration, and validation of medical record documentation, which are outside the UAP's scope of practice. Communication with the family who is requesting an urgent consult with the physician should not be delegated. The UAP should not need to ask the client to wait for an analgesic as the LPN can administer analgesics and should be assigned that task. The nurse should not prioritize the client with pain over the client with a new onset of itching, as itching may be a sign of an anaphylactic reaction.

Test-taking Tip: *Use Maslow's Hierarchy of Needs to establish priorities, selecting the physiological problem of itching as the first priority. You can also use the ABCs (airway, breathing, circulation), recognizing itching is a sign of a possible medication reaction. Then use the five rights of delegation for appropriate delegation.*

Content Area: Management of Care; *Category of Health Alteration:* Leadership and Management; *Integrated Processes:* Nursing Process Assessment; *Client Need:* Safe and Effective Care Environment/Management of Care/Delegation; *Cognitive Level:* Application

References: Berman, A., Snyder, S., Kozier, B., & Erb, G. (2008). *Kozier & Erb's Fundamentals of Nursing: Concepts, Process, and Practice* (8th ed., pp. 517–520). Upper Saddle River, NJ: Pearson Education; Harkreader, H., Hogan, M., & Thobaben, M. (2007). *Fundamentals of Nursing* (3rd ed., p. 301). St. Louis, MO: Saunders/Elsevier.

Sao_2, HCO_3)], serum creatinine (SCr) and blood urea nitrogen (BUN), serum total cholesterol, glucose, hematocrit (Hct), hemoglobin (Hgb), glycosylated hemoglobin (Hb A_{1C}), platelets (Plt), potassium (K), red blood cells (RBCs), sodium (Na), white blood cells (WBCs), and coagulation values. Table 3.7 provides normal adult laboratory value ranges for the essential laboratory values on the NCLEX-RN® examination. You will find that laboratory value ranges vary slightly from source to source. However, laboratory values included on the NCLEX-RN® examination and in the practice items will either be within the typical normal ranges or be significantly abnormal.

Besides knowing certain laboratory values, you should be able to recognize deviations from the normal. Table 3.8 provides normal laboratory value ranges for the laboratory values identified in the 2010 NCLEX-RN® Test Plan that you should be able to recognize when taking the NCLEX-RN® examination. Knowing the normal ranges and significance before you start the test will increase your ability to pass the licensure examination. Also, being able to correlate certain

TABLE 3.7 Laboratory Normal Values for Adults to Know for the NCLEX-RN® Examination

Laboratory Values and Normal Ranges
Arterial Blood Gases (ABGs)
pH (7.35–7.45)
Pco_2 (32–42 mm Hg)
HCO_3 (Bicarb 22–26 mEq/L)
Po_2 (75–100 mm Hg)
Serum Tests of Renal Function
BUN (10–20 mg/dL)
SCr (0.5–1.5 mg/dL)
Serum Chemistry
Glucose (70–110 mg/dL)
Hb A_{1C} (4%–6%)
Na (135–145 mEq/L)
K (3.5–5.0 mEq/L)
Lipid Profile
Total Cholesterol (140–200 mg/dL)
Complete Blood Count (CBC)
WBC (4–11 K/μL or 4–11 × 10^3/μL)
RBC (4.5–5.5 mil/μL or 4.5–5.5 × 10^6/μL)
Male (4.5–6.2 mil/μL or 4.5–6.2 × 10^6/μL)
Female (4.2–5.4 mil/μL or 4.2–5.4 × 10^6/μL)
Hgb (13.1–17.1 g/dL)
Male (13.5–18 g/dL)
Female (12–16 g/dL)
Hct (40%–45%)
Male (40%–54%)
Female (38%–47%)
Plt (150–400 K/μL or 150,000–400,000/mm^3)
Coagulation Tests
Bleeding time (3.0–9.5)
Prothrombin time (PT: 10–14 sec)
International normalized ratio (INR: 0.9–1.1 sec)
Activated partial thromboplastin time (aPTT: 24–36 sec)

Adapted from Lewis, S., Heitkemper, M., Dirksen, S., O'Brien, P., Bucher, L. (2007). *Medical-Surgical Nursing: Assessment and Management of Clinical Problems* (7th ed., pp. 1855–1863). St. Louis: MO: Mosby.

TABLE 3.8 Deviations From Normal Adult Laboratory Values to Recognize for the NCLEX-RN® Examination

Laboratory Values and Normal Ranges
Other Serum Electrolytes
Total calcium (9–11 mg/dL)
Magnesium (Mg: 1.5–2.5 mEq/L)
Phosphorus, inorganic (2.8–4.5 mg/dL)
Chloride (Cl: 95–105 mEq/L)
Carbon dioxide (CO_2: 20–30 mEq/L)
Lipid Profile
Total cholesterol (140–200 mg/dL)
High-density lipoprotein (HDL)
Male (>45 mg/dL)
Female (>55 mg/dL)
Low-density lipoprotein (LDL: <130 mg/dL)
Triglycerides (40–150 mg/dL)
Liver Enzymes
Albumin (3.5–5.0 g/dL)
Alanine aminotransferase (ALT/SGPT: 5–36 U/L)
Aspartate aminotransferase (AST/SGOT: 7–40 U/L)
Ammonia (30–70 mcg/dL)
Total bilirubin (0.2–1.3 mg/dL)
Alkaline phosphatase (30–120 U/L)
Nutrition Panel
Total protein (6–8 g/dL)
Hematology: WBC Differential
Neutrophils (43–70%)
Lymphocytes (20–40%)
Monocytes (4–8%)
Eosinophils (EOS: 0–4%)
Basophils (0–2%)
Hematology: Erythrocyte Sedimentation Rate
(ESR: 15–30 mm/hr; age and gender dependent)
Male ≤50 yr (<15 mm/hr)
Male >50 yr (<20 mm/hr)
Female ≤50 yr (<20 mm/hr)
Female >50 yr (<30 mm/hr)
Therapeutic Blood Levels
Digoxin (0.8–2 ng/mL)
Lithium (0.6–1.2 mEq/L)
Urine
pH (4–8)
Albumin (negative)
White blood cells (WBCs: Negative)
Urine Specific Gravity
1.003–1.030

Adapted from Lewis, S., Heitkemper, M., Dirksen, S., O'Brien, P., & Bucher, L. (2007). *Medical-Surgical Nursing: Assessment and Management of Clinical Problems* (7th ed., pp. 1855–1863). St. Louis: MO: Mosby.

laboratory values with various illnesses will help you answer the more complex questions.

Throughout this book, practice items are presented that will give you an opportunity to improve your skills at analyzing laboratory values. Box 3.15 provides an example of a practice item with both essential laboratory values and those you need to recognize for deviations from normal.

MNEMONICS TO REMEMBER KEY INFORMATION

Mnemonics are techniques that help us to remember information. For example, the classic triad for preeclampsia can be remembered by the **pre** in preeclampsia, which refers to **p**roteinuria, **r**ising blood pressure, and **e**dema. To remember the number of vertebrae, just remember the times people typically eat meals: breakfast is at **7** a.m. and there are **7** cervical vertebrae; lunch is at **12** p.m. and there are **12** thoracic vertebrae; and dinner is at **5** p.m. and there are **5** lumbar vertebrae.

An acrostic, a type of mnemonic, uses a phrase, motto, or verse in which a letter (usually the first letter) prompts your memory to retrieve information. An example of an acrostic presented in the test-taking tips is the phrase "**a**ll **p**oints **e**ssential **t**o **m**emorize" to remember the names of the heart valves and auscultation points of the heart: **a**ortic, **p**ulmonic, **E**rb's point, **t**ricuspid, and **m**itral.

Throughout this book, a variety of mnemonics, acronyms, and acrostics are presented in the test-taking tips to assist you in remembering key information. The practice question in Box 3.15 provides a memory aid to remember the essential laboratory tests for liver function.

BOX 3.15
Laboratory Value Practice Item

A nurse reports that a preoperative client has normal liver function. Which liver function laboratory values should the nurse note to be within the normal ranges? SELECT ALL THAT APPLY.

1. Hemoglobin 14 g/dL
2. Total bilirubin 1.0 mg/dL
3. White blood cells (WBCs) 8 K/μL
4. Serum creatinine (SCr) 0.7 mg/dL
5. Alanine aminotransferase (ALT) 18 U/L
6. Aspartate aminotransferase (AST) 25 U/L

ANSWER: 2, 5, 6

ALT (normal = 5–36 U/L) and AST (normal = 7–40 U/L) are two enzymes found in the liver and other organs and are elevated in most liver disorders. The total bilirubin normal is 0.2–1.3 mg/dL. Bilirubin is conjugated and excreted by the liver and is used in the evaluation of liver and biliary function. Other lab values used to evaluate liver function include alkaline phosphatase (ALP, normal = 30–120 U/L) and albumin (normal = 3.5–5.0 g/dL). Hemoglobin is the main protein in erythrocytes and is used to evaluate the ability to carry oxygen to and remove carbon dioxide from red blood cells (normal = 13.5–18 g/dL for males and 12–16 g/dL for females). WBCs (normal = 4–11 K/μL or 4–11 × 10^3/μL) evaluate the presence of inflammation or infection. Serum creatinine (normal 0.5–1.5 mg/dL) evaluates kidney function.

▸ *Test-taking Tip: While all laboratory values are within the normal ranges, only three of the laboratory values presented are used to evaluate liver function. A memory cue to remember two of the liver function tests is to associate the liver function tests with AA. You may know the "AA" acronym as alcoholic anonymous, but in this situation it is alanine aminotransferase (**A**LT) and aspartate aminotransferase (**A**ST). This tip can also be used to remember the other two laboratory values that begin with the letter A, albumin and alkaline phosphatase (ALP). The letter B follows in the alphabet and can be used to remember bilirubin.*

Content Area: Adult Health; *Category of Health Alteration:* Perioperative Management; *Integrated Processes:* Nursing Process Evaluation; *Client Need:* Physiological Integrity/Reduction of Risk Potential/Laboratory Values; *Cognitive Level:* Analysis

Reference: Lewis, S., Heitkemper, M., Dirksen, S., O'Brien, P., & Bucher, L. (2007). *Medical-Surgical Nursing: Assessment and Management of Clinical Problems* (7th ed., pp. 1855–1863). St. Louis: MO: Mosby.

MEDICAL TERMINOLOGY

Medical terminology is another easy way to understand questions or answer options. By knowing the meaning of common suffixes and prefixes, it is easier to understand what is being addressed in a question or an option. Review common terminology before taking the NCLEX-RN® examination. Some common prefixes and suffixes are included in Table 3-9. The test-taking tips within this book will also highlight some other common medical terminology prefixes and suffixes.

PHARMACOLOGY QUESTIONS

Use medical terminology to also identify unfamiliar medications. Certain classifications of medications will have common suffixes for the generic names of the medications. For example, the generic names of the beta blocker medications will end in "-lol." Table 3.10 includes common identifiers for pharmacology questions. Unfortunately, not all medications for treating a certain condition or within a medication classification have common suffixes. Therefore, the table of medication suffixes is not inclusive

TABLE 3.9
Common Prefixes and Suffixes in Medical Terminology

Prefix	Meaning	Suffix	Meaning
A(n)-	No, not, without	-algia	Pain
Ab-	Away from	-ase	Enzyme
Ante-	Before	-ation	Action or process
Brady-	Slow	-cele	Hernia
De-	Down, remove	-cyte	Cell
Endo-	Inside	-eal	Pertaining to
Intra-	Within	-ectomy	Excision
Mal-	Bad	-emia	Blood
Post-	After, behind	-ia, -iasis	Condition
Pre-	Before	-itis	Inflammation of
Tachy-	Fast	-oma	Tumor

TABLE 3.10
Common Suffixes Pertaining to Pharmacology Questions

Suffix	Medication Classification	Suffix	Medication Classification
-amide	Sulfonylureas antidiabetics	-lol	Beta-adrenergic antagonists (beta blockers)
-ase	Thrombolytic agents	-mycin	Aminoglycoside or macrolide antibiotics
-avir; -ivir; -ovir	Antivirals	-navir	Protease inhibitors (treatment of HIV and AIDS)
-azine	Typical antipsychotics	-pam; -lam	Benzodiazepines; antianxiety; sedative
-azole	Antifungal; antiprotozoans or antihelminthics (parasitic infections)	-parin	Anticoagulant
-bital	Barbiturates	-pramine or -triptyline	Tricyclic antidepressants
-caine	Local anesthetic agents	-pril	Angiotensin-converting enzyme inhibitors (ACE inhibitors)
-choline	Cholinergic agonists (direct acting muscarinic agonists)	-profen	Nonsteroidal anti-inflammatory drugs (NSAIDs): Prostaglandin synthetase inhibitors
-cillin	Penicillin antibiotics	-sartans	Angiotensin II receptor blockers (ARBs)

TABLE 3.10
Common Suffixes Pertaining to Pharmacology Questions (continued)

Suffix	Medication Classification	Suffix	Medication Classification
-curium; -curonium	Neuromuscular blocking agents	-setron	Antiemetics
-cycline	Tetracycline antibiotics	-statin	Antihyperlipidemic: Statins
-dipine	Calcium channel blockers; antiarrhythmics	-suximide	Antiepileptics
-dronate	Antihypercalcemics	-terol	Bronchodilators
-floxacin	Quinolone/fluoroquinolone antibiotics	-thiazide	Thiazide diuretics
-fungin	Antifungals	-tidine	H_2 receptor blockers
-glinide	Meglitinide antidiabetics	-triptan	NSAIDs: Serotonin-selective agonists
-grastin	Colony-stimulating factors	-urane	Inhalation anesthetic agents
-idone	Atypical antipsychotics	-vudine	Nucleoside/nucleotide reverse transcriptase inhibitors (treatment of HIV and AIDS)
Interferon	Cytokines (affecting immune response)	-ximab; -zumab	Antibodies affecting immune response
-isone; -asone; or -solone	Corticosteroids	-zolamide	Diuretics: Carbonic anhydrase inhibitors
-line	Xanthine bronchodilators	-zoline	Topical decongestants
		-zosin; -eride	Alpha-adrenergic antagonists (alpha blockers)

of all medication classifications or medications used in the disease treatment. Box 3.16 provides an example of a pharmacology practice item.

VISUALIZATION AND ASSOCIATION

Visualization can be used not only as a relaxation technique in preparing for the NCLEX-RN® examination but also in answering test items. This can be accomplished by visualizing yourself performing the nursing action in the test item or associating the item to a client for whom you have provided care.

Visualization works exceptionally well for prioritization items, for which you will prioritize nursing actions or place items in sequence. These items may include tasks or skills that need to be sequenced in an appropriate order for what should be done first, second, and so forth. First, read the question and understand what is expected of you when completing the item. Then, visualize performing the skill or completing the task addressed. Finally, carefully read the options to prevent missing essential information and then begin sequencing. Besides visualization, the previously mentioned strategies of using the ABCs, Maslow's Hierarchy of Needs, and the nursing process can also be applied to prioritization items. Box 3.17 provides a practice item for using the skill of visualization.

THINGS TO AVOID

Avoid answering NCLEX-RN® examination questions according to real-life experiences that may be different from the textbook content. The NCLEX-RN® examination is designed so that the content of the examination is directly related to content in textbooks that you have used during your education and on national standards of care and best nursing practices. Remember that this examination is supported by information in these sources and sometimes what you may have experienced in "real-life situations" may not be what is currently being taught; rather, your experiences could be based on time-saving shortcuts, old information, or procedures and practices specific to a health-care agency. Studying is the key to success because the licensure examination is based in "NCLEX land" where everything is performed by the book and the nurse in the test items has the time and resources to complete responsibilities, unless it is

BOX 3.16
Pharmacology Practice Item

A client diagnosed with chronic obstructive pulmonary disease (COPD) is hospitalized due to increasing dyspnea. The client is anxious and requesting an antianxiety medication. A nurse notes the current time as 1000 hours and reviews the client's medication administration record. Which actions should the nurse take? SELECT ALL THAT APPLY.

Date: Today — **Medication Administration Record**

Client: J. Jones | **Account Number:** 246810 | **Allergies:** Benzodiazepines
Sex: Male
Height: 68 in. | **Weight:** 70 kg | **Date of Birth:** 01-31-1950

Medication	0001–0730	0731–1530	1531–2400
Furosemide (Lasix®) 20 mg oral bid		0800 ABC	2000 _____
Salmeterol (Serevent Diskus®) 50 mcg q12h per diskus inhaler		0800 ____	2000 _____
Alprazolam (Xanax®) 0.25–0.5 mg oral tid prn			
Ondansetron (Zofran®) 2–4 mg IV q4–6h prn	0500 NNN		
Temazepam (Restoril®) 15 mg oral HS prn			

1. Administer alprazolam (Xanax®) 0.25 mg orally
2. Administer temazepam (Restoril®) 15 mg orally
3. Administer the salmeterol, which was due at 0800
4. Administer ondansetron (Zofran®) 4 mg IV
5. Contact the client's physician

ANSWER: 3, 5

Salmeterol is a bronchodilator. Dyspnea can increase anxiety. The medication should be given now because it was missed at 0800. The client's physician should be notified because the client is allergic to benzodiazepines and both alprazolam and temazepam are benzodiazepines. The orders for the alprazolam and temazepam should be discontinued and another medication for anxiety should be ordered. Ondansetron is an antiemetic.

➧ ***Test-taking Tip:*** *First, carefully review the MAR before answering the question. If unsure of the medications, consider the client's diagnosis of COPD and use the cue of the "diskus inhaler" as a clue that this is a bronchodilator. Use the suffixes "–lam and –pam" to determine that both Alprazolam (Xanax®) and Temazepam (Restoril®) are benzodiazepines. In carefully reviewing the MAR, you should see that the client is allergic to benzodiazepines.*

Content Area: Adult Health; *Category of Health Alteration:* Pharmacology & Parenteral Therapies; *Integrated Processes:* Nursing Process Implementation; *Client Need:* Physiological Integrity/Pharmacological & Parenteral Therapies/Adverse Effects/Contradictions/Interactions; *Cognitive Level:* Analysis

Reference: Aschenbrenner, D., & Venable, S. (2009). *Drug Therapy in Nursing* (3rd ed., p. 971). Philadelphia: Lippincott Williams & Wilkins.

BOX 3.17
Visualization and Association Practice Item

A nurse is teaching new parents about the best method of bathing their newborn. Prioritize the steps for the newborn's bath in the order that the nurse should teach them to the parents.

______ Wash around the umbilical cord
______ Wash the face with clear water
______ Wash the newborn's upper body and then dry
______ Wipe the newborn's eyes with clear water from the inner canthus outward
______ Wash and dry the perineal area
______ Wash the legs and dry
______ Assemble needed equipment
______ Wash the newborn's hair with a gentle soap

ANSWER: 6, 3, 5, 2, 8, 7, 1, 4

Before beginning a bath, the parents should first assemble the needed equipment. This will help the parents avoid leaving their infant exposed or unattended while gathering the equipment. Bathing should proceed from the cleanest area first to the most soiled areas of the body. Therefore, the bath should start at the eyes, and then wash the face with clear water, the newborns hair, upper body, the umbilical cord, the legs, and end at the diaper area. As each area is washed, it should be dried and covered to protect the infant from becoming chilled.

Test-taking Tip: First, visualize performing the newborn's bath and then visualize teaching the parents. Recall the principle of working from the cleanest to the most soiled areas when performing the newborn's bath.

Content Area: Childbearing Families; *Category of Health Alteration:* Neonatal and High-Risk Neonatal Management; *Integrated Processes:* Teaching/Learning; *Client Need:* Physiological Integrity/Basic Care and Comfort/Personal Hygiene; Health Promotion and Maintenance/Ante/Intra/Postpartum and Newborn Care; *Cognitive Level:* Application

Reference: Pillitteri, A. (2007). *Maternal & Child Health Nursing: Care of the Childbearing & Childrearing Family* (5th ed., p. 712). Philadelphia: Lippincott Williams & Wilkins.

stated otherwise in the situation described. Also, unless otherwise stated, the nurse will always have all the supplies needed within reach and does not need to call or leave the room. The nurse should be able to complete most of the tasks independently, without calling for help or assigning the task to someone else, unless the task or responsibility is not within the scope of registered nursing practice.

Avoid reading meaning into the questions. When reading a question and the answer options, simply read what is written. Often, the situation provides more information than needed to answer the specific question. Avoid asking, "What if . . . ?" Focus on the information provided and do not add more details. Although you should not read meaning into the question, make sure that you are reading the entire question and not missing pertinent information. You may select the wrong option if an important piece of information is missed in either the situation or the options. Box 3.18 provides an example of avoiding reading meaning into a practice item.

Avoid becoming frustrated or anxious. Use visualization often, seeing yourself as the competent nurse performing professional nursing care. Expect that there may be information that you do not know and use all the strategies that you have learned to arrive at the best option among the items.

DIFFICULT QUESTIONS ARE A GOOD SIGN

As you are answering questions on the actual NCLEX-RN® examination and it seems that the test questions are getting increasingly harder, this is a good sign. Answering questions correctly will cue the Computerized Adaptive Testing (CAT) to present more difficult questions. As the number of difficult questions you answer correctly increases, the number of actual test items that you will need to complete decreases. However, do not focus on the difficulty level and the number of items you complete. Items may seem difficult to you because you do not know the content, but these could actually be easier items. Therefore, although the questions may seem to be getting harder, continue to focus on using the test-taking strategies to select the best answer for each item.

This book is designed such that the majority of items are at the more difficult cognitive levels so that you gain experience with these types of questions. The rationales to both the answers and the incorrect options are sometimes lengthy, providing you with the content necessary to strengthen your knowledge base and prepare you for the actual NCLEX-RN® examination. Like the NCLEX-RN® examination, questions may seem hard initially, but as you progress through this question-and-answer book, you should find that items get easier to answer. Practice in answering the NCLEX-RN®-style questions, understanding the rationales for the answers and the incorrect options, and using a question drill process in which you complete multiple questions during one sitting and analyzing your results provide the best opportunity to develop your test-taking skills. At the completion of this book, you should feel confident in your abilities to answer the more complex questions using the test-taking strategies you have learned

BOX 3.18
Avoiding Reading Meaning Into a Question Practice Item

A client has an automatic blood pressure cuff and the same number is displayed for 11 hours of a 12-hour shift. A nurse documents the reading, thinking it is a new blood pressure measurement each hour. When the nurse working the next shift takes the client's blood pressure, the client is hypotensive. The nurse manager speaks with the nurse about the event and concludes that the nurse failed to assess the client's blood pressure (BP) for 11 hours of a 12-hour shift. Due to a similar event with a new nurse, the standards and protocols were reviewed with all nurses at a required department meeting the previous week. Which intervention by the nurse manager with the involved nurse is most appropriate?

1. Terminating the nurse's employment immediately
2. Reviewing the operation of the blood pressure machine with the nurse
3. Providing the nurse with a notice of intent to terminate if further incidents occur
4. Informing the nurse of the unsafe action and expectations related to BP assessment

ANSWER: 3

The nurse manager is responsible for ensuring safe client care and to discipline the employee to prevent further occurrences. A notice of intent to terminate is a form of discipline with the intent to improve job performance. Employees are required to conform to rules and regulations. The first step in the disciplinary process is generally not termination. Nurses may be terminated for flagrant errors; however, the most supportive approach is to discipline if necessary and allow time for the nurse to improve practice. Although the nurse may need to relearn how to operate the blood pressure machine, the issue is lack of client assessment. Educating the nurse and not taking disciplinary action may result in another incident of unsafe client care. The nurse manager is responsible for client safety.

▶ ***Test-taking Tip:*** *The key words are "most appropriate." Carefully read the situation and question to avoid missing important points. Avoid reading into the question and asking whether or not the nurse attended the department meeting. Even if the meeting had not been attended by the nurse, the meeting was required, and information covered at the meeting would be expected of the employee. Also, avoid thinking as if you were the involved nurse in the situation and what action you would prefer to be taken. Rather, answer the question focusing on the employee disciplinary process, which includes remediation, warning, and then termination.*

Content Area: Management of Care; *Category of Health Alteration:* Leadership and Management; *Integrated Processes:* Nursing Process Implementation; *Client Need:* Safe and Effective Care Environment/Management of Care/Supervision; *Cognitive Level:* Analysis

References: Harkreader, H. Hogan, M., & Thobaben, M. (2007). *Fundamentals of Nursing* (3rd ed., pp. 40–41). St. Louis, MO: Saunders/Elsevier; Jones, R. (2007). *Nursing Leadership and Management: Theories, Processes and Practice* (p. 310). Philadelphia: F. A. Davis.

and should be well prepared for the actual licensure examination.

NCLEX-RN® PREPARATION: GENERAL TIPS

PQRST Approach

Use the **PQRST approach** to master studying for the NCLEX-RN® examination and be successful on your first attempt. Remember that the PQRST mnemonic is used both for assessing pain and for analyzing the rhythm of an electrocardiogram (EKG) monitor strip. While the licensure examination can be painful, using strategic interventions can reduce the pain and keep you in a healthy rhythm to achieve your life goal of becoming a registered nurse. The **PQRST approach** includes having a positive mindset, questions to assess and build your knowledge, review of strengths and weaknesses, stress reduction, and finally taking the NCLEX-RN® test.

Positive Mindset

The first step in preparing for the NCLEX-RN® examination is having a positive mindset. "I can do it! I will pass the NCLEX-RN® exam!" Use positive self-talk and self-reassurance. Acknowledge what you already know and use self-congratulation for your success thus far: graduation (or near graduation) from a registered nurse program. You have accomplished much and you are ready for the final step.

Study with enthusiasm, sincerity, and determination, keeping your goal in mind. Visualizing your goal can keep you motivated. Smile. You know what you are doing! Smiling reduces facial tension and stress and can help you feel better about yourself.

Questions

Did you know that mastering test-taking strategies and being ready to take the NCLEX-RN® exam successfully requires completing from 2,000 to 4,000 questions? This book and the accompanying CD provide you with more than 5,000 questions to hone your test-taking skills and review the content. Use the strategies from this chapter to answer the questions. Because rationales for all answers are provided with each question, you will be maximizing your study time to learn new information as well as enhancing your test-taking abilities. Using practice questions improves your testing performance; you become test-wise in learning how to read a question and eliminate incorrect options!

The cognitive level of questions will also boost the likelihood of success on the NCLEX-RN® exam. The majority of questions in this book and accompanying CD are at the application and analysis level. Practicing with these more difficult questions should make it easier for you to answer the less difficult knowledge and comprehension level questions that may appear on the actual NCLEX-RN® exam.

Develop a Plan

Before you begin to take the tests in this book, you need to develop a plan. There are over 2,000 questions in this book and an additional 3,000 plus questions on the CD. Nearly all of the items from the book also appear on the CD, totaling more than 5,000 questions. Determine your approach to studying the questions in this book and accompanying CD. For example, answering 25 to 30 questions per day will allow you to complete all of the questions in about 180 days, that is, about 30 to 45 minutes per day that you allocate to answering questions for about a 6-month time period. Answering 50 to 60 questions per day will allow you to complete all 5,000 questions in about 90 days, that is, studying 60 to 90 minutes per day for a 90-day time period. If planning to study less than 90 days or 3 months, consider that completing 5,000 questions may take about 100 hours or more of study time. Be sure to allow yourself enough time for taking practice questions!

Schedule a Consistent Study Time

After developing a study plan, determine the time of day that works best for you. Some prefer breaking the study period into time blocks of an hour or less to avoid fatigue and boredom. Others prefer longer study periods to allow for greater concentration. Still others prefer to accomplish a certain number of questions once or twice daily rather than setting aside a certain amount of time. Whichever you choose, you should be consistent and diligent. Remember to reward yourself daily for your consistency and accomplishments.

At some point in your schedule, you should plan times to answer 75 questions during one sitting. This is the minimum number of questions on the exam. In addition, you should plan times to answer 265 items during one sitting. This is the maximum number of items. During these study sessions, time yourself to determine how long it takes you to answer all of the questions.

Study Space

Determine your best study space where you can concentrate. Be consistent with this space if possible. Stay focused and do not try to do two things at the same time, such as watching television and studying.

Computer Practice

Although you should be consistent in your study space, you should allocate time at the computer for completing questions from the accompanying CD. You will be taking the NCLEX-RN® exam at the computer from 1 to 5 hours. Thus, at some point in your studying you should practice at the computer from 1 to 5 hours, completing questions on the accompanying CD. Do this a few times during your review, varying the time periods. This practice allows acclimating yourself to the rigors of taking the NCLEX-RN® exam at the computer.

In addition, complete some practice questions using headphones. Although not intentional, others can be distracting at the actual NCLEX-RN® exam. If you are easily distracted, you will have the option of using headphones. Your practice using headphones will ease your anxiety if you elect to use these during the actual exam.

Practice taking the chapter and comprehensive tests using a timer so that you can determine how many questions you can correctly answer in a specified amount of time. Practice taking items at a steady pace so that you do not rush through the test.

Review of Strengths and Weaknesses

Your goal should be to achieve a correct response rate of 75% to 80% on the practice and comprehensive tests. If you are unsuccessful, determine if the problem is in a traditional content area, for example, pharmacology, fundamentals, or nursing care of children and families; the integrated processes; or a specific content area on the NCLEX-RN® Test Plan. Use the unique features of the CD to review questions in the area in which you are weak. For example, the features of the CD will allow you to select a traditional content area, and you will be presented with questions in only the area you select. The unique features also allow you to select subcontent areas of the Client Needs categories to ensure your success when taking the NCLEX-RN® exam.

When reviewing your strengths and weaknesses, reflect back on your self-discipline. Consider what has worked for you in studying and staying focused and what seems to be a deterrent to concentration. If you find that you are lacking motivation to study, consider studying with a friend. Self-discipline is about setting priorities and saying "no" to things that will hinder accomplishment of your developed time plan. For some, using self-rewards can be successful in maintaining motivation.

Stress Reduction

As you study, focus on using stress-reduction strategies. These include but are not limited to positive self-talk, mental rehearsal, progressive muscle relaxation, deep breathing, and repositioning.

Positive Self-Talk

As you study, continue with positive self-talk. Rather than thinking, "I don't know this information" or "I never learned this," tell yourself, "I can use the test-taking strategies to figure this out." Remember to tell yourself often, "I can do this!" Erase negative thoughts as they come to mind and replace them with positive thoughts. Positive thoughts can help keep you motivated. Avoid frustration that comes with negative thinking; this can sap you of the energy you need to study.

Mental Rehearsal

Visualize yourself in the room taking the test in a relaxed pose, concentrating on the questions. Focus on sensations of being calm and in control. Do this each time you start a study session. During the study session, if an unfamiliar question appears, visualize yourself reducing your anxiety and rehearse what you will do to control your anxiety. For example, you might take a deep breath or perform positive self-talk, "I can do it; I can use the strategies I've learned." Finally, anticipate the sights and sounds in the actual testing environment. Unless you are requesting special accommodations due to a disability, you can anticipate that you will be taking the test on the computer. Visualize yourself at the computer, in control of the computer mouse or keyboard arrows, and moving through questions at a steady pace.

Progressive Muscle Relaxation

Progressive muscle relaxation involves tensing and then relaxing various muscles throughout the body. It can progress from either the face and neck to the toes or vice versa (see Table 4.1). While studying, practice using progressive muscle relaxation. With advance practice you will be ready to use this strategy should you feel tense or experience test-taking anxiety during the exam.

Deep Breathing

Deep breathing involves taking a deep breath, slowly inhaling to the count of 5, and then slowly exhaling to the count of 10. Performing deep breathing 5 to 10 times increases oxygen to the brain and can improve thinking. It also helps to relieve tension by refocusing your thoughts on your breathing and not on your concerns.

Repositioning

Think of how repositioning a client relieves stress on body parts and improves circulation. Use this strategy during studying to improve blood flow to your brain. Change your sitting position, relieving pressure on your bony prominences by leaning from one side to the other side. Flex and perform neck circumduction. Move your feet or stand. Repositioning can also relieve the boredom of long study periods.

Exercise Regularly

Although you usually cannot exercise while studying, do not forget to exercise at least 30 minutes daily. Beside keeping you healthy, walking, running, or other physical exercise will reduce tension and stress by expending nervous energy. Maintaining balance in your life with exercise and healthy eating is just as important to keeping your mind alert and your stress level under control as is studying and using stress reduction strategies. Why not use the natural endorphins produced during exercise to give yourself a boost of energy just before a study session!

Taking the NCLEX-RN® Test

The day before the test, do something you enjoy and avoid last-minute cramming. Keep your usual routine. Avoid alcoholic beverages and excess amounts of caffeine. Alcohol is a depressant and can reduce your ability to think clearly. Caffeine can reduce your concentration and attention span by overstimulating your body. Plan to get at least 8 hours of sleep, going to bed at your regular time. Use a relaxation strategy that you found successful during your preparation. Give yourself positive affirmation that you are ready and believe that you will be successful!

If driving to the testing site, be sure your gas tank is filled the night before and tires checked. Plan the driving route and know where you can park. Plan to arrive early and allow time for potential events that could cause a delay, such as excessive traffic.

The morning of the test, eat a healthy breakfast that includes a protein. Carbohydrate loading, though recommended by some, should be avoided if this is not your usual routine. While it may give you an immediate energy boost, it can cause a rebound effect of fatigue once the carbohydrates have been metabolized. Dress for comfort, in layers that can be easily removed or added based on the environmental temperature.

Finally, during the exam remain focused and concentrate on the exam. Use the headphones if easily distracted. Do not be concerned if others finish before you. Each person has his or her own speed for taking tests. The computer will stop anywhere between 75 and 265 items, depending on your performance. Continue to use positive self-talk during the exam. You have prepared and studied. You can pass the NCLEX-RN® exam!

References

Aschenbrenner, D., & Venable, S. (2009). *Drug Therapy in Nursing* (3rd ed.). Philadelphia: Lippincott Williams & Wilkins.

Aucoin, J., & Treas, L. (2005). Assumptions and Realities of the NCLEX-RN. *Nursing Education Perspectives,* 26, 268–271.

Ball, J., & Bindler, R. (2008). *Pediatric Nursing: Caring for Children* (4th ed.). Upper Saddle River, NJ: Pearson Education.

Ball, J., & Bindler, R. (2006). *Child Health Nursing: Partnering with Children and Families*. Upper Saddle River, NJ: Pearson Education.

Beare, P., & Thompson, P. (1998). *Davis's Q & A for the NCLEX-RN®*. Philadelphia: F. A. Davis.

Berman, A., Snyder, S., Kozier, B., & Erb, G. (2008). *Kozier & Erb's Fundamentals of Nursing: Concepts, Process, and Practice* (8th ed.). Upper Saddle River, NJ: Pearson Education.

Billings, D. (2008). *Lippincott's Q&A Review for NCLEX-RN®* (9th ed.). Philadelphia: Lippincott Williams & Wilkins.

Bonis, S., Taft, L., & Wendler, M. (2007). Strategies to promote success on the NCLEX-RN: An evidence-based approach using the ACE Star Model of Knowledge Transformation. *Nursing Education Perspectives*, 28(2), 82–87.

Clark, A., Giuliano, K., & Chen, H. (2006). Legal and ethical: Pulse oximetry revisited: "But his O_2 sat was normal!" *Clinical Nurse Specialist: The Journal for Advanced Nursing Practice,* 20, 268–272.

Craven, R., & Hirnle, C. (2009). *Fundamentals of Nursing: Human Health and Function* (6th ed.). Philadelphia: Lippincott Williams & Wilkins.

Davidson, M., London, M., & Ladewig, P. (2008). *Olds' Maternal-Newborn Nursing & Women's Health Across the Lifespan* (8th ed.). Upper Saddle River, NJ: Prentice Hall Health.

Harkreader, H., Hogan, M., & Thobaben, M. (2007). *Fundamentals of Nursing* (3rd ed.). St. Louis, MO: Saunders/Elsevier.

Jones, R. (2007). *Nursing Leadership and Management: Theories, Processes and Practice.* Philadelphia: F. A. Davis.

Lewis, S., Heitkemper, M., Dirksen, S., O'Brien, P., & Bucher, L. (2007). *Medical-Surgical Nursing: Assessment and Management of Clinical Problems* (7th ed.). St. Louis, MO: Mosby.

McDowell, B. (2008). KATTS: A Framework for Maximizing NCLEX-RN Performance. *Journal of Nursing Education,* 47(4), 183–186.

Mohr, W. (2006). *Psychiatric-Mental Health Nursing* (6th ed.). Philadelphia: Lippincott Williams & Wilkins.

National Council of State Boards of Nursing. *2009 NCLEX® Examination Candidate Bulletin.* Available at: www.ncsbn.org/2009_NCLEX_Candidate_Bulletin.pdf

National Council of State Boards of Nursing. (2009). *2010 NCLEX-RN® Detailed Test Plan, Effective April 2010.* Chicago: Author.

Nugent, P., & Vitale, B. (2008). *Test Success: Test-taking Techniques for Beginning Nursing Students* (5th ed.). Philadelphia: F. A. Davis.

Pillitteri, A. (2007). *Maternal & Child Health Nursing: Care of the Childbearing & Childrearing Family* (5th ed.). Philadelphia: Lippincott Williams & Wilkins.

Potter, P., & Perry, A. (2009). *Fundamentals of Nursing* (7th ed.). St. Louis, MO: Mosby Elsevier.

Saxton, D., Nugent, P., & Pelikan, P. (2003). *Mosby's Comprehensive Review of Nursing for NCLEX-RN* (17th ed.). St. Louis, MO: Mosby/Elsevier.

Siegel, J., Rhinehart, E., Jackson, M., Chiarello, L., & the Healthcare Infection Control Practices Advisory Committee. (2007). *Guideline for Isolation Precautions: Preventing Transmission of Infectious Agents in Healthcare Settings.* Atlanta, GA. Available at: www.apic.org/AM/Template.cfm?Section=Guidelines&TEMPLATE=/CM/ContentDisplay.cfm&CONTENTID=1174

Silvestri, L. (2008). *Saunders Comprehensive Review for the NCLEX-RN® Examination.* (4th ed.). St. Louis, MO: Saunders/Elsevier.

Smeltzer, S., Bare, B., Hinkle, J., & Cheever, K. (2008). *Brunner and Suddarth's Textbook of Medical-Surgical Nursing* (11th ed.). Philadelphia: Lippincott Williams & Wilkins.

Springhouse. (2000). *NCLEX-RN® Questions & Answers Made Incredibly Easy!* Springhouse, PA: Springhouse Corporation.

Wilkinson, J., & Van Leuven, K. (2007). *Fundamentals of Nursing: Theory, Concepts and Applications* (Vol. 1). Philadelphia: F. A. Davis.

Williams, L., & Hopper, P. (2007). *Understanding Medical-Surgical Nursing* (3rd ed.). Philadelphia: F. A. Davis.

Wong, D., Hockenberry, M., Wilson, D., Perry, S., & Lowdermilk, D. (2006). *Maternal Child Nursing Care* (3rd ed.). Philadelphia: Lippincott Williams & Wilkins.

Chapter Four

Tips for International and Repeat Test-Takers

The first part of this chapter is intended for individuals who have completed their nursing education outside the United States and are planning to work as registered nurses (RNs) in the United States. The second part of this chapter is intended for individuals who are studying to retake the NCLEX-RN® examination because of an unsuccessful attempt.

THE LICENSING REQUIREMENTS FOR FOREIGN EDUCATED NURSES

The U.S. Citizenship and Immigration Law (section 343 of the Illegal Immigration Reform and Immigrant Responsibility Act [IIRIRA] of 1996) requires that internationally educated health-care professionals, including RNs, successfully complete a screening process and seek a temporary or permanent occupational visa. This two-step screening process is *separate* from that necessary for obtaining a work visa. The processes are addressed below.

Commission on Graduates of Foreign Nursing Schools (CGFNS International)

The Commission on Graduates of Foreign Nursing Schools (CGFNS International) is named in the law as an organization qualified to offer the federal screening program for foreign health-care professionals. CGFNS, a not-for-profit, immigration-neutral organization, is internationally recognized as an authority on credential evaluation pertaining to the education, practice standards, registration, and licensure of nurses and other health-care professionals worldwide.

Thus, the first step in the process to establish eligibility to practice as a registered nurse in the United States is to contact the CGFNS. CGFNS prescreens foreign-educated nurses wishing to practice in the United States through its VisaScreen® program. Information about the VisaScreen® program administered through CGFNS is available at www.cgfns.org/sections/programs/vs/.

The VisaScreen® components include a review of the nurse's education, licensure verification in the home country, English language proficiency testing, and a predictor examination that tests nursing knowledge and provides an indicator of the nurse's ability to pass the U.S. national licensure examination (NCLEX-RN®). The CGFNS examination is a qualifying examination taken before the NCLEX-RN® test. The CGFNS Qualifying Exam is offered three times a year at various locations within and outside the United States. These sites are listed at the CGFNS Web site, www.cgfns.org.

The following states require foreign-educated registered nurses to pass the CGFNS examination before taking the NCLEX-RN®: Alabama, Alaska, Arizona, Arkansas, Colorado, Connecticut, District of Columbia, Florida, Georgia, Hawaii, Idaho, Indiana, Iowa, Kansas, Kentucky, Louisiana, Maine, Maryland, Massachusetts, Michigan, Minnesota, Missouri, Montana, Nebraska, Nevada, New Hampshire, New Jersey, North Carolina, North Dakota, Oklahoma, Pennsylvania, Rhode Island, South Carolina, South Dakota, Texas, Vermont, Virginia, Washington, West Virginia, and Wyoming. If seeking licensure in those states not listed, be sure to contact the state's board of nursing for requirements (see state requirements below).

Specifics about each of the components of the VisaScreen® may be obtained from CGFNS International, *2008 Visascreen® Applicant Handbook 2008*, available at www.cgfns.org/sections/programs/vs/ or by contacting the Commission on Graduates of Foreign Nursing Schools, 3600 Market Street, Suite 400, Philadelphia, PA 19104-2651, USA; 215-222-8454.

Applicants who successfully complete VisaScreen® receive a CGFNS/International Commission on Healthcare Professions (ICHP) VisaScreen® Certificate, which satisfies all federal screening requirements and is required for the visa application. The CGFNS/ICHP VisaScreen® Certificate must be received before the Department of Homeland Security, U.S. Citizenship and Immigration Services (USCIS) will issue an occupational visa or Trade NAFTA status to an applicant to work as a registered nurse in the United States. For information regarding temporary or permanent visas, contact the U.S. Department of State and the U.S. Immigration and Naturalization Service at www.uscis.gov/portal/site/uscis.

State Requirements

In the United States, each state has its own board of nursing and requirements for practicing as a registered nurse within that state. A foreign-educated nurse must meet the requirements established by the board of nursing in the state in which licensure is being sought. Upon an applicant meeting the requirements, the board of nursing in that state will issue a registered nurse license for practicing within that state. Therefore, a second step in the screening process is to contact the specific board of nursing in the state in which licensure is being sought to determine that state's requirements to practice as a registered nurse. This can be completed simultaneously while completing the VisaScreen® program.

The boards of nursing vary by state in their requirements for foreign-educated nurses to practice as a registered nurse. Some state boards of nursing require the VisaScreen® Certificate, and many require completion of the CGFNS Certification Program in order to be eligible to take the NCLEX-RN® examination. There are some states in which the board of nursing accepts the Canadian Nurses Association Testing Service (CNATS) or the Canadian Registered Nurses Examination (CRNE). There are also a few state boards of nursing that endorse foreign-educated nurses without requiring completion of the NCLEX-RN® examination. Because requirements can change and do vary, it is necessary to contact the state board of nursing to determine requirements, such as CGFNS certification, completion of the CGFNS Qualifying Exam prior to the NCLEX-RN® examination, successful completion of the NCLEX-RN® examination, or a policy regarding direct endorsement for foreign-educated nurses.

For contact information for a specific state board of nursing, contact National Council of State Boards of Nursing, 676 N. St. Clair, Suite 550, Chicago, IL 60611-2921, USA; 312-787-6555; https://www.ncsbn.org/515.htm.

National Council of State Boards of Nursing

Regardless of the variation in state requirements, the National Council of State Boards of Nursing (NCSBN) posits that international nurses should receive comparable nursing education from a government-approved school (current federal requirements); possess effective English skills to safely practice in the U.S. health-care environment; and have no current or previous disciplinary actions related to their international or domestic licenses in order to practice as a registered nurse in the United States. Specific information from NCSBN for international nurses can be found at the following Web address: www.ncsbn.org/08_Manual_for_International_nurses.pdf.

If passing the NCLEX-RN® licensing examination is a requirement of the state in which a foreign-educated nurse wishes to practice as a registered nurse, the person must first be made eligible by the board of nursing of that state before an examination can be administered. Eligibility is determined when a foreign-educated nurse contacts a state board of nursing regarding the specific registration process for licensure in that state. Once a foreign-educated nurse is made eligible by the specified state board of nursing, an authorization to test (ATT) is mailed to the candidate, and the candidate can then register for the NCLEX-RN® examination.

The NCLEX-RN® examination is administered by Pearson VUE at 18 different international Pearson Professional Centers (on behalf of NCSBN) and in over 220 Pearson Professional Centers in the United States. International locations include Seoul, South Korea; London, England; and Hong Kong, China. Taking the NCLEX-RN® at an international site does not remove state requirements for licensure or make it easier to become a nurse in the United States. It does, however, reduce the time it takes to travel to testing centers and allows an opportunity for a nurse to pass the NCLEX-RN® licensure examination before traveling to the United States. Information about applying for the NCLEX-RN® and a list of available NCLEX-RN® foreign testing centers may be found in the NCLEX-RN® Candidate Bulletin at www.ncsbn.org/2009_NCLEX_Candidate_Bulletin.pdf. For additional information about the NCLEX-RN® licensure examination and test structure, refer to Chapter 1.

NCLEX-RN® PREPARATION: TIPS FOR FOREIGN-EDUCATED NURSES

The NCLEX-RN® is intended to test basic nursing knowledge required for entry-level RN practice in the United States. Language and cultural differences, however, may present challenges for foreign-educated students in passing the NCLEX-RN®. The key to success is in adequate preparation.

One of the components of the VisaScreen® program administered through CGFNS is testing English language proficiency. It is important that this testing be completed early so that you have an understanding of your ability to read and comprehend English. Should you have difficulty in this area, you should consider taking courses in English as a second language (ESL) before completing NCLEX-RN® practice questions. Taking an English medical terminology course may also be helpful. Although the test items on the NCLEX-RN® examination are written at a 10th-grade reading level, the terms used in the examination will be terms used in the health-care field.

Once you feel confident in your ability to read and comprehend English and have an understanding of medical terminology, begin taking NCLEX-RN®-type practice questions to assess your knowledge of nursing practice in the United States and to prepare for the NCLEX-RN® examination. Using this book and the accompanying CD with more than 5,000 questions will provide you with the experience necessary to become proficient at taking multiple-choice and alternate item format questions. The more items you complete, the more skillful you will become at deciphering questions, identifying key information in an item, and choosing the best option.

The beginning chapters of this book on the licensure exam, NCLEX-RN® questions, and test-taking strategies will assist you in learning about the structure and content of the examination. Review the test plan illustrated because it will assist you in identifying the scope of practice of the registered nurse in the United States. Pay particular attention to the test-taking strategies in Chapter 3. These are most helpful when the content of an item may be unfamiliar to you or when you need to eliminate options when some or all seem to be correct.

Begin to review questions from one entire content area before moving to the next content area. If it seems that you are answering many book items incorrectly, answer the questions from the CD in that particular content area before beginning the next content area. Be sure to read the rationales provided, which include the rationale for both the correct and incorrect options. The rationale should aid you in learning why an option may be correct or incorrect and help to build your knowledge base or enhance recall of content. As you complete the questions, with the assistance of the CD you should be able to identify content areas that you may need to study in more depth. The comprehensive test located on the CD will serve as an assessment guide to help you determine the need for further study. Your goal is to achieve 80% mastery on questions. The references provided with the questions will direct you to common nursing textbooks or resources that are used in formulating questions for the NCLEX-RN® examination should additional study be needed.

As you review questions, you should think about your experiences, skills, and knowledge and compare them to those of nursing candidates educated in the United States. In many countries, registered nurses may actually prescribe medications and treatments. In the United States, however, registered nurses anticipate, plan, and administer medications and treatments that are prescribed by a physician or other licensed health-care providers. Be sure to read the rationales carefully to assist in identifying the scope of registered nursing practice in the United States. The test on prioritization and delegation will be particularly helpful in this area.

Cultural differences may exist in your perception of the client needs and the nursing responses or actions. The more items that you are able to complete before taking the NCLEX-RN® exam, the better you will be able to identify client needs and responses of not only an American culture but also those of various cultural groups. You will also become more accustomed to reading questions and selecting options for nursing responses and actions based on nursing practice within the United States. Because items within the book and accompanying CD have been written to all content areas published in the *2010 NCLEX-RN® Detailed Test Plan-Candidate Version*, you should be building your knowledge of cultural practices within the United States as you complete questions. An electronic copy of the *2010 NCLEX-RN® Detailed Test Plan-Candidate Version* is available free of charge from the NCSBN at www.ncsbn.org.

Finally, use the CD, which contains over 5,000 questions, to assess your knowledge of all the areas identified in the test plan. The features of the CD will provide you with information about how well you do in each of the content areas, integrated processes, client needs, and subareas of the client needs. This feature will allow you to identify areas that you have mastered and to focus your study on your most problematic areas. Once you have achieved 80% mastery, you should be well-prepared and ready to pass the NCLEX-RN® examination.

NCLEX-RN® PREPARATION: TIPS FOR REPEAT TEST-TAKERS

In most states, candidates who were unsuccessful on the NCLEX-RN® exam must wait a minimum of 45 days before retesting. Georgia, Guam, and Washington have different requirements, however, with Washington requiring 91 days before retesting. Use this waiting period to enhance your success on the retake exam by applying relaxation skills, focusing your review, and then learning and applying the test-taking strategies presented in this book.

First, establish a positive mindset: "I can do it! I will pass the NCLEX-RN® exam!" Use positive self-talk and self-reassurance: acknowledge what you already know and congratulate yourself for this. What you already know has been presented in the Candidate Performance Report (CPR), a report sent to you with your NCLEX-RN® exam results. This individualized, two-page document identifies the content areas of the exam, the percentage of the test represented by that content area, a statement of your performance (your ability in that content area), and a description of the content area with a list of topics related to it. Your performance in each content area is described as **Above the Passing Standard**, **Near the Passing Standard**, or **Below the Passing Standard**. Look at the content areas that are **Above the Passing Standard**. Congratulate yourself because you have mastered this information.

Now, take a deep breath, and perform a visualization and self-relaxation exercise. Imagine yourself in a location or in an activity you absolutely love. Incorporate the color blue (a blue sky, a blue lake, a blue room, etc.). With your eyes closed and focusing on your image, begin head-to-toe relaxation. If you have forgotten the steps, refer to Table 4.1. After completing the steps, stay seated for a minute or two, then open your eyes. Stand up and stretch. Congratulate yourself for being able to relax before you begin studying. *Perform this activity each time before starting your review of practice questions.*

Begin your review by identifying your content area or areas of weakness on the NCLEX-RN® CPR so you can focus your review. For example, if the content area on Pharmacological and Parenteral Therapies is **Below the Passing Standard**, then this is a content area on which you should focus. However, if the content area on Reduction of Risk

TABLE 4.1
Progressive Muscle Relaxation

Instructions
1. Sit in a quiet, undisturbed place and get comfortable. 2. Keep your legs and arms uncrossed. 3. Close your eyes and keep them closed during the entire exercise. 4. Become aware of your body and notice any areas that feel especially tense. 5. Breathe in deeply to the count of four and then exhale to the count of four. 6. Begin by frowning and tensing the muscles of your forehead, eyes, face, and neck. Hold 5 to 10 seconds, and become aware of the feeling of tension. 7. Let your facial muscles relax the same amount of time, and become aware of the feeling of relaxation. 8. Bend your neck forward to your chin and tense. Hold for 5 to 10 seconds, and become aware of the feeling of tension. 9. Return your head to a neutral position and relax. Hold for 5 to 10 seconds, and become aware of the feeling of relaxation. 10. Now, bring your shoulders toward your head and tense the muscles. Hold for 5 to 10 seconds, and become aware of the feeling of tension. 11. Relax your shoulders. Hold for 5 to 10 seconds, and become aware of the feeling of relaxation. 12. Continue this process with all muscle groups for the rest of the body, including the arms, hands, chest, abdomen and pelvis, small of the back, buttocks, legs, thighs, calves, ankles, feet, toes, and then the entire body. 13. Relax and mentally search for any tense areas of the body. If you notice tense muscles, relax them. 14. Finally, breathe in deeply to the count of four and then exhale to the count of four. 15. Continue to breathe slowly and deeply. 16. Feel the sensations of relaxation or heaviness. 17. Remain relaxed for a few minutes, open your eyes, and slowly stretch.

Adapted from Harkreader, H., Hogan, M., & Thobaben, M. (2007). *Fundamentals of Nursing* (3rd ed., p. 1129). St. Louis, MO: Saunders/Elsevier.

Potential is **Above the Passing Standard**, this is an area in which minimal review is necessary.

Next, read Chapter 3 on test-taking strategies carefully. Focus on understanding these strategies to select the correct option. Remember to prioritize the options in the following order: actual threats to safety, physiological integrity, psychosocial integrity, and finally, health maintenance. When choosing the correct answer for the practice questions, ask yourself, "What part of the nursing process is this question addressing: assessment, analysis, planning, implementation, or evaluation?" Avoid selecting options that include "all," "always," "never," or "none." Look for options that are different. If three options state the same information, but in different words, choose the option that is different. When given options that are pharmacologically based or nonpharmacologically based, read the question carefully because the nonpharmacological intervention is likely the answer.

After establishing an understanding of the test-taking strategies, go to the tests in the book that focus on the content areas in which you are weak. Table 4.2 identifies the NCLEX-RN® content areas included in the CPR and the applicable tests within this book. Although the majority of the questions in the tests will focus on a respective NCLEX-RN® content area, some questions within a test will pertain to other content areas and will help you refresh your knowledge in these other areas. As you answer questions, focus on using the test-taking strategies. Carefully read the rationales to determine why an option is either correct or incorrect.

Next, use the unique features of the CD to review questions in the content areas in which you are weak. The features of the CD will allow you to select the content areas of Client Needs and the subcontent areas and will present questions only in those areas. This feature will allow you to master each subcontent area and ensure your success the next time you take the NCLEX-RN® exam.

Finally, complete the comprehensive tests in the book and on the CD. Once you have achieved a score of 80% correct, you should be well-prepared and ready to pass the NCLEX-RN® Examination. The night before the exam, use the relaxation strategy that you have been using during your preparation and plan for 8 hours of sleep. Give yourself positive affirmation that you are ready, and believe that you will be successful!

TABLE 4.2
NCLEX-RN® Content Areas From the CPR and Applicable Tests in the Q&A Book

Content Area	TESTS
Management of Care (18%–22% of the test)	1–4, and integrated in all tests
• Providing and directing nursing care that enhances the care delivery setting to protect clients, family/significant others, and health-care personnel. • Related content includes but is not limited to Advance Directives, Advocacy, Case Management, Client Rights, Collaboration with Interdisciplinary Team, Concepts of Management, Confidentiality/Information Security, Consultation, Continuity of Care, Delegation, Establishing Priorities, Ethical Practice, Informed Consent, Information Technology, Legal Rights and Responsibilities, Performance Improvement (Quality Improvement), Referrals, Supervision.	
Safety and Infection Control (8%–14% of the test)	1, 5, 6, 7, 46
• Protecting clients, family/significant others, and health-care personnel from health and environmental hazards. • Related content includes but is not limited to Accident/Injury Prevention, Emergency Response Plan, Ergonomic Principles, Error Prevention, Handling Hazardous and Infectious Materials, Home Safety, Reporting of Incident/Event/Irregular Occurrence/Variance, Safe Use of Equipment, Security Plan, Standard/Transmission-based Precautions/Surgical Asepsis, Use of Restraints/Safety Devices.	
Basic Care and Comfort (6%–12% of the test)	5, 15–26, 29–36, 45, 48
• Providing comfort and assistance in the performance of activities of daily living. • Related content includes but is not limited to Assistive Devices, Elimination, Mobility/Immobility, Nonpharmacological Comfort Interventions, Nutrition and Oral Hydration, Personal Hygiene, Rest and Sleep.	
Health Promotion and Maintenance (6%–12% of the test)	8–14, 28
• Provides and directs nursing care of the client and family/significant others that incorporates the knowledge of expected growth and development principles, prevention and/or early detection of health problems, and strategies to achieve optimal health. • Related content includes but is not limited to Aging Process, Antepartum/Intrapartum/Postpartum and Newborn Care, Developmental Stages and Transitions, Health and Wellness, Health Promotion/Disease Prevention, Health Screening, High-risk Behaviors, Lifestyle Choices, Principles of Teaching/Learning, Self-Care, Techniques of Physical Assessment.	
Reduction of Risk Potential (10%–16% of the test)	15–27, 29–37, 45–48
• Reducing the likelihood that clients will develop complications or health problems related to existing conditions, treatments, or procedures. • Related content includes but is not limited to Changes/Abnormalities in Vital Signs, Diagnostic Tests, Laboratory Values, Potential for Alterations in Body Systems, Potential for Complications of Diagnostic Tests/Treatments/Procedures, Potential for Complications from Surgical Procedures and Health Alterations, System-specific Assessments, Therapeutic Procedures.	
Physiological Adaptation (11%–17% of the test)	15–27, 29–37, 45–48
• Managing and providing care for clients with acute, chronic, or life-threatening physical health conditions. • Related content includes but is not limited to Alterations in Body Systems, Fluid and Electrolyte Imbalances, Hemodynamics, Illness Management, Medical Emergencies, Pathophysiology, Unexpected Response to Therapies.	

TABLE 4.2

NCLEX-RN® Content Areas From the CPR and Applicable Tests in the Q&A Book (continued)

Content Area	TESTS
Psychosocial Integrity (6%–12% of the test)	4, 38–44
• Provides and directs nursing care that promotes and supports the emotional, mental, and social well-being of the client and family/significant others experiencing stressful events, as well as clients with acute or chronic mental illness. • Related content includes but is not limited to Abuse/Neglect, Behavioral Interventions, Chemical and Other Dependencies, Coping Mechanisms, Crisis Intervention, Cultural Diversity, End of Life Care, Family Dynamics, Grief and Loss, Mental Health Concepts, Religious and Spiritual Influences on Health, Sensory/Perceptual Alterations, Stress Management, Support Systems, Therapeutic Communications, Therapeutic Environment.	
Pharmacological and Parenteral Therapies (13%–19% of the test)	6, 12, 27, 37, 44, and integrated in all tests
• Providing care related to the administration of medications and parenteral therapies. • Related content includes but is not limited to Adverse Effects/Contraindications/Side Effects/ Interactions, Blood and Blood Products, Central Venous Access Devices, Dosage Calculation, Expected Actions/Outcomes, Medication Administration, Parenteral/Intravenous Therapies, Pharmacological Pain Management, Total Parenteral Nutrition.	

Adapted from National Council of State Boards of Nursing. (2008). *NCLEX-RN® Performance Candidate Report National Council Licensure Examination for Registered Nurses.* Available at: www.ncsbn.org/1223.htm

References

American Nurses Association. (2008). *Foreign Educated Nurses.* Available at: www.nursingworld.org/MainMenuCategories/ThePracticeofProfessionalNursing/workplace/ForeignNurses.aspx

Commission on Graduates of Foreign Nursing Schools (CGFNS International). (2008). *VisaScreen® Program.* Available at: www.cgfns.org/sections/programs/vs/

Commission on Graduates of Foreign Nursing Schools (CGFNS International). (2008). *CGFNS Certification Program.* Available at: www.cgfns.org/sections/programs/cp/

Embassy of the United States, U.S. Department of State. (2008). *Immigrant Visas.* Available at: newdelhi.usembassy.gov/employment_based_visas.html

Harkreader, H., Hogan, M., & Thobaben, M. (2007). *Fundamentals of Nursing* (3rd ed., p. 1129). St. Louis: Saunders/Elsevier.

Lagerquist, S., McMillin, J., Nelson, R., & Snider, K. (2006). *Davis's NCLEX-RN® Success* (2nd ed.). Philadelphia: F. A. Davis.

National Council of State Boards of Nursing. (2009). *2010 NCLEX-RN® Detailed Test Plan Candidate, Effective April 2010.* Available at: www.ncsbn.org/2010_NCLEX_RN_Detailed_Test_Plan_Candidate.pdf

National Council of State Boards of Nursing. (2008). *Contact a Board of Nursing.* Available at: www.ncsbn.org/515.htm

National Council of State Boards of Nursing. (2008). Home Page. Available at: www.ncsbn.org.

National Council of State Boards of Nursing. (2008). *Resource Manual for International Nurses.* Available at: www.ncsbn.org/08_Manual_for_International_nurses.pdf

National Council of State Boards of Nursing. (2009). *NCLEX® Examination Candidate Bulletin.* Available at: www.ncsbn.org/2009_NCLEX_Candidate_Bulletin.pdf

National Council of State Boards of Nursing. (2008). *NCLEX-RN® Performance Candidate Report National Council Licensure Examination for Registered Nurses.* Available at: www.ncsbn.org/1223.htm.

National Council of State Boards of Nursing. (2008). *You've Completed the NCLEX-RN® Examination but Still have Questions.* Available at: www.ncsbn.org/Youve_Completed_2007.pdf

Pendergast, J. (2006). Know the federal requirements for foreign-educated nurses. *Nursing Management,* 37(11), 13–14, 55.

Silvestri, L. A. (2008). *Saunders Comprehensive Review for the NCLEX-RN® Examination* (4th ed.). St. Louis, MO: Saunders/Elsevier.

Section

II

PRACTICE TESTS

Chapter Five

Safe and Effective Care Environment: Management of Care

Test 1: Management of Care: Ethical, Legal, and Safety Issues in Nursing

1. A hospitalized client diagnosed with end-stage cancer has suddenly decided to discontinue treatment. The client requests no additional treatment, such as antibiotics, tube feedings, and mechanical ventilation. When acting as the client's advocate, which action should a nurse take?

   1. Respect the client's wishes and indicate those wishes on the plan of care
   2. Encourage the client to share the decision with the family and the client's physician
   3. Clarify other treatments that the client wishes to withhold
   4. Wait until additional treatment is required and then decide what to do based on the client's condition

ANSWER: 2

In advocating for the client, the nurse should encourage the client to share the decision with family and the physician. To advocate for someone means to speak for that person when the person is unable to speak for him- or herself. The client is still able to make his or her own decisions, which will be better supported when the client shares with the family and physician. Although the wishes should be indicated on the plan of care, this nurse action does not demonstrate advocating for the client. A physician order is required to limit treatment. Although additional treatments should be discussed, the priority at this time is the discussion with the family and physician.

▶ ***Test-taking Tip:*** *Use the process of elimination. Note the key word "suddenly," which indicates the decision is new.*

Content Area: Management of Care; *Category of Health Alteration:* Ethical, Legal, and Safety Issues in Nursing; *Integrated Processes:* Caring; *Client Need:* Safe and Effective Care Environment/Management of Care/Advocacy; *Cognitive Level:* Application

Reference: Harkreader, H., Hogan, M., & Thobaben, M. (2007). *Fundamentals of Nursing* (3rd ed., pp. 12–21). St. Louis, MO: Saunders/Elsevier.

2. An experienced nurse is orienting a new nurse caring for multiple clients on an oncology nursing unit. The experienced nurse explains to the new nurse that to advocate for clients, a nurse must be able to identify ethical issues and communicate the clients' wishes to others. Which *primary* role of the nurse advocate should the experienced nurse also explain to the new nurse?

   1. Safeguard clients against abuse and violation of their rights.
   2. Make decisions for clients based on the nurse's knowledge and relationship.
   3. Assist clients in expressing their rights.
   4. Have knowledge of the clients' values so the nurse can assist in decision making.

ANSWER: 1

The primary role in advocacy is to keep the client safe—to safeguard clients against abuse and violation of their rights. Clients may not be able to advocate for themselves. The professional role of the nurse is to defend clients' autonomy in decision making. The nurse must never make a treatment decision for clients. However, the nurse should keep clients informed about their treatment orders and their rights. Although it is important to know the clients' values, it is not the primary role of the nurse advocate.

▶ ***Test-taking Tip:*** *"Primary role" are key words. Recall that advocacy focuses on clients' rights, thus eliminate options 2 and 4. Of the remaining two options, select the option that demonstrates a stronger nursing role.*

Content Area: Management of Care; *Category of Health Alteration:* Ethical, Legal, and Safety Issues in Nursing; *Integrated Processes:* Nursing Process Planning; *Client Need:* Safe and Effective Care Environment/ Management of Care/Advocacy; *Cognitive Level:* Application

Reference: Wilkinson, J., & Van Leuven, K. (2007). *Fundamentals of Nursing* (pp. 1048, 1068–1069). Philadelphia: F. A. Davis.

3. A surgical client tells a nurse that he/she has been in significant pain since surgery earlier in the day. The nurse reviews the medication administration record (MAR) and notes that hydrocodone plus acetaminophen (Vicodin®) has been administered at the highest possible dose and at regular intervals since surgery. The nurse brings the client two Vicodin® tablets. The client states, "That isn't what I had before. I only had one pink pill." Which action should be taken by the nurse?

1. Call the pharmacy and ask the pharmacist to send the pink hydrocodone and acetaminophen
2. Complete a variance report because the MAR is incorrect
3. Report the event to the supervisor
4. Confront the nurse on the previous shift with the suspicion that the nurse took the Vicodin®

ANSWER: 3

Reporting the event to the supervisor allows the supervisor to investigate the situation before action is initiated. If the formulation prescribed is not available, a medication request to the pharmacy should include the name of the medication, dose, route, and frequency. Requesting a pink hydrocodone and acetaminophen is inappropriate; the pharmacy would not change medication suppliers without prior notification. What may have occurred previously is speculation, so completing a variance report or confronting the nurse is premature.

▶ ***Test-taking Tip:*** *Remember that illegal and unsafe practice must be reported.*

Content Area: Management of Care; *Category of Health Alteration:* Ethical, Legal, and Safety Issues in Nursing; *Integrated Processes:* Nursing Process Analysis; *Client Need:* Safe and Effective Care Environment/ Management of Care/Ethical Practice; *Cognitive Level:* Application

Reference: Wilkinson, J., & Van Leuven, K. (2007). *Fundamentals of Nursing* (pp. 525–526). Philadelphia: F. A. Davis.

4. A nurse is told by a client of an advance health-care directive that was completed 8 years ago. The nurse looks in the medical record for the advance directive to review its content. Which content should the nurse expect the advance health-care directive to include? SELECT ALL THAT APPLY.

1. Preference for health-care treatment
2. Preference for hospitalization
3. Violation of client confidentiality
4. Do-not-resuscitate orders
5. Notification of next of kin
6. Durable power of attorney for health care

ANSWER: 1, 2, 4, 6

An advance directive is a written document that provides direction for health care in the future, when clients may be unable to make personal treatment choices. Client confidentiality and next-of-kin notification does not pertain to direction for health care.

▶ ***Test-taking Tip:*** *Select options that address wishes pertaining to health care.*

Content Area: Management of Care; *Category of Health Alteration:* Ethical, Legal, and Safety Issues in Nursing; *Integrated Processes:* Nursing Process Assessment; *Client Need:* Safe and Effective Care Environment/Management of Care/Ethical Practice; *Cognitive Level:* Comprehension

Reference: Harkreader, H., Hogan, M., & Thobaben, M. (2007). *Fundamentals of Nursing* (3rd ed., pp. 37–38). St. Louis, MO: Saunders/ Elsevier.

5. After a car/pedestrian accident, a pedestrian client is brought to the emergency room. The client is alert and oriented but complains of dyspnea. Oxygen saturation (SpO_2) levels vary from 88% to 90%. Oxygen is applied at 2 liters per nasal cannula with no improvement in SpO_2. Oxygen per mask is initiated at 40% with little improvement. Radiograph films reveal no obvious injury or fractures. Suddenly the client loses consciousness, has a respiratory arrest, and subsequently dies. During the respiratory arrest resuscitation, it is determined that a nurse failed to open the valve to the oxygen tank and the client had not been receiving oxygen. What is the key ethical principle involved in this situation?

1. Nonmaleficence
2. Fidelity
3. Beneficence
4. Justice

ANSWER: 1

Nonmaleficence is the requirement that health-care providers do no harm to their clients, either intentionally or unintentionally. Fidelity is the obligation of an individual to be faithful; beneficence is doing good for clients, and justice is the obligation to be fair to all people.

▶ ***Test-taking Tip:*** *Focus on the nurse's actions. A memory aid is remembering "**nonmaleficence**" is "**not** harm."*

Content Area: Management of Care; *Category of Health Alteration:* Ethical, Legal, and Safety Issues in Nursing; *Integrated Processes:* Nursing Process Analysis; *Client Need:* Safe and Effective Care Environment/Management of Care/Ethical Practice; *Cognitive Level:* Application

Reference: Catalano, J. (2006). *Nursing Now! Today's Issues, Tomorrow's Trends* (4th ed., pp. 118–120). Philadelphia: F. A. Davis.

6. In the Laotian culture, pain may be severe before relief is requested. Traditionally, the oldest male makes health care decisions and may answer questions for female clients. A nurse is caring for a female Laotian client who is in severe pain, rating an 8 on a scale of 0 to 10. Her spouse will not allow the nurse to give any analgesics. What is the nurse's best course of action?

1. Administer the analgesic when the client's spouse leaves the room.
2. Educate the client's spouse on the reason for the pain and the action of analgesics.
3. Respect the Laotian culture and do not administer the analgesic.
4. Report the issue to the supervisor.

ANSWER: 2

The first stage of ethical decisionmaking is to collect, analyze, and interpret the data. The spouse may not have enough information about pain and pain management. Education may provide the information to assist him in making a decision without compromising his cultural beliefs. Administering the analgesic without the spouse present would be unethical. It would violate the Laotian culture. Not treating the pain would also be unethical. Promoting comfort is a nursing responsibility. Reporting to the supervisor may result in an action to relieve pain, although it would cause delay.

▶ ***Test-taking Tip:*** *The nurse should advocate for the client while still respecting the wishes of all involved.*

Content Area: Management of Care; *Category of Health Alteration:* Ethical, Legal, and Safety Issues in Nursing; *Integrated Processes:* Nursing Process Assessment; *Client Need:* Safe and Effective Care Environment/Management of Care/Ethical Practice; *Cognitive Level:* Application

References: Catalano, J. (2006). *Nursing Now! Today's Issues, Tomorrow's Trends* (4th ed., pp. 130–131). Philadelphia: F. A. Davis; D'Avanzo, C., & Geissler, E. (2003). *Cultural Health Assessment* (3rd ed., pp. 436–440). St. Louis, MO: Mosby.

---

7. A nurse gives a medication without checking the medication administration record (MAR). When the nurse documents the medication given, the nurse notices that the medication was also given 15 minutes earlier by another nurse, resulting in the client receiving a double dose. The nurse notifies a supervisor and a physician of the event. Which action should the nurse who administered the second medication dose expect?

1. Assignment of fewer clients at one time
2. Disciplinary action to the first nurse for giving the first dose
3. Disciplinary action possibly including suspension or termination
4. Completion of a variance report that would be reviewed by management

ANSWER: 4

The nurse who made the error should expect the completion of a variance report with review by management. A complete review of the situation needs to occur, including the type of medication, dose, outcome of the client, and steps of medication administration, including documentation. The nurse should not expect a change in client assignments. Although disciplinary action varies by organization, generally a pattern of incompetent actions must be demonstrated for suspension or termination.

▶ ***Test-taking Tip:*** *Use the process of elimination. Focus on the professional responsibility of the nurse. Look for the strategic words "variance" and "reviewed."*

Content Area: Management of Care; *Category of Health Alteration:* Ethical, Legal, and Safety Issues in Nursing; *Integrated Processes:* Communication and Documentation; *Client Need:* Safe and Effective Care Environment/Management of Care/Ethical Practice; *Cognitive Level:* Analysis

Reference: Catalano, J. (2006). *Nursing Now! Today's Issues, Tomorrow's Trends* (4th ed., p. 117). Philadelphia: F. A. Davis.

---

8. **EBP** A client, admitted with abdominal pain, smokes cigarettes. The client is complaining about not being able to smoke in the hospital. A nurse would like to provide support and assist the client in managing a craving for cigarettes. Which actions should be taken by the nurse to educate the client about the effects of cigarette smoking? SELECT ALL THAT APPLY.

1. Review the smoking-cessation information for client education on the hospital's Web site.
2. Use the Internet to find the latest evidence for supporting smoking cessation during hospitalization.
3. Ask the supervisor to check in the library for client education materials on smoking cessation.
4. Discourage the client from smoking during hospitalization due to the risk of fire.
5. Check the American Lung Association Web site for their latest guidelines on smoking cessation.
6. Go to the library, conduct a literature search, and write a policy on smoking cessation.

ANSWER: 1, 2, 3, 5

Using informatics from the hospital Web site and library and the Internet will result in obtaining the most current information to assist the client, as well as being the most expedient. Discouraging the client from smoking is not a supported strategy for smoking cessation. Conducting a literature search and writing a policy will not be done in time to assist this client.

▶ ***Test-taking Tip:*** *Eliminate options that would not educate the client.*

Content Area: Management of Care; *Category of Health Alteration:* Ethical, Legal, and Safety Issues in Nursing; *Integrated Processes:* Caring; *Client Need:* Safe and Effective Care Environment/Management of Care/Information Technology; *Cognitive Level:* Application

EBP Reference: National Institute for Health and Clinical Excellence (NICE). (2006). *Brief Interventions and Referral for Smoking Cessation in Primary Care and Other Settings*. London, UK: Author. Available at: www.guideline.gov/summary/summary.aspx?ss=15&doc_id=9740&nbr=5214

9. A nurse plans to access a client's electronic health record for documentation of a medication. Which steps should be taken by the nurse to access a client's electronic health record? Place each step in the correct sequence.

______ Enter the user ID and password.
______ Select the correct client from the list of clients.
______ Document the medication on the electronic medical administration record (MAR).
______ Log out of the program.
______ Select the correct list of clients.
______ Access the MAR.
______ Open the electronic record computer program.

ANSWER: 2, 4, 6, 7, 3, 5, 1

The nurse should first open the electronic record computer program and then enter the user ID and password. The next step should be to select the correct list of clients and then the correct client from the list. The nurse should then access the MAR and document the medication. Finally, the nurse should log out of the program.

Test-taking Tip: *Use visualization to focus on the steps in the process prior to placing items in the correct order. Prioritizing is placing items in the correct sequence.*

Content Area: Management of Care; *Category of Health Alteration:* Ethical, Legal, and Safety Issues in Nursing; *Integrated Processes:* Communication and Documentation; *Client Need:* Safe and Effective Care Environment/Management of Care/Information Technology; *Cognitive Level:* Application

Reference: Wilkinson, J., & Van Leuven, K. (2007). *Fundamentals of Nursing* (pp. 980–981). Philadelphia: F. A. Davis.

---

10. EBP A nurse calls a physician regarding a change in a client's condition. The physician gives orders over the telephone for arterial blood gases (ABGs) to be drawn stat. Which is the most important safety consideration when obtaining the order?

1. Writing the order down and reading it back to the physician
2. Calling the respiratory therapist stat to draw the ABGs
3. Giving the order stat to the health unit coordinator to place in the computer
4. Writing down the order for ABGs immediately

ANSWER: 1

The Joint Commission National Patient Safety Goals requires telephone orders to be written down and read back. This action will validate the accuracy of the order received. Although the order is stat, calling the respiratory therapist or giving the order to the health unit coordinator is not the most important safety consideration. Writing down the order without reading it back does not meet the Joint Commission safety goal requirements.

Test-taking Tip: *The key words are "most important safety consideration." Select the option that would ensure that the nurse's understanding of the order is correct.*

Content Area: Management of Care; *Category of Health Alteration:* Ethical, Legal, and Safety Issues in Nursing; *Integrated Processes:* Communication and Documentation; *Client Need:* Safe and Effective Care Environment/Management of Care/Information Technology; *Cognitive Level:* Application

Reference: Berman, A., Snyder, S., Kozier, B., & Erb, G. (2008). *Kozier & Erb's Fundamentals of Nursing: Concepts, Process, and Practice* (8th ed., pp. 263–264). Upper Saddle River, NJ: Pearson Education.

EBP Reference: The Joint Commission. (2008). *2008 National Patient Safety Goals*. Available at: www.jointcommission.org/NR/rdonlyres/82B717D8-B16A-4442-AD00-CE3188C2F00A/0/08_HAP_NPSGs_Master.pdf

---

11. A client has an advance health care directive on file at a hospital that identifies a friend as the legal health-care agent. A nurse is to obtain informed consent for the client to have an exploratory laparotomy. Because of sedation, the client is unable to sign the form or give verbal consent. Who should provide consent for this client?

1. The client's spouse
2. The client's oldest adult child
3. Since the client is unable to give consent, the surgery cannot be performed
4. The client's durable power of attorney (DPA) for health care

ANSWER: 4

Since the client has a DPA for health care (health-care agent), that person is designated to make health-care decisions when the client is unable to do so. The client's spouse and oldest adult child would not be able to give consent. Even though the client is unable to provide consent, the surgery may be performed by following the legal process for obtaining informed consent.

Test-taking Tip: *Apply knowledge of informed consent and the use of an advance health-care directive. Recall that the health-care directive specifies the wishes of the client when the client is unable to make decisions related to health care.*

Content Area: Management of Care; *Category of Health Alteration:* Ethical, Legal, and Safety Issues in Nursing; *Integrated Processes:* Nursing Process Implementation; *Client Need:* Safe and Effective Care Environment/Management of Care/Informed Consent; *Cognitive Level:* Analysis

Reference: Harkreader, H., Hogan, M., & Thobaben, M. (2007). *Fundamentals of Nursing* (3rd ed. pp. 37–38). St. Louis, MO: Saunders/Elsevier.

12. A nurse is instructing a Somali client about a lung resection scheduled for tomorrow. The client does not speak English. What is the best method of instruction for this client?

1. Obtaining a translator who can restate the words used to describe the surgery
2. Asking an English-speaking family member to translate what the nurse states
3. Obtaining an interpreter over the telephone
4. Using diagrams and pictures to describe a lung resection

ANSWER: 4

The best method of instruction is to use nonverbal communication, such as illustrations, when unable to understand the language. Whenever possible, obtain an interpreter rather than a translator. An interpreter will decode the words and provide the meaning behind the message. Avoid using relatives who may distort information or not be objective. An interpreter over the telephone is an option; however, it would be best to have the interpreter present.

▶ ***Test-taking Tip:*** *The key words are "best method." Apply knowledge of communicating with non–English-speaking clients.*

Content Area: Management of Care; *Category of Health Alteration:* Ethical, Legal, and Safety Issues in Nursing; *Integrated Processes:* Teaching and Learning; *Client Need:* Safe and Effective Care Environment/Management of Care/Informed Consent; *Cognitive Level:* Analysis

Reference: Catalano, J. (2006). *Nursing Now! Today's Issues, Tomorrow's Trends* (4th ed., p. 424). Philadelphia: F. A. Davis.

---

13. EBP A nurse took several courses in Spanish and studied in Central America for one semester. A supervisor asks the nurse to serve as an interpreter during orientation of a new Spanish-speaking nurse. Which information is most important for the nurse to know prior to agreeing to be an interpreter?

1. The facility policy on client interpretation services
2. The state mandates on the requirements of interpretation
3. The confirmation of interpreter skill level through test-taking
4. The need to support a new nurse since it was requested by the supervisor

ANSWER: 2

Requirements for interpretation may be state mandated, or there may also be a facility policy. The prudent nurse should investigate the legal requirements and risks of interpretation before agreeing to be an interpreter. Client interpretation policies would not apply. No test is required to determine interpreter skill level. Although it is important to support a new nurse, the nurse should not feel obligated to perform this task just because the supervisor requested the interpretation.

▶ ***Test-taking Tip:*** *The key words are "most important." Recall that legal and facility policies are typically developed for high-risk situations.*

Content Area: Management of Care; *Category of Health Alteration:* Ethical, Legal, and Safety Issues in Nursing; *Integrated Processes:* Nursing Process Analysis; *Client Need:* Safe and Effective Care Environment/Management of Care/Informed Consent; *Cognitive Level:* Application

Reference: Berman, A., Snyder, S., Kozier, B., & Erb, G. (2008). *Kozier & Erb's Fundamentals of Nursing: Concepts, Process, and Practice* (8th ed., pp. 319–320). Upper Saddle River, NJ: Pearson Education.

EBP Reference: University of Iowa College of Nursing, Gerontological Nursing Interventions Research Center Research Dissemination Core. (2001). *Interpreter Proficiency for Persons with Limited English Proficiency.* Available at: www.nursing.uiowa.edu/products_services/evidence_based.htm

---

14. A nurse is caring for a client diagnosed with cystic fibrosis who is refusing to take a recommended nebulizer treatment. The client's refusal of treatment is classified as which of the following?

1. A moral obligation
2. A legal obligation
3. An ethical right
4. A basic human right

ANSWER: 3

Rights are generally defined as something owed to an individual. Ethical rights are based on an ethical principle and are often privileges allotted to individuals. A legal obligation would be one required by law. A moral obligation would be taking the treatment based on an ethical principle. Basic human rights are rights based on the fundamental belief in the dignity and freedom of humans.

▶ ***Test-taking Tip:*** *Apply knowledge of client rights and eliminate the options related to obligation. Of options 3 and 4, determine which best fits the situation.*

Content Area: Management of Care; *Category of Health Alteration:* Ethical, Legal, and Safety Issues in Nursing; *Integrated Processes:* Nursing Process Assessment; *Client Need:* Safe and Effective Care Environment/Management of Care/Client Rights; *Cognitive Level:* Application

Reference: Catalano, J. (2006). *Nursing Now! Today's Issues, Tomorrow's Trends.* (4th ed., pp. 123–124). Philadelphia: F. A. Davis.

15. A client informs a nurse that a physician is recommending a kidney biopsy. The client fears the result will be cancer and would not want treatment. The client feels it would be better just "not to know." Which action should be taken by the nurse to determine if the client understands his/her client rights?

1. Explain to the client that the physician is doing what is best for the client.
2. Inform the client of his/her right to make decisions based on personal values and beliefs.
3. Encourage the client to talk with family and let the family decide.
4. Talk with the physician about the client's fear of having the biopsy.

ANSWER: 2

Clients have the right to make decisions based on personal values and beliefs. Physicians cannot make treatment decisions without the consent of the client, nor may the family. It is important to notify the physician about the client's fear of the biopsy; however, it does not address the client's understanding of client rights.

➧ ***Test-taking Tip:*** *Key words are "best action." Select the option that would support client rights.*

Content Area: Management of Care; *Category of Health Alteration:* Ethical, Legal, and Safety Issues in Nursing; *Integrated Processes:* Caring; *Client Need:* Safe and Effective Care Environment/Management of Care/Client Rights; *Cognitive Level:* Analysis

Reference: Chulay, M., & Burns, S. (2007). *AACN Essentials of Progressive Care Nursing* (p. 176). New York: McGraw-Hill.

16. A client is experiencing increased dyspnea and chest pain. A physician is notified and orders an electrocardiogram (ECG) to be done stat. The nurse has not done an ECG before and there is no ECG technician in the hospital at this time. Which steps should be taken by the nurse in performing an ECG? Place each answer option into the correct order.

______ Obtain the ECG machine
______ Place the ECG tracing in the medical record
______ Contact an experienced nurse or supervisor for assistance
______ Ask an experienced nurse or supervisor to teach the procedure for performing an ECG
______ Observe the experienced nurse or supervisor do the ECG
______ Call the physician to notify that the ECG is completed
______ Review the hospital policy on doing ECGs

ANSWER: 4, 7, 2, 3, 5, 6, 1

The nurse should first review the hospital policy on doing ECGs and ask a nurse with experience for assistance. The new nurse should learn how to do an ECG, as it may be needed in the future, and should ask to learn from the experienced nurse. The nurse should obtain the ECG machine and observe the experienced nurse doing the ECG. The physician should then be notified that the ECG is complete. Finally, the nurse should place the ECG in the medical record.

➧ ***Test-taking Tip:*** *Always follow organizational policies. Know that the nurse is at a legal risk when performing a task that has not been learned.*

Content Area: Management of Care; *Category of Health Alteration:* Ethical, Legal, and Safety Issues in Nursing; *Integrated Processes:* Nursing Process Implementation; *Client Need:* Safe and Effective Care Environment/Management of Care/Legal Rights and Responsibilities; *Cognitive Level:* Application

Reference: Catalano, J. (2006). *Nursing Now! Today's Issues, Tomorrow's Trends* (4th ed., p. 166). Philadelphia: F. A. Davis.

17. A client is admitted to a surgical unit. The client has multiple rings, a watch, and $65 in cash. What is the safest action for a nurse to take regarding the valuables?

1. Allowing the client to keep the items so they will be safeguarded by the client
2. Collecting the items and placing them in the client's room closet
3. Giving the money to the client's spouse and allowing the client to keep the jewelry
4. Collecting the items according to hospital policy for safekeeping

ANSWER: 4

Hospital policy will determine if the items were handled appropriately in the case of loss. Although the hospital policy may allow the items to stay with the client, to be in the room, or to be sent home with the spouse, the safest action is to follow hospital policy.

➧ ***Test-taking Tip:*** *The key word is "safest." Use the process of elimination to determine the correct answer.*

Content Area: Management of Care; *Category of Health Alteration:* Ethical, Legal, and Safety Issues in Nursing; *Integrated Processes:* Communication and Documentation; *Client Need:* Safe and Effective Care Environment/Management of Care/Legal Rights and Responsibilities; *Cognitive Level:* Application

References: Berman, A., Snyder, S., Kozier, B., & Erb, G. (2008). *Kozier & Erb's Fundamentals of Nursing: Concepts, Process, and Practice* (8th ed., p. 71). Upper Saddle River, NJ: Pearson Education; Catalano, J. (2006). *Nursing Now! Today's Issues, Tomorrow's Trends* (4th ed., p. 166). Philadelphia: F. A. Davis.

18. EBP An adolescent client enters a clinic alone and discloses that he/she is human immunodeficiency virus (HIV) positive. The client has a productive cough and low-grade fever. Which is the best action by the nurse?

1. Nothing can be done without the consent of the parents.
2. Educate the client concerning birth control, safe sex, and partner disclosure.
3. Draw an HIV titer to confirm the HIV positive status of the client.
4. Obtain a sexual risk history and notify the parents.

ANSWER: 2

The best action by the nurse is to educate the client concerning birth control, safe sex, and partner disclosure. Individuals diagnosed with HIV may receive treatment, including education and counseling, without consent of the parents. It is not necessary to redraw the HIV titer. Although it is important to obtain an updated sexual risk history, the parents do not need to be notified of the client's clinic visit.

▶ ***Test-taking Tip:*** *Note that options 1 and 4 both involve the parents, so either one or both of these options must be wrong. Of options 2 and 3, determine which demonstrates the role of the nurse.*

Content Area: Management of Care; *Category of Health Alteration:* Ethical, Legal, and Safety Issues in Nursing; *Integrated Processes:* Teaching and Learning; *Client Need:* Safe and Effective Care Environment/Management of Care/Legal Rights and Responsibilities; *Cognitive Level:* Analysis

EBP Reference: New York State Department of Health. (2004). *Identification and Ambulatory Care of HIV-Exposed and -Infected Adolescents.* Available at: www.guideline.gov/summary/summary.aspx?doc_id=10979&nbr=005759&string=legal+AND+issues

19. EBP A nurse is working in a busy emergency department with multiple admissions. Which clients would meet the requirement for mandatory reporting? SELECT ALL THAT APPLY.

1. A client who has a gunshot wound
2. A client who has meningitis
3. A child who has cigarette burns
4. A child who has respiratory syntactial virus (RSV)
5. A vulnerable adult who is admitted for dehydration
6. An adult client who has a broken hip from a fall

ANSWER: 1, 2, 3, 4, 5

A gunshot wound, a communicable disease, an abused child, and a vulnerable adult all require mandatory reporting through the Health and Human Services Your Health Information Privacy Rights law. An injury from a fall is not a situation for mandatory reporting.

▶ ***Test-taking Tip:*** *Recall that injuries with weapons, communicable diseases, child abuse, and vulnerable adults are reportable.*

Content Area: Management of Care; *Category of Health Alteration:* Ethical, Legal, and Safety Issues in Nursing; *Integrated Processes:* Nursing Process Implementation; *Client Need:* Safe and Effective Care Environment/Management of Care/Legal Rights and Responsibilities; *Cognitive Level:* Application

EBP Reference: U.S. Department of Health & Human Services Office for Civil Rights. (2004). *Your Health Information Privacy Rights.* Available at: www.hhs.gov/ocr/hipaa/consumer_rights.pdf

20. A nurse assists a physician with the placement of a central venous catheter. The nurse notices the physician brush his sterile glove against the client's bedspread. Which action by the nurse demonstrates professional conduct?

1. Inform the physician of the break in sterile procedure and provide new sterile gloves
2. Inform the physician of the break in sterile procedure after the procedure is completed and observe for a central venous catheter line infection
3. Notify the supervisor of the break in sterile procedure
4. Report the event to the Infection Control Nurse to educate the physician on proper sterile procedure

ANSWER: 1

The physician should be notified immediately of the break in sterile procedure to reduce risk of infection to the client. To wait until after the procedure is completed to talk with the physician or to report the event to someone else will not prevent this client from a hospital-acquired infection.

▶ ***Test-taking Tip:*** *The key words are "professional conduct." Select the option that protects the safety of the client. Note that only option 1 deals with the break in sterile technique immediately.*

Content Area: Management of Care; *Category of Health Alteration:* Ethical, Legal, and Safety Issues in Nursing; *Integrated Processes:* Nursing Process Implementation; *Client Need:* Safe and Effective Care Environment/Management of Care/Legal Rights and Responsibilities; *Cognitive Level:* Analysis

Reference: Catalano, J. (2006). *Nursing Now! Today's Issues, Tomorrow's Trends* (4th ed., pp. 164–165). Philadelphia: F. A. Davis.

21. A nurse is reviewing a client's electronic medical record. The nurse allows a colleague, who is not caring for the client, to view the screen. Place an X on the areas of the computer screen that violate the Health Insurance Portability and Accountability Act (HIPAA) if viewed by a non-care provider.

Electronic Medical Record: Maple, John

Summary | H&P | Notes | Flowsheets | Imaging | Lab | Surgery | Allergies

John Maple	**MRN**	**DOB**	**Age**	**Gender**	**Physician**
	12345	11/25/36	71	male	Nelson

Date: 1/14/08	0400	0800	1015	1200	1400	1600	1800	2000	2200	2359
BP Systole	120	132		134						
BP Diastole	86	80		72						
Pulse	84	90		72						
Respirations	16	20		16						
Temperature	98.6	99.4		98.2						
SpO_2	97	98		98						
Oxygen	21									
Oxygen Source	NC									
Pain (0-10)	2	2	5	1	1					

Notes:
0400 Awake. Pain rating of 2. Refuses analgesic. Ambulated to bathroom independently.
0800 Increase in temperature of 99.4. Wife called and updated with current status. Will be in mid-morning.
1015 Increase in pain rating to 5. One Vicodin given.
1045 Pain rating 2.
1200 Wife here. Resting comfortably.

ANSWER:

Electronic Medical Record: Ma[X] John

Summary | H&P | Notes | Flowsheets | Imaging | Lab | Surgery | Allergies

Joh[X]aple	**[X]**	**[X]**	**Age**	**Gender**	**Physician**
	12345	11/25/36	71	male	Nelson

Date: 1/14/08	0400	0800	1015	1200	1400	1600	1800	2000	2200	2359
BP Systole	120	132		134						
BP Diastole	86	80		72						
Pulse	84	90		72						
Respirations	16	20		16						
Temperature	98.6	99.4		98.2						
SpO_2	97	98		98						
Oxygen	21									
Oxygen Source	NC									
Pain (0-10)	2	2	5	1	1					

Notes:
0400 Awake. Pain rating of 2. Refuses analgesic. Ambulated to bathroom independently
0800 Increase in temperature of 99.4. Wife called and updated with current status. Will be in mid-morning.
1015 Increase in pain rating to 5. One Vicodin given.
1045 Pain rating 2.
1200 Wife here. Resting comfortably.

Client names, medical record numbers, birth dates, and other identifiers cannot be viewable to non–health-care providers, according to HIPAA. Room number, age, physician, and other information displayed cannot be linked to an individual client for identification.

▸ ***Test-taking Tip:*** *Apply knowledge of HIPAA. Note that the word "areas" is plural, indicating that more than one X should be placed.*

Content Area: Management of Care; *Category of Health Alteration:* Ethical, Legal, and Safety Issues in Nursing; *Integrated Processes:* Communication and Documentation; *Client Need:* Safe and Effective Care Environment/Management of Care/Confidentiality; *Cognitive Level:* Analysis

Reference: Wilkinson, J., & Van Leuven, K. (2007). *Fundamentals of Nursing* (p. 1073). Philadelphia: F. A. Davis.

22. Two clients are in a semi-private room on a medical unit. A physician is about to inform client A of a cancer diagnosis. Which statement by the nurse is best when attempting to maintain client confidentiality?

1. To client B: "This would be a good time to go for a walk. The doctor needs to tell your roommate something confidential."
2. To the physician: "For privacy, could you please wait to tell client A about his cancer? His roommate will be going home in a couple of hours."
3. To client B: "The doctor needs to talk to your roommate. Could you please turn on your TV and not listen to what they say?"
4. To client B: "I would like to take you in a wheelchair or have you walk down to the lobby for 10 or 15 minutes. It's good for your lungs to do some deep breathing with activity. Do you feel like getting up for a little while?"

ANSWER: 4

Offering client B to get out of bed for his benefit completely eliminates the need to share any information about client A. Sharing with client B that client A will be receiving confidential information is not appropriate, nor is expecting client B to turn on his TV and not listen to the conversation. Asking the physician to return later may not be realistic for the physician's schedule and the client may have another roommate by that time.

Test-taking Tip: *The key words are "best" and "maintain confidentiality." The word best indicates that two or more options would be acceptable but one is better than the others are.*

Content Area: Management of Care; *Category of Health Alteration:* Ethical, Legal, and Safety Issues in Nursing; *Integrated Processes:* Nursing Process Planning; *Client Need:* Safe and Effective Care Environment/Management of Care/Confidentiality; *Cognitive Level:* Analysis

Reference: Wilkinson, J., & Van Leuven, K. (2007). *Fundamentals of Nursing* (p. 1073). Philadelphia: F. A. Davis.

23. A nurse sees a physician reviewing a medical record. After the physician leaves, the nurse picks up the chart and notices that this physician is not involved in this client's care. Which professional action should be taken by the nurse?

1. Report the event to the nurse's supervisor
2. Call the physician and confront him or her with reading the medical record
3. Report the physician to the chief of staff
4. No action is required; all physicians may look at any client records

ANSWER: 1

Breaches in confidentiality are serious offenses. Typically, such issues are handled by management. It would be best to report the event to the nursing supervisor. Confronting the physician may not result in appropriate follow-up action related to Health Insurance Portability and Accountability Act (HIPAA) violations. A nurse should always use the chain of command and report to the immediate supervisor, not the chief of staff. This is a potential breach and must be evaluated. Physicians are also required to be compliant with HIPAA laws.

Test-taking Tip: *The key words are "professional action." Use the chain of command when selecting the correct action. Recognize that the physician's action is illegal.*

Content Area: Management of Care; *Category of Health Alteration:* Ethical, Legal, and Safety Issues in Nursing; *Integrated Processes:* Communication and Documentation; *Client Need:* Safe and Effective Care Environment/Management of Care/Confidentiality; *Cognitive Level:* Analysis

Reference: Wilkinson, J., & Van Leuven, K. (2007). *Fundamentals of Nursing* (p. 1073). Philadelphia: F. A. Davis.

24. EBP A client has a peripheral intravenous (IV) line with a piggyback line, oxygen at 2 liters per nasal cannula, an as needed (prn) nebulizer treatment, and a chest tube connected to a chest drainage system. Several family members are present, wanting to be very helpful, and have been placing the oxygen back on when the nasal cannula slips, turning the IV pump off when it alarms, and placing the nebulizer tubing in the mouthpiece of the nebulizer. Which action by the nurse is required for the safe care of the client?

1. Inform the family that they are not allowed to touch any medical equipment
2. Inform the family that they must get help from clinical staff when there is a need to connect tubing or devices
3. Thank the family for noticing when tubing is disconnected and getting the client the treatment required
4. Inform the family that they are only allowed to turn off the IV pump alarm

ANSWER: 2

The nurse should inform nonclinical staff, clients, and their families that they must get help from clinical staff whenever there is a real or perceived need to connect or disconnect devices or infusions. The family may touch the equipment; however, they should not operate any client care equipment including answering alarms and reconnecting tubing. The potential for incorrect reconnection exists. Tubing misconnections have resulted in death.

Test-taking Tip: *Apply knowledge of safety policies and guidelines. Note that only option 2 informs the family of the actions to take for tubing disconnections or devices that are alarming.*

Content Area: Management of Care; *Category of Health Alteration:* Ethical, Legal, and Safety Issues in Nursing; *Integrated Processes:* Teaching and Learning; *Client Need:* Safe and Effective Care Environment/Safety and Infection Control/Accident Prevention; *Cognitive Level:* Analysis

EBP Reference: The Joint Commission. (2006). Tubing misconnections: A persistent and potentially deadly occurrence. *Sentinel Event Alert Issue #36.* Available at: www.jointcommission.org/SentinelEvents/SentinelEventAlert/sea_36.htm

25. EBP A nurse is preparing to administer medications to a client. Which two unique client identifiers must be checked prior to administration?

1. Client name and room number
2. Client birth date and primary physician
3. Client telephone number and place of birth
4. Client name and medical record number

ANSWER: 4

Client name, birth date, medical record number, and telephone number are all examples of unique identifiers. The intent is to reliably identify the individual as the person for whom the medication administration is intended. Room number, primary physician, and place of birth are not unique to one individual. Bar coding that includes two or more person-specific identifiers (not room number) is an acceptable means of identification.

Test-taking Tip: *"Unique client identifiers" are key words. Identify the two identifiers unlikely to change.*

Content Area: Management of Care; *Category of Health Alteration:* Ethical, Legal, and Safety Issues in Nursing; *Integrated Processes:* Nursing Process Assessment; *Client Need:* Safe and Effective Care Environment/Safety and Infection Control/Error Prevention; *Cognitive Level:* Application

EBP Reference: The Joint Commission. (2007). *2007 National Patient Safety Goals.* Available at: www.jointcommission.org/PatientSafety/NationalPatientSafetyGoals/07_hap_cah_npsgs.htm

---

26. A nurse is caring for a client who has a sudden onset of symptoms including itchy eyes, runny nose, coughing, and shortness of breath. The client is now complaining of chest pain. The client has a history of several surgeries during childhood and spina bifida. The nurse suspects a latex allergy. Which order should the nurse carry out first?

1. Transfer to the cardiac care unit
2. Remove all allergens from the room
3. Place in contact isolation
4. Administer epinephrine subcutaneously

ANSWER: 4

The symptoms of itchy eyes, runny nose, coughing, and shortness of breath are indicators of an allergic reaction. Clients with spina bifida are at high risk for latex allergies. The addition of chest pain indicates the reaction is severe and epinephrine needs to be administered immediately to relax the bronchial muscles. All other actions would be carried out, but epinephrine is the priority.

Test-taking Tip: *Use the ABCs (airway, breathing, circulation) to determine priority. Airway is priority and to maintain the airway epinephrine must be administered.*

Content Area: Management of Care; *Category of Health Alteration:* Ethical, Legal, and Safety Issues in Nursing; *Integrated Processes:* Nursing Process Assessment and Implementation; *Client Need:* Safe and Effective Care Environment/Safety and Infection Control/Error Prevention; *Cognitive Level:* Analysis

Reference: Harkreader, H., Hogan, M., & Thobaben, M. (2007). *Fundamentals of Nursing* (3rd ed., pp. 433–434). St. Louis, MO: Saunders/Elsevier.

27. EBP A client is on a heparin protocol preoperatively. Postoperatively a surgeon writes "Resume heparin at 1600, do not bolus." Then a cardiologist writes an order: "Restart heparin protocol no bolus previous rate at 0700 tomorrow if OK with surgeon." Later, an on-call surgeon writes "Clarification: Resume heparin drip tonight—no bolus at previous rate." At what rate should the heparin be started and why?

Heparin Protocol

1. aPTT/PT; INR; daily CBC.
2. Initiate IV of 500 mL D5W with 25,000 units heparin at 25 mL/hr.
3. Give IV bolus of 2,500 units heparin (or ______units heparin).
4. Repeat aPTT/PT in 6 hours from time IV heparin infusion is initiated.
5. Adjust IV rate of heparin and repeat a PTT/PT per protocol
6. Notify physician if aPTT >129 sec.

aPTT (sec)	IV Bolus (units)	Hold (minutes)	IV Rate (mL/hr)	Repeat aPTT/PT
<50	5,000	0	31	6 hr
50 – <60	0	0	28	6 hr
60 – <86	0	0	25	Next AM
86 – <96	0	0	23	Next AM
96 – 120	0	30	21	6 hr
>120	0	60	17	6 hr

1. Start the heparin at 25 mL/hr because that is the initiation rate on the protocol.
2. Bolus with 5,000 units and begin the drip at 31 mL/hr because that is the first line of the protocol.
3. Contact the surgeon to determine the rate at which the heparin drip should be started because the order is not clear.
4. Start the heparin at 28 mL/hr per protocol and obtain an activated partial thromboplastin time (aPTT) in 6 hours to reestablish the baseline.

ANSWER: 3

The order is not clear as to what rate to start the heparin. Use critical-thinking skills to evaluate the orders. Determine which physician is managing the heparin protocol. Continue to ask questions until the orders are completely clarified. If it is change of shift and the orders have not been clarified, make sure the handoff communication includes the need to clarify orders before administration of heparin. Never guess or assume what the physician meant to write. Nurses can expect clearly written orders.

***Test-taking Tip:** Carefully read the directions from the physicians. Note there is no clear direction.*

Content Area: Management of Care; *Category of Health Alteration:* Ethical, Legal, and Safety Issues in Nursing; *Integrated Processes:* Communication and Documentation; *Client Need:* Safe and Effective Care Environment/Safety and Infection Control/Error Prevention; *Cognitive Level:* Analysis

Reference: Wilkinson, J., & Van Leuven, K. (2007). *Fundamentals of Nursing* (pp. 497–498). Philadelphia: F. A. Davis.

EBP Reference: The National Coordinating Council for Medication Error Reporting and Prevention. (2005). *Recommendations to Enhance Accuracy of Administration of Medications.* Available at: www.nccmerp.org/council/council1999-06-29.html

28. EBP A nurse is hanging an intravenous (IV) solution of D5NS with 20 mEq of KCL. The nurse notices the label from the pharmacy is correct as indicated; however, the solution is D5W. Which actions should be taken by the nurse to safely administer the IV infusion? SELECT ALL THAT APPLY.

1. Check for one unique client identifier before administration
2. Consult the supervisor
3. Administer the IV solution
4. Call the pharmacist
5. First, initiate the new stat orders for another client
6. Know the organization's policy for medication administration

ANSWER: 2, 4, 6

Safe medication practices include knowing the organization's policy for medication administration and knowing what actions to take in the event of a potential error. This includes consulting the supervisor or calling the pharmacist. Although it is important to always check for two unique identifiers, that action will not prevent the medication error. The IV solution should not be administered since it is not the correct solution. Distractions, such as the assignment of another client with stat orders, may result in forgetting to clarify the IV solution.

***Test-taking Tip:** Note that the IV solution is incorrect; identify actions to prevent the error.*

Content Area: Management of Care; *Category of Health Alteration:* Ethical, Legal, and Safety Issues in Nursing; *Integrated Processes:* Nursing Process Implementation; *Client Need:* Safe and Effective Care Environment/Safety and Infection Control/Error Prevention; *Cognitive Level:* Analysis

EBP Reference: The National Coordinating Council for Medication Error Reporting and Prevention. (2005). *Recommendations to Enhance Accuracy of Administration of Medications.* Available at: www.nccmerp.org/council/council1999-06-29.html

29. A nurse is totaling the 8-hour shift intake and output for a client with an intravenous (IV) infusion on an IV pump. The IV is infusing at 125 mL/hr. The total IV intake is 900 mL. Based on this information, which conclusion should the nurse make?

1. The IV pump is not functioning correctly and should be sequestered for inspection and replaced.
2. The IV infusion was stopped for 2 hours during a procedure and the intake is correct.
3. The total intake is correct.
4. The IV pump has malfunctioned. The IV should be run off the pump at 125 mL/hr.

ANSWER: 1

The pump should have infused 1,000 mL in 8 hours. The pump is not functioning and should be replaced with a functioning IV pump. Malfunctioning equipment should be sequestered so it will not be used on another client. The IV pump must be inspected by a professional who is trained in equipment repair. If the IV infusion was stopped for 2 hours the total intake would be 850 mL, thus 900 mL would be an incorrect IV total. IV fluids should not be run off an IV pump. A new pump should be obtained.

Test-taking Tip: *Multiply 8 hours times 125 mL/hr to determine the amount the client should have received in 8 hours. Then, eliminate option 3 because this option indicates that the volume is correct. Of the remaining options, select the one that maintains the client's IV fluids and prevents future errors.*

Content Area: Management of Care; *Category of Health Alteration:* Ethical, Legal, and Safety Issues in Nursing; *Integrated Processes:* Nursing Process Analysis; *Client Need:* Safe and Effective Care Environment/Safety and Infection Control/Injury Prevention; *Cognitive Level:* Analysis

Reference: Wilkinson, J., & Van Leuven, K. (2007). *Fundamentals of Nursing* (p. 433). Philadelphia: F. A. Davis.

30. A nurse admits a client who is experiencing nausea and vomiting to the emergency department. The client is alone. The nurse completes an assessment and prepares to leave the room. Which is the safest instruction for the client?

1. "If you need to vomit, here is a basin for you. I don't want you to get up on your own."
2. "I will be in the room next door. I'll check back in about 10 minutes."
3. "I will go update the doctor about you. Do you need anything before I go?"
4. "Here is the nurse call light. Press this button if you need me."

ANSWER: 4

A newly admitted client should be oriented to the new environment. One of the most important features of safety is teaching the client how to use the call light; a mechanism to signal staff members at all times is essential to client safety. Making sure there is a basin available in the case of an emesis is also important to safety; however, the client may need a nurse for other reasons. Checking back later with the client and offering assistance before leaving the room are important actions but are not the best answers.

Test-taking Tip: *The key word is "safest."*

Content Area: Management of Care; *Category of Health Alteration:* Ethical, Legal, and Safety Issues in Nursing; *Integrated Processes:* Nursing Process Planning; *Client Need:* Safe and Effective Care Environment/Safety and Infection Control/Injury Prevention; *Cognitive Level:* Application

Reference: Harkreader, H., Hogan, M., & Thobaben, M. (2007). *Fundamentals of Nursing* (3rd ed., pp. 552–553). St. Louis, MO: Saunders/Elsevier.

31. A charge nurse receives a phone call from the emergency room where a client is being admitted. The admission diagnosis of the client is renal failure. The client is also confused and restless. Which is the safest room assignment for this client?

1. A semi-private room 50 feet from the nurse's station
2. A small, private room at the end of the hallway
3. A seclusion room that is monitored by a camera for client safety
4. A large private room within view of the nurse's station

ANSWER: 4

Large, uncluttered areas tend to promote safety for most confused clients. Being in close proximity to monitor client activity will also contribute to client safety. Rooms far away will not allow frequent observations. A small, private room at the end of the hallway is not the best place for frequent observations. A seclusion room is inappropriate for a confused client unless the client's behavior warrants the seclusion.

Test-taking Tip: *The key word is "safest." Note that the client is confused and restless.*

Content Area: Management of Care; *Category of Health Alteration:* Ethical, Legal, and Safety Issues in Nursing; *Integrated Processes:* Nursing Process Assessment; *Client Need:* Safe and Effective Care Environment/Safety and Infection Control/Injury Prevention; *Cognitive Level:* Application

Reference: Harkreader, H., Hogan, M., & Thobaben, M. (2007). *Fundamentals of Nursing* (3rd ed., pp. 556–559, 1091–1092). St. Louis, MO: Saunders/Elsevier.

32. EBP A postoperative client is pulling at intravenous (IV) lines and a drainage tube. The client is disoriented to time, place, and person. A decision is made to place wrist restraints on the client to prevent tube removal. Which statement is true regarding the regulatory guidelines of restraint application and monitoring?

1. A registered nurse (RN) is a licensed independent practitioner and therefore may decide to apply restraints.
2. An order to apply a restraint may come from the physician's standing orders.
3. Restraint application may be trialed for up to 2 hours before a physician order is required.
4. Ongoing assessment and monitoring of the client's condition are crucial for prevention of injury or death.

ANSWER: 4

The improper use of restraints may result in injury or death. Ongoing assessment and monitoring of the client will reduce this risk. A RN is not a licensed, independent practitioner. Standing orders may not be used to apply restraints. A physician order is required within 24 hours of application in the hospital setting. Restraint trials violate client rights.

Test-taking Tip: *Apply knowledge of regulatory practices related to restraint and seclusion. Use the nursing process to decide that assessment is priority for this question.*

Content Area: Management of Care; *Category of Health Alteration:* Ethical, Legal, and Safety Issues in Nursing; *Integrated Processes:* Nursing Process Assessment; *Client Need:* Safe and Effective Care Environment/Safety and Infection Control/Use of Restraints/Safety Devices; *Cognitive Level:* Application

Reference: Harkreader, H., Hogan, M., & Thobaben, M. (2007). *Fundamentals of Nursing* (3rd ed., pp. 554–562). St. Louis, MO: Saunders/Elsevier.

EBP Reference: Department of Health and Human Services: Centers for Medicare & Medicaid Services. (2006). Medicare and Medicaid Programs; Hospital Conditions of Participation: Patients' Rights; Final Rule. (DHHS Publication 42 CFR Part 482). Available at: www.cms.hhs.gov/CertificationandCompliance/Downloads/PatientsRights.pdf

---

33. A client is agitated and restless. Physical restraints are applied. A decision is made to begin chemical restraints with intravenous (IV) sedatives. For which common side effect of chemical sedation/restraint should the client be monitored?

1. Hypotension
2. Ability to remove physical restraints
3. Respiratory depression
4. Pain level less than 3 on a 0 to 10 scale

ANSWER: 3

Clients receiving chemical sedation/restraint should be monitored for excessive drowsiness or respiratory depression. Care must be taken with long-acting sedation, as the effect is not seen for up to 1 hour after administration. The blood pressure may decrease; however, hypotension should not occur from the sedation. Physical restraints may also be necessary if the client is significantly agitated until the cause of the agitation is resolved. Pain may accompany restlessness; however, it is not a side effect of chemical restraints.

Test-taking Tip: *Use the ABCs (airway, breathing, circulation) to prioritize the common side effect of chemical sedation for which a client should be monitored.*

Content Area: Management of Care; *Category of Health Alteration:* Ethical, Legal, and Safety Issues in Nursing; *Integrated Processes:* Nursing Process Assessment; *Client Need:* Safe and Effective Care Environment/Safety and Infection Control/Use of Restraints/Safety Devices

Reference: Chulay, M., & Burns, S. (2007). *AACN Essentials of Progressive Care Nursing* (p. 140). New York: McGraw-Hill.

---

34. A nursing home client is confused and trying to get out of bed. The client suffered a broken hip from a fall 6 months ago and is unable to walk independently. Alternatives to restraints have been tried; however, the client continues to try to get out of bed. A decision has been made to apply restraints. Which type of restraint would be best for this client to prevent getting out of bed?

1. Jacket restraint
2. Bilateral ankle restraints
3. Mitten restraints
4. Belt restraint

ANSWER: 1

A jacket restraint is the best restraint to prevent the client from getting out of bed as it secures both the shoulder and the waist and yet allows the client to turn from side to side. The client would still be able to sit up and try to get out of bed with ankle restraints. Mitten restraints prevent the use of hands but still allow free arm movement. A belt restraint is less restrictive than a jacket.

Test-taking Tip: *The key phrase is "would be best." Focus on the activity of the client to select the correct option.*

Content Area: Management of Care; *Category of Health Alteration:* Ethical, Legal, and Safety Issues in Nursing; *Integrated Processes:* Nursing Process Assessment; *Client Need:* Safe and Effective Care Environment/Safety and Infection Control/Use of Restraints; *Cognitive Level:* Application

Reference: Harkreader, H., Hogan, M., & Thobaben, M. (2007). *Fundamentals of Nursing* (3rd ed., pp. 556–557). St. Louis, MO: Saunders/Elsevier.

35. A nurse is assisting a physician with a cardioversion procedure. The client is anxious and fears the pain associated with the countershock. Conscious sedation is given. Monitoring of the client is especially important in conscious sedation due to which of the following?

1. Risk of hypertensive response
2. Potential loss of airway
3. Allergic reaction to sedatives
4. Change in level of consciousness

ANSWER: 2

The client's ability to maintain a patent airway is central to the decision to use conscious sedation. Oversedation may result in the loss of the airway. A hypertensive response is not associated with conscious sedation. Although an allergic reaction may occur, the loss of airway is a more common complication. A change in level of consciousness is expected.

Test-taking Tip: *Use the ABCs (airway, breathing, circulation) to answer this question. Remember that the airway is especially important.*

Content Area: Management of Care; *Category of Health Alteration:* Ethical, Legal, and Safety Issues in Nursing; *Integrated Processes:* Nursing Process Assessment; *Client Need:* Physiological Integrity/ Reduction of Risk Potential/System Specific Assessments; *Cognitive Level:* Application

Reference: Chulay, M., & Burns, S. (2007). *AACN Essentials of Progressive Care Nursing* (p. 138). New York: McGraw-Hill.

36. A nurse is assisting a physician who is performing an endoscopy on a client. The nurse instructs the client and family about the procedure, including conscious sedation. What is the purpose of conscious sedation during the procedure?

1. To have the client asleep with a sluggish response
2. To produce deep sleep due to potential agitation and oxygenation problems
3. To keep the client cooperative, oriented, and tranquil
4. To keep the client comfortable and responsive

ANSWER: 4

The goal of conscious sedation is to minimize discomfort while ensuring that the client is able to communicate throughout the procedure. The client should not sleep or have a sluggish response. A deep sleep would be considered anesthesia. Although it is good to have the client cooperative, oriented, and tranquil, that is not the purpose of conscious sedation.

Test-taking Tip: *The key word is "purpose." Apply knowledge of conscious sedation.*

Content Area: Management of Care; *Category of Health Alteration:* Ethical, Legal, and Safety Issues in Nursing; *Integrated Processes:* Nursing Process Implementation; *Client Need:* Physiological Integrity/Reduction of Risk Potential/System Specific Assessments; *Cognitive Level:* Analysis

Reference: Chulay, M., & Burns, S. (2007). *AACN Essentials of Progressive Care Nursing* (pp. 138–139). New York: McGraw-Hill.

37. A client is having a computerized tomography (CT) scan for a needle-guided pancreatic biopsy. A short-term sedative is administered to the client. Clients receiving short-term sedatives should receive which monitoring?

1. Pulse oximetry
2. Electroencephalography
3. Central venous pressure
4. Intracranial pressure

ANSWER: 1

A client should be monitored with pulse oximetry while receiving short-term sedatives. Pulse oximetry will provide early warning signs of a decrease in oxygenation due to potential oversedation. Electroencephalography (EEG) monitoring and intracranial pressure monitoring are not necessary for conscious sedation. Central venous pressure monitoring measures cardiovascular pressures, which are not significantly affected by conscious sedation.

Test-taking Tip: *Focus on the effects of a sedative. Use the ABCs (airway, breathing, circulation) to determine an appropriate intervention.*

Content Area: Management of Care; *Category of Health Alteration:* Ethical, Legal, and Safety Issues in Nursing; *Integrated Processes:* Nursing Process Assessment; *Client Need:* Physiological Integrity/ Reduction of Risk Potential/System Specific Assessments; *Cognitive Level:* Application

Reference: Chulay, M., & Burns, S. (2007). *AACN Essentials of Progressive Care Nursing* (pp. 138–139). New York: McGraw-Hill.

38. A client has multiple pieces of electrical equipment in a room, including a cardiac monitor, three intravenous (IV) pumps, a mechanical ventilator, and sequential stockings. Which nursing action decreases the client's risk for an electrical injury?

1. Places multiple electrical plugs into one electrical outlet
2. Pulls the IV pump plug from the socket by the cord
3. Plugs grounded equipment into a three-prong outlet
4. Uses an extension cord with multiple electrical plugs

ANSWER: 3

Electrical safety is maintained by using grounded equipment with a three-prong outlet. Overloading outlets, pulling on an electrical cord to remove it from the socket, and using an extension cord should be avoided with the use of medical equipment due to potential shortages.

➧ ***Test-taking Tip:*** *The key word is "decrease." Select the statement that is true. Use Maslow's Hierarchy of Needs to prioritize for safety and security.*

Content Area: Management of Care; *Category of Health Alteration:* Ethical, Legal, and Safety Issues in Nursing; *Integrated Processes:* Nursing Process Assessment; *Client Need:* Safe and Effective Care Environment/Safety and Infection Control/Safe Use of Equipment; *Cognitive Level:* Application

Reference: Harkreader, H., Hogan, M., & Thobaben, M. (2007). *Fundamentals of Nursing* (3rd ed., pp. 551–552). St. Louis, MO: Saunders/Elsevier.

39. A client is receiving patient-controlled analgesia (PCA). The client complains to a nurse that the button has been pushed several times but there is no pain relief. On examination of the PCA pump, it appears no analgesic has been delivered for 3 hours. Which is the safest action for the nurse to take?

1. Replace the old pump with a new one. Place the old pump in soiled receiving.
2. Check the programming on the pump to ensure it is programmed correctly.
3. Replace the old pump with a new one. Sequester the old pump.
4. Report the pump malfunction to the supervisor.

ANSWER: 3

Since no analgesic has been delivered for 3 hours, the pump is not working, and it should be replaced. Sequestering the pump will prevent other clients from receiving the malfunctioning pump. Placing the old pump in soiled receiving risks another user taking the pump for a client. Checking the programming will not get the pump to work. Reporting the pump malfunction to the supervisor will delay a replacement pump for the client and is not the safest action.

➧ ***Test-taking Tip:*** *The key phrase is "safest action." A safe action would include ensuring that the client receives the medication and that the equipment is not the cause of another error.*

Content Area: Management of Care; *Category of Health Alteration:* Ethical, Legal, and Safety Issues in Nursing; *Integrated Processes:* Nursing Process Assessment; *Client Need:* Safe and Effective Care Environment/Safety and Infection Control/Safe Use of Equipment; *Cognitive Level:* Application

Reference: Guido, G. (2006). *Legal and Ethical Issues in Nursing* (4th ed., pp. 396–397). Upper Saddle River, NJ: Pearson Education.

40. A client will be going home with a vacuum-assisted closure (VAC) dressing. A nurse is preparing the client for discharge. Which statement best supports the safe use of equipment at home?

1. "The home care nurse will come check on the dressing tomorrow."
2. "If you notice that the suction is released, place a piece of tape over the loose area which may help resume the suction."
3. "The sales representative who rents the VAC will visit before you leave to make sure you know how to use it."
4. "I will observe you change the dressing and place the VAC on correctly."

ANSWER: 4

Having the client do a return demonstration is the best method for evaluating a new skill. Having the home care nurse check the dressing tomorrow will not address any equipment issues that arise between discharge and the visit. Giving a tip on device malfunction does not support the need for full understanding of the function of the VAC. Never rely on a non-hospital employee to provide your client's education.

➧ ***Test-taking Tip:*** *The key phrase is "supports safe use of equipment at home," indicating a need to instruct the client on the operation of the equipment before discharge.*

Content Area: Management of Care; *Category of Health Alteration:* Ethical, Legal, and Safety Issues in Nursing; *Integrated Processes:* Teaching and Learning; *Client Need:* Safe and Effective Care Environment/Safety and Infection Control/Safe Use of Equipment; *Cognitive Level:* Application

Reference: Harkreader, H., Hogan, M., & Thobaben, M. (2007). *Fundamentals of Nursing* (3rd ed., pp. 285–288). St. Louis, MO: Saunders/Elsevier.

Test 2: **Management of Care: Leadership and Management**

41. An 84-year-old client wishes to be discharged to home status postkyphoplasty. The client has a medical history, including thrombocytopenia and emphysema, which requires oxygen therapy at night. To ensure discharge to home is appropriate, which is most important for the nurse to assess?

1. Home care resources
2. Pain management plan
3. Self-care deficits
4. Medication regime

ANSWER: 3

Assessment of the client's self-care deficits will determine if additional resources or client education is necessary. The client may have pain related to the surgical procedure and may be taking medications; however, if the nursing assessment demonstrates that the client has no self-care deficits, the client will be able to be discharged safely without further intervention. Home-care resources may be necessary if the nursing assessment demonstrates that the client has a self-care deficit.

➧ ***Test-taking Tip:*** *The key phrase is "most important." Apply knowledge of discharge planning and basic physiological needs.*

Content Area: Management of Care; *Category of Health Alteration:* Leadership and Management; *Integrated Processes:* Nursing Process Assessment; *Client Need:* Safe and Effective Care Environment/ Management of Care/Case Management; *Cognitive Level:* Application

Reference: Wilkinson, J., & Van Leuven, K. (2007). *Fundamentals of Nursing* (p. 297). Philadelphia: F. A. Davis.

---

42. A client is admitted for coronary artery bypass surgery (CABG) with an anticipated admission to the coronary care unit (CCU). In preparation for the client's admission to the hospital, which action will best predict the sequence and timing of care and direct the course of the client's hospital stay?

1. Implementation of a clinical pathway
2. Initiation of a client education plan
3. Implementation of physician-initiated interventions
4. Initiation of discharge planning at the time of admission

ANSWER: 1

A clinical pathway is a standardized multidisciplinary care plan that projects the client goals, expected course of the client's treatment, and progress over the client's hospital stay. A client education plan will include the information required for the client to understand the care and treatment related to the surgical procedure but is not a comprehensive plan for their care. A physician-initiated intervention is an individual treatment initiated by a physician related to a medical diagnosis that is then carried out by a nurse. Although discharge planning helps establish client goals and should be started at the time of admission, it will not predict the client's course during the hospital stay.

➧ ***Test-taking Tip:*** *The key words are "predict" and "direct." Apply knowledge of clinical pathways, care maps, clinical paths, collaborative care plans, or multidisciplinary care plans, all of which provide a timeline with projected client goals, expected course of the client's treatment, and progress over the client's hospital stay.*

Content Area: Management of Care; *Category of Health Alteration:* Leadership and Management; *Integrated Processes:* Nursing Process Planning; *Client Need:* Safe and Effective Care Environment/Management of Care/Case Management; *Cognitive Level:* Analysis

Reference: Harkreader, H., Hogan, M., & Thobaben, M. (2007). *Fundamentals of Nursing* (3rd ed., pp. 219–220). St. Louis, MO: Saunders/Elsevier.

43. A 72-year-old client with a deep vein thrombosis in the left leg and a history of a brain tumor is hospitalized for 3 days. The client's care plan indicates a nursing diagnosis of *Imbalanced nutrition: less than body requirements related to poor appetite and decreased oral intake*. Which assessment finding would best indicate a need to revise the care plan related to the nursing diagnosis?

1. Oral mucous membranes are dry due to dehydration.
2. Daily intake and output reveals that daily caloric intake is inadequate.
3. Client is not receptive to education regarding nutrition.
4. Client states that he/she is not hungry.

ANSWER: 1

If the client has an impaired oral mucous membrane, it may be uncomfortable to chew and swallow food, therefore exacerbating the underlying condition. To help the client achieve the goal of balanced nutrition, addressing the problem on the care plan will alert caregivers to the issue and facilitate appropriate interventions. Although the other three answers may also support the client's nutrition needs, revising the care plan to address the impaired oral mucous membrane is the best action to take related to the diagnosis.

➧ ***Test-taking Tip:*** *The key words are "best indicate." Select an option that would exacerbate the nursing diagnosis.*

Content Area: Management of Care; *Category of Health Alteration:* Leadership and Management; *Integrated Processes:* Nursing Process Evaluation; *Client Need:* Safe and Effective Care Environment/Management of Care/Case Management; *Cognitive Level:* Application

Reference: Harkreader, H., Hogan, M., & Thobaben, M. (2007). *Fundamentals of Nursing* (3rd ed., pp. 220, 224). St. Louis, MO: Saunders/Elsevier.

44. A pediatric client is being discharged to home with a new diagnosis of cystic fibrosis. The client's parents are anxious about going home and frequently ask questions relating to the child's nutrition, medication regimen, nebulizer treatments, and chest percussion. They also express concern regarding the high cost of care and potential financial hardship. To adequately address the client and client family needs, a multidisciplinary care conference is held. Which health-care disciplines should be included in the client care conference? SELECT ALL THAT APPLY.

1. Nurse
2. Pharmacist
3. Dietitian
4. Social worker
5. Nursing assistant
6. Respiratory therapist

ANSWER: 1, 2, 3, 4, 6

Comprehensive discharge planning involves significant collaboration. A client's postdischarge needs often call for services from an interdisciplinary team. The nurse should coordinate care, the pharmacist should manage medication, the dietitian should provide diet counseling, the social worker should address finances, and the respiratory therapist should instruct on chest percussion and nebulizer treatments. All disciplines, except for the nursing assistant, are needed to assist in developing a comprehensive discharge plan that addresses both the client and client family needs.

➧ ***Test-taking Tip:*** *Apply knowledge of interdisciplinary discharge planning. Recall that care conferences are multidisciplinary.*

Content Area: Management of Care; *Category of Health Alteration:* Leadership and Management; *Integrated Processes:* Nursing Process Planning; *Client Need:* Safe and Effective Care Environment/Management of Care/Collaboration with Interdisciplinary Team; *Cognitive Level:* Application

References: Harkreader, H., Hogan, M., & Thobaben, M. (2007). *Fundamentals of Nursing* (3rd ed., p. 304). St. Louis, MO: Saunders/Elsevier; Wilkinson, J., & Van Leuven, K. (2007). *Fundamentals of Nursing* (p. 85). Philadelphia: F. A. Davis.

45. A nurse reviews the plan of care for an elderly client diagnosed with chronic obstructive pulmonary disease (COPD) and limited mobility. The nurse notes that the physical therapist has indicated a change in the plan of care to progress ambulation from 100 to 200 feet twice a day. Which action is necessary to ensure that the client's needs are met?

1. Instructing the physical therapist not to ambulate the client without the nurse present
2. Informing the physical therapist of the client's respiratory status prior to progressing ambulation
3. Cancelling the physical therapy referral
4. Informing the physician about the physical therapist's plan to progress ambulation

ANSWER: 2

Collaborating with other health-care professionals is crucial for facilitating outcome attainment. Using an interdisciplinary approach to meet the client's needs will expedite recovery. The nurse is responsible for overseeing the client's care. Therefore the nurse should inform the physical therapist of the client's respiratory status. The importance of communication regarding the respiratory status of the patient and a discussion of an alteration in the plan of care would be necessary to meet the needs of the client. The physical therapist may independently ambulate the client; however, the nurse may want to give instructions such as "stop ambulation if the respiratory rate exceeds 30 beats per minute." The physical therapy referral should not be cancelled as the client needs assistance in progressing ambulation. Although it would have been preferable for the physical therapist to tell the nurse about the plan to progress ambulation, the plan of care reflects the change; it is unnecessary to notify the physician.

▶ ***Test-taking Tip:*** *The key phrases are "which action is necessary" and "to meet the needs of the client." Focus on the respiratory status of the client and the responsible person for the overall care of the client.*

Content Area: Management of Care; *Category of Health Alteration:* Leadership and Management; *Integrated Processes:* Nursing Process Evaluation; *Client Need:* Safe and Effective Care Environment/ Management of Care/Collaboration with Interdisciplinary Team; *Cognitive Level:* Analysis

Reference: Harkreader, H., Hogan, M., & Thobaben, M. (2007). *Fundamentals of Nursing* (3rd ed., pp. 61–62, 208, 304). St. Louis, MO: Saunders/Elsevier.

---

46. A client diagnosed with chronic renal failure is placed on a restricted renal diet. The diet requires the client to limit protein and dairy intake. After reviewing a list of allowed, limited, and restricted foods, the client reports to a nurse a dislike for all the food choices that can be eaten. Which collaborative action would best meet the needs of the client?

1. Reviewing the list with the client and compromising on which foods are acceptable
2. Identifying the primary meal preparer in the family and reviewing the list with that person
3. Reporting the client's noncompliance to the physician so medications may be adjusted
4. Contacting the dietitian to counsel the client on acceptable foods

ANSWER: 4

The nurse collaborates with other health professionals to meet client health needs. It is essential for nurses to rely on the expertise of other disciplines to assist in meeting client needs; therefore the nurse should collaborate with the dietitian to assist this client. Renal failure diets are very specialized, and the nurse should not independently compromise with the client without consulting the dietitian, as this is the dietitian's area of expertise. Working with the primary meal preparer does not involve the client; therefore the outcome may not be successful. The client is not indicating noncompliance. Changing the medication regimen may not be an alternative to following the renal diet.

▶ ***Test-taking Tip:*** *The key words are "collaborative action," which means working with another discipline.*

Content Area: Management of Care; *Category of Health Alteration:* Leadership and Management; *Integrated Processes:* Teaching and Learning; *Client Need:* Safe and Effective Care Environment/Management of Care/Collaboration with Interdisciplinary Team; *Cognitive Level:* Application

References: Harkreader, H., Hogan, M., & Thobaben, M. (2007). *Fundamentals of Nursing* (3rd ed., p. 304). St. Louis, MO: Saunders/Elsevier; American Nurses Association. (2005). *Code of Ethics for Nurses*. Available at: http://nursingworld.org/ethics/code/protected_nwcoe813.htm

---

47. A new nurse notices that the client's pulse oximeter is frequently alarming. The nurse enters the room and notices the probe is off the finger and replaces it. The alarm is heard again and the nurse finds the reading to be 84 with the number quickly changing to 92. The client's pulse oximeter continues to vary, causing the machine to alarm five more times within the next 30 minutes. Which action will help the nurse to establish a safe and accurate pulse oximeter reading?

1. Replace the oximeter with a functioning machine
2. Consult with a more experienced nurse to determine how to obtain accurate readings
3. Turn the alarm off since it is not functioning properly
4. Notify the physician of the low oximeter readings

ANSWER: 2

Consulting with a more experienced nurse will improve client care. Alarms from both inaccurate pulse oximeter operation and incorrect sensing of the client's pulse are common. The new nurse may not be familiar with techniques to improve the operation of the machine. Turning off the alarm is an unsafe practice and should never be done. It would be inappropriate to notify the physician of the low pulse oximeter reading as an accurate reading has not been established.

▶ ***Test-taking Tip:*** *Apply knowledge of consultation. Remember that you are working as a part of a team and to use resources when necessary.*

Content Area: Management of Care; *Category of Health Alteration:* Leadership and Management; *Integrated Processes:* Nursing Process Analysis; *Client Need:* Safe and Effective Care Environment/Management of Care/Consultation; *Cognitive Level:* Application

Reference: Harkreader, H., Hogan, M., & Thobaben, M. (2007). *Fundamentals of Nursing* (3rd ed., p. 208). St. Louis, MO: Saunders/Elsevier.

48. EBP A client diagnosed with delirium tremens is receiving periodic intravenous (IV) sedation. A nursing assessment indicates that the client is becoming increasingly agitated. Upon reviewing the medical administration record (MAR); the nurse notes there are orders for diazepam (Valium®), lorazepam (Ativan®), and propofol (Diprovan®). The nurse is unclear regarding which medication would be most effective. Which action by the nurse will improve the client's outcome?

1. Giving the same medication given by the previous nurse, knowing it will provide temporary relief of agitation
2. Contacting the physician for different medication orders, knowing these medications will not reduce agitation
3. Administering propofol, because the client's agitation may lead to client harm
4. Consulting with the pharmacist on the medications previously given and the actions of the prescribed medications, requesting a recommendation for which medication to administer.

ANSWER: 4

Consulting with specialists and experts provides optimal care for each client by helping to solve difficult problems. Pharmacists are experts in medication actions and indications. Continuing to give the same medication as the previous nurse does not demonstrate critical thinking skills in analyzing the complex needs of managing alcohol withdrawal. Current evidence does not indicate that a particular sedative is most effective in treatment of delirium tremens. The three medication options are recommended as best practice and should be used appropriately until the desired affect is achieved. Propofol is an IV anesthetic and should only be considered if the diazepam and lorazepam have been demonstrated to be ineffective. If propofol is administered, the client should be intubated and mechanically ventilated for safety.

➧ ***Test-taking Tip:*** *Apply knowledge of best practice related to alcohol withdrawal and consultation practices.*

Content Area: Management of Care; *Category of Health Alteration:* Leadership and Management; *Integrated Processes:* Nursing Process Analysis; *Client Need:* Safe and Effective Care Environment/Management of Care/Continuity of Care; *Cognitive Level:* Analysis

Reference: Harkreader, H., Hogan, M., & Thobaben, M. (2007). *Fundamentals of Nursing* (3rd ed., p. 208). St. Louis, MO: Saunders/Elsevier.

EBP Reference: American Society of Addiction Medicine. (2004). *Management of Alcohol Withdrawal Delirium. An Evidence-Based Practice Guideline.* Available at: www.guideline.gov/summary/summary.aspx?doc_id=6543&nbr=004109&string=delirium+AND+tremens

49. EBP A client returns from surgery performed 2 hours ago. A nurse expects the client to be more alert and notices intermittent apnea. The client's blood pressure had been in the low 100s and is now 90/54 mm Hg. The client is difficult to awaken. Which steps should be taken by the nurse to obtain immediate assistance? Prioritize the nurse's actions by placing each step in the correct order.

______ Assist in the reassessment of the client
______ Contact the surgeon
______ Request the rapid response team
______ Prepare necessary equipment including an oximeter and noninvasive BP monitor
______ Communicate using a handoff method such as SBAR
______ Be present to answer questions and obtain supplies and medications
______ Contact the client's family

ANSWER: 4, 5, 1, 2, 3, 6, 7

To obtain immediate assistance, request the rapid-response team before the client deteriorates further into respiratory arrest. Prepare necessary equipment, including an oximeter and noninvasive BP monitor, so supplies are available for the team. Communicate using a handoff method such as SBAR (situation, background, assessment, and recommendation) so the team has clear information to treat the client. Assist in the reassessment of the client so the team may clearly identify recent changes in the client's condition. Contact the surgeon for notification of the presence of the rapid-response team. Be present to answer questions and obtain supplies and medications for the team. Contact the client's family to update them regarding the changes in the client's condition.

➧ ***Test-taking Tip:*** *Knowledge of consultation in emergency situations. The key words are "immediate assistance." Use the steps of the nursing process and the ABCs (airway, breathing, circulation) of emergency management to prioritize the nurse's actions.*

Content Area: Management of Care; *Category of Health Alteration:* Leadership and Management/Consultation; *Integrated Processes:* Nursing Process Evaluation; *Client Need:* Safe and Effective Care Environment/Management of Care/Consultation; *Cognitive Level:* Synthesis

Reference: Harkreader, H., Hogan, M., & Thobaben, M. (2007). *Fundamentals of Nursing* (3rd ed., pp. 208–210). St. Louis, MO: Saunders/Elsevier.

EBP Reference: Institute for Healthcare Improvement. (2003). *Establish a Rapid Response Team.* Available at: www.ihi.org/IHI/topics/criticalcare/intensivecare/changes/establisharapidresponseteam.htm

50. A new client is admitted to a facility and requires an initial admission assessment. Which should be included in the admission assessment? SELECT ALL THAT APPLY.

1. Collection of subjective data
2. Vital signs
3. Development of the care plan
4. Functional ability assessment
5. Documentation of education completed

ANSWER: 1, 2, 4

Collecting subjective data, vital signs, and functional ability assessment is an essential component of an admission assessment. The development of the care plan and documentation of any education completed are done following the admission assessment.

Test-taking Tip: *The key words are "should be included." Focus on what is included in an initial admission assessment. Use the nursing process to eliminate options.*

Content Area: Management of Care; *Category of Health Alteration:* Leadership and Management; *Integrated Processes:* Nursing Process Assessment; *Client Need:* Safe and Effective Care Environment/ Management of Care/Continuity of Care; *Cognitive Level:* Application

Reference: Wilkinson, J., & Van Leuven, K. (2007). *Fundamentals of Nursing* (p. 45). Philadelphia: F. A. Davis.

51. A client is transferring from a hospital setting to a long-term care facility. What is the primary objective of maintaining continuity of care between health-care facilities?

1. Communicating treatments, medications, and plans of care to meet client needs
2. Communicating treatment information per the regulatory requirements from the Center for Medicare Services
3. Communicating Health Insurance Portability and Accountability Act (HIPAA) regulations between health-care facilities
4. Completing a transfer checklist, which will ensure that all pertinent client information is forwarded to the next facility

ANSWER: 1

Well-coordinated continuity of care through collaborative practice will ensure that providers of services work together to meet client needs. National patient safety goals of the Joint Commission and the Medication Reconciliation law provide guidance related to what must be communicated between levels of care and health-care facilities. Communicating information through a communication format such as SBAR (situation, background, assessment, and recommendation) also ensures continuity of care. There are no regulatory requirements from the Center for Medicare Services related to what must be communicated between health-care facilities when moving clients from a higher level of care to a lower level of care. HIPAA regulations are well-known and do not need to be communicated between members of the care team. A transfer checklist may be helpful but will not ensure all pertinent information is included.

Test-taking Tip: *The key words are "primary objective." Select an option that is the most inclusive.*

Content Area: Management of Care; *Category of Health Alteration:* Leadership and Management; *Integrated Processes:* Communication and Documentation; *Client Need:* Safe and Effective Care Environment/ Management of Care/Continuity of Care; *Cognitive Level:* Analysis

References: Whitehead, D., Weiss, S., & Tappen, R. (2007). *Essentials of Nursing Leadership and Management.* (p. 147). Philadelphia: F. A. Davis; The Joint Commission. (2008). *2009 National Patient Safety Goals.* Available at: www.jointcommission.org/PatientSafety/NationalPatientSafetyGoals/

52. A nurse is giving a change-of-shift report to another nurse. Which are essential components of a change-of-shift report? SELECT ALL THAT APPLY.

1. Reporting the client diagnosis
2. Sharing new orders, medications, and treatments
3. Sharing personal opinions about treatment options
4. Discussing the effectiveness of analgesics
5. Sharing routine turning schedule for the client
6. Informing about client progress toward goals and areas for priority focus on the next shift

ANSWER: 1, 2, 4, 6

During change-of-shift report, pertinent information related to events that occurred is conveyed to individuals responsible for providing continuity of care. This includes the client diagnosis, new orders, medications and treatments, and effectiveness of analgesics. Use SBAR (situation, background, assessment, and recommendation) to communicate information, especially information that requires follow-up action or is a priority in progressing the client toward meeting goals. Personal opinions not pertinent to providing client care should be omitted. The turning schedule can be reviewed in documentation and is not necessary in shift report.

Test-taking Tip: *Apply knowledge of essential shift report information.*

Content Area: Management of Care; *Category of Health Alteration:* Leadership and Management; *Integrated Processes:* Communication and Documentation; *Client Need:* Safe and Effective Care Environment/ Management of Care/Continuity of Care; *Cognitive Level:* Application

Reference: Whitehead, D., Weiss, S., & Tappen, R. (2007). *Essentials of Nursing Leadership and Management* (pp. 83–84). Philadelphia: F. A. Davis.

53. EBP An elderly client, diagnosed with a cardiovascular accident several weeks ago, has been receiving feedings via a nasogastric feeding tube for 3 weeks. The tube feedings are stopped because the client is able to swallow. However, the client gags periodically and tires easily while eating. Which action should be taken by the nurse to prevent aspiration?

1. Remove the feeding tube as it interferes with the ability to swallow
2. Refer the client for a swallow evaluation
3. Stop all oral intake
4. Permit only health-care personnel to feed the client

ANSWER: 2

The best practice to prevent aspiration is to obtain a referral with a speech therapist for a swallow evaluation. The speech therapist can determine if the client is able to swallow safely. Removing the feeding tube may improve the ability to swallow, but until the client's nutrition needs are met, the feeding tube should stay in place. Consideration for placement of a gastrostomy tube would allow removal of the nasogastric feeding tube. Oral intake should not be stopped unless aspiration has occurred and the client is unable to manage the secretions. Permitting only health-care personnel to feed the client may reduce the likelihood of aspiration but will not prevent aspiration from occurring if the client is not able to swallow effectively.

➧ ***Test-taking Tip:*** *Apply the ABCs (airway, breathing, circulation) and the method to determine if the client's airway is being compromised.*

Content Area: Management of Care; *Category of Health Alteration:* Leadership and Management; *Integrated Processes:* Nursing Process Evaluation; *Client Need:* Safe and Effective Care Environment/ Management of Care/Referrals; *Cognitive Level:* Analysis

References: Harkreader, H., Hogan, M., & Thobaben, M. (2007). *Fundamentals of Nursing* (3rd ed., pp. 548, 596–601). St. Louis, MO: Saunders/Elsevier; Craven, R., & Hirnle, C. (2009). *Fundamentals of Nursing: Human Health and Function* (6th ed., p. 967). Philadelphia: Lippincott Williams & Wilkins.

EBP Reference: American College of Chest Physicians. (2006). *Cough and Aspiration of Food and Liquids Due to Oral-Pharyngeal Dysphagia: ACCP Evidence-Based Clinical Practice Guidelines.* Available at: www.guideline.gov/summary/summary.aspx?doc_id=8664&nbr=004829&string=swallowing

54. EBP A client diagnosed with an unknown bleeding dyscrasia is urgently transferred to another facility to receive a higher level of care. Which documents are essential to provide to the receiving facility? SELECT ALL THAT APPLY.

1. Emergency Medical Treatment and Active Labor Act (EMTALA) form, which includes information related to client status prior to transfer
2. Client teaching record
3. Transfer note
4. History and physical
5. Progress notes
6. Activity flowsheet

ANSWER: 1, 3, 4, 5

The EMTALA form (required by law from the Health Care Financing Administration), transfer note, history and physical, and progress notes are essential documentation for the receiving facility to continue client care. The transfer note should include the reason for and method of transfer and condition of the client. The client teaching record and activity flowsheet are all legal parts of the medical record; however, they are not required for ongoing urgent care. Each facility determines what should be included in transfer documentation.

➧ ***Test-taking Tip:*** *The key word is "essential." Review each option and determine if the document is necessary to continue with care or if the information on that form may be included elsewhere in the documentation.*

Content Area: Management of Care; *Category of Health Alteration:* Leadership and Management; *Integrated Processes:* Communication and Documentation; *Client Need:* Safe and Effective Care Environment/ Management of Care/Referrals; *Cognitive Level:* Analysis

References: Craven, R., & Hirnle, C. (2009). *Fundamentals of Nursing: Human Health and Function* (6th ed., pp. 215, 219–221). Philadelphia: Lippincott Williams & Wilkins; Harkreader, H., Hogan, M., & Thobaben, M. (2007). *Fundamentals of Nursing* (3rd ed., p. 303). St. Louis, MO: Saunders/Elsevier; Killion, S., & Dempski, K. (2006). *Quick Look Nursing: Legal and Ethical Issues* (p. 71). Sudbury, MA: Jones and Bartlett.

EBP Reference: U.S. Department of Health and Human Services. (2006). *Center for Medicare and Medicaid Services: EMTALA*. Available at: www.cms.hhs.gov/EMTALA/

55. An elderly male client with newly diagnosed end-stage chronic obstructive pulmonary disease (COPD) is being discharged to home. The client's wife is his sole caregiver. The client is unable to provide self-care and requires continuous assistance. Which service would provide the greatest assistance to the client's wife?

1. Skilled nursing care
2. Respite care
3. Hospice care
4. Physical therapy

ANSWER: 2

Respite care is the service that provides relief care for family caregivers. Skilled nursing care and physical therapy would provide direct care for the client but not the client's caregiver. Hospice care provides end-of-life services for both the client and family.

➧ ***Test-taking Tip:*** *The key words are "greatest assistance to the client's wife." Read the question thoroughly so that you do not miss any information.*

Content Area: Management of Care; *Category of Health Alteration:* Leadership and Management; *Integrated Processes:* Caring; *Client Need:* Safe and Effective Care Environment/Management of Care/Referrals; *Cognitive Level:* Analysis

Reference: Wilkinson, J., & Van Leuven, K. (2007). *Fundamentals of Nursing* (p. 1035). Philadelphia: F. A. Davis.

---

56. A client is scheduled to have a chest x-ray and a pulmonary function test (PFT). The client tires easily. Which action should be taken by the nurse to coordinate the client's care?

1. Have the PFT rescheduled for tomorrow
2. Have the chest x-ray changed to a portable x-ray
3. Accompany the client to both tests so the client can be returned to the unit if excessively tired
4. Contact the radiology department and request the chest x-ray be done right before the PFT

ANSWER: 4

Coordinating care and advocating for the client may include ensuring that two departments work together to provide for the best and most convenient care for the client. It is possible that the radiology department is not aware that the PFT is scheduled on the same day or that the client tires easily. The nurse is responsible for acting as a liaison between the client and other health-care team members. Rescheduling the PFT may not be consistent with the physician's treatment plan and should not be decided by the nurse. A portable chest x-ray may not produce that same quality as a standing chest x-ray in the radiology department. It is the physician's decision to change to a portable view. It is unrealistic for the nurse to accompany the client to both of these tests as other clients will need nursing care during this time.

➧ ***Test-taking Tip:*** *The key words are "to coordinate the client's care." Read each option carefully and consider which option would allow expedient treatment of the client's problem.*

Content Area: Management of Care; *Category of Health Alteration:* Leadership and Management; *Integrated Processes:* Nursing Process Planning; *Client Need:* Safe and Effective Care Environment/Management of Care/Concepts of Management; *Cognitive Level:* Analysis

Reference: Wilkinson, J., & Van Leuven, K. (2007). *Fundamentals of Nursing* (p. 126). Philadelphia: F. A. Davis.

---

57. **EBP** A nurse is aware of the American Nurses Association's nursing-sensitive quality indicators regarding the management and prevention of hospital-acquired infections. Which nursing action is most likely to reduce hospital-acquired infection rates?

1. Ensuring appropriate nurse-to-client ratios
2. Improving team functioning
3. Monitoring medication safety events
4. Ensuring adequate supplies are available for care delivery

ANSWER: 1

The American Nurses Association has identified that the appropriate numbers and mix of nursing personnel (registered nurses, licensed practical nurses, and unlicensed staff) are imperative for the delivery of safe, cost-effective quality care. This includes the reduction of hospital-acquired infections. Although important for quality client care, improving team functioning, monitoring medication safety events, and ensuring that adequate supplies are available have not demonstrated an impact on infection rates. While nurse-to-client ratios are imperative to positive patient outcomes, team functioning, hand hygiene, and appropriateness of supplies should not be understated.

➧ ***Test-taking Tip:*** *Apply knowledge of the impact of nurse-to-client ratios.*

Content Area: Management of Care; *Category of Health Alteration:* Leadership and Management; *Integrated Processes:* Nursing Process Evaluation; *Client Need:* Safe and Effective Care Environment/Management of Care/Concepts of Management; *Cognitive Level:* Application

Reference: Whitehead, D., Weiss, S., & Tappen, R. (2007). *Essentials of Nursing Leadership and Management* (pp. 151–153). Philadelphia: F. A. Davis.

EBP Reference: American Nurses Association. (2008). *Nursing Quality Indicators.* Available at: http://nursingworld.org/MainMenuCategories/ANAPoliticalPower/State/2006/quality12763.aspx

58. A nurse has a conflict with another staff member regarding a perceived lack of teamwork and negative attitude. The nurse has a choice among effective conflict-resolution strategies. Which are useful conflict resolution strategies? SELECT ALL THAT APPLY.

1. Ignore the conflict
2. Postpone the conflict
3. Oppose the conflict
4. Confront the conflict
5. Smooth the conflict

ANSWER: 1, 2, 4, 5

To ignore, postpone, confront, or smooth the conflict are strategies of conflict resolution. Opposing the conflict is not a strategy that facilitates conflict resolution.

Test-taking Tip: *The key word is "resolution." Eliminate options that would not resolve the conflict.*

Content Area: Management of Care; *Category of Health Alteration:* Leadership and Management; *Integrated Processes:* Communication and Documentation; *Client Need:* Safe and Effective Care Environment/Management of Care/Concepts of Management; *Cognitive Level:* Application

References: Catalano, J. (2006). *Nursing Now! Today's Issues, Tomorrow's Trends* (4th ed., p. 282), Philadelphia: F. A. Davis; Marquis, B., & Huston, C. (2009). *Leadership Roles and Management Functions in Nursing* (6th ed., pp. 494–495). Philadelphia: Wolters Kluwer Health/Lippincott Williams & Wilkins.

---

59. A nurse is providing hospice care to a client diagnosed with cancer. The client is in the last hours of life and is experiencing significant pain. The client expresses a desire to be alert in order to spend time with family members. Which strategy will address this problem?

1. Standardized care
2. Client education
3. Therapeutic judgment
4. Reassessment

ANSWER: 3

Using therapeutic judgment allows the nurse to consider giving smaller increments of morphine to keep the client comfortable while being alert enough to be with family members. Standardized care means giving a usual morphine dose and it is the standard way of managing pain, but the usual dose may cause somnolence. Client education will not address pain management or the desire to be with family. Reassessment is the process of determining whether a problem still exists.

Test-taking Tip: *Visualize the nurse performing each action noted in the options. Select the option that would apply principles of strategic problem solving.*

Content Area: Management of Care; *Category of Health Alteration:* Leadership and Management; *Integrated Processes:* Caring; *Client Need:* Safe and Effective Care Environment/Management of Care/Concepts of Management; *Cognitive Level:* Analysis

Reference: Wilkinson, J., & Van Leuven, K. (2007). *Fundamentals of Nursing* (pp. 109–110). Philadelphia: F. A. Davis.

---

60. A nurse is responsible for supervising staff on a unit that includes registered nurses (RNs), licensed practical nurses (LPNs), and unlicensed assistive personnel (UAP). Which statement is related to the supervision of staff as opposed to the delegation of tasks?

1. Statement to another RN: "Please start an IV on Mr. Smith in room 458."
2. Statement to a health unit coordinator: "There are new orders on Mr. Jones's chart that need to be entered."
3. Statement to a UAP: "Please answer the call light for the client in 321."
4. Statement to a LPN: "Please give 8:00 a.m. medications to the client in 322."

ANSWER: 2

Supervision is the initial direction and periodic evaluation of a person performing an assigned task to ensure that he or she is meeting the standards of care. The RN is supervising the health unit coordinator to perform the task of completing orders. Delegation includes understanding that the authorized person is acting in the place of the RN and carrying out tasks such as starting an IV, answering a call light, or giving medications.

Test-taking Tip: *Think about the difference between supervision and delegation and the role of each team member. Remember what tasks can be performed by different staff members.*

Content Area: Management of Care; *Category of Health Alteration:* Leadership and Management; *Integrated Processes:* Nursing Process Implementation; *Client Need:* Safe and Effective Care Environment/Management of Care/Supervision; *Cognitive Level:* Analysis

Reference: Catalano, J. (2006). *Nursing Now! Today's Issues, Tomorrow's Trends* (4th ed., pp. 290–291), Philadelphia: F. A. Davis.

61. A client diagnosed with hyperglycemia is receiving a continuous intravenous (IV) insulin drip. Blood glucose measures are being taken every 1 to 2 hours. A nurse checks the client's blood glucose, and the reading is 32 mg/dL. The client, who was previously alert, is now lethargic and does not respond to questions. The nurse administers 25 mL of D50W per protocol. The client begins to respond. Which additional risk-management action should be taken by the nurse?

1. Continue the insulin drip
2. Report the event to the nurse manager
3. Recheck the blood glucose measure in 1 hour
4. Administer a second dose of 25 mL of D50W

ANSWER: 2

Safety events must be reported to the nurse manager. Risk management seeks to identify and eliminate potential safety hazards. The monitoring and medication protocol may need revision based on changes in the client's status and correlating blood glucose results. Reporting the client's hypoglycemia to the nurse manager will result in the monitoring of patterns and trends, and possibly regulatory reporting. Some states require reporting of hypoglycemia that leads to client injury or death. To continue the insulin drip would result in client injury. Waiting 1 hour is too long to determine if the client is still hypoglycemic. A second dose of D50W should not be given without first assessing the client's response and taking another blood glucose measurement.

***Test-taking Tip:** The key words "risk management action" include appropriate follow-up and reporting. Eliminate options that pertain only to the client.*

Content Area: Management of Care; *Category of Health Alteration:* Leadership and Management; *Integrated Processes:* Nursing Process Evaluation; *Client Need:* Safe and Effective Care Environment/ Management of Care/Performance Improvement; *Cognitive Level:* Analysis

Reference: Chitty, K., & Black, B. (2007). *Professional Nursing: Concepts and Challenges* (2nd ed., p. 105). St. Louis, MO: Saunders.

---

62. **EBP** Prior to medication administration, a hospital policy requires a double check of two unique client identifiers against the medical administration record (MAR). A nurse manager forms a performance improvement team with the goal of improving nursing compliance with this important safety check. Which activity, related to checking two unique identifiers, should be the responsibility of the performance improvement team?

1. Hold staff accountable for the practice of checking two unique identifiers
2. Discipline staff members who fail to comply with checking two unique identifiers
3. Observe and report the practice of medication administration
4. Change the practice of two unique identifiers to a more compliant practice

ANSWER: 3

Individual clinical units must be active and independent in monitoring their adherence to client safety initiatives. The role of a performance improvement team is to observe and report measures within the initiative. It is the responsibility of the nurse manager to hold staff members accountable for their practice as well as disciplining staff if appropriate. Performance improvement is focused on education and system changes for client safety, which create a blame-free environment. Evidence-based practice supports improved client safety by checking two unique identifiers; therefore, changing this practice would be unsafe.

***Test-taking Tip:** Read the scenario carefully before selecting options. Apply knowledge of the performance improvement process.*

Content Area: Management of Care; *Category of Health Alteration:* Leadership and Management; *Integrated Processes:* Nursing Process Analysis; *Client Need:* Safe and Effective Care Environment/ Management of Care/Performance Improvement; *Cognitive Level:* Application

Reference: Wachter, R.M. (2008). *Understanding Patient Safety* (p. 243). New York: McGraw-Hill.

EBP Reference: The Joint Commission. (2008). *2008 National Patient Safety Goals*. Available at: www.jointcommission.org/NR/rdonlyres/ 82B717D8-B16A-4442-AD00-CE3188C2F00A/0/08_HAP_NPSGs_ Master.pdf

---

63. **EBP** A hospital recently formed a rapid-response team (RRT) with the goal of reducing unexpected cardiopulmonary arrests. Which measures should be used to evaluate the performance of the RRT? SELECT ALL THAT APPLY.

1. The number of cardiopulmonary arrests
2. The types of supplies used during the RRT call
3. Evaluation of the team's actions
4. The outcome of the client following the RRT call
5. The types of medications given during the RRT call

ANSWER: 1, 3, 4

Performance improvement requires that the process used to deliver services receives close and constant scrutiny. Monitoring outcomes, including the number of cardiopulmonary arrests, evaluation of the team's actions, and outcome of the client, will all serve to improve the RRT process. Determining the types of supplies and medications used by the RRT on each call will not improve the performance of the RRT.

***Test-taking Tip:** Apply knowledge of performance/quality improvement processes. The key word is "performance."*

Content Area: Management of Care; *Category of Health Alteration:* Leadership and Management; *Integrated Processes:* Nursing Process Evaluation; *Client Need:* Safe and Effective Care Environment/ Management of Care/Performance Improvement (Quality Improvement); *Cognitive Level:* Analysis

Reference: Catalano, J.T. (2006). *Nursing Now! Today's Issues, Tomorrow's Trends.* (4th ed., p. 330). Philadelphia: F. A. Davis.

EBP Reference: Institute for Healthcare Improvement. (2005). Building rapid response teams. Available at: www.ihi.org/IHI/Topics/CriticalCare/IntensiveCare/ImprovementStories/BuildingRapidResponseTeams.htm

64. A nurse manager is developing next year's equipment budget. Which factors should be considered when deciding how many oxygen flow meters should be purchased next year? SELECT ALL THAT APPLY.

1. Staff request for more flow meters
2. Cost of nasal cannulas
3. Cost of flow meters
4. Current number of flow meters
5. Predicted client days for next year
6. Number of mechanical ventilators

ANSWER: 1, 3, 4, 5

Nurse managers must be able to project and justify supplies and equipment needed and must be able to provide a reasoned argument that quality nursing care is affected by the lack of equipment. Many methods may be used for this assessment, including staff request, cost, volume, and projected need. Although the cost of nasal cannulas and number of mechanical ventilators pertain to oxygen therapy, it is not information that will help the nurse manager predict the number of oxygen flow meters needed.

Test-taking Tip: *Eliminate options that are irrelevant to the question about oxygen flow meters.*

Content Area: Management of Care; *Category of Health Alteration:* Leadership and Management; *Integrated Processes:* Nursing Process Assessment; *Client Need:* Safe and Effective Care Environment/Management of Care/Concepts of Management; *Cognitive Level:* Analysis

Reference: Harkreader, H., Hogan, M., & Thobaben, M. (2007). *Fundamentals of Nursing* (3rd ed., p. 297). St. Louis, MO: Saunders/Elsevier.

65. At a staff meeting, a nurse manager shares that the unit is over budget by 2% and needs to reduce costs. A staff nurse suggests that report could be shortened so that nurses could finish their shifts on time. How should the nurse manager measure the success of this idea?

1. Observe the change-of-shift report to determine how many nurses are leaving on time at the end of the shift
2. Delegate end-of-shift monitoring to the charge nurses
3. Review the capital budget on a monthly basis
4. Monitor for a reduction in hours per client day

ANSWER: 4

Monitoring hours per client day will allow the nurse manager to determine if staff members are reducing clinical hours by finishing closer to the end of their shift. A reduction in client hours per day may indicate that reducing the duration of the end-of-shift report is effective. Observing the shift report will not measure the success, nor will delegating the monitoring to the charge nurses. The capital budget includes only equipment with a minimum dollar cost and includes no labor costs.

Test-taking Tip: *The key words are "measure the success." Apply knowledge of budgeting based on hours per client day.*

Content Area: Management of Care; *Category of Health Alteration:* Leadership and Management; *Integrated Processes:* Nursing Process Evaluation; *Client Need:* Safe and Effective Care Environment/Management of Care/Concepts of Management; *Cognitive Level:* Analysis

Reference: Jones, R. (2007). *Nursing Leadership and Management: Theories, Processes and Practice* (pp. 270–271). Philadelphia: F. A. Davis.

66. A nurse notices a posting on a bulletin board for a continuing education (CE) offering on the prevention of pressure ulcers. Which is the most compelling reason for the nurse to attend?

1. The unit has experienced an increase in pressure ulcers.
2. The nurse wants continuing education in order to keep up with current clinical knowledge.
3. The nurse needs one more CE unit for state license renewal.
4. The nurse is able to attend by coming in 1 hour earlier than the next scheduled shift.

ANSWER: 2

To stay current with evidence-based practice after completing a nursing program, nurses must participate in ongoing education. EBP changes rapidly, and advances in health care have a strong influence on nursing practice. The other options are all reasons to attend, but the most compelling is for professional growth.

Test-taking Tip: *The key words are "most compelling reason." Think about what would motivate you to attend a CE offering.*

Content Area: Management of Care; *Category of Health Alteration:* Leadership and Management; *Integrated Processes:* Nursing Process Assessment; *Client Need:* Safe and Effective Care Environment/Management of Care/Performance Improvement; *Cognitive Level:* Application

Reference: Wilkinson, J., & Van Leuven, K. (2007). *Fundamentals of Nursing* (p. 15). Philadelphia: F. A. Davis.

67. EBP A nurse educator is responsible for teaching staff members about the prevention of central line–associated bloodstream infections. To prevent infection, a central line dressing change procedure has been changed. The staff needs to be informed of the change in procedure. Which method of education would best enhance the staff's retention of this information?

1. In-service education
2. Certification
3. Informal education
4. Contact hour

ANSWER: 1

In-service education is offered at the work site and may focus on new equipment or policies. Certification is a formal validation of a high level of knowledge in a defined area of practice, typically administered by a certifying organization in nursing. Informal education is typically from one person to another to enhance current knowledge. Contact hour is the measure of continuing education credit.

➧ ***Test-taking Tip:*** *The key words are "best methods of education."*

Content Area: Management of Care; *Category of Health Alteration:* Leadership and Management; *Integrated Processes:* Teaching and Learning; *Client Need:* Safe and Effective Care Environment/Management of Care/Performance Improvement; *Cognitive Level:* Application

Reference: Chitty, K., & Black, B. (2007). *Professional Nursing: Concepts and Challenges* (2nd ed., pp. 178–181). St. Louis, MO: Saunders.

EBP Reference: Hadaway, L. (2006). Best-practice interventions: Keeping central line infection at bay. *Nursing 2008,* 36(4), 58–63. Available at: www.nursing2006.com/pt/re/nursing/fulltext.00152193-200604000-00042.htm;jsessionid=HmJCQ2TQfkW1fmGcxGp5XRvmntlLN02jlVC2gWyGKndZvv9JvHtQ!-1108188142!181195628!8091!-1

68. Following a same-day surgical procedure, a client and his or her family are preparing to go home. At change of shift, a nurse enters the room and the family complains about the previous nurse. They indicate relief that another nurse has taken over and state that discharge instructions were confusing and were not correct. The family indicates that they do not know how to perform dressing changes or what level of activity is appropriate for the client. After meeting the needs of the client and family, which action should the oncoming nurse take to prevent this situation from happening again?

1. Ask other nursing staff if they have encountered similar situations while working with the nurse cited by the family
2. Review the discharge documentation to determine if the previous nurse provided the education
3. Report the client and family complaint to the risk manager
4. Report the incident of the previous nurse's incompetence to the nurse manager

ANSWER: 4

One of the most common reasons for malpractice lawsuits is failing to report another health-care provider's incompetence or negligence. Supervision includes ensuring safety and completeness of care. If care for a client was not complete, the oncoming nurse has a responsibility to report the previous nurse to the nurse manager within the context of supervision. The nurse manager, not the oncoming nurse, is responsible for collecting data regarding the nurse cited by the family and in evaluating competence. Although it is a client complaint, it is not an issue to be brought forward to the risk manager because the nurse in question has an opportunity to resolve the dilemma.

➧ ***Test-taking Tip:*** *The key words are "prevent this from happening again." Note the verbs in each of the options. Select an option that ensures follow-up action.*

Content Area: Management of Care; *Category of Health Alteration:* Leadership and Management; *Integrated Processes:* Nursing Process Evaluation; *Client Need:* Safe and Effective Care Environment/Management of Care/Supervision; *Cognitive Level:* Analysis

Reference: Catalano, J. (2006). *Nursing Now! Today's Issues, Tomorrow's Trends* (4th ed., p. 166). Philadelphia: F. A. Davis.

69. A nurse manager is evaluating a new nurse's time-management skills. Which statement made by the new nurse may indicate potential concerns with time management?

1. "I am late in giving the antibiotic because I needed to assist with a dressing change."
2. "I completed the physical assessment before checking for morning medications to be given."
3. "I didn't get out on time because I admitted a client who came 15 minutes before the end of my shift."
4. "I would like to leave but I still need to document all the medications I gave today."

ANSWER: 4

Adequate time-management skills will reduce anxiety for nurses. Documentation should be done as soon as possible, especially for medication administration. With the constantly changing environment of client care, individual components of care may be delayed or nurses may not finish their assigned shift on time due to outside factors. This does not mean a nurse does not have good time-management skills.

➧ ***Test-taking Tip:*** *Read the question and answers carefully to make sure that all information is understood before choosing an answer. Note that all options provide a rationale for time management except one.*

Content Area: Management of Care: *Category of Health Alteration:* Leadership and Management; *Integrated Processes:* Nursing Process Evaluation; *Client Need:* Safe and Effective Care Environment/Management of Care/Supervision; *Cognitive Level:* Application

Reference: Jones, R. (2007). *Nursing Leadership and Management: Theories, Processes and Practice* (p. 366). Philadelphia: F. A. Davis.

70. A nurse observes the following situations. Which situations would require the nurse to complete a variance (or incident) report? SELECT ALL THAT APPLY.

1. A daily medication given 2 hours later than scheduled
2. A physician who is angry with a delayed laboratory report
3. An incorrect narcotic count at the end of the shift
4. An incomplete laboratory draw ordered for the morning
5. A client falling out of bed and suffering an ankle fracture
6. A new nurse arriving late to work for the third time

ANSWER: 1, 3, 4, 5

A variance report, also called an incident or occurrence report, is completed when a standard of care is breached or an unusual incident occurs. It is used for quality improvement in the agency and should not be used to discipline staff members or be placed in an employee's file. A physician becoming angry or a nurse arriving late for work does not directly impact failure to provide client care.

Test-taking Tip: *Think about the purpose and requirements of completing a variance report. Recall that a variance report is completed when a standard of care is breached or an unusual incident occurs.*

Content Area: Management of Care; *Category of Health Alteration:* Leadership and Management; *Integrated Processes:* Nursing Process Evaluation; *Client Need:* Safe and Effective Care Environment/Safety and Infection Control/Reporting of Incident/Event/Irregular Occurrence/Variance; *Cognitive Level:* Application

References: Craven, R., & Hirnle, C. (2009). *Fundamentals of Nursing: Human Health and Function* (6th ed., pp. 216–217). Philadelphia: Lippincott Williams & Wilkins; Wilkinson, J., & Van Leuven, K. (2007). *Fundamentals of Nursing* (p. 1084). Philadelphia: F. A. Davis.

---

71. A nurse is caring for a client who had colorectal surgery on the client's first postoperative day. The nurse is expecting to administer an antibiotic but the medication is not on the medication administration record (MAR). In reviewing the physician orders, an antibiotic was ordered but it has not been administered since surgery. Based on the order, the client has missed three doses. Which action should minimize the nurse's malpractice risk?

1. Contact the previous nurse and determine the source of the omission
2. Complete an incident report
3. Contact the physician and request a new antibiotic order
4. Document the reason for the error in the medical record

ANSWER: 2

An incident report, also called an occurrence or variance report, is a formal record of an unusual occurrence or accident. Submitting an incident report will best document the error and minimize the nurse's malpractice risk. Investigating the source of the error for agency follow-up should include contacting previous care nurses so that future errors can be prevented. The physician should also be contacted, but requesting a new antibiotic may not minimize the malpractice risk. The report is for the agency and not a part of the client's record.

Test-taking Tip: *The key phrase is "minimize the nurse's malpractice risk." Think about the purpose of the incident report.*

Content Area: Management of Care; *Category of Health Alteration:* Leadership and Management; *Integrated Processes:* Nursing Process Evaluation; *Client Need:* Safe and Effective Care Environment/Safety and Infection Control/Reporting of Incident/Event/Irregular Occurrence/Variance; *Cognitive Level:* Analysis

References: Craven, R., & Hirnle, C. (2009). *Fundamentals of Nursing: Human Health and Function* (6th ed., pp. 216–217). Philadelphia: Lippincott Williams & Wilkins; Wilkinson, J., & Van Leuven, K. (2007). *Fundamentals of Nursing* (p. 298). Philadelphia: F. A. Davis.

---

72. EBP An error occurs and an admission order for a client to be on a venous thromboembolic protocol is not processed. Two days later, a nurse notices the omitted order for heparin 5,000 units subcutaneous every 8 hours. Which statement best describes appropriate follow-up?

1. "I am so glad I didn't make that mistake, that other nurse is going to be in trouble."
2. "I am too busy to complete a variance report. I'll do it next week."
3. "I need to contact the physician and complete a variance report."
4. "I will contact the supervisor immediately about this error."

ANSWER: 3

Reporting systems rely on nurses to recognize and report errors. Recent emphasis has been placed on making error reporting "blame-free" and determining how the system can be used to reduce errors. Variance reports should be completed right away for appropriate follow-up. It may be appropriate to contact the supervisor also, but it is the responsibility of the nurse to first notify the physician and document the event in a variance report.

Test-taking Tip: *Focus on "appropriate follow-up." Eliminate options that do not demonstrate follow-up. Of the remaining options, determine which is best.*

Content Area: Management of Care; *Category of Health Alteration:* Leadership and Management; *Integrated Processes:* Nursing Process Evaluation; *Client Need:* Safe and Effective Care Environment/Safety and Infection Control/Reporting of Incident/Event/Irregular Occurrence/Variance; *Cognitive Level:* Application

Reference: Craven, R., & Hirnle, C. (2009). *Fundamentals of Nursing: Human Health and Function* (6th ed., pp. 216–217). Philadelphia: Lippincott Williams & Wilkins.

EBP References: Fitzpatrick, J., Stone, P., & Walker, P. (2006). *Annual Review of Nursing Research, Focus on Patient Safety* (p. 33). New York: Springer; Medicare Quality Improvement Community. (2006). DVT order set tools. Available at: www.medqic.org/dcs/ContentServer?cid=1147808149675&pagename=Medqic%2FMQTools%2FToolTemplate&siteVersion=null&c=MQTools

73. EBP A client falls from a bed, and a nurse documents the incident. Based on the following documentation of the client's fall, what time did the nurse make a risk-management error related to the client's medical record?

2100 Noise heard from the client's room. Client found lying on the floor. States she hit her head. Alert and oriented X3. PEARLA. No visible injuries, but moaning and holding head. Returned back to bed (see physical findings flowsheet). Will continue to monitor. Client instructed on use of call light for help with getting out of bed.
_______________ KAO

2115 Charge nurse A. Smith, RN, and Dr. Brown notified of client fall. Dr. Brown states he will come in to assess the client.
_______________ KAO

2130 Dr. Brown here. Client sent for CT of the head with RN monitoring. See physical findings flowsheet. No change in client status.
_______________ KAO

2145 Variance form completed and filed in the client's medical record.
_______________ KAO

2200 Return from head CT. Voided 300 mL while on bedside commode. Returned to bed with bed exit alarm on. Reminder given on use of call light for help with getting out of bed. Neuro reassessment completed. No change in neuro status.
_______________KAO

1. At 2100
2. At 2115
3. At 2130
4. At 2145
5. At 2200

ANSWER: 4

An incident, occurrence, or variance report should be completed for the purpose of reviewing patterns and trends and allowing the agency to identify prevention measures. For legal reasons, a copy should not be included in the client's medical record. When an incident occurs, the documentation in the client's medical record should accurately describe what occurred but not highlight any mistakes that could result in litigation or refer to the filing of an incident report. The other time periods show correct documentation.

➧ ***Test-taking Tip:*** *Focus on the procedure for reporting an incident.*

Content Area: Management of Care; *Category of Health Alteration:* Leadership and Management; *Integrated Processes:* Nursing Process Evaluation; *Client Need:* Safe and Effective Care Environment/Safety and Infection Control/Reporting of Incident/Event/Irregular Occurrence/Variance; *Cognitive Level:* Analysis

References: Craven, R., & Hirnle, C. (2009). *Fundamentals of Nursing: Human Health and Function* (6th ed., p. 217). Philadelphia: Lippincott Williams & Wilkins; Harkreader, H., Hogan, M., & Thobaben, M. (2007). *Fundamentals of Nursing* (3rd ed., pp. 39–40, 232). St. Louis, MO: Saunders/Elsevier.

EBP Reference: Fitzpatrick, J., Stone, P., & Walker, P. (2006). *Annual Review of Nursing Research, Focus on Patient Safety* (p. 40). New York: Springer.

74. A client is admitted with a positive culture for methicillin-resistant *Staphylococcus aureus* (MRSA). Contact precautions are implemented to prevent the infection from spreading to health-care workers and other clients. Which are components of contact precautions?

1. Wearing a mask when working within 3 feet of the client
2. Placing the client in a private room
3. Wearing an N-95 respirator
4. Placing the client in a negative-air-pressure room

ANSWER: 2

The client should be placed in a private room or in a room with a client with an active infection caused by the same organism and no other infections. A mask, N-95 respirator, or negative-air-pressure room are included in airborne precautions and are not necessary for contact precautions.

➧ ***Test-taking Tip:*** *Note the similarities in options 1, 3, and 4 related to air, whereas option 2 is related to placing a client in a private room. When an option is different, it is usually correct.*

Content Area: Management of Care; *Category of Health Alteration:* Leadership and Management; Occurrence/Variance; *Integrated Processes:* Nursing Process Implementation; *Client Need:* Safe and Effective Care Environment/Safety and Infection Control/Standard/Transmission-based/Other Precautions; *Cognitive Level:* Application

Reference: Wilkinson, J., & Van Leuven, K. (2007). *Fundamentals of Nursing* (p. 412). Philadelphia: F. A. Davis.

75. EBP A staff nurse educator is focusing on the prevention of infection. Place an X on the picture that displays the best measure to prevent infection when caring for clients on a nursing unit.

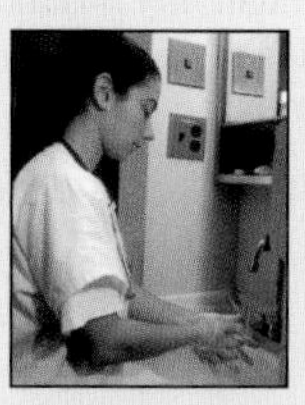
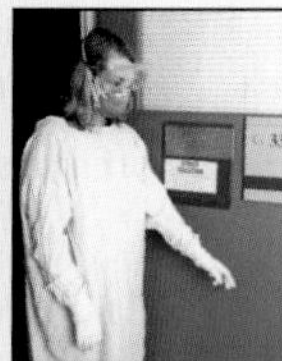
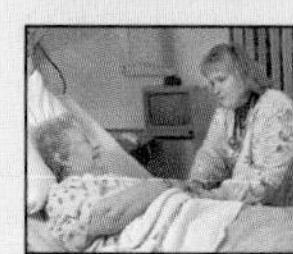
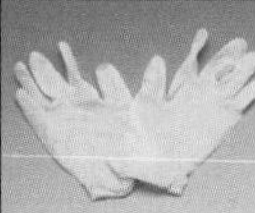
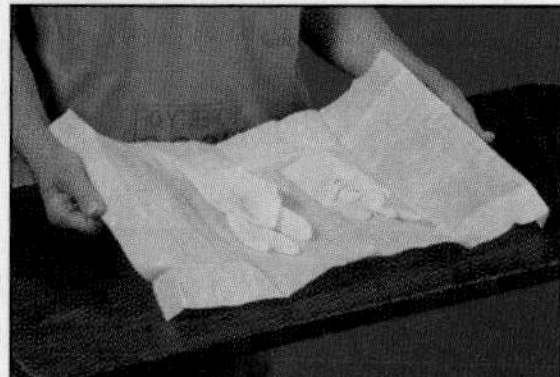

ANSWER:

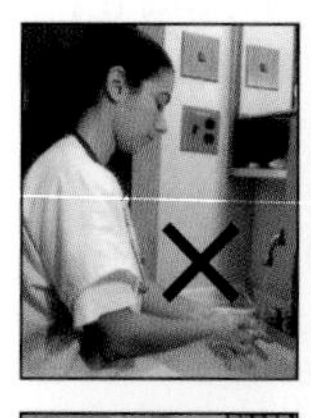
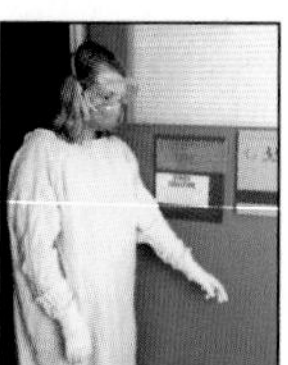
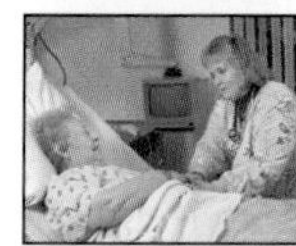
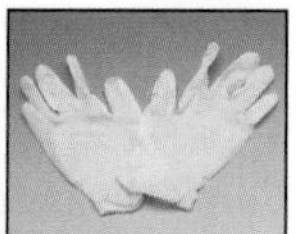
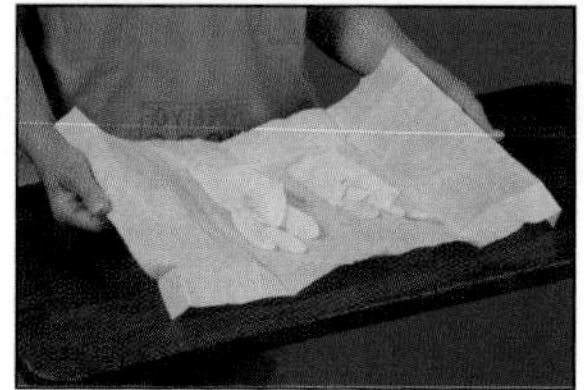

The best and first line of defense in medical asepsis is good hand hygiene. Friction or rubbing increases the amount of soil and microorganisms removed. Isolation, maintaining a 3-foot distance, or using examination or sterile gloves are not required in every client-care situation.

➧ ***Test-taking Tip:*** *Focus on the key word "best" and read the scenario carefully.*

Content Area: Management of Care; *Category of Health Alteration:* Leadership and Management; *Integrated Processes:* Nursing Process Implementation; *Client Need:* Safe and Effective Care Environment/Safety and Infection Control/Standard/Transmission-based/Other Precautions; *Cognitive Level:* Application

References: Williams, L., & Hopper, P. (2007). *Understanding Medical-Surgical Nursing* (3rd ed.). Philadelphia: F. A. Davis; Wilkinson, J., & Van Leuven, K. (2007). *Fundamentals of Nursing: Thinking & Doing*. Philadelphia: F. A. Davis; Harkreader, H., Hogan, M., & Thobaben, M. (2007). *Fundamentals of Nursing* (3rd ed., pp. 510–513). St. Louis, MO: Saunders/Elsevier.

EBP Reference: National Institute for Clinical Excellence. (2003). *Infection Control. Prevention of Healthcare-Associated Infection in Primary and Community Care.* Available at: www.guideline.gov/summary/summary.aspx?doc_id=5069&nbr=003553&string=hand+AND+hygiene

76. EBP A client is scheduled for a hysterectomy tomorrow morning. The client will be admitted from home on the same day as the surgical procedure. According to Medicare's Surgical Care Improvement Project, what instruction is important for the client to receive prior to arrival at the hospital to prevent postoperative infection?

1. Arrive in time to receive an antibiotic before surgery
2. Notify the nurse of any antibiotic allergies
3. Be sure to wash your hands before coming to the hospital
4. Do not shave hair from the surgical site area

ANSWER: 4

Shaving the surgical site with a razor induces small skin lacerations, creating a potential site of infection. Shaving disturbs hair follicles, which are often colonized with *Staphylococcus aureus*. The greatest threat for infection occurs when shaving is done the night before surgery. Clipping of hair should be done the day of surgery. Ensure that clients are aware of the risks associated with shaving a surgical site prior to arriving at the hospital. It is important that clients receive an antibiotic within 1 hour of the incision time; however, preoperative preparations will easily allow the 1-hour time frame to be met. Notifying the nurse of antibiotic allergies is important information for the team but will not prevent infection, nor will the client washing hands before arrival to the hospital.

➧ ***Test-taking Tip:*** *Apply knowledge of the Medicare Surgical Care Improvement Project to prevent postoperative infections.*

Content Area: Management of Care; *Category of Health Alteration:* Leadership and Management; *Integrated Processes:* Teaching and Learning; *Client Need:* Safe and Effective Care Environment/ Management of Care/Performance Improvement; *Cognitive Level:* Application

Reference: Harkreader, H., Hogan, M., & Thobaben, M. (2007). *Fundamentals of Nursing* (3rd ed., p. 1290). St. Louis, MO: Saunders/ Elsevier.

EBP Reference: Medicare Quality Improvement Community. (2006). *Surgical Care Improvement Project.* Available at: www.medqic.org/dcs/ ContentServer?cid=1137346750659&pagename=Medqic%2FContent% 2FParentShellTemplate&parentName=TopicCat&c=MQParents

Test 3: **Management of Care: Prioritization and Delegation**

77. A nurse receives a change-of-shift report for four assigned clients. Which clients should the nurse attend to first? Prioritize the nurse's actions by placing each client in the correct order.

_____ A 44-year-old client who has questions about how to empty the Jackson-Pratt drain at home after being discharged tomorrow
_____ A 33-year-old client who has a new order to insert a nasogastric (NG) tube and connect to low intermittent suction
_____ A usually oriented 76-year-old client diagnosed with thrombophlebitis who has new-onset confusion
_____ A 58-year-old client requesting a pain medication for abdominal incision pain rated at a 6 on a 0–10 scale

ANSWER: 4, 3, 1, 2
The client who is confused needs immediate assessment because confusion may be a sign of a complication, such as a stroke or pulmonary embolism. The client in pain should be attended to next because pain can interfere with necessary postoperative activities, such as deep breathing, coughing, and ambulating. The client who has an order for a NG tube insertion should be attended to next. There is no information indicating that this client is nauseated or the purpose of the NG. The last client to be seen is the client who needs teaching.

Test-taking Tip: Use the ABCs (airway, breathing, circulation) to establish the priority client who should be attended to first. Confusion can be indicative of a breathing or circulatory problem. Then follow Maslow's Hierarchy of Needs to address comfort and psychosocial concerns.

Content Area: Management of Care; *Category of Health Alteration:* Prioritization and Delegation; *Integrated Processes:* Nursing Process Planning; *Client Need:* Safe and Effective Care Environment/Management of Care/Establishing Priorities; *Cognitive Level:* Analysis

Reference: Berman, A., Snyder, S., Kozier, B., & Erb, G. (2008). *Kozier & Erb's Fundamentals of Nursing: Concepts, Process, and Practice* (8th ed., pp. 217–218). Upper Saddle River, NJ: Pearson Education.

---

78. Two hours after admitting a client to a postsurgical unit following a nephrectomy, the client states feeling nauseated. A nurse notes minimal drainage from the nasogastric (NG) tube. Which action should the nurse take *first*?

1. Notify the physician
2. Administer an antiemetic medication listed on the client's medication record
3. Pull the NG tube out about an inch to release it suctioning against the wall of the stomach
4. Irrigate the NG and check to see if the fluid returns to the drainage-collection container

ANSWER: 4
Nausea and minimal returns from the NG tube suggest possible occlusion of the tube. The tube should be irrigated per agency policy or physician's order, especially if the surgical area involved the gastrointestinal system. It is unnecessary to notify the physician as the first action; nurses are responsible for maintaining the patency of the tube. Administering an antiemetic is important with nausea, but is not the first action because a functioning NG should relieve the nausea by decompressing the stomach contents. In a Salem sump-type NG with a vent lumen, air may need to be injected to release the tube from suctioning against the wall of the stomach, but the tube should not be partially withdrawn unless it has been determined that intestinal and not gastric drainage is returning.

Test-taking Tip: Focus on the situation and the type of surgery to determine the appropriate action.

Content Area: Management of Care; *Category of Health Alteration:* Prioritization and Delegation; *Integrated Processes:* Nursing Process Implementation; *Client Need:* Safe and Effective Care Environment/Management of Care/Establishing Priorities; *Cognitive Level:* Analysis

Reference: Berman, A., Snyder, S., Kozier, B., & Erb, G. (2008). *Kozier & Erb's Fundamentals of Nursing: Concepts, Process, and Practice* (8th ed., pp. 1267–1268). Upper Saddle River, NJ: Pearson Education.

79. A nurse notes that a client has dyspnea and red blotches on the face and arms and appears anxious following exposure to latex. The nurse calls the acute response team (ART) who initiate emergency treatment per protocol. Of all the emergency treatments available, which action should be taken *first* by ART?

1. Start oxygen at 1 liter per minute via nasal cannula (NC)
2. Start an intravenous (IV) access with a large-bore IV catheter
3. Administer diphenhydramine (Benadryl®) 25 mg intramuscularly
4. Administer epinephrine hydrochloride (Adrenalin®) 0.4 mL subcutaneously

ANSWER: 4

Epinephrine is a sympathomimetic that acts rapidly to prevent or reverse cardiovascular collapse, airway narrowing from bronchospasm, and inflammation. Oxygen should be initiated at the onset, but 1 liter per NC is too low. Generally emergency oxygen is administered using a nonrebreather mask at 90% to 100% oxygen concentration. Obtaining IV access will take longer, so it should not be the first action. Intramuscular administration of diphenhydramine (Benadryl®) has an onset of 20 to 30 minutes.

➧ ***Test-taking Tip:*** *Select option 4, noting the key word "first" and considering the amount of time it takes to complete the other actions.*

Content Area: Management of Care; *Category of Health Alteration:* Prioritization and Delegation; *Integrated Processes:* Nursing Process Implementation; *Client Need:* Safe and Effective Care Environment/ Management of Care/Establishing Priorities; *Cognitive Level:* Application

Reference: Black, J., & Hokanson Hawks, J. (2009). *Medical-Surgical Nursing: Clinical Management for Positive Outcomes* (8th ed., p. 283). St. Louis, MO: Saunders/Elsevier.

---

80. During the emergency insertion of a central venous line in a client diagnosed with hepatitis B (HBV), a nurse suffers a needle-stick injury from a blood-contaminated needle. The nurse goes directly to the hospital's occupational health service. Which immediate treatment should the nurse anticipate receiving?

1. Administration of hepatitis B immune globulin (HBIG) and initiation of the hepatitis vaccine if the nurse has not been previously vaccinated
2. Administration of hepatitis B immune globulin (HBIG)
3. Blood tests for the presence of hepatitis B antigens and administration of HBIG 1 week later
4. Blood tests for the presence of hepatitis B antigens and treatment with HBIG if the tests are positive

ANSWER: 1

For postexposure prophylaxis, hepatitis immune globulin along with the HBV vaccine is given (if the nurse has not had it previously). The HBIG contains antibodies against HBV and confers temporary passive immunity. HBIG should be given within 24 hours of exposure. If the nurse has previously been vaccinated for HBV, HBIG is still given, plus a booster dose of HBV vaccine, and blood tests are drawn for the presence of anti-HBs. Administration of just HBIG is insufficient treatment if the vaccination status is unknown. The incubation period of HBV is 1 to 6 months. HBIG should be administered as soon as possible, not 1 week later or when blood tests are positive.

➧ ***Test-taking Tip:*** *Focus on the properties of immune globulins. They offer passive immunity and thus need to be administered as soon as possible after exposure to be effective. This knowledge would enable elimination of options 3 and 4.*

Content Area: Management of Care; *Category of Health Alteration:* Prioritization and Delegation; *Integrated Processes:* Nursing Process Planning; *Client Need:* Safe and Effective Care Environment/Safety and Infection Control/Standard/Transmission-based/Other Precautions; *Cognitive Level:* Application

References: Lewis, S., Heitkemper, M., Dirksen, S., O'Brien, P., & Bucher, L. (2007). *Medical-Surgical Nursing: Assessment and Management of Clinical Problems* (7th ed., p. 1096). St. Louis, MO: Mosby; Monahan, F., Sands, J., Neighbors, M., Marek, J., & Green, C. (2007). *Phipps' Medical-Surgical Nursing: Health and Illness Perspectives* (8th ed., p. 1339). St. Louis, MO: Mosby.

81. A nurse working in the obstetrical unit receives reports on four clients. Prioritize the order in which the nurse should assess the clients.

______ A 19-year-old primigravida at term admitted 2 hours ago after membranes were ruptured at home; dilated to 3 cm with contractions every 5 to 6 minutes lasting 20 to 30 seconds
______ A 25-year-old primigravida at 35 weeks gestation on electronic fetal/maternal monitoring with a new order to administer ampicillin 2-g loading dose followed by 1 g q4hr to treat an acute streptococcal infection
______ A 35-year-old woman at 37 weeks gestation on electronic fetal/maternal monitoring with a blood pressure of 130/90 mm Hg, 2+ protein in the urine, and edema of the hands and face just started on oxytocin (Pitocin®) intravenous infusion
______ A 28-year-old female with contractions every 2 to 3 minutes lasting from 60 to 90 seconds; just put on the light and states she feels rectal pressure

ANSWER: 4, 3, 2, 1

The 28-year-old female, with contractions every 2 to 3 minutes lasting from 60 to 90 seconds with rectal pressure should be assessed first because the signs suggest that birth could be imminent and the woman has started the second stage of labor. The second client to be assessed should be the 35-year-old woman; she is exhibiting signs of preeclampsia and the oxytocin infusion can hasten her labor. The 25-year-old client with primigravida, who has a new order for ampicillin, should be assessed next and the ampicillin initiated. The physician has just likely assessed this woman. The last client to be assessed should be the 19-year-old in the latent phase of labor.

➧ ***Test-taking Tip:*** *Situations in which birth could be imminent are priority.*

Content Area: Management of Care; *Category of Health Alteration:* Prioritization and Delegation; *Integrated Processes:* Nursing Process Planning; *Client Need:* Safe and Effective Care Environment/ Management of Care/Establishing Priorities; *Cognitive Level:* Analysis

Reference: Pillitteri, A. (2007). *Maternal & Child Health Nursing: Care of the Childbearing & Childrearing Family* (5th ed., pp. 351, 429, 505–507, 609–611). Philadelphia: Lippincott Williams & Wilkins.

---

82. A nurse assesses that a laboring client receiving an oxytocin (Pitocin®) infusion has a contraction occurring 1 minute after the previous contraction and remains strong after 70 seconds. Which should be the nurse's *first* action?

1. Notify the physician
2. Reassess the fetal heart tones
3. Stop the oxytocin (Pitocin®) infusion
4. Prepare to administer terbutaline sulfate (Brethine®)

ANSWER: 3

A contraction that occurs more frequently than every 2 minutes and remains strong for 70 seconds or more suggests hyperstimulation and approaching tetany, which could lead to uterine rupture. Because oxytocin stimulates contractions, it should be stopped. Only after stopping the infusion should the nurse monitor the fetal heart tones and notify the physician. Terbutaline sulfate, a beta-adrenergic receptor medication, stops the hyperstimulation and may be ordered to decrease myometrial activity.

➧ ***Test-taking Tip:*** *Note that all options suggest an unsafe situation; this should cue you to the correct option.*

Content Area: Management of Care; *Category of Health Alteration:* Prioritization and Delegation/Childbearing; *Integrated Processes:* Nursing Process Implementation; *Client Need:* Safe and Effective Care Environment/Management of Care/Establishing Priorities; *Cognitive Level:* Analysis

Reference: Pillitteri, A. (2007). *Maternal & Child Health Nursing: Care of the Childbearing & Childrearing Family* (5th ed., pp. 609–610). Philadelphia: Lippincott Williams & Wilkins.

83. A nurse has just initiated an intravenous piggyback (IVPB) of cefuroxime sodium (Zinacef®) for a woman diagnosed with a postpartum infection. Within 5 minutes, the client is experiencing dyspnea, wheezing, and stridor. Prioritize the nurse's actions by placing each intervention in the correct order.

_____ Shout for help
_____ Call the health-care provider (HCP)
_____ Turn off the antibiotic
_____ Ask another nurse to set up new IV maintenance solution and tubing and aspirate the IV port before initiating the new solution.
_____ Administer the ordered emergency medications intravenously
_____ Maintain the airway and administer oxygen

ANSWER: 2, 5, 1, 4, 6, 3

The nurse should turn off the antibiotic immediately since it is the cause of the problem. The next step would be to call for help. Then, administer oxygen. The nurse should then ask another nurse to obtain new solution and tubing and aspirate the IV port until blood returns. This will remove any remaining antibiotic in the port. It is necessary to keep the IV open for the administration of emergency medications. Finally, the nurse should call the HCP and administer the ordered medications. In some settings, the call for help may be to an emergency response team, and a physician often responds as part of this team. The client's primary HCP should also be notified.

➧ ***Test-taking Tip:*** *Visualize the steps in responding to an emergency: remove from immediate danger (stopping the IV in this situation), call for help, and maintain the airway. Prioritizing is placing items in the correct sequence.*

Content Area: Management of Care; *Category of Health Alteration:* Prioritization and Delegation; *Integrated Processes:* Nursing Process Implementation; *Client Need:* Physiological Integrity/Physiological Adaptation/Unexpected Response to Therapies; *Cognitive Level:* Application

References: Lewis, S., Heitkemper, M., Dirksen, S., O'Brien, P., & Bucher, L. (2007). *Medical-Surgical Nursing: Assessment and Management of Clinical Problems* (7th ed., p. 230). St. Louis, MO: Mosby; Institute for Clinical Systems Improvement. (2008). *Diagnosis and Treatment of Respiratory Illness in Children and Adults.* Available at: www.guideline.gov/summary/summary.aspx?view_id=1&doc_id=12294

---

84. A nurse assesses heavy bleeding with large clots for a postpartum client 2 hours after delivery of a 10-pound infant. Which action should the nurse take initially?

1. Perform fundal massage
2. Notify the primary health-care provider
3. Start a dilute oxytocin (Pitocin®) infusion intravenously
4. Offer a bedpan or assist the woman in ambulating to the bathroom

ANSWER: 1

Because uterine atony is the most frequent cause of postpartum hemorrhage, initial management is fundal massage. If the uterus does not remain contracted with fundal massage, the primary health-care provider should be notified. A dilute intravenous infusion of oxytocin helps the uterus maintain tone. The bladder should be kept empty to prevent a full bladder from pushing an uncontracted uterus into an even more uncontracted state.

➧ ***Test-taking Tip:*** *The key word is "initially." Because the client is hemorrhaging, use the ABCs (airway, breathing, circulation) to identify the correct option to control bleeding.*

Content Area: Management of Care; *Category of Health Alteration:* Prioritization and Delegation; *Integrated Processes:* Nursing Process Implementation; *Client Need:* Safe and Effective Care Environment/Management of Care/Establishing Priorities; *Cognitive Level:* Analysis

Reference: Pillitteri, A. (2007). *Maternal & Child Health Nursing: Care of the Childbearing & Childrearing Family* (5th ed., pp. 656–659). Philadelphia: Lippincott Williams & Wilkins.

85. A nurse, working on a pediatric unit, has the following medications to administer at 1000 hours: (1) oral pain medication for a child with burn injuries who will be undergoing a débridement at 1045; (2) an intravenous (IV) antibiotic to a child with aspiration pneumonia secondary to a near-drowning experience; (3) oral antitussive to a child with a cough; and (4) oral acetaminophen to a child with a fever of 102°F (38.9°C) due to an infection secondary to a motor vehicle accident. To which child should the nurse administer medication first?

1. The child with a cough receiving an antitussive
2. The child with burn injuries receiving a pain medication
3. The child with aspiration pneumonia receiving an IV antibiotic
4. The child with a fever of 102°F (38.9°C) receiving acetaminophen

ANSWER: 2

Because the child will be undergoing a débridement in 45 minutes and the medication is oral, it will take approximately 30 to 45 minutes for effects of the medication to occur. The nurse should be cognizant of the time needed to assure optimum pain relief during this procedure. The IV antibiotic and the oral medications can be given after the pain medication because there is a half-hour window for medication administration. Although giving acetaminophen is not the top priority, it should be administered in a timely manner.

➧ ***Test-taking Tip:*** *Identify which child is most at risk for negative implications if the nurse does not prioritize medication administration.*

Content Area: Management of Care; *Category of Health Alteration:* Prioritization and Delegation; *Integrated Processes:* Nursing Process Implementation; *Client Need:* Safe and Effective Care Environment/Management of Care/Establishing Priorities; *Cognitive Level:* Analysis

Reference: Wilson, B., Shannon, M., & Stang, C. (2006). *Nurse's Drug Guide 2006* (pp. 9–11, 808–809). Upper Saddle River, NJ: Pearson Education.

---

86. A nurse is assessing a 4-year-old female client on admission to a pediatric unit for pneumonia. During the assessment, the child asks, "Are you going to look where my daddy puts his fingers?" What should be the nurse's next priority action?

1. Contact the primary physician
2. Refer to social services
3. Obtain more information from the child
4. Confront the parent/caregiver regarding information provided by the child

ANSWER: 3

The child apparently felt comfortable telling the nurse about what is occurring between her and her daddy. Because a relationship has begun to be formed between the nurse and the child, the nurse should obtain more information. A 4-year-old should be able to explain what is occurring. Though the nurse should communicate with the physician prior to the physician's examination, the nurse has already developed a trusting relationship, so obtaining more information is priority. Referral to social services, when deemed appropriate, can be done by either professional, but it is not the next priority. It is not the role or responsibility of the professional nurse to investigate allegations of abuse.

➧ ***Test-taking Tip:*** *The key words are "next priority." Think about the relationship between the child and the nurse.*

Content Area: Management of Care; *Category of Health Alteration:* Prioritization and Delegation; *Integrated Processes:* Nursing Process Evaluation; *Client Need:* Psychological Integrity/Abuse/Neglect; *Cognitive Level:* Analysis

References: Pillitteri, A. (2007). *Maternal and Child Health Nursing* (5th ed., pp. 1753–1756). Philadelphia: Lippincott Williams & Wilkins; Hockenberry, M., & Wilson, D. (2007). *Wong's Nursing Care of Infants and Children* (8th ed., pp. 699–700). St. Louis, MO: Mosby/Elsevier.

---

87. A nurse assesses that the pulse of a 2-year-old hospitalized toddler is 120 beats per minute (bpm). What should be the nurse's priority based on this finding?

1. Notify the physician
2. Apply oxygen by face mask
3. Document the toddler's pulse
4. Reassess the toddler's vital signs in 15 minutes

ANSWER: 3

Because the pulse rate is within the normal range of 80 to 130 bpm for a 2-year-old child, it should be documented. Notifying the physician, applying oxygen, and reassessing the vital signs are unnecessary actions.

➧ ***Test-taking Tip:*** *Recall that the adult's pulse rate is between 60 to 100 bpm. To help remember a normal value for a 2-year-old child, double the low range of 60 for the adult.*

Content Area: Management of Care; *Category of Health Alteration:* Prioritization and Delegation; *Integrated Processes:* Nursing Process Implementation; *Client Need:* Physiological Integrity/Reduction of Risk Potential/Vital Signs; *Cognitive Level:* Application

Reference: Pillitteri, A. (2007). *Maternal & Child Health Nursing: Care of the Childbearing & Childrearing Family* (5th ed., p. 1814). Philadelphia: Lippincott Williams & Wilkins.

88. A nurse is planning care for four clients. Prioritize the order in which the nurse should plan to attend to the clients.

____ A 13-year-old client waiting to be admitted from the emergency department after receiving stitches for facial lacerations from a dog bite

____ A 9-year-old client whose mother is present to receive teaching about wound care for her child's left leg skin graft in anticipation of discharge tomorrow

____ A 5-year-old client with an infected leg wound who is scheduled for a dressing change now

____ A 2-year-old client who's temperature has risen to 103.8°F (39.9°C)

ANSWER: 3, 4, 2, 1

The 2-year-old client with an elevated temperature should be assessed first. This is the most life-threatening situation. The next action should be to change the leg dressing for the 5-year-old client. Delaying the dressing change increases the risk of sepsis. The child can then be admitted from the emergency department. The child should still be monitored while in the emergency room, and it is appropriate to delay admission to the unit if other interventions are priority. The last action by the nurse should be to teach the 9-year-old child's mother on wound care. This client is being discharged tomorrow, which means that the wound care teaching, while important, can be delayed.

➧ ***Test-taking Tip:*** *Immediate physiological needs should be attended to first.*

Content Area: Management of Care; *Category of Health Alteration:* Prioritization and Delegation; *Integrated Processes:* Nursing Process Planning; *Client Need:* Safe and Effective Care Environment/ Management of Care/Establishing Priorities; *Cognitive Level:* Analysis

Reference: Berman, A., Snyder, S., Kozier, B., & Erb, G. (2008). *Kozier & Erb's Fundamentals of Nursing: Concepts, Process, and Practice* (8th ed., pp. 217–218). Upper Saddle River, NJ: Pearson Education.

---

89. A 3-year-old child is on mechanical ventilation, which has been effective in treating oxygenation problems secondary to hypovolemic shock. When developing the plan of care for this child, which nursing diagnosis should the nurse consider a priority at this time?

1. Impaired gas exchange
2. Fear
3. Risk for infection
4. Risk for impaired skin integrity

ANSWER: 3

Critical illness and mechanical ventilation increase the risk for infection. This child is already compromised from the inadequate tissue perfusion that occurred with hypovolemic shock, so the priority at this time is to prevent an infection that would further compromise the child's physical condition. Impaired gas exchange would be an appropriate diagnosis if the child's blood gases were not within normal limits while on mechanical ventilation. Otherwise, the mechanical ventilation is effective in treating the impaired gas exchange as noted in the situation. A child of 3 years of age would be afraid. The standard of practice is to sedate a child who requires ventilator support. This should have been initiated when the child was placed on mechanical ventilation. Typically children, unless there are other risk factors, are not at high risk for impaired skin integrity. However, the nurse should be extremely mindful of assessing for areas of pressure.

➧ ***Test-taking Tip:*** *Look for clues in the stem, especially when there are multiple correct answers. The key phrase is "priority at this time."*

Content Area: Management of Care; *Category of Health Alteration:* Prioritization and Delegation; *Integrated Processes:* Nursing Process Analysis; *Client Need:* Safe and Effective Care Environment/ Management of Care/Establishing Priorities; *Cognitive Level:* Application

References: Doenges, M., Moorhouse, M., & Murr, A. (2006). *Nursing Care Plans* (pp. 171–175). Philadelphia: F. A. Davis; Craven, R., & Hirnle, C. (2007). *Fundamentals of Nursing: Human Health and Function* (5th ed., pp. 176–181). Philadelphia: Lippincott Williams & Wilkins.

90. A triage nurse, working in an emergency department, receives four admissions. Prioritize the order in which the nurse should assess the clients.

______ A 40-year-old client who is diaphoretic and is feeling chest pressure
______ An 18-year-old client who thinks he might have a broken ankle
______ A 35-year-old client who cut her hand with a knife while preparing food
______ A 60-year-old client who is dyspneic and has swollen lips after being stung by a bee

ANSWER: 2, 4, 3, 1

The client with dyspnea and swollen lips should be assessed first and is likely experiencing an anaphylactic reaction. Airway maintenance and medication administration are required to prevent death. Next, the 40-year-old client should be assessed. The client could be experiencing a myocardial infarction, and "time is muscle." Ideally, a nurse should be able to delegate actions for this client while assessing the first client. The client with a cut hand is a priority because of the potential blood loss but should be assessed third because it is not as life threatening as either the client with a possible anaphylactic reaction or the client with a possible myocardial infarction. The last client to be assessed should be the client with the possible ankle fracture. An x-ray is needed to confirm a fracture, but the client is stable and does not have a life-threatening problem.

➧ ***Test-taking Tip:*** *Use the ABCs (airway, breathing, circulation) to establish priority and select the client that needs immediate airway protection as the first client to be assessed.*

Content Area: Management of Care; *Category of Health Alteration:* Prioritization and Delegation; *Integrated Processes:* Nursing Process Analysis; *Client Need:* Safe and Effective Care Environment/Management of Care/Establishing Priorities; *Cognitive Level:* Analysis

References: Berman, A., Snyder, S., Kozier, B., & Erb, G., (2008). *Kozier & Erb's Fundamentals of Nursing: Concepts, Process, and Practice* (8th ed., pp. 217–218). Upper Saddle River, NJ: Pearson Education; LaCharity, L., Kumagai, C., & Bartz, B. (2006). *Prioritization, Delegation Assignment: Practice Exercises For Medical-Surgical Nursing* (pp. 4–5). St. Louis, MO: Mosby.

91. EBP A 30-year-old client is brought to an emergency trauma center with a hand injury from a nail gun sustained while remodeling an old barn. There is a strong odor of alcohol and the client admits to having three beers during a 3-hour period. Which assessment finding is most important for the nurse to evaluate *first*?

1. Blood type
2. Time of last voiding
3. Current blood alcohol level
4. Date of last tetanus immunization

ANSWER: 4

There is a strong risk of infection with *Clostridium tetani.* The spores are present in soil, garden mold, and manure and enter the body through a traumatic or suppurative wound. Tetanus immune globulin is recommended when the client's history of tetanus immunization is not known. Tetanus toxoid, 0.5 mL given intramuscularly, enhances acquired immunity to *C. tetani* if the client has not had an immunization within 10 years. If blood replacement is needed, blood typing would be completed. There usually is not a large blood loss from a hand injury. A urinal should be provided for the client to void. A level may be drawn; however, alcohol is metabolized at a constant rate of approximately one drink (or 12 oz of beer) per hour.

➧ ***Test-taking Tip:*** *Focus on the situation and note the key words "hand injury," "barn," and "most important." Select option 4 using knowledge of infectious diseases.*

Content Area: Management of Care; *Category of Health Alteration:* Prioritization and Delegation; *Integrated Processes:* Nursing Process Assessment; *Client Need:* Physiological Integrity/Reduction of Risk Potential/Potential for Complications from Surgical Procedures and Health Alterations; *Cognitive Level:* Analysis

Reference: Ignatavicius, D., & Workman, M. (2006). *Medical-Surgical Nursing: Critical Thinking for Collaborative Care* (5th ed., p. 373). St. Louis, MO: Saunders/Elsevier.

EBP Reference: Kretsinger, K., Broder, K., Cortese, M., et al. (2006). Preventing tetanus, diphtheria, and pertussis among adults: use of tetanus toxoid, reduced diphtheria toxoid and acellular pertussis vaccine. *Morbidity and Mortality Weekly Report,* 55(17). Available at: www.cdc.gov/mmwr/preview/mmwrhtml/rr5517a1.htm.

92. EBP A postanesthesia care nurse is planning care for a client immediately following lengthy abdominal surgery with the general anesthetic agent isoflurane (Forane®). Which nursing diagnosis should the nurse plan to address *first*?

1. Acute Pain related to surgical procedure
2. Anxiety related to lack of knowledge of surgical outcomes
3. Risk for Urinary Retention related to fear of pain
4. Risk for Impaired Physical Mobility related to incisional discomfort

ANSWER: 1

Planning care during the immediate postoperative phase focuses on pain after managing the ABCs (airway, breathing, circulation). General anesthetic agents are expired quickly through the lungs, and, as the client wakens, the need for postoperative analgesia increases. Anxiety, risk for urinary retention, and risk for impaired physical mobility are important, but not the priority in the immediate postoperative period.

▶ ***Test-taking Tip:*** *Note the key word "first." Concentrate on the components of initial postanesthesia care.*

Content Area: Management of Care; *Category of Health Alteration:* Prioritization and Delegation; *Integrated Processes:* Nursing Process Planning; *Client Need:* Physiological Integrity/Pharmacological and Parenteral Therapies/Pharmacological Pain Management; *Cognitive Level:* Application

References: Adams, M., Holland, L., & Bostwick, P. (2008). *Pharmacology for Nurses: A Pathophysiologic Approach* (2nd ed., p. 253). Upper Saddle River, NJ: Prentice Hall; Monahan, F., Sands, J., Neighbors, M., et al. (2007). *Phipps' Medical-Surgical Nursing: Health and Illness Perspectives* (8th ed., pp. 321–327). St. Louis, MO: Mosby.

EBP Reference: Layzell, M. (2008). Current interventions and approaches to postoperative pain management. *British Journal of Nursing, 17*(7), 414–419.

93. An older client with osteoarthritis is taking celecoxib (Celebrex®). After reviewing the client's laboratory values for the past 3 months, what should be a clinic nurse's priority when assessing the client?

Serum Laboratory Test	6 Months Ago	3 Months Ago	Today
BUN	13 mg/dL	19 mg/dL	28 mg/dL
Creatinine	0.8 mg/dL	1.2 mg/dL	1.8 mg/dL

1. Review urinalysis results
2. Measure the client's blood pressure
3. Ask the client if there has been any weight gain
4. Auscultate the client's heart sounds

ANSWER: 2

Adverse effects of long-term use of Cox-2 inhibitors include renal impairment, which can be manifested by edema and elevated blood pressure. The progressive elevation of the serum creatinine and blood urea nitrogen suggest renal impairment. The urinalysis provides additional information, but is not the priority. Weight measurement and auscultation of the heart are part of normal health assessment.

▶ ***Test-taking Tip:*** *Note the key word "priority." Apply knowledge of the adverse effects of celecoxib to answer this question.*

Content Area: Management of Care; *Category of Health Alteration:* Prioritization and Delegation; *Integrated Processes:* Nursing Process Assessment; *Client Need:* Physiological Integrity/Pharmacological and Parenteral Therapies/Adverse Effects/Contraindications; *Cognitive Level:* Analysis

Reference: Abrams, A., Lammon, C., & Pennington, S. (2007). *Clinical Drug Therapy: Rationales for Nursing Practice* (8th ed., p. 108). Philadelphia: Lippincott Williams & Wilkins.

94. When assessing the appropriateness of a self-help group for a 20-year-old client recently diagnosed with an eating disorder, a nurse should pay initial attention to which of the following?

1. The average age of the group's membership.
2. Ratio of clients to involved health-care professionals.
3. How compatible the group's meeting schedule is with the client's expectations.
4. The group's ability to promote positive adaptive responses among clients similar to this one.

ANSWER: 4

Because self-help groups may employ various philosophies that govern their approach to client care, it is initially important to assess the effectiveness of the treatment as it relates to clients that share the characteristics of this client. Option 1 reflects a consideration that may affect the client's comfort with the group, but it is not the initial consideration. Option 2 reflects a consideration that may affect the client's comfort with the group as well as its management of clients, but it is not the initial consideration. Option 3 reflects a consideration that may affect the client's comfort with the group and ultimate attendance, but it is not the initial consideration.

▶ ***Test-taking Tip:*** *Focus on the information presented in the item's stem while noting the key word "priority." Use your understanding of the goals of a self-help group and the variables that naturally exist between similar groups.*

Content Area: Management of Care; *Category of Health Alteration:* Prioritization and Delegation; *Integrated Processes:* Caring; *Client Need:* Psychosocial Integrity/Stress Management; *Cognitive Level:* Analysis

Reference: Stuart, G. (2009). *Principles and Practices of Psychiatric Nursing* (9th ed., pp. 458–476). St. Louis, MO: Elsevier/Mosby.

95. Which statement made by a client, who is being treated for severe depression and receiving information regarding self-help groups, best reflects understanding of the priority goal for crisis intervention?

1. "I'm going to attend a self-help group to learn how to best cope with stress."
2. "Stress causes my depression, and I must learn to deal with it effectively."
3. "I know to take my medication regularly as prescribed by my physician."
4. "I really think I can learn how to cope so I can get my old life back."

ANSWER: 4

The priority goal for crisis intervention should be the client's return to a precrisis level of functioning. Option 1 reflects an outcome of crisis intervention, but it is not the initial goal of crisis intervention. Option 2 reflects an understanding of the role of stress in the development and management of depression, but it is not the initial goal of crisis intervention. Option 3 reflects an understanding of the role medication compliance plays in the prevention of relapse, but it is not the initial goal of crisis intervention

Test-taking Tip: *Focus on the information presented in the item's stem while noting the key word "priority." Use your understanding of crisis intervention focusing on the goal and being able to identify outcomes as well as teaching topics.*

Content Area: Management of Care; *Category of Health Alteration:* Prioritization and Delegation; *Integrated Processes:* Nursing Process Evaluation; *Client Need:* Psychosocial Integrity/Support Systems; *Cognitive Level:* Analysis

Reference: Stuart, G. (2008). *Principles and Practices of Psychiatric Nursing* (9th ed., pp. 283–312). St. Louis, MO: Mosby.

---

96. Which intervention should be implemented *initially* when providing crisis intervention for a client being treated for exacerbation of depression who states, "Caring for all my children is just too hard!"?

1. Encouraging grandparents to assume temporary responsibility for the children's care
2. Providing one-on-one nurse-client time to reinforce the nurse's commitment to help
3. Arranging for the client to attend a self-help group that focuses on the stressors of parenting
4. Facilitating the client's ability to identify the stressors that initially preceded this particular crisis

ANSWER: 1

There are four levels of crisis intervention. Changing environmental factors that affect the situation should be initially addressed (Environmental Manipulation). Arranging for appropriate, alternative child care would be considered such an intervention in this case. One-on-one nurse-client time reflects an intervention that is more appropriately implemented during level 2 (General Support). A self-help group reflects an intervention that is more appropriately implemented during level 4 (Individual Approach). Identifying stressors reflects an intervention that is more appropriately implemented during level 3 (Generic Approach).

Test-taking Tip: *Focus on the information presented in the item's stem while noting the key word "initial." Use your understanding of crisis intervention focusing on the four levels of crisis intervention to identify the action most reflective of level 1's focus.*

Content Area: Management of Care; *Category of Health Alteration:* Prioritization and Delegation; *Integrated Processes:* Nursing Process Implementation; *Client Need:* Psychosocial Integrity/Crisis Intervention; *Cognitive Level:* Analysis

Reference: Stuart, G. (2008). *Principles and Practices of Psychiatric Nursing* (9th ed., pp. 282–312). St. Louis, MO: Mosby.

---

97. A registered nurse (RN) assesses that a client is pale, diaphoretic, dyspneic, and experiencing chest pain. Which actions are best for the nurse to take?

1. Stay with the client, call the charge nurse for help, and call the patient care assistant (PCA) to bring an automatic vital signs machine to the room immediately.
2. Call the PCA to take the client's vital signs while the RN leaves to obtain a narcotic analgesic for administration and notify the charge nurse.
3. Apply oxygen, call the PCA to bring an automatic vital signs machine, and call the charge nurse for help and ask to bring the chart and morphine sulfate noted on the medication record.
4. Activate the emergency system for a code to get immediate help, apply oxygen, and send responders for needed equipment and medication.

ANSWER: 3

Because the client is in distress, the RN should stay with the client, apply oxygen, and obtain help from other members of the health-care team. Asking the charge nurse to bring the chart and morphine sulfate, or other medications noted in the chart, will save time in responding to the situation. The charge nurse should delegate locating the chart and obtaining the medication to another nurse. In option 1 the charge nurse is responding, but then either the nurse or the charge nurse would need to leave the room to obtain needed medication, causing a loss of time in treating the client's pain. In option 2 the RN leaves the room but should have stayed, as the client is in distress. In option 4, the code system should only be activated if the client's pulse or respirations are absent because activation will bring members from multiple departments. Some facilities have an acute response team (ART), which has a different composition of personnel who can respond in emergency situations.

Test-taking Tip: *Read each option carefully and systematically. Eliminate any options that allow the nurse to leave the room. Use the ABCs (airway, breathing, circulation) to establish the priority intervention for the RN.*

Content Area: Management of Care; *Category of Health Alteration:* Prioritization and Delegation; *Integrated Processes:* Nursing Process Implementation; *Client Need:* Safe and Effective Care Environment/ Management of Care/Delegation; *Cognitive Level:* Application

Reference: Marquis, B., & Huston, C. (2009). *Leadership Roles and Management Functions in Nursing* (6th ed., pp. 473–482). Philadelphia: Wolters Kluwer Health/Lippincott Williams & Wilkins.

98. EBP A nurse is working with a certified nursing assistant (CNA) and a licensed practical nurse (LPN) in providing care to a group of clients. Which tasks should the nurse assign to the CNA and LPN?

1. CNA to perform simple dressing changes; LPN to assess and care for two noncomplex clients
2. CNA to empty and record urinary catheter bag drainage; LPN to administer oral and intramuscular medications
3. CNA to assist clients with hygiene; LPN to provide postmortem care and meet with a deceased client's family
4. CNA to take and document vital signs on all clients; LPN to complete the discharge paperwork to be reviewed with two clients

ANSWER: 2

The scope of practice for a CNA includes measuring and recording intake and output and for the LPN to administer oral and intramuscular medications. A CNA is able in some facilities to perform a simple dressing change, but if the registered nurse (RN) changes it the RN would be able to assess the incision. An LPN should not be assessing clients. A CNA is able to assist with hygiene, but meeting with the family of a deceased client should be completed by the RN and not the LPN. A CNA is able to take and document vital signs, but the RN should be completing discharge paperwork to be reviewed with the clients. The discharge paperwork often includes a review of the care plan and addressing unmet needs of the client.

Test-taking Tip: *Eliminate options that include aspects of the RN role that should not be delegated, including assessment, evaluation, and education.*

Content Area: Management of Care; *Category of Health Alteration:* Prioritization and Delegation; *Integrated Processes:* Nursing Process Planning; *Client Need:* Safe and Effective Care Environment/ Management of Care/Delegation; *Cognitive Level:* Application

Reference: Berman, A., Snyder, S., Kozier, B., & Erb, G. (2008). *Kozier & Erb's Fundamentals of Nursing: Concepts, Process, and Practice* (8th ed., pp. 518–520). Upper Saddle River, NJ: Pearson Education.

EBP Reference: National Council of State Boards of Nursing (2005). *Working with Others: A Position Paper.* Available at: https://www.ncsbn.org/Working_with_Others.pdf

99. EBP A charge nurse is reviewing documentation completed by a registered nurse (RN) and evaluating delegation abilities to a licensed practical nurse (LPN) and nursing assistant (NA). Which medical record documentation should the charge nurse determine may have occurred because of inappropriate delegation?

Client Narrative Notes		
1	0800	BP elevated at 150/90 mm Hg (obtained per J. Brown, NA). Client rates right shoulder incisional pain at 10/10. Morphine sulfate given intravenously for pain control. ________ M. Drew, RN.
2	1000	Assisted up to the bathroom per J. Brown, NA. Voided cloudy, foul-smelling urine. Urine output 20 mL/hr for past 4 hr. Dr. Peters notified. ________ M. Drew, RN.
3	1200	Fingerstick blood glucose 55 mg/dL (taken per J. Brown, NA). Given 4 units lispro (Humalog®) insulin subcut as ordered before lunch. ________ A. Smith, LPN
4	1400	Ambulated 100 feet in hallway. Assisted with hygiene while sitting in chair per RN direction. Hygienic care refused earlier due to fatigue. ________ J. Brown, NA

ANSWER: 3

Appropriate delegation includes assessing the knowledge and skill of the delegate. A glucose level of 55 mg/dL is low (normal = 70–110 mg/dL) and rapid-acting lispro insulin should not have been administered. There is no indication that the LPN notified the RN of the abnormal findings. Taking a blood pressure and reporting the findings to the RN is evident in option 1. Administering intravenous medications is within the RN scope of practice. Assisting a client to the bathroom is an appropriate task for the NA, reporting to the RN the findings is evident, and the RN's role in calling the physician is appropriate. Assisting a client with activity and hygienic care is appropriate NA tasks and reporting of refused hygienic care is evident. Documenting completion of tasks is appropriate for the NA. The location of documentation of task completion may vary by facility and may include only a flowsheet or narrative documentation.

Test-taking Tip: *Carefully read each option. Consider the RN's responsibility in assessing the knowledge and skills of the delegate.*

Content Area: Management of Care; *Category of Health Alteration:* Prioritization and Delegation; *Integrated Processes:* Communication and Documentation; *Client Need:* Safe and Effective Care Environment/ Management of Care/Delegation; *Cognitive Level:* Analysis

References: Potter, P., & Perry, A. (2009). *Fundamentals of Nursing* (7th ed., pp. 287, 309–311). St. Louis, MO: Mosby/Elsevier; Smeltzer, S., Bare, B., Hinkle, J., & Cheever, K. (2008). *Brunner & Suddarth's Textbook of Medical-Surgical Nursing* (11th ed., pp. 1392, 2586). Philadelphia: Lippincott Williams & Wilkins.

EBP Reference: Standing, T., & Anthony, M. (2008). Delegation: What it means to acute care nurses. *Applied Nursing Research*, 21(1), 8–14.

100. A nurse is supervising an experienced nursing assistant (NA) who is new to the unit. Which question is best to evaluate the NA's knowledge and skill in obtaining a client's fingerstick blood glucose, which is a permissible NA-performed skill within the agency?

1. "How many times did you perform a fingerstick blood glucose measurement on the unit in which you previously worked?"
2. "How would you obtain a blood specimen and perform the procedure for measuring the client's blood glucose?"
3. "When was the last time you were observed by a RN performing a blood glucose measurement on the client?"
4. "When was the last time you obtained a blood glucose measurement that was out of the normal ranges and what did you do about this?"

ANSWER: 2

The NA describing the procedure is one method of evaluating the NA's knowledge and skill. Using an open-ended question elicits conversation and details. It is better if the nurse observes the NA performing this skill. Asking the NA the number of times the skill has been performed, the last time it was performed, or when last observed by a RN does not evaluate knowledge and abilities. Even if performed numerous times, in the recent past, and under another RN's supervision, the NA could be performing the procedure incorrectly. Asking what the NA did when obtaining abnormal results may provide information about the NA's ability to follow through with information, but it does not evaluate the procedure.

➧ ***Test-taking Tip:*** *Select an option with an open-ended question.*

Content Area: Management of Care; *Category of Health Alteration:* Prioritization and Delegation; *Integrated Processes:* Communication and Documentation; *Client Need:* Safe and Effective Care Environment/Management of Care/Supervision; *Cognitive Level:* Application

Reference: Potter, P., & Perry, A. (2009). *Fundamentals of Nursing* (7th ed., pp. 287, 309–310). St. Louis, MO: Mosby/Elsevier.

---

101. In caring for a postpartum mother experiencing perineal pain and discomfort, which task is most appropriate for a nurse to delegate to a nursing assistant?

1. Checking the perineum for degree of edema
2. Preparing a sitz bath
3. Evaluating relief after applying an ice pack
4. Teaching the client how to apply an anesthetic agent after perineal care

ANSWER: 2

A nursing assistant is able to assist a client with hygiene and should be aware of safety and comfort concerns with a sitz bath. Assessing the client, evaluation, and teaching are RN responsibilities that cannot be delegated.

➧ ***Test-taking Tip:*** *Consider the role of the nursing assistant and the aspects of care in the options that do not involve assessment, teaching, or evaluation.*

Content Area: Management of Care; *Category of Health Alteration:* Prioritization and Delegation; *Integrated Processes:* Nursing Process Implementation; *Client Need:* Safe and Effective Care Environment/Management of Care/Delegation; *Cognitive Level:* Application

References: Davidson, M., London, M., & Ladewig, P. (2008). *Olds' Maternal-Newborn Nursing & Women's Health Across the Lifespan* (8th ed., pp. 1078–1080). Upper Saddle River, NJ: Prentice Hall Health; Berman, A., Snyder, S., Kozier, B., & Erb, G. (2008). *Kozier & Erb's Fundamentals of Nursing: Concepts, Process, and Practice* (8th ed., pp. 518–520). Upper Saddle River, NJ: Pearson Education.

---

102. A patient care assistant (PCA) is assisting a registered nurse (RN) in providing care to mothers and babies on the maternal-newborn unit. A charge nurse recognizes the RN's need for further education regarding appropriate delegation of client care when overhearing the RN make which statement to the nursing assistant?

1. "I've observed you feeding a newborn; you hold and feed infants safely and accurately."
2. "Prepare a sitz bath for Mrs. Jones who has a perineal laceration and is uncomfortable."
3. "When checking the infants temperature, look at the umbilical cord and tell me what you see."
4. "Mrs. Smith's baby just died. You need to prepare the baby for the family's viewing."

ANSWER: 3

The scope of practice for ancillary staff does not include the management of client care. Assessing the umbilical cord is not a responsibility that the RN can delegate to the ancillary staff. Observing a skill and providing feedback indicates appropriate evaluation of the PCA's skill prior to delegation. Hygienic care, taking vital signs, and postmortem care are responsibilities that can be safely delegated to ancillary staff.

➧ ***Test-taking Tip:*** *The key phrase "needs further education" indicates that this is a false-response item. Select the option that indicates incorrect delegation—which includes assessment, planning, evaluation, or teaching; these are responsibilities that the RN cannot delegate.*

Content Area: Management of Care; *Category of Health Alteration:* Prioritization and Delegation; *Integrated Processes:* Nursing Process Evaluation; *Client Need:* Safe and Effective Care Environment/Management of Care/Delegation; *Cognitive Level:* Application

References: Berman, A., Snyder, S., Kozier, B., & Erb, G. (2008). *Kozier & Erb's Fundamentals of Nursing: Concepts, Process, and Practice* (8th ed., pp. 518–520). Upper Saddle River, NJ: Pearson Education; Potter, P., & Perry, A. (2009). *Fundamentals of Nursing* (7th ed., pp. 287, 309–311). St. Louis, MO: Mosby/Elsevier.

103. Before delegating the task of bottle feeding a 6-hour-old term newborn to a nursing assistant, a nurse should evaluate the nursing assistant's knowledge of this task by asking the assistant:

1. how many times she/he has fed an infant previously.
2. how long she/he has worked in the newborn nursery.
3. how she/he would position the infant for the feeding.
4. if she/he has children of her/his own.

ANSWER: 3

Asking open-ended questions about the specific task to be delegated will help the nurse to determine if the nursing assistant has the knowledge to perform the assigned task. Knowing how many times the assistant has performed the task previously does not tell the nurse about the assistant's actual abilities in the particular area. This reasoning would also apply to the question about the length of time the assistant has worked in the newborn nursery. Knowing the number of children the assistant has would not necessarily provide any information about the assistant's ability to bottle feed a newborn.

➧ ***Test-taking Tip:*** *Review each option individually and select the option that would provide the most information about the specific activity to be delegated.*

Content Area: Management of Care; *Category of Health Alteration:* Prioritization and Delegation; *Integrated Processes:* Nursing Process Evaluation; *Client Need:* Safe and Effective Care Environment/ Management of Care/Delegation; *Cognitive Level:* Analysis

Reference: Potter, P., & Perry, A. (2009). *Fundamentals of Nursing* (7th ed., pp. 287, 309–310). St. Louis, MO: Mosby/Elsevier.

104. EBP A patient care assistant (PCA), who usually works on an adult unit, reports to a nurse that a 2-year-old child's blood glucose level is normal at 82 mg/dL. The nurse's response to the PCA is based on knowing that the target blood glucose for a toddler is:

1. 60–100 mg/dL.
2. 80–120 mg/dL.
3. 90–150 mg/dL.
4. 100–180 mg/dL.

ANSWER: 4

A blood glucose of 82 mg/dL is low. A normal preprandial target blood glucose is 100 to 180 mg/dL. Toddlers have a very high vulnerability to hypoglycemia and are unable to recognize symptoms. Any attempt to control the child at levels less than 100 mg/dL is risky. The ranges for target blood glucose for a toddler in options 1, 2, and 3 are too low.

➧ ***Test-taking Tip:*** *Recall that the ranges for children's blood glucose levels are different from adults and are much higher. They also vary by age of the child.*

Content Area: Child Health; *Category of Health Alteration:* Endocrine Management; *Integrated Processes:* Nursing Process Evaluation; *Client Need:* Physiological Integrity/Reduction of Risk Potential/Diagnostic Tests; *Cognitive Level:* Comprehension

Reference: Hockenberry, M., & Wilson, D. (2007). *Wong's Nursing Care of Infants and Children* (8th ed., pp. 1705–1711). St. Louis, MO: Mosby.

EBP Reference: Silverstein, J., Klingensmith, G., Copeland, K., Plotnick, L., Kaufman, F., et al. (2005). Care of children and adolescents with type 1 diabetes: A statement of the American Diabetes Association. *Diabetes Care*, 28(1), 186–212. Available at: www.guideline.gov/summary/summary.aspx?doc_id=6826

105. EBP A 4-month-old infant with no previous health problems is brought to an ambulatory care clinic by a parent for a routine well-child appointment. A senior student nurse, working with a registered nurse (RN), completes the infant's physical assessment and reports to the RN that the baby's pulse rate is 165 beats per minute and the infant is awake and calm. Which action should the nurse take *first* in evaluating the accuracy of this measurement?

1. Immediately retake the infant's vital signs and perform a complete assessment
2. Notify the physician of the abnormal findings
3. Advise the student to ask the parent if there is a family history of cardiovascular disease
4. Direct the student to determine how the heart rate compares with readings from previous clinic visits

ANSWER: 4

The first action is to compare the value to both the norms for the infant's age group and to the infant's previous readings. A normal heart rate for an infant 1 to 11 months is 80 to 160 beats per minute. Environmental changes and stressors can cause temporary increases in heart rate. Even though the RN delegates the action to the student, the RN is still accountable for the outcome, so the RN must also follow up as necessary. Because the heart rate is near the normal range, an immediate reassessment of the infant is unnecessary, as is notifying the physician, until further information is collected. The physician would not be notified if findings are normal. Infants rarely have hereditary cardiac problems. Cardiovascular diseases commonly seen in adults are atypical of this young age group.

➧ ***Test-taking Tip:*** *Read the situation carefully, focusing on the age of the infant, the level of student, and the findings to select the correct option.*

Content Area: Management of Care; *Category of Health Alteration:* Prioritization and Delegation; *Integrated Processes:* Nursing Process Implementation; *Client Need:* Safe and Effective Care Environment/ Management of Care/Delegation; *Cognitive Level:* Analysis

Reference: Berman, A., Snyder, S., Kozier, B., & Erb, G. (2008). *Kozier & Erb's Fundamentals of Nursing: Concepts, Process, and Practice* (8th ed., pp. 518–520). Upper Saddle River, NJ: Pearson Education.

EBP Reference: Li, S., & Kenward, K. (2006). *A National Survey on Elements of Nursing Education*. Available at: www.ncsbn.org/vol_24_web.pdf

106. A registered nurse's (RN) findings upon assessment of a 2-year-old diagnosed with meningitis include an altered level of consciousness, decreased urine output, and temperature of 103.4°F (39.7°C). A licensed practical nurse (LPN) who works on an adult oncology unit arrives to assist in "any way possible." Which task should the RN delegate to the LPN?

1. Notifying the health-care provider
2. Checking the size of the child's pupils
3. Administering an acetaminophen suppository
4. Removing extra blankets from the child's bed and extra clothing

ANSWER: 4

Measures should be taken to lower the child's temperature, including removing extra blankets and clothing. The RN should be communicating with health-care providers. In most health-care facilities, only RNs can accept health-care provider verbal orders. Assessment of the child, including pupils, is the responsibility of the RN and should not be delegated. The LPN would not have a frame of reference for the normal size of a 2-year-old child's pupils. Although the LPN may be experienced on an oncology unit, the LPN may not have the experience of administering a suppository to a 2-year-old child, which would include the use of a smaller finger and shorter depth, and the RN would not have the time to assess the LPN's ability.

***Test-taking Tip:** Focus on the child's health problem and the immediacy of the situation to determine appropriate delegation.*

Content Area: Management of Care; *Category of Health Alteration:* Prioritization and Delegation; *Integrated Processes:* Nursing Process Planning; *Client Need:* Safe and Effective Care Environment/ Management of Care/Delegation; *Cognitive Level:* Analysis

Reference: Berman, A., Snyder, S., Kozier, B., & Erb, G. (2008). *Kozier & Erb's Fundamentals of Nursing: Concepts, Process, and Practice* (8th ed., pp. 518–520). Upper Saddle River, NJ: Pearson Education.

107. A registered nurse (RN) is acting as preceptor for a new graduate nurse during the new nurse's second week of orientation. Which clients should a charge nurse assign to the graduate nurse under the supervision of the experienced RN? SELECT ALL THAT APPLY.

1. A 16-year-old client with moderate chronic asthma to be discharged in 24 hours
2. A 5-year-old with a tracheostomy needing trach care every shift
3. A 12-year-old client who had surgery for a ruptured appendix with a temperature of 99°F (37.2°C)
4. An 8-year-old just admitted with a new diagnosis of leukemia
5. A 4-year-old diagnosed with hemophilia and admitted for a blood transfusion

ANSWER: 1, 3

Because the new nurse is at an early point in orientation, the new nurse should be assigned to clients who are stable and have routine care needs. The new nurse may also be assigned to the older children. While tracheostomy care may be a routine skill, a more experienced nurse should perform this care due to the age of the child. The child with a new diagnosis of leukemia should have an experienced nurse because the parents will likely have multiple questions and a comprehensive admission assessment will be required. A blood transfusion has a high potential for error and should be performed by an experienced nurse.

***Test-taking Tip:** Consider the ages of the children in addition to the diagnoses when making assignments.*

Content Area: Management of Care; *Category of Health Alteration:* Prioritization and Delegation; *Integrated Processes:* Nursing Process Planning; *Client Need:* Safe and Effective Care Environment/ Management of Care/Delegation; *Cognitive Level:* Application

Reference: Finkelman, A. (2006). *Leadership and Management in Nursing* (pp. 224–233). Upper Saddle River, NJ: Pearson Education.

108. A client on a telemetry unit has a blood pressure (BP) of 88/40 mm Hg, a heart rate of 44 beats per minute, feels faint, and is pale and confused. When caring for this client, which tasks should a registered nurse (RN) delegate to a patient care assistant (PCA)? SELECT ALL THAT APPLY

1. Paging for the charge nurse
2. Paging for a respiratory therapist
3. Applying oxygen per protocol
4. Securing an automatic BP machine
5. Completing a head-to-toe assessment
6. Obtaining a cardiac rhythm strip that the nurse has sent for printing at a central location

ANSWER: 1, 4, 6

Because the client's condition is deteriorating, additional assistance is needed. The PCA should be able to page for the charge nurse, secure an automatic BP machine, and obtain a printed rhythm strip. There is no indication of respiratory distress, so it is unnecessary to page for a respiratory therapist. The RN should apply the oxygen and complete a focused assessment, not a complete head-to-toe assessment.

***Test-taking Tip:** Focus on the client's symptoms to eliminate options that do not pertain, such as paging a respiratory therapist. RN-only responsibilities, including assessment and evaluation of information, should not be delegated to the PCA.*

Content Area: Management of Care; *Category of Health Alteration:* Prioritization and Delegation; *Integrated Processes:* Nursing Process Planning; *Client Need:* Safe and Effective Care Environment/ Management of Care/Delegation; *Cognitive Level:* Application

References: Berman, A., Snyder, S., Kozier, B., & Erb, G. (2008). *Kozier & Erb's Fundamentals of Nursing: Concepts, Process, and Practice* (8th ed., pp. 518–520). Upper Saddle River, NJ: Pearson Education; Finkelman, A. (2006). *Leadership and Management in Nursing* (pp. 224–233). Upper Saddle River, NJ: Pearson Education.

109. A nursing assistant's (NA) job responsibilities include totaling the intake and output (I&O) records for clients at the end of an 8-hour shift. Near the end of the shift, a licensed practice nurse (LPN) reports to the registered nurse (RN) that a new NA on the unit has not completed the task. What is the RN's best action?

1. Ask the LPN to complete this task because the information is needed to give report
2. Remind the NA that the task needs to be completed as quickly as possible
3. Notify the charge nurse that the NA needs additional orientation on job responsibilities
4. Ask the NA what instruction was given on job responsibilities and ask the NA to state how to total I&O records

ANSWER: 4

Delegation of assigned tasks includes determining the delegate's knowledge and ability to perform the task correctly. Asking what instruction was given may also clarify what the NA was told and what the RN perceives to be the task. It may be that the RN or LPN must give the NA the appropriate forms to be completed after recording the amount for intravenous infusions. Delegation of the NA-assigned job responsibilities is inappropriate and can create tension between team members. Reminding the NA may be insufficient if the NA does not know how to total I&O records. Notifying the charge nurse may be premature. Additional information is needed regarding the reason the NA is not performing the task.

➧ ***Test-taking Tip:*** *Focus on the tasks of delegation, assuring that the delegate has the knowledge to perform the task.*

Content Area: Management of Care; *Category of Health Alteration:* Prioritization and Delegation; *Integrated Processes:* Nursing Process Implementation; *Client Need:* Safe and Effective Care Environment/ Management of Care/Delegation; *Cognitive Level:* Application

References: Berman, A., Snyder, S., Kozier, B., & Erb, G. (2008). *Kozier & Erb's Fundamentals of Nursing: Concepts, Process, and Practice* (8th ed., pp. 518–520). Upper Saddle River, NJ: Pearson Education; Potter, P., & Perry, A. (2009). *Fundamentals of Nursing* (7th ed., pp. 287, 309–311). St. Louis, MO: Mosby/Elsevier.

110. EBP A registered nurse (RN) is informed by a nursing assistant (NA) that a client, hospitalized last evening with chest pain, plans to leave right now because the pain is gone and "nobody has done anything anyway." Which is the nurse's best action?

1. Thank the NA for the information and then call the client's doctor regarding the situation
2. Tell the NA that the client has the right to leave and send the NA to help the client pack
3. Talk with the client to discuss the client's concerns and explain the plan of care
4. Tell the NA to inform the client that it is unsafe to leave and that the RN will review the test results with the client shortly

ANSWER: 3

Seeing the client provides an opportunity for further assessment and client teaching. The nurse's responsibility is to inform clients of the status of their care. Unjustifiable detention is false imprisonment. The client has a right to leave. Sending the NA to assist the client to pack or to speak to the client is inappropriate delegation of the nurse's responsibilities. Telling the client it is unsafe to leave does not explain why the client should remain in the hospital. Calling the physician is premature.

➧ ***Test-taking Tip:*** *Focus on the option that uses therapeutic communication techniques and correct decision making regarding the RN's responsibility.*

Content Area: Management of Care; *Category of Health Alteration:* Prioritization and Delegation; *Integrated Processes:* Communication and Documentation; *Client Need:* Safe and Effective Care Environment/ Management of Care/Client Rights; *Cognitive Level:* Application

Reference: Berman, A., Snyder, S., Kozier, B., & Erb, G. (2008). *Kozier & Erb's Fundamentals of Nursing: Concepts, Process, and Practice* (8th ed., pp. 69, 518–520). Upper Saddle River, NJ: Pearson Education.

EBP Reference: Conway, J., & Kearin, M. (2007). The contribution of the patient support assistant to direct patient care: An exploration of nursing and PSA role perceptions. *Contemporary Nurse,* 24(2), 175–188.

111. A nurse manager has six new graduate registered nurses beginning work on a busy oncology unit. The nurse manager's role in orienting the new graduate nurses to the clinical unit is ensuring which of the following? SELECT ALL THAT APPLY

1. That each new graduate develops expertise in the client population cared for on the clinical unit
2. That each new graduate is socialized into the clinical unit
3. That each new graduate has successfully completed the licensure process before beginning the unit position
4. That each new graduate participates in the orientation program
5. That each new graduate completes the competency verification process
6. That each new graduate becomes a productive, contributing member of the clinical unit

ANSWERS: 2, 4, 5, 6

The nurse manager's role is management of the unit, which includes ensuring that new nurses are socialized into the clinical unit; verifying that the new nurses are participating in orientation; ensuring that the new nurses are completing the competency verification process; and ensuring that the new nurses are being productive, contributing members of the clinical unit. Expertise will not be developed during the orientation period. Responsibilities for assuring licensure registration are not the responsibility of a unit-based manager but rather those of a centralized department, such as human resources, because this is a condition of employment.

➧ ***Test-taking Tip:*** *Focus on just the orientation period. Eliminate any options that would be a condition of employment.*

Content Area: Management of Care; *Category of Health Alteration:* Prioritization and Delegation; *Integrated Processes:* Nursing Process Evaluation; *Client Need:* Safe and Effective Care Environment/ Management of Care/Concepts of Management; *Cognitive Level:* Application

Reference: Barker, A., Sullivan, D., & Emery, M. (2006). *Leadership Competencies for Clinical Managers: The Renaissance of Transformational Leadership* (pp. 200–201). Sudbury, MA: Jones and Bartlett.

---

112. A nurse manager is reviewing assignments for an evening shift. The nurse manager should intervene if an experienced licensed practical nurse (LPN) is assigned to which action?

1. Complete a foot soak for a 55-year-old client who has an infected heel ulcer
2. Assist a 44-year-old client who is 6 hours postoperative following a vaginal hysterectomy to sit at the edge of the bed and then ambulate
3. Discharge a 34-year-old client with a wound drain following a right mastectomy 4 days ago who still needs instruction regarding the wound drain
4. Perform intermittent urinary catheterizations for residual urine for a 55-year-old client who had an abdominal hysterectomy 2 days ago

ANSWER: 3

The 34-year-old client preparing for discharge will need teaching related to the care of the wound drain and will have other psychosocial and physical needs. The registered nurse (RN) should assess the client's readiness for discharge. Nursing tasks for stable clients with expected outcomes should be assigned to the LPN.

➧ ***Test-taking Tip:*** *Focus on the role of the RN and abilities that should not be delegated.*

Content Area: Management of Care; *Category of Health Alteration:* Prioritization and Delegation; *Integrated Processes:* Nursing Process Analysis; *Client Need:* Safe and Effective Care/Management of Care/Delegation; *Cognitive Level:* Application

Reference: Finkelman, A. (2006). *Leadership and Management in Nursing* (pp. 224–233). Upper Saddle River, NJ: Pearson Education.

---

113. Which intervention should a registered nurse (RN), who is managing a mental health unit, delegate to an unlicensed ancillary staff member?

1. Implementing an as needed (prn) order for physical restraints on a 35-year-old client with a history of aggressive behavior who is threatening to "tear the place apart!"
2. Transporting a group of clients diagnosed with chronic alcoholism to an off-unit Alcoholics Anonymous meeting
3. Explaining to a client, diagnosed with obsessive compulsive disorder, why he or she is not permitted in another client's room
4. Evaluating a depressed client's ability to self-monitor blood glucose levels

ANSWER: 2

The RN may deem it appropriate to delegate noninvasive interventions to an unlicensed ancillary staff member. The RN is responsible for all assessment, planning, and analyzing of client information; implementing and evaluating of client care; supervising care; initiating teaching; and administering medications intravenously. The only intervention that may be appropriately delegated to unlicensed ancillary staff would be the transportation of clients to off-site treatments since the remaining options require more involved nursing judgments. Interventions that are physically invasive, involve evaluation of client information or behaviors (need for restraints or ability to use glucose monitor), or teaching (explanation of unit requirement) are within the RN scope of practice and should not be delegated.

➧ ***Test-taking Tip:*** *Look at the verb in each of the options: implement, transport, explain, and evaluate, respectively. Select the option that would require the least amount of critical thinking.*

Content Area: Management of Care; *Category of Health Alteration:* Prioritization and Delegation; *Integrated Processes:* Nursing Process Planning; *Client Need:* Safe and Effective Care Environment/ Management of Care/Continuity of Care; *Cognitive Level:* Application

References: Berman, A., Snyder, S., Kozier, B., & Erb, G. (2008). *Kozier & Erb's Fundamentals of Nursing: Concepts, Process, and Practice* (8th ed., pp. 518–520). Upper Saddle River, NJ: Pearson Education; Potter, P., & Perry, A. (2009). *Fundamentals of Nursing* (7th ed., pp. 287, 309–311). St. Louis, MO: Mosby/Elsevier.

---

114. A client is returning to a unit after electroconvulsive therapy (ECT) treatment. Which intervention should a nurse delegate to an unlicensed ancillary staff member?

1. Evaluating the client's level of consciousness
2. Observing the client for restlessness or agitated behavior and reporting it to the nurse
3. Assisting with the client's first food and beverage intake after the treatment
4. Assuring the client's family that the client's memory loss is generally temporary

ANSWER: 2

While all of the options are appropriate when implementing post-ECT care, the nurse should only delegate care that is noninvasive and does not require nursing judgment. Asking the ancillary staff member to observe the client's behavior and report any changes is appropriate. Evaluation of the level of consciousness is a nursing responsibility that may not be delegated. Since this client is a possible risk for aspiration due to an absent gag reflex, being present when the client eats or drinks for the first time after the treatment is again not a task that the nurse should delegate. Teaching the family should not be delegated.

➧ ***Test-taking Tip:*** *Focus on the information presented in the item's stem and in the options and the scope of practice of the ancillary staff. Recall that the five rights of delegation include the right situation. Ask yourself if assisting the client to eat after ECT is the right situation for delegation.*

Content Area: Management of Care; *Category of Health Alteration:* Prioritization and Delegation; *Integrated Processes:* Nursing Process Planning; *Client Need:* Safe and Effective Care Environment/Management of Care/Continuity of Care; *Cognitive Level:* Application

References: Potter, P., & Perry, A. (2009). *Fundamentals of Nursing* (7th ed., pp. 287, 309–311). St. Louis, MO: Mosby/Elsevier; Stuart, G. (2008). *Principles and Practices of Psychiatric Nursing* (9th ed., pp. 535–548). St. Louis, MO: Mosby.

---

115. A registered nurse (RN) recognizes the need to provide further education regarding the scope of practice for an ancillary staff member when the staff member offers to take which action?

1. Facilitate the smoking breaks earned by the various clients on the unit
2. Transport a 25-year-old client diagnosed with schizophrenia to an off-site eye appointment
3. Provide visual observation every 15 minutes for a client who expresses suicidal ideations
4. Determine whether restraints may be removed from a client who was acting aggressively

ANSWER: 4

The scope of practice for ancillary staff does not include evaluation of client status/condition/behavior. Determining whether the removal of physical restraints is therapeutic is not within the scope of ancillary staff. The other interventions may be assumed by ancillary staff as deemed appropriate by the RN.

➧ ***Test-taking Tip:*** *Focus on the information presented in the item's stem and in the options. Using your understanding of the appropriate delegation of interventions to unlicensed ancillary staff will assist in the elimination of any interventions that are physically invasive or that involve client evaluation, assessment, planning, or teaching.*

Content Area: Management of Care; *Category of Health Alteration:* Prioritization and Delegation; *Integrated Processes:* Nursing Process Planning; *Client Need:* Safe and Effective Care Environment/Management of Care/Continuity of Care; *Cognitive Level:* Application

References: Berman, A., Snyder, S., Kozier, B., & Erb, G. (2008). *Kozier & Erb's Fundamentals of Nursing: Concepts, Process, and Practice* (8th ed., pp. 518–520). Upper Saddle River, NJ: Pearson Education; Potter, P., & Perry, A. (2009). *Fundamentals of Nursing* (7th ed., pp. 287, 309–311). St. Louis, MO: Mosby/Elsevier.

116. A registered nurse (RN), caring for an elderly client diagnosed with dementia as a result of metastatic brain cancer, is delegating actions to a nursing assistant (NA). Which action is inappropriately delegated to the NA?

1. Toileting the client prior to settling the client in bed for the night
2. Informing the family that the client will need a follow-up brain scan
3. Accompanying the client on a walk in the gardens on the hospital grounds
4. Reinforcing the client's orientation by frequently stating the year, month, and day

ANSWER: 2

The scope of practice for ancillary staff does not include the management of client care. Discussing the client's diagnostic needs is not a responsibility that the RN can delegate to the ancillary staff. Assisting with basic cares, such as toileting, ambulation, and communicating with a client to assist in the client's orientation are appropriate actions to delegate.

Test-taking Tip: *Focus on the information presented in the item's stem and in the options. Eliminating options of appropriate delegation to unlicensed ancillary staff will assist in identifying an inappropriate action to delegate because it involves client teaching.*

Content Area: Management of Care; *Category of Health Alteration:* Prioritization and Delegation; *Integrated Processes:* Nursing Process Planning; *Client Need:* Safe and Effective Care Environment/ Management of Care/Delegation; *Cognitive Level:* Application

References: Berman, A., Snyder, S., Kozier, B., & Erb, G. (2008). *Kozier & Erb's Fundamentals of Nursing: Concepts, Process, and Practice* (8th ed., pp. 518–520). Upper Saddle River, NJ: Pearson Education; Potter, P., & Perry, A. (2009). *Fundamentals of Nursing* (7th ed., pp. 287, 309–311). St. Louis, MO: Mosby/Elsevier.

---

117. A nurse is admitting a client, diagnosed with obsessive-compulsive disorder (OCD), who has ordering issues. Which intervention should the nurse delegate to ancillary staff?

1. Assisting the client to store personal belongings so as to minimize the client's anxiety
2. Asking the client to identify someone who can be notified regarding the client's admission
3. Providing the client with the general "unit rules" that the client will be expected to follow
4. Encouraging the client to "talk to someone" if feeling anxious or excited

ANSWER: 1

The scope of practice for ancillary staff does not include the management of client care or the performance of invasion procedures. A client, diagnosed with OCD, who focuses on ordering items may find storing belongings stressful if not done in a particular manner. Facilitating the client in storing belongings in a fashion that does not produce stress is an intervention that the RN can delegate to the ancillary staff. The other interventions may not be assumed by ancillary staff since they involve some aspect of care management.

Test-taking Tip: *Focus on the tasks presented in the options. Note that options 2, 3, and 4 involve communicating with the client, whereas option 1 is different in that it involves helping the client.*

Content Area: Management of Care; *Category of Health Alteration:* Prioritization and Delegation; *Integrated Processes:* Nursing Process Planning; *Client Need:* Safe and Effective Care Environment/ Management of Care/Delegation; *Cognitive Level:* Application

References: Potter, P., & Perry, A. (2009). *Fundamentals of Nursing* (7th ed., pp. 287, 309–311). St. Louis, MO: Mosby/Elsevier; Videbeck, S. (2008). *Psychiatric–Mental Health Nursing* (4th ed., pp. 257–259). Philadelphia: Wolters Kluwer/Lippincott Williams & Wilkins.

Test 4: **Management of Care: Teaching and Learning, Communication, and Cultural Diversity**

118. A community health nurse is planning prenatal teaching for pregnant adolescents who intend to keep their babies. Which teaching strategy would be most effective for the nurse to use in teaching the adolescents?

1. Inviting mothers and daughters for one-to-one teaching sessions
2. Preparing group sessions for teaching the pregnant adolescents together
3. Offering open sessions for the pregnant adolescents and anyone else who wants to attend
4. Designing poster boards that the girls can view individually in the school nurse's office

ANSWER: 2

Peer groups are important for adolescents, so group teaching sessions are effective. Inviting mothers and daughters for individual teaching sessions would be more effective for teaching the mothers. Prenatal teaching, especially the topic of body changes with pregnancy, could threaten the adolescent's self-esteem and body image if it is discussed in open sessions where anyone could attend. Young adults have a strong need for independence. Poster boards could be an effective strategy for young adults, but not adolescents.

▶ ***Test-taking Tip:*** *Focus on the issue: teaching strategies appropriate to adolescents.*

Content Area: Management of Care; *Category of Health Alteration:* Teaching and Learning, Communication, and Cultural Diversity; *Integrated Processes:* Nursing Process Planning; *Client Need:* Health Promotion and Maintenance/Principles of Teaching and Learning; *Cognitive Level:* Application

Reference: Harkreader, H., Hogan, M., & Thobaben, M. (2007). *Fundamentals of Nursing* (3rd ed., p. 286). St. Louis, MO: Saunders/Elsevier.

---

119. A nurse, working in a school, is planning an educational program to prevent accidental poisonings. The targeted audience is school-aged children, specifically fifth- and sixth-grade students. Which developmental task is most important for the nurse to consider when developing this program?

1. Willingness to try new things
2. Reasoning ability
3. Adherence to group rules
4. Increasing independence

ANSWER: 3

The development of the school-aged child is characterized by Erikson's theory of "industry versus inferiority." Developmentally, children ages 10 to 12 years need to succeed at tasks and be acknowledged for adhering to group rules. The accidental poisonings that occur in school-aged children are mostly caused by ingesting nonprescription drugs or alcohol. The Drug Abuse Resistance Education (D.A.R.E.) program is a successful program with school-aged children because it incorporates the developmental task of adhering to group rules. School-aged children also seek to do the "right thing" to secure approval. Trying something new and incorporating reasoning and independence are both part of the developmental stage of "industry versus inferiority," but none would impact as greatly the design of the educational program as incorporating the developmental task of adhering to group rules.

▶ ***Test-taking Tip:*** *Focus on the issue: developmental tasks of school-aged children. The key words are "most important." When "most important" is used in a question, all the options are likely correct, but one option may be inclusive of some of the others.*

Content Area: Management of Care; *Category of Health Alteration:* Teaching and Learning, Communication, and Cultural Diversity; *Integrated Processes:* Nursing Process Planning; *Client Need:* Health Promotion and Maintenance/Principles of Teaching and Learning; *Cognitive Level:* Analysis

References: Harkreader, H., Hogan, M., & Thobaben, M. (2007). *Fundamentals of Nursing* (3rd ed., p. 286). St. Louis, MO: Saunders/Elsevier; Hockenberry, M. & Wilson, D. (2007). *Wong's Nursing Care of Infants and Children* (8th ed., pp. 714–715). St. Louis, MO: Mosby/Elsevier.

120. A nurse is instructing parents, who are of Mexican origin, on administering their toddler's oral medication. What is the best method for the nurse to use to ensure that the toddler will get the prescribed amount of medicine at the appropriate times?

1. Have an interpreter available to translate information to the parents
2. Have a parent demonstrate the medication administration process prior to discharge
3. Initiate a referral to a home health-care agency for a follow-up visit
4. Provide written instructions to the parents on how to administer the medication

ANSWER: 2

Accidental overdoses or poisonings can occur when parents are not effectively educated in administrating medication to young children. In adult learning theory, return demonstration or demonstrating ability to do the task is the most effective means of evaluating performance. Having an interpreter may be warranted, but there is no indication that the parents are unable to speak English. Initiating a referral would not be warranted unless there are other health-care or parenting concerns. Providing written instructions is a supplemental resource for the parents but would require evaluation of reading and comprehension skills.

➧ ***Test-taking Tip:*** *The key word is "best." Consider adult learning theory as it relates to parent education. Also carefully take into account cultural differences when dealing with families.*

Content Area: Management of Care; *Category of Health Alteration:* Teaching and Learning, Communication, and Cultural Diversity; *Integrated Processes:* Teaching and Learning; *Client Need:* Health Promotion and Maintenance/Principles of Teaching and Learning; *Cognitive Level:* Application

References: Craven, R., & Hirnle, C. (2007). *Fundamentals of Nursing: Human Health and Function* (5th ed., p. 400). Philadelphia: Lippincott Williams & Wilkins; McGoldrick, M., Giordano, J., & Garcia-Preto, N. (2005). *Ethnicity and Family Therapy* (3rd ed., pp. 229–238). New York: Guilford Press.

121. A nurse is preparing a campaign for teachers who are teaching the seventh and eighth grades. The purpose of the campaign is to decrease and, subsequently, eliminate bullying at school. Which strategy should the nurse utilize to most effectively present this information?

1. Panel presentation and small-group discussion
2. Case studies with time for discussion
3. Lecture
4. Educational videos

ANSWER: 1

According to adult learning theory, the older the learner, the more increased is the need for self-direction. Adults also learn when the topic is of immediate value. Adults see themselves as doers; therefore interactive sessions are most effective when dealing with issues in which the targeted audience has variable knowledge and/or experience. Case studies, lecture, and educational videos may be useful, but are not as interactive as a panel presentation and small-group discussion.

➧ ***Test-taking Tip:*** *This is a session for the teachers (not the junior high students). Apply concepts of adult learning theory identifying the method that would be the most interactive and provide the most discussion.*

Content Area: Management of Care; *Category of Health Alteration:* Teaching and Learning, Communication, and Cultural Diversity; *Integrated Processes:* Nursing Process Planning; Teaching and Learning; *Client Need:* Health Promotion and Maintenance/Principles of Teaching and Learning; *Cognitive Level:* Analysis

References: Craven, R., & Hirnle, C. (2007). *Fundamentals of Nursing: Human Health and Function* (5th ed., pp. 398–401). Philadelphia: Lippincott Williams & Wilkins; Pillitteri, A. (2007). *Maternal and Child Health Nursing* (5th ed., p. 1051). Philadelphia: Lippincott Williams & Wilkins.

122. A nurse is evaluating teaching for a client who has diabetes and is beginning insulin therapy. Which behavior suggests that the teaching about medications was effective?

1. The nurse showing the client a video that explains the effects of insulin and mechanism of action
2. The client reading a handout that describes the different types of insulin
3. The nurse demonstrating the correct procedure for drawing medication from a vial
4. The client withdrawing insulin from the vial and injecting self correctly on the second attempt

ANSWER: 4

The client correctly demonstrating withdrawing and administering insulin suggests that the teaching about medication was effective. Options 1 and 3 are teaching strategies. Option 2 does not demonstrate that learning has occurred.

➧ ***Test-taking Tip:*** *Focus on what the question is asking. Select the option that best demonstrates that learning has occurred.*

Content Area: Management of Care; *Category of Health Alteration:* Teaching and Learning, Communication, and Cultural Diversity; *Integrated Processes:* Nursing Process Evaluation; *Client Need:* Health Promotion and Maintenance/Principles of Teaching and Learning; *Cognitive Level:* Application

Reference: Harkreader, H., Hogan, M., & Thobaben, M. (2007). *Fundamentals of Nursing* (3rd ed., p. 284). St. Louis, MO: Saunders/Elsevier.

123. A nurse performs discharge teaching for an elderly client who is fully dressed and watching a television program while waiting for family to arrive. The nurse sits in a chair facing the client and shows the client a handout. The client squints while reading the paper and periodically looks at the television. When the nurse is about to review the information and determine if the client understood the discharge instructions, the family enters the room. The nurse determines that there is need for further education due to barriers in learning. Which barriers have affected the client's ability to comprehend the discharge information? SELECT ALL THAT APPLY.

1. The client is watching a television program.
2. The client is elderly.
3. The client is fully dressed.
4. The client squints while reading the handout.
5. The family enters the room during teaching.

ANSWER: 1, 4, 5

The television is a distracter. The client squinting suggests that the lettering is too small or the client does not understand. The family entering the room is a distraction. Just because the client is elderly and fully dressed does not mean that the client cannot comprehend the information being taught. There is no statement indicating that the client may have a cognitive dysfunction.

➧ ***Test-taking Tip:*** *Focus on factors that could inhibit learning.*

Content Area: Management of Care; *Category of Health Alteration:* Teaching and Learning, Communication, and Cultural Diversity; *Integrated Processes:* Nursing Process Evaluation; *Client Need:* Health Promotion and Maintenance/Principles of Teaching and Learning; *Cognitive Level:* Analysis

Reference: Harkreader, H., Hogan, M., & Thobaben, M. (2007). *Fundamentals of Nursing* (3rd ed., pp. 280–281). St. Louis, MO: Saunders/Elsevier.

---

124. A nurse brings a client's morning medications and attempts to teach the client about the medications. The client says to the nurse, "Just tell my wife. She gives me all my pills." Which is the best response by the nurse?

1. "You also need to learn about your medications. What will you do if something happens to your wife?"
2. "Because your wife manages your medications, I will write out a list for her with instructions for how and when they should be given."
3. "Let me know when your wife will be visiting next and then I can go over the medications with both of you."
4. "This sounds like a good plan. You are fortunate to have a caring wife."

ANSWER: 3

Psychological and situational stressors can interfere with concentration and learning. If the wife will be administering the medications, then both the husband and wife should be included in the teaching. The statement in option 1 is nontherapeutic and inappropriate. While the nurse may also write out a list of medications for the client and his wife, option 2 is not the best option. Option 4 is not the best option because it does not involve the client in learning about his own medications.

➧ ***Test-taking Tip:*** *Focus on using both therapeutic communication techniques and principles of teaching and learning. Note the key word "best."*

Content Area: Management of Care; *Category of Health Alteration:* Teaching and Learning, Communication, and Cultural Diversity; *Integrated Processes:* Communication and Documentation; *Client Need:* Health Promotion and Maintenance/Self-Care; *Cognitive Level:* Application

Reference: Harkreader, H., Hogan, M., & Thobaben, M. (2007). *Fundamentals of Nursing* (3rd ed., pp. 271–272, 281). St. Louis, MO: Saunders/Elsevier.

---

125. A nurse is providing discharge teaching to a client who has recently been diagnosed with type 2 diabetes mellitus. Which steps should be taken by the nurse when teaching this client? Prioritize the nurse's actions by placing each step in the correct order.

______ Implement the teaching plan
______ Collect and analyze data about the client's knowledge of type 2 diabetes mellitus
______ Formulate an educational nursing diagnosis
______ Reassess as needed
______ Develop a teaching plan
______ Evaluate client learning based on the objectives
______ Identify learning needs

ANSWER: 5, 1, 3, 7, 4, 6, 2

The nurse should first collect and analyze data about the client's knowledge of type 2 diabetes mellitus. Next, the nurse should identify client-specific learning needs and formulate an educational nursing diagnosis. Examples of nursing diagnoses include deficient knowledge, ineffective health maintenance, or health-seeking behaviors. The nurse should then develop a teaching plan that includes objectives, content, time frame, and teaching format and methodology. Next, the nurse should implement the teaching plan and then evaluate client learning based on the objectives. Finally, the nurse should reassess the client as needed.

➧ ***Test-taking Tip:*** *The teaching process is similar to the nursing process. Use the steps of the nursing process to guide placing the options for teaching in the correct sequence.*

Content Area: Management of Care; *Category of Health Alteration:* Teaching and Learning, Communication, and Cultural Diversity; *Integrated Processes:* Nursing Process Planning; *Client Need:* Health Promotion and Maintenance/Principles of Teaching and Learning; *Cognitive Level:* Synthesis

Reference: Harkreader, H., Hogan, M., & Thobaben, M. (2007). *Fundamentals of Nursing* (3rd ed., p. 277). St. Louis, MO: Saunders/Elsevier.

126. A nurse is caring for a client who has been repeatedly hospitalized in hypertensive crisis for failing to take prescribed antihypertensive medications. The client states, "I stop taking the blood pressure medication when my blood pressure is okay because I can't afford the medications." Which nursing diagnosis is the best for the nurse to include in the client's plan of care?

1. Knowledge deficit related to medication actions
2. Ineffective health maintenance related to repeated hospital admissions
3. Ineffective therapeutic regimen management related to poor blood pressure control
4. Noncompliance related to the cost of medications

ANSWER: 4

The goal of client teaching should be considered before selecting a nursing diagnosis. Because the goal of teaching should be to remove barriers to complying with the treatment plan, the nursing diagnosis is noncompliance. Though options 1, 2, and 3 may be appropriate, option 4 is best because the client is not taking the medication due to its cost.

➧ ***Test-taking Tip:*** *The key word is "best." Focus on the information provided in the situation and match it with the second half of the nursing diagnosis to select the best option.*

Content Area: Management of Care; *Category of Health Alteration:* Teaching and Learning, Communication, and Cultural Diversity; *Integrated Processes:* Nursing Process Analysis; *Client Need:* Health Promotion and Maintenance/Principles of Teaching and Learning; *Cognitive Level:* Analysis

Reference: Harkreader, H., Hogan, M., & Thobaben, M. (2007). *Fundamentals of Nursing* (3rd ed., p. 282). St. Louis, MO: Saunders/Elsevier.

127. EBP A new nurse is planning to change a central-line dressing. An experienced nurse, who is assisting, asks the new nurse to describe the steps to be taken to complete the dressing change. Which statement by the new nurse would indicate that further teaching is needed?

1. "I will wash my hands before and after the dressing change."
2. "I will put on clean gloves prior to removing the dressing."
3. "I will ask the client to turn his or her face away from the dressing while I am changing it."
4. "I will cleanse the site with an antiseptic solution before applying the new dressing."

ANSWER: 2

The nurse should put on sterile gloves prior to removing the dressing on a central line to prevent contamination of the catheter and site. Once the dressing is removed, the nurse should don a new set of sterile gloves to complete the dressing change. The other statements are correct regarding the central line dressing change. Washing hands before and after the dressing change, asking the client to face away from the site, and cleaning the site with an antiseptic solution all limit the spread of microorganisms and are used to prevent catheter related bloodstream infections.

➧ ***Test-taking Tip:*** *The key words are "further teaching needed." Choose the statement that is incorrect.*

Content Area: Management of Care; *Category of Health Alteration:* Teaching and Learning, Communication, and Cultural Diversity; *Integrated Processes:* Nursing Process Evaluation; *Client Need:* Health Promotion and Maintenance/Principles of Teaching and Learning; *Cognitive Level:* Application

EBP Reference: Rupp, E., & Craig, R. (2004). Nosocomial infection: Prevention of central venous catheter related blood stream infections. *Infections in Medicine,* 21(3), 123–127.

128. A nurse is working in a clinic with a 16-year-old client who is in the first trimester of a pregnancy. While collecting information to complete the history form, the nurse learns that the client drinks four to six alcoholic beverages, three to four times a week. Based on the client's current developmental stage, what should be the nurse's *initial* focus of care?

1. Establishing a trusting relationship with the client
2. Educating the client about the risk for developing fetal alcohol syndrome
3. Informing the client about the personal health risks of continuing with excessive drinking
4. Seeking further information about her home life and the friends with whom she spends time

ANSWER: 1

According to Erikson's theory, the developmental task of adolescence (age 16) is "identity versus identity confusion." Adolescents are very egocentric, and peers are a strong influence. Because it is very important to be a part of a group, many will do whatever is necessary, believing that "nothing bad will ever happen" to them. The short-term effects of drinking with friends may far outweigh concerns about the physiological effects of alcohol on the fetus or her own body. Adolescents are quick to reject individuals who attempt to impose personal values on them and those whose interests appear ingenuous or are perceived to have little or no respect for their thoughts or ideas. Although options 2, 3, and 4 are topics for the future, only with a trusting relationship will the nurse be able to gather more data and provide education that can protect the fetus.

➧ ***Test-taking Tip:*** *The key word is "initial." Be cognizant of the client's developmental stage and how to best provide information that will impact future choices and protect the fetus.*

Content Area: Management of Care; *Category of Health Alteration:* Teaching and Learning, Communication, and Cultural Diversity; *Integrated Processes:* Communication and Documentation; *Client Need:* Health Promotion and Maintenance/Developmental Stages and Transitions; *Cognitive Level:* Analysis

References: Pillitteri, A. (2007). *Maternal and Child Health Nursing* (5th ed., p. 942). Philadelphia: Lippincott Williams & Wilkins; Hockenberry, M., & Wilson, D. (2007). *Wong's Nursing Care of Infants and Children* (8th ed., pp. 818–819). St. Louis, MO: Mosby/Elsevier.

129. A 5-year-old client has died due to internal injuries. One parent is rocking the child back and forth and sobbing, and the other parent is sitting nearby. Which is the best response by the nurse?

1. "I will certainly remember your child. What things will you recall when you think of him?"
2. "I know this is hard, so why don't you go spend some time alone while I prepare for the funeral director."
3. "Let me contact the physician to see if there is something that can be prescribed to help calm you."
4. "What can I do to help you say goodbye?"

ANSWER: 1

The death of a child is an extremely difficult event. Parents need time to say goodbye to the child and will need the assistance of the nurse to do so. Allowing reminiscence can facilitate parental coping and provide the parents with an opportunity to say goodbye. To rush the process will not give the parents time to comprehend what has happened. The nurse should be present in the room but be as unobtrusive as possible. The parents should be provided adequate time to understand that their child has died. Option 2 attempts to move the parents out of the room without consideration as to where the parents are in the process of saying goodbye. Option 3 is not appropriate because the parent's grief is real. Option 4 is acceptable because the nurse is there to support the parents; but typically grieving parents are unable to articulate what they need.

➧ ***Test-taking Tip:*** *The key word is "best." Select the option that responds to the parents' grief and provides support. Eliminate options 2 and 3 because the parents would be separated from the nurse. Eliminate option 4 because the focus is on the nurse rather than on the deceased child and his parents.*

Content Area: Management of Care; *Category of Health Alteration:* Teaching and Learning, Communication, and Cultural Diversity; *Integrated Processes:* Communication and Documentation; Caring; *Client Need:* Psychosocial Integrity/Grief and Loss; *Cognitive Level:* Analysis

References: Ball, J., & Binder, R. (2006). *Child Health Nursing: Partnering with Children and Families* (p. 718). Upper Saddle River, NJ: Pearson Education; Pillitteri, A. (2007). *Maternal and Child Health Nursing* (5th ed., pp. 1781–1782). Philadelphia: Lippincott Williams & Wilkins.

130. A nurse admits a client, who has a tracheostomy, to a medical unit. The client's spouse reports that the client does not use a speaking valve at home. A nurse is planning to assess the client and obtain a medical history of present symptoms. Which actions should be taken by the nurse to communicate with the client? SELECT ALL THAT APPLY.

1. Make eye contact and speak to the client directly
2. Only ask the spouse for information
3. Supply the client with a writing board
4. Place a Passy-Muir® speaking valve over the tracheostomy
5. Assess the client's preferred communication method
6. Ask the client only "yes" and "no" questions

ANSWER: 1, 3, 5

Making eye contact and speaking to the client directly convey an interest in the client and are essential to facilitate communication. Supplying the client with a writing board allows the client to answer and ask questions about care. Assessing the client's preferred communication method allows the client to participate in the development of the plan of care and shows that the client's needs are valued. Only asking the spouse information excludes the client from the conversation and does not facilitate trust between the nurse and client. Placing a Passy-Muir® speaking valve over the tracheostomy should not be done until the client has been assessed further for ability to tolerate cuff deflation without aspiration or respiratory distress. Asking the client only "yes" and "no" questions does not allow the client to provide any descriptions, can be frustrating for the client, and also does not allow the client to ask any questions.

➧ ***Test-taking Tip:*** *Eliminate the responses that do not encourage communication between client and nurse.*

Content Area: Management of Care; *Category of Health Alteration:* Teaching and Learning, Communication, and Cultural Diversity; *Integrated Processes:* Communication and Documentation; *Client Need:* Psychosocial Integrity/Therapeutic Communications; *Cognitive Level:* Application

Reference: Lewis, S., Heitkemper, M., Dirksen, S., O'Brien, P., & Bucher, L. (2007). *Medical-Surgical Nursing: Assessment and Management of Clinical Problems* (7th ed., pp. 580–581). St. Louis, MO: Mosby.

131. A nurse is having a conversation with a client who is beginning hemodialysis. How many different therapeutic communication techniques does the nurse use in conversing with the client?

Interaction Number	Interaction
1	Nurse: "Tell me what I can teach you about your dialysis treatments."
	Client: "I don't know much about it except what my doctor told me."
2	Nurse: "Maybe you can explain what the doctor told you so I can be more helpful."
	Client: "Since my kidneys aren't working I will need to go for treatments three times weekly."
3	Nurse: "What will it be like for you going for the treatments?"
	Client: "I don't know. My husband can't drive anymore with his failing eyesight."
4	Nurse: "Your husband can't drive anymore because of his failing eyesight?"
	Client: "That's right."
5	Nurse: "Oh." *Sits quietly.*
	Client: "I don't know how I'm going to get to the center for my treatments."
6	Nurse: "You should have one of your children drive you for treatments. You told me they live nearby."
	Client: "Both of my children work during the day."
7	Nurse: "Well, don't worry. I'll have a social worker make transportation arrangements."
	Client: "You are so kind."

1. One technique
2. Two techniques
3. Three techniques
4. Four techniques

ANSWER: 4

In interaction 1, the nurse uses a broad opening. In interaction 2, the nurse is asking for clarification. In interaction 3, the nurse is reflecting. In interaction 5, the nurse is using silence to allow time to think about what to say next or allow the client to further express concerns. The nurse uses nontherapeutic techniques in the remaining interaction. In interaction 4, the nurse is "parroting." If it were restating, the nurse would paraphrase the message back to the client. In interaction 6, the nurse is advising. In interaction 7, the nurse is belittling the client's feeling by telling her not to worry.

➧ ***Test-taking Tip:*** *The key word is "therapeutic." Eliminate the interactions in which the nurse uses nontherapeutic techniques and count the remaining options to determine the answer.*

Content Area: Management of Care; *Category of Health Alteration:* Teaching and Learning, Communication, and Cultural Diversity; *Integrated Processes:* Communication and Documentation; *Client Need:* Psychosocial Integrity/Therapeutic Communications; *Cognitive Level:* Analysis

Reference: Harkreader, H., Hogan, M., & Thobaben, M. (2007). *Fundamentals of Nursing* (3rd ed., pp. 266–272). St. Louis, MO: Saunders/Elsevier.

132. A clinic nurse is communicating with various clients during clinic visits. An observing nurse notices that the clinic nurse uses the therapeutic communication technique of reflection well. Which interaction did the observing nurse likely overhear that demonstrates the use of reflection?

1. *Child:* "Don't turn out the light. I don't like the dark." *Nurse:* "I will have your mommy hold you while I turn out the light to check your eye."
2. *Adolescent:* "My mom won't let me pierce my tongue." *Nurse:* "What would it be like to have a pierced tongue?"
3. *Adult:* "My blood sugar was really out of control yesterday." *Nurse:* "Was your blood sugar high or low yesterday?"
4. *Older Adult:* "My life means nothing anymore." *Nurse:* "Socializing more allows you to reflect back on the good times and will help you feel better about your life."

ANSWER: 2

In using reflection, the nurse selects one or two words said by the client to reflect back to the client for consideration. This technique strengthens client confidence. Option 1 is presenting reality, but offering support to the child to boost confidence in handling the dark. Option 3 seeks clarification. Option 4 demonstrates advising, a nontherapeutic communication technique.

***Test-taking Tip:** Focus on selecting the option in which the nurse uses the communication technique of reflection.*

Content Area: Management of Care; *Category of Health Alteration:* Teaching and Learning, Communication, and Cultural Diversity; *Integrated Processes:* Communication and Documentation; *Client Need:* Psychosocial Integrity/Therapeutic Communications; *Cognitive Level:* Analysis

Reference: Harkreader, H., Hogan, M., & Thobaben, M. (2007). *Fundamentals of Nursing* (3rd ed., pp. 266–269). St. Louis, MO: Saunders/Elsevier.

133. A nurse is completing a home-care visit with an elderly client who is ready to be discharged from home-care services. This is the nurse's last visit. Each time that the nurse attempts to leave, the client offers a new subject and attempts to delay the nurse's departure. Which is the best action by the nurse?

1. Abruptly tell the client that the session has ended and that the nurse must leave
2. Set up an appointment for an additional home-care visit
3. Plan to meet the client for coffee the following Sunday
4. Be firm and clear about the termination of the relationship and solicit feedback from the client

ANSWER: 4

Being firm and clear about the termination of the relationship maintains professional boundaries, while soliciting feedback helps the client maintain a positive attitude about the interaction. Abruptly telling the client that the session has ended does not leave room for feedback from the client and may also leave the client with negative feelings about the interaction. The client may feel as though he or she did or said something wrong to cause the nurse to leave abruptly. Setting up an additional home-care visit only prolongs the termination phase and may allow the client to become manipulating. Planning to meet the client for a social visit is inappropriate and may violate professional and ethical codes of conduct.

***Test-taking Tip:** Read each response carefully and select the response that allows for termination of the interaction while maintaining a positive interaction.*

Content Area: Management of Care; *Category of Health Alteration:* Teaching and Learning, Communication and Cultural Diversity; *Integrated Processes:* Communication and Documentation; *Client Need:* Psychosocial Integrity/Therapeutic Communications; *Cognitive Level:* Analysis

Reference: Craven, R., & Hirnle, C. (2007). *Fundamentals of Nursing: Human Health and Function* (5th ed., p. 369). Philadelphia: Lippincott Williams & Wilkins.

134. An experienced nurse overhears four conversations between a new nurse and a client. Which exhibit best demonstrates active listening by the new nurse when communicating with the client?

Client A

Client: "I just learned I have cancer."
Nurse: "I wonder how you are feeling about this." *Leans forward with a concerned expression.*
Client: "I'm afraid I will die."
Nurse: "Dying feels like a real possibility to you."
Client: "My dad died of cancer when I was 9 and my son is 9 years old."
Nurse: "The age similarities seem especially worrisome for you."

Client B

Client: "My doctor told me I need a transplant."
Nurse: "I see."
Client: "I'm afraid there won't be a donor in time."
Nurse: "Hmm. Maybe a family member will be a tissue match."
Client: "I doubt it. I have a small family."
Nurse: "Don't be discouraged. Usually an organ is available in time."

Client C

Client: "I just want to go home."
Nurse: "Tell me what you know about caring for your incision at home."
Client: "I don't want to talk about that now; my family is waiting to take me home."
Nurse: "Then let's review the hip precautions and your medications before you leave."
Client: "My family is in a hurry. I don't have time for this."
Nurse: "Okay. Here are the materials you need to read when you get home."

Client D

Client: "It's no use; I just can't seem to lose weight."
Nurse: "You seem pretty discouraged."
Client: "Oh, I am! Nothing works."
Nurse: "Have you thought about joining Weight Watchers?"
Client: "That's one of the things I have tried. Do you think a gastric bypass is a good idea?"
Nurse: "For some people. You should ask your physician about it."

1. Client A
2. Client B
3. Client C
4. Client D

ANSWER: 1

Active listening involves the use of verbal cues, nonverbal cues, and therapeutic communication techniques. Nonverbal cues are lacking in the interactions with clients B, C, and D.

➧ ***Test-taking Tip:*** *Recall that active listening also includes nonverbal cues.*

Content Area: Management of Care; *Category of Health Alteration:* Teaching and Learning, Communication, and Cultural Diversity; *Integrated Processes:* Communication and Documentation; *Client Need:* Psychosocial Integrity/Therapeutic Communications; *Cognitive Level:* Analysis

Reference: Harkreader, H., Hogan, M., & Thobaben, M. (2007). *Fundamentals of Nursing* (3rd ed., pp. 266–269). St. Louis, MO: Saunders/Elsevier.

135. A nurse is setting up supplies to complete a dressing change at 2000 hours on a client's stump following a below-the-knee amputation of the right leg. The client looks away and angrily says, "I don't want to look at that thing. Can't you come back later?" Which is the best action by the nurse?

1. Putting the supplies away and reattempt the dressing change in 1 hour
2. Completing the dressing change because it is ordered for 2000
3. Asking the client, "Why don't you want your dressing changed?"
4. Restating to the client, "You don't want to look at your leg?" and allow time for a response

ANSWER: 4

Restating to the client provides an opportunity for the client to clarify further and encourages discussion of the client's feelings about their amputation. Putting the supplies away and reattempting in 1 hour avoids discussing the client's feelings about the amputation when the client is clearly upset and the opportunity is there for establishing a relationship. Completing the dressing change despite the client's request, because it is ordered for 2000, takes the control away from the client and violates any trust between nurse and client. Asking the client a why question can be interrogating and does not address the client's feelings about the amputation.

***Test-taking Tip:** Eliminate the answers that do not promote communication between the nurse and client.*

Content Area: Management of Care; *Category of Health Alteration:* Teaching and Learning, Communication, and Cultural Diversity; *Integrated Processes:* Communication and Documentation; *Client Need:* Psychosocial Integrity/Therapeutic Communications; *Cognitive Level:* Analysis

Reference: Craven, R., & Hirnle, C. (2007). *Fundamentals of Nursing: Human Health and Function* (5th ed., p. 376). Philadelphia: Lippincott Williams & Wilkins.

136. A new nurse is told by experienced unit nurses that the nurse manager is an empowering manager. Which statements made by the nurse manager should lead the new nurse to agree with the experienced nurses' opinions? SELECT ALL THAT APPLY.

1. "You hardly ever complete your documentation during work hours. I'll have the charge nurse work on making better assignments for you."
2. "The team worked well together on the pain documentation project. Through your efforts, there were improvements in client satisfaction scores for pain control on client surveys."
3. "I observed that you managed all your clients' care today, but most days you stay overtime to complete the documentation. Is there something we can do to help you accomplish the expected goal of completing all duties within the scheduled work time?"
4. "The charge nurse told me that you didn't complete some of your client care today. What was the problem?"
5. "We are at peak census. For the next shift, I need one more nurse than usual. Our options include a volunteer, calling in an off-duty staff, or mandating someone. Is there a volunteer?"
6. "I've arranged for a new staffing schedule because no one working part-time will volunteer for extra shifts and administration won't allow me to pay nurses overtime anymore."

ANSWER: 2, 3, 5

The statements in options 2, 3, and 5 are empowering because the nurse manager's statements indicate personal ownership of beliefs, values, and needs while communicating expectations about values and goals. The nurse manager uses a variation of "I want" or "I need" rather than "you must" or "you didn't." Options 1, 4, and 6 are not empowering statements because each statement uses a variation of "you didn't."

***Test-taking Tip:** Recall that empowering means giving power to another person. Read each option carefully to determine if the nurse manager's statements give power to the nurse or staff.*

Content Area: Management of Care; *Category of Health Alteration:* Teaching and Learning, Communication, and Cultural Diversity; *Integrated Processes:* Nursing Process Evaluation; *Client Need:* Safe and Effective Care Environment/Management of Care/Concepts of Management; *Cognitive Level:* Analysis

Reference: Harkreader, H., Hogan, M., & Thobaben, M. (2007). *Fundamentals of Nursing* (3rd ed., pp. 297–298). St. Louis, MO: Saunders/Elsevier.

137. A registered nurse (RN), working on a telemetry unit for 2 years, is discharged for jeopardizing client safety by consistently failing to notify the physician when the health status of a client has changed. The RN applies at another health-care facility and the facility calls the nurse manager for a reference check. Which statement by the nurse manager is most appropriate?

1. "The RN resigned due to safety concerns such as failure to notify the physician when the health status of clients changed."
2. "The RN is uncomfortable communicating with physicians. Otherwise, the nurse's work meets standards of care."
3. "I need to consult with the hospital attorney to determine if any information can be provided."
4. "The nurse worked at this facility on the telemetry unit for 2 years but was discharged."

ANSWER: 4

Only factual information should be provided. The former employee has not consented to provide additional information. Option 1 is incorrect information. The RN was discharged. Option 2 suggests that the employee's failure to notify is related to discomfort with communication which could be an incorrect conclusion. Option 3 is inappropriate. The nurse manager should know the policies of the agency.

➧ ***Test-taking Tip:*** *Select the option that provides the most factual information.*

Content Area: Management of Care; *Category of Health Alteration:* Teaching and Learning, Communication, and Cultural Diversity; *Integrated Processes:* Communication and Documentation; *Client Need:* Safe and Effective Care Environment/Management of Care/Legal Rights and Responsibilities; *Cognitive Level:* Analysis

Reference: Catalano, J. (2006). *Nursing Now! Today's Issues, Tomorrow's Trends* (4th ed., p. 227). Philadelphia: F. A. Davis.

138. EBP A charge nurse informs a nurse manager that a new nurse is demonstrating strong, caring behaviors when providing care to clients. Which actions by the new nurse resulted in the charge nurse making this conclusion? SELECT ALL THAT APPLY.

1. Carefully performed procedures according to agency policy and guarded against client harm
2. Clocked in and out on time during assigned shifts
3. Demonstrated concern for the client and ensured that client needs are met
4. Remained optimistic when caring for a verbally abusive client
5. Supported family members when one of the new nurse's clients died
6. Volunteered to serve on a unit committee completing chart audits

ANSWER: 1, 3, 4, 5

Caring embodies human service to another person and encompasses "taking care of" the needs of another, a caring emotion or attitude, and caution in the performance of duties. Brilowski and Wendler (2005) also suggested that the core attributes of caring are relationship, action, attitude, acceptance, and variability. Options 2 and 5 do not demonstrate human service to another person.

➧ ***Test-taking Tip:*** *Think about human service behaviors when selecting correct options. Eliminate options that do not include service to another person.*

Content Area: Management of Care; *Category of Health Alteration:* Teaching and Learning, Communication, and Cultural Diversity; *Integrated Processes:* Caring; *Client Need:* Safe and Effective Care Environment/Management of Care/Ethical Practice; *Cognitive Level:* Analysis

Reference: Harkreader, H., Hogan, M., & Thobaben, M. (2007). *Fundamentals of Nursing* (3rd ed., pp. 81–83). St. Louis, MO: Saunders/Elsevier.

EBP Reference: Brilowski, G., & Wendler, M. (2005). An evolutionary concept analysis of caring. *Journal of Advanced Nursing,* 50(6), 641–650.

139. A pediatric nurse is providing a change-of-shift report to an oncoming shift nurse for a client diagnosed with gastroenteritis. Which information should the nurse include in a typical shift report? SELECT ALL THAT APPLY.

1. Client name and room number
2. Brief medical history of the current problem
3. Client-family dynamics and client psychosocial concerns
4. Surgery, tests, or procedures for the next 24 hours
5. New orders completed and those remaining
6. The client's satisfaction with the nurse's care that shift
7. The status of tubes and intravenous (IV) infusions
8. The telephone number of the nurse giving report if questions arise

ANSWER: 1, 2, 3, 4, 5, 7

Information to include in shift report includes the name, room number, physician, and date of admission or date of surgery; medical diagnosis or surgery performed; brief medical history of the current problem; surgery tests or procedures scheduled for the next 24 hours; vital signs or abnormal findings; information reported to the physician; tube and equipment status, including IVs; treatments; assistance needed with activities of daily living; new orders, special problems; needed teaching; and family/client dynamics. Additionally, some agencies include an evaluation of how the client is progressing on the plan of care. A typical end-of-shift report does not include the client's satisfaction with the nurse's care and telephone numbers of where the nurse can be reached. The nurse's work is done with the client when responsibility for the care of the client is passed to another nurse.

➧ ***Test-taking Tip:*** *The key word is "typical."*

Content Area: Management of Care; *Category of Health Alteration:* Teaching and Learning, Communication, and Cultural Diversity; *Integrated Processes:* Communication and Documentation; *Client Need:* Safe and Effective Care Environment/Management of Care/Continuity of Care; *Cognitive Level:* Synthesis

Reference: Harkreader, H., Hogan, M., & Thobaben, M. (2007). *Fundamentals of Nursing* (3rd ed., p. 300). St. Louis, MO: Saunders/Elsevier.

140. A nurse manager, reviewing the electronic medical record for a client who fell, notes that an employed licensed practical nurse (LPN) documented in the client's medical record on a day that the LPN was not scheduled to work. The nurse manager determines that, on that day, the LPN was attending the registered nursing program and assigned to care for the client as a registered nurse student. Based on this information, which action should the nurse manager take?

1. Report the incident to the student's clinical instructor and request that the clinical instructor assist the LPN in making the correction
2. Instruct the LPN to make the correction
3. Discuss the incident with the LPN and advise the LPN to leave the medical record untouched because it is a legal document
4. Advise the LPN to delete the incorrect entry and use the registered student nurse log-in ID to re-enter the information
5. Make a notation in the client's medical record that the LPN was functioning in the registered nurse student role when the client fell

ANSWER: 1

While in the student nurse role, the LPN is not considered an employee of the agency. The clinical instructor is responsible for clinical supervision. Options 2, 3, and 4 involve the nurse manager instructing or advising the LPN. Although the LPN should be instructed to make a correction entry, the person discussing the incident with the LPN should be the clinical instructor. The nurse manager should not make a notation in the client's medical record, but should complete an incident (unusual occurrence) report because the nurse manager found the documentation error.

➧ ***Test-taking Tip:*** *First look at the options that are opposite and then eliminate either one or both of these. Then read each option carefully. Think carefully about who was providing supervision in the situation.*

Content Area: Management of Care; *Category of Health Alteration:* Teaching and Learning, Communication, and Cultural Diversity; *Integrated Processes:* Communication and Documentation; *Client Need:* Safe and Effective Care Environment/Management of Care/Information Technology; *Cognitive Level:* Analysis

References: Berman, A., Snyder, S., Kozier, B., & Erb, G. (2008). *Fundamentals of Nursing: Concepts, Process, and Practice* (8th ed., pp. 74–75). Upper Saddle River, NJ: Pearson Education; Harkreader, H., Hogan, M., & Thobaben, M. (2007). *Fundamentals of Nursing* (3rd ed., pp. 251–253). St. Louis, MO: Saunders/Elsevier.

141. EBP A new nurse is being oriented to the electronic medical record (EMR) on a nursing unit. Which points should be included in the new nurse's orientation session? SELECT ALL THAT APPLY.

1. Any entries into the computer will be credited to the person who is logged into the computer
2. Leaving a computer without first logging off can be a breach of client confidentiality
3. Orders entered into the computer system can enhance work flow
4. For the experienced EMR user, the EMR enhances time efficiency and accuracy of data
5. If data are entered incorrectly, the entry can be opened and edited, thus keeping the original date.
6. Most agencies using EMR incorporate a system for tracking computer printouts

ANSWER: 1, 2, 3, 4, 6

The log-in access includes an electronic signature with the name of the person to whom the log-in access is assigned. Information displayed on the monitor can be viewed by others. Orders entered in the EMR are automatically routed to the correct departments. Studies have shown that EMR enhances time efficiency, direct client-care time, user satisfaction, accuracy of data, and completeness of the medical record. Both computer printouts and log-ins are tracked by most agencies. Computer printouts are tracked to prevent indiscriminate duplication or distribution. Entered data cannot be changed; incorrect entries are noted by making a correction entry. The date of the entry will be the log-in date at the time of the correction entry.

➧ ***Test-taking Tip:*** *Read each option carefully and think about whether these could be features on an EMR.*

Content Area: Management of Care; *Category of Health Alteration:* Teaching and Learning, Communication, and Cultural Diversity; *Integrated Processes:* Communication and Documentation; *Client Need:* Safe and Effective Care Environment/Management of Care/Information Technology; *Cognitive Level:* Synthesis

Reference: Harkreader, H., Hogan, M., & Thobaben, M. (2007). *Fundamentals of Nursing* (3rd ed., pp. 236, 251–254). St. Louis, MO: Saunders/Elsevier.

EBP Reference: Bakken, S. (2006). Informatics for patient safety: A nursing research perspective. *Annual Review of Nursing Research*, 24, 219–254.

142. A nurse is preparing teaching materials for highly educated, self-directed adult clients on a cardiac step-down unit at a major medical center. Which methods of instruction should the nurse consider when preparing the instruction materials? SELECT ALL THAT APPLY.

1. Computer-assisted instruction
2. Videotapes
3. Closed-circuit television programs
4. Group sessions presented by hospitalized clients
5. Printed materials for handouts
6. Poster boards strategically placed on the unit

ANSWER: 1, 2, 3, 5, 6

The teaching methods depend on the subject matter and the client's background, personality, and needs. Computer-assisted instruction, videotapes, closed-circuit television programs, handouts, and poster boards allow motivated, self-directed learners to learn at their own pace. Professionals should lead group sessions and not hospitalized clients who are in the hospital for health reasons.

➧ ***Test-taking Tip:*** *Read each option carefully. Consider that many health-care facilities have computer capabilities.*

Content Area: Management of Care; *Category of Health Alteration:* Teaching and Learning, Communication, and Cultural Diversity; *Integrated Processes:* Communication and Documentation; *Client Need:* Safe and Effective Care Environment/Management of Care/Information Technology; *Cognitive Level:* Synthesis

Reference: Harkreader, H., Hogan, M., & Thobaben, M. (2007). *Fundamentals of Nursing* (3rd ed., pp. 236, 251–254). St. Louis, MO: Saunders/Elsevier.

---

143. An experienced nurse is orienting a new nurse to essential documentation when caring for clients through a home health-care agency. Which statement should be made by the experienced nurse regarding home health documentation?

1. "During each visit, an assessment is performed and then documented similarly to hospital documentation."
2. "Your documentation must show the need for professional medical services."
3. "Reimbursements for visits are directly related to the accuracy and wording of documentation."
4. "The assistance you provide with activities of daily living (ADLs) can be documented on a flowsheet."

ANSWER: 3

With each visit, the need for a professional nurse must be noted. Reimbursement for a visit is directly related to the documentation showing a need for professional assistance. Documentation is often different from an acute-care facility because of the need to justify the visit by a professional nurse. Nurses justify the need for nursing, not medical services. A professional nurse would not be performing ADLs during a visit. These are completed by a home health aid.

➧ ***Test-taking Tip:*** *Think about how home health nursing differs from acute-care nursing.*

Content Area: Management of Care; *Category of Health Alteration:* Teaching and Learning, Communication, and Cultural Diversity; *Integrated Processes:* Communication and Documentation; *Client Need:* Safe and Effective Care Environment/Management of Care/Continuity of Care; *Cognitive Level:* Application

Reference: Harkreader, H., Hogan, M., & Thobaben, M. (2007). *Fundamentals of Nursing* (3rd ed., pp. 242–243). St. Louis, MO: Saunders/Elsevier.

---

144. A nurse makes a documentation error by documenting the wrong vital signs (VS) in a client's written medical record. Which procedure should the nurse follow to correct the error?

1. Draw a line through the error, initial and date the line, and then document a corrected entry.
2. Circle the error and note above the error that it was an incorrect entry, and then date and initial the entry.
3. Use a highlighter to highlight the error, write the correct VS above the entry, and date and initial the line.
4. Cover the incorrect VS with the correct VS in such a manner that these are clearly readable.

ANSWER: 1

Agency policy should be followed for correcting a documentation error. Common policies include drawing a single line through the entry, dating and initialing the entry, then adding the correct information. Writing void in the space above the entry is sometimes included in agency policy. While agency policy may include circling the error, option 2 does not include entering the correct vital signs. If medical records are copied for any reason, the highlighted information may not show up as being highlighted. Writing over (covering) an existing entry is not permitted because of the implication of covering up an error or mistake.

➧ ***Test-taking Tip:*** *Read each option carefully and determine which option would both correct the error and include the correct information.*

Content Area: Management of Care; *Category of Health Alteration:* Teaching and Learning, Communication, and Cultural Diversity; *Integrated Processes:* Communication and Documentation; *Client Need:* Safe and Effective Care Environment/Management of Care/Continuity of Care; *Cognitive Level:* Application

Reference: Harkreader, H., Hogan, M., & Thobaben, M. (2007). *Fundamentals of Nursing* (3rd ed., p. 235). St. Louis, MO: Saunders/Elsevier.

145. A client is admitted to a neurological unit with a suspected stroke. What information should the nurse include in the admission note documentation? SELECT ALL THAT APPLY.

1. Client's assigned room number and orientation to the room
2. Admitting diagnosis
3. Nurse's assessment findings or reference to a flowsheet assessment
4. Allergies
5. That the client is wearing a 1-carat diamond ring
6. Physician who was notified of client's admission

ANSWER: 1, 2, 3, 4, 6

All listed elements, except the description of the ring, should be included in an admission note entry. Additional information should include any laboratory work or orders that have been completed, such as intravenous fluids initiated, teaching completed, and psychosocial information about the family or significant others and their presence. Valuables such as jewelry should be described in general terms, such as a "yellow ring with a clear stone."

➧ ***Test-taking Tip:*** *An admit note is the first note acknowledging the arrival of a new client. It should be one of the most complete documentations to ensure continuity of care.*

Content Area: Management of Care; *Category of Health Alteration:* Teaching and Learning, Communication, and Cultural Diversity; *Integrated Processes:* Communication and Documentation; *Client Need:* Safe and Effective Care Environment/Management of Care/Continuity of Care; *Cognitive Level:* Application

Reference: Harkreader, H., Hogan, M., & Thobaben, M. (2007). *Fundamentals of Nursing* (3rd ed., pp. 236–237). St. Louis, MO: Saunders/Elsevier.

---

146. **EBP** A client who does not speak or understand English has an interpreter at the bedside assisting a nurse with an admission interview and assessment. Which action is most appropriate for the nurse while utilizing the interpreter?

1. Asking the questions directly to the interpreter
2. Asking the questions directly to the client
3. Asking the interpreter to step out of the room while completing the physical assessment
4. Allowing the interpreter to rephrase questions and responses instead of interpreting each word

ANSWER: 2

Asking the questions directly to the client allows the client and nurse to develop a relationship and allows the client to feel included in their plan of care. Asking the questions directly to the interpreter excludes the client and may make the client feel that his or her statements are unimportant. The nurse should not ask the interpreter to step out of the room while doing a physical assessment because the nurse would need to ask the client questions and explain directions to the client. The client should also be allowed to ask questions during the physical assessment. The interpreter should not be allowed to rephrase questions and responses as it may change the meanings of the response and may also provide inaccurate information.

➧ ***Test-taking Tip:*** *Eliminate the responses that decrease the client's ability to be active in the conversation.*

Content Area: Management of Care; *Category of Health Alteration:* Teaching and Learning, Communication, and Cultural Diversity; *Integrated Processes:* Communication and Documentation; *Client Need:* Psychosocial Integrity/Therapeutic Communications; *Cognitive Level:* Application

EBP Reference: Lehna, C. (2005). Interpreter services in pediatric nursing. *Pediatric Nursing,* 31(4), 292–296.

147. EBP A nurse is working in an emergency department when a Hmong family arrives with a sick child. Upon examination, the nurse sees the markings illustrated on the child's back. Which interpretation of the clinical finding is correct?

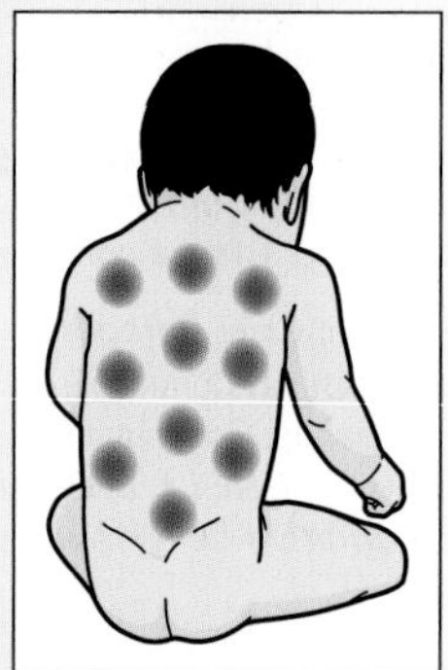

1. Consistent with findings of abuse and should be reported immediately
2. Consistent with cultural practices but need to be reported as possible abuse
3. Insignificant because they are not related to the infant's illness
4. Consistent with the practice of coining

ANSWER: 4

The Hmong practice alternative forms of medicine for illnesses, including coining. Coining involves rubbing heated oil on the skin and then vigorously rubbing a coin over the area until a red mark is seen. Coining is believed to allow a path by which a "bad wind" (cause of the illness) can be released from the body. Coining has led to false reporting of child abuse because the practice does leave marks. The marks are significant because it provides information to the nurse about the use of alternative forms of medicine.

➧ ***Test-taking Tip:*** *Apply knowledge of alternative forms of medicine.*

Content Area: Management of Care; *Category of Health Alteration:* Teaching and Learning, Communication, and Cultural Diversity; *Integrated Processes:* Nursing Process Analysis; *Client Need:* Psychosocial Integrity/Cultural Diversity; *Cognitive Level:* Application

EBP References: University of Hawaii. (2004). *Brief Overview of Hmong Culture.* Available at: www.hawaii.edu/hivandaids/brief_overview_of_hmong_culture.pdf; Clinics and Departments: Resources and Educational Materials, Children's Hospitals and Clinics of Minnesota (2007). *Cultural and Medical Traditions.* Available at: http://xpedio02.childrensmn.org/stellent/groups/public@xcp/@web/@clinicsanddepts/documents/policyreferenceprocedure/web025019.asp

148. While assessing a Chinese American male who had Billroth I surgery for gastric cancer 2 days ago, a nurse observes the client grimace and moan in pain when moving. The nurse's planned intervention should be based on the knowledge that Chinese culture expects:

1. clients to utilize only Chinese medications.
2. that a person will exert self-control at all times.
3. that the female member of the family determines when and if medications are needed.
4. that suffering must be endured for healing to occur.

ANSWER: 2

The teachings of Confucius are very important in Chinese culture. Confucianism teaches self-control and self-reliance. Nursing interventions should address the health concern while allowing the client to maintain self-control. Chinese Americans will use both Western and Eastern medicine. Husbands and elders have authority over wives and children. Suffering is not considered to be of primary importance for healing.

➧ ***Test-taking Tip:*** *Focus on the specific norms of the Chinese culture.*

Content Area: Management of Care; *Category of Health Alteration:* Teaching and Learning, Communication, and Cultural Diversity; *Integrated Processes:* Nursing Process Planning; *Client Need:* Psychosocial Integrity/Cultural Diversity; *Cognitive Level:* Application

Reference: Harkreader, H., Hogan, M., & Thobaben, M. (2007). *Fundamentals of Nursing* (3rd ed., pp. 54–56). St. Louis, MO: Saunders/Elsevier.

149. A nurse is planning care for multiple clients who have various cultural and religious beliefs. Which clients have cultural and religious beliefs characteristic of their cultures that may pose a potential conflict with the dominant American health-care system? SELECT ALL THAT APPLY.

1. A Native American woman who values large body size
2. The spouse of a terminally ill Hispanic client who refuses to allow health-care personnel to inform the client of the prognosis
3. A client of Jehovah's Witness faith who will not accept blood transfusions
4. A client who is an Orthodox Sikhs who refuses to have any body hair cut or shaved
5. An Amish client who wants to wait until the community has had prayer before giving consent for surgery
6. A client from the Hopi nation who wants to wear a scapula for spiritual protection

ANSWER: 1, 2, 3, 4, 5

Native American women value large body size and may be resistant to weight control. The family of Hispanics and Asians may prevent informing a client of the diagnosis or prognosis, which can impact whether the client is able to receive hospice care. Members of the Jehovah's Witness faith do not accept blood transfusions, which can affect their need to receive emergency treatment. Orthodox Sikhs do not cut their hair, which can conflict with the need to shave the skin for medical procedures. The Amish bishop and healers are consulted about a member's hospitalization for prayer for healing. A member of the Hopi nation may wear a thunderbird for spiritual protection and good luck. A person of the Catholic faith may wear a scapula.

➧ ***Test-taking Tip:*** *Examine each cultural or religious group and determine whether these are practices or beliefs of that group.*

Content Area: Management of Care; *Category of Health Alteration:* Teaching and Learning, Communication, and Cultural Diversity; *Integrated Processes:* Nursing Process Planning; *Client Need:* Psychosocial Integrity/Cultural Diversity; *Cognitive Level:* Analysis

Reference: Harkreader, H., Hogan, M., & Thobaben, M. (2007). *Fundamentals of Nursing* (3rd ed., pp. 54–56). St. Louis, MO: Saunders/Elsevier.

150. A married woman, who upholds Amish beliefs and practices, is brought to a hospital in an ambulance after being hit by a car. In caring for the woman, an emergency nurse should do which of the following? SELECT ALL THAT APPLY.

1. Select the newest, brightly colored gown available for the woman
2. Speak to both the husband and client regarding health-care decisions
3. Consider that the woman will most likely have group insurance coverage
4. Anticipate that the church bishop will be consulted about the woman's hospitalization
5. Ask about alternative health-care practices including the use of healers, herbs, and massage
6. Provide a videotape about care after discharge for the client and spouse to view at home

ANSWER: 2, 4, 5

Speaking to both the husband and wife regarding health-care decisions is necessary because they consider themselves partners in family life. The bishop and community members are consulted regarding hospitalization because the community pays for its cost. The Amish use both traditional health care and alternative health care. A simple, plain gown should be selected. Amish women avoid vanity and dress in handmade, unadorned clothing. Usually, Amish choose not to have health insurance because it may suggest a lack of faith in God's healing power. A videotape would not be useful. Many Amish reject materialism and worldliness, avoiding technology, such as electricity and television.

➧ ***Test-taking Tip:*** *Focus on the issue: respecting cultural and religious beliefs of an Amish client.*

Content Area: Management of Care; *Category of Health Alteration:* Teaching and Learning, Communication, and Cultural Diversity; *Integrated Processes:* Nursing Process Implementation; *Client Need:* Psychosocial Integrity/Cultural Diversity; *Cognitive Level:* Analysis

References: Berman, A., Snyder, S., Kozier, B., & Erb, G. (2008). *Fundamentals of Nursing: Concepts, Process, and Practice* (8th ed., p. 1052). Upper Saddle River, NJ: Pearson Education; Harkreader, H., Hogan, M., & Thobaben, M. (2007). *Fundamentals of Nursing* (3rd ed., p. 960). St. Louis, MO: Saunders/Elsevier.

151. A nurse is caring for a Hispanic-American client who has just been diagnosed with gallbladder cancer. The nurse plans interventions that would provide emotional support and comfort for this client. As part of the plan of care, the nurse should:

1. offer to pray with the client.
2. offer to open the window in the hospital room to allow fresh air to enter.
3. ask the client to describe thoughts about the external cause of this illness.
4. not mention the diagnosis unless the client discusses it first.

ANSWER: 1

During times of crisis, Hispanic Americans turn to religion and prayer. Chinese Americans emphasize maintaining harmonious relationships with the environment and they believe fresh air is important. Native Americans do not subscribe to the germ theory and believe illness is a result of some external cause. Irish Americans may cope with illness by using denial for a time and may want to ignore the diagnosis initially.

➧ ***Test-taking Tip:*** *Recall the connection of Hispanic Americans to the Catholic faith and religious beliefs.*

Content Area: Management of Care; *Category of Health Alteration:* Teaching and Learning, Communication, and Cultural Diversity; *Integrated Processes:* Nursing Process Planning; *Client Need:* Psychosocial Integrity/Coping Mechanisms; *Cognitive Level:* Analysis

References: Berman, A., Snyder, S., Kozier, B., & Erb, G. (2008). *Fundamentals of Nursing: Concepts, Process, and Practice* (8th ed., pp. 315–318). Upper Saddle River, NJ: Pearson Education; Harkreader, H., Hogan, M., & Thobaben, M. (2007). *Fundamentals of Nursing* (3rd ed., pp. 52–56). St. Louis, MO: Saunders/Elsevier.

152. A nurse is admitting a client who is in labor with her first child. The client states that she was born in Somalia. When performing a cultural assessment, what should be the nurse's *first* action?

1. Ask the client about any particular ethnic or religious beliefs that could impact care
2. Obtain the client's vital signs and compare them against the norm for people from Somalia
3. Request that the spouse be present in the room when interviewing the woman
4. Document any cultural remedies that the client currently uses

ANSWER: 1

An initial action in performing a cultural assessment is to determine whether the client identifies with any cultural group or has particular ethnic or religious beliefs that could impact care. The normal vital sign ranges are standard among all ethnic groups. In some ethnic groups, the male speaks for the woman. Asking the spouse to be present may be appropriate if the client does identify with ethnic or religious beliefs of a particular culture. Documenting cultural remedies is important but not the first action.

➧ ***Test-taking Tip:*** *The key word is "first." Obtaining a brief history is the initial component in performing a physical assessment.*

Content Area: Management of Care; *Category of Health Alteration:* Teaching and Learning, Communication, and Cultural Diversity; *Integrated Processes:* Nursing Process Assessment; *Client Need:* Psychosocial Integrity/Cultural Diversity; *Cognitive Level:* Application

Reference: Lewis, S., Heitkemper, M., Dirksen, S., O'Brien, P., & Bucher, L. (2007). *Medical-Surgical Nursing: Assessment and Management of Clinical Problems* (7th ed., p. 29). St. Louis, MO: Mosby.

Chapter Six

Safety and Infection Control: Fundamental Concepts of Nursing

Test 5: Fundamentals: Basic Care and Comfort

153. A nurse is discussing hearing aids with a client who began wearing hearing aids 5 weeks earlier. Which statement demonstrates that the client is successfully adapting to the hearing aids?

1. "I just wear the hearing aids when I go out in public."
2. "I take a cotton-tipped swab and clean out my ear canals before I insert the hearing aids."
3. "I store the hearing aids in the protective box."
4. "I use mild soap and water weekly to soak the plastic parts of the hearing aids after I remove the batteries."

ANSWER: 3

Hearing aids are expensive and delicate, and they should be stored in a protective container in a dry safe place. Clients should adjust to hearing aids by wearing them on a daily basis and by gradually increasing the wearing time. Noisy public situations are difficult for persons with hearing aids in many circumstances. Small objects including cotton-tipped swabs should not be inserted into any person's ear canal due to possible injury and infection. Hearing aids should be kept dry except when cleaning the ear mold with mild soap and water.

Test-taking Tip: *The key phrase in the stem is "successfully adapting to the hearing aids," and the question calls for a true response. Read the stem carefully and consider the criteria for the use and care of hearing aids.*

Content Area: Fundamentals; *Category of Health Alteration:* Basic Care and Comfort; *Integrated Processes:* Nursing Process Evaluation; *Client Need:* Physiological Integrity/Basic Care and Comfort/Assistive Devices; *Cognitive Level:* Analysis

Reference: Ignatavicius, D., & Workman, M. (2006). *Medical-Surgical Nursing: Critical Thinking for Collaborative Care* (5th ed., pp. 1137–1138). St. Louis, MO: Elsevier/Saunders.

---

154. A nurse is caring for a client who is unable to perform oral hygiene. The client has dentures, including both upper and lower plates. Which technique should the nurse use to correctly perform oral hygiene for this client?

1. Don sterile gloves before removing the dentures.
2. Use a foam swab to pry the upper plate loose before removing it.
3. Loosen the upper plate by grasping it at the front teeth with a piece of gauze and moving the plate up and down to loosen it prior to removal.
4. Leave the dentures in the client's mouth and use a toothbrush to brush the plates.

ANSWER: 3

Grasping the upper plate and moving it breaks the suction that holds the plate on the roof of the client's mouth. Removing denture plates is a clean procedure and sterile gloves are not necessary. Removing the upper plate with a foam swab to pry the plate could injure the client. Dentures must be removed to properly clean the client's mouth and the dentures.

Test-taking Tip: *Visualize the procedure of removing the dentures and performing oral hygiene on a client. Consider each option and evaluate whether it is consistent with the correct procedure. Use the process of elimination to rule out incorrect options.*

Content Area: Fundamentals; *Category of Health Alteration:* Basic Care and Comfort; *Integrated Processes:* Nursing Process Planning; *Client Need:* Physiological Integrity/Basic Care and Comfort/Personal Hygiene; *Cognitive Level:* Application

Reference: Berman, A., Snyder, S., Kozier, B., & Erb, G. (2008). *Kozier & Erb's Fundamentals of Nursing: Concepts, Process, and Practice* (8th ed., p. 771). Upper Saddle River, NJ: Pearson Education.

155. A nurse is caring for a client who has had an amputation of the right leg. The client reports pain in the right leg. Which complementary therapy should the nurse use to control the phantom pain associated with the client's amputation?

1. A small dose of alprazolam (Xanax®) at 8-hour intervals in addition to prescribed oxycodone and acetaminophen (Percocet®) ordered every 6 hours as needed
2. A diet rich in fiber and a fluid intake of 2,000 mL in 24 hours while the client is taking hydromorphone (Dilaudid®) at 4- to 6-hour intervals as needed
3. Progressive relaxation exercises three times daily in addition to use of a transdermal patch of fentanyl (Duragesic®)
4. A local anesthetic as a nerve block in addition to prescribed long-acting oxycodone (OxyContin®).

ANSWER: 3

Complementary interventions are those holistic therapies used in addition to conventional medicinal interventions to achieve effective treatment and symptom control. Progressive relaxation therapy, used along with prescribed analgesic medication to control phantom pain, is an example of complementary therapy. Combining antianxiety medication with analgesics, combining dietary interventions to control constipation associated with opioids, and use of nerve blocks with analgesics are all examples of conventional or allopathic medical practice.

➧ ***Test-taking Tip:*** *The key words in the stem are "complementary medicine." Consider the definition of complementary medicine. Evaluate each option and select the option that describes a holistic intervention used in addition to traditional treatment.*

Content Area: Fundamentals; *Category of Health Alteration:* Basic Care and Comfort; *Integrated Processes:* Nursing Process Implementation; *Client Need:* Physiological Integrity/Basic Care and Comfort/Nonpharmacological Comfort Interventions; *Cognitive Level:* Application

Reference: Taylor, C., Lillis, C., LeMone, P., & Lyn, P. (2008). *Fundamentals of Nursing: The Art and Science of Nursing Care* (6th ed., p. 747). Philadelphia: Lippincott Williams & Wilkins.

156. A client who underwent surgery for colon cancer 6 weeks earlier has an appointment with a wound care nurse. After correctly demonstrating the changing of the stoma pouch, the client asks the nurse for advice regarding how to deal with gas coming from the stoma. To respond to the client's concern, the nurse should ask the client to do which of the following? SELECT ALL THAT APPLY.

1. Describe the usual dietary intake, including types of foods
2. Include cruciferous vegetables in the diet daily
3. Decrease fluid intake to 1,200 mL per 24 hours
4. Prick the colostomy stoma pouch with a pin
5. Limit intake of gas-producing beverages such as carbonated sodas
6. Go to the restroom to release the gas that collects in the colostomy stoma pouch by opening the pouch clamp

ANSWER: 1, 5, 6

The nurse assesses the client's usual dietary intake for foods known to produce gas. Limiting carbonated beverage limits gas formation in the intestinal tract. Gas that collects in the pouch should be released from the pouch in a restroom environment. Cruciferous vegetables, which include vegetables of the cabbage family, are known to cause gas formation. The client needs at least 2,000 mL of fluid on a daily basis to maintain proper function of the colostomy. Pricking the colostomy pouch with a pin leads to constant gas release associated with unpleasant odor.

➧ ***Test-taking Tip:*** *Read the scenario in the stem carefully. Focus on the issue: helping a client with a colostomy deal with gas from the stoma. Evaluate each option regarding a positive or negative effect on gas from the stoma.*

Content Area: Fundamentals; *Category of Health Alteration:* Basic Care and Comfort; *Integrated Processes:* Nursing Process Implementation; *Client Need:* Physiological Integrity/Basic Care and Comfort/Elimination; *Cognitive Level:* Analysis

Reference: Taylor, C., Lillis, C., LeMone, P., & Lyn, P. (2008). *Fundamentals of Nursing: The Art and Science of Nursing Care* (6th ed., pp. 1581–1585). Philadelphia: Lippincott Williams & Wilkins.

157. A male client undergoes surgery for a hernia repair. The client has orders to be discharged to home when stable. The client has tried several times to urinate into the urinal while in bed without success. Which interventions are appropriate to promote voiding for this client? SELECT ALL THAT APPLY.

1. Apply an external catheter
2. Assist the client to stand at the bedside to attempt to void
3. Assess the pain level of the client and administer medication appropriately if in pain
4. Assist the client to the bathroom and turn on running water within hearing distance of the client while the client attempts to void
5. Discuss relaxation techniques and ask the client to imagine being at home and voiding in his own home bathroom
6. Explain that the client should void within 8 hours of surgery or return to the hospital for catheterization.

ANSWER: 2, 3, 4, 5

The nurse should try to assist the client to void by assisting him to the normal position of standing, treating pain that may be interfering with the ability to urinate, using the sound of running water to stimulate the voiding reflex, and teaching the client relaxation techniques, including guided imagery. Use of an external catheter will not assist the client to void. Threatening the client with catheterization or staying in the hospital is not appropriate since it belittles the client.

Test-taking Tip: *The issue of the question is "appropriate measures to promote voiding for a male client." Evaluate each option regarding whether it is an appropriate way to promote urination.*

Content Area: Fundamentals; *Category of Health Alteration:* Basic Care and Comfort; *Integrated Processes:* Nursing Process Implementation; *Client Need:* Physiological Integrity/Basic Care and Comfort/Elimination; *Cognitive Level:* Application

Reference: Berman, A., Snyder, S., Kozier, B., & Erb, G. (2008). *Kozier & Erb's Fundamentals of Nursing: Concepts, Process, and Practice* (8th ed., p. 1299). Upper Saddle River, NJ: Pearson Education.

---

158. A client who was treated for constipation 1 month earlier comes to a primary care provider's office for an appointment. A nurse interviews the client and obtains information from the client about bowel function and the effectiveness of the prescribed treatments. The nurse determines that the client is no longer constipated based on which statement?

1. The client drinks 2,000 mL of fluids daily; including 4 ounces of prune juice.
2. The client has had a soft, formed bowel movement without straining every other day for the past 2 weeks.
3. The client self-administered one disposable enema the day of last month's appointment.
4. The client has minor discomfort from hemorrhoids during bowel movements.

ANSWER: 2

Constipation is defined as having fewer than three bowel movements per week. The fact that the client now has a bowel movement without straining every other day establishes that the client is no longer constipated. The fluid intake, which includes prune juice, shows the client is taking action to prevent constipation. The client used the disposable enema to stimulate bowel function after the last appointment. The client may still have some hemorrhoid irritation from straining due to past constipation.

Test-taking Tip: *Consider the clinical definition of constipation when answering the question.*

Content Area: Fundamentals; *Category of Health Alteration:* Basic Care and Comfort; *Integrated Processes:* Nursing Process Evaluation; *Client Need:* Physiological Integrity/Basic Care and Comfort/Elimination; *Cognitive Level:* Analysis

Reference: Berman, A., Snyder, S., Kozier, B., & Erb, G. (2008). *Kozier & Erb's Fundamentals of Nursing: Concepts, Process, and Practice* (8th ed., p. 1328). Upper Saddle River, NJ: Pearson Education.

---

159. A client who is recovering from orthopedic surgery keeps an appointment at a clinic and uses a walker to ambulate with partial weight-bearing as instructed. Which observation should lead the nurse to conclude that the client is using the correct technique?

1. Has elbows bent at a 30-degree angle
2. Is bent over the walker
3. Lifts the walker while walking; holding it about 2 inches above the floor
4. Has a walker that has four wheels in place

ANSWER: 1

The client is demonstrating correct technique when the elbows are bent at a 30-degree angle; indicating that the walker is at the proper height for the client. The client should stand erect while using the walker. The client cannot be ambulating with partial weight-bearing if the client lifts the walker off the floor or is using a walker with four wheels.

Test-taking Tip: *The issue of the question is the correct use of a walker with partial weight-bearing. Evaluate each option as to whether it correctly describes the use of a walker with partial weight-bearing.*

Content Area: Fundamentals; *Category of Health Alteration:* Basic Care and Comfort; *Integrated Processes:* Nursing Process Evaluation; *Client Need:* Physiological Integrity/Basic Care and Comfort/Mobility/Immobility; *Cognitive Level:* Analysis

Reference: Taylor, C., Lillis, C., LeMone, P., & Lyn, P. (2008). *Fundamentals of Nursing: The Art and Science of Nursing Care* (6th ed., p. 1305). Philadelphia: Lippincott Williams & Wilkins.

160. A nurse reviews the record of a client who has been immobile because of a degenerative neurological condition. The nurse reads that the client has bilateral foot drop. Which finding during the nurse's assessment supports the presence of foot drop?

1. The great toe is dorsiflexed and the other toes are fanned out.
2. The feet are unable to be maintained perpendicular to the legs.
3. The client is unable to move feet into a position of plantar flexion.
4. The client is only able to dorsiflex the feet bilaterally.

ANSWER: 2

A client with foot drop is unable to hold the feet up in dorsiflexion or in a perpendicular position to the leg. A positive Babinski's sign occurs when the great toe dorsiflexes and the toes fan out in response to stroking the lateral surface of the foot. With foot drop, the feet stay in plantar flexion and the client is unable to dorsiflex the feet.

Test-taking Tip: *The issue of the question is the definition of foot drop. Define foot drop in terms of dorsal or plantar flexion.*

Content Area: Fundamentals; *Category of Health Alteration:* Basic Care and Comfort; *Integrated Processes:* Nursing Process Assessment; *Client Need:* Physiological Integrity/Basic Care and Comfort/Mobility/Immobility; *Cognitive Level:* Analysis

Reference: Taylor, C., Lillis, C., LeMone, P., & Lyn, P. (2008). *Fundamentals of Nursing: The Art and Science of Nursing Care* (6th ed., p. 1289). Philadelphia: Lippincott Williams & Wilkins.

---

161. EBP A home health nurse visits an 82-year-old client who has experienced multiple strokes and is unable to change position independently in bed. The nurse teaches family caregivers techniques to move and reposition the client, who is in a hospital bed. Which technique should be included in the teaching plan for this client?

1. Before moving the client, family caregivers should raise the hospital bed to the level of their waists. After completing the move, the bed must be returned to the lowest level.
2. The pillow should be removed from under the client's head when positioned in a dorsal recumbent position.
3. Family members should tighten their abdominal muscles and buttocks while keeping their feet about 12 inches apart when using a lift sheet to pull the client up in bed.
4. The client's heels should rest on the bed surface and feet kept in a position perpendicular to the legs when the client is lying on the back.

ANSWER: 1

Family members should be instructed in how to use the hospital bed correctly. By raising the bed to waist level, caregivers put the client near their centers of gravity. This improves the stability of the caregivers during the move and lessens the risk for injury. Moving the bed to the lowest position decreases the risk of injury if the client falls out of bed. A client in dorsal recumbent position should have a pillow under the head to prevent hyperextension of the neck. Family members should assume a broad stance to improve balance when moving the client. The heels of the client should be kept off the bed to eliminate pressure on the heels while feet are maintained perpendicular to the legs to avoid foot drop.

Test-taking Tip: *Read the scenario in the stem carefully. The issue of the question includes proper methods of moving clients and body mechanics. Evaluate each option and eliminate those that describe techniques that are unsafe or lead to injury.*

Content Area: Fundamentals; *Category of Health Alteration:* Basic Care and Comfort; *Integrated Processes:* Teaching and Learning; *Client Need:* Safe and Effective Care Environment/Safety and Infection Control/Accident/Injury Prevention; *Cognitive Level:* Analysis

Reference: Berman, A., Snyder, S., Kozier, B., & Erb, G. (2008). *Kozier & Erb's Fundamentals of Nursing: Concepts, Process, and Practice* (8th ed., pp. 723, 1128–1129, 1133, 1136). Upper Saddle River, NJ: Pearson Education.

EBP Reference: Springhouse Publishing Company Staff. (2006). *Best Practices: Evidence-Based Nursing Procedures* (2nd ed., p. 75). Philadelphia: Lippincott Williams & Wilkins.

---

162. A hospitalized client, identified to be at risk for thromboembolic disease, has anti-embolism hose ordered. A nurse discusses the correct use of the stockings. Which direction should the nurse include in teaching this client?

1. If ambulating 10 times daily for 5 minutes at a time, wearing the hose is unnecessary.
2. The most appropriate time to apply the hose is before standing to get out of bed in the morning.
3. If the hose becomes painful to the skin underneath, notify the nurse and request pain medication.
4. Only cross the legs while wearing the antiembolism hose; otherwise keep the legs uncrossed.

ANSWER: 2

The most appropriate time to apply anti-embolism stockings is before the client arises from bed. This maximizes the compression effect, thus lessening venous distension and development of edema. Frequent ambulation is a positive intervention to prevent thromboembolic disease but should be used in addition to wearing the anti-embolism stockings. If the stockings cause skin discomfort to the client, the stockings and skin underneath must be assessed. The stockings may need to be removed and then reapplied without twisting or wrinkles in the stockings. Crossing the legs impedes circulation and should be avoided with or without the elastic stockings.

Test-taking Tip: *The issue of the question is the correct use of anti-embolism stockings. Evaluate each option regarding safe use. Eliminate option 1 since it contradicts use of the elastic stockings.*

Content Area: Fundamentals; *Category of Health Alteration:* Basic Care and Comfort; *Integrated Processes:* Teaching and Learning; *Client Need:* Physiological Integrity/Basic Care and Comfort/Mobility/Immobility; *Cognitive Level:* Analysis

Reference: Berman, A., Snyder, S., Kozier, B., & Erb, G. (2008). *Kozier & Erb's Fundamentals of Nursing: Concepts, Process, and Practice* (8th ed., pp. 950–952). Upper Saddle River, NJ: Pearson Education.

163. A client reports pain at an intravenous infusion site that has infiltrated. When a nurse applies a warm, moist compress to the site, the client asks how the treatment will help the condition. The nurse answers the client based on the understanding that the application of moist heat will:

1. alter tissue sensitivity by producing numbness.
2. decrease the metabolic needs of the involved tissues.
3. stop the local release of histamine in the tissues.
4. increase blood flow and improve capillary permeability.

ANSWER: 4

Application of the warm moist compress dilates the blood vessels, thus increasing local blood flow and capillary permeability. This accelerates the inflammatory response and promotes healing to the involved tissues. Application of cold alters the sensitivity of nerves in the area and causes numbness. Heat causes an increase in tissue metabolism. Cold application decreases the inflammatory response including the release of histamine from the inflamed tissues.

➧ ***Test-taking Tip:*** *The issue of the question is the effect of heat on an area of sustained inflammation. Recall the effects of heat on tissues. Evaluate each option to determine whether it accurately describes the effect of heat.*

Content Area: Fundamentals; *Category of Health Alteration:* Basic Care and Comfort; *Integrated Processes:* Nursing Process Analysis; *Client Need:* Physiological Integrity/Basic Care and Comfort/Non-Pharmacological Interventions; *Cognitive Level:* Analysis

Reference: Taylor, C., Lillis, C., LeMone, P., & Lyn, P. (2008). *Fundamentals of Nursing: The Art and Science of Nursing Care* (6th ed., p. 1222). Philadelphia: Lippincott Williams & Wilkins.

164. EBP A nurse is caring for a client who has experienced a first-degree sprain of the ankle. A primary care provider writes a prescription for an analgesic medication. Which intervention, beside the analgesic, should the nurse advise the client to utilize for the first 24 hours after the injury?

1. Applying ice directly to the ankle
2. Soaking the foot in warm water for 20 minutes, three times per day
3. Applying ice continuously to the ankle
4. Resting and elevating the limb as much as possible

ANSWER: 4

When a sprain occurs, there is excessive stretching of a ligament. With a first-degree sprain, some fibers of the ligament are torn, but there is no impaired joint function. Resting and elevating the limb will decrease the inflammation and associated swelling in the tissues. Ice should be applied to the injury during the first 24 hours to limit inflammation and swelling. The ice source should be covered to protect the skin, and the ice application should be limited to 30 minutes with an hour between applications for maximum therapeutic effect. Heat is contraindicated because it will increase swelling and bleeding in the injured area.

➧ ***Test-taking Tip:*** *The issue of the question involves interventions to limit inflammation during the first 24 hours postinjury. Eliminate option 2 since heat will increase swelling to the area. Recall the safety and therapeutic application of cold and eliminate options 1 and 3. Select option 4, which limits activity and decreases effect of gravity.*

Content Area: Fundamentals; *Category of Health Alteration:* Basic Care and Comfort; *Integrated Processes:* Nursing Process Intervention; *Client Need:* Physiological Integrity/Basic Care and Comfort/Non-Pharmacological Interventions; *Cognitive Level:* Application

References: Berman, A., Snyder, S., Kozier, B., & Erb, G. (2008). *Kozier & Erb's Fundamentals of Nursing: Concepts, Process, and Practice* (8th ed., pp. 932–933). Upper Saddle River, NJ: Pearson Education; Ignatavicius, D., & Workman, M. (2006). *Medical-Surgical Nursing: Critical Thinking for Collaborative Care* (5th ed., p. 1226). St. Louis, MO: Elsevier/Saunders; Taylor, C., Lillis, C., LeMone, P., & Lyn, P. (2008). *Fundamentals of Nursing: The Art and Science of Nursing Care* (6th ed., p. 1225). Philadelphia: Lippincott Williams & Wilkins.

EBP Reference: Institute for Clinical Systems Improvement (ICSI). (2008). *Assessment and Management of Acute Pain.* Available at: www.guideline.gov/summary/summary.aspx?view_id=1&doc_id=12302

165. A nurse is caring for a female client who is 65 inches tall and has a small body frame. Based on the information provided in the chart, what is the approximate ideal body weight for this client?

Approximating Ideal Body Weight

Rule of 5 for Females	Rule of 6 for Males
105 lb for 5 ft of height + 5 lb for each inch over 5 ft ± 10% for body-frame size	106 lb for 5 ft of height + 6 lb for each inch over 5 ft ± 10% for body-frame size

Add 10% for large body-frame size, and subtract 10% for small body-frame size.

1. 105 lb
2. 117 lb
3. 125 lb
4. 130 lb

ANSWER: 2

To determine the client's ideal body weight, first calculate the client's height in feet and inches. Since 1 foot equals 12 inches, the client's height is 5 feet, 5 inches (65/12 = 5 remainder of 5).

Apply the formula from the chart: 105 lb for 5 feet height

$$5 \text{ lb} \times 5 = 25$$
$$105 + 25 = 130 \text{ lb}$$

Since the client has a small body-frame size, calculate 10% of 130 lb.

$$10\% = 0.1$$
$$0.1 \times 130 = 13 \text{ lb}$$

Subtract the 10% due to small body-frame size: 130 − 13 = 117 lb.

▶ ***Test-taking Tip:*** *Focus on the information in the question. Utilize the formula given in the chart. Verify your calculation, especially if it seems like an unusual amount.*

Content Area: Fundamentals; *Category of Health Alteration:* Basic Care and Comfort; *Integrated Processes:* Nursing Process Analysis; *Client Need:* Physiological Integrity/Basic Care and Comfort/Nutrition and Oral Hydration; *Cognitive Level:* Application

Reference: Berman, A., Snyder, S., Kozier, B., & Erb, G. (2008). *Kozier & Erb's Fundamentals of Nursing: Concepts, Process, and Practice* (8th ed., p. 1236). Upper Saddle River, NJ: Pearson Education.

166. An elderly client residing in a nursing home has bilaterally weak handgrips and has difficulty with self-feeding. Which nursing interventions should be implemented to promote independence for this client? SELECT ALL THAT APPLY.

1. Ask the client for permission to open all containers, remove lids from items on the food tray, and cut up meats
2. Obtain built-up silverware for the client to use
3. Observe the client but do not provide assistance if the client is having difficulty
4. Feed the client if the client is eating too slowly
5. Ensure that the client is wearing prescribed dentures, eye glasses, or hearing aids before starting to eat

ANSWER: 1, 2, 5

Interventions that promote client independence include those that foster self-care and maximize interaction with the activity of eating. The nurse should observe the client and assist with specific obstacles to limit client frustration. Feeding the client will tend to extinguish independent behaviors.

▶ ***Test-taking Tip:*** *Select interventions that promote client independence in eating. Consider each option as to whether it will assist clients to overcome sensory or mobility deficits and promote independence.*

Content Area: Fundamentals; *Category of Health Alteration:* Basic Care and Comfort/Nutrition and Oral Hydration; *Integrated Processes:* Nursing Process Implementation; *Client Need:* Physiological Integrity/Basic Care and Comfort/Nutrition and Oral Hydration; *Cognitive Level:* Analysis

Reference: Taylor, C., Lillis, C., LeMone, P., & Lyn, P. (2008). *Fundamentals of Nursing: The Art and Science of Nursing Care* (6th ed., p. 1445). Philadelphia: Lippincott Williams & Wilkins.

167. A dietitian, who is consulted to see a hospitalized client because of nutritional concerns, orders a calorie count. The nurse should participate in this intervention by:

1. asking the client to recall the food and beverages consumed on a normal day.
2. asking the client to recall the food and beverages consumed on the day the calorie count is initiated.
3. informing the client that a record is being maintained of food and beverages consumed.
4. asking the client to approximate how many times per week certain food groups, such as cereals and breads, are eaten.

ANSWER: 3

A calorie count is actual documentation of all the foods and beverages consumed by a client. In a hospital, a calorie count involves the observation and documentation of food eaten from meal trays and snacks. Option 1 asks the client to describe usual intake in general terms. The 24-hour recall method asks clients to recall foods and beverages taken in for a specific day. A food frequency record gives a general picture of the usual nutritional intake.

▶ ***Test-taking Tip:*** *Consider the process of completing a calorie count. Select the option that best matches the definition of a calorie count. Note that options 1, 2, and 4 are similar and option 3 is different.*

Content Area: Fundamentals; *Category of Health Alteration:* Basic Care and Comfort; *Integrated Processes:* Nursing Process Implementation; *Client Need:* Physiological Integrity/Basic Care and Comfort/Nutrition and Oral Hydration; *Cognitive Level:* Analysis

Reference: Taylor, C., Lillis, C., LeMone, P., & Lyn, P. (2008). *Fundamentals of Nursing: The Art and Science of Nursing Care* (6th ed., pp. 1436–1437). Philadelphia: Lippincott Williams & Wilkins.

168. A hospitalized client has daily weights ordered. The client is able to stand, and the nursing unit has an electronic digital scale to use for client weights. Which intervention best ensures that the client's daily weight is accurate?

1. Asking the client to wear supportive shoes before stepping on the scale
2. Ensuring that the scale is calibrated and "zeroed" before a weight is obtained
3. Weighing the client by moving the sliding indicator until the scale balances
4. Weighing the client at different times of the day

ANSWER: 2

Electronic digital scales should be calibrated and "zeroed" before weighing the client to ensure accuracy. The client should not wear shoes since this will add to the weight. The nurse moves a slide indicator until the scale balances with a balancing arm scale. For accuracy, it is best to weigh clients at the same time each day.

➧ ***Test-taking Tip:*** *Visualize the process of weighing a client using an electronic digital scale. Evaluate each option and consider if it is correct in describing the process.*

Content Area: Fundamentals; *Category of Health Alteration:* Basic Care and Comfort/Nutrition and Oral Hydration; *Integrated Processes:* Nursing Process Implementation; *Client Need:* Physiological Integrity/Basic Care and Comfort/Nutrition and Oral Hydration; *Cognitive Level:* Analysis

References: Berman, A., Snyder, S., Kozier, B., & Erb, G. (2008). *Kozier & Erb's Fundamentals of Nursing: Concepts, Process, and Practice* (8th ed., p. 575). Upper Saddle River, NJ: Pearson Education; Taylor, C., Lillis, C., LeMone, P., & Lyn, P. (2008). *Fundamentals of Nursing: The Art and Science of Nursing Care* (6th ed., p. 611). Philadelphia: Lippincott Williams & Wilkins.

169. EBP A nurse plans guidelines to assist nursing personnel in meeting the hygiene needs of adult clients with dementia. Which guidelines are appropriate for the nurse to include? SELECT ALL THAT APPLY.

1. Utilizing two staff members to bathe the client quickly while limiting the client's ability to physically resist
2. Creating a calm environment during a bed bath by including music and dimmed lighting
3. Allowing clients, who are willing and able, to participate in some of the hygiene activities
4. Assessing and treating clients for pain before initiating hygiene activities
5. Washing the hair and body separately if either activity causes distress or is overwhelming to the client
6. Keeping the temperature of the bathing area warm and limiting body exposure of clients during bathing

ANSWER: 2, 3, 4, 5, 6

Research findings indicate that hygiene activities can be improved for clients with dementia and their caregivers by providing a calm bathing environment and keeping clients warm with limited exposure. Clients are more likely to cooperate with hygiene activities when pain is adequately controlled and they are allowed to participate in the process. Separating hair washing from bathing limits the stress of activity on the client with dementia. Quick and routine institutional bathing practices, which emphasize efficiency, can add to agitation and lack of cooperation in clients with dementia.

➧ ***Test-taking Tip:*** *Consider interventions to improve hygiene practices for clients with dementia. Evaluate each option and choose those that limit distress to the client.*

Content Area: Fundamentals; *Category of Health Alteration:* Basic Care and Comfort; *Integrated Processes:* Nursing Process Planning; *Client Need:* Physiological Integrity/Basic Care and Comfort/Personal Hygiene; *Cognitive Level:* Analysis

Reference: Harkreader, H., Hogan, M., & Thobaben, M. (2007). *Fundamentals of Nursing* (3rd ed., pp. 793–806). St. Louis, MO: Saunders/Elsevier.

EBP Reference: Rader, J., Barrick, A., Hoeffer, B., Sloane, P., McKenzie, et al. (2006). The bathing of older adults with dementia. *American Journal of Nursing,* 106(4), 40–49.

170. A client is transferred to a medical center from a local hospital and undergoes emergency treatment related to acute coronary syndrome. The client has slept little over the past 24 hours. Which assessment finding is consistent with sleep deprivation?

1. Periods of apnea lasting greater than 5 seconds
2. Slowing of thought processes
3. Hyperventilation
4. Cool extremities

ANSWER: 2

Clients who become sleep-deprived often show signs of impaired cognitive functioning. The other assessment findings are not associated with sleep deprivation.

➧ ***Test-taking Tip:*** *Focus on the issue: sleep deprivation. Evaluate each option and select option 2 because it relates to brain function.*

Content Area: Fundamentals; *Category of Health Alteration:* Basic Care and Comfort; *Integrated Processes:* Analysis; *Client Need:* Physiological Integrity/Basic Care and Comfort/Rest and Sleep; *Cognitive Level:* Analysis

Reference: Taylor, C., Lillis, C., LeMone, P., & Lyn, P. (2008). *Fundamentals of Nursing: The Art and Science of Nursing Care* (6th ed., p. 1348). Philadelphia: Lippincott Williams & Wilkins.

171. A nurse should inform a nursing assistant to avoid taking a rectal temperature for which client?

1. The adult client who underwent ileostomy surgery because of a perforated bowel
2. The adult client who has a frequent, productive cough and is receiving oxygen by nasal cannula
3. The adult client who developed thrombocytopenia after receiving chemotherapy
4. The adult client with hypothermia

ANSWER: 3

Clients with thrombocytopenia have lower than normal levels of platelets and are at increased risk of bleeding. Measuring the temperature rectally exposes the client to the risk of rectal bleeding. There are no contraindications for using the rectal method to assess temperature in the other clients. In fact, monitoring rectal temperature is often used in clients with hypothermia since the temperature is too low to be measured orally.

➧ ***Test-taking Tip:*** *The question calls for a negative answer. Evaluate each option and consider whether taking a temperature rectally would harm the client.*

Content Area: Fundamentals; *Category of Health Alteration:* Basic Care and Comfort; *Integrated Processes:* Nursing Process Analysis; *Client Need:* Physiological Integrity/Reduction of Risk Potential/Vital Signs; *Cognitive Level:* Application

Reference: Ignatavicius, D., & Workman, M. (2006). *Medical-Surgical Nursing: Critical Thinking for Collaborative Care* (5th ed., p. 906). St. Louis, MO: Elsevier/Saunders.

---

172. EBP A nursing assistant (NA), who is taking routine vital signs, tells a nurse that the small adult cuff is nowhere to be found and that a client's arm is too small to use an adult-size cuff. In response to the NA's report, which direction should the nurse give to the NA?

1. Document the other vital signs and note that proper blood pressure (BP) equipment is not available
2. Contact the nursing supervisor, obtain a small, adult BP cuff, and take the client's BP with the small, adult-size cuff
3. Use the adult size BP cuff to obtain the blood pressure, add 10 to both the diastolic and systolic readings, and document on the client's record the BP was obtained with an adult cuff
4. Take the client's BP using any available cuff

ANSWER: 2

The BP must be taken with the correct BP cuff. The NA should not omit the BP or adjust the numbers of the reading from an improperly sized cuff. Palpating a BP with an improperly sized cuff will not obtain the correct measurement.

➧ ***Test-taking Tip:*** *Read the scenario in the stem carefully. Consider that a correct measurement is the only acceptable option and select option 2.*

Content Area: Fundamentals; *Category of Health Alteration:* Basic Care and Comfort; *Integrated Processes:* Nursing Process Implementation; *Client Need:* Physiological Integrity/Reduction of Risk Potential/Vital Signs; *Cognitive Level:* Analysis

Reference: Berman, A., Snyder, S., Kozier, B., & Erb, G. (2008). *Kozier & Erb's Fundamentals of Nursing: Concepts, Process, and Practice* (8th ed., p. 551). Upper Saddle River, NJ: Pearson Education.

EBP Reference: Springhouse Publishing Company Staff. (2006). *Best Practices: Evidence-Based Nursing Procedures* (2nd ed., p. 26). Philadelphia: Lippincott Williams & Wilkins.

---

173. A nurse takes a client's blood pressure with an automatic blood pressure machine. The blood pressure is 86/56 mm Hg with a pulse rate of 64 beats per minute. Which action should the nurse do *first*?

1. Assess the client for dizziness and assess the skin on the extremities for warmth
2. Obtain a manual blood pressure cuff and retake the client's blood pressure
3. Elevate the head of the client's bed
4. Read the client's medical record and determine the client's normal range of blood pressure

ANSWER: 1

Initially, the nurse should assess the condition of the client and ascertain if there are physical signs consistent with hypotension resulting in decreased perfusion to the brain and peripheral circulation. After assessing the client's condition, the nurse should recheck the blood pressure to verify the accuracy of the reading. The nurse should not elevate the head of the client's bed since this action would further lower the blood pressure. Determining the normal range of blood pressure is indicated after condition assessment and verification of the reading.

➧ ***Test-taking Tip:*** *Read the scenario in the stem carefully. The key word is "first." Use the nursing process; assessment is the first step in the process.*

Content Area: Fundamentals; *Category of Health Alteration:* Basic Care and Comfort; *Integrated Processes:* Nursing Process Implementation; *Client Need:* Physiological Integrity/Reduction of Risk Potential/Vital Signs; *Cognitive Level:* Synthesis

Reference: Taylor, C., Lillis, C., LeMone, P., & Lyn, P. (2008). *Fundamentals of Nursing: The Art and Science of Nursing Care* (6th ed., p. 575). Philadelphia: Lippincott Williams & Wilkins.

174. **EBP** A nurse is using a tympanic thermometer to measure a client's temperature. When using a tympanic thermometer, the nurse should:

1. check the setting to know the type of measurement reading, such as oral or core temperature.
2. irrigate the ear canal with sterile saline 6 hours before obtaining the temperature.
3. pull downward on the pinna in an adult when inserting the thermometer.
4. hold the thermometer loosely in the ear until the thermometer sounds that the reading is finished.

ANSWER: 1

The nurse should check the setting on the thermometer, since the tympanic temperature is a core temperature and the thermometer can be set to either a core or an oral temperature, which vary in readings. Irrigating the ear canal is not indicated before taking the temperature, which is not affected by ear wax. The pinna of the ear should be pulled slightly upward on an adult to straighten the ear canal. The thermometer should be snugly inside the external ear to accurately record the temperature.

➧ ***Test-taking Tip:*** *Understand that the tympanic thermometer measures the temperature by sensing the heat given off from the tympanic membrane (ear drum). Eliminate option 2 since ear irrigation is unreasonable to perform before monitoring temperatures. Eliminate option 3 because it incorrectly describes the technique to straighten the ear canal in an adult.*

Content Area: Fundamentals; *Category of Health Alteration:* Basic Care and Comfort; *Integrated Processes:* Nursing Process Implementation; *Client Need:* Physiological Integrity/Reduction of Risk Potential/Vital Signs; *Cognitive Level:* Application

Reference: Taylor, C., Lillis, C., LeMone, P., & Lyn, P. (2008). *Fundamentals of Nursing: The Art and Science of Nursing Care* (6th ed., pp. 582–583). Philadelphia: Lippincott Williams & Wilkins.

EBP Reference: Springhouse Publishing Company Staff. (2006). *Best Practices: Evidence-Based Nursing Procedures* (2nd ed., p. 74). Philadelphia: Lippincott Williams & Wilkins.

---

175. **EBP** A client who underwent a surgical procedure the preceding day has a normal assessment with an oral temperature of 99.7°F (37.6°C) at 0800 hours. The client is to be discharged later in the day if the client's condition is stable. Based on the client's current temperature, which action should be taken by the nurse?

1. Inform the surgeon since the discharge should be cancelled
2. Instruct the client to use the incentive spirometer 10 times every hour and drink plenty of fluids and then recheck the temperature in 2 hours
3. Administer the dose of aspirin 81 mg earlier than the scheduled time
4. Realize that the temperature is only mildly elevated and was taken during the time of day when temperatures are highest according to normal diurnal deviations

ANSWER: 2

A temperature of 99.7°F (37.6°C) is only mildly elevated. The client should be encouraged to follow activities that promote recovery from surgery and lower fever. The nurse is prudent to monitor the temperature in 2 hours and reassess the client and the situation. It is premature to notify the surgeon to delay the discharge of the client. A dose of 81 mg of aspirin is given for antiplatelet agglutination effect and is unlikely to lower a fever. Normally, the diurnal deviation of temperatures results in the highest readings between 1600 and 2000 hours.

➧ ***Test-taking Tip:*** *Read the scenario in the stem carefully. Recognize that the client's temperature is slightly elevated. Evaluate the options and select option 2, which focuses on improving the client's condition with a planned reevaluation.*

Content Area: Fundamentals; *Category of Health Alteration:* Basic Care and Comfort; *Integrated Processes:* Nursing Process Analysis; *Client Need:* Physiological Integrity/Reduction of Risk Potential/Vital Signs; *Cognitive Level:* Analysis

Reference: Berman, A., Snyder, S., Kozier, B., & Erb, G. (2008). *Kozier & Erb's Fundamentals of Nursing: Concepts, Process, and Practice* (8th ed., p. 551). Upper Saddle River, NJ: Pearson Education.

EBP Reference: Springhouse Publishing Company Staff. (2006). *Best Practices: Evidence-Based Nursing Procedures* (2nd ed., p. 73). Philadelphia: Lippincott Williams & Wilkins.

176. EBP A nurse is preparing to provide phototherapy to a 4-day-old newborn who was admitted with hyperbilirubinemia. The nurse instructs the parents on how to care for their baby while receiving phototherapy in the hospital. The nurse's teaching should include:

1. keeping the baby fully clothed to prevent hypothermia.
2. covering the baby's eyes with eye shields to prevent retinal damage.
3. decreasing the number of feedings for their baby to reduce the number of soiled diapers.
4. discontinuing the phototherapy if a mild skin rash develops.

ANSWER: 2

Covering the baby's eyes with eye shields will protect the baby's eyes from the transmission of light, which could be damaging to the retinas. Keeping the baby fully clothed is incorrect because the mechanism of phototherapy is designed to convert the bilirubin in the superficial capillaries in the skin. Maximum skin exposure is desired to achieve the ideal effect of bilirubin conversion and excretion. Decreasing the number of feedings is incorrect because bilirubin is excreted in the urine and stool, and excretion can be increased with increased feedings. Discontinuing the phototherapy if a mild skin rash develops is incorrect because the rash can be caused by capillary dilation and is not harmful to the baby.

▶ ***Test-taking Tip:*** *Recall the goals and mechanism of action of phototherapy.*

Content Area: Fundamentals; *Category of Health Alteration:* Basic Care and Comfort; *Integrated Processes:* Teaching and Learning; *Client Need:* Physiological Integrity/Physiological Adaptation/Alterations in Body Systems; *Cognitive Level:* Analysis

Reference: Pillitteri, A. (2007). *Maternal & Child Health Nursing: Care of the Childbearing & Childrearing Family* (5th ed., p. 786). Philadelphia: Lippincott Williams & Wilkins.

EBP Reference: Stokowski, L., Short, M., & Witt, C. (2006). Fundamentals of phototherapy for neonatal jaundice. *Advances in Neonatal Care*, 6, 303–312.

177. When using a hypothermia blanket for a febrile client, which findings should lead the nurse to suspect hypothermia? SELECT ALL THAT APPLY.

1. Increased urine output
2. Drowsiness
3. Decreased heart rate (HR)
4. Decreased blood pressure (BP)
5. Increased BP
6. Increased HR

ANSWER: 2, 3, 4

When using a hypothermia blanket to reduce temperature, a nurse should monitor the client for signs of hypothermia, which include a decreased heart rate, decreased blood pressure, and drowsiness. The low cardiac output from the decreased BP and HR affect the central nervous system producing drowsiness. Urine output is decreased in a hypothermic client as a result of decreased perfusion.

▶ ***Test-taking Tip:*** *Carefully read each option. Note that some options are opposite.*

Content Area: Fundamentals; *Category of Health Alteration:* Basic Care and Comfort; *Integrated Processes:* Nursing Process Analysis; *Client Need:* Physiological Integrity/Physiological Adaptation/Alterations in Body Systems; *Cognitive Level:* Application

Reference: Wilkinson, J., & Van Leuven, K. (2007). *Fundamentals of Nursing: Theory, Concepts & Applications* (Vol. 1, p. 317). Philadelphia: F. A. Davis.

178. EBP Which signs should indicate to a nurse that a client is experiencing a surgical site infection? SELECT ALL THAT APPLY.

1. Temperature of 100.4°F (38°C)
2. Localized pain and tenderness
3. Well-approximated wound edges
4. Redness or warmth at the affected site
5. Purulent drainage at the incision site
6. Thick, white drainage in the Jackson-Pratt (JP) tubing

ANSWER: 1, 2, 4, 5, 6

Fever, localized pain, and redness are results of an inflammatory response to an infection. Purulent drainage at the site and thick, white drainage in the JP would contain white blood cells and microorganisms that would indicate the presence of infection. Well-approximated wound edges are a desired outcome and indicate a healing incision.

▶ ***Test-taking Tip:*** *Eliminate the option with a normal finding. Apply knowledge of the inflammatory response to answer this question.*

Content Area: Fundamentals; *Category of Health Alteration:* Basic Care and Comfort; *Integrated Processes:* Nursing Process Assessment; *Client Need:* Physiological Integrity/Physiological Adaptation/Alterations in Body Systems; *Cognitive Level:* Analysis

Reference: Craven, R., & Hirnle, C. (2009). *Fundamentals of Nursing: Human Health and Function* (6th ed., pp. 1046–1049). Philadelphia: Lippincott Williams & Wilkins.

EBP Reference: Pinto, S. (2006). *Infections, Surgical Site: Prevention* (Evidence-Based Care Sheet). Available at: http://web.ebscohost.com/ehost/pdf?vid=27&hid=114&sid=ee304e15-dea3-4d4b-8edf-438bd10613be%40sessionmgr108

179. A nurse is assessing a wound while completing a dressing change. The nurse documents the pressure ulcer as stage III. Which is the best description of the stage III pressure ulcer?

1. Partial-thickness skin loss involving the epidermis, dermis, or both
2. Full-thickness skin loss involving damage to subcutaneous tissue
3. Redness with intact skin that client reports as "itchy"
4. Full-thickness skin loss with undermining and sinus tracks

ANSWER: 2

Full-thickness skin loss involving damage to subcutaneous tissue is a description of a stage III pressure ulcer. Partial-thickness skin loss involving the epidermis, dermis, or both describes a stage II pressure ulcer. Redness with intact skin that a client reports as "itchy" describes a stage I pressure ulcer. Full-thickness skin loss with undermining and sinus tracks describes a stage IV pressure ulcer.

***Test-taking Tip:** Review staging descriptions of pressure ulcers.*

Content Area: Fundamentals; *Category of Health Alteration:* Basic Care and Comfort; *Integrated Processes:* Nursing Process Assessment; *Client Need:* Physiological Integrity/Physiological Adaptation/Alterations in Body Systems; *Cognitive Level:* Application

Reference: Lewis, S., Heitkemper, M., Dirksen, S., O'Brien, P., & Bucher, L. (2007). *Medical-Surgical Nursing: Assessment and Management of Clinical Problems* (7th ed., p. 226). St. Louis, MO: Mosby.

180. EBP Which actions should a nurse plan when caring for a client with a stage III pressure ulcer to the right lower-extremity heel? SELECT ALL THAT APPLY.

1. Monitor the client's nutritional intake
2. Assess for pain and premedicate prior to dressing changes
3. Monitor pedal pulses and capillary refill of affected extremity
4. Use hydrogen peroxide for cleaning of ulcer wound
5. Turn and reposition client every 1 to 2 hours
6. Elevate the extremity on pillows

ANSWER: 1, 2, 3, 5, 6

Monitoring the client's nutritional intake is essential to promote wound healing. Assessing and medicating for pain, prior to dressing changes, promotes client comfort. Monitoring pedal pulses and capillary refill of the affected extremity alerts the nurse to further vascular compromise as a result of the wound. Repositioning the client is also important to promote circulation and to prevent further skin breakdown. Elevation reduces edema, but care must be taken to avoid putting pressure on the ulcer. The use of hydrogen peroxide or acetic acid solutions is incorrect because they can be excoriating to the wound and will not promote healing.

***Test-taking Tip:** Use the process of elimination to rule out incorrect options. Eliminate any options that would worsen wound healing.*

Content Area: Fundamentals; *Category of Health Alteration:* Basic Care and Comfort; *Integrated Processes:* Nursing Process Planning; *Client Need:* Physiological Integrity/Physiological Adaptation/Alterations in Body Systems; *Cognitive Level:* Application

Reference: Craven, R., & Hirnle, C. (2009). *Fundamentals of Nursing: Human Health and Function* (6th ed., pp. 282–287). Philadelphia: Lippincott Williams & Wilkins.

EBP Reference: Registered Nurses Association of Ontario. (2007). *Assessment and Management of Stage I to IV Pressure Ulcers*. Available at: www.rnao.org/Storage/29/2371_BPG_pressure_ulcers_I_to_IV.pdf

181. A nurse is assessing a client who was just admitted to a surgical unit following abdominal surgery. Which assessment finding would require an immediate intervention by the nurse?

1. A nasogastric tube (NG) to low intermittent suction with small amounts of dark bloody returns
2. A compressed Jackson-Pratt (JP) drain with 30 mL bright red blood
3. A NG tube to low intermittent suction with pale green returns
4. A round JP drain with 20 mL serosanguineous drainage

ANSWER: 4

A round JP drain requires immediate intervention because the drain needs to be compressed to create suction and collect fluid. Suction is lost when there is a leak in the system or if there is too much drainage. A compressed JP drain with bright red blood is considered a normal finding immediately after surgery. A NG tube to low intermittent suction with pale green returns is also a normal finding due to drainage of the stomach contents. A NG tube to low intermittent suction with small amounts of dark bloody returns would be normal immediately after surgery if there were any trauma associated with insertion of tube; thus no intervention would be required.

***Test-taking Tip:** The key phrase is "immediate intervention." Think about which response needs to be corrected to improve client outcomes.*

Content Area: Fundamentals; *Category of Health Alteration:* Basic Care and Comfort; *Integrated Processes:* Nursing Process Assessment; *Client Need:* Physiological Integrity/Physiological Adaptation/Alterations in Body Systems; *Cognitive Level:* Assessment

Reference: Craven, R., & Hirnle, C. (2007). *Fundamentals of Nursing: Human Health and Function* (5th ed., p. 1033). Philadelphia: Lippincott Williams & Wilkins.

182. A nurse is teaching a client, who is 24 hours post–abdominal surgery, how to use an incentive spirometer. Which instructions should the nurse include in the teaching? SELECT ALL THAT APPLY.

1. Inhale slowly and deeply through mouth
2. Seal lips tightly around mouthpiece
3. After inhaling, hold breath for 2 to 3 seconds
4. Sit with head of bed down and bed almost flat
5. Splint incision with pillows
6. Exhale forcefully, fast, and hard

ANSWER: 1, 2, 3, 5

Inhaling slowly and deeply through the mouth and holding the breath prevent hyperventilation and provides maximal inflation of the alveoli. Sealing the lips around the mouthpiece prevents leakage of air. Splinting of the incision promotes comfort and encourages the client to take larger volume breaths. Exhaling forcefully, fast, and hard may lead to hyperventilation and is the technique used to measure peak expiratory flow rate. Sitting with the head of bed down or flat does not promote lung expansion. The desired position for maximum lung expansion is a high Fowler's position or a sitting position.

Test-taking Tip: *Use process of elimination to rule out incorrect options. Recall the physiology of lung expansion.*

Content Area: Fundamentals; *Category of Health Alteration:* Basic Care and Comfort; *Integrated Processes:* Teaching and Learning; *Client Need:* Physiological Integrity/Physiological Adaptation/Alterations in Body Systems; *Cognitive Level:* Application

Reference: Craven, R., & Hirnle, C. (2007). *Fundamentals of Nursing: Human Health and Function* (5th ed., pp. 842–846). Philadelphia: Lippincott Williams & Wilkins.

183. A nurse approaches a client who needs nasotracheal suctioning. The nurse explains the procedure to the client and washes hands. Which steps should be taken by the nurse when performing nasotracheal suctioning? Prioritize the nurse's actions by placing each step in the correct order.

______ Prepare suction equipment; open water-soluble lubricant
______ Place finger over suction control port of catheter and suction intermittently while withdrawing the catheter
______ Put on sterile gloves
______ Lubricate catheter, insert into nare, and advance into pharynx
______ When client inhales, advance catheter into trachea
______ Pick up suction catheter with dominant hand and attach it to connection tubing
______ Place tip into sterile saline container while applying suction to clear secretions from the tubing

ANSWER: 1, 6, 2, 4, 5, 3, 7

The nurse would prepare equipment first and then put on sterile gloves. The nurse would then connect the suction tubing to the catheter, lubricate the end of the catheter, and insert the catheter into the nare and then the pharynx. The nurse should wait for the client to inhale and then advance the catheter into the trachea. The nurse would then apply suction by placing a finger over the suction-control port and withdraw the catheter while suctioning intermittently. After the catheter is withdrawn from the nare, the tip should be placed in sterile saline, with suction applied, to clear the catheter.

Test-taking Tip: *Visualize the steps required to perform nasotracheal suctioning.*

Content Area: Fundamentals; *Category of Health Alteration:* Basic Care and Comfort; *Integrated Processes:* Nursing Process Implementation; *Client Need:* Physiological Integrity/Physiological Adaptation/Alterations in Body Systems; *Cognitive Level:* Application

Reference: Wilkinson, J., & Van Leuven, K. (2007). *Fundamentals of Nursing: Thinking & Doing* (Vol. 2, p. 835). Philadelphia: F. A. Davis.

184. A nurse is caring for an 11-month-old infant diagnosed with bronchopulmonary dysplasia. The infant has a tracheostomy with 30% supplemental oxygen being provided via the tracheostomy. The infant has a decline in oxygen saturations from 96% to 87% and appears anxious and restless. Which action should be taken by the nurse?

1. Obtain arterial blood gases (ABGs)
2. Increase oxygen rate from 30% to 50%
3. Suction the tracheostomy tube
4. Medicate for anxiety and pain

ANSWER: 3

Suctioning the tracheostomy should be the first priority in caring for this infant. Many tracheostomies require frequent suctioning to remove secretions and mucous plugs. Increasing the oxygen rate will not be effective if the airway is occluded by secretions. Obtaining ABGs may be helpful if oxygen saturations remain low after suctioning and the infant remains in distress, but clearing the airway should be priority. Medicating for anxiety and pain would not improve oxygen saturations if the airway is not patent due to secretions. Medicating the infant may reduce respiratory drive and cause further distress.

Test-taking Tip: *Think about the ABCs: airway, breathing circulation. Airway management is priority.*

Content Area: Fundamentals; *Category of Health Alteration:* Basic Care and Comfort; *Integrated Processes:* Nursing Process Implementation; *Client Need:* Physiological Integrity/Physiological Adaptation/Alterations in Body Systems; *Cognitive Level:* Analysis

Reference: Lewis, S., Heitkemper, M., Dirksen, S., O'Brien, P., & Bucher, L. (2007). *Medical-Surgical Nursing: Assessment and Management of Clinical Problems* (7th ed., pp. 575–585). St. Louis, MO: Mosby.

185. A 33-year-old client reports left leg pain, right-sided chest pain, and a sudden onset of shortness of breath. Which action should be taken immediately by the nurse?

1. Take the client's temperature
2. Auscultate the client's the lung sounds
3. Percuss the client's abdomen
4. Request a stat chest x-ray

ANSWER: 2

Auscultation of lung sounds should be one of the first assessments performed by the nurse to determine the cause of the client's shortness of breath. Chest x-ray would be helpful in assessing the cause of shortness of breath but would need a physician's order and would not be the first priority. Percussion of abdomen and measurement of the client's temperature are helpful tools when completing a full assessment but are not priority in this situation.

Test-taking Tip: *Think about the ABCs: airway, breathing, circulation. Airway is priority.*

Content Area: Fundamentals; *Category of Health Alteration:* Basic Care and Comfort/Techniques of Physical Assessment; *Integrated Processes:* Nursing Process Assessment; *Client Need:* Health Promotion and Maintenance/Techniques of Physical Assessment; *Cognitive Level:* Application

Reference: Lewis, S., Heitkemper, M., Dirksen, S., O'Brien, P., & Bucher, L. (2007). *Medical-Surgical Nursing: Assessment and Management of Clinical Problems* (7th ed., pp. 544–558). St. Louis, MO: Mosby.

186. A nurse is assessing a client who has new onset atrial fibrillation and reports shortness of breath. The client has a history of rheumatic fever as a child and also reports increased exercise intolerance. Place an X where the nurse would best be able to assess the heart murmur associated with these symptoms.

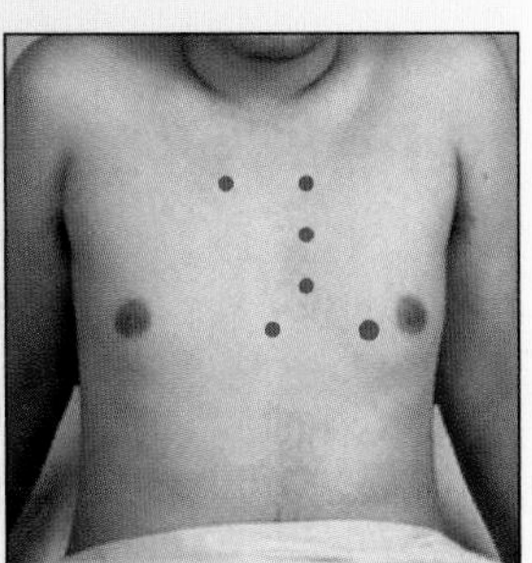

ANSWER:

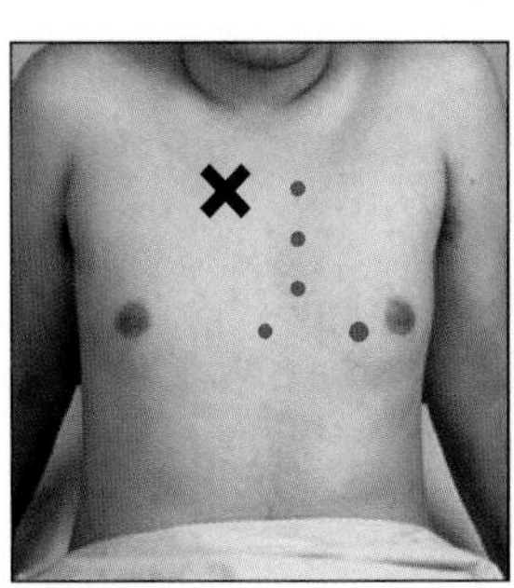

The "X" should be placed on the second intercostal space at the right sternal border to hear a murmur associated with aortic regurgitation. Shortness of breath, atrial fibrillation, and exercise intolerance are often associated with aortic regurgitation, especially in clients with a history of rheumatic fever.

Test-taking Tip: *Use the memory aid "all points essential to memorize" to remember the names of the heart valves and auscultation points: aortic, pulmonic, Erb's point, tricuspid, and mitral valve. Note the formation of a "2" on the chest and that the aortic valve is located at the first point.*

Content Area: Fundamentals; *Category of Health Alteration:* Basic Care and Comfort; *Integrated Processes:* Nursing Process Assessment; *Client Need:* Health Promotion and Maintenance/Techniques of Physical Assessment; *Cognitive Level:* Analysis

Reference: Rhoads, J., & Meeker, B. (2008). *Davis's Guide to Clinical Nursing Skills.* Philadelphia: F. A. Davis.

187. Which rationale should a nurse use to explain the reason for oxygen being bubbled through a humidifier to a client receiving 2 liters of oxygen by nasal cannula?

1. Prevents the burning sensation of direction oxygen
2. Prevents drying of the nasal passages
3. Prevents a chemical reaction between the tubing and oxygen
4. Prevents contamination with environmental gases

ANSWER: 2

Humidification of the oxygen prevents drying of the clients nasal passages. Oxygen does not cause a burning sensation, but it is combustible. Oxygen does not produce a chemical reaction with the tubing and is not contaminated by environmental gases.

Test-taking Tip: *Focus on the key word "humidifier." Look for the option that is similar.*

Content Area: Fundamentals; *Category of Health Alteration:* Basic Care and Comfort; *Integrated Processes:* Teaching and Learning; *Client Need:* Safe and Effective Care Environment/Safety and Infection Control/Safe Use of Equipment; *Cognitive Level:* Application

Reference: Lewis, S., Heitkemper, M., Dirksen, S., O'Brien, P., & Bucher, L. (2007). *Medical-Surgical Nursing: Assessment and Management of Clinical Problems* (7th ed., p. 1807). St. Louis, MO: Mosby/Elsevier.

Test 6: **Fundamentals: Medication Administration**

188. EBP A nurse, checking newly written physician orders, determines that which orders require the nurse to contact the physician to clarify the order? SELECT ALL THAT APPLY.

1. Aspirin 325 mg orally qd
2. MS 4 mg IV q1hr prn
3. Furosemide (Lasix®) 40 mg IV now
4. D5W with 20 mEq KCL IV at 125 mL/hr
5. Heparin 5,000 u subcutaneously bid

ANSWER: 1, 2, 5

The abbreviations "qd," "MS," and "u" are disallowed by the Joint Commission (formerly the Joint Commission on Accreditation of Healthcare Organizations [JCAHO]). Responses 3 and 4 are incorrect choices because these responses have the essential components of a medication order—medication name, dose, frequency, and route—and use of acceptable abbreviations.

➧ ***Test-taking Tip:*** *Read each order carefully to identify the disallowed abbreviations.*

Content Area: Fundamentals; *Category of Health Alteration:* Medication Administration; *Integrated Processes:* Nursing Process Analysis; *Client Need:* Physiological Integrity/Pharmacological and Parenteral Therapies/Medication Administration; *Cognitive Level:* Analysis

Reference: Wilkinson, J., & Van Leuven, K. (2007). *Fundamentals of Nursing: Theory, Concepts & Applications* (Vol. 1, pp. 492–494). Philadelphia: F. A. Davis.

EBP Reference: The Joint Commission. (2005). *Patient Safety Do Not Use List.* Available at: www.jointcommission.org/NR/rdonlyres/2329F8F5-6EC5-4E21-B932-54B2B7D53F00/0/06_dnu_list.pdf

---

189. EBP A nurse receives a medication order for an adult client to administer ferrous sulfate 300 mg PO bid. After thinking critically about this order, the nurse should:

1. administer the medication as ordered.
2. contact the physician to clarify the route of the medication.
3. contact the physician to question the twice daily administration of the medication.
4. withhold the medication because the dosage is not within acceptable ranges.

ANSWER: 1

The medication order contains all essential information using approved abbreviations. The abbreviation "PO" is an acceptable abbreviation for the oral route. The abbreviation "bid" is acceptable for twice daily administration. The dose is within acceptable ranges.

➧ ***Test-taking Tip:*** *First, determine if the order contains the essential information and the dosage of the medication is acceptable. Then read each option carefully.*

Content Area: Fundamentals; *Category of Health Alteration:* Medication Administration; *Integrated Processes:* Nursing Process Implementation; *Client Need:* Physiological Integrity/Pharmacological and Parenteral Therapies/Medication Administration; *Cognitive Level:* Analysis

Reference: Berman, A., Snyder, S., Kozier, B., & Erb, G. (2008). *Kozier & Erb's Fundamentals of Nursing: Concepts, Process, and Practice* (8th ed., p. 840). Upper Saddle River, NJ: Pearson Education.

EBP Reference: The Joint Commission. (2005). *Patient Safety Do Not Use List.* Available at: www.jointcommission.org/NR/rdonlyres/2329F8F5-6EC5-4E21-B932-54B2B7D53F00/0/06_dnu_list.pdf

---

190. EBP Before a child's hospital discharge, a nurse is teaching the parents how to administer an oral medication to the child. Which nurse instruction would be most appropriate?

1. Administer the medication and then follow it with a small glass of milk
2. Give the child a flavored ice pop just before the medication
3. Tell the child that the medication will taste good
4. Open all capsules and mix the contents with applesauce

ANSWER: 2

The cold from the ice pop will help to numb the taste buds and weaken the taste of the medication. Options 1, 3, and 4 are incorrect. Essential foods, such as milk, should be avoided because the child may later refuse the food that he/she associates with the medicine. If the child is old enough, warn the child that the medication is objectionable, but then praise the child after the medication is swallowed. Some capsules are extended release and should not be opened.

➧ ***Test-taking Tip:*** *Note the key words "most appropriate." Recall that cold has a numbing effect. Therefore, select option 2.*

Content Area: Fundamentals; *Category of Health Alteration:* Medication Administration; *Integrated Processes:* Teaching and Learning; *Client Need:* Health Promotion and Maintenance/Self-Care; *Cognitive Level:* Analysis

Reference: Wilkinson, J., & Van Leuven, K. (2007). *Fundamentals of Nursing: Theory, Concepts & Applications* (Vol. 1, p. 501). Philadelphia: F. A. Davis.

EBP Reference: Stucky, E. (2003). Prevention of medication errors in the pediatric inpatient setting. *Pediatrics*, 112(2), 431–436.

191. A nurse is administering oral medications to a client. Which steps should be taken by the nurse to safely administer oral medications? Prioritize the nurse's actions by placing each step in the correct order.

______ Document administering the medication
______ Check the label after preparing the medication
______ Check the client's name band and another identifier
______ Review the medication order on the administration medication record (MAR)
______ Check the label on the medication against the MAR
______ Give the medication to the client with a glass of water
______ Check the medication at the bedside

ANSWER: 7, 3, 4, 1, 2, 6, 5

The nurse should first review the medication order on the MAR. The next step should be to check the label on the medication against the MAR before preparing the medication. Then the nurse should check the label again after preparing the medication. The nurse should then check the client's name band and check the medication again at the bedside. The medication should then be given to the client with a glass of water. Finally, the nurse should document administering the medication. These are the steps for the nurse to administer oral medications safely.

➧ ***Test-taking Tip:*** *Use visualization to focus on the information in the question and then visualize the steps of the procedure. Prioritizing is placing items in the correct sequence.*

Content Area: Fundamentals; *Category of Health Alteration:* Medication Administration; *Integrated Processes:* Nursing Process Implementation; *Client Need:* Physiological Integrity/Pharmacological and Parenteral Therapies/Medication Administration; *Cognitive Level:* Application

Reference: Wilkinson, J., & Van Leuven, K. (2007). *Fundamentals of Nursing: Theory, Concepts & Applications* (Vol. 1, pp. 495–499). Philadelphia: F. A. Davis.

192. A nurse is evaluating whether a client on multiple oral medications is taking the medications correctly. Which finding should be most concerning to the nurse because the absorption rate of medications can be increased?

1. Taking afternoon oral medications with a carbonated soft drink
2. Drinking a glass of milk with the tetracycline antibiotic oral medication
3. Taking morning oral medications with water and consuming 2,500 mL of water daily
4. Taking mealtime oral medications with a meal low in fiber and high in fatty foods

ANSWER: 1

Carbonated beverages can cause oral medications to dissolve faster, be neutralized, or experience a change in absorption rate in the stomach. When dairy products are taken with an antibiotic, such as tetracycline, there is decreased drug absorption in the stomach. Medications should be taken with a full glass of water. Foods low in fiber and high in fat will delay stomach emptying and medication absorption by up to 2 hours.

➧ ***Test-taking Tip:*** *Focus on key words "most concerning" and the focus of the question: increases rate of absorption. Then use the process of elimination to select option 1. Although options 2 and 4 are concerning, these do not increase medication absorption rate.*

Content Area: Fundamentals; *Category of Health Alteration:* Medication Administration; *Integrated Processes:* Nursing Process Evaluation; *Client Need:* Physiological Integrity/Pharmacological and Parenteral Therapies/Medication Administration; *Cognitive Level:* Analysis

Reference: Wilkinson, J., & Van Leuven, K. (2007). *Fundamentals of Nursing: Theory, Concepts & Applications* (Vol. 1, p. 491). Philadelphia: F. A. Davis.

193. EBP A nurse is observing a nursing student prepare and administer medications to adult clients. Which action by the nursing student warrants intervention by the nurse?

1. Injecting air into a vial before withdrawing 20 mg furosemide (Lasix®) from a vial labeled 20 mg/mL
2. Selecting a 1-mL syringe with a ⅝-inch needle to be used for administering 0.5 mL of heparin subcutaneously
3. Instructing a client to place a buccal medication under the client's tongue and allowing it to absorb
4. Pouring the ordered medication "Robitussin® 2 tsp now" to the 10 mL mark on a medication cup

ANSWER: 3

Buccal medications should be held in the cheek rather than under the tongue. Air should be injected into a vial before withdrawing the medication. A needle size of ½ to ⅝ inch in length should be used for adult subcutaneous injections. A teaspoon is equivalent to 5 mL; thus 2 teaspoons is 10 mL.

➧ ***Test-taking Tip:*** *This is a false-response item. Look for the student nurse's incorrect action.*

Content Area: Fundamentals; *Category of Health Alteration:* Medication Administration; *Integrated Processes:* Nursing Process Implementation; *Client Need:* Safe and Effective Care Environment/ Management of Care/Supervision; *Cognitive Level:* Application

Reference: Wilkinson, J., & Van Leuven, K. (2007). *Fundamentals of Nursing: Theory, Concepts & Applications* (Vol. 1, p. 506). Philadelphia: F. A. Davis.

EBP Reference: Harding, L., & Petrick, T. (2008). Nursing student medication errors: A retrospective review. *Journal of Nursing Education*, 47(1), 43–47.

194. A nurse has taught a client to self-administer a nasal medication. Which conclusions should the nurse make when observing the client administering the medication as illustrated? SELECT ALL THAT APPLY.

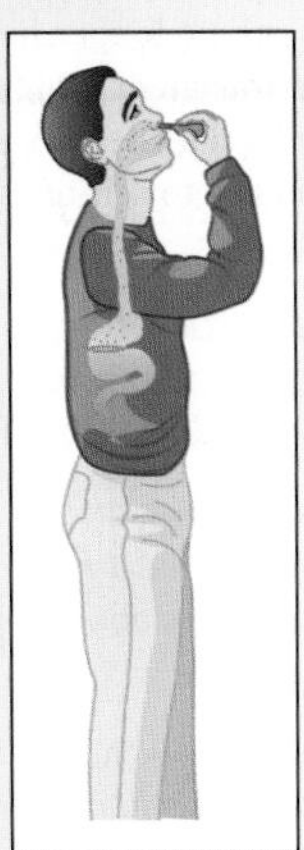

1. The client needs additional instruction about the correct procedure for administering a nasal medication.
2. The client is able to correctly demonstrate the procedure for administering a nasal medication.
3. The client should have his head titled further back to distribute the medication into the sinuses.
4. The client should not be placing the medication dispenser into the nostrils.
5. The client should have his head bent down and leaning forward to administer the medication and then tilt his head back to distribute the medication.
6. The client has his head at the appropriate angle to administer and distribute the medication.

ANSWER: 1, 5

Because this position is incorrect for administering nasal medications, the client needs additional instructions. The correct position for administering nasal medications is assuming a head down and forward position, if the client can assume this position. Once the medication is administered, the client should tilt the head back to distribute the medication. The client did not correctly demonstrate administering medications by the nasal route. Having the head titled further back is not a correct position for administering medications by the nasal route. The medication dispenser should be placed in the nostril for administration and washed after use. The head should be tilted forward for administration. Studies have shown that administering nasal sprays or drops while the client is sitting and leaning the head back causes poor distribution into the nasal complex and sinuses.

▶ ***Test-taking Tip:*** *Use the illustration as a clue to selecting the correct options. Note that the gastrointestinal tract is illustrated rather than the respiratory tract. This suggests that the position is incorrect.*

Content Area: Fundamentals; *Category of Health Alteration:* Medication Administration; *Integrated Processes:* Nursing Process Evaluation; *Client Need:* Physiological Integrity/Pharmacological and Parenteral Therapies/Medication Administration; *Cognitive Level:* Application

Reference: Wilkinson, J., & Van Leuven, K. (2007). *Fundamentals of Nursing: Thinking & Doing* (Vol. 2, p. 466). Philadelphia: F. A. Davis.

195. A nurse is planning to administer medications through a nasogastric (NG) tube. Which interventions should the nurse plan after checking the medications, checking client identification, and verifying tube placement? SELECT ALL THAT APPLY.

1. Crush together all medications that are acceptable for crushing
2. Pour crushed medications into one medication cup and mix with water
3. Withdraw all medications and water solution from the medication cup with a syringe and administer
4. Crush each medication separately
5. Pour each individual crushed medication into individual medication cups and mix with water
6. With a syringe, withdraw the single dose of medication from the medication cup and administer.
7. Flush the tubing with water between medications

ANSWER: 4, 5, 6, 7

Medications to be administered NG should be crushed and administered separately. The NG tube should be flushed with water between each medication. Some medications are less effective when combined with other medications. Therefore, medications should be placed in individual medication cups and administered individually. Options 1, 2, and 3 are incorrect because these actions combine the medications for crushing and administration.

▶ ***Test-taking Tip:*** *Visualize the sequence to administer medications through a NG tube. Remember to administer medications separately.*

Content Area: Fundamentals; *Category of Health Alteration:* Medication Administration; *Integrated Processes:* Nursing Process Planning; *Client Need:* Physiological Integrity/Pharmacological and Parenteral Therapies/Medication Administration; *Cognitive Level:* Application

Reference: Wilkinson, J., & Van Leuven, K. (2007). *Fundamentals of Nursing: Theory, Concepts & Applications* (Vol. 1, p. 500). Philadelphia: F. A. Davis.

196. A nurse is teaching a client to self-administer a medication dose through a metered-dose inhaler (MDI). Which steps should be taken by the nurse when instructing the client? Prioritize the nurse's actions by placing each step in the correct order.

_____ Press the top of the canister
_____ Shake the canister several times
_____ Close your teeth and lips tightly around the mouthpiece
_____ Exhale slowly through pursed lips
_____ Take a deep breath and exhale until you cannot exhale any more air
_____ Insert the mouthpiece into the mouth over the tongue
_____ Inhale deeply and hold the breath for 10 seconds
_____ Sit upright

ANSWER: 6, 2, 4, 8, 5, 3, 7, 1

After sitting upright, the client should first shake the canister several times. The next step is to have the client insert the mouthpiece into the mouth over the tongue. Then, the client should secure the teeth and lips tightly around the mouthpiece. Next, the client should take a deep breath and exhale until air can no longer be exhaled. The top of the canister is then pressed and the client inhales deeply and holds the breath for 10 seconds. Finally, the client exhales slowly through pursed lips. This is the correct sequence to self-administer medication through an MDI with a spacer.

➧ ***Test-taking Tip:*** *Use visualization to focus on the data in the question and then visualize the remaining steps of the procedure. Prioritizing is placing items in the correct sequence.*

Content Area: Fundamentals; *Category of Health Alteration:* Medication Administration; *Integrated Processes:* Nursing Process Analysis; *Client Need:* Health Promotion and Maintenance/Self-Care; *Cognitive Level:* Analysis

Reference: Wilkinson, J., & Van Leuven, K. (2007). *Fundamentals of Nursing: Theory, Concepts & Applications* (Vol. 1, p. 506). Philadelphia: F. A. Davis.

---

197. A nurse is observing a nursing student administering a clonidine (Catapres®) transdermal patch to a client diagnosed with hypertension. Which action requires the nurse to intervene?

1. Applies gloves
2. Asks the client to state name and also checks the client's name band
3. Applies patch, rubbing the patch against the skin, and then securing it in place
4. Folds old patch with medication to the inside and discards in a medication disposal receptacle

ANSWER: 3

The medication should not be rubbed into the skin. Patches are designed to allow constant, controlled amounts of medication to be released over 24 hours or more. Options 1, 2, and 4 follow the correct procedure for applying a transdermal patch.

➧ ***Test-taking Tip:*** *Note the key phrase "requires the nurse to intervene." Look for the incorrect action, which is option 3.*

Content Area: Fundamentals; *Category of Health Alteration:* Medication Administration; *Integrated Processes:* Teaching and Learning; *Client Need:* Safe and Effective Care Environment/Management of Care/Supervision; *Cognitive Level:* Analysis

Reference: Wilkinson, J., & Van Leuven, K. (2007). *Fundamentals of Nursing: Theory, Concepts & Applications* (Vol. 1, p. 502). Philadelphia: F. A. Davis.

---

198. A nurse administers a prochlorperazine (Compazine®) suppository to an adult client. Which action by the nurse best ensures that the medication is correctly administered?

1. Positioning the client on the left side
2. Lubricating the suppository prior to insertion
3. Feeling the sensation of the suppository pulling away when inserted against the rectal wall past the internal anal sphincter
4. Noting soft, formed stool 30 minutes after the suppository

ANSWER: 3

Rectal suppositories should be inserted past the internal anal sphincter and against the rectal wall. Stimulation of the bowel, once past the internal anal sphincter, will draw the medication inward. Stool in the bowel could cause incorrect placement of the suppository. Although the client should be positioned on the left side, this does not indicate whether the medication is in the correct position. Lubrication makes passage easier, but does not ensure the correct placement against the rectal wall and past the sphincter. Prochlorperazine is an antiemetic medication. It does not produce bowel peristalsis. Digital stimulation may cause passage of stool that is in the bowel, but this does not ensure correct administration.

➧ ***Test-taking Tip:*** *Focus on the issue: correct administration of a rectal suppository. The key word is "best," suggesting that more than one option could be correct, but one is best.*

Content Area: Fundamentals; *Category of Health Alteration:* Medication Administration; *Integrated Processes:* Nursing Process Evaluation; *Client Need:* Physiological Integrity/Pharmacological and Parenteral Therapies/Medication Administration; *Cognitive Level:* Application

Reference: Craven, R., & Hirnle, C. (2007). *Fundamentals of Nursing: Human Health and Function* (5th ed., p. 572). Philadelphia: Lippincott Williams & Wilkins.

199. A new clinic nurse is teaching the mother of a 2-year-old child how to administer ear drops while an experienced nurse is observing. The new nurse is using an illustration of a child's ear to teach the mother and states the following actions while pointing to the picture: clean the child's ear, warm the solution, pull the child's ear up and back, instill the medication, depress on the tragus of the ear, keep the child side-lying for about 5 minutes, and then insert a small cotton fluff loosely in the auditory canal for about 20 minutes. Which action should the experienced nurse take during or following the teaching?

1. Suggest to the new nurse that the mother return demonstrate instilling ear drops
2. Confirm with the new nurse and mother that the procedure was correctly described
3. Interrupt to state that the child's ear should be pulled down and back
4. Praise the new nurse for the thorough teaching provided to the mother

ANSWER: 3

For children under 3 years of age, the ear canal should be gently pulled down and back because the ear canal is directed upward. The experienced nurse should interrupt so the mother is not taught an incorrect procedure. Suggesting a return demonstration would be appropriate, but it is not the best option because the procedure was taught incorrectly and the mother would demonstrate it incorrectly. The experienced nurse cannot confirm an incorrectly taught procedure, nor should the nurse praise the new nurse for the thorough teaching. Praise should be given for selecting an illustration for learning enhancement.

➧ ***Test-taking Tip:*** *Carefully read the situation provided. Take note of the age of the child.*

Content Area: Fundamentals; *Category of Health Alteration:* Medication Administration; *Integrated Processes:* Teaching and Learning; *Client Need:* Physiological Integrity/Pharmacological and Parenteral Therapies/Medication Administration; *Cognitive Level:* Application

References: Berman, A., Snyder, S., Kozier, B., & Erb, G. (2008). *Kozier & Erb's Fundamentals of Nursing: Concepts, Process, and Practice* (8th ed., pp. 890–892). Upper Saddle River, NJ: Pearson Education; Craven, R., & Hirnle, C. (2007). *Fundamentals of Nursing: Human Health and Function* (5th ed., p. 572). Philadelphia: Lippincott Williams & Wilkins.

200. An experienced nurse is supervising a new registered nurse who is administering medications to adult clients. Which action by the new registered nurse requires the experienced nurse to intervene?

1. Withdraws 1 mL of purified protein derivative (PPD) from a vial for intradermal injection
2. Pinches the abdominal tissue of a thin adult and inserts the needle at a 45-degree angle to administer insulin subcutaneously
3. Measures three finger-breadths below the acromion process to inject codeine 15 mg/0.5 mL in the deltoid muscle
4. Administers 5,000 units heparin subcutaneously in the abdomen without aspirating for a blood return

ANSWER: 1

Only small amounts are administered in intradermal injections, usually no more than 0.1 mL. Options 2, 3, and 4 demonstrate the correct procedures for administering the medications by other routes.

➧ ***Test-taking Tip:*** *Note the key phrase "requires the experienced nurse to intervene." Select the action by the new registered nurse that is incorrect.*

Content Area: Fundamentals; *Category of Health Alteration:* Medication Administration; *Integrated Processes:* Nursing Process Evaluation; Teaching and Learning; *Client Need:* Safe and Effective Care Environment/Management of Care/Supervision; *Cognitive Level:* Application

References: Wilkinson, J., & Van Leuven, K. (2007). *Fundamentals of Nursing: Theory, Concepts & Applications* (Vol. 1, pp. 513–516). Philadelphia: F. A. Davis; Craven, R., & Hirnle, C. (2007). *Fundamentals of Nursing: Human Health and Function* (5th ed., p. 580). Philadelphia: Lippincott Williams & Wilkins.

201. A nurse, who is working the evening shift, is planning to administer insulin subcutaneously to a hospitalized child. Which statement made by the nurse to the mother would be *inappropriate*?

1. "It is okay for your child to say 'ouch,' cry, or even scream when receiving an injection."
2. "I can give the injection while your child is sleeping; then the injection won't be noticed."
3. "I will apply lidocaine/prilocaine (EMLA®) cream, a topical analgesic, 1 hour before the injection to reduce pain."
4. "The child will need to be lying, but after the injection you can hold and comfort your child."

ANSWER: 2

Injections should never be administered to a sleeping child because the injection is painful and the child will wake up and be terrified. Giving approval for the child to vent his or her feelings provides the child with a better sense of control. EMLA® cream can reduce the pain with insertion, but pain may still be felt as the medication is injected. The child can be lying flat during the injection.

➧ ***Test-taking Tip:*** *The key word is "inappropriate."*

Content Area: Fundamentals; *Category of Health Alteration:* Medication Administration; *Integrated Processes:* Communication and Documentation; *Client Need:* Physiological Integrity/Pharmacological and Parenteral Therapies/Medication Administration; *Cognitive Level:* Analysis

References: Craven, R., & Hirnle, C. (2007). *Fundamentals of Nursing: Human Health and Function* (5th ed., p. 600). Philadelphia: Lippincott Williams & Wilkins; Pillitteri, A. (2007). *Maternal & Child Health Nursing: Care of the Childbearing & Childrearing Family* (5th ed., pp. 1148–1149). Philadelphia: Lippincott Williams & Wilkins.

202. EBP A client with a diagnosis of multiple sclerosis is hospitalized due to a pressure ulcer. The client provides to the admitting nurse a handwritten list of medications, which includes interferon beta-1b (Betaseron®) 25 mg subcutaneously daily. Which nursing actions are correct related to the client's medication list? SELECT ALL THAT APPLY.

1. Rewrite the medications on official facility documents as written and file per agency policy
2. Inquire about vitamins, herbals, and over-the-counter medications that may not be on the list
3. Verify the Betaseron® dose with the prescribing physician
4. Verify the Betaseron® with the pharmacy in which the medication was last filled
5. Insert an unaltered copy of the handwritten list into the client's medical record
6. Tell the client that only the physician prescribing medications will need to see the list
7. Ask a family member to bring the container with the prescription noted for verification

ANSWER: 2, 3, 4, 7

Vitamins, herbals, and over-the-counter medications can affect the action of other medications. The usual dose and frequency of Betaseron® is 0.25 mg (8 million IU) every other day, so the dose and frequency should be verified. Medications can be verified by contacting the prescribing physician or pharmacy where the medication was last filled, reviewing medical records, or by asking a family member to bring the container that has the prescribing information. Medication reconciliation (verifying medications) is an important safety procedure and is a Joint Commission requirement for health-care facilities. Rewriting the medications or inserting an unaltered copy into the client's medical record without verifying the dose and frequency can result in a medication overdose. The nurse admitting the client should review the medication list with the client and verify the accuracy of the medications listed.

➧ ***Test-taking Tip:*** *Focus on the issue: the nursing actions involved in medication reconciliation.*

Content Area: Fundamentals; *Category of Health Alteration:* Medication Administration; *Integrated Processes:* Nursing Process Implementation; *Client Need:* Physiological Integrity/Pharmacological and Parenteral Therapies/Medication Administration; *Cognitive Level:* Analysis

Reference: Craven, R., & Hirnle, C. (2007). *Fundamentals of Nursing: Human Health and Function* (5th ed., pp. 559–560). Philadelphia: Lippincott Williams & Wilkins.

EBP Reference: Rogers, G. (2006). Reconciling medications at admission: Safe practice recommendations and implementation strategies. *Joint Commission Journal on Quality and Patient Safety*, 32(1), 37–50. Available at: www.jointcommission.org/SentinelEvents/SentinelEventAlert/sea_35.htm

203. A nurse plans to administer an intramuscular injection into the left dorsogluteal muscle for a client positioned prone because of anterior body burns. On the illustration below, place an X on the area where the nurse should plan to administer the injection.

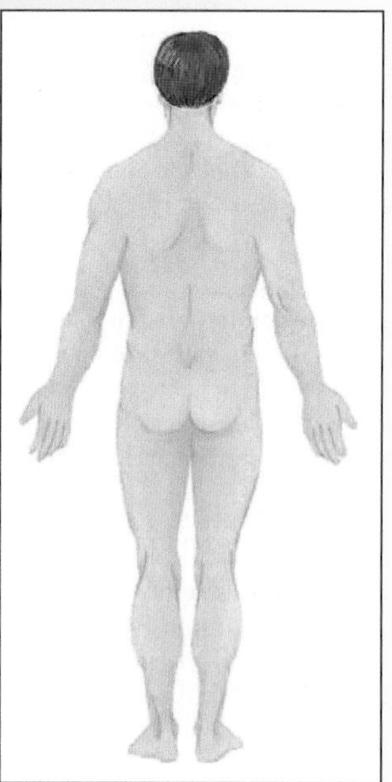

ANSWER:

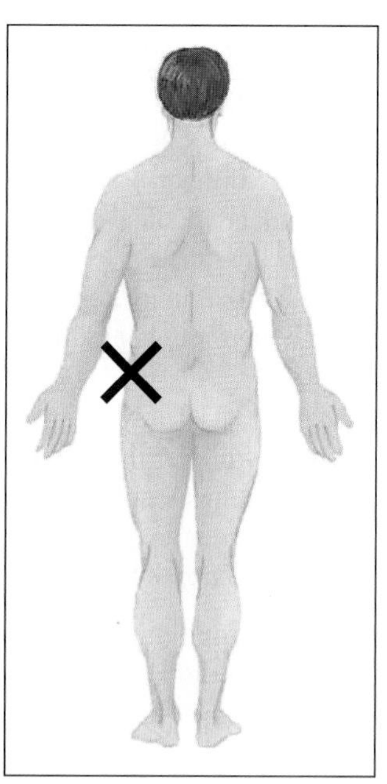

The left dorsogluteal muscle is best located above and outside a line drawn from the left posterior superior iliac spine to the left greater trochanter of the femur. An alternative method is to divide the buttock into four quadrants and make the injection in the upper outer quadrant, about 2 to 3 (5–7.6 cm) below the iliac crest. A combination of these methods is often used to identify the correct location and avoid the sciatic nerve. The needle should be inserted at a 90-degree angle.

➧ ***Test-taking Tip:*** *Read the stem carefully, noting the term "left dorsogluteal muscle." Knowledge of underlying anatomy is needed to answer this question.*

Content Area: Fundamentals; *Category of Health Alteration:* Medication Administration; *Integrated Processes:* Nursing Process Planning; *Client Need:* Physiological Integrity/Pharmacological and Parenteral Therapies/Medication Administration; *Cognitive Level:* Application

Reference: Craven, R., & Hirnle, C. (2007). *Fundamentals of Nursing: Human Health and Function* (5th ed., pp. 589–593). Philadelphia: Lippincott Williams & Wilkins.

204. EBP A nurse receives an order to administer hydroxyzine (Vistaril®) 25 mg intramuscularly (IM) to a client. Before injecting the medication, which statements should the nurse make to the client? SELECT ALL THAT APPLY.

1. "You will feel minimal pain at the injection site."
2. "Expect to experience relief from nausea within about 10 minutes."
3. "You will feel me pull the skin to the side at the site before I inject the medication."
4. "Tense your muscle as I make the injection to avoid focusing on the injection itself."
5. "I will select your deltoid muscle because use of the muscles with turning increases absorption."
6. "You will feel a cold sensation as I cleanse your skin with the alcohol swab."

ANSWER: 3, 6

Hydroxyzine is an antiemetic and sedative/hypnotic. The injection can be extremely painful, so it is administered by the Z-track IM method. In the Z-track method, the skin is pulled away from the injection site, the injection made, the medication is administered, and the nurse waits 10 seconds before the needle is withdrawn and the skin is released. The skin is disinfected with alcohol prior to administration, which will feel cool when applied. Medications administered by the IM route generally take 20 to 30 minutes to become effective. Tensing muscles increase pain. A large muscle such as the ventrogluteal, not the deltoid muscle, should be used for the injection. Literature suggests the ventrogluteal site is safer than the dorsogluteal site for intramuscular injections.

Test-taking Tip: *Note the issue of the question, an IM injection of hydroxyzine. Apply knowledge of IM injections and hydroxyzine to answer this question.*

Content Area: Fundamentals; *Category of Health Alteration:* Medication Administration; *Integrated Processes:* Nursing Process Implementation; *Client Need:* Physiological Integrity/Pharmacological and Parenteral Therapies/Medication Administration; *Cognitive Level:* Application

Reference: Craven, R., & Hirnle, C. (2007). *Fundamentals of Nursing: Human Health and Function* (5th ed., pp. 590–591). Philadelphia: Lippincott Williams & Wilkins.

EBP Reference: Small, S. (2004). Preventing sciatic nerve injury from intramuscular injections: Literature review. *Journal of Advanced Nursing*, 47(3), 287–296.

205. EBP A clinic nurse is administering monovalent HepB (hepatitis B vaccine) intramuscularly to a newborn prior to hospital discharge. Which site is best for the nurse to plan to administer the injection?

1. Deltoid
2. Ventrogluteal
3. Dorsogluteal
4. Vastus lateralis

ANSWER: 4

The anterolateral thigh muscle is recommended as the site for HebB administration for neonates (age less than 1 month). The deltoid and dorsogluteal muscles are not well-developed in neonates. Although 0.5 mL of medication can be administered into the ventrogluteal muscle of neonates, it is not a recommended site.

Test-taking Tip: *Think about the largest muscle in neonates before reviewing the options. The key word is "best."*

Content Area: Fundamentals; *Category of Health Alteration*: Medication Administration; *Integrated Processes:* Nursing Process Planning; *Client Need:* Physiological Integrity/Pharmacological and Parenteral Therapies/Medication Administration; *Cognitive Level:* Application

Reference: Craven, R., & Hirnle, C. (2007). *Fundamentals of Nursing: Human Health and Function* (5th ed., p. 588). Philadelphia: Lippincott Williams & Wilkins.

EBP References: Centers for Disease Control and Prevention. (2008). *Recommendations and Guidelines: 2008 Child & Adolescent Immunization Schedules for Persons Aged 0–6 Years.* Available at: www.cdc.gov/vaccines/recs/schedules/downloads/child/2008/08_0-6yrs_schedule_pr.pdf; Centers for Disease Control and Prevention. (2005, December 23). Appendix B Immunization Management Issues. *MMWR* 54(RR16), 27–30. Available at: www.cdc.gov/MMWR/preview/mmwrhtml/rr5416a3.htm

206. A nurse is caring for a client who has 0.9% NaCl infusing intravenously (IV). An order had been written the previous day to change the IV solution to 0.9% NaCl with 10 mEq KCL. Which action should the nurse initiate *first*?

1. Notify the client's physician
2. Complete an incident report
3. Check the client's serum potassium level
4. Replace 0.9% NaCl with the ordered solution

ANSWER: 3

Because the order was written the previous day and not implemented, the nurse should first check the client's serum potassium level and then notify the physician. The nurse should determine if there are order changes before replacing the solution. The physician may change the amount of KCL in the IV solution based on the client's serum potassium level and other client data. An incident report should be completed by the nurse after caring for the client.

Test-taking Tip: *Note the key word "first." Remember that KCL is potassium chloride.*

Content Area: Fundamentals; *Category of Health Alteration:* Medication Administration; *Integrated Processes:* Nursing Process Implementation; *Client Need:* Safe and Effective Care Environment/ Management of Care/Establishing Priorities; *Cognitive Level:* Application

Reference: Wilkinson, J., & Van Leuven, K. (2007). *Fundamentals of Nursing: Theory, Concepts & Applications* (Vol. 1, p. 1085). Philadelphia: F. A. Davis.

207. EBP A nurse plans to administer an antibiotic intravenous piggyback (IVPB) to a client who is on a fluid restriction and strict intake and output. On the illustration below, which port on the 0.9% NaCl IV line would it be best for the nurse to add a secondary line for the antibiotic?

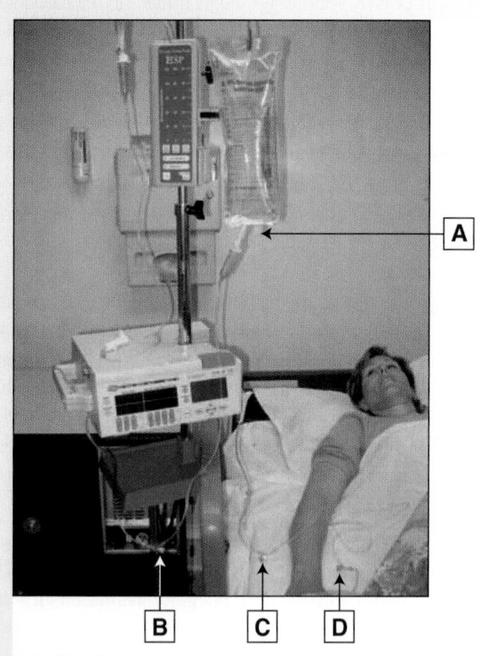

1. A
2. B
3. C
4. D

ANSWER: 2

The IVPB secondary line should be inserted at the port immediately distal to the back-check valve on the tubing and before the pump. The antibiotic should run through the IV infusion pump to control the rate and ensure that the medication is delivered. Tubing misconnections can result in client injury and are an important and underreported problem in health-care organizations.

Test-taking Tip: *Note the key words "strict intake and output." The volume delivered is best controlled by delivering the medication through the pump.*

Content Area: Fundamentals; *Category of Health Alteration:* Medication Administration; *Integrated Processes:* Nursing Process Planning; *Client Need:* Physiological Integrity/Pharmacological and Parenteral Therapies/Intravenous Therapies; *Cognitive Level:* Application

Reference: Phillips, L. (2005). *Manual of I.V. Therapeutics* (4th ed., p. 211). Philadelphia: F. A. Davis.

EBP Reference: The Joint Commission. (2006). Tubing misconnections—A persistent and potentially deadly occurrence. *Sentinal Event Alert*, 36. Available at: www.jointcommission.org/SentinelEvents/SentinelEventAlert/sea_36.htm

208. EBP An experienced nurse is supervising a new nurse caring for a hospitalized child who is receiving intravenous (IV) therapy. Which action should indicate to the experienced nurse that the new nurse needs additional orientation regarding IV therapy for children?

1. Determines that the current solution has been infusing for 24 hours and should be changed
2. Selects a 1,000-mL bag of the prescribed IV solution and checks it against the orders
3. Prepares new tubing and the prescribed IV solution 1 hour before it is due to be changed
4. Removes the plastic cover, spikes the bag with the tubing spike, and squeezes the drip chamber

ANSWER: 2

IV solutions in 250- and 500-mL containers should be selected to guard against circulatory overload. IV solutions are considered medications and errors in administration can have negative consequences. IV solutions open longer than 24 hours are no longer considered sterile. Tubing is changed every 72 to 96 hours, depending on agency policy. The procedure for spiking the bag is correct. The bag could be either hung first or after being spiked.

➧ *Test-taking Tip: The key words are "needs additional orientation." Read each option carefully to determine which option has the greatest potential for producing harm.*

Content Area: Fundamentals; *Category of Health Alteration:* Medication Administration; *Integrated Processes:* Nursing Process Evaluation; *Client Need:* Safe and Effective Care Environment/ Management of Care/Supervision; *Cognitive Level:* Analysis

Reference: Craven, R., & Hirnle, C. (2007). *Fundamentals of Nursing: Human Health and Function* (5th ed., pp. 621–623). Philadelphia: Lippincott Williams & Wilkins.

EBP Reference: Carlton, G. (2006). Medication-related errors: A literature review of incidence and antecedents. *Annual Review of Nursing Research*, 24, 19–38.

---

209. EBP To maintain patency of a peripheral intravenous (IV) access device for an infant, a physician has ordered intermittent flushing of the access device. Which action should be taken by the nurse?

1. Consult the physician and request an order for a continuous infusion at a "to keep open rate"
2. Flush the IV access device with 5 mL 0.9% NaCl
3. Verify the amount and type of solution that should be used to flush the access device
4. Flush the IV access device with 10 units heparin

ANSWER: 3

The standard of practice is to verify the amount and type of solution, either by consulting the physician's order or agency protocols. Research has shown that intermittent flushes are not associated with a decreased cannula life, or any other disadvantages, thus lending some support for the use of intermittent flushing rather than maintaining a continuous infusion. Although saline is the typical flush solution, 5 mL is unnecessary. Heparin may be used to maintain patency of central lines.

➧ *Test-taking Tip: Select the option that would be safest for the client and use the process of elimination.*

Content Area: Fundamentals; *Category of Health Alteration:* Medication Administration; *Integrated Processes:* Nursing Process Implementation; *Client Need:* Physiological Integrity/Pharmacological and Parenteral Therapies/Intravenous Therapies; *Cognitive Level:* Application

Reference: Pillitteri, A. (2007). *Maternal & Child Health Nursing: Care of the Childbearing & Childrearing Family* (5th ed., p. 1155). Philadelphia: Lippincott Williams & Wilkins.

EBP Reference: Flint, A., McIntosh, D., & Davies, M. (2005). Continuous infusion versus intermittent flushing to prevent loss of function of peripheral intravenous catheters used for drug administration in newborn infants. *Cochrane Database of Systematic Reviews* 2005, Issue 4, Art. No. CD004593. DOI: 10.1002/14651858.CD004593.pub2. Available at: www.cochrane.org/reviews/en/ab004593.html

---

210. A nurse receives the following medication orders while caring for multiple clients. Which medication should the nurse plan to administer *first*?

1. Nitroglycerin (Nitrostat®) 0.4 mg sublingually (SL) stat for the client experiencing chest pain
2. Morphine sulfate 4 mg intravenously (IV) now for the client experiencing incisional pain
3. Lorazepam 2 mg IV now for the client experiencing restlessness and picking at tubing
4. One unit packed red blood cells stat for the client with a hemoglobin of 9.5 g

ANSWER: 1

Nitroglycerin increases coronary blood flow by dilating coronary arteries and improving collateral flow to ischemic areas of the heart. Increasing collateral blood flow reduces anginal pain and the potential of myocardial infarction. This action has the greatest potential of changing client outcomes and can be performed more quickly than the other actions. Both morphine and lorazepam are controlled substances, requiring the nurse to retrieve and sign these out from a secure location. Administering IV medications takes longer than SL medications. Obtaining blood from the blood bank will take longer than the time it takes to administer a SL medication.

➧ *Test-taking Tip: Use the ABCs (airway, breathing, circulation) and the time it takes to implement each action to establish the priority. Because nitroglycerine affects the circulatory system, this action should be first.*

Content Area: Fundamentals; *Category of Health Alteration:* Medication Administration; *Integrated Processes:* Nursing Process Planning; *Client Need:* Safe and Effective Care Environment/ Management of Care/Establishing Priorities; *Cognitive Level:* Analysis

References: Craven, R., & Hirnle, C. (2007). *Fundamentals of Nursing: Human Health and Function* (5th ed., p. 209). Philadelphia: Lippincott Williams & Wilkins; Deglin, J., & Vallerand, A. (2007). *Davis's Drug Guide for Nurses* (10th ed., p. 868). Philadelphia: F. A. Davis.

211. A nurse's assessment finding for a client at 0800 hours includes blood pressure (BP) 180/88 mm Hg, heart rate (HR) 96 beats per minute, respiratory rate (RR) 24 breaths per minute, and temperature 102.6°F (39.2°C). The last bowel movement for the client was 6 days ago. The client is due to receive multiple medications, but prefers to take medications one at a time due to difficulty swallowing. Currently the client is lying flat in bed. In which order should the nurse administer the medications to this client?

______ Timolol (Blocadren®) 2 gtts OD
______ Labetalol (Normodyne®) 20 mg IVP for SBP greater than 160 mm Hg
______ Ramiapril (Altace®) 2.5 mg oral daily
______ Propantheline (Pro-Banthine®) 15 mg oral tid
______ Ducosate sodium (Docusate®) rectal suppository this a.m.
______ Cefazoline sodium (Ancef®) 1 g IVSP

ANSWER: 3, 1, 4, 5, 6, 2

Labetalol is a beta-blocker that will lower the BP. This should be administered first because the client's blood pressure is elevated and the onset of action is 2 to 5 minutes. Next, the cetazoline sodium, which is a cephalosporin antibiotic, should be administered because the nurse is working with the intravenous (IV) lines and the client's temperature is also elevated, suggesting an infection. Because the client is lying flat in bed, timolol should be administered next. It is used for treating glaucoma; OD is the abbreviation for right eye. Next, the oral medications should be administered, with ramipril first. It is an ace inhibitor with an onset of 1 to 2 hours, and the client's BP is already elevated. Propantheline is used in the treatment of peptic ulcer disease and is administered next. Finally, the client should resume a side-lying position and the rectal suppository administered. It is used to soften stool and promote defecation. It should be retained as long as possible.

▶ ***Test-taking Tip:*** *Use the ABCs (airway, breathing, circulation) to determine the priority action; the focus is on using aseptic technique, starting with the cleanest areas first.*

Content Area: Fundamentals; *Category of Health Alteration:* Medication Administration; *Integrated Processes:* Nursing Process Analysis; *Client Need:* Physiological Integrity/Pharmacological and Parenteral Therapies/Medication Administration; *Cognitive Level:* Analysis

References: Craven, R., & Hirnle, C. (2007). *Fundamentals of Nursing: Human Health and Function* (5th ed., pp. 209, 524). Philadelphia: Lippincott Williams & Wilkins; Deglin, J., & Vallerand, A. (2007). *Davis's Drug Guide for Nurses* (10th ed., pp. 147–152, 199–201, 253–256, 689–691, 1331). Philadelphia: F. A. Davis.

212. A nurse notes that a hospital coworker omits treatments for clients, experiences mood swings, makes frequent requests for help with assignments, and has an increased number of requests to witness the waste of controlled substances. Which nursing action is most appropriate?

1. Report the findings to the nurse's immediate supervisor
2. Tell the coworker that drug abuse is suspected and offer support
3. Notify the police, who will investigate because drug abuse is a legal offense
4. Complete an incident report, noting the times the coworker has wasted controlled substances

ANSWER: 1

The findings should be reported to the coworker's supervisor, who should collect additional data and approach the coworker with the concern. Telling the coworker of suspicions may cause the coworker to hide the problem, if one exists, and could jeopardize client safety. The immediate supervisor should be collecting additional data to either support or refute the nurse's suspicions. The nurse should document suspicions, but completing an incident report is unnecessary because there are no data to support that an incident has occurred.

▶ ***Test-taking Tip:*** *Identify the focus of the question from the behaviors described, which suggest suspected drug abuse. Then, note the key words "most appropriate." Eliminate options 2, 3, and 4 because these actions are inappropriate until additional information is collected to eliminate other potential problems.*

Content Area: Fundamentals; *Category of Health Alteration:* Medication Administration; *Integrated Processes:* Communication and Documentation; *Client Need:* Safe and Effective Care Environment/ Management of Care/Legal Rights and Responsibilities; *Cognitive Level:* Analysis

Reference: Wilkinson, J., & Van Leuven, K. (2007). *Fundamentals of Nursing: Theory, Concepts & Applications* (Vol. 1, pp. 1087–1088). Philadelphia: F. A. Davis.

213. EBP A client is to receive oxycodone 5 mg with acetaminophen 325 mg (Percocet®), two tablets orally for pain rated as 4 out of 10 on a numeric pain scale. Which nursing actions, observed by a coworker, suggest that a new nurse planning to administer the medication needs additional orientation? SELECT ALL THAT APPLY.

1. Obtains apple juice for the client to drink with the medication
2. Unlocks the medication box in the client's room to retrieve the medication
3. Checks the client's medication record for the first time and then documents administering the two tablets
4. Identifies the client by name and medical record number
5. Informs the client to expect some pain relief within 10 to 15 minutes
6. Tells the client to place the tablets under the tongue for faster pain relief

ANSWER: 2, 3, 6

Percocet® is a schedule II controlled substance. The Controlled Substances Act requires facilities to keep controlled substances in a locked drawer, box, or automated dispensing machine in a location that is inaccessible to clients. A count of all controlled medications is performed at specified times (usually at the end of a shift). Medication should not be documented as administered until it is actually given to the client. A medication is to be administered by the route it was ordered. Percocet® can be taken with apple juice. Two client identifiers should be used to administer medications safely. The time of onset for analgesic effect from Percocet® is 10 to 15 minutes.

▶ ***Test-taking Tip:*** *The key words are "needs additional orientation." Select the nursing actions that are incorrect.*

Content Area: Fundamentals; *Category of Health Alteration:* Medication Administration; *Integrated Processes:* Nursing Process Evaluation; *Client Need:* Physiological Integrity/Pharmacological and Parenteral Therapies/Medication Administration; *Cognitive Level:* Application

References: Craven, R., & Hirnle, C. (2007). *Fundamentals of Nursing: Human Health and Function* (5th ed., pp. 555–556). Philadelphia: Lippincott Williams & Wilkins; Deglin, J., & Vallerand, A. (2007). *Davis's Drug Guide for Nurses* (10th ed., p. 1283). Philadelphia: F. A. Davis.

EBP References: Food and Drug Administration. (n.d.). *Controlled Substances Act: Part C - Registration of Manufacturers, Distributors, and Dispensers of Controlled Substances.* Available at: www.fda.gov/opacom/laws/cntrlsub/cntlsbc.htm; The Joint Commission. (2007). *Joint Commission National Patient Safety Goals 2007.* Available at: www.jointcommission.org/PatientSafety/

214. The son of a client with advanced lung cancer asks a hospice nurse to administer larger doses of pain medication so the client will sleep more and "peacefully slip away." The client is adamantly refusing increased doses of medication, despite experiencing pain. The client's wish to not receive medication that causes increased loss of awareness and inability to recognize people is noted in health-care directives. By withholding the undesired medication, the nurse demonstrates ethical practice guided by which principle?

1. Nonmaleficence
2. Autonomy
3. Beneficence
4. Fidelity

ANSWER: 2

Autonomy refers to the client's right to make individual choices and have those choices honored by the nurse. Each client with lung cancer should be asked if he or she has an advance directive, and, if so, this should be placed in the client's chart. Only the client or, if so designated in the directive, the health-care agent has the right to change the wishes identified in a health-care directive. Beneficence is the promotion of good. The good actions must be weighed against any possible harm. Nonmaleficence requires the practitioner to do no harm. The nurse's actions should not cause the client harm. Fidelity means keeping promises.

▶ ***Test-taking Tip:*** *Focus on the definition of the ethical principles in the option choices.*

Content Area: Fundamentals; *Category of Health Alteration:* Medication Administration; *Integrated Processes:* Caring; *Client Need:* Safe and Effective Care Environment/Management of Care/Ethical Practice; *Cognitive Level:* Application

Reference: Wilkinson, J., & Van Leuven, K. (2007). *Fundamentals of Nursing: Theory, Concepts & Applications* (Vol. 1, pp. 1052–1056). Philadelphia: F. A. Davis.

215. EBP A client adamantly refuses to take an oral dose of cephalexin (Keflex®) despite implementing measures to treat the client's nausea. What is the action by the nurse?

1. Administer the medication 1 hour after repeating the dose of antiemetic
2. Have the client suck on ice chips for several minutes before taking the medication
3. Crush the medication and mix it with applesauce for administration
4. Report the information to the client's physician and request a different medication order

ANSWER: 4

In this situation, the client has the right to refuse medications and treatments regardless of the reasons and the consequences. Options 1, 2, and 3 include administering the medication against the client's wishes. The stem indicates the nurse has already tried measures to relieve the client's nausea.

▶ ***Test-taking Tip:*** *Eliminate options 1, 2, and 3 noting that these options are similar. Option 4 is different.*

Content Area: Fundamentals; *Category of Health Alteration:* Medication Administration; *Integrated Processes:* Nursing Process Implementation; *Client Need:* Safe and Effective Care Environment/Management of Care/Client Rights; *Cognitive Level:* Application

Reference: Wilkinson, J., & Van Leuven, K. (2007). *Fundamentals of Nursing: Theory, Concepts & Applications* (Vol. 1, p. 499). Philadelphia: F. A. Davis.

EBP Reference: Baston, S. (2007). The right to refuse. *Emergency Nurse*, 14(10), 12–18.

---

216. EBP A nurse is administering metoclopramide (Reglan®) 10 mg intravenously (IV) to a client with decreased peristalsis. Which nursing action would result in a medication error?

1. Pushing the medication intravenously over 1 minute
2. Administering the medication 30 minutes after meals
3. Noting a Y-site incompatibility of metoclopramide and furosemide
4. Injecting the medication into the D5W with 0.45 NaCl IV in the Y-site closest to the IV insertion site

ANSWER: 2

Metoclopramide is well absorbed in the gastrointestinal (GI) tract and should be administered 30 minutes before meals to increase gastrointestinal motility and prevent nausea at mealtime. The other nurse actions are all correct.

Test-taking Tip: *Note the key word "error." Look for the action that is incorrect.*

Content Area: Fundamentals; *Category of Health Alteration:* Medication Administration; *Integrated Processes:* Nursing Process Implementation; *Client Need:* Physiological Integrity/Pharmacological and Parenteral Therapies/Medication Administration; *Cognitive Level:* Application

References: Wilkinson, J., & Van Leuven, K. (2007). *Fundamentals of Nursing: Theory, Concepts & Applications* (Vol. 1, p. 506). Philadelphia: F. A. Davis; Deglin, J., & Vallerand, A. (2007). *Davis's Drug Guide for Nurses* (10th ed., pp. 782–784). Philadelphia: F. A. Davis.

EBP Reference: Carlton, G. (2006). Medication-related errors: A literature review of incidence and antecedents. *Annual Review of Nursing Research*, 24, 19–38.

---

217. A mother calls a clinic to determine how much cough medicine she should administer to her child who has a cough. The bottle states to give 5 mL using the dropper provided. The mother wants to use a teaspoon because the dropper was destroyed in the dishwasher. The nurse should tell the mother to administer _______ teaspoon(s).

ANSWER: 1

Use the formula for converting medication doses from one medication measurement system to another.

Formula:

5 mL = 1 teaspoon

Test-taking Tip: *Focus on what the question is asking: converting milliliters to teaspoon(s). Verify your response, especially if it seems like an unusual amount.*

Content Area: Fundamentals; *Category of Health Alteration:* Medication Administration; *Integrated Processes:* Communication and Documentation; *Client Need:* Health Promotion and Maintenance/Self-Care; *Cognitive Level:* Analysis

Reference: Berman, A., Snyder, S., Kozier, B., & Erb, G. (2008). *Kozier & Erb's Fundamentals of Nursing: Concepts, Process, and Practice* (8th ed., p. 844). Upper Saddle River, NJ: Pearson Education.

218. An adult client is to receive chlordiazepoxide HCL (Librium®) 25 mg intramuscularly (IM) q6 hours prn for agitation. A vial of the medication supplies 100 mg of sterile, powdered Librium® that needs to be reconstituted with 2 mL of diluent that is packaged with the Librium®. After the medication has been reconstituted, how many milliliters of medication should the nurse withdraw into the syringe illustrated to administer the correct dose of Librium®?

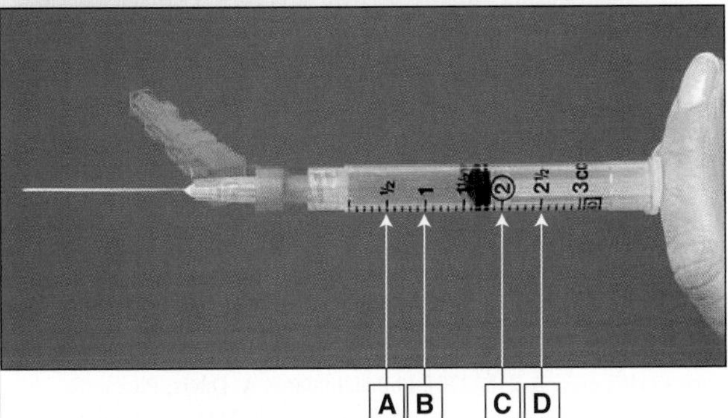

1. A
2. B
3. C
4. D

ANSWER: 1

The line is pointing to the 1/2 mL or 0.5 mL mark on the syringe. Use a proportion formula to calculate the correct dose.
100 mg : 2 mL :: 25 mg : X mL
Multiply the extremes and then the means.
100X = 50
X = 50/100 or 0.5 mL

➧ ***Test-taking Tip:*** *Carefully read what the question is asking.*

Content Area: Fundamentals; *Category of Health Alteration:* Medication Administration; *Integrated Processes:* Nursing Process Implementation; *Client Need:* Physiological Integrity/Pharmacological and Parenteral Therapies/Medication Administration; *Cognitive Level:* Application

Reference: Pickar, G. (2007). *Dosage Calculations: A Ratio-Proportion Approach* (2nd ed., p. 269). Clifton Park, NY: Thomson Delmar Learning.

219. A nurse is to administer promethazine (Phenergan®) 12.5 mg intramuscularly (IM) stat to a client. The medication is supplied in an ampule of 50 mg/mL. How many milliliters should the nurse administer to the client?

1. 0.125 mL
2. 0.25 mL
3. 0.3 mL
4. 1 mL

ANSWER: 2

Use a proportion formula:
50 mg : 1 mL :: 12.5 mg : X mL
Multiple the extremes and then the means and solve for X:
50X = 12.5 mg
X = 12.5/50 = 0.25
Medication is always expressed with a 0 preceding the decimal.

➧ ***Test-taking Tip:*** *Think about the dose; 12.5 mg is less than 50 mg, so the answer obtained should be less than 1 mL. In medication dosing, the number is never rounded to the nearest whole number.*

Content Area: Fundamentals; *Category of Health Alteration:* Medication Administration; *Integrated Processes:* Nursing Process Implementation; *Client Need:* Physiological Integrity/Pharmacological and Parenteral Therapies/Dosage Calculation; *Cognitive Level:* Application

Reference: Pickar, G. (2007). *Dosage Calculations: A Ratio-Proportion Approach* (2nd ed., pp. 46, 344). Clifton Park, NY: Thomson Delmar Learning.

220. A client is to receive esomeprazole (Nexium®) 40 mg oral daily. The medication is supplied in 20-mg capsules. In order to give the correct dose, a nurse should administer ____ capsules to the client.

ANSWER: 2

20 mg : 1 capsule :: 40 mg : X capsules
20X = 40
X = 2 capsules

➧ ***Test-taking Tip:*** *Use a formula to calculate the correct dose and verify the answer if it seems unusually large.*

Content Area: Fundamentals; *Category of Health Alteration:* Medication Administration; *Integrated Processes:* Nursing Process Planning; *Client Need:* Physiological Integrity/Pharmacological and Parenteral Therapies/Dosage Calculation; *Cognitive Level:* Application

Reference: Pickar, G. (2007). *Dosage Calculations: A Ratio-Proportion Approach* (2nd ed., p. 314). Clifton Park, NY: Thomson Delmar Learning.

221. EBP On admission to a hospital, a client provides a nurse with a handwritten medication list on which is listed bupropion (Wellbutrin XL®) 150 mg daily. The client also shows to the nurse the medication bottle that is labeled Wellbutrin XL® 300-mg tablets. Which questions should the nurse ask the client? SELECT ALL THAT APPLY.

1. "Has your dosage of medication increased or decreased recently?"
2. "Were you able to halve the tablets to safely give yourself the correct dose?"
3. "Did you take two tablets daily from this bottle?"
4. "Are you taking the medication for smoking cessation, treating depression, or for another reason?"
5. "When was the last time you took medication from this bottle?"
6. "Have you experienced headaches, tremors, or a dry mouth while taking this medication?"

ANSWER: 1, 4, 5, 6

The handwritten medication list is half the strength of the tablets in the bottle. Either the dose was increased and this is the correct bottle, or the dose was decreased and the handwritten medication list is correct and this is the wrong bottle. Bupropion is used for smoking cessation or in the treatment of depression, attention deficit-hyperactivity disorder (ADHD) in adults, or to increase sexual desire in women. The last time a dose was taken from the bottle will help determine the amount the client is taking and to verify if it is the correct amount. Major side effects of bupropion include headaches, tremors, and dry mouth. If the client is taking a higher dose than prescribed, the client could be experiencing side effects. Wellbutrin XL® is sustained release; tablets should not be halved for safe administration. This is the wrong question to ask; taking two tablets will result in a 600 mg dose.

***Test-taking Tip:** Carefully read the client's medication list and compare it against the medication label to answer the question. Recall that XL means sustained release.*

Content Area: Fundamentals; *Category of Health Alteration:* Medication Administration; *Integrated Processes:* Communication and Documentation; *Client Need:* Physiological Integrity/Pharmacological and Parenteral Therapies/Dosage Calculation; *Cognitive Level:* Analysis

References: Deglin, J., & Vallerand, A. (2007). *Davis's Drug Guide for Nurses* (10th ed., pp. 218–220). Philadelphia: F. A. Davis; Pickar, G. (2007). *Dosage Calculations: A Ratio-Proportion Approach* (2nd ed., pp. 170–180). Clifton Park, NY: Thomson Delmar Learning.

EBP Reference: Health Care Association of New Jersey (HCANJ). (2006). *Medication Management Guideline*. Hamilton, NJ: Author.

222. A client is to receive a systemic cephalosporin, cephalexin (Keflex®) 500 mg in 50 mL of normal saline intravenous piggyback (IVPB). The medication is to be infused over 20 minutes. To correctly infuse the medication, the nurse should set the pump rate at_______ mL/hr.

ANSWER: 150

50 mL : 20 min :: X mL/hr: 60 min/hr

Multiple the means (inside values) and then the extremes (outside values) to solve for X.

20X = 3,000

X = 150 mL/hr

***Test-taking Tip:** Use a formula to calculate the correct dose and verify the answer if it seems unusually large.*

Content Area: Fundamentals; *Category of Health Alteration:* Medication Administration; *Integrated Processes:* Nursing Process Analysis; *Client Need:* Physiological Integrity/Pharmacological and Parenteral Therapies/Dosage Calculation; *Cognitive Level:* Application

Reference: Pickar, G. (2007). *Dosage Calculations: A Ratio-Proportion Approach* (2nd ed., pp. 46, 362). Clifton Park, NY: Thomson Delmar Learning.

Test 7: **Fundamentals: Safety, Disaster Preparedness, and Infection Control**

223. A charge nurse is observing staff nurses who are ambulating and transferring clients. Which activity, illustrated below, would put a nurse at risk for back injury and require intervention by the charge nurse?

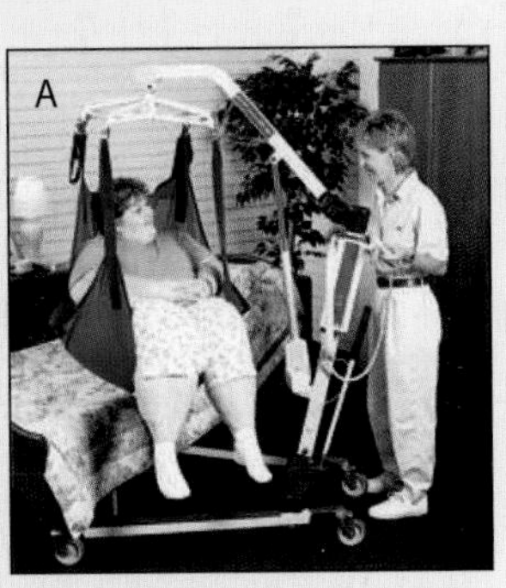

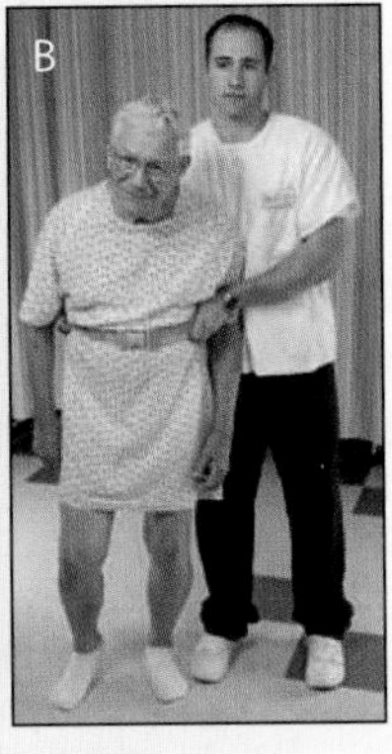

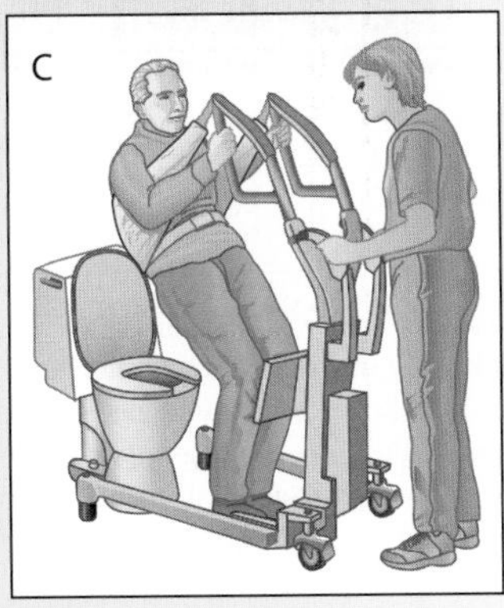

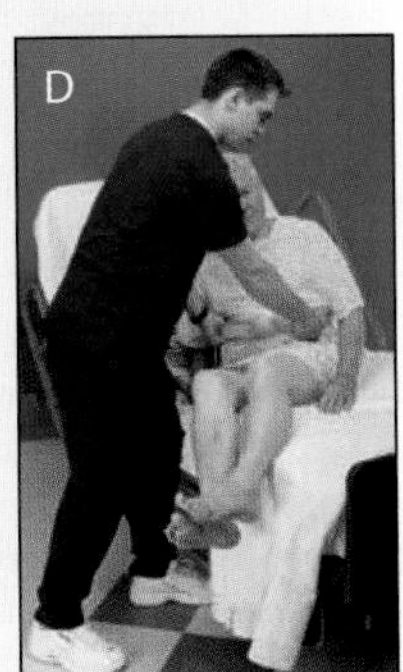

1. Activity A
2. Activity B
3. Activity C
4. Activity D

ANSWER: 4

Bending and twisting the torso can cause back injury if the nurse does not use correct body mechanics. A nurse has reduced the risk by using a transfer belt and proper body mechanics, but the risk for injury exists because the client could easily grab the nurse's shoulder or arm with his left hand, altering the nurse's stance. The nurse in activity A is using a mechanical lift to move the client. Because another person is not present in the illustration to assist, there is a perceived increased risk for injury to the client. Ambulating a client with a transfer belt also increases the nurse's risk for a back injury should the client fall, but it is less of a risk than the twisting and bending illustrated in activity D. In activity C, the nurse is using a standing assist device to help the client move from a sitting to a standing position and vice versa. Using assistive devices minimizes the risk for injury to the client and nurse.

Test-taking Tip: *Examine each illustration carefully and focus on the position of the client and nurse to determine the nurse's risk for injury.*

Content Area: Fundamentals; *Category of Health Alteration:* Safety, Disaster Preparedness, and Infection Control; *Integrated Processes:* Nursing Process Assessment; *Client Need:* Safe and Effective Care Environment/Safety and Infection Control/Ergonomic Principles; *Cognitive Level:* Analysis

Reference: Wilkinson, J., & Van Leuven, K. (2007). *Fundamentals of Nursing: Theory, Concepts & Applications* (Vol. 1, pp. 437, 755–756). Philadelphia: F. A. Davis.

224. A client with a left-sided weakness is to be discharged to home, where the client has an electrical bed. In preparation for discharge, a nurse assesses the client's ability to get out of bed independently. Which client actions indicate that further instruction is needed? SELECT ALL THAT APPLY.

1. Places the bed in the lowest position
2. Raises the head of the bed (HOB)
3. Rolls onto the left side
4. Pushes against the mattress with the weak elbow and stronger hand to rise to a sitting position
5. Slides legs off the bed while pushing against the mattress to raise the body off the bed
6. Once in a sitting position, sits at the edge of the bed for a few minutes before standing

ANSWER: 3, 4

With a left-sided weakness, the client should turn onto the stronger side. The stronger elbow, hand, and leg can then be used to push off the bed into a sitting position. A low bed position prevents a fall from the feet not touching the floor. Raising the HOB decreases the distance to a sitting position. The body does not bend to a sitting position without changing the position of the legs and the weight of the legs dangling will decrease the effort required to push into a sitting position. Sudden position changes can cause orthostatic hypotension. Sitting awhile assures that the client is not dizzy prior to standing.

Test-taking Tip: *Note that the client has a left-sided weakness. Visualizing the steps that the client should use to transfer when the left side is weak should direct you to the correct actions.*

Content Area: Fundamentals; *Category of Health Alteration:* Safety, Disaster Preparedness, and Infection Control; *Integrated Processes:* Nursing Process Evaluation; *Client Need:* Safe and Effective Care Environment/Safety and Infection Control/Ergonomic Principles; *Cognitive Level:* Analysis

Reference: Harkreader, H., Hogan, M., & Thobaben, M. (2007). *Fundamentals of Nursing* (3rd ed., p. 846). St. Louis, MO: Saunders/Elsevier.

225. A nurse assesses a client's balance and ability to use crutches safely before allowing the client to ambulate independently. The nurse documents in the client's medical record: "Client uses a three-point gait correctly to maintain non-weight-bearing on left foot when ambulating with crutches. Maintains steady balance and keeps eyes focused ahead." On the illustration, place an X in the tripod position box for the column that most accurately illustrates the gait documented by the nurse.

4. Advance right foot and left crutch	4. Advance right foot	4. Advance right foot	4. Lift both feet; swing them forward, landing feet next to the crutches	4. Lift both feet; swing them forward, landing feet in front of the crutches
3. Advance left foot and right crutch	3. Advance left foot and both crutches	3. Advance left crutch	3. Advance both crutches	3. Advance both crutches
2. Advance right foot and left crutch	2. Advance right foot	2. Advance left foot	2. Lift both feet; swing them forward, landing feet next to the crutches	2. Lift both feet; swing them forward, landing feet in front of the crutches
1. Advance left foot and right crutch	1. Advance left foot and both crutches	1. Advance right crutch	1. Advance both crutches	1. Advance both crutches
Tripod position	Tripod position	Tripod position	Tripod position	Tripod position

ANSWER:

4. Advance right foot and left crutch	4. Advance right foot	4. Advance right foot	4. Lift both feet; swing them forward, landing feet next to the crutches	4. Lift both feet; swing them forward, landing feet in front of the crutches
3. Advance left foot and right crutch	3. Advance left foot and both crutches	3. Advance left crutch	3. Advance both crutches	3. Advance both crutches
2. Advance right foot and left crutch	2. Advance right foot	2. Advance left foot	2. Lift both feet; swing them forward, landing feet next to the crutches	2. Lift both feet; swing them forward, landing feet in front of the crutches
1. Advance left foot and right crutch	1. Advance left foot and both crutches	1. Advance right crutch	1. Advance both crutches	1. Advance both crutches
Tripod position	Tripod position X	Tripod position	Tripod position	Tripod position

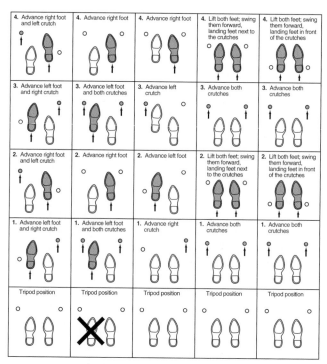

A three-point gait should be used for non-weight-bearing ambulation. Both the crutches and the weaker leg move forward first. Then, the stronger leg advances. Column 1 illustrates a two-point gait. Column 3 illustrates a four-point gait. Column 4 illustrates a swing-to gate. Column 5 illustrates a swing-through gait. The two-point and four-point gait are partial weight-bearing gaits and the swing-to and swing-through gaits are weight-bearing gaits.

▶ ***Test-taking Tip:*** *If unsure of the types of gaits, focus on the illustration and try to determine which illustration depicts a non-weight-bearing gait.*

Content Area: Fundamentals; *Category of Health Alteration:* Safety, Disaster Preparedness, and Infection Control; *Integrated Processes:* Communication and Documentation; *Client Need:* Safe and Effective Care Environment/Safety and Infection Control/Ergonomic Principles; *Cognitive Level:* Application

Reference: Harkreader, H., Hogan, M., & Thobaben, M. (2007). *Fundamentals of Nursing* (3rd ed., p. 855). St. Louis, MO: Saunders/Elsevier.

226. A lightweight client, diagnosed with chronic obstructive pulmonary disease and an ulcer on the sole of the foot, slides down in bed. Pressure is being exerted to the client's foot from the bottom bed guard. Due to an emergency on the unit, no one is available to assist a nurse with repositioning the client. Which action by the nurse is best?

1. Wait until sufficient help is available to reposition the client
2. Place pillows over the bed guard and elevate both of the client's legs on the pillows
3. Place the bed in Tredelenburg's position to relieve the pressure and then wait for help
4. Use the slight Trendelenburg's position to pull the client up in bed and place the client in a Fowler's position

ANSWER: 4

The force of gravity, created by the slight Trendelenburg's position, increases the ability to move a lightweight client up in bed safely while alone. Waiting for help delays relieving the pressure and can increase pain and tissue damage. Placing pillows over the bed guard and elevating the client's legs increases the risk of the client sliding off of the bed when unattended. Leaving the client in the Trendelenburg's position can compromise the client's respiratory status.

***Test-taking Tip:** Select the option that applies ergonomic principles and maintains the safety of the client.*

Content Area: Fundamentals; *Category of Health Alteration:* Safety, Disaster Preparedness, and Infection Control; *Integrated Processes:* Nursing Process Implementation; *Client Need:* Safe and Effective Care Environment/Safety and Infection Control/Ergonomic Principles; *Cognitive Level:* Analysis

Reference: Harkreader, H., Hogan, M., & Thobaben, M. (2007). *Fundamentals of Nursing* (3rd ed., pp. 881–882). St. Louis, MO: Saunders/Elsevier.

227. EBP A nurse is providing educational materials to parents of a full-term newborn at discharge. When discussing the infant's transportation in a vehicle, which information should the nurse provide to the parent? SELECT ALL THAT APPLY

1. The infant should be restrained in a car seat located in the front seat facing the rear of the car.
2. The infant should be restrained in a car seat located in the back seat facing the rear of the car.
3. The infant should be restrained in a car seat located in the back seat facing the front of the car.
4. Because some infant car seat restraints are designed only for infants, another one will need to be obtained when the infant reaches the weight limit for that model.
5. Some states and provinces in the United States and Canada have mandated the use of infant and child restraints.
6. A car seat should have a certification label stating that it complies with federal motor vehicle safety standards.

ANSWER: 2, 4, 6

The infant should be restrained in a car seat located in the back seat, facing the rear of the car to provide protection should an accident occur. Infants and toddlers should be in the child-restraint device (car seat) appropriate for the infant's weight and size. Some models are for infants only; others convert for toddler use. Parents should only purchase a car seat that has a certification label stating that it complies with federal motor vehicle safety standards. An infant should never be placed in the front seat of cars equipped with air bags because the infant could be seriously injured if the airbag were released. If the infant is in the front or back facing forward, if an accident should occur, the force of the crash would whip the infant's head forward, causing tremendous neck stress. In the United States and Canada, all states and provinces have mandated the use of child restraints while traveling in a car.

***Test-taking Tip:** Consider the disproportionally heavy head and weak neck muscles of the infant and then select the options that are safest for the infant.*

Content Area: Fundamentals; *Category of Health Alteration:* Safety, Disaster Preparedness, and Infection Control; *Integrated Processes:* Teaching and Learning; Caring; *Client Need:* Safe and Effective Care Environment/Safety and Infection Control/Accident Prevention; *Cognitive Level:* Application

References: Hockenberry, M., & Wilson, D. (2007). *Wong's Nursing Care of Infants and Children* (8th ed., pp. 304–305). St. Louis, MO: Mosby/Elsevier; Pillitteri, A. (2007). *Maternal and Child Health Nursing* (5th ed., pp. 480–481). Philadelphia: Lippincott Williams & Wilkins.

EBP Reference: Department of Health and Human Services: Centers for Disease Control and Prevention. (2006). *Child Passenger Safety: Fact Sheet.* Washington, DC: U.S. Government Printing Office. Available at: www.cdc.gov/ncipc/factsheets/childpas.htm

228. Which nursing diagnosis is most appropriate for safety needs of school-aged children?

1. Risk for injury related to risk-taking behavior and lack of supervision
2. Deficient diversional activities related to lack of appropriate toys or peers
3. Risk for imbalanced nutrition less than body requirements related to chronic illness
4. Anxiety related to change in health status

ANSWER: 1

Risk for injury related to risk-taking behavior and lack of supervision addresses the safety needs of children. Nursing's role is to educate the parents on the safety needs of children and should focus on injury prevention. The other diagnoses may be applicable to the client but do not address the safety needs.

***Test-taking Tip:** Select the option that can be associated with the key word in the question: "safety."*

Content Area: Fundamentals; *Category of Health Alteration:* Safety, Disaster Preparedness, and Infection Control; *Integrated Processes:* Nursing Process Analysis; *Client Need:* Safe and Effective Care Environment/Safety and Infection Control/Injury Prevention; *Cognitive Level:* Analysis

References: Hockenberry, M., & Wilson, D. (2007). *Wong's Nursing Care of Infants and Children* (8th ed., p. 743). St. Louis, MO: Mosby/Elsevier; Pillitteri, A. (2007). *Maternal & Child Health Nursing: Care of the Childbearing & Childrearing Family* (5th ed., p. 1091). Philadelphia: Lippincott Williams & Wilkins.

229. EBP An experienced nurse is observing a new nurse providing care to a client. Which action requires the experienced nurse to intervene to ensure client safety?

1. Turning on the client's bathroom light and turning out the room lights after settling the client for sleep
2. Checking the client's room number and name on the client's name band to verify client identity prior to administering medications
3. Taking a telephone order from a physician, writing the order, and reading it back to the physician before implementing the order
4. Delaying an on-coming physician from performing a right thoracentesis scheduled by a previous physician by calling "a timeout" to verify the client's identity, consent, procedure, and site

ANSWER: 2

The client's room number is not one of the two unique client identifiers that should be used prior to medication administration. The usual identifiers are the client's name on the name band and the medical record number on the name band. Keeping a light on can prevent confusion about the surroundings if the client should waken during the night. The person taking a verbal or telephone order should "read back" the complete order to be sure it is accurate. A final verification process to confirm the correct client, procedure, and site should be conducted prior to the start of any invasive procedure. This "timeout" also allows verification that the necessary supplies and documents are available.

➧ ***Test-taking Tip:*** *The key phrase is "ensure client safety." Read each option carefully to identify the situation that increases the risk for the nurse to cause an error.*

Content Area: Fundamentals; *Category of Health Alteration:* Safety, Disaster Preparedness, and Infection Control; *Integrated Processes:* Nursing Process Evaluation; *Client Need:* Safe and Effective Care Environment/Safety and Infection Control/Error Prevention; *Cognitive Level:* Analysis

Reference: Berman, A., Snyder, S., Kozier, B., & Erb, G. (2008). *Fundamentals of Nursing: Concepts, Process, and Practice* (8th ed., p. 715). Upper Saddle River, NJ: Pearson Education.

EBP References: The Joint Commission. (2009). *National Patient Safety Goals Hospital Program.* Available at: www.jointcommission.org/patientsafety/nationalpatientsafetygoals/; www.jointcommission.org/NR/rdonlyres/31666E86-E7F4-423E-9BE8-F05BD1CB0AA8/0/HAP_NPSG.pdf; The Joint Commission. (2003). *Universal Protocol for Preventing Wrong Site, Wrong Procedure, Wrong Person Surgery.* Available at: www.jointcommission.org/patientsafety/universalprotocol/

230. A nurse is caring for multiple clients in a nursing home. The nurse knows that a competent client's right to autonomy will be limited by health-care providers when the client is diagnosed with which of the following?

1. Medication-resistant tuberculosis and refuses treatment at the nearest health-care facility
2. Entering the end stage of renal failure and refuses to continue dialysis treatments
3. Severe anemia and refuses blood transfusions based upon religious beliefs
4. Having metastases from breast cancer to the brain and refuses chemotherapy

ANSWER: 1

A client's autonomy is limited when the client has a communicable disease that can endanger others. The client must undergo treatment as directed. Pursuant to a client's rights under the Self-Determination Act of 1990, a client's refusal of treatment must be respected unless it endangers others.

➧ ***Test-taking Tip:*** *Read the situation carefully. Use the process of elimination to eliminate options in which refusal of treatment would not endanger others.*

Content Area: Fundamentals; *Category of Health Alteration:* Safety, Disaster Preparedness, and Infection Control; *Integrated Processes:* Nursing Process Analysis; *Client Need:* Safe and Effective Care Environment/Safety and Infection Control/Injury Prevention; *Cognitive Level:* Analysis

References: Harkreader, H., Hogan, M., & Thobaben, M. (2007). *Fundamentals of Nursing* (3rd ed., p. 37). St. Louis, MO: Saunders/Elsevier; Potter, P., & Perry, A. (2009). *Fundamentals of Nursing* (7th ed., pp. 328–329). St. Louis, MO: Mosby.

231. A client presents to an emergency department after experiencing a seizure at home. A nurse pads the client's side rails, lowers the client's bed, and ensures that suction equipment is available while waiting for the serum laboratory results. Place an X in the right-hand column to indicate the laboratory value indicative of a condition that could lead to a seizure.

Serum Laboratory Test	Client's Value	Normal	Laboratory Value Indicative of a Condition that Could Lead to a Seizure
BUN	26	5–25 mg/dL	
Creatinine	2.4	0.5–1.5 mg/dL	
Na	119	135–145 mEq/L	
K	3.5	3.5–5.3 mEq/L	
Cl	95	95–105 mEq/L	
CO_2	23	22–30 mEq/L	
Phosphate	1.8	1.7–2.6 mEq/L	
Calcium	9.5	9–11 mg/dL	
Hgb	13.1	13.5–17 g/dL	
Hct	39.8	40%–54%	
PTH	15	11–54 pg/mL	

ANSWER:

Serum Laboratory Test	Client's Value	Normal	Laboratory Value Contributing to Seizures
Na	119	135–145 mEq/L	X

Serum sodium is dangerously below normal values. Hyponatremia, when severe, can cause cellular swelling in the brain and lead to seizures. An elevated blood urea nitrogen (BUN) and serum creatinine level indicates renal impairment. The level is not high enough to induce seizures. The serum potassium is on the low side of normal and would not contribute to seizures. Chloride, serum CO_2, phosphate, calcium, hematocrit, and parathyroid hormone are within normal limits and would not contribute to seizure activity. Slightly below-normal hemoglobin will not contribute to seizures.

▶ ***Test-taking Tip:*** *Knowledge of laboratory values and imbalances are essential to respond to this question. Eliminate the laboratory values that are within the normal ranges.*

Content Area: Fundamentals; *Category of Health Alteration:* Safety, Disaster Preparedness, and Infection Control; *Integrated Processes:* Nursing Process Assessment; *Client Need:* Safe and Effective Care Environment/Safety and Infection Control/Injury Prevention; *Cognitive Level:* Analysis

Reference: Lewis, S., Heitkemper, M., Dirksen, S., O'Brien, P., & Bucher, L. (2007). *Medical-Surgical Nursing: Assessment and Management of Clinical Problems* (7th ed., pp. 340–341). St. Louis, MO: Mosby.

232. A nurse is ambulating an elderly client using a transfer belt for support. The client begins to experience signs and symptoms of orthostatic hypotension. Which steps should be taken by the nurse to prevent the client from falling? Prioritize the nurse's actions by placing each step in the correct order.

______ Support and ease the client to the floor, allowing the client to slide down the forward leg
______ Call for help
______ Bend at the knees
______ Assess the client for injuries
______ Use the transfer belt to pull the client toward the forward leg
______ Protect the client's head from hitting objects on the floor
______ Assume a broad stance with the stronger leg somewhat behind the other leg

ANSWER: 5, 1, 3, 7, 4, 6, 2

First, call for help. Then assume a broad stance with the stronger leg somewhat behind the other leg and bend at the knees. This position forms a solid base of support for bearing the weight on the stronger leg. Using the transfer belt, pull the client toward the forward leg. Next, support and ease the client to the floor, allowing the client to slide down the forward leg. Protect the client's head from hitting objects on the floor. Finally, assess the client for injuries. A minor fall can result in a hip fracture for an older adult with osteoporosis.

▶ ***Test-taking Tip:*** *Visualize the steps prior to placing them in the correct order.*

Content Area: Fundamentals; *Category of Health Alteration:* Safety, Disaster Preparedness, and Infection Control; *Integrated Processes:* Nursing Process Implementation; *Client Need:* Safe and Effective Care Environment/Safety and Infection Control/Injury Prevention; *Cognitive Level:* Synthesis

Reference: Harkreader, H., Hogan, M., & Thobaben, M. (2007). *Fundamentals of Nursing* (3rd ed., p. 851). St. Louis, MO: Saunders/Elsevier.

233. An 82-year-old client has a right total hip arthroplasty with a hip prosthesis and is planning to move in with his son following discharge. A nurse is discussing home modifications with the son. Which modifications should the nurse recommend? SELECT ALL THAT APPLY.

1. Pad bed side rails
2. Install safety bars around the toilet and shower
3. Install an elevated toilet seat in the bathroom
4. Plan for the client's bed to be in a main floor room
5. Place a nonskid bathmat in the bathtub and have the client bathe daily
6. Remove scatter rugs and secure electrical cords against baseboards

ANSWER: 2, 3, 4, 6

Safety bars around the toilet and shower are useful for support and fall prevention. An elevated toilet seat is necessary because the client should avoid a 90-degree hip flexion for 4 to 6 weeks postoperatively. A main floor bedroom will prevent unnecessary stair climbing that could cause a fall. Scatter rugs can cause tripping and falls. Padded side rails are unnecessary; these are used for injury prevention with seizure activity or agitation. The client should shower rather than bathe. Tub baths are not allowed for 4 to 6 weeks to avoid a 90-degree hip flexion.

➧ ***Test-taking Tip:*** *Focus on both the age of the client and the type of surgery when selecting the answer options.*

Content Area: Fundamentals; *Category of Health Alteration:* Safety, Disaster Preparedness, and Infection Control; *Integrated Processes:* Nursing Process Implementation; *Client Need:* Safe and Effective Care Environment/Safety and Infection Control/Home Safety; *Cognitive Level:* Application

References: Lewis, S., Heitkemper, M., Dirksen, S., O'Brien, P., & Bucher, L. (2007). *Medical-Surgical Nursing: Assessment and Management of Clinical Problems* (7th ed., p. 1663). St. Louis, MO: Mosby; Potter, P., & Perry, A. (2009). *Fundamentals of Nursing* (7th ed., pp. 830–831). St. Louis, MO: Mosby.

234. EBP A nurse is teaching a client diagnosed with a latex allergy about home safety. Which points will be important for the nurse to emphasize? SELECT ALL THAT APPLY.

1. Identify items in the home that are made from synthetic materials
2. Keep emergency telephone numbers readily accessible
3. Have someone remove items such as latex balloons and rubber bands from the home
4. Increase intake of foods high in potassium, such as kiwi, bananas, avocados, and chestnuts
5. Remove certain plants in the home, such as poinsettia plants, which can initiate an allergic reaction
6. Before purchasing items for the home, determine if they are likely to contain latex

ANSWER: 2, 3, 5, 6

Persons with a latex allergy react to either contact with or aerosolized particles of natural latex rubber; emergency telephone numbers should be available because an anaphylactic reaction can occur. Latex balloons, rubber bands, and plants such as poinsettia can initiate an allergic reaction. A multitude of items contain latex, and items should be checked for latex prior to purchase. Foods such as kiwi, bananas, avocados, and chestnuts should be avoided because these increase the risk of an allergic reaction.

➧ ***Test-taking Tip:*** *Recall that foods, plants, and many other items in the home can initiate an allergic response.*

Content Area: Fundamentals; *Category of Health Alteration:* Safety, Disaster Preparedness, and Infection Control; *Integrated Processes:* Teaching and Learning; *Client Need:* Safe and Effective Care Environment/Safety and Infection Control/Home Safety; *Cognitive Level:* Analysis

Reference: Harkreader, H., Hogan, M., & Thobaben, M. (2007). *Fundamentals of Nursing* (3rd ed., p. 1284). St. Louis, MO: Saunders/Elsevier.

EBP Reference: Grier, T. (2007). *Literature Review on Latex-Food Cross-Reactivity 1991–2006.* Greer Laboratories Inc., Research and Development. Available at: www.latexallergyresources.org/FileDownloads/Latex-food%20cross-reactivity%20review.pdf.

235. A client, diagnosed with diabetes mellitus, is receiving care in the home for a foot ulcer. A home health nurse documents in the client's medical record the narrative note illustrated. Which nursing diagnosis should be the nurse's priority on the return visit?

Progress Notes

Date	Time	Entry
6-20-09	0900	Client visited in home. Left foot ulcer showing signs of healing with granulation tissue. Wet-to-dry dressing change completed. Instructed on wearing nonskid slipper on left foot and shoe on right after noting client wearing white socks for ambulation. Blood pressure 140/86 mm Hg; states has not yet taken morning dose of medication; "Can't stomach breakfast if eaten before the dressing change." Plan to return in AM for further assessment. -----------------------------B. Green, RN

1. Impaired skin integrity related to left foot ulcer
2. Potential for injury related to improper footwear
3. Potential altered nutrition: less than body requirements related to nausea
4. Ineffective therapeutic regimen management related to not taking medications as prescribed

ANSWER: 2

The risk for injury should be the nurse's priority. A client with diabetes may have decreased sensation to the feet. Trauma to the foot can result in injury that may not be felt by the client. Falling is also a concern because the client's mobility is impaired due to the foot ulcer. A fall could be life-threatening. The impaired skin integrity is not currently health-threatening because the wound is showing signs of healing. Nutrition is not currently health-threatening, but it could be if it persists. Though the blood pressure is slightly elevated, there is no indication that the client does not plan to take the medication.

➧ ***Test-taking Tip:*** *Use Maslow's Hierarchy of Needs theory to establish priority. Actual or potential life-threatening situations are priority.*

Content Area: Fundamentals; *Category of Health Alteration:* Safety, Disaster Preparedness, and Infection Control; *Integrated Processes:* Nursing Process Analysis; *Client Need:* Safe and Effective Care Environment/Safety and Infection Control/Home Safety; *Cognitive Level:* Analysis

Reference: Berman, A., Snyder, S., Kozier, B., & Erb, G. (2008). *Fundamentals of Nursing: Concepts, Process, and Practice* (8th ed., pp. 217–218, 711). Upper Saddle River, NJ: Pearson Education.

---

236. A client makes the following statements to a home health nurse. Which statement requires the nurse to intervene immediately?

1. "I can't lift pans from the back burners, but I can manage just fine using the front burners of my stove."
2. "My home is less costly to heat when I use my gas oven with the oven door open to heat just my living areas."
3. "I almost fell down the stairs so I bought myself a pair of slippers with nonskid soles."
4. "The grass near the sidewalk will be dead because my son insists on putting salt on the icy sidewalk."

ANSWER: 2

Using a gas oven or range to heat the home can result in carbon monoxide accumulation and poisoning. Inability to lift pans from the back burners poses a safety concern for burns and scalds. While further assessment is required, this does not require immediate intervention. Wearing nonskid slippers and applying salt to icy sidewalks promotes client safety.

➧ ***Test-taking Tip:*** *Eliminate the statements that promote client safety. Of the remaining options, determine which needs further assessment and which needs immediate intervention.*

Content Area: Fundamentals; *Category of Health Alteration:* Safety, Disaster Preparedness, and Infection Control; *Integrated Processes:* Communication and Documentation; *Client Need:* Safe and Effective Care Environment/Safety and Infection Control/Home Safety; *Cognitive Level:* Analysis

Reference: Wilkinson, J., & Van Leuven, K. (2007). *Fundamentals of Nursing: Theory, Concepts & Applications* (Vol. 1, pp. 424–426). Philadelphia: F. A. Davis.

237. A nurse asks a nursing assistant (NA) to apply a mitten restraint for a client seated in the wheelchair next to the bed. Which observation by the nurse indicates that the NA needs further instructions on applying restraints?

1. Restraint strap is tied to the bed frame
2. Restraint straps are secured using a half bow slip knot
3. Mitten restraint is secured at wrists so that two fingers can be inserted between the restraint and client's skin
4. Mesh portion of the mitten restraint is on the back of the hand

ANSWER: 1

When seated in the wheelchair, the mitten restraint should be secured to the frame of the wheelchair. Client injury can occur if the wheelchair is pulled away from the bed. A half bow slip knot should be used for quick release. Allowing room for two fingerbreadths between the restraint and client's skin prevents circulatory constriction. The mesh portion of the mitten restraint should be on the back of the hand to observe hand and finger color while the mitten restraint is in place.

➧ ***Test-taking Tip:*** *Focus on client safety. Select the option that could result in client injury if the wheelchair is moved.*

Content Area: Fundamentals; *Category of Health Alteration:* Safety, Disaster Preparedness, and Infection Control; *Integrated Processes:* Nursing Process Evaluation; *Client Need:* Safe and Effective Care Environment/Safety and Infection Control/Use of Restraints/Safety Devices; *Cognitive Level:* Analysis

Reference: Harkreader, H., Hogan, M., & Thobaben, M. (2007). *Fundamentals of Nursing* (3rd ed., pp. 558–559). St. Louis, MO: Saunders/Elsevier.

---

238. An older adult, hospitalized with chest trauma following a motor vehicle accident, has a right femoral arterial line. Because the client has been thrashing about in bed, a physician writes an order for wrist restraints to be applied. Based on this information, which action by a nurse is correct?

1. Apply the wrist restraints as ordered
2. Request an order for a right ankle restraint also
3. Request an order for sedation instead of restraints
4. Question the order because restraints will increase the client's agitation

ANSWER: 2

An ankle restraint will help prevent dislodgement of the arterial catheter and bleeding and injury that could occur from thrashing in bed. While applying wrist restraints will prevent side-to-side movement, it will not keep the client's right leg straight to prevent catheter dislodgement. The client has chest trauma. Sedation may compromise the client's respiratory status. While restraints can increase agitation, especially for an older adult, keeping one leg unrestrained may prevent this from occurring. Safety of the client is priority.

➧ ***Test-taking Tip:*** *Focus on the information provided in the scenario. The issue is an appropriate restraint for a client with chest trauma who also has a femoral arterial catheter. Select the option that protects the client from injury.*

Content Area: Fundamentals; *Category of Health Alteration:* Safety, Disaster Preparedness, and Infection Control; *Integrated Processes:* Nursing Process Implementation; *Client Need:* Safe and Effective Care Environment/Safety and Infection Control/Use of Restraints/Safety Devices *Cognitive Level:* Analysis

Reference: Harkreader, H., Hogan, M., & Thobaben, M. (2007). *Fundamentals of Nursing* (3rd ed., p. 557). St. Louis, MO: Saunders/Elsevier.

---

239. A nurse sees smoke coming from a client's hospital room. When entering the room, the nurse notes that the client is standing on the far side of the room with clothing on fire. Which action should be taken by the nurse immediately?

1. Go find the nearest fire alarm box
2. Tell the client to drop and roll on the floor
3. Grab a blanket to smother the fire
4. Obtain water to douse the clothes

ANSWER: 2

Rolling on the ground will smother the flames and put the fire out. The client is priority. Those responding can locate and activate the alarm box. Smothering the fire is the next action. Finding and obtaining water is too time-consuming and the fire will continue to burn.

➧ ***Test-taking Tip:*** *Remember the key phrase "Stop, drop, and roll."*

Content Area: Fundamentals; *Category of Health Alteration:* Safety, Disaster Preparedness, and Infection Control; *Integrated Processes:* Nursing Process Implementation; *Client Need:* Safe and Effective Care Environment/Safety and Infection Control/Emergency Response Plan; *Cognitive Level:* Application

Reference: Potter, P., & Perry, A. (2009). *Fundamentals of Nursing* (7th ed., pp. 839–840). St. Louis, MO: Mosby.

240. What should a nurse do *first* when a hospitalized client tells the nurse about feeling a strong shock when turning on an electric hairdryer?

1. Assess the client's apical pulse
2. Disconnect the hairdryer from the electrical outlet
3. Assess the client's skin for signs of an electrical burn
4. Send the hairdryer to the maintenance department for inspection

ANSWER: 1

Because body fluids (consisting of sodium chloride) are an excellent conductor of electricity, an electric shock can be transmitted through the body. The electrical charge may interfere with the heart's electrical conduction system, causing a dysrhythmia. Disconnecting the hairdryer is contraindicated because it may place the nurse at risk. Assessing the client's skin is not the priority; depending on the voltage, electrical burns may or may not be evident. Although sending the hairdryer for inspection should be done eventually, it is not the priority at this time.

▶ ***Test-taking Tip:*** *Use the nursing process to establish priority. Assessment is the first step and should be priority. Focus on the client's safety.*

Content Area: Fundamentals; *Category of Health Alteration:* Safety, Disaster Preparedness, and Infection Control; *Integrated Processes:* Nursing Process Assessment; *Client Need:* Safe and Effective Care Environment/Safety and Infection Control/Injury Prevention; *Cognitive Level:* Analysis

Reference: Potter, P., & Perry, A. (2009). *Fundamentals of Nursing* (7th ed., p. 842). St. Louis, MO: Mosby.

---

241. A power outage occurs at a hospital and a backup generator, supplying power to a telemetry unit fails. After obtaining a flashlight, what is a nurse's next best action?

1. Call the nursing supervisor
2. Assess the most critically ill clients
3. Obtain oxygen tanks for clients on oxygen
4. Delegate which clients a nursing assistant should monitor

ANSWER: 3

When power is interrupted, the oxygen sources in the room will also fail. Oxygen will need to be delivered by oxygen tanks. A call to the nursing supervisor may be necessary for assistance on the unit, but is not the next action. Assessment of the most critical clients is also a priority, but those in need of oxygen are the priority. A nurse should delegate activities, but rather than monitoring clients, the nurse should delegate retrieving oxygen tanks.

▶ ***Test-taking Tip:*** *Use the ABCs (airway, breathing, circulation) to determine the priority action. In emergency situations, an intervention (oxygen) is priority over assessment.*

Content Area: Fundamentals; *Category of Health Alteration:* Safety, Disaster Preparedness, and Infection Control; *Integrated Processes:* Nursing Process Implementation; *Client Need:* Safe and Effective Care Environment/Safety and Infection Control/Emergency Response Plan; *Cognitive Level:* Analysis

Reference: Berman, A., Snyder, S., Kozier, B., & Erb, G. (2008). *Fundamentals of Nursing: Concepts, Process, and Practice* (8th ed., p. 1372). Upper Saddle River, NJ: Pearson Education.

---

242. An expectant mother asks a nurse, "With all the newborn babies in the nursery, how will I know that the nurse is bringing me my baby? I have heard that babies have gotten mixed up." What is the nurse's best response?

1. "The baby has a plastic bracelet with permanent locks that must be cut for removal."
2. "If taken from the unit, your baby's security band will set off an alarm and lock exits."
3. "A number that corresponds to your hospital number and your full name is also printed on your baby's identification band."
4. "After an identification band is applied to your infant, the footprints are taken and kept on record."

ANSWER: 3

The nurse's best response answers the mother's question directly. Identification numbers and the mother's full name on both the mother's and infant's bands must match. Some agencies require the application of two bands, one on the wrist and another on an ankle in the event that one slides off. Some agencies also have bands that can be scanned for proper identification. Although the plastic band must be cut for removal, a security band may be in place, and the infants footprints are on file, these are extra security measures and not the main means for identifying the infant.

▶ ***Test-taking Tip:*** *Read the scenario carefully and focus on the issue: the method for identifying newborns.*

Content Area: Fundamentals; *Category of Health Alteration:* Safety, Disaster Preparedness, and Infection Control; *Integrated Processes:* Communication and Documentation; Caring; *Client Need:* Safe and Effective Care Environment/Safety and Infection Control/Security Plan; *Cognitive Level:* Application

Reference: Pillitteri, A. (2007). *Maternal & Child Health Nursing: Care of the Childbearing & Childrearing Family* (5th ed., p. 708). Philadelphia: Lippincott Williams & Wilkins.

243. A nurse has been asked to be a member of a hospital's Emergency Operations Committee, which is working on reviewing the components of the emergency plan in place. When reviewing the plan, which components should the nurse expect to be included? SELECT ALL THAT APPLY.

1. Calling 911 to activate an emergency response
2. An internal and external communication plan
3. Identification of external resources
4. A plan for practice drills.
5. Identification of anticipated expendable resources needed
6. Methods for educating personnel

ANSWER: 2, 3, 4, 5, 6

Communication to and from the prehospital arena and to all parties involved is needed for a rapid and orderly response to a disaster. Local, state, and federal resources should be identified as well as how to activate these resources. Practice drills with community participation allows for troubleshooting problems before an event happens and gives persons an opportunity to practice their roles. Food, water, and supplies must be available and sources for these identified. Educating personnel allows for improved readiness and additional input for refining the process. An activation response defines where, how, and when the response is initiated. Calling 911 would not be an appropriate activation.

Test-taking Tip: *Read each option carefully to determine if the option is a necessary component for a health-care facility to respond to a disaster.*

Content Area: Fundamentals; *Category of Health Alteration:* Safety, Disaster Preparedness, and Infection Control; *Integrated Processes:* Communication and Documentation; *Client Need:* Safe and Effective Care Environment/Safety and Infection Control/Security Plan; *Cognitive Level:* Comprehension

Reference: Smeltzer, S., Bare, B., Hinkle, J., & Cheever, K. (2008). *Brunner & Suddarth's Textbook of Medical-Surgical Nursing* (11th ed., p. 2561). Philadelphia: Lippincott Williams & Wilkins.

244. At 2000 hours, a mother calls a nurse to ask when her newborn should be returned to her room to finish feeding. The mother states that a doctor came about 30 minutes ago to take the baby for an examination and has not returned with her baby. Which action should be taken by the nurse *first*?

1. Check the unit for the infant
2. Initiate procedures for possible newborn abduction
3. Ask other staff if they saw any physicians on the unit
4. Check to see if the physician is still examining the infant

ANSWER: 2

The circumstances are suspicious enough to warrant initiating procedures for possible newborn abduction to retrieve the newborn as soon as possible. Checking the unit or checking with other staff and the physician will delay getting the help needed to search the hospital and notify authorities.

Test-taking Tip: *Read the situation carefully to ascertain if a physician is likely to retrieve a newborn at 2000 hours, in the middle of a feeding, for an examination when the baby could be examined while with the mother.*

Content Area: Fundamentals; *Category of Health Alteration:* Safety, Disaster Preparedness, and Infection Control; *Integrated Processes:* Nursing Process Implementation; *Client Need:* Safe and Effective Care Environment/Safety and Infection Control/Security Plan; *Cognitive Level:* Application

Reference: Pillitteri, A. (2007). *Maternal & Child Health Nursing: Care of the Childbearing & Childrearing Family* (5th ed., p. 708). Philadelphia: Lippincott Williams & Wilkins.

245. A hospital is overloaded with victims from a tornado that leveled a nearby community of 75,000 people, and the hospital is short staffed. Which actions might be necessary in this situation? SELECT ALL THAT APPLY.

1. Nurses performing duties outside of the nurses' area of expertise
2. Family members providing nonskilled interventions for their loved ones
3. Giving care to persons with extensive injuries and little chance of survival first
4. Setting up a hospital ward in a community shelter
5. Asking if anyone can interpret for clients that only speak a foreign language
6. Leaving victims to perform rituals required by another victim's religion and culture

ANSWER: 1, 2, 4, 5

Nurses may be asked to take on responsibilities normally held by physicians or advanced practice nurses. When insufficient health-care personnel are available, family members may take on nonskilled responsibilities. Care may need to be provided outside of the hospital setting. Although client confidentially is important, a medical emergency may require the services of lay persons. Victims with extensive injuries and unlikely to survive should be triaged and treated as the last priority. Nursing care in a disaster focuses on essential care from the perspective of what is best for all persons. Treating physical injures should take priority over partaking in cultural rituals.

Test-taking Tip: *In a disaster, atypical roles occur for health-care personnel, victims, and families.*

Content Area: Fundamentals; *Category of Health Alteration:* Safety, Disaster Preparedness, and Infection Control; *Integrated Processes:* Nursing Process Implementation; *Client Need:* Safe and Effective Care Environment/Safety and Infection Control/Emergency Response Plan; *Cognitive Level:* Application

Reference: Smeltzer, S., Bare, B., Hinkle, J., & Cheever, K. (2008). *Brunner & Suddarth's Textbook of Medical-Surgical Nursing* (11th ed., pp. 2562–2563). Philadelphia: Lippincott Williams & Wilkins.

246. EBP Which statement, if made by a community nurse teaching disaster-preparedness to a group of community members, is accurate?

1. "Change stored bottled water every year."
2. "Keep on hand a 3-day supply of water, 1 gallon per person per day."
3. "Animals will be able to fend for themselves in a disaster."
4. "Beside water, include in the disaster supply kit a 1-day supply of food and other necessities for each person in the household."

ANSWER: 2

The amount of water to keep on hand is calculated according to family size (1 gallon per person per day) for a 3-day supply of water. Food that will not spoil should also be stored. Bottled water that is stored for use in the event of an emergency should be replaced before it expires or, if self-prepared, every 6 months. A disaster kit should also contain water, food, and other necessary items for household pets. The disaster kit should contain a 3-day supply of food and necessities.

➧ ***Test-taking Tip:*** *Focus on the issue, disaster preparedness, and the information that would be most helpful to know.*

Content Area: Fundamentals; *Category of Health Alteration:* Safety, Disaster Preparedness, and Infection Control; *Integrated Processes:* Teaching and Learning; *Client Need:* Safe and Effective Care Environment/Safety and Infection Control/Emergency Response Plan; *Cognitive Level:* Analysis

Reference: Stanhope, M., & Lancaster, J. (2008). *Community and Public Health Nursing* (7th ed., pp. 457–462). St. Louis, MO: Mosby.

EBP Reference: Federal Emergency Management Agency. (2008). *FEMA Are You Ready Guide*. Available at: www.fema.gov/areyouready/assemble_disaster_supplies_kit.shtm

247. An emergency trauma center receives a call to expect to receive the infant illustrated. Which precautions should a nurse plan when preparing for the infant's care? SELECT ALL THAT APPLY.

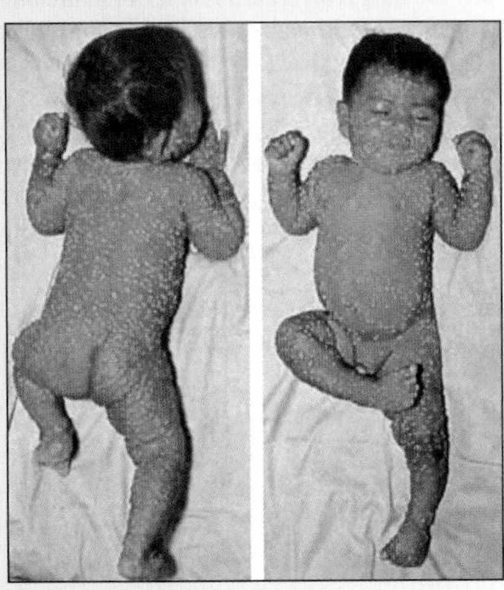

1. Placing the infant in a negative-air-pressure isolation room
2. Wearing a surgical mask when in contact with the infant
3. Wearing a N-95 (HEPA) particulate mask when in contact with the infant
4. Wearing gloves and a gown when entering the room to assess the infant
5. Taking measures to notify the Centers for Disease Control and Prevention (CDC) of a suspected act of bioterrorism
6. Decontaminating the infant because of suspected smallpox exposure

ANSWER: 2, 3, 4

The lesions are characteristic of smallpox, which is highly contagious. Smallpox is transmitted via both large and small respiratory droplets. Person-to-person transmission is likely from airborne and droplet exposure and by contact with skin lesions or secretions. Airborne, contact, and standard precautions should be used. Airborne precautions require wearing respiratory protection that protects against airborne droplet nuclei smaller than 5 microns. Contact precautions include wearing a gown and gloves when in contact with the infant or environmental surfaces that could be contaminated. Though the CDC should be notified, there is no indication that this is an act of bioterrorism. Smallpox does not require decontamination.

➧ ***Test-taking Tip:*** *Recognize that this is smallpox and select options that include airborne, contact, and standard precautions.*

Content Area: Fundamentals; *Category of Health Alteration:* Safety, Disaster Preparedness, and Infection Control; *Integrated Processes:* Nursing Process Planning; *Client Need:* Safe and Effective Care Environment/Safety and Infection Control/Emergency Response Plan; *Cognitive Level:* Analysis

Reference: Berman, A., Snyder, S., Kozier, B., & Erb, G. (2008). *Fundamentals of Nursing: Concepts, Process, and Practice* (8th ed., pp. 688–690). Upper Saddle River, NJ: Pearson Education.

248. A school nurse is planning a school-based intervention program for children who lost their homes due to a tornado and are now residing in temporary housing. With which group should the nurse initially focus the intervention program because they are more likely to experience symptoms of mental health distress?

1. Older age female children of higher socioeconomic status
2. Older age male children of higher socioeconomic status
3. Younger age female children of lower socioeconomic status
4. Younger age male children of lower socioeconomic status

ANSWER: 3

Posttraumatic stress syndrome is experienced more frequently in children than adults. According to research conducted by members of the Department of Psychiatry and Pediatrics of Mount Sinai School of Medicine and the National Center for Posttraumatic Stress Disorder, clients who are female, younger age, and lower socioeconomic status are more likely to experience symptoms of mental health distress. School-based intervention programs after disasters are considered to be cost-effective and valid. While all individuals may experience symptoms of mental health distress, the initial focus should be on the age and gender group that is most likely to be affected.

➧ ***Test-taking Tip:*** *The key word is "initial." Focus on the most vulnerable age group in which the threat of safety and security are most likely to cause mental health distress.*

Content Area: Fundamentals; *Category of Health Alteration:* Safety, Disaster Preparedness, and Infection Control; *Integrated Processes:* Nursing Process Planning; *Client Need:* Safe and Effective Care Environment/Safety and Infection Control/Emergency Response Plan; *Cognitive Level:* Application

References: Smeltzer, S., Bare, B., Hinkle, J., & Cheever, K. (2008). *Brunner & Suddarth's Textbook of Medical-Surgical Nursing* (11th ed., p. 2564). Philadelphia: Lippincott Williams & Wilkins; Stanhope, M., & Lancaster, J. (2008). *Community and Public Health Nursing* (7th ed., p. 475). St. Louis, MO: Mosby.

249. EBP A nurse enters a client's hospital room at the beginning of the shift. A nurse surveys the client and the care area for potential sources of infection. Which options represent potential sources of infection to this client? SELECT ALL THAT APPLY.

1. A bottle of saline irrigation solution has the cap tightly closed and a label identifying that it was opened 10 hours previously.
2. The client's abdominal dressing has three different areas of moist drainage saturating the dressing and soiling the client's gown.
3. The tubing of the client's intravenous (IV) fluid is not labeled with the date of the last tubing change.
4. The bathroom contains a calibrated graduate used to measure urine that is labeled with the word *urine* and the client's initials.
5. An opened package of gauze sponges is present on the window sill.

ANSWER: 2, 3, 5

The saturated dressing represents a risk for contamination since microorganisms can move through the moist environment through the dressing to the wound and back. Recommendations for IV tubing changes are every 72 to 96 hours. Unlabeled IV tubing represents a potential infection risk. An opened package of dressing supplies is considered contaminated and should not be used for dressing changes. Open bottles of solutions for wound care are considered aseptic and suitable for use with wound care for 24 hours. Care equipment, especially items contaminated with body fluids should be labeled and used for just one client.

➧ ***Test-taking Tip:*** *Read the stem carefully and determine that the question calls for a negative response. Recall the guidelines for infection control in health-care settings. Select the options that are incorrect and describe potential risks for infection.*

Content Area: Fundamentals; *Category of Health Alteration:* Safety, Disaster Preparedness, and Infection Control; *Integrated Processes:* Nursing Process Assessment; *Client Need:* Safe and Effective Care Environment/Safety and Infection Control/Medical Surgical Asepsis; *Cognitive Level:* Analysis

Reference: Taylor, C., Lillis, C., LeMone, P., & Lyn, P. (2008). *Fundamentals of Nursing: The Art and Science of Nursing Care* (6th ed., pp. 719, 1209, 1238, 1693, 1728). Philadelphia: Lippincott Williams & Wilkins.

EBP Reference: Centers for Disease Control and Prevention. (2007). *Guideline for Isolation Precautions: Preventing Transmission of Infectious Agents in Healthcare Settings* [Excerpt]. Available at: www.cdc.gov/ncidod/dhqp/gl_isolation_standard.html

250. A nurse is preparing a sterile field for a dressing change using surgical aseptic technique. The nurse gathers the supplies and prepares the sterile field using a packaged sterile drape. Which option correctly describes how the nurse should set up the sterile field?

1. Donning sterile gloves before opening the packaged sterile drape
2. Cleansing the bottle of irrigating solution with alcohol before placing the bottle on the field
3. Holding items 6 inches above the field and dropping them on the sterile field inside the 1-inch border along the edge of the drape
4. Leaving the sterile field unattended to obtain supplies not in the area

ANSWER: 3

Holding the item 6 inches above the surface of the sterile field prevents contamination of the field and avoids dropping items too close to the edge of or off the sterile field. The sterile drape should be opened before donning sterile gloves, utilizing a technique of just touching the outer inch of the drape. The irrigation solution should be poured into a sterile container on the field. Only sterile items should be added to the sterile field. A sterile field should be considered contaminated if not visualized.

➧ ***Test-taking Tip:*** *Read the stem carefully and recall the principles of surgical asepsis. Visualize performing each option to set up a sterile field. Select the option that is consistent with the criteria.*

Content Area: Fundamentals; *Category of Health Alteration:* Safety, Disaster Preparedness, and Infection Control; *Integrated Processes:* Nursing Process Implementation; *Client Need:* Safe and Effective Care Environment/Safety and Infection Control/Medical Surgical Asepsis; *Cognitive Level:* Analysis

Reference: Taylor, C., Lillis, C., LeMone, P., & Lyn, P. (2008). *Fundamentals of Nursing: The Art and Science of Nursing Care* (6th ed., pp. 719, 732–737). Philadelphia: Lippincott Williams & Wilkins.

---

251. EBP A client with a wound infection is ordered contact precautions based on culture results. When should a nurse caring for the client don disposable medical examination gloves?

1. Upon entering the client's room
2. When anticipating contact with drainage from the wound
3. When determining a potential for contamination with blood or body fluids of the client
4. When providing care within 3 feet of the client

ANSWER: 1

Gloves should be donned by caregivers upon entry into the room of a client requiring contact precautions. Gloves are also worn in the other actions described in the other options.

➧ ***Test-taking Tip:*** *Recall the use of personal protective equipment with clients who require contact precautions. Read the options carefully and select option 1, which is comprehensive and includes the other options.*

Content Area: Fundamentals; *Category of Health Alteration:* Safety, Disaster Preparedness, and Infection Control; *Integrated Processes:* Nursing Process Planning; *Client Need:* Safe and Effective Care Environment/Safety and Infection Control/Medical Surgical Asepsis; *Cognitive Level:* Application

EBP Reference: National Guideline Clearinghouse. (2007). *Guideline for Isolation Precautions: Preventing Transmission of Infectious Agents in Healthcare Settings* [Excerpt]. Available at: www.guideline.gov/summary/summary.doc

---

252. A nurse cares for a hospitalized client and inspects the client's bedside table. Which of the items on the table pose a potential risk of infection for the client and should be removed? SELECT ALL THAT APPLY.

1. The menu from the last meal
2. A half-full cup of water without a cover
3. An empty urinal that was rinsed out with water after being used
4. A sealed package of soda crackers
5. A box of paper tissues
6. A pitcher of water covered with a lid

ANSWER: 2, 3

The urinal on the bedside table is a vehicle for microorganism transmission and potential source for nosocomial infection. The cup of water and all fluid containers should be covered because prolonged exposure leads to contamination and promotes microbial growth. The other options do not pose a specific infection risk.

➧ ***Test-taking Tip:*** *Read the stem carefully and determine that the question calls for a negative answer. Evaluate each response as a possible source for contamination or growth of pathogens. Eliminate the options that pose no potential infection risk.*

Content Area: Fundamentals; *Category of Health Alteration:* Safety, Disaster Preparedness, and Infection Control; *Integrated Processes:* Nursing Process Assessment; *Client Need:* Safe and Effective Care Environment/Safety and Infection Control/Medical Surgical Asepsis; *Cognitive Level:* Analysis

Reference: Berman, A., Snyder, S., Kozier, B., & Erb, G. (2008). *Kozier & Erb's Fundamentals of Nursing: Concepts, Process, and Practice* (8th ed., pp. 672, 683). Upper Saddle River, NJ: Pearson Education.

253. EBP A nurse is working in a clinic and encounters a client who has a congested cough and rhinorrhea. The nurse follows respiratory hygiene/cough protocol by doing which of the following? SELECT ALL THAT APPLY

1. Offering the client disposable tissues
2. Wearing a mask while examining the client
3. Offering the client water to drink while waiting
4. Instructing the client about the importance of covering the mouth when coughing and frequent handwashing.
5. Performing hand hygiene before and after contact with the client
6. Separating the client by at least 3 feet from other persons in the area

ANSWER: 1, 2, 4, 5, 6

Respiratory hygiene/cough protocol measures include assisting and educating clients and families about source control measures, separating ill persons 3 feet from others, and utilization of droplet precautions (wearing a mask, frequent handwashing) by health-care workers caring for the clients. Clients with upper respiratory infections should increase their fluid intake, but this will not limit transmission of pathogens.

➧ ***Test-taking Tip:*** *Recall the pathophysiology involved with upper respiratory infections. Evaluate each option regarding the effect to minimize the transmission of pathogens. Evaluate each option and select the options that are consistent with standard and droplet precautions.*

Content Area: Fundamentals; *Category of Health Alteration:* Safety, Disaster Preparedness, and Infection Control; *Integrated Processes:* Nursing Process Implementation; *Client Need:* Safe and Effective Care Environment/Safety and Infection Control/Standard/Transmission-based/Other Precautions; *Cognitive Level:* Analysis

EBP Reference: Centers for Disease Control and Prevention. (2007). *Guideline for Isolation Precautions: Preventing Transmission of Infectious Agents in Healthcare Settings* [Excerpt]. Available at: www.cdc.gov/ncidod/dhqp/gl_isolation_standard.html

---

254. EBP A nurse admits a male client to a hospital with exacerbation of asthma. During the admission history, the nurse learns that the client has a history of chronic hepatitis C. Which precautions should the nurse plan to implement based on the transmission of the hepatitis C virus?

1. Airborne
2. Contact
3. Droplet
4. Standard

ANSWER: 4

Standard precautions are infection preventive practices that protect against infectious agents present in body fluids, including the blood. Hepatitis C is transmitted through body fluids, principally the blood. Hepatitis C is not transmitted via the respiratory tract. Further precautions included in contact precautions are not necessary.

➧ ***Test-taking Tip:*** *Recall the cycle of infection and that hepatitis C is transmitted primarily through infected blood. Consider the protective measures involved with each type of precautions and determine that standard precautions are indicated and sufficient.*

Content Area: Fundamentals; *Category of Health Alteration:* Safety, Disaster Preparedness, and Infection Control; *Integrated Processes:* Nursing Process Planning; *Client Need:* Safe and Effective Care Environment/Safety and Infection Control/Standard/Transmission-based/Other Precautions; *Cognitive Level:* Application

Reference: Craven, R., & Hirnle, C. (2009). *Fundamentals of Nursing: Human Health and Function* (6th ed., p. 476). Philadelphia: Lippincott Williams & Wilkins.

EBP References: Centers for Disease Control and Prevention. (2007). *Guideline for Isolation Precautions: Preventing Transmission of Infectious Agents in Healthcare Settings* [Excerpt]. Available at: www.cdc.gov/ncidod/dhqp/gl_isolation_standard.html; Strader, D., Wright, T., Thomas, D., & Seeff, L. (2004). Diagnosis, management, and treatment of hepatitis C. *Hepatology,* 39(4), 1147–1171.

255. EBP A client who is receiving total parenteral nutrition (TPN) through a subclavian triple lumen catheter expresses concern to a nurse about bacteria entering the blood through the catheter. The nurse explains that the risk of catheter-related infections can be decreased by doing which of the following?

1. Applying an antibiotic ointment at the catheter insertion site
2. Changing the dressing over the catheter insertion site daily
3. Designating one port of the triple lumen catheter exclusively for the TPN solution
4. Instilling an antibiotic solution daily into each port of the triple lumen catheter

ANSWER: 3

Consistently utilizing one port for TPN solution minimizes the risk of infection. Unless loose, soiled, or bloody, the dressing should be changed weekly or every 10 days depending on the cleansing solution used. Using antibiotic ointment and instilling antibiotic solution do not decrease the risk of infection and may predispose to the development of antibiotic-resistant bacteria.

➧ ***Test-taking Tip:*** *Focus on the nutrient content of the TPN, which is high in dextrose, and the relationship to increased infection risk.*

Content Area: Fundamentals; *Category of Health Alteration:* Safety, Disaster Preparedness, and Infection Control; *Integrated Processes:* Nursing Process Implementation; *Client Need:* Safe and Effective Care Environment/Safety and Infection Control/Medical and Surgical Asepsis; *Cognitive Level:* Application

Reference: Cresci, G. (2005). *Nutrition Support for the Critically Ill Patient: A Guide to Practice.* (p. 307). Boca Raton, FL: CRC Press.

EBP Reference: National Guideline Clearinghouse. (n.d.). *Guidelines for the Prevention of Intravascular Catheter-Related Infections.* Available at: www.guideline.gov/summary/summary.aspx?doc_id=3387&nbr=002613&string=guidelines+AND+prevention+AND+intravascular+AND+catheter-related+AND+infections

---

256. EBP A hospitalized client has protective precautions in place because of severe neutropenia. Which statement by a nurse is correct regarding the use of protective precautions?

1. "Caregivers should don gloves as soon as they enter the client's room."
2. "The client should minimize the time spent outside the room."
3. "The client should be in a private room with negative air pressure."
4. "All persons entering the client's room should wear a mask."

ANSWER: 2

The client should remain in the room as much as possible to minimize exposure to pathogens. Barrier precautions including gloves and masks are not necessary if the client does not have a suspected or actual infection. The client room should be private with positive air pressure.

➧ ***Test-taking Tip:*** *Key words in the stem are "protective precautions" and "neutropenia." Recall the client has decreased resistance against infection and is being protected from pathogens in the environment. Eliminate options 1 and 4 because these are interventions included in contact precautions, preventing transmission of pathogens from the client. Eliminate option 3 since negative pressure in the room would draw air from the hospital environment (possibly containing pathogens) into the client's room.*

Content Area: Fundamentals; *Category of Health Alteration:* Safety, Disaster Preparedness, and Infection Control; *Integrated Processes:* Nursing Process Implementation; *Client Need:* Safe and Effective Care Environment/Safety and Infection Control/Standard/Transmission-based/Other Precautions; *Cognitive Level:* Analysis

EBP Reference: Centers for Disease Control and Prevention. (2007). *Guideline for Isolation Precautions: Preventing Transmission of Infectious Agents in Healthcare Settings* [Excerpt]. Available at: http://www.cdc.gov/ncidod/dhqp/gl_isolation_standard.html

257. EBP A charge nurse of a step-down unit in a hospital plans bed placement for five male clients transferring from a critical care unit. The clients will be transferred into the three open rooms on the unit. The beds are available in two 2-bed rooms and one private room. Which room assignments should be made by the charge nurse?

Client	Diagnosis/Medical Information
A	Client with infected postoperative abdominal wound, cultured positive for methicillin-resistant *Staphylococcus aureus*
B	Client admitted with ketoacidosis, history of chronic hepatitis C
C	Client has history of bloody sputum, night sweats; airborne precautions currently in place
D	Client postoperative from vascular surgery, leg ulcers cultured positive for methicillin-resistant *Staphylococcus aureus*
E	1 day postoperative small bowel resection; had postoperative hypotension issues

1. Client B: private room; clients C and E in same room; clients A and D in same room.
2. Client C: private room; clients A and D in same room; clients B and E in same room.
3. Client E: private room; clients B and C in same room; clients A and D in same room.
4. Client C: private room; clients A and B in same room; clients D and E in same room.

ANSWER: 2

Client C has airborne precautions and requires a private room. Clients A and D have the same organism, may be roomed together, and require contact precautions. Clients B and E may be roomed together since both require only the standard precautions. Transmission of hepatitis C occurs mainly with blood and this is addressed with the standard precautions. The other options list client placements that are not as sound in preventing infection transmission.

Test-taking Tip: *Read the chart carefully. Client C with airborne precautions may have infectious tuberculosis and definitely requires a private room. This eliminates options 1 and 3. Determine that clients A and D require contact precautions for the same organism and clients B and E both require standard precautions and select option 2.*

Content Area: Fundamentals; *Category of Health Alteration:* Safety, Disaster Preparedness, and Infection Control; *Integrated Processes:* Nursing Process Planning; *Client Need:* Safe and Effective Care Environment/Safety and Infection Control/Standard/Transmission-based/Other Precautions; *Cognitive Level:* Synthesis

Reference: Craven, R., & Hirnle, C. (2009). *Fundamentals of Nursing: Human Health and Function* (6th ed., pp. 472–477). Philadelphia: Lippincott Williams & Wilkins.

EBP Reference: Centers for Disease Control and Prevention. (2007). *Guideline for Isolation Precautions: Preventing Transmission of Infectious Agents in Healthcare Settings* [Excerpt]. Available at: www.cdc.gov/ncidod/dhqp/gl_isolation_standard.html

258. EBP A nurse instructs a client on safe disposal of insulin syringes and needles when at home. Which statement by the client indicates that additional teaching is needed?

1. "After I draw up my insulin, I scoop the cap to cover it while I cleanse my skin."
2. "I have a needle destruction device that breaks the needles from the syringes so that others won't get stuck by the needles."
3. "I plan to use this plastic milk container to discard my used needles and syringes and take it to the clinic for disposal."
4. "Because the needles are capped, the syringes are safe to dispose of with my household trash."

ANSWER: 4

Used needles and syringes should not be placed in the household trash because of the risk of needlestick injuries to waste management personnel. Scooping the cap to cover the needle protects others from needlestick injuries. The U.S. Environmental Protection Agency (2004) recommends that at-home syringes and needles be disposed of through use of needle destruction devices, sharps mail-back programs, community drop-off programs, or household hazardous waste facilities.

Test-taking Tip: *The key phrase is "additional teaching is needed." Select the statement that is incorrect.*

Content Area: Fundamentals; *Category of Health Alteration:* Safety, Disaster Preparedness, and Infection Control; *Integrated Processes:* Nursing Process Evaluation; *Client Need:* Safe and Effective Care Environment/Safety and Infection Control/Handling Hazardous and Infectious Materials; *Cognitive Level:* Application

Reference: Harkreader, H., Hogan, M., & Thobaben, M. (2007). *Fundamentals of Nursing* (3rd ed., pp. 459–460). St. Louis, MO: Saunders/Elsevier.

EBP References: Environmental Protection Agency. (2004). *Disposal of Medical Sharps.* Available at: www.epa.gov/epaoswer/non-hw/househld/hhw/han-care.pdf; Environmental Protection Agency. (2004). *Protect Yourself, Protect Others: Safe Options for Home Needle Disposal.* Available at: www.epa.gov/epaoswer/other/medical/med-home.pdf.

259. A nurse is using contact precautions for a client diagnosed with *Clostridium difficile.* While transferring the client from the bed to the commode, the client has loose stool that falls on the floor. After positioning the client on the commode, how should the nurse proceed to cleanse the floor?

1. Wipe up the stool with toilet paper and then clean the area with soap and water
2. Wipe up the stool with toilet paper and then clean the area with a 1:10 bleach-water solution
3. Call housekeeping personnel to come clean the floor now with the unit's mop and bucket
4. Wipe up the stool and apply the alcohol-based hand wash to clean the area of stool

ANSWER: 2

The nurse should wipe up the stool and clean the area with a bleach solution to adequately disinfect the area and prevent transmission of the microorganism. To maintain the dignity of the client, the nurse should stay with the client and avoid having housekeeping personnel present while the client is using the commode. Using the unit's mop and bucket could cause transmission to other areas of the unit. Soap and water will not adequately disinfect the area. The alcohol-based hand wash is ineffective against the spores of *C. difficile.*

➧ ***Test-taking Tip:*** *Recall that C. difficile is a spore-forming microbe and is relatively resistant to disinfectants.*

Content Area: Fundamentals; *Category of Health Alteration:* Safety, Disaster Preparedness, and Infection Control; *Integrated Processes:* Nursing Process Implementation; *Client Need:* Safe and Effective Care Environment/Safety and Infection Control/Handling Hazardous and Infectious Materials; *Cognitive Level:* Application

Reference: Smeltzer, S., Bare, B., Hinkle, J., & Cheever, K. (2008). *Brunner & Suddarth's Textbook of Medical-Surgical Nursing* (11th ed., p. 2482). Philadelphia: Lippincott Williams & Wilkins.

---

260. A nurse is caring for a client who received afterload internal radiotherapy (brachytherapy) for treatment of uterine cancer. A nurse manager evaluates that the nurse uses correct hazardous material precautions when noting that the nurse does which of the following?

1. Double-bags linens before removing them from the client's room
2. Minimizes the amount of time spent in contact with the client
3. Maintains a distance of 1 foot away from the client
4. Wears lead gloves and apron and a dosimetry badge when in contact with the client

ANSWER: 2

In afterload radiation therapy, the radioactive substance is inserted in the client's private hospital room after prepared applicators have been placed in surgery. Exposure to radiation is controlled by minimizing the time spent with the client. Linens should be kept in the room until the radioactive source is removed and the room is swept with a radiation detector to assess for spills or contamination. After clearance, the linens may be sent to the laundry. A 1-foot distance increases the nurse's chance of exposure to the radiation. A nurse standing 2 feet away from the source of radiation receives only ¼ as much exposure as when standing only 1 foot away. Lead gloves and aprons are insufficient to block gamma rays during brachytherapy. Dosimetry badges measure the amount of radiation exposure and is not a precaution.

➧ ***Test-taking Tip:*** *The key phrase is "hazardous material precautions." Read each option carefully and eliminate options that would not protect the nurse from radiation exposure.*

Content Area: Fundamentals; *Category of Health Alteration:* Safety, Disaster Preparedness, and Infection Control; *Integrated Processes:* Nursing Process Evaluation; *Client Need:* Safe and Effective Care Environment/Safety and Infection Control/Handling Hazardous and Infectious Materials; *Cognitive Level:* Analysis

References: Berman, A., Snyder, S., Kozier, B., & Erb, G. (2008). *Fundamentals of Nursing: Concepts, Process, and Practice* (8th ed., p. 729). Upper Saddle River, NJ: Pearson Education; Craven, R., & Hirnle, C. (2009). *Fundamentals of Nursing: Human Health and Function* (6th ed., p. 670). Philadelphia: Lippincott Williams & Wilkins.

---

261. A health-care agency has different receptacles for the various categories of institutional waste. Into which container should a nurse dispose of a suction canister used to collect drainage from a client's nasogastric tube?

1. Injurious waste receptacle
2. Hazardous waste receptacle
3. Infectious waste receptacle
4. Wastebasket in the client's bathroom

ANSWER: 3

Blood and body fluids are considered infectious waste. Therefore, the suction canister should be placed in the infectious waste receptacle. Injurious wastes would include items such as needles, scalpel blades, lancets, or other objects that could injure another person. Hazardous waste includes radioactive material, chemotherapy agents, or caustic chemicals. Regular waste that does not pose a health hazard to others can be placed in a regular wastebasket.

➧ ***Test-taking Tip:*** *Think about the likely contents of the canister, and then review each option.*

Content Area: Fundamentals; *Category of Health Alteration:* Safety, Disaster Preparedness, and Infection Control; *Integrated Processes:* Nursing Process Implementation; *Client Need:* Safe and Effective Care Environment/Safety and Infection Control/Handling Hazardous and Infectious Materials; *Cognitive Level:* Application

Reference: Craven, R., & Hirnle, C. (2009). *Fundamentals of Nursing: Human Health and Function* (6th ed., p. 470). Philadelphia: Lippincott Williams & Wilkins.

262. A clinic has taught its employees to recognize the hazards of various chemicals using the National Fire Protection Association's (NFPA) diamond label and coding system. What should a nurse determine about the substance that has the label illustrated?

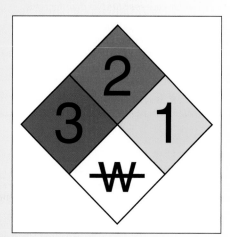

NFPA Coding System

Red: Fire Hazard
- 0 – Will not burn
- 1 – Must be preheated for ignition; flashpoint above 200°F (93°C)
- 2 – Must be moderately heated for ignition, flashpoint above 100°F (38°C)
- 3 – Ignition may occur under most ambient conditions, flashpoint below 100°F (38°C)
- 4 – Extremely flammable and will readily disperse through air under standard conditions, flashpoint below 73°F (23°C)

Blue: Health Hazard
- 0 – Hazard no greater than ordinary material
- 1 – May cause irritation; minimal residual injury
- 2 – Intense or prolonged exposure may cause incapacitation; residual injury may occur if not treated
- 3 – Exposure could cause serious injury even if treated
- 4 – Exposure may cause death

Yellow: Reactivity Hazard
- 0 – Stable
- 1 – May become unstable at elevated temperatures and pressures, may be mildly water reactive
- 2 – Unstable; may undergo violent decomposition, but will not detonate. May form explosive mixtures with water
- 3 – Detonates with strong ignition source
- 4 – Readily detonates

White: Special Hazard
- OX – Strong Oxidizer
- W – Water reactive

From: *Hazardous Material Classification System.* Available at: atsdr.cdc.gov/MHMI/mhmi-v1-a.pdf.

1. It is extremely flammable.
2. It can become explosive if mixed with water.
3. It has no special hazard.
4. It could cause a serious health injury.

ANSWER: 4

The blue diamond indicates a health hazard, with the number 3 indicating that it could cause serious injury even if treated. Red is flammability, with number 2 indicating that it must be preheated for flammability. The flash point is above 200°F (93.3°C). Yellow is the level of reactivity hazard, with a number 1 indicating that it may cause irritation. The symbol "W" indicates the substance has a special hazard of reacting when mixed with water.

Test-taking Tip: *Examine the illustration and then read the NFPA coding system and the options. The easiest method is to start with a color on the illustration, find the meaning of the number in the coding system illustrated, and then read the options.*

Content Area: Fundamentals; *Category of Health Alteration:* Safety, Disaster Preparedness, and Infection Control; *Integrated Processes:* Nursing Process Analysis; *Client Need:* Safe and Effective Care Environment/Safety and Infection Control/Handling Hazardous and Infectious Materials; *Cognitive Level:* Application

References: Craven, R., & Hirnle, C. (2009). *Fundamentals of Nursing: Human Health and Function* (6th ed., p. 654). Philadelphia: Lippincott Williams & Wilkins.

Chapter Seven

Health Promotion and Maintenance: Care of Childbearing Families

Test 8: Childbearing Families: Prenatal and Antepartal Management

263. A nurse is in the room during a physician's examination of a client who thinks that she may be pregnant. Which findings during the examination support a possibility of pregnancy?

1. Increased hyperplasia and hypertrophy in the breasts
2. Vaginal atrophy
3. Decrease in respiratory tidal volume
4. Increase in hemoglobin

ANSWER: 1

The breasts increase in size and weight because of hyperplasia and hypertrophy of the breast tissue in preparation for lactation. Vaginal hypertrophy occurs from the increase in estrogen levels. Tidal volume increases throughout pregnancy because of a small degree of hyperventilation that occurs during pregnancy. Hemoglobin typically decreases as the pregnancy progresses, with some women developing pregnancy-induced anemia.

Test-taking Tip: *Apply knowledge of the standards of practice for assessing fetal growth and development.*

Content Area: Childbearing Families; *Category of Health Alteration:* Prenatal and Antepartal Management; *Integrated Processes:* Nursing Process Assessment; *Client Need:* Physiological Integrity/Physiological Adaptation/Pathophysiology; *Cognitive Level:* Application

Reference: Davidson, M., London, M., & Ladewig, P. (2008). *Olds' Maternal-Newborn Nursing & Women's Health Across the Lifespan* (8th ed., p. 316). Upper Saddle River, NJ: Prentice Hall Health.

---

264. A 22-year-old woman tells a clinic nurse that her last menstrual period was 3 months ago, which began on 11/21. She has a positive urine pregnancy test. Using Nagele's rule, which date should the nurse calculate to be the woman's estimated date of confinement (EDC)?

1. 8/28
2. 1/28
3. 8/15
4. 1/15

ANSWER: 1

To calculate the EDC using Nagele's rule, subtract 3 months, and add 7 days. This makes the EDC 8/28.

Test-taking Tip: *Focus on the issue: using Nagele's rule to calculate EDC.*

Content Area: Childbearing Families; *Category of Health Alteration:* Prenatal and Antepartal Management; *Integrated Processes:* Nursing Process Assessment; *Client Need:* Health Promotion and Maintenance/Ante/Intra/Postpartum and Newborn Care; *Cognitive Level:* Analysis

Reference: Davidson, M., London, M., & Ladewig, P. (2008). *Olds' Maternal-Newborn Nursing & Women's Health Across the Lifespan* (8th ed., p. 344). Upper Saddle River, NJ: Prentice Hall Health.

265. EBP A nurse is caring for a 32-week-pregnant client. The client asks how the nurse will monitor the baby's growth and determine if the baby is "really okay." Based on current evidence, during the third trimester, which assessment should the nurse perform to evaluate the fetus for adequate growth and viability?

1. Auscultate maternal heart tones
2. Measure fundal height
3. Measure the woman's abdominal girth
4. Complete a third-trimester ultrasound

ANSWER: 2

Current evidence suggests that the presence of fetal (not maternal) heart tones and adequate growth evaluated by measuring the fundal height are the standard to assess fetal growth and viability. Measurement of the woman's abdominal circumference does not provide information about the growth of the fetus. The increase in abdominal girth could be due to weight gain or fluid retention, not just growth of the baby Third-trimester ultrasound is not routine nor advised for routine prenatal care because of the added cost and potential risk to the fetus.

➧ ***Test-taking Tip:*** *Read each option carefully. Use the standards of practice for assessing fetal growth and development to answer the question.*

Content Area: Childbearing Families; *Category of Health Alteration:* Prenatal and Antepartal Management; *Integrated Processes:* Nursing Process Assessment; *Client Need:* Health Promotion and Maintenance/ Growth and Development; *Cognitive Level:* Analysis

Reference: Pillitteri, A. (2007). *Maternal & Child Health Nursing: Care of the Childbearing & Childrearing Family* (5th ed., pp. 204–206). Philadelphia: Lippincott Williams & Wilkins.

EBP Reference: Bricker, L., Neilson J., & Dowswell, T. (2008). Routine ultrasound in late pregnancy (after 24 weeks gestation). *Cochrane Database of Systematic Reviews*, Issue 4, Art. No. CD001451. DOI: 10.1002/ 14651858.CD001451.pub3. Available at: www.cochrane.org/reviews/en/ ab001451.html

---

266. A nurse is caring for a 24-year-old client whose pregnancy history is as follows: elective termination in 1998, spontaneous abortion in 2001, term vaginal delivery in 2003, and currently pregnant again. Which documentation by the nurse of the client's gravity and parity is correct?

1. G4P1
2. G4P2
3. G3P1
4. G2P1

ANSWER: 1

The woman has been pregnant four times in all (gravity). Each time a woman is pregnant it counts as a pregnancy, regardless of the outcome. Parity is counted once a woman delivers a fetus over 20 weeks old, regardless of whether the fetus survives. This woman has delivered once and is currently pregnant, so the parity is 1.

➧ ***Test-taking Tip:*** *Review the definitions of gravity and parity.*

Content Area: Childbearing Families; *Category of Health Alteration:* Prenatal and Antepartal Management; *Integrated Processes:* Communication and Documentation; *Client Need:* Health Promotion and Maintenance/Ante/Intra/Postpartum and Newborn Care; *Cognitive Level:* Analysis

Reference: Davidson, M., London, M., & Ladewig, P. (2008). *Olds' Maternal-Newborn Nursing & Women's Health Across the Lifespan* (8th ed., p. 338). Upper Saddle River, NJ: Prentice Hall Health.

---

267. If a pregnant woman is at 20 weeks gestation, at what level should a clinic nurse expect to palpate the woman's uterine height?

1. Two finger-breadths above the symphysis pubis
2. Halfway between the symphysis pubis and the umbilicus
3. At the umbilicus
4. Two finger-breadths above the umbilicus

ANSWER: 3

At 20 gestational weeks, the uterus should be at the umbilicus. The uterus should be approximately two finger-breadths above the symphysis pubis at 13 weeks and halfway between the umbilicus and symphysis pubis at 16 weeks. At 22 weeks, the uterus would be two finger-breadths above the umbilicus.

➧ ***Test-taking Tip:*** *Eliminate one of the options with duplicate words first, "symphysis pubis" and "umbilicus," then choose the best answer.*

Content Area: Childbearing Families; *Category of Health Alteration:* Prenatal and Antepartal Management; *Integrated Processes:* Nursing Process Assessment; *Client Need:* Health Promotion and Maintenance/ Growth and Development; *Cognitive Level:* Application

Reference: Davidson, M., London, M., & Ladewig, P. (2008). *Olds' Maternal-Newborn Nursing & Women's Health Across the Lifespan* (8th ed., p. 352). Upper Saddle River, NJ: Prentice Hall Health.

268. A nurse is assessing the fundal height for multiple pregnant clients. For which client should the nurse conclude that a fundal height measurement is most accurate?

1. A pregnant client with uterine fibroids
2. A pregnant client who is obese
3. A pregnant client with polyhydramnios
4. A pregnant client experiencing fetal movement

ANSWER: 4

Excessive fetal movement may make it difficult to measure a woman's fundal height; however, it should not cause an inaccuracy in the measurement. Fibroids, obesity, and polyhydramnios can all increase fundal height and give a false measurement.

Test-taking Tip: *Consider what factors would increase the fundal height measurement and eliminate these options.*

Content Area: Childbearing Families; *Category of Health Alteration:* Prenatal and Antepartal Management; *Integrated Processes:* Nursing Process Analysis; *Client Need:* Physiological Integrity/Physiological Adaptation/Alterations in Body Systems; *Cognitive Level:* Analysis

Reference: Davidson, M., London, M., & Ladewig, P. (2008). *Olds' Maternal-Newborn Nursing & Women's Health Across the Lifespan* (8th ed., p. 352). Upper Saddle River, NJ: Prentice Hall Health.

269. Which physiological cervical changes associated with pregnancy should a nurse expect to find during a physical assessment of a pregnant woman? SELECT ALL THAT APPLY.

1. Formation of mucous plug
2. Chadwick's sign
3. Presence of colostrum
4. Goodell's sign
5. Cullen's sign

ANSWER: 1, 2, 4

Cervical changes associated with pregnancy include the formation of the mucous plug, softening of the cervix (Goodell's sign), and a bluish-purple discoloration of the cervix (Chadwick's sign). Colostrum does occur with pregnancy but is a physiological change associated with the breasts. Cullen's sign is a bluish discoloration of the periumbilical skin caused by intraperitoneal hemorrhage. It can occur with a ruptured ectopic pregnancy or acute pancreatitis.

Test-taking Tip: *The key words are "cervical changes." Use the process of elimination to eliminate a breast change or a sign of an ectopic pregnancy.*

Content Area: Childbearing Families; *Category of Health Alteration:* Prenatal and Antepartal Management; *Integrated Processes:* Nursing Process Assessment; *Client Need:* Health Promotion and Maintenance/Developmental Stages and Transitions; *Cognitive Level:* Analysis

Reference: Davidson, M., London, M., & Ladewig, P. (2008). *Olds' Maternal-Newborn Nursing & Women's Health Across the Lifespan* (8th ed., p. 315). Upper Saddle River, NJ: Prentice Hall Health.

270. When assessing pregnant clients, during which time frames should a nurse expect clients to report frequent urination throughout the night? SELECT ALL THAT APPLY.

1. Before the first missed menstrual period
2. During the first trimester
3. During the second trimester
4. During the third trimester
5. One week following delivery

ANSWER: 2, 4

Urinary frequency is most likely to occur in the first and third trimesters. First-trimester urinary frequency occurs as the uterus enlarges in the pelvis and begins to put pressure on the bladder. In the third trimester, urinary frequency returns due to the increased size of the fetus and uterus placing pressure on the bladder. During the second trimester, the uterus moves into the abdominal cavity, putting less pressure on the bladder. Urinary frequency is not a sign of impending labor. Women do not typically experience urinary changes before the first missed menstrual period. Nocturnal frequency a week after delivery may be a sign of a urinary tract infection.

Test-taking Tip: *Consider urinary changes that occur as a result of pregnancy. Use this information to eliminate incorrect options. Think about how uterine changes would influence your answer choice.*

Content Area: Childbearing Families; *Category of Health Alteration:* Prenatal and Antepartal Management; *Integrated Processes:* Nursing Process Assessment; *Client Need:* Physiological Integrity/Physiological Adaptation/Pathophysiology; *Cognitive Level:* Application

Reference: Davidson, M., London, M., & Ladewig, P. (2008). *Olds' Maternal-Newborn Nursing & Women's Health Across the Lifespan* (8th ed., p. 317). Upper Saddle River, NJ: Prentice Hall Health.

271. A pregnant woman asks a nurse, who is teaching a prepared childbirth class, when she should expect to feel fetal movement. The nurse responds that fetal movement usually can be first felt between which time frame?

1. 8 and 12 weeks of pregnancy
2. 12 and 16 weeks of pregnancy
3. 18 and 20 weeks of pregnancy
4. 22 and 26 weeks of pregnancy

ANSWER: 3

Subtle fetal movement (quickening) can be felt as early as 18 to 20 weeks of gestation, and it gradually increases in intensity. Options 1 and 2 are too early to expect the first fetal movement to be felt and option 4 is later than expected.

Test-taking Tip: *The key phrase is "usually . . . first felt." Think about each option and the growth of the fetus during each week.*

Content Area: Childbearing Families; *Category of Health Alteration:* Prenatal and Antepartal Management; *Integrated Processes:* Nursing Process Assessment; *Client Need:* Physiological Integrity/Physiological Adaptation/Pathophysiology; *Cognitive Level:* Comprehension

Reference: Pillitteri, A. (2007). *Maternal & Child Health Nursing: Care of the Childbearing Families & Childrearing Family* (5th ed., p. 200). Philadelphia: Lippincott Williams & Wilkins.

272. EBP Which universal screenings should a nurse complete during the initial prenatal visit? SELECT ALL THAT APPLY.

1. Taking the blood pressure
2. Testing the urine for protein
3. Testing the urine for glucose
4. Screening for domestic violence
5. Screening for smoking

ANSWER: 1, 4, 5

Blood pressure screening, domestic violence screening, and screening for smoking should all be performed at the initial prenatal visit to determine fetal and maternal risk. The use of routine urine dip assessments are unreliable in detecting proteinuria and glycosuria and are not always considered accurate.

Test-taking Tip: *Differentiate between which interventions may be done in practice and which ones are supported by evidence-based practice.*

Content Area: Childbearing Families; *Category of Health Alteration:* Prenatal and Antepartal Management; *Integrated Processes:* Nursing Process Implementation; *Client Need:* Health Promotion and Maintenance/Techniques of Physical Assessment; *Cognitive Level:* Application

Reference: Pillitteri, A. (2007). *Maternal & Child Health Nursing: Care of the Childbearing Families & Childrearing Family* (5th ed., p. 266). Philadelphia: Lippincott Williams & Wilkins.

EBP Reference: Kirkham, C., Harris, S., & Grzybowski, S. (2005). Evidence-based prenatal care: Part I. General prenatal care and counseling issues. *American Family Physician, 71*(7), 1307–1326.

273. A nurse is assessing a prenatal client. Which findings should be most concerning to the nurse? Prioritize the nurse's assessment findings at the first prenatal visit from the most significant finding to the least significant finding.

_____ Current bleeding and cramping
_____ Previous varicella infection
_____ Current smoking
_____ Intense pelvic pain

ANSWER: 2, 4, 3, 1

Intense pelvic pain is always the most concerning symptom, because it can represent a variety of serious medical conditions (abortion, ectopic pregnancy, appendicitis). This symptom represents a possible pathology that could warrant immediate surgical intervention, which is what makes it the most concerning. Bleeding and cramping in any pregnant woman are also extremely concerning. Smoking in the pregnancy can put the woman at risk for multiple adverse outcomes and should be addressed, although it is not an immediately concerning factor. A previous history of varicella is important to document but poses no risk to the woman or the fetus, so it is the least important factor within this scenario.

Test-taking Tip: *Consider the possible etiology for each listed abnormal finding. Prioritize the most serious as first and proceed to rank the symptoms by the seriousness of each one.*

Content Area: Childbearing Families; *Category of Health Alteration:* Prenatal and Antepartal Management; *Integrated Processes:* Nursing Process Assessment; *Client Need:* Physiological Integrity/Physiological Adaptation/Alterations in Body Systems; *Cognitive Level:* Analysis

Reference: Pillitteri, A. (2007). *Maternal & Child Health Nursing: Care of the Childbearing & Childrearing Family* (5th ed., pp. 267–268). Philadelphia: Lippincott Williams & Wilkins.

274. Which laboratory test results, performed during the 15th to 18th week of pregnancy, should a nurse plan to review for a pregnant woman?

1. Quadruple screen
2. Nuchal translucency testing
3. 1-hour glucose screen
4. Indirect Coombs' testing

ANSWER: 1

The quadruple screen is performed between 15 to 18 weeks and assesses for trisomies 13, 18, and 21 and for neural tube defects. The nuchal translucency testing is performed between 11 and 13 weeks and screens for trisomies 13, 18, and 21. The 1-hour glucose screen is performed between 24 and 28 weeks, and the indirect Coombs' testing is routinely performed at 28 weeks.

➧ ***Test-taking Tip:*** *Review the timing of the listed tests to determine the appropriate answer.*

Content Area: Childbearing Families; *Category of Health Alteration:* Prenatal and Antepartal Management; *Integrated Processes:* Nursing Process Planning; *Client Need:* Health Promotion and Maintenance/ Techniques of Physical Assessment; *Cognitive Level:* Application

Reference: Davidson, M., London, M., & Ladewig, P. (2008). *Olds' Maternal-Newborn Nursing & Women's Health Across the Lifespan* (8th ed., p. 357). Upper Saddle River, NJ: Prentice Hall Health.

275. A nurse is reviewing the laboratory report from the first prenatal visit of a newly admitted client. Which laboratory result should the nurse most likely question?

1. Hematocrit: 36.5%
2. White blood cells (WBCs): 7,000/mm^3
3. Pap smear: Negative; human papillomavirus (HPV) changes noted
4. Urine pH: 7.4

ANSWER: 3

A pap smear with HPV changes reflects an abnormal result. HPV changes are a risk factor for cervical cancer and require ongoing assessment and follow-up. A hematocrit of 36.5% is within normal limits for a pregnant woman (normal hematocrit value = 38% to 44%; this decreases by 4% to 7% in pregnancy). A WBC count of 7,000/mm^3 is normal (normal = 5,000 to 15,000/mm^3). A urine pH of 7.4 is normal (normal = 4.6 to 8.0).

➧ ***Test-taking Tip:*** *Review the laboratory results and determine which ones are correct or in normal range. Based on this information, eliminate correct options and make the best choice.*

Content Area: Childbearing Families; *Category of Health Alteration:* Prenatal and Antepartal Management; *Integrated Processes:* Nursing Process Evaluation; *Client Need:* Health Promotion and Maintenance/ Health Screening; *Cognitive Level:* Analysis

Reference: Davidson, M., London, M., & Ladewig, P. (2008). *Olds' Maternal-Newborn Nursing & Women's Health Across the Lifespan* (8th ed., p. 349). Upper Saddle River, NJ: Prentice Hall Health.

276. A nurse is taking the health history of a new, pregnant client. Which medical conditions are most likely to be risk factors for complications during pregnancy? SELECT ALL THAT APPLY.

1. Diabetes
2. Previous pregnancy
3. Controlled chronic hypertension
4. Anemia
5. Hemorrhage with a previous pregnancy

ANSWER: 1, 3, 4, 5

Diabetes, hypertension, anemia, and previous pregnancy complications are all risk factors for complications. Having a previous pregnancy is not a risk factor for a current pregnancy.

➧ ***Test-taking Tip:*** *Focus on the question, risk factors for complications. Select options that are medical problems.*

Content Area: Childbearing Families; *Category of Health Alteration:* Prenatal and Antepartal Management; *Integrated Processes:* Communication and Documentation; *Client Need:* Physiological Integrity/Reduction of Risk Potential/Potential for Alterations in Body Systems; *Cognitive Level:* Application

Reference: Davidson, M., London, M., & Ladewig, P. (2008). *Olds' Maternal-Newborn Nursing & Women's Health Across the Lifespan* (8th ed., pp. 340–342). Upper Saddle River, NJ: Prentice Hall Health.

277. EBP A nurse working in a prenatal clinic is asked which testing regimen is recommended by the Center for Disease Control and Prevention (CDC) regarding HIV testing. What is the correct 2006 CDC recommendation upon which the nurse should base a response?

1. All women should be encouraged to have the HIV test and sign a separate consent form.
2. All women with risk factors should be tested after consent for HIV testing has been obtained.
3. All pregnant women should have an HIV test included in the prenatal panel after obtaining a general consent form for all screening tests.
4. HIV testing may be done on all pregnant women without obtaining consent because the fetus is at risk.

ANSWER: 3

According to the CDC (2006), all pregnant women should have HIV testing included in the prenatal panel. A separate consent is not needed. The other options are incorrect.

Test-taking Tip: *Think about which option provides the broadest approach to HIV test, but still protects the client's rights.*

Content Area: Childbearing Families; *Category of Health Alteration:* Prenatal and Antepartal Management; *Integrated Processes:* Nursing Process Analysis; *Client Need:* Health Promotion and Maintenance/Health Screening; *Cognitive Level:* Application

References: Pillitteri, A. (2007). *Maternal & Child Health Nursing: Care of the Childbearing & Childrearing Family* (5th ed., pp. 251–252). Philadelphia: Lippincott Williams & Wilkins; March of Dimes. (2006). HIV and AIDS in pregnancy. Available at: www.marchofdimes.com/professionals/14332_1223.asp

EBP Reference: Branson, B., Handsfield, H., Lampe, M., Jannsen, R., Taylor, A., et al. (2006). Revised recommendations for HIV testing of adults, adolescents, and pregnant women in health care settings. *Morbidity & Mortality Weekly Reports*, *55*(R140), 1–17.

---

278. EBP Multiple clients are being seen in a clinic. Which clients should a nurse prepare to receive a group beta streptococcus (GBS) culture? SELECT ALL THAT APPLY.

1. Women experiencing preterm labor
2. Women who had a previous neonatal death
3. All pregnant women between 35 to 37 weeks gestation
4. Women with a history of spontaneous abortion
5. Women with a history of an abortion for an unwanted pregnancy

ANSWER: 1, 3

All pregnant women, regardless of risk status, should be screened for GBS infection. Ten to 30% of all women are colonized for GBS. There is no indication that a woman with a previous neonatal death is pregnant. A woman would not be screened for GBS solely because of a history of spontaneous or an elective abortion.

Test-taking Tip: *Determine the management of GBS in pregnant women. Eliminate options that do not indicate whether the women are pregnant.*

Content Area: Childbearing Families; *Category of Health Alteration:* Prenatal and Antepartal Management; *Integrated Processes:* Nursing Process Implementation; *Client Need:* Health Promotion and Maintenance/Health Screening; *Cognitive Level:* Analysis

Reference: Davidson, M., London, M., & Ladewig, P. (2008). *Olds' Maternal-Newborn Nursing & Women's Health Across the Lifespan* (8th ed., p. 533). Upper Saddle River, NJ: Prentice Hall Health.

EBP Reference: Kirkham, C., Harris, S., & Grzybowski, S. (2005). Evidence-based prenatal care: Part II. Third trimester care and prevention of infectious diseases. *American Family Physician*, *71*(8), 1555–1560.

---

279. A nurse is caring for a client who has a positive quadruple screen for Down's syndrome at 16 weeks. Which diagnostic test can be used to confirm the diagnosis?

1. Chorionic villus sampling (CVS)
2. Amniocentesis
3. Level II ultrasound
4. Nuchal translucency testing

ANSWER: 2

The amniocentesis is the only diagnostic test that can be performed at this time during the pregnancy to confirm diagnosis of Down's syndrome. CVS and nuchal translucency testing are both done during the first trimester and cannot be performed at 16 weeks. An ultrasound can be performed after 16 weeks but is not a diagnostic test. It is also considered a screening test and does not offer a definitive diagnosis.

Test-taking Tip: *Think about the timing of the tests listed to determine the correct selection along with which tests are considered screening tests and which ones are diagnostic.*

Content Area: Childbearing Families; *Category of Health Alteration:* Prenatal and Antepartal Management; *Integrated Processes:* Nursing Process Implementation; *Client Need:* Health Promotion and Maintenance/Health Screening; *Cognitive Level:* Analysis

Reference: Pillitteri, A. (2007). *Maternal & Child Health Nursing: Care of the Childbearing Families & Childrearing Family* (5th ed., p. 174). Philadelphia: Lippincott Williams & Wilkins.

280. A pregnant client has an abnormal 1-hour glucose screen and completes a 3-hour, 100-gram oral glucose tolerance test. Which test result should a nurse interpret as being abnormal?

1. Fasting blood sugar = 84 mg/dL
2. 1 hr = 186 mg/dL
3. 2 hr = 146 mg/dL
4. 3 hr = 129 mg/dL

ANSWER: 2

A 1-hour value of 186 is abnormal. All other options are at or less than the normal expected values for a glucose tolerance test: fasting blood sugar = 95 mg/dL; 1 hr = 180 mg/dL; 2 hr = 155 mg/dL; 3 hr = 140 mg/dL.

➧ ***Test-taking Tip:*** *To answer this question, you must know the criteria of normal values for diagnosing gestational diabetes.*

Content Area: Childbearing Families; *Category of Health Alteration:* Prenatal and Antepartal Management; *Integrated Processes:* Nursing Process Assessment; *Client Need:* Physiological Integrity/Physiological Adaptation/Alterations in Body Systems; *Cognitive Level:* Analysis

Reference: Ward, S., & Hisley, S. (2009). *Maternal-Child Nursing Care* (p. 335). Philadelphia: F. A. Davis.

281. A nurse is reviewing the laboratory test results of a pregnant client. Which lab value is outside the normal range for a pregnant woman?

Laboratory test	Result
Hemoglobin	10.6 g/dL
Indirect Coombs' test	Negative
50 gram 1-hour glucose test	137
Glucosuria	Negative
Proteinuria	Trace
Group beta streptococcus (GBS)	Negative

1. Hemoglobin
2. 50-gram, 1-hour glucose test
3. Glucosuria
4. Proteinuria

ANSWER: 1

The normal hemoglobin level should be 12–16 g/dL in a pregnant woman. The indirect Coombs' test should be negative; a positive result is an indication of maternal sensitization. The 50-gram 1-hour glucose test should be less than 140. Values over 140 warrant a 3-hour glucose screen to determine if the woman has gestational diabetes. Proteinuria in trace amounts is common in pregnant women although higher protein concentrations should be evaluated. Group beta streptococcus cultures should be negative. A positive culture indicates maternal infection and possible transmission to the infant during the birth process.

➧ ***Test-taking Tip:*** *Evaluate each laboratory result and identify normal pregnancy levels. Evaluate which lab result is abnormal and select the appropriate levels.*

Content Area: Childbearing Families; *Category of Health Alteration:* Prenatal and Antepartal Management; *Integrated Processes:* Nursing Process Assessment; *Client Need:* Physiological Integrity/Reduction of Risk Potential/Laboratory Values; *Cognitive Level:* Analysis

Reference: Davidson, M., London, M., & Ladewig, P. (2008). *Olds' Maternal-Newborn Nursing & Women's Health Across the Lifespan* (8th ed., p. 349). Upper Saddle River, NJ: Prentice Hall Health.

282. A nurse is caring for a 34-week pregnant client (G2P1) with the following symptoms. Which manifestations should be most concerning to the nurse? Prioritize the abnormal findings for a pregnant woman in the third trimester from the most significant (1) to the least significant (4).

______ +3 pedal edema
______ BP 144/94 mm Hg
______ Group beta streptococcus-positive vaginal culture
______ Fundal height increase of 4.5 cm in 1 week

ANSWER: 3, 1, 4, 2

Preeclampsia is a condition that can progress to serious complications. A woman suspected of having preeclampsia needs immediate inpatient evaluation. A blood pressure (BP) of 144/94 warrants immediate evaluation. A fundal height increase of 1 to 2 cm per week is considered normal fundal growth. An increase in fundal size can be related to gestational diabetes, large for gestational age fetus, fetal anomalies, or polyhydramnios. Further assessment is warranted. Excessive pedal edema can be a normal physiological process if it is an isolated finding. Pedal edema warrants further assessment because it can be a symptom of preeclampsia. A positive group beta streptococcus culture warrants antibiotic treatment in labor but does not warrant intervention during the pregnancy.

➧ ***Test-taking Tip:*** *Consider the possible etiology for each listed abnormal finding. Prioritize the most serious as first and proceed to rank the abnormalities by the seriousness of each condition.*

Content Area: Childbearing Families; *Category of Health Alteration:* Prenatal and Antepartal Management; *Integrated Processes:* Nursing Process Assessment; *Client Need:* Physiological Integrity/Physiological Adaptation/Alterations in Body Systems; *Cognitive Level:* Application

Reference: Davidson, M., London, M., & Ladewig, P. (2008). *Olds' Maternal-Newborn Nursing & Women's Health Across the Lifespan* (8th ed., p. 379). Upper Saddle River, NJ: Prentice Hall Health.

283. EBP A pregnant client tells a nurse that she thinks she is carrying twins. In reviewing the client's history and medical records, the nurse should determine that which factors are associated with a multiple gestation? SELECT ALL THAT APPLY.

1. Elevated serum alpha-fetoprotein
2. Use of reproductive technology
3. Maternal age greater than 40
4. Family history
5. Elevated hemoglobin

ANSWER: 1, 2, 4

An elevated serum alpha-fetoprotein level (an oncofetal protein normally produced by the fetal liver and yolk sac), use of reproductive technology, and family history are all associated with a multiple gestation. Maternal age greater than 40 and an elevated hemoglobin are not associated with multiple gestation.

➧ ***Test-taking Tip:** Focus on the issue: the factors that can indicate or lead to multiple gestation.*

Content Area: Childbearing Families; *Category of Health Alteration:* Prenatal and Antepartal Management; *Integrated Processes:* Nursing Process Assessment; *Client Need:* Physiological Integrity/Physiological Adaptation/Pathophysiology; *Cognitive Level:* Application

Reference: Pillitteri, A. (2007). *Maternal & Child Health Nursing: Care of the Childbearing Families & Childrearing Family* (5th ed., p. 433). Philadelphia: Lippincott Williams & Wilkins.

EBP Reference: Fleischer, A., Andreotti, R., Bohm-Velez, M., Horrow, M., Hricak, H., et al. (2005). *Expert Panel on Women's Imaging: Multiple Gestations*. Reston, VA: American College of Radiology.

---

284. A 22-year-old client, who is experiencing vaginal bleeding in the first trimester of pregnancy, fears that she has lost her baby at 8 weeks. Which definitive test result should indicate to a nurse that the client's fetus has been lost?

1. Falling beta human chorionic gonadotropin (BHCG) measurement
2. Low progesterone measurement
3. Ultrasound demonstrating lack of fetal cardiac activity
4. Ultrasound determining crown–rump length

ANSWER: 3

Ultrasound is used to determine if the fetus has died. The lack of fetal heart activity in a pregnancy over 6 weeks determines a fetal loss. Crown–rump length determines only the fetal gestational age. Falling BHCG levels and low progesterone levels do not conclusively diagnose fetal demise.

➧ ***Test-taking Tip:** Prioritize the above options to determine which choice offers the most definitive diagnosis.*

Content Area: Childbearing Families; *Category of Health Alteration:* Prenatal and Antepartal Management; *Integrated Processes:* Nursing Process Analysis; *Client Need:* Physiological Integrity/Physiological Adaptation/Pathophysiology; *Cognitive Level:* Analysis

Reference: Davidson, M., London, M., & Ladewig, P. (2008). *Olds' Maternal-Newborn Nursing & Women's Health Across the Lifespan* (8th ed., p. 482). Upper Saddle River, NJ: Prentice Hall Health.

---

285. A new pregnant client (G1P0) presents at a clinic and states that she is anxious regarding her pregnancy, her prenatal care, and her labor and birth. Which teaching need is priority during the first trimester?

1. Sexual relations with her spouse
2. Fetal growth and development
3. Labor and delivery options
4. Completion of preparations for the baby

ANSWER: 2

Information about fetal growth and development is important to cover during the first trimester. There is no indication that sexual relations is a concern for the woman. Labor and delivery options and completion of preparations for the baby are priorities in the third trimester. Birth control methods are priorities in the postpartum period.

➧ ***Test-taking Tip:** The priorities for teaching should focus on the learning needs of each trimester and the concerns of the client.*

Content Area: Childbearing Families; *Category of Health Alteration:* Prenatal and Antepartal Management; *Integrated Processes:* Nursing Process Implementation; *Client Need:* Health Promotion and Maintenance/Principles of Teaching and Learning; *Cognitive Level:* Application

Reference: Davidson, M., London, M., & Ladewig, P. (2008). *Olds' Maternal-Newborn Nursing & Women's Health Across the Lifespan* (8th ed., pp. 368–369). Upper Saddle River, NJ: Prentice Hall Health.

---

286. EBP A nurse is teaching a woman who wishes to travel by airplane during the first 36 weeks of her pregnancy. Which is the primary risk of air travel for this woman that the nurse should address?

1. Preterm labor
2. Deep vein thrombosis
3. Spontaneous miscarriage
4. Nausea and vomiting

ANSWER: 2

The most significant medical risk that can occur with air travel during pregnancy is deep vein thrombosis, because pregnancy increases the risk of blood coagulation and prolonged sitting produces venous stasis. Although nausea and vomiting can occur, they are not dangerous. Preterm labor and spontaneous abortion are not associated with air travel.

➧ ***Test-taking Tip:** Review both the physiological process and changes associated with pregnancy and implications of air travel to choose the best answer.*

Content Area: Childbearing Families; *Category of Health Alteration:* Prenatal and Antepartal Management; *Integrated Processes:* Nursing Process Planning; *Client Need:* Safe and Effective Care Environment/Safety and Infection Control/Injury Prevention; *Cognitive Level:* Application

Reference: Pillitteri, A. (2007). *Maternal & Child Health Nursing: Care of the Childbearing & Childrearing Family* (5th ed., pp. 360–361). Philadelphia: Lippincott Williams & Wilkins.

EBP Reference: Kirkham, C., Harris, S., & Grzybowski, S. (2005). Evidence-based prenatal care: Part I. General prenatal care and counseling issues. *American Family Physician, 71*(7), 1307–1326.

---

287. EBP A first-trimester pregnant woman asks a nurse if the activities in which she participates are safe in the first trimester. Which activity should the nurse verify as a safe activity during the client's first trimester?

1. Hair coloring
2. Hot tub use
3. Sauna use
4. Sexual activity

ANSWER: 4

Sexual activity is not contraindicated in pregnancy unless a specific risk factor is identified. Hair coloring and hot tub and sauna use should be avoided in the first trimester of pregnancy because of the dangers to the developing fetus and pregnant woman.

➧ ***Test-taking Tip:*** *Determine the best answer based on your knowledge of which activities could pose a direct threat to a developing fetus.*

Content Area: Childbearing Families; *Category of Health Alteration:* Prenatal and Antepartal Management; *Integrated Processes:* Nursing Process Planning; *Client Need:* Safe and Effective Care Environment/Safety and Infection Control/Injury Prevention; *Cognitive Level:* Application

Reference: Pillitteri, A. (2007). *Maternal & Child Health Nursing: Care of the Childbearing Families & Childrearing Family* (5th ed., pp. 274–276). Philadelphia: Lippincott Williams & Wilkins.

EBP Reference: Kirkham, C., Harris, S., & Grzybowski, S. (2005). Evidence-based prenatal care: Part I. General prenatal care and counseling issues. *American Family Physician, 71*(7), 1307–1326.

---

288. EBP Which is the *first* intervention that should be recommended to a pregnant woman complaining of hemorrhoid pain?

1. Steroid-based creams
2. Diet modifications
3. Surgery
4. Oral medications

ANSWER: 2

A high-fiber diet is the first intervention that should be attempted when counseling a woman on the management of hemorrhoids. Steroid-based creams are frequently used, although evidence does not support their effectiveness. Oral medications, such as flavonoids, are found to aid in symptom relief, although they are not recommended as the first line of treatment. Surgical intervention to remove hemorrhoids is not recommended in pregnancy because they frequently resolve after pregnancy.

➧ ***Test-taking Tip:*** *Determine the intervention that is the least invasive and has supportive evidence based on the research literature.*

Content Area: Childbearing Families; *Category of Health Alteration:* Prenatal and Antepartal Management; *Integrated Processes:* Nursing Process Implementation; *Client Need:* Physiological Integrity/Physiological Adaptation/Alterations in Body Systems; *Cognitive Level:* Analysis

Reference: Pillitteri, A. (2007). *Maternal & Child Health Nursing: Care of the Childbearing & Childrearing Family* (5th ed., pp. 280–281). Philadelphia: Lippincott Williams & Wilkins.

EBP Reference: National Institute of Clinical Excellence. (2003). *Antenatal Care: Routine Care for the Healthy Pregnant Woman.* London: Royal College of Obstetricians and Gynecologists.

289. EBP A nurse should recommend which preconceptual supplement as a preventative measure to decrease the incidence of neural tube defects?

1. Folic acid supplementation
2. Iron supplements
3. Vitamin C supplementation
4. Vitamin B_6 supplementation

ANSWER: 1

Folic acid supplementation when taken at the time of conception has been found to decrease the incidence of neural tube defects. Iron supplements are used to treat anemia that is associated with pregnancy.

Test-taking Tip: Review nutritional interventions to determine the best answer.

Content Area: Childbearing Families; *Category of Health Alteration:* Prenatal and Antepartal Management; *Integrated Processes:* Nursing Process Implementation; *Client Need:* Health Promotion and Maintenance/Disease Prevention; *Cognitive Level:* Application

Reference: Pillitteri, A. (2007). *Maternal & Child Health Nursing: Care of the Childbearing Families & Childrearing Family* (5th ed., p. 1205). Philadelphia: Lippincott Williams & Wilkins.

EBP Reference: National Institute of Clinical Excellence. (2003). *Antenatal Care: Routine Care for the Healthy Pregnant Woman.* London: Royal College of Obstetricians and Gynecologists.

290. A nurse should recommend which suggested weight gain for a woman who is in the ideal weight range before becoming pregnant?

1. Less than 15 lb
2. 15–25 lb
3. 25–35 lb
4. 35–45 lb

ANSWER: 3

A woman, who is in the ideal weight range prior to pregnancy, is typically advised to gain 25 to 35 lb during pregnancy. The increased uterine size and its contents, breasts, intravascular fluid, excess fat, water, and protein make up the maternal reserves.

Test-taking Tip: Recall the suggested weight gain for pregnant women and use this information to make your best choice.

Content Area:: Childbearing Families; *Category of Health Alteration:* Prenatal and Antepartal Management; *Integrated Processes:* Nursing Process Implementation; *Client Need:* Health Promotion and Maintenance/Developmental Stages and Transitions; *Cognitive Level:* Comprehension

Reference: Davidson, M., London, M., & Ladewig, P. (2008). *Olds' Maternal-Newborn Nursing & Women's Health Across the Lifespan* (8th ed., p. 362). Upper Saddle River, NJ: Prentice Hall Health.

291. EBP A pregnant woman, who has a previous surgical history of bariatric surgery, should be counseled by a nurse to supplement her diet with which of the following? SELECT ALL THAT APPLY.

1. Vitamin B_{12}
2. Folate
3. Iron
4. Vitamin A
5. Calcium

ANSWER: 1, 2, 3, 5

Women who have had any type of bariatric surgery should supplement their diets with vitamin B_{12}, folate, iron, and calcium because the surgery decreases the absorption of these vitamins and minerals. Vitamin A excess can lead to fetal defects and should not be supplemented unless specifically indicated.

Test-taking Tip: Recall knowledge of nutrition and the digestive process to determine which vitamins or minerals are not well absorbed after bariatric surgery. Eliminate a fat soluble vitamin.

Content Area: Childbearing Families; *Category of Health Alteration:* Prenatal and Antepartal Management; *Integrated Processes:* Nursing Process Implementation; *Client Need:* Health Promotion and Maintenance/Health Promotion Programs; *Cognitive Level:* Application

Reference: Pillitteri, A. (2007). *Maternal & Child Health Nursing: Care of the Childbearing & Childrearing Family* (5th ed., pp. 304–305). Philadelphia: Lippincott Williams & Wilkins.

EBP References: Moliterno, J., DiLuna, M., Sood, S., Roberts, K., & Duncan, C. (2008). Gastric bypass: A risk factor for neural tube defects? Case report. *Journal of Neurosurgery: Pediatrics, 1*(5), 406–409; American College of Obstetrics and Gynecology (ACOG). (2005). *Obesity in Pregnancy.* (ACOG Committee Opinion No. 315). Washington, DC: Author.

292. A nurse is working in a government nutritional education program. The nurse is counseling a young pregnant woman who is a vegan. Based on the nurse's knowledge of vegetarianism, which definition of vegan is correct?

1. An individual who does not eat meat
2. An individual who does not eat eggs
3. An individual who does not eat animal products
4. An individual who prefers vegetables

ANSWER: 3

A vegan is an individual who does not eat any animal products, including meat, eggs, and milk. A lacto-ovo vegetarian does not eat meat, but does eat eggs and drink milk. A lacto-vegetarian drinks milk, but does not eat eggs.

Test-taking Tip: *Determine the different types of vegetarianism based on which types of animal products are consumed in each classification.*

Content Area: Childbearing Families; *Category of Health Alteration:* Prenatal and Antepartal Management; *Integrated Processes:* Nursing Process Assessment; *Client Need:* Health Promotion and Maintenance/ Health and Wellness; *Cognitive Level:* Application

Reference: Davidson, M., London, M., & Ladewig, P. (2008). *Olds' Maternal-Newborn Nursing & Women's Health Across the Lifespan* (8th ed., p. 431). Upper Saddle River, NJ: Prentice Hall Health.

---

293. A woman presents with vaginal bleeding at 7 weeks. What is the primary nursing intervention for a woman who is bleeding during the first trimester?

1. Monitor vital signs
2. Prepare equipment for examination
3. Have oxygen available
4. Assess family's response to the situation

ANSWER: 1

Assessing the woman's vital signs is the most important nursing intervention. Preparing equipment, having oxygen available, and assessing the family's responses are also important nursing interventions.

Test-taking Tip: *Determine which intervention is the highest priority and select that answer.*

Content Area: Childbearing Families; *Category of Health Alteration:* Prenatal and Antepartal Management; *Integrated Processes:* Nursing Process Implementation; *Client Need:* Physiological Integrity/ Physiological Adaptation/Alteration in Body Systems; *Cognitive Level:* Analysis

Reference: Davidson, M., London, M., & Ladewig, P. (2008). *Olds' Maternal-Newborn Nursing & Women's Health Across the Lifespan* (8th ed., pp. 481–482). Upper Saddle River, NJ: Prentice Hall Health.

---

294. A woman who is actively bleeding due to a spontaneous abortion asks a nurse why this is happening. The nurse advises the woman that the majority of first-trimester losses are related to which of the following?

1. Cervical incompetence
2. Chronic maternal disease
3. Poor implantation
4. Chromosomal abnormalities

ANSWER: 4

Chromosomal abnormalities account for the majority of first-trimester spontaneous abortions. The other options also can result in spontaneous abortion, but do not account for the majority.

Test-taking Tip: *Review causes of spontaneous abortion to determine the correct answer.*

Content Area: Childbearing Families; *Category of Health Alteration:* Prenatal and Antepartal Management; *Integrated Processes:* Nursing Process Assessment; *Client Need:* Physiological Integrity/Physiological Adaptation/Pathophysiology; *Cognitive Level:* Application

Reference: Davidson, M., London, M., & Ladewig, P. (2008). *Olds' Maternal-Newborn Nursing & Women's Health Across the Lifespan* (8th ed., pp. 481–483). Upper Saddle River, NJ: Prentice Hall Health.

---

295. A nurse is providing emotional support for a woman who experienced a recent miscarriage during her second trimester. The nurse's care of the woman should be based on knowing which cause of spontaneous abortions is most common in the second trimester?

1. Maternal factors
2. Chromosomal abnormalities
3. Fetal death
4. Alcoholism

ANSWER: 1

The most common causes of second-trimester losses are maternal factors, such as incompetent cervix. Often, the fetal death may not precede the onset of the abortion.

Test-taking Tip: *Consider the causes of second-trimester abortion and determine which cause is the most prevalent to make your selection.*

Content Area: Childbearing Families; *Category of Health Alteration:* Prenatal and Antepartal Management; *Integrated Processes:* Nursing Process Assessment; *Client Need:* Physiological Integrity/Physiological Adaptation/Pathophysiology; *Cognitive Level:* Analysis

Reference: Davidson, M., London, M., & Ladewig, P. (2008). *Olds' Maternal-Newborn Nursing & Women's Health Across the Lifespan* (8th ed., pp. 481–483). Upper Saddle River, NJ: Prentice Hall Health.

296. A pregnant client presents with vaginal bleeding and increasing cramping. Her exam reveals that the cervical os is open. Which term should the nurse expect to see in the client's chart notation to most accurately describe the client's condition?

1. Ectopic pregnancy
2. Complete abortion
3. Imminent abortion
4. Incomplete abortion

ANSWER: 3

In imminent abortion, the woman's bleeding and cramping increase and the cervix is open, which indicates that abortion is imminent or inevitable. In ectopic pregnancy, the pregnancy is outside of the uterus and intervention is indicated to resolve the pregnancy. A complete abortion indicates that the contents of the pregnancy have been passed. In an incomplete abortion, a portion of the pregnancy has been expelled and a portion remains in the uterus.

▶ ***Test-taking Tip:*** *Review the definitions of the above diagnoses to determine the best answer.*

Content Area: Childbearing Families; *Category of Health Alteration:* Prenatal and Antepartal Management; *Integrated Processes:* Communication and Documentation; *Client Need:* Physiological Integrity/Physiological Adaptation/Pathophysiology; *Cognitive Level:* Comprehension

Reference: Davidson, M., London, M., & Ladewig, P. (2008). *Olds' Maternal-Newborn Nursing & Women's Health Across the Lifespan* (8th ed., pp. 481–483). Upper Saddle River, NJ: Prentice Hall Health.

---

297. A pregnant client (G7P5) presents after being advised she has a missed abortion. She tells a nurse that she wants to wait and let the pregnancy pass "naturally." Which length of time should the nurse tell the client is the longest she can wait before having a dilatation and curettage (D&C) after being diagnosed with a missed abortion?

1. 24 hours
2. 72 hours
3. 4–6 weeks
4. 6–8 weeks

ANSWER: 3

In missed abortions, a D&C, or suction evacuation, should be performed by 4 to 6 weeks if expulsion of the fetal products has not occurred. Pregnancies that progress beyond 6 weeks put the mother at risk for developing disseminated intravascular coagulation disorder (DIC).

▶ ***Test-taking Tip:*** *Identify the consequences of delaying a D&C. Based on this information, make the best selection of the possible options.*

Content Area: Childbearing Families; *Category of Health Alteration:* Prenatal and Antepartal Management; *Integrated Processes:* Nursing Process Implementation; *Client Need:* Physiological Integrity/Physiological Adaptation/Pathophysiology; *Cognitive Level:* Application

Reference: Davidson, M., London, M., & Ladewig, P. (2008). *Olds' Maternal-Newborn Nursing & Women's Health Across the Lifespan* (8th ed., p. 483). Upper Saddle River, NJ: Prentice Hall Health.

---

298. A nurse is caring for a woman with decreased fetal movement at 35 weeks gestation. Interventions have been ordered by the physician. Prioritize the prescribed interventions in the order in which they should be performed.

____ Prepare for nonstress test
____ Prepare for biophysical profile
____ Palpate for fetal movement
____ Apply and explain the external fetal monitor

ANSWER: 3, 4, 1, 2

Women who present with a decrease in fetal movement should be evaluated by first palpating for fetal movement externally. Next, the fetal monitor should be placed and the fetus should be monitored for heart rate changes. A nonstress test should be conducted to determine fetal well-being. A biophysical profile, which may or may not be performed in addition to the nonstress test, is the final test performed to determine fetal well-being.

▶ ***Test-taking Tip:*** *Consider which testing is most in-depth and which testing is used for initial screening. Use this information to prioritize nursing care.*

Content Area: Childbearing Families; *Category of Health Alteration:* Prenatal and Antepartal Management; *Integrated Processes:* Nursing Process Assessment; *Client Need:* Physiological Integrity/Physiological Adaptation/Alterations in Body Systems; *Cognitive Level:* Application

Reference: Davidson, M., London, M., & Ladewig, P. (2008). *Olds' Maternal-Newborn Nursing & Women's Health Across the Lifespan* (8th ed., pp. 551–552). Upper Saddle River, NJ: Prentice Hall Health.

299. EBP A nurse is screening prenatal clients who may be carriers for potential genetic abnormalities. Which ethnic group should the nurse identify as having the lowest risk for hemoglobinopathies, such as sickle cell disease and thalassemia?

1. African descent
2. Southeast Asian descent
3. Scandinavian descent
4. Mediterranean descent

ANSWER: 3

Individuals of Scandinavian descent are not an identified risk group for hemoglobinopathies. Individuals of African, Southeast Asian, or Mediterranean descent are all at risk for hemoglobinopathies and should be offered carrier screening.

➧ ***Test-taking Tip:*** *Review which conditions can be linked to specific ethnic groups to choose the best answer. If uncertain, consider the geographic proximity of ancestors from each ethnic group.*

Content Area: Childbearing Families; *Category of Health Alteration:* Prenatal and Antepartal Management; *Integrated Processes:* Nursing Process Planning; *Client Need:* Health Promotion and Maintenance/ Health Screening; *Cognitive Level:* Application

Reference: Pillitteri, A. (2007). *Maternal & Child Health Nursing: Care of the Childbearing & Childrearing Family* (5th ed., pp. 264–265). Philadelphia: Lippincott Williams & Wilkins.

EBP Reference: American College of Obstetricians and Gynecologists (ACOG). (2007). Hemoglobinopathies in pregnancy. *ACOG Practice Bulletin,* No. 78. Available at: www.guideline.gov/summary/summary.aspx?doc_id=10920&nbr=005700&string=Hemoglobinopathies+AND+pregnancy.

300. EBP A pregnant woman is suspected of having a hemoglobinopathy. Which test should a nurse anticipate that the health-care provider would order to appropriately diagnose a hemoglobinopathy?

1. Complete blood count (CBC)
2. Solubility test
3. Hemoglobin electrophoresis
4. CBC and hemoglobin electrophoresis

ANSWER: 4

CBC and hemoglobin electrophoresis are both appropriate tests for diagnosing hemoglobinopathies. Both are necessary to determine a specific diagnosis for hemoglobinopathies. Solubility testing is not recommended because it fails to identify the transmissible hemoglobin gene abnormalities.

➧ ***Test-taking Tip:*** *If uncertain, select the most global option.*

Content Area: Childbearing Families; *Category of Health Alteration:* Prenatal and Antepartal Management; *Integrated Processes:* Nursing Process Planning; *Client Need:* Health Promotion and Maintenance/ Health Screening; *Cognitive Level:* Application

Reference: Pillitteri, A. (2007). *Maternal & Child Health Nursing: Care of the Childbearing & Childrearing Family* (5th ed., pp. 264–265). Philadelphia: Lippincott Williams & Wilkins.

EBP Reference: American College of Obstetricians and Gynecologists (ACOG). (2005). Hemoglobinopathies in pregnancy. *ACOG Practice Bulletin,* No. 64.

301. EBP A nurse is caring for a pregnant woman who states she smokes two packs per day (PPD) of cigarettes. She states she has smoked in other pregnancies and has never had any problems. What is the nurse's best response?

1. "I am glad to hear your other pregnancies went well. Smoking can cause a variety of problems in pregnancies and it would be best if you could quit smoking with this pregnancy."
2. "You need to stop smoking for the baby's sake."
3. "Smoking can lead to having a large baby which can make it difficult for delivery. You may even need a cesarean section."
4. "Smoking less would eliminate the risk for your baby."

ANSWER: 1

The mother should be advised that there are adverse effects associated with smoking. including small for gestational age size, smaller fetal head, spontaneous abortion, placental abruption, neural tube defects, and increase risk of sudden infant death syndrome (SIDS). Secondhand smoke is also associated with adverse health effects for the fetus, including a risk for neural tube defects. Telling the woman to stop smoking for the baby's sake is confrontational, making the woman less likely to listen to the nurse's teaching. Decreasing her smoking intake should be suggested; however, it does not eliminate the risk to the baby completely.

➧ ***Test-taking Tip:*** *First eliminate option 3 because it contains incorrect information. Then eliminate options 2 and 4 because these statements do not use therapeutic communication techniques.*

Content Area: Childbearing Families; *Category of Health Alteration:* Prenatal and Antepartal Management; *Integrated Processes:* Teaching and Learning; *Client Need:* Health Promotion and Maintenance/High-Risk Behaviors; *Cognitive Level:* Analysis

Reference: Davidson, M., London, M., & Ladewig, P. (2008). *Olds' Maternal-Newborn Nursing & Women's Health Across the Lifespan* (8th ed., pp. 445–446). Upper Saddle River, NJ: Prentice Hall Health.

EBP Reference: Suarez, L., Felkner, M., Brender, J., Canfield, M., & Hendricks, K. (2007). Maternal exposures to cigarette smoke, alcohol, and street drugs and neural tube defect: Occurrence in offspring. *Maternal Child Health Journal, 12*(3), 394–401.

302. A nurse is caring for a woman who had a miscarriage 2 months ago. The woman is a heavy drinker (more than four drinks per day), and she has been advised that her recent miscarriage may have been associated with her alcohol use. Which additional problems related to prolonged alcohol abuse should the woman be informed about by the nurse? SELECT ALL THAT APPLY.

1. Malnutrition
2. Bone marrow suppression
3. Liver disease
4. Hepatitis B infection
5. Neurological damage to a developing fetus

ANSWER: 1, 2, 3, 5

Alcohol use is associated with malnutrition, bone marrow suppression, and liver disease. Fetuses cannot remove the breakdown products of alcohol. The large buildup of these byproducts leads to vitamin B deficiency and accompanying neurologic damage. Alcoholism is not associated with hepatitis B; although hepatitis B can also cause liver disease.

➧ ***Test-taking Tip:*** *Consider the physiological changes associated with alcoholism and use the process of elimination.*

Content Area: Childbearing Families; *Category of Health Alteration:* Prenatal and Antepartal Management; *Integrated Processes:* Nursing Process Analysis; *Client Need:* Physiological Integrity/Physiological Adaptation/Pathophysiology; *Cognitive Level:* Analysis

References: Davidson, M., London, M., & Ladewig, P. (2008). *Olds' Maternal-Newborn Nursing & Women's Health Across the Lifespan* (8th ed., pp. 445–446). Upper Saddle River, NJ: Prentice Hall Health; Pillitteri, A. (2007). *Maternal & Child Health Nursing: Care of the Childbearing Families & Childrearing Family* (5th ed., p. 292). Philadelphia: Lippincott Williams & Wilkins.

303. EBP A 28-year-old pregnant client (G3P2) has just been diagnosed with gestational diabetes at 30 weeks. The client asks what types of complications may occur with this diagnosis. Which complications should the nurse identify as being associated with gestational diabetes? SELECT ALL THAT APPLY.

1. Seizures
2. Large for gestational age infant
3. Low birth weight infant
4. Congenital anomalies
5. Preterm labor

ANSWER: 2, 4

Infants of diabetic mothers can be large as a result of excess glucose to the fetus. Congenital anomalies are more common in diabetic pregnancies. Seizures do not occur as a result of diabetes but can be associated with preeclampsia, another pregnancy complication. Preterm labor is not typically associated with maternal diabetes.

➧ ***Test-taking Tip:*** *Focus on the issue: risk factors and complications related to diabetic pregnancies. Seizures are associated with another type of complication. Remove this option and consider the other options.*

Content Area: Childbearing Families; *Category of Health Alteration:* Prenatal and Antepartal Management; *Integrated Processes:* Nursing Process Analysis; *Client Need:* Physiological Integrity/Physiological Adaptation/Pathophysiology; *Cognitive Level:* Application

Reference: Pillitteri, A. (2007). *Maternal & Child Health Nursing: Care of the Childbearing & Childrearing Family* (5th ed., pp. 378–383). Philadelphia: Lippincott Williams & Wilkins.

EBP Reference: Virally, M., Laloi-Michelin, M., Meas, T., Ciraru, N., Ouled, N., et al. (2007). Occurrence of gestational diabetes mellitus, maternal and fetal outcomes beyond the 28th week of gestation in women at high risk of gestational diabetes. A prospective study. *Diabetes & Metabolism, 33*(4), 290–295.

304. EBP A nurse informs a pregnant woman that her laboratory test indicates she has iron-deficiency anemia. Based on this diagnosis, for which problems should the nurse monitor this client? SELECT ALL THAT APPLY.

1. Susceptibility to infection
2. Fatigue
3. Increased risk of preeclampsia
4. Increased risk of diabetes
5. Congenital defects

ANSWER: 1, 2, 3

Iron-deficiency anemia is associated with susceptibility to infection, fatigue, and risk of preeclampsia because oxygen is not transported effectively. It is not associated with an increased risk of diabetes or congenital defects.

➧ ***Test-taking Tip:*** *Consider which conditions could be caused from a reduction in the hemoglobin and hematocrit levels that occur with iron-deficiency anemia.*

Content Area: Childbearing Families; *Category of Health Alteration:* Prenatal and Antepartal Management; *Integrated Processes:* Nursing Process Assessment; *Client Need:* Health Promotion and Maintenance/Disease Prevention; *Cognitive Level:* Analysis

Reference: Pillitteri, A. (2007). *Maternal & Child Health Nursing: Care of the Childbearing Families & Childrearing Family* (5th ed., p. 362). Philadelphia: Lippincott Williams & Wilkins.

EBP Reference: Rioux, F., & LeBlanc, C. (2007). Iron supplementation during pregnancy: What are the risks and benefits of current practices? *Applied Physiological Nutrition & Metabolism, 32*(2), 282–288.

305. EBP A nurse is caring for a woman who is 9 weeks pregnant and has a past medical history of anemia during pregnancy and postpartum hemorrhage after her last delivery. In which order should interventions be implemented by the nurse? Prioritize the nurse's actions by placing each intervention in the correct sequence.

______ Obtaining serum hemoglobin and hematocrit levels
______ Starting an iron supplement of 27 mg of iron daily
______ Increasing iron supplementation to 120 mg daily
______ Providing dietary counseling for prevention
______ Notifying client of iron deficiency
______ Obtaining serum iron studies (ferritin, serum iron, total iron binding capacity) if no improvement

ANSWER: 3, 2, 5, 1, 4, 6

The initial step is to provide dietary counseling at the first prenatal visit. A supplement of 27 mg of iron is recommended for all pregnant women. Obtaining serum hemoglobin and hematocrit levels are next. The woman should then be notified of the results and increase her iron supplement to 120 mg per day. If her level does not increase, serum iron studies may be warranted.

Test-taking Tip: *Mentally provide teaching for a client in this scenario and determine the order in which you would advise each item.*

Content Area: Childbearing Families; *Category of Health Alteration:* Prenatal and Antepartal Management; *Integrated Processes:* Nursing Process Analysis; *Client Need:* Safe and Effective Care Environment/Management of Care/Establishing Priorities; *Cognitive Level:* Analysis

EBP References: Rioux, F., & LeBlanc, C. (2007). Iron supplementation during pregnancy: what are the risks and benefits of current practices? *Applied Physiological Nutrition & Metabolism, 32*(2), 282–288; Shersten, K., Bennett, J., & Chambers, M. (2007). Iron deficiency anemia. *American Family Physician, 75*(5), 112–123.

306. EBP A pregnant client presents to a clinic with ongoing nausea, vomiting, and anorexia at 29 weeks gestation. Her medical record reveals a hemoglobin level of 5 g/dL. A blood smear reveals that newly formed red blood cells are macrocytic. The nurse determines that the client is most likely experiencing:

1. sickle cell anemia.
2. folic acid deficiency anemia.
3. beta thalassemia minor.
4. beta thalassemia major.

ANSWER: 2

These symptoms and lab findings are indicative of folic acid deficiency. It is usually seen in the third trimester and coexists with iron-deficiency anemia. Sickle cell anemia is an inherited disorder in which the hemoglobin is abnormally formed. The chief complaint among individuals with sickle cell anemia is pain. Thalassemia is another inherited hematological disorder in which there is a defect in the synthesis of the beta chain within the hemoglobin molecule. Beta-thalassemia minor typically results in mild anemia, whereas beta-thalassemia major is much more severe. Pregnancy in individuals with beta-thalassemia major is rare. Symptoms are usually severe anemia that warrants transfusion therapy.

Test-taking Tip: *Review the different types of anemia. Focus on the timing of anemia in the pregnancy and the signs and symptoms presented in the scenario.*

Content Area: Childbearing Families; *Category of Health Alteration:* Prenatal and Antepartal Management; *Integrated Processes:* Nursing Process Analysis; *Client Need:* Physiological Integrity/Physiological Adaptation/Pathophysiology; *Cognitive Level:* Analysis

Reference: Davidson, M., London, M., & Ladewig, P. (2008). *Olds' Maternal-Newborn Nursing & Women's Health Across the Lifespan* (8th ed., pp. 462–465). Upper Saddle River, NJ: Prentice Hall Health.

EBP Reference: Tamura, T., & Picciano, M. (2006). Folate and human reproduction. *American Journal of Clinical Nutrition, 83*(5), 993–1016.

307. EBP A 42-year-old woman who had a partial hydatidiform molar pregnancy 3 months ago, asks a nurse whether she and her husband can try conceiving again. Which response by the nurse is incorrect and warrants follow-up action by an observing nurse manager?

1. "You will need serial beta human chorionic gonadotropin (BHCG) levels every 1 to 2 weeks until negative, and then every 1 to 2 months for 6 to 12 months."
2. "You cannot conceive again because of the risk of choriocarcinoma."
3. "You should not become pregnant for 6 to 12 months."
4. "Your risk of hydatidiform molar pregnancy reoccurrence is low."

ANSWER: 2

Women who have had a molar pregnancy can conceive again once their BHCG levels are normal and remain normal for a certain time period, usually 6 to 12 months. Women undergo serial serum BHCG testing after a hydatidiform molar pregnancy. These women are at risk for choriocarcinoma and need careful follow-up; however, in the absence of this malignancy, pregnancy is not contraindicated. Couples with a past history of molar pregnancy have the same statistical chance of conceiving again and having a normal pregnancy as those without.

➧ ***Test-taking Tip:*** *Review your knowledge related to both molar pregnancy and choriocarcinoma. Use that information to choose the correct option.*

Content Area: Childbearing Families; *Category of Health Alteration:* Prenatal and Antepartal Management; *Integrated Processes:* Teaching and Learning; *Client Need:* Health Promotion and Maintenance/Self-Care; *Cognitive Level:* Application

Reference: Pillitteri, A. (2007). *Maternal & Child Health Nursing: Care of the Childbearing & Childrearing Family* (5th ed., pp. 164, 401). Philadelphia: Lippincott Williams & Wilkins.

EBP Reference: Sebire, N., Foskett, M., Short, D., Savage, P., Stewart, W., et al. (2007). Shortened duration of human chorionic gonadotropin surveillance following complete or partial hydatidiform mole: Evidence for revised protocol of a UK regional trophoblastic disease unit. *British Journal of Obstetrics & Gynecology, 114*(6), 760–762.

308. A pregnant woman presents to the emergency department with a large amount painless of bright red bleeding. She looks to be about 30 to 34 weeks pregnant based on her uterine size. She speaks limited English and is unable to communicate with the staff. Which interventions are appropriate for this client? SELECT ALL THAT APPLY.

1. Calling for an interpreter for this client
2. Establishing intravenous access
3. Obtaining fetal heart tones
4. Positioning the client into a lithotomy position with her legs in stirrups
5. Performing a vaginal examination to determine the cause of the bleeding

ANSWER: 1, 2, 3

Calling for an interpreter, establishing intravenous access, and obtaining fetal heart tones should all be performed by the nurse. Positioning the client in a lithotomy position can cause abdominal pain and there is no indication that birth is imminent for delivery in the emergency department. A pregnant woman who presents in later pregnancy should never have a digital pelvic exam because this could cause additional bleeding in a woman with placenta previa.

➧ ***Test-taking Tip:*** *Review the etiology for bleeding in the third trimester.*

Content Area: Childbearing Families; *Category of Health Alteration:* Prenatal and Antepartal Management; *Integrated Processes:* Nursing Process Implementation; *Client Need:* Physiological Integrity/Physiological Adaptation/Alterations in Body Systems; Psychosocial Integrity/Cultural Diversity; *Cognitive Level:* Analysis

References: Pillitteri, A. (2007). *Maternal & Child Health Nursing: Care of the Childbearing & Childrearing Family* (5th ed., pp. 400–402). Philadelphia: Lippincott Williams & Wilkins; Sakornbut, E., Leeman, L., & Fontaine, P. (2007). Late pregnancy bleeding. *American Family Physician, 75*(8), 1199–1206.

309. A nurse admits a woman with a diagnosis of placenta previa. Which symptom is the nurse most likely to assess in a woman with this diagnosis?

1. Painful vaginal bleeding
2. Painless vaginal bleeding
3. Contractions
4. Absence of fetal movement

ANSWER: 2

Placenta previa is characterized by painless vaginal bleeding. Painful vaginal bleeding is often associated with placental abruption. Contractions are associated with preterm labor. An absence of fetal movement is always cause for concern but is not a primary symptom of placenta previa.

➧ ***Test-taking Tip:*** *Focus on the symptoms, bright red vaginal bleeding, and absence of pain or contractions. Eliminate options 1 and 4 because pain is present with placenta abruption and preterm labor. Note that options 1 and 2 are opposite, so either one or both are incorrect options.*

Content Area: Childbearing Families; *Category of Health Alteration:* Prenatal and Antepartal Management; *Integrated Processes:* Nursing Process Assessment; *Client Need:* Physiological Integrity/Physiological Adaptation/Alterations in Body Systems; *Cognitive Level:* Application

References: Pillitteri, A. (2007). *Maternal & Child Health Nursing: Care of the Childbearing & Childrearing Family* (5th ed., p. 413). Philadelphia: Lippincott Williams & Wilkins; Sakornbut, E., Leeman, L., & Fontaine, P. (2007). Late pregnancy bleeding. *American Family Physician, 75*(8), 1199–1206.

310. A client presents with moderate vaginal bleeding and intense abdominal pain at 38 weeks gestation. The fetal heart rate is 90 beats per minute with no variability. A sonogram completed at 20 weeks reveals no evidence of a previa and an anterior placenta. The nurse determines that the most likely cause of her bleeding and pain is:

1. class 0 placenta abruption.
2. class 2 placenta abruption.
3. late-onset placenta previa.
4. spontaneous abortion.

ANSWER: 2

Placenta abruption is characterized by painful vaginal bleeding. A class 2 (not class 0) placenta abruption is characterized by moderate vaginal bleeding with non-reassuring fetal status. Placenta previa does not occur in the third trimester but instead is an ongoing physiological finding once the placenta has implanted. Spontaneous abortions occur in the beginning of pregnancy. The term spontaneous abortion is not used in late pregnancy.

Test-taking Tip: *Focus on the stage of pregnancy. Based on the physiological events described, eliminate the options that do not occur in the third trimester. Next, identify which symptoms are associated with the causes of vaginal bleeding.*

Content Area: Childbearing Families; *Category of Health Alteration:* Prenatal and Antepartal Management; *Integrated Processes:* Nursing Process Analysis; *Client Need:* Physiological Integrity/Physiological Adaptation/Alterations in Body Systems; *Cognitive Level:* Analysis

References: Pillitteri, A. (2007). *Maternal & Child Health Nursing: Care of the Childbearing & Childrearing Family* (5th ed., pp. 415–417). Philadelphia: Lippincott Williams & Wilkins; Sakornbut, E., Leeman, L., & Fontaine, P. (2007). Late pregnancy bleeding. *American Family Physician, 75*(8), 1199–1206.

311. A nurse is caring for a young woman who presents to a hospital with a severe headache at 32 weeks gestation. The client has not been seen by her obstetrician in 3 weeks. Her admission blood pressure is 184/104 mm Hg. She is requesting pain medications. The physician orders a nonstress test and laboratory studies. Based on the findings of the serum laboratory report, the nurse suspects that the woman is experiencing:

Serum Laboratory Test	Client Results
Serum bilirubin	2.1 mg/dL
LDH	782 IU/L
AST (SGOT)	84 IU/L
ALT (SGPT)	51 IU/L
PLT	99,000 per mm^3
Hgb	12.1 g/dL
Hct	42.8%

1. renal failure.
2. liver failure.
3. preeclampsia.
4. HELLP syndrome.

ANSWER: 4

The clinical laboratory values support the diagnosis of HELLP syndrome, a variation of pregnancy-induced hypertension characterized by hemolysis, elevated liver enzymes, and low platelets. The laboratory results involved both renal and liver alterations, making either liver or renal failure unlikely. The diagnosis of preeclampsia commonly coexists with HELLP; however, these laboratory findings show worsening symptoms that are associated with HELLP syndrome.

Test-taking Tip: *Review the laboratory findings to identify which condition is most likely.*

Content Area: Childbearing Families; *Category of Health Alteration:* Prenatal and Antepartal Management; *Integrated Processes:* Nursing Process Analysis; *Client Need:* Physiological Integrity/Physiological Adaptation/Alterations in Body Systems; *Cognitive Level:* Analysis

Reference: Pillitteri, A. (2007). *Maternal & Child Health Nursing: Care of the Childbearing Families & Childrearing Family* (5th ed., p. 1833). Philadelphia: Lippincott Williams & Wilkins.

312. Another nurse is caring for a 29-weeks-pregnant woman who presents with decreased fetal movement. Her initial blood pressure (BP) reading is 140/90 mm Hg. She states she "doesn't feel well" and her vision is "blurry." Additional assessment data include +3 reflexes, +2 proteinuria, +2 pedal edema, and puffy face and hands. What is the most important information that the nurse should obtain from the client's prenatal record?

1. BP at 20 weeks
2. BP at her first prenatal visit
3. Urine dip stick from last visit
4. Weight gain pattern

ANSWER: 2

A pregnant woman with a BP that is greater than 140/90 mm Hg with the presence of proteinuria is diagnosed with preeclampsia. The BP at 20 weeks, urine dip from the last visit, and weight gain pattern should all be reviewed, but are not the most important to review.

Test-taking Tip: *Recite the parameters needed for the diagnosis of preeclampsia.*

Content Area: Childbearing Families; *Category of Health Alteration:* Prenatal and Antepartal Management; *Integrated Processes:* Nursing Process Assessment; *Client Need:* Physiological Integrity/Reduction of Risk Potential/Vital Signs; *Cognitive Level:* Analysis

References: Pillitteri, A. (2007). *Maternal & Child Health Nursing: Care of the Childbearing & Childrearing Family* (5th ed., pp. 427–428). Philadelphia: Lippincott Williams & Wilkins; Blackburn, S. (2007). *Maternal, Fetal & Neonatal Physiology: A Clinical Perspective* (3rd ed., p. 474). St. Louis, MO: Saunders.

313. An office nurse is evaluating a 32-weeks-pregnant client. The client presents for her routine visit with an elevated blood pressure of 142/89 mm Hg. Her urine is negative for protein and her weight gain is 2 pounds since her last routine visit at 30 weeks. She has trace pedal edema. Based on this information, the nurse should conclude that the client is most likely experiencing:

1. gestational hypertension.
2. chronic hypertension.
3. preeclampsia.
4. eclampsia.

ANSWER: 1

Gestational hypertension is defined as an elevation of maternal blood pressure with normal urine findings. Chronic hypertension occurs before 20 weeks and is a preexisting condition. Preeclampsia is marked by an elevated blood pressure with proteinuria. Eclampsia is characterized by the addition of nonepileptic seizures that coexist with preeclampsia.

➧ ***Test-taking Tip:*** *Focus on the woman's symptoms. Review the definition of each of the options*

Content Area: Childbearing Families; *Category of Health Alteration:* Prenatal and Antepartal Management; *Integrated Processes:* Nursing Process Analysis; *Client Need:* Physiological Integrity/Physiological Adaptation/Alterations in Body Systems; *Cognitive Level:* Analysis

References: Pillitteri, A. (2007). *Maternal & Child Health Nursing: Care of the Childbearing & Childrearing Family* (5th ed., pp. 426–427). Philadelphia: Lippincott Williams & Wilkins; Gibson, P., & Carson, M. (2007). Hypertension and pregnancy. *E-Medicine from WebMD*. Available at: www.emedicine.com/med/TOPIC3250.HTM.

314. A nurse caring for a woman with preeclampsia should monitor for which complications associated with preeclampsia? SELECT ALL THAT APPLY.

1. Abruption
2. Hyperbilirubinemia
3. Nonreassuring fetal status
4. Eclampsia
5. Gestational diabetes

ANSWER: 1, 2, 3, 4

Abruption, hyperbilirubinemia, nonreassuring fetal status, and eclampsia can all occur as a complication of preeclampsia. Gestational diabetes is not associated with preeclampsia.

➧ ***Test-taking Tip:*** *Consider the pathophysiological aspects of preeclampsia to determine the appropriate options.*

Content Area: Childbearing Families; *Category of Health Alteration:* Prenatal and Antepartal Management; *Integrated Processes:* Nursing Process Implementation; *Client Need:* Physiological Integrity/ Physiological Adaptation/Alterations in Body Systems; *Cognitive Level:* Analysis

Reference: Pillitteri, A. (2007). *Maternal & Child Health Nursing: Care of the Childbearing Families & Childrearing Family* (5th ed., pp. 426–433). Philadelphia: Lippincott Williams & Wilkins.

315. A nurse is caring for a client who is Rh negative at 13 weeks gestation. The client is having cramping and has moderate vaginal bleeding. Which physician order should the nurse question?

1. Administer Rho(D) immune globulin (RhoGAM®).
2. Obtain a beta human chorionic gonadotropin level (BHCG).
3. Schedule an ultrasound.
4. Assess for fetal heart tones.

ANSWER: 2

Obtaining the BHCG level is not indicated at this late stage in pregnancy. BHCG levels are followed in early pregnancy before a fetal heart can be confirmed. RhoGAM® is indicated for any pregnant woman with bleeding who is Rh negative. An ultrasound can identify the cause of bleeding and confirm viability. A Doppler can be used to confirm a fetal heartbeat.

➧ ***Test-taking Tip:*** *Consider at what stage in pregnancy each of the interventions can be used. Remember that the client in the scenario is at 13 weeks gestation.*

Content Area: Childbearing Families; *Category of Health Alteration:* Prenatal and Antepartal Management; *Integrated Processes:* Nursing Process Implementation; *Client Need:* Safe and Effective Care Environment/Management of Care/Legal Rights and Responsibilities; *Cognitive Level:* Analysis

References: Pillitteri, A. (2007). *Maternal & Child Health Nursing: Care of the Childbearing & Childrearing Family* (5th ed., pp. 200–206). Philadelphia: Lippincott Williams & Wilkins; American College of Obstetricians & Gynecologists (ACOG). (2004). Ultrasonography in pregnancy. *ACOG Practice Bulletin,* No. 58.

316. The nurse is caring for an antepartal client with a velamentous cord insertion. The client asks what symptom she would most likely experience first if one of the vessels should tear. The nurse responds that the most likely symptom to occur is:

1. vaginal bleeding.
2. cramping.
3. uterine contractions.
4. placenta abruption.

ANSWER: 1

In a velamentous cord insertion, vessels of the cord divide some distance from the placenta in the placental membrane. Thus, the most likely symptom would be vaginal bleeding. Cramping and contractions are unlikely to occur because it is not related to uterine activity. An abruption, when the placenta comes off the uterine wall, results in severe abdominal pain.

Test-taking Tip: *Apply knowledge of medical terminology of a velamentous cord insertion and eliminate options 2, 3, and 4, because bleeding would be the common symptom when vessels divide.*

Content Area: Childbearing Families; *Category of Health Alteration:* Prenatal and Antepartal Management; *Integrated Processes:* Teaching and Learning; *Client Need:* Physiological Integrity/Physiological Adaptation/Alterations in Body Systems; *Cognitive Level:* Analysis

Reference: Davidson, M., London, M., & Ladewig, P. (2008). *Olds' Maternal-Newborn Nursing & Women's Health Across the Lifespan* (8th ed., p. 749). Upper Saddle River, NJ: Prentice Hall Health.

317. A 38-year-old pregnant woman has just been told she has hydramnios after undergoing a sonogram for size greater than dates. For which conditions, associated with hydramnios, should the nurse assess? SELECT ALL THAT APPLY.

1. Presence of major congenital anomaly
2. Gestational diabetes
3. Chronic hypertension
4. Infections
5. Preeclampsia

ANSWER: 1, 2, 4

Infants with congenital anomalies and mothers who are affected by gestational diabetes or infected with toxoplasmosis, rubella, cytomegalovirus, or herpes simplex virus infection (TORCH) are more likely to have hydramnios (excess amniotic fluid). Chronic hypertension and preeclampsia are not associated with excess amniotic fluid.

Test-taking Tip: *Focus on the issue: causes of hydramnios. Apply knowledge of medical terminology (hydramnios) and then think about possible causes.*

Content Area: Childbearing Families; *Category of Health Alteration:* Prenatal and Antepartal Management; *Integrated Processes:* Nursing Process Assessment; *Client Need:* Physiological Integrity/Reduction of Risk Potential/System Specific Assessment; *Cognitive Level:* Analysis

References: Davidson, M., London, M., & Ladewig, P. (2008). *Olds' Maternal-Newborn Nursing & Women's Health Across the Lifespan* (8th ed., p. 752). Upper Saddle River, NJ: Prentice Hall Health; Pillitteri, A. (2007). *Maternal & Child Health Nursing: Care of the Childbearing Families & Childrearing Family* (5th ed., p. 288). Philadelphia: Lippincott Williams & Wilkins.

Test 9: **Childbearing Families: Intrapartal Management**

318. A nurse is assessing a laboring client who is morbidly obese. The nurse is unable to determine the fetal position. Which is the most accurate method of determining fetal position in this client?

1. Inspection of the fetal abdomen
2. Palpation of the abdomen
3. Vaginal examination
4. Ultrasound

ANSWER: 4

The most accurate assessment measure is ultrasound. Inspection of the abdomen, palpation of the abdomen, and vaginal examination are all assessment techniques that can be used to determine fetal position. It is not uncommon to have difficulty assessing the fetal presentation in obese women or when the fetal part is not engaged.

➧ ***Test-taking Tip:*** *Determine the accuracy and ease of use of each of the methods to determine the best option. The key words are "most accurate."*

Content Area: Childbearing Families; *Category of Health Alteration:* Intrapartal Management; *Integrated Processes:* Nursing Process Implementation; *Client Need:* Health Promotion and Maintenance/ Techniques of Physical Assessment; *Cognitive Level:* Application

Reference: Davidson, M., London, M., & Ladewig, P. (2008). *Olds' Maternal-Newborn Nursing & Women's Health Across the Lifespan* (8th ed., p. 551). Upper Saddle River, NJ: Prentice Hall Health.

---

319. A nurse caring for multiple clients determines that which woman would be a candidate for intermittent monitoring during labor?

1. A woman with a previous cesarean birth
2. A 41-weeks primigravida
3. A woman with preeclampsia
4. A woman with gestational diabetes

ANSWER: 2

A woman who is overdue by 7 days, but has a reassuring fetal heart rate pattern, is able to have intermittent fetal monitoring. Women with a previous cesarean birth are at an increased risk for uterine rupture. Women with preeclampsia and gestational diabetes are at an increased risk for placental insufficiency and need continuous monitoring during labor.

➧ ***Test-taking Tip:*** *The key words are "intermittent monitoring." Eliminate any incorrect options by determining which options involve a risk factor that could negatively affect the birth outcome and would require more frequent monitoring.*

Content Area: Childbearing Families; *Category of Health Alteration:* Intrapartal Management; *Integrated Processes:* Nursing Process Analysis; *Client Need:* Physiological Integrity/Reduction of Risk Potential for Complications of Diagnostic Tests/Treatments/Procedures; *Cognitive Level:* Analysis

Reference: Davidson, M., London, M., & Ladewig, P. (2008). *Olds' Maternal-Newborn Nursing & Women's Health Across the Lifespan.* (8th ed., p. 622). Upper Saddle River, NJ: Prentice Hall Health.

---

320. A client who is 39-weeks pregnant presents to the birthing facility with a complaint of uterine contractions. Her contractions are mild, infrequent, and every 9 to 12 minutes; however, she is having variable decelerations. A physician orders a sonogram to determine if her amniotic fluid index (AFI) is adequate. The nurse interprets that which AFI is normal at 39 weeks?

1. 4.75 cm
2. 5.0 cm
3. 10.5 cm
4. 26 cm

ANSWER: 3

The normal AFI for a term pregnancy is greater than 5 and less than 25 cm. The abdomen is divided into four quadrants. The fluid volume is assessed by measuring the largest vertical pocket in each quadrant and adding these four measurements. Fluid levels less than 5 or greater than 25 are outside of normal limits.

➧ ***Test-taking Tip:*** *Select an option that is between 5 cm and 25 cm.*

Content Area: Childbearing Families; *Category of Health Alteration:* Intrapartal Management; *Integrated Processes:* Nursing Process Assessment; *Client Need:* Physiological Integrity/Reduction of Risk Potential for Complications of Diagnostic Tests/Treatments/Procedures; *Cognitive Level:* Analysis

Reference: Davidson, M., London, M., & Ladewig, P. (2008). *Olds' Maternal-Newborn Nursing & Women's Health Across the Lifespan* (8th ed., p. 560). Upper Saddle River, NJ: Prentice Hall Health.

321. A nurse determines that a gestationally diabetic client in preterm labor has a reactive nonstress test (NST) when which findings are noted?

1. Two fetal heart rate (FHR) accelerations of 15 beats per minute (bpm) above baseline for at least 15 seconds in a 20-minute period
2. A FHR acceleration of 15 bpm above baseline for at least 15 seconds in a 20-minute period
3. Two FHR accelerations of 20 bpm above baseline for at least 20 seconds in a 20-minute period
4. The absence of decelerations in a 20-minute period

ANSWER: 1

The criterion for a reactive NST is the presence of 2 accelerations of 15 bpm above baseline lasting 15 seconds or longer in a 20-minute period.

➧ ***Test-taking Tip:*** *Review the criteria for determining if an NST is reactive or nonreactive.*

Content Area: Childbearing Families; *Category of Health Alteration:* Intrapartal Management; *Integrated Processes:* Nursing Process Assessment; *Client Need:* Physiological Integrity/Reduction of Risk Potential/Diagnostic Tests; *Cognitive Level:* Analysis

Reference: Davidson, M., London, M., & Ladewig, P. (2008). *Olds' Maternal-Newborn Nursing & Women's Health Across the Lifespan* (8th ed., p. 552). Upper Saddle River, NJ: Prentice Hall Health.

---

322. A 39-year-old client, diagnosed with type 1 diabetes mellitus, presents at 36 weeks gestation with regular contractions. A physician decides to do an amniocentesis. Which statement best supports why a nurse should prepare the client for an amniocentesis now?

1. Diabetic women have a higher incidence of birth defects, and the physician wants to determine if a birth defect is present.
2. The woman is over 35 and is at risk for chromosomal disorders.
3. Infants of diabetic mothers are less likely to have mature lung capacity at this gestational age, and determination of lung maturity can influence whether delivery should proceed.
4. The amniocentesis is more accurate than the fetal fibronectin test in determining if delivery is imminent.

ANSWER: 3

An amniocentesis performed at this stage is most commonly done to determine if the fetal lungs have matured. In midpregnancy, the cells in amniotic fluid can be studied for genetic abnormalities such as Down's syndrome and birth defects. Many women over the age of 35 have amniocentesis done for this reason, but not this late in the pregnancy. Fetal fibronectin testing is used to determine if a preterm birth is likely (not amniocentesis), but it cannot be used to determine lung maturity.

➧ ***Test-taking Tip:*** *Focus on the issue: reason for amniocentesis with a woman in premature labor. Recall that the normal gestation is 38 to 42 weeks.*

Content Area: Childbearing Families; *Category of Health Alteration:* Intrapartal Management; *Integrated Processes:* Nursing Process Analysis; *Client Need:* Physiological Integrity/Physiological Adaptation/Alteration in Body Systems; *Cognitive Level:* Analysis

Reference: Davidson, M., London, M., & Ladewig, P. (2008). *Olds' Maternal-Newborn Nursing & Women's Health Across the Lifespan.* (8th ed., p. 564). Upper Saddle River, NJ: Prentice Hall Health.

---

323. EBP A 35-year-old client, who is now 1 week past her due date, presents to a labor and birth unit. She had an ultrasound at 6 weeks for vaginal bleeding and another scan at 20 weeks. She believes that, according to her last menstrual period (LMP), she should be 3 days before her due date; however, she has a history of irregular periods. The estimated date of confinement (EDC) is off by 11 days on the second sonogram. Her fundal height is 43 centimeters. Based on this information, the nurse determines that which method would be the most accurate for dating this pregnancy?

1. The crown–rump length on the 6-week sonogram
2. Her last menstrual period
3. Head circumference on a second-trimester sonogram
4. Her fundal height measurement obtained today

ANSWER: 1

The 6-week ultrasound offers the most accurate dating. Because she has irregular periods, the client's LMP is not a good measure of gestational age. Second-trimester ultrasound is less accurate than first-trimester ultrasound. Fundal height can be varied by multiple factors, including amount of amniotic fluid, maternal weight, fetal size, and fetal position.

➧ ***Test-taking Tip:*** *The key phrase is "most accurate." Use the process of elimination, eliminate option 2 because her menses are irregular. From the remaining options, choose the option that offers the best dating of this pregnancy.*

Content Area: Childbearing Families; *Category of Health Alteration:* Intrapartal Management; *Integrated Processes:* Nursing Process Evaluation; *Client Need:* Health Promotion and Maintenance/Techniques of Physical Assessment; *Cognitive Level:* Synthesis

Reference: Davidson, M., London, M., & Ladewig, P. (2008). *Olds' Maternal-Newborn Nursing & Women's Health Across the Lifespan* (8th ed., pp. 722–723). Upper Saddle River, NJ: Prentice Hall Health.

EBP Reference: American College of Obstetricians and Gynecologists (ACOG). (2004). Management of postterm pregnancy. *ACOG Practice Bulletin,* No. 55.

324. A laboring client is experiencing dyspnea, diaphoresis, tachycardia, and hypotension. A nurse suspects aortocaval compression. Which intervention should the nurse implement immediately?

1. Turning the client onto her left side
2. Turning the client onto her right side
3. Positioning the bed in reverse Trendelenburg's position
4. Positioning the client in a supine position

ANSWER: 1

When a laboring woman lies flat on her back, the gravid uterus completely occludes the inferior vena cava and laterally displaces the subrenal aorta. This aortocaval compression reduces maternal cardiac output, producing dyspnea, diaphoresis, tachycardia, and hypotension. Other symptoms include air hunger, nausea, and weakness. Lying on the right side, reverse Trendelenburg's position, and the supine positions all increase aortocaval compression.

➧ ***Test-taking Tip:*** *Apply knowledge of medical terminology for aortocaval compression. If unsure, think of the maternal structures that would result in decreased cardiac output when compressed by the gravid uterus.*

Content Area: Childbearing Families; *Category of Health Alteration:* Intrapartal Management; *Integrated Processes:* Nursing Process Implementation; *Client Need:* Physiological Integrity/Physiological Adaptation/Medical Emergencies; *Cognitive Level:* Application

References: Davidson, M., London, M., & Ladewig, P. (2008). *Olds' Maternal-Newborn Nursing & Women's Health Across the Lifespan* (8th ed., p. 595). Upper Saddle River, NJ: Prentice Hall Health; Kharazmi, E., Kaaja, R., Fallah, M., & Luoto, R. (2007). Pregnancy-related factors and the risk of isolated systolic hypertension. *Blood Pressure, 16*(1), 50–55.

325. A nurse receives notification that a client is to be admitted for labor induction for suspected macrosomia. For which risk factors should the nurse assess the client upon admission? SELECT ALL THAT APPLY.

1. Maternal obesity
2. Post-term pregnancy
3. Female sex of the fetus
4. Previous macrosomic infant
5. Past history of anorexia
6. Large for gestational age (LGA) infant delivered at 30 weeks

ANSWER: 1, 2, 4

Maternal obesity, post-term pregnancy, and previous macrosomic infant are all associated with macrosomic infants. Male infants are more likely to be macrosomic than infants who are female. Women with anorexia (and those with a past history) may be at risk to deliver an infant that is small for gestational age (SGA). An infant can be classified as LGA at any gestational age; however, only infants that are greater than 4,500 grams are classified as macrosomic.

➧ ***Test-taking Tip:*** *Consider which factors would predispose an infant to being macrosomic (greater than 4,500 grams).*

Content Area: Childbearing Families; *Category of Health Alteration:* Intrapartal Management; *Integrated Processes:* Nursing Process Assessment; *Client Need:* Safe and Effective Care Environment/Management of Care/Continuity of Care; *Cognitive Level:* Application

References: Davidson, M., London, M., & Ladewig, P. (2008). *Olds' Maternal-Newborn Nursing & Women's Health Across the Lifespan* (8th ed., p. 733). Upper Saddle River, NJ: Prentice Hall Health; Lowdermilk, D., & Perry, S. (2007). *Maternity and Women's Health Care* (9th ed., p. 831). St. Louis, MO: Mosby/Elsevier.

326. A primigravida client has been pushing for 2 hours when the head emerges. The fetus fails to deliver, and the physician notes that the turtle sign has occurred. Which should be a nurse's interpretation of this information?

1. Cephalopelvic disproportion
2. Shoulder dystocia
3. Persistent occiput posterior position
4. Cord prolapse

ANSWER: 2

Shoulder dystocia is a significant complication when the head is born but the fetal shoulders are unable to deliver. Cephalopelvic disproportion occurs when the head is too large to fit through the pelvis. In that case, fetal descent ceases. Persistent occiput posterior results in prolonged pushing; however, once the head is born, the remainder of the birth occurs without difficulty. A cord prolapse occurs when the umbilical cord enters the cervix before the fetal presenting part and is considered a medical emergency.

➧ ***Test-taking Tip:*** *Apply knowledge of medical terminology. Recall that the turtle sign is associated with a complication.*

Content Area: Childbearing Families; *Category of Health Alteration:* Intrapartal Management; *Integrated Processes:* Nursing Process Analysis; *Client Need:* Physiological Integrity/Physiological Adaptation/Alterations in Body Systems; *Cognitive Level:* Application

Reference: Davidson, M., London, M., & Ladewig, P. (2008). *Olds' Maternal-Newborn Nursing & Women's Health Across the Lifespan* (8th ed., p. 734). Upper Saddle River, NJ: Prentice Hall Health.

327. A nurse is caring for a woman who is being evaluated for a suspected malpresentation. The fetus's long axis is lying across the maternal abdomen, and the contour of the abdomen is elongated. Which should be the nurse's documentation of the lie of the fetus?

1. Vertex
2. Breech
3. Transverse
4. Brow

ANSWER: 3

A transverse lie occurs in 1 in 300 births and is marked by the fetus's lying in a side-lying position across the abdomen. Both vertex and breech presentations result in the lie being vertical. A brow presentation is also a vertical lie.

➧ ***Test-taking Tip:*** *Review the definition of lie, position, and presentation to help identify the correct option.*

Content Area: Childbearing Families; *Category of Health Alteration:* Intrapartal Management; *Integrated Processes:* Communication and Documentation; *Client Need:* Physiological Integrity/Physiological Adaptation/Pathophysiology; *Cognitive Level:* Application

Reference: Davidson, M., London, M., & Ladewig, P. (2008). *Olds' Maternal-Newborn Nursing & Women's Health Across the Lifespan* (8th ed., p. 724). Upper Saddle River, NJ: Prentice Hall Health.

---

328. A nurse is caring for a client who just gave birth vaginally. The nurse indicates that the presenting part was vertex and a hand. What should the proper documentation read in this woman's chart?

1. "Client gave birth via vertex presentation with a second-degree perineal laceration."
2. "Client gave birth via compound presentation of vertex and hand with a second-degree perineal laceration."
3. "Client gave birth via breech presentation."
4. "Client gave birth via cesarean section with a hand presentation and breech part presenting."

ANSWER: 2

A compound presentation occurs when there is more than one presenting part and occurs when the presenting part is not completely filling the pelvic inlet. The typical compound part is the occiput and a hand. When a compound presentation is noted, the 2 parts should be identified. By stating it was a vertex presentation, there is no indication that a compound presentation occurred. The question indicates it was a vertex (head presentation). A breech presentation indicates the buttocks, knees, or foot would be the presenting part.

➧ ***Test-taking Tip:*** *Recall the definitions of different malpresentations that can occur at birth.*

Content Area: Childbearing Families; *Category of Health Alteration:* Intrapartal Management; *Integrated Processes:* Communication and Documentation; *Client Need:* Health Promotion and Maintenance/Ante/Intra/Postpartum and Newborn Care; *Cognitive Level:* Application

Reference: Davidson, M., London, M., & Ladewig, P. (2008). *Olds' Maternal-Newborn Nursing & Women's Health Across the Lifespan* (8th ed., p. 726). Upper Saddle River, NJ: Prentice Hall Health.

---

329. A nurse is caring for a client who wants minimal intervention in terms of pain relief. A physician recommends a procedure of injecting perineal anesthesia into the pudendal plexus for pain relief for the second stage of labor, birth, and episiotomy repair. Which type of anesthesia should the nurse anticipate that the health-care provider will likely request?

1. Epidural anesthesia
2. Systemic analgesia
3. Pudendal bloc
4. Local infiltration anesthesia

ANSWER: 3

Pudendal anesthesia involves injecting perineal anesthesia into the pudendal plexus for pain relief for the second stage of labor, birth, and episiotomy repair. Epidural anesthesia is injected into a space between the vertebrae of the spine. Systemic analgesics are intravenous or intramuscular anesthesia that is given to the mother to provide pain relief. Local infiltration anesthesia is used to repair the perineal and vaginal area after an episiotomy or laceration has occurred.

➧ ***Test-taking Tip:*** *Identify the different types of anesthesia that can be used to provide pain relief in the second stage of labor and birth and during an episiotomy or laceration repair.*

Content Area: Childbearing Families; *Category of Health Alteration:* Intrapartal Management; *Integrated Processes:* Nursing Process Planning; *Client Need:* Physiological Integrity/Pharmacological and Parenteral Therapies/Pharmacological Pain Management; *Cognitive Level:* Application

Reference: Davidson, M., London, M., & Ladewig, P. (2008). *Olds' Maternal-Newborn Nursing & Women's Health Across the Lifespan* (8th ed., p. 708). Upper Saddle River, NJ: Prentice Hall Health.

330. A nurse is caring for a client who has been in the second stage of labor for the last 12 hours. The nurse should monitor for which cardiovascular change that occurs during labor?

1. An increase in maternal heart rate
2. A decrease in cardiac output
3. An increase in peripheral vascular resistance
4. A decrease in the uterine artery blood flow during contractions

ANSWER: 1

Maternal heart rate is normally increased due to pain resulting from increased catecholamine secretion, fear, anxiety, and increased blood volume. During the second stage of labor, the maternal intravascular volume is increased by 300 to 500 mL of blood from the contracting uterus. Following delivery, this autotransfusion compensates for blood losses during delivery, resulting in increased cardiac output, increased stroke volume, and a decreased heart rate. A 30% increase in cardiac output occurs during labor.

➧ ***Test-taking Tip:*** *Consider the cardiovascular changes associated with pregnancy and determine which changes are most likely to occur in the intrapartum period.*

Content Area: Childbearing Families; *Category of Health Alteration:* Intrapartal Management; *Integrated Processes:* Nursing Process Assessment; *Client Need:* Physiological Integrity/Physiological Adaptation/Pathophysiology; *Cognitive Level:* Application

References: Davidson, M., London, M., & Ladewig, P. (2008). *Olds' Maternal-Newborn Nursing & Women's Health Across the Lifespan* (8th ed., pp. 594–595). Upper Saddle River, NJ: Prentice Hall Health; Kharazmi, E., Kaaja, R., Fallah, M., & Luoto, R. (2007). Pregnancy-related factors and the risk of isolated systolic hypertension. *Blood Pressure*, *16*(1), 50–55.

331. A client presents with regular contractions that she describes as strong in intensity. Her cervical exam indicates that she is dilated to 3 cm. This information should suggest to a nurse that the client is experiencing:

1. early labor.
2. false labor.
3. cervical ripening.
4. lightening.

ANSWER: 1

Early labor is a pattern of labor that occurs when contractions become regular and the cervix dilates to 3 cm. False labor occurs when Braxton-Hicks contractions are strong enough for the woman to believe she is in actual labor. The contractions are infrequent or do not have a definite pattern. The lack of cervical change is also consistent with false labor. The latent phase is characterized by regular contractions, although fetal descent may not occur. Lightening is settling or lowering of the fetus into the pelvis. Lightening can occur a few weeks or a few hours before labor.

➧ ***Test-taking Tip:*** *Recall the definitions of each of the types of labor and make the best choice based on your knowledge of these definitions.*

Content Area: Childbearing Families; *Category of Health Alteration:* Intrapartal Management; *Integrated Processes:* Nursing Process Analysis; *Client Need:* Physiological Integrity/Physiological Adaptation/Pathophysiology; *Cognitive Level:* Analysis

Reference: Davidson, M., London, M., & Ladewig, P. (2008). *Olds' Maternal-Newborn Nursing & Women's Health Across the Lifespan* (8th ed., p. 720). Upper Saddle River, NJ: Prentice Hall Health.

332. A nurse is reviewing laboratory values for a client who is in the early stage of labor. Based on these findings, which condition should the nurse conclude that the client is experiencing?

Serum Laboratory Test	Client's Value
RBC	4.2 x 10^6/µL
WBC	10,420 cells/µL
MCHC	28.2%
MCV	78 femtoliter (fL)
Hgb	11.1 g/dL
Hct	30.4%
Fe (total)	7 µmol/L
TIBC	85 µmol/L
PLT	182,000/µL

1. Megaloblastic anemia
2. Thalassemia minor
3. Folate anemia
4. Iron-deficiency anemia

ANSWER: 4

Iron-deficiency anemia is marked by decreased hemoglobin and hematocrit levels. In iron-deficiency anemia, the mean corpuscular volume (MCV), or average red blood cell size, is typically less than 80 fL, the mean corpuscular hemoglobin concentration (MCHC, or hemoglobin concentration per red blood cell), is less than 30%, the serum iron is decreased, and the total iron-binding capacity (TIBC) is increased. Normal values are MCV 82–88 fL, MCHC 32%–36%, serum Fe 9–26 µmol/L, and TIBC 45–73 µmol/L. Megaloblastic anemia is a vitamin B_{12} deficiency. Persons with thalassemia minor have a defective production of hemoglobin and (at most) mild anemia with slight lowering of the hemoglobin level. This can very closely resemble mild iron-deficiency anemia, except the person will have a normal serum iron level. Folate-deficiency anemia is a decrease in red blood cells (RBCs) caused by folate deficiency. Normal RBCs for adult females is 4.2 to 5.0 million, with normal values being slightly lower in pregnancy.

► ***Test-taking Tip:*** *Consider normal levels for pregnant women and then consider what the abnormal values indicate.*

Content Area: Childbearing Families; *Category of Health:* Intrapartal Management; *Integrated Processes:* Nursing Process Assessment; *Client Need:* Physiological Integrity/Reduction of Risk Potential/Laboratory Values; *Cognitive Level:* Analysis

Reference: Gabbe, S., Niebyl, J., & Simpson, J. (2007). *Obstetrics: Normal and Problem Pregnancies* (5th ed., p. 1053). Philadelphia: Churchill Livingstone.

333. A 39-year-old client presents in active labor. The client is breathing rapidly and having difficulty coping with the contractions. Based on this assessment, what would a nurse predict should occur if interventions are not initiated immediately?

1. Respiratory acidosis
2. Respiratory alkalosis
3. Metabolic acidosis
4. Metabolic alkalosis

ANSWER: 2

Women who are hyperventilating have a decrease in the $PaCO_2$ levels, which leads to respiratory alkalosis. Respiratory acidosis occurs because of hypoventilation, which does not routinely occur in labor. Metabolic acidosis occurs when there is an excessive acidity in the blood and most commonly occurs in kidney failure, diabetic ketoacidosis, and cases of shock. Although it could occur in women with severe diabetes or in a client who has had a considerable obstetric hemorrhage and is in shock, it is not a normal occurrence in pregnancy or labor. Metabolic alkalosis is primarily related to kidney and gastrointestinal disorders and is not a normal physiological process that occurs in labor.

► ***Test-taking Tip:*** *Determine the physiological processes of each of the options to determine the best choice.*

Content Area: Childbearing Families; *Category of Health Alteration:* Intrapartal Management; *Integrated Processes:* Nursing Process Analysis; *Client Need:* Physiological Integrity/Physiological Adaptation/Pathophysiology; *Cognitive Level:* Analysis

Reference: Davidson, M., London, M., & Ladewig, P. (2008). *Olds' Maternal-Newborn Nursing & Women's Health Across the Lifespan* (8th ed., p. 595). Upper Saddle River, NJ: Prentice Hall Health.

334. A nurse's client, who is in labor, is waiting for laboratory results to come back so epidural anesthesia can be administered. Which result is abnormal and should be reported to a physician?

1. White blood cells (WBCs): 24,000/mm^3
2. Glucose: 78 gm/dL
3. Hemoglobin: 13.2 g/dL
4. Platelets: 112,000/mm^3

ANSWER: 4

The normal platelet count is 150,000 to 450,000/mm^3. Counts less than 150,000 should be evaluated because they can contribute to bleeding. Counts less than 100,000 may interfere with the woman's choice to receive epidural anesthesia. The normal WBC count in labor is increased and can be as high as 25,000/mm^3 to 30,000/mm^3. The normal glucose level falls during labor because of an expenditure in labor. Anemia or a reduction in the hemoglobin and hematocrit are common in pregnancy. Hemoglobin levels less than 10 g/dL are considered abnormal in pregnancy.

► ***Test-taking Tip:*** *Focus on the situation. Determine which laboratory value will affect the use of epidural anesthesia and then use the process of elimination to eliminate options 1 and 2. Then between options 3 and 4, determine which is abnormal. Review your knowledge of laboratory data to determine which laboratory value is outside of the normal range for a pregnant woman. The NCLEX-RN® will include critical laboratory values.*

Content Area: Childbearing Families; *Category of Health Alteration:* Intrapartal Management; *Integrated Processes:* Nursing Process Analysis; *Client Need:* Physiological Integrity/Reduction of Risk Potential/Laboratory Values; *Cognitive Level:* Analysis

Reference: Davidson, M., London, M., & Ladewig, P. (2008). *Olds' Maternal-Newborn Nursing & Women's Health Across the Lifespan* (8th ed., pp. 594–595). Upper Saddle River, NJ: Prentice Hall Health.

335. A nurse's laboring client presents with ruptured membranes, frequent contractions, and bloody show. She reports a greenish discharge for 2 days. Which actions should be taken by the nurse when caring for this client? Prioritize the nurse's actions by placing each step in the correct order.

_____ Perform a sterile vaginal exam
_____ Assess the woman thoroughly
_____ Obtain fetal heart tones
_____ Notify the health-care provider (HCP)

ANSWER: 2, 3, 1, 4

The nurse should first obtain the heart tones to determine the status of the fetus. Because the woman has ruptured membranes with greenish fluid, the fetus could be experiencing nonreassuring fetal status. Once the heart tones have been obtained, a vaginal examination should be performed. The woman should be fully assessed before notifying the HCP. The woman should then be moved into an inpatient room.

Test-taking Tip: *Focus on the issue: the significance of the greenish discharge and the viability of the fetus.*

Content Area: Childbearing Families; *Category of Health Alteration:* Intrapartal Management; *Integrated Processes:* Nursing Process Planning; *Client Need:* Safe and Effective Care Environment/ Management of Care/Establishing Priorities; *Cognitive Level:* Analysis

Reference: Davidson, M., London, M., & Ladewig, P. (2008). *Olds' Maternal-Newborn Nursing & Women's Health Across the Lifespan* (8th ed., p. 653). Upper Saddle River, NJ: Prentice Hall Health.

336. A nurse is about to obtain a fetal heart rate (FHR) on a client in triage for evaluation of possible labor. When preparing to auscultate the FHR, what information is needed to determine where to find the correct placement?

1. Fetal position
2. Position of the placenta
3. Presence of contractions
4. Whether ultrasonic gel should be used

ANSWER: 1

The nurse should first perform Leopold's maneuvers to determine the fetal position, which will enable proper placement of the Doppler device over the location of the FHR. The position of the placenta can provide important information. However, if the Doppler device is placed over the placenta, the nurse will hear a swishing sound and not the FHR. The FHR is still assessed regardless of the presence of contractions. The nurse who has difficulty obtaining a FHR because of a contraction can listen again once the contraction has concluded. Ultrasonic gel is used with any ultrasound device and allows for the conduction of sound and continuous contact of the device with the maternal abdomen.

Test-taking Tip: *The key word in both the stem and options is "fetal." Carefully read the question to determine what is being asked.*

Content Area: Childbearing Families; *Category of Health Alteration:* Intrapartal Management; *Integrated Processes:* Nursing Process Planning; *Client Need:* Health Promotion and Maintenance/Techniques of Physical Assessment; *Cognitive Level:* Analysis

Reference: Davidson, M., London, M., & Ladewig, P. (2008). *Olds' Maternal-Newborn Nursing & Women's Health Across the Lifespan* (8th ed., p. 650). Upper Saddle River, NJ: Prentice Hall Health.

337. EBP A nurse is monitoring a laboring client, who has ruptured membranes and is 4 cm dilated. The client has been having intermittent decelerations for the last hour. There is a decrease in variability, although the fetal heart rate (FHR) remains in the 140s. The decelerations are now becoming more regular. What is the most accurate means to monitor the FHR in this client?

1. Fetal electrocardiography
2. Continuous external fetal monitoring
3. Cardiotocography
4. Fetal electrocardiography and cardiotocography

ANSWER: 4

Evidenced-based research indicates that the combination of fetal electrocardiography and cardiotocography provides the most accurate assessment, results in less surgical intervention, and ensures better oxygen levels. Although all of these methods can provide a means of assessing the FHR, options 1, 2, and 3 are not the most accurate of the options.

Test-taking Tip: *Select the most inclusive option. Only option 4 provides two means of monitoring and is different from the other options. An option that is different is likely the answer.*

Content Area: Childbearing Families; *Category of Health Alteration:* Intrapartal Management; *Integrated Processes:* Nursing Process Planning; *Client Need:* Physiological Integrity/Reduction of Risk Potential/Diagnostic Tests; *Cognitive Level:* Analysis

Reference: Davidson, M., London, M., & Ladewig, P. (2008). *Olds' Maternal-Newborn Nursing & Women's Health Across the Lifespan* (8th ed., p. 630). Upper Saddle River, NJ: Prentice Hall Health.

EBP Reference: Neilson, J. (2006). Fetal electrocardiogram (ECG) for fetal monitoring during labour. *Cochrane Database of Systematic Reviews,* Issue 2, Art. No. CD000116. DOI: 10.1002/14651858.CD000116.pub2. Available at: www.cochrane.org/reviews/en/ab000116.html

338. A nurse is caring for a Hispanic woman who is in the active stage of labor. What is the most crucial assessment parameter that should be assessed related to the client's ethnicity and stage of labor?

1. Choice of pain-control measures
2. Desire for hot or cold fluids
3. Selection of support persons in the room during the labor and birth
4. Desire for circumcision if a male infant is born

ANSWER: 1

Because cultural variations exist in pain-control measures used and pain tolerance, the most crucial assessment in the active stage of labor is the client's choice of pain-control measures. A desire for hot or cold fluids and selection of support persons are both important aspects that should be determined during the early stage of labor. The desire for circumcision is also an important consideration; however, it is not the primary need during the active stage of labor. All of the factors have cultural implications that require the nurse to have an understanding of cultural diversity and needs.

Test-taking Tip: *The key phrase is "active stage of labor." Use the process of elimination to eliminate options that would be inappropriate during this stage such as options 2, 3, and 4.*

Content Area: Childbearing Families; *Category of Health Alteration:* Intrapartal Management; *Integrated Processes:* Nursing Process Assessment; *Client Need:* Physiological Integrity/Pharmacological and Parenteral Therapies/Pharmacological Pain Management; *Cognitive Level:* Analysis

Reference: Darby, S. (2007). Pre- and perinatal care of Hispanic families: Implications for nurses. *Nursing for Women's Health, 11,* 160–169.

339. EBP A nurse's client has requested an epidural for pain management during delivery. Which factor is associated with epidural anesthesia?

1. Need for medications to stimulate contractions
2. Decrease in incidence of vaginal operative deliveries
3. Decrease in second stage of labor
4. Increase in cesarean births

ANSWER: 1

Epidural anesthesia is associated with less pain during the intrapartum period. Women who receive epidural anesthesia are more likely to require stimulation of uterine contractions. There is an increase, not decrease, in incidence of a vaginal operative delivery, such as forceps or vacuum extraction. There is no association between cesarean births and epidural anesthesia.

Test-taking Tip: *Focus on the issue: risk associated with epidural anesthesia. Note that three options are similar (decrease and increase). Select the option that is different.*

Content Area: Childbearing Families; *Category of Health Alteration:* Intrapartal Management; *Integrated Processes:* Nursing Process Planning; *Client Need:* Safe and Effective Care Environment/ Management of Care/Intra/Ante/Postpartum and Newborn Care; *Cognitive Level:* Analysis

Reference: Davidson, M., London, M., & Ladewig, P. (2008). *Olds' Maternal-Newborn Nursing & Women's Health Across the Lifespan* (8th ed., p. 706). Upper Saddle River, NJ: Prentice Hall Health.

EBP Reference: Anim-Somuah, M., Smyth, R., & Howell, C. (2005). Epidural versus non-epidural or no analgesia in labour. *Cochrane Database of Systematic Reviews, 2005,* Issue 4 Art. No. CD000331. DOI: 10.1002/14651858.CD000331.pub2. Available at: www.cochrane.org/reviews/en/ab000331.html

340. EBP A laboring client is experiencing problems, and a nurse is concerned about possible side effects from the epidural anesthetic just administered. Which problems should the nurse attribute to the epidural anesthetic? SELECT ALL THAT APPLY.

1. Uncontrolled pain
2. Postpartum hemorrhage
3. Period of inability to move lower extremities
4. Inability to urinate
5. Maternal fever

ANSWER: 1, 3, 4, 5

Epidural anesthesia is associated with less pain during the intrapartum period. Women who receive epidural anesthesia are more likely to experience an inability to move the lower extremities, inability to urinate, and maternal fever. Postpartum hemorrhage is not associated with epidural anesthesia.

➧ ***Test-taking Tip:*** *Focus on the issue: side effects of epidural anesthesia. Select the option that is not a side effect.*

Content Area: Childbearing Families; *Category of Health Alteration:* Intrapartal Management; *Integrated Processes:* Nursing Process Analysis; *Client Need:* Safe and Effective Care Environment/ Management of Care/Intra/Ante/Postpartum and Newborn Care; *Cognitive Level:* Analysis

Reference: Davidson, M., London, M., & Ladewig, P. (2008). *Olds' Maternal-Newborn Nursing & Women's Health Across the Lifespan* (8th ed., p. 706). Upper Saddle River, NJ: Prentice Hall Health.

EBP Reference: Anim-Somuah, M., Smyth, R., & Howell, C. (2005). Epidural versus non-epidural or no analgesia in labour. *Cochrane Database of Systematic Reviews, 2005,* Issue 4, Art. No. CD000331. DOI: 10.1002/14651858.CD000331.pub2. Available at: www.cochrane.org/reviews/en/ab000331.html

341. EBP A nurse's laboring client is becoming increasingly uncomfortable during labor and requests to labor in a tub of water. Which factors are true regarding laboring in the water? SELECT ALL THAT APPLY.

1. Clients who labor in a tub of water perceive less pain than women who do not use water therapy in early labor.
2. Women who labor in a tub have a prolonged first stage of labor because of uterine relaxation.
3. Women who labor in water report greater satisfaction during the second stage of labor.
4. Neonates who deliver after being submerged in water show no differences in adverse outcomes when compared to neonates whose mothers have not labored in water.
5. Clients who labor in water have a reduced incidence of feces being expelled while pushing during the second stage of labor.

ANSWER: 1, 3, 4

Women who labor in water perceive less pain and report greater satisfaction with the pushing stage of labor. Neonates born to mothers who have labored or given birth in a tub bath do not show differences in adverse outcomes. Differences in the length of labor have not been reported in women who use hydrotherapy in labor. Laboring in water has no effect on whether feces are expelled with pushing during the second stage of labor. A concern with laboring in water is that the water can become contaminated with feces expelled with pushing during the second stage of labor, thus increasing the mother's risk of uterine infection and the fetus's risk of aspiration pneumonia.

➧ ***Test-taking Tip:*** *Look for positive key phases in each option: "less pain," "greater satisfaction," and "no differences."*

Content Area: Childbearing Families; *Category of Health Alteration:* Intrapartal Management; *Integrated Processes:* Nursing Process Evaluation; *Client Need:* Safe and Effective Care Environment/ Management of Care/Intra/Ante/Postpartum and Newborn Care; *Cognitive Level:* Analysis

Reference: Pillitteri, A. (2007). *Maternal & Child Health Nursing: Care of the Childbearing & Childrearing Family* (5th ed., pp. 341–342). Philadelphia: Lippincott Williams & Wilkins.

EBP Reference: Thoeni, A., Zech, N., Moroder, L., & Ploner, F. (2005). Review of 1600 water births. Does water birth increase the risk of neonatal infection? *Journal of Maternal-Fetal & Neonatal Medicine, 17*(5), 357–361.

342. A nurse is admitting a client who has been in labor for 32 hours at home. Which factor is associated with delayed admission to a labor and delivery unit?

1. A reduction in use of pain medications
2. A sense of loss of control
3. Higher rates of maternal infection
4. Higher rates of unplanned out-of-hospital births

ANSWER: 1

Delayed admission to labor and delivery units have been associated with less use of pain medication. A greater sense of control (rather than loss of control) and shorter overall hospital stays are also associated with delayed admission. There is no increase in out-of-hospital births or maternal and neonatal complications.

➧ ***Test-taking Tip:*** *Review your experiences with women who are admitted in very early labor and later labor to determine which characteristics are common in those groups. Read each option carefully, noting that option 1 is different from the other options. When an option is different it is usually the answer.*

Content Area: Childbearing Families; *Category of Health Alteration:* Intrapartal Management; *Integrated Processes:* Nursing Process Evaluation; *Client Need:* Safe and Effective Care Environment/ Management of Care/Intra/Ante/Postpartum and Newborn Care; *Cognitive Level:* Analysis

Reference: Pillitteri, A. (2007). *Maternal & Child Health Nursing: Care of the Childbearing & Childrearing Family* (5th ed., pp. 341–342). Philadelphia: Lippincott Williams & Wilkins.

343. A nurse practitioner informs a new nurse that a client in the last delivery room is having a prolonged deceleration on the monitor. The new nurse interprets this to mean that there is a fetal heart rate (FHR) decrease of:

1. 30 beats per minute (bpm) below baseline for greater than 30 seconds.
2. 15 bpm or more below baseline that occurs for at least 2 minutes but not more than 5 minutes.
3. 15 bpm or more below baseline that occurs for at least 2 minutes but not more than 10 minutes.
4. 15 bpm or more below baseline that occurs for 10 minutes and then resolves spontaneously or with interventions.

ANSWER: 3

A prolonged deceleration occurs when the FHR decreases 15 bpm or more below baseline for at least 2 minutes but not more than 10 minutes. The prolonged deceleration may resolve spontaneously or with the aid of interventions.

➧ ***Test-taking Tip:*** *Focus on the bpm and length of time of FHR reduction with prolonged deceleration.*

Content Area: Childbearing Families; *Category of Health Alteration:* Intrapartal Management; *Integrated Processes:* Nursing Process Analysis; *Client Need:* Safe and Effective Care Environment/ Management of Care/Collaboration with Interdisciplinary Team; *Cognitive Level:* Application

Reference: Davidson, M., London, M., & Ladewig, P. (2008). *Olds' Maternal-Newborn Nursing & Women's Health Across the Lifespan* (8th ed., p. 634). Upper Saddle River, NJ: Prentice Hall Health.

344. EBP A nurse's laboring client is being monitored electronically during her labor. The baseline fetal heart rate (FHR) throughout the labor has been in the 130s. In the last 2 hours, the baseline has decreased to the 100s. How should the nurse document this heart rate pattern?

1. Tachycardia
2. Bradycardia
3. Prolonged deceleration
4. Acceleration

ANSWER: 2

An FHR baseline less than 110 is classified as bradycardia. Tachycardia occurs when the baseline is greater than 160 beats per minute. A prolonged deceleration is defined as a change from the baseline FHR that occurs for 2 to 10 minutes before returning to baseline. An "acceleration" is an increase in the FHR.

➧ ***Test-taking Tip:*** *Recall that the normal FHR is 120 to 160 bpm.*

Content Area: Childbearing Families; *Category of Health Alteration:* Intrapartal Management; *Integrated Processes:* Communication and Documentation; *Client Need:* Health Promotion and Maintenance/ Ante/Intra/Postpartum and Newborn Care; *Cognitive Level:* Application

Reference: Pillitteri, A. (2007). *Maternal & Child Health Nursing: Care of the Childbearing & Childrearing Family* (5th ed., p. 524). Philadelphia: Lippincott Williams & Wilkins.

EBP Reference: American College of Obstetricians and Gynecologists (ACOG). (2005). Intrapartum fetal heart rate monitoring. *ACOG Practice Bulletin,* No. 70.

345. A nurse's client has had recurrent variable decelerations for the last 2 hours. For which intervention should the nurse plan?

1. Continuous electronic fetal monitoring
2. Maternal position changes
3. Amnioinfusion
4. Cesarean delivery

ANSWER: 3

Amnioinfusion is sterile fluid instillation into the amniotic cavity through a catheter to supplement the amniotic fluid and prevent further cord compression. It is usually performed transcervically during the intrapartum period. Amnioinfusion has been found to be effective in the treatment of severe variable decelerations and decreases the need for cesarean births. Continuous electronic fetal monitoring is not a treatment for variable decelerations. Position changes may be effective, although the evidence supports the use of amnioinfusion as an intervention that decreases the need for cesarean section birth.

➧ ***Test-taking Tip:*** *Focus on the key words "intervention" and "treatment." Use the nursing process and eliminate option 1 because it is not an intervention and eliminate option 2 because it is not a treatment. Of the other two options, think about an intervention that is supported by research.*

Content Area: Childbearing Families; *Category of Health Alteration:* Intrapartal Management; *Integrated Processes:* Nursing Process Planning; *Client Need:* Physiological Integrity/Physiological Adaptation/ Alterations in Body Systems; *Cognitive Level:* Analysis

Reference: Pillitteri, A. (2007). *Maternal & Child Health Nursing: Care of the Childbearing & Childrearing Family* (5th ed., p. 524). Philadelphia: Lippincott Williams & Wilkins.

346. A nurse is caring for a pregnant client whose fetal heart rate tracing reveals a reduction in variability over the last 40 minutes. The client has been having occasional decelerations that are now appearing to occur after the onset of the contraction and not resolve until after the contraction is over. Suddenly, the client has a prolonged deceleration that does not resolve. Which steps should the nurse take to provide immediate care to this client? Prioritize the nurse's actions by placing each step in the correct order.

______ Administer oxygen via facemask.
______ Call for assistance and page the health-care provider.
______ Place an indwelling Foley catheter in anticipation for emergency cesarean birth.
______ Increase intravenous fluids.
______ Assist the woman into a different position.
______ Prepare for a vaginal exam and scalp stimulation.

ANSWER: 2, 4, 6, 3, 1, 5

The first step is to assist in changing the maternal position in an attempt to increase the fetal heart rate in case of cord obstruction. Next, the nurse should apply oxygen by facemask to increase oxygenation to the fetus. IV fluids should be increased to treat possible hypotension, the most common cause of fetal bradycardia. The health-care provider should be paged, and additional nursing personnel should be called for assistance. A vaginal exam should be performed to rule out a cord prolapse and to provide stimulation to the fetal head. If the heart rate remains low, an indwelling Foley should be placed in anticipation of a possible cesarean birth.

➧ ***Test-taking Tip:*** *Prioritize which steps should be done initially and which steps are dependent on previous steps to properly order your answer. Use the ABCs (airway, breathing, circulation) to establish that promoting oxygenation is the initial action.*

Content Area: Childbearing Families; *Category of Health Alteration:* Intrapartum Management; *Integrated Processes:* Nursing Process Planning; *Client Need:* Safe and Effective Care Environment/ Management of Care/Establishing Priorities; *Cognitive Level:* Synthesis

Reference: Davidson, M., London, M., & Ladewig, P. (2008). *Olds' Maternal Newborn Nursing & Women's Health Across the Lifespan* (8th ed., p. 1233). Upper Saddle River, NJ: Prentice Hall Health.

347. A nurse has been advised by a laboring client that she wants to avoid an episiotomy if possible. The nurse's response should be based on which recommendation related to an episiotomy?

1. Restricted use of episiotomy is preferred.
2. Routine use of episiotomy reduces prolonged pushing and perineal trauma.
3. Routine episiotomy can prevent pelvic floor damage.
4. Episiotomies should not be performed in modern clinical practice.

ANSWER: 1

The restricted use of episiotomies should guide modern clinical practice, although they may be used in some circumstances. Routine use of episiotomy to decrease the incidence of perineal trauma or prolonged pushing has been determined to increase perineal trauma and healing time. Routine episiotomy is not associated with a decrease in pelvic floor damage and may increase the severity of the trauma. Episiotomies are sometimes indicated in cases of nonreassuring fetal status or in dystocias to facilitate the delivery process.

➧ ***Test-taking Tip:*** *Note the similarities between options 1 and 4, and 2 and 3. Think about each option. Eliminate option 4 because "not" is absolute; eliminate options 2 and 3 because these both address routine use.*

Content Area: Childbearing Families; *Category of Health Alteration:* Intrapartal Management; *Integrated Processes:* Nursing Process Analysis; *Client Need:* Safe and Effective Care Environment/ Management of Care/Intra/Ante/Postpartum and Newborn Care; *Cognitive Level:* Application

Reference: Davidson, M., London, M., & Ladewig, P. (2008). *Olds' Maternal-Newborn Nursing & Women's Health Across the Lifespan* (8th ed., pp. 774–775). Upper Saddle River, NJ: Prentice Hall Health.

348. A nurse is performing a vaginal exam on a client who is being evaluated in triage for possible labor. The client's contractions are every 3 to 4 minutes, 60 to 70 seconds in duration, and moderate by palpation. Her cervical exam in the office is illustration 1. Her current exam is illustration 2. What conclusions should the nurse draw from illustration 2?

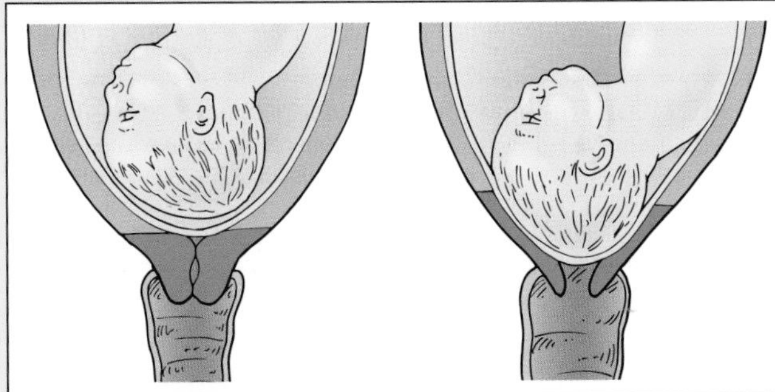

1. The woman is not dilated or effaced.
2. The woman is completely dilated but not effaced.
3. The woman has minimal dilatation but is completely effaced.
4. The woman is completely effaced but not dilated.

ANSWER: 3

Effacement refers to a thinning of the cervix, whereas dilatation refers to the opening of the cervix. In illustration 1, the woman is not effaced or dilated. In illustration 2, she is completely effaced and has some dilatation.

➧ ***Test-taking Tip:*** *Review the definitions of effacement and dilatation and compare them to the illustrations.*

Content Area: Childbearing Families; *Category of Health Alteration:* Intrapartal Management; *Integrated Processes:* Nursing Process Assessment; *Client Need:* Physiological Integrity/Physiological Adaptation/Pathophysiology; *Cognitive Level:* Analysis

Reference: Gabbe, S., Niebyl, J., & Simpson, J. (2007). *Obstetrics: Normal and Problem Pregnancies* (5th ed., p. 220). Philadelphia: Churchill Livingstone.

349. A nurse's laboring client has decided to try to get through labor without an epidural. The client is requesting intravenous pain medication instead. The nurse determines that which factor would contraindicate the administration of nalbuphine hydrochloride (Nubain®)?

1. Transition stage of labor
2. Fetal heart rate (FHR) of 110 beats per minute
3. Presence of variability
4. Presence of variable decelerations

ANSWER: 1

Systemic medications should not be administered when advanced dilation is present because they can lead to respiratory depression if administered too close to the time of delivery. A FHR of 110 beats per minute with variability is reassuring. If mild variable decelerations are present but the FHR pattern remains reassuring, Nubain® can still be administered.

➧ ***Test-taking Tip:*** *Eliminate the correct options first to determine which option represents a contraindication to Nubain® administration.*

Content Area: Childbearing Families; *Category of Health Alteration:* Intrapartal Management; *Integrated Processes:* Nursing Process Analysis; *Client Need:* Physiological Integrity/Pharmacological and Parenteral Therapies/Pharmacological Pain Management; *Cognitive Level:* Analysis

Reference: Davidson, M., London, M., & Ladewig, P. (2008). *Olds' Maternal-Newborn Nursing & Women's Health Across the Lifespan* (8th ed., p. 686). Upper Saddle River, NJ: Prentice Hall Health.

350. A nurse's client has been experiencing frequent, painful contractions for the last 6 hours. The contractions are of poor quality, and there has been no cervical change. Which nursing interventions should be initiated? SELECT ALL THAT APPLY.

1. Maintain bedrest
2. Administer a sedative
3. Administer pain medications
4. Prepare for amniotomy
5. Prepare for cesarean delivery
6. Administer oxytocin (Pitocin®)

ANSWER: 1, 2, 3, 6

This woman is experiencing a hypertonic labor pattern in which her contractions are frequent and painful but no cervical change has occurred. This woman should be encouraged to rest often with the aid of a sedative. Pain medication can also be administered to help the woman relax and cope more effectively. If the hypertonic labor pattern continues, augmentation, with either amniotomy or oxytocin infusion, should be initiated. A cesarean birth is not a treatment for a hypertonic labor pattern unless a nonreassuring fetal heart rate pattern is present.

➧ ***Test-taking Tip:*** *Consider the options for the management of this type of labor pattern.*

Content Area: Childbearing Families; *Category of Health Alteration:* Intrapartal Management; *Integrated Processes:* Nursing Process Implementation; *Client Need:* Physiological Integrity/Reduction of Risk Potential/Therapeutic Procedures; *Cognitive Level:* Analysis

Reference: Davidson, M., London, M., & Ladewig, P. (2008). *Olds' Maternal-Newborn Nursing & Women's Health Across the Lifespan* (8th ed., p. 719). Upper Saddle River, NJ: Prentice Hall Health.

351. A nurse enters a room to perform an assessment of a laboring client before stimulating labor because of a hypertonic labor pattern. Which findings would be contraindications to stimulating labor in the woman and should be reported to the health-care provider? SELECT ALL THAT APPLY.

1. Cephalopelvic disproportion (CPD)
2. Fetal malposition
3. Lack of cervical change
4. Nonreassuring FHR pattern
5. Previous classical incision
6. Presence of an undocumented previous uterine scar

ANSWER: 1, 2, 4, 5, 6

CPD, fetal malposition, and nonreassuring FHR pattern are all contraindications for stimulation of labor. Women with a previous classical incision or an undocumented uterine scar should not be stimulated because both factors are contraindications for a vaginal birth and warrant an immediate repeat cesarean birth. Lack of cervical change is an indication to initiate stimulation of labor.

➧ ***Test-taking Tip:*** *Focus on the issue of "contraindications to stimulating labor in a woman with a hypertonic labor pattern." Eliminate situations in which it is acceptable to stimulate labor.*

Content Area: Childbearing Families; *Category of Health Alteration:* Intrapartal Management; *Integrated Processes:* Nursing Process Analysis; *Client Need:* Physiological Integrity/Physiological Adaptation/Alterations in Body Systems; *Cognitive Level:* Application

Reference: Davidson, M., London, M., & Ladewig, P. (2008). *Olds' Maternal-Newborn Nursing & Women's Health Across the Lifespan* (8th ed., p. 719). Upper Saddle River, NJ: Prentice Hall Health.

352. A nurse is caring for a client who has been in labor for 21 hours. The client has made little progress and is now dilated 5 cm. There has been no fetal descent since her induction was started 16 hours ago. The woman has been diagnosed with cephalopelvic disproportion (CPD). For which mode of delivery should the nurse plan?

1. Vaginal delivery
2. Forceps-assisted delivery
3. Vacuum-assisted delivery
4. Cesarean section delivery

ANSWER: 4

A fetus, diagnosed with CPD, is unable to be delivered vaginally and requires a cesarean section birth. A vaginal, forceps, and vacuum delivery are all contraindicated once a diagnosis of CPD has been given.

➧ ***Test-taking Tip:*** *Consider the definition of CPD and the safety of the fetus and mother when selecting an option.*

Content Area: Childbearing Families; *Category of Health Alteration:* Intrapartal Management; *Integrated Processes:* Nursing Process Planning; *Client Need:* Physiological Integrity/Physiological Adaptation/Alterations in Body Systems; *Cognitive Level:* Application

Reference: Davidson, M., London, M., & Ladewig, P. (2008). *Olds' Maternal-Newborn Nursing & Women's Health Across the Lifespan* (8th ed., p. 753). Upper Saddle River, NJ: Prentice Hall Health.

353. A primigravida client is being induced for a post-term pregnancy. A nurse closely monitors the client knowing which facts about post-term pregnancy? SELECT ALL THAT APPLY.

1. It increases the need for a vacuum or forceps birth.
2. It increases the risk of perineal trauma.
3. It increases the risk of hemorrhage.
4. It prolongs labor.
5. It is associated with a precipitous labor and birth.
6. It increases the risk of lung immaturity in the fetus.

ANSWER: 1, 2, 3

Post-term pregnancies are commonly associated with large for gestational age fetuses. This presents multiple maternal risks, including use of vacuum or forceps, perineal trauma, and hemorrhage. Prolonged labor or precipitous labor and birth are not commonly associated with post-term pregnancies. Fetuses that are preterm are at risk for immature lung capabilities.

➧ ***Test-taking Tip:*** *Consider the impact of a post-term pregnancy in terms of risk factors and adverse consequences for the mother.*

Content Area: Childbearing Families; *Category of Health Alteration:* Intrapartal Management; *Integrated Processes:* Nursing Process Implementation; *Client Need:* Physiological Integrity/Reduction of Risk Potential/Potential for Complications from Surgical Procedures and Health Alterations; *Cognitive Level:* Application

Reference: Davidson, M., London, M., & Ladewig, P. (2008). *Olds' Maternal-Newborn Nursing & Women's Health Across the Lifespan* (8th ed., p. 723). Upper Saddle River, NJ: Prentice Hall Health.

354. A laboring client just had a convulsion after being given regional anesthesia. Which interventions should a nurse initiate? SELECT ALL THAT APPLY.

1. Establish an airway.
2. Position the client on her side.
3. Provide 100% oxygen.
4. Administer diazepam (Valium®).
5. Page the anesthesiologist stat.
6. Initiate cardiopulmonary resuscitation (CPR) immediately.

ANSWER: 1, 3, 4, 5

The woman experiencing a convulsion related to anesthesia should first have an airway established and receive 100% oxygen. Small doses of diazepam or thiopental can be administered to stop the convulsions. The anesthesiologist should be stat paged to provide assistance. The woman's head should be turned to the side if vomiting occurs, but the woman typically remains in a left lateral tilt position so an airway can be maintained. CPR should only be initiated if respiratory or cardiac arrest is present.

➧ ***Test-taking Tip:*** *Use the ABCs (airway, breathing, circulation) to establish the most important physical aspects that should be maintained for this client. Consider how each of the options can affect the woman's physiological status and choose those as your correct options.*

Content Area: Childbearing Families; *Category of Health Alteration:* Intrapartal Management; *Integrated Processes:* Nursing Process Implementation; *Client Need:* Physiological Integrity/Physiological Adaptation/Medical Emergencies; *Cognitive Level:* Application

Reference: Davidson, M., London, M., & Ladewig, P. (2008). *Olds' Maternal-Newborn Nursing & Women's Health Across the Lifespan* (8th ed., p. 707). Upper Saddle River, NJ: Prentice Hall Health.

355. A pregnant client has been pushing for 2.5 hours and a large fetus is suspected. After some difficulty, the fetal head emerges. The physician attempts to deliver the shoulders without success. Which actions should be taken by a nurse for a client who is experiencing shoulder dystocia? Prioritize the nurse's actions by placing each step in the correct order.

______ Apply suprapubic pressure per direction of physician.
______ Place the woman in exaggerated lithotomy position.
______ Catheterize the woman's bladder to make more room.
______ Call for the neonatal resuscitation team to be present.
______ Prepare for an emergency cesarean birth.

ANSWER: 3, 2, 4, 1, 5

When a problem is anticipated, the neonatal team should be immediately notified. The woman should be placed in exaggerated lithotomy position so the McRobert's maneuver can be performed (flexing her thighs sharply on her abdomen may widen the pelvic outlet and let the anterior shoulder be delivered). The nurse should apply suprapubic pressure in an effort to dislodge the shoulder from under the pubic bone. If that is unsuccessful, the bladder should be emptied to make more room for the fetal head. If all efforts for a vaginal birth fail, the woman should be prepared for an emergency cesarean section.

➧ ***Test-taking Tip:*** *Identify the most crucial steps in order of importance. Recall that calling for help should be priority if this is provided as an option.*

Content Area: Childbearing Families; *Category of Health Alteration:* Intrapartal Management; *Integrated Processes:* Nursing Process Implementation; *Client Need:* Safe and Effective Care Environment/Management of Care/Establishing Priorities; *Cognitive Level:* Synthesis

References: Pillitteri, A. (2007). *Maternal & Child Health Nursing: Care of the Childbearing & Childrearing Family* (5th ed., p. 606). Philadelphia: Lippincott Williams & Wilkins; Varney, H., Kriebs, J., & Gegor, C. (2004). *Varney's Midwifery* (4th ed., p. 489). Boston: Jones & Bartlett.

356. A nurse's laboring client is experiencing decelerations that occur after the onset of the contraction and do not end until after the contraction is completed. The variability is minimal. Which interventions should the nurse initiate? SELECT ALL THAT APPLY.

1. Reposition the woman.
2. Provide oxygen via facemask.
3. Discontinue oxytocin (Pitocin®).
4. Reassess in 30 minutes.
5. Increase oxytocin.
6. Increase intravenous fluids.

ANSWER: 1, 2, 3, 6

The nurse should reposition the woman, provide oxygen, and discontinue oxytocin in order to decrease the contraction frequency. The woman should be given a bolus of fluid in case the decelerations are related to maternal hypotension. This fetus is experiencing nonreassuring fetal status. The oxytocin should not be increased because this can lead to further nonreassuring fetal status.

➧ ***Test-taking Tip:*** *Focus on the issue: late decelerations that require immediate intervention. Note that options 3 and 5 are opposites, so one or both of these must be wrong.*

Content Area: Childbearing Families; *Category of Health Alteration:* Intrapartal Management; *Integrated Processes:* Nursing Process Implementation; *Client Need:* Physiological Integrity/Reduction of Risk Potential/Potential for Complications from Surgical Procedures and Health Alterations; *Cognitive Level:* Analysis

Reference: Davidson, M., London, M., & Ladewig, P. (2008). *Olds' Maternal-Newborn Nursing & Women's Health Across the Lifespan* (8th ed., p. 632). Upper Saddle River, NJ: Prentice Hall Health.

357. A client (G9P7) presents to a labor and delivery unit and her labor is progressing quickly. Which intervention is most important when caring for a woman experiencing a precipitous delivery?

1. Supporting the infant during the birth
2. Preventing the perineum from tearing
3. Promoting delivery of an intact placenta
4. Cutting the umbilical cord

ANSWER: 1

The most important intervention is preventing injury to the infant during the delivery. Other aspects of care include preventing the perineum from trauma and cutting the umbilical cord. The placenta can be left in place until the physician or nurse midwife arrives.

➧ ***Test-taking Tip:*** *Consider which factor is the most important aspect of the delivery and which has the most potential for harm to the mother and baby.*

Content Area: Childbearing Families; *Category of Health Alteration:* Intrapartal Management; *Integrated Processes:* Nursing Process Implementation; *Client Need:* Safe and Effective Care Environment/ Safety and Infection Control/Injury Prevention; *Cognitive Level:* Analysis

Reference: Davidson, M., London, M., & Ladewig, P. (2008). *Olds' Maternal-Newborn Nursing & Women's Health Across the Lifespan* (8th ed., p. 722). Upper Saddle River, NJ: Prentice Hall Health.

358. A nurse is admitting a full-term pregnant client presenting with bright red, vaginal bleeding and intense abdominal pain. Her blood pressure on admission is 150/96 mm Hg and her pulse is 109 beats per minute. Which problem should the nurse suspect that the client is likely experiencing?

1. Placenta previa
2. Placenta abruption
3. Bloody show
4. Succenturiate placenta

ANSWER: 2

Placenta abruption occurs when the placenta separates from the uterine wall before the birth of the fetus. It is commonly associated with preeclampsia. Placenta previa is marked by painless vaginal bleeding. Bloody show is a normal physiological sign associated with normal labor progression and is marked by bloody mucous-like consistency. Succenturiate placenta is the presence of one or more accessory lobes that develop on the placenta with vascular connections of fetal origin.

➧ ***Test-taking Tip:*** *Consider the definitions and symptoms associated with each of the options to make the best selection.*

Content Area: Childbearing Families; *Category of Health Alteration:* Intrapartal Management; *Integrated Processes:* Nursing Process Analysis; *Client Need:* Physiological Integrity/Physiological Adaptation/Alterations in Body Systems; *Cognitive Level:* Analysis

Reference: Davidson, M., London, M., & Ladewig, P. (2008). *Olds' Maternal-Newborn Nursing & Women's Health Across the Lifespan* (8th ed., p. 741). Upper Saddle River, NJ: Prentice Hall Health.

359. A nurse's laboring client suddenly experiences a dramatic drop in the fetal heart rate (FHR) from the 150s to the 110s. A vaginal exam reveals the presence of the fetal cord that has protruded through the cervix. What is the initial step the nurse should take?

1. Provide continuous pressure to hold the presenting part off the cord
2. Place the client in Trendelenburg's position
3. Insert and fill a Foley catheter
4. Continue to monitor the FHR

ANSWER: 1

The nurse should first exert continuous pressure on the presenting part to prevent further cord compression. This is continued until birth is achieved, usually by cesarean section birth. The bed should then be placed in Trendelenburg's position to further prevent pressure on the cord. A Foley catheter may be inserted with 500 mL of warmed saline to help float the head and prevent further compression. The fetus is continually monitored throughout until birth is accomplished.

➧ ***Test-taking Tip:*** *Consider the first intervention needed for a fetus that is diagnosed with a prolapsed umbilical cord. Use the ABCs (airway, breathing, circulation) to determine priority and eliminate options.*

Content Area: Childbearing Families; *Category of Health Alteration:* Intrapartal Management; *Integrated Processes:* Nursing Process Implementation; *Client Need:* Safe and Effective Care Environment/ Management of Care/Establishing Priorities; *Cognitive Level:* Analysis

Reference: Davidson, M., London, M., & Ladewig, P. (2008). *Olds' Maternal-Newborn Nursing & Women's Health Across the Lifespan* (8th ed., pp. 748–750). Upper Saddle River, NJ: Prentice Hall Health.

360. A nurse is caring for a client who has come to a unit in active labor. The client is contracting every 2 minutes with contractions that last 60 to 70 seconds. The contractions are moderate to strong by palpation. The woman notes extreme pain in the small of her back. Her abdomen reveals a small depression under the umbilicus. Which fetal position should the nurse document?

1. Occiput anterior.
2. Occiput posterior.
3. Left occiput anterior.
4. Right occiput anterior.

ANSWER: 2

An occiput posterior position is characterized by intense back pain (back labor). A depression under the umbilicus occurs as a result of the posterior shoulder. When a fetus presents anterior, it is uncommon for the mother's chief complaint to be back pain and the uterus appears smooth.

▶ ***Test-taking Tip:*** *Remember when the fetal back (occiput posterior) is against the mother's spine, back pain is the chief complaint. Note that all options except 2 include the word anterior. Thus, eliminate options 1, 3, and 4.*

Content Area: Childbearing Families; *Category of Health Alteration:* Intrapartal Management; *Integrated Processes:* Communication and Documentation; *Client Need:* Safe and Effective Care Environment/Management of Care/Continuity of Care; *Cognitive Level:* Analysis

References: Pillitteri, A. (2007). *Maternal & Child Health Nursing: Care of the Childbearing & Childrearing Family* (5th ed., p. 521). Philadelphia: Lippincott Williams & Wilkins; Varney, H., Kriebs, J., & Gegor, C. (2004). *Varney's Midwifery* (4th ed., p. 477). Boston: Jones & Bartlett.

361. EBP A night nurse has admitted multiple maternity clients with various fetal presentations. Which fetal presentations, if unchanged, would require the nurse to prepare for cesarean sections? SELECT ALL THAT APPLY.

1. Brow presentation
2. Face presentation (with posterior mentum)
3. Single footling breech
4. Double footling breech
5. Frank breech
6. Shoulder presentation

ANSWER: 1, 2, 3, 4, 6

A brow presentation with complete flexion that does not rotate or change position could not deliver vaginally. A face presentation can only be delivered if the mentum is anterior. Footling breeches and shoulder presentations are all delivered via cesarean section. A frank breech (buttocks alone presented to the cervix) is not a contraindication to vaginal birth, although many practitioners do not perform any breech vaginal deliveries.

▶ ***Test-taking Tip:*** *Think about the risk to the mother and neonate. Identify which types of presentations must be delivered via cesarean section and eliminate those options.*

Content Area: Childbearing Families; *Category of Health Alteration:* Intrapartal Management; *Integrated Processes:* Nursing Process Planning; *Client Need:* Safe and Effective Care Environment/Safety and Infection Control/Injury Prevention; *Cognitive Level:* Analysis

Reference: Vialle, R., Pietin-Vialle, C., Vinchon, M., Dauger, S., Ilharreborde, B., et al. (2008). Birth-related spinal cord injuries: A multicentric review of 9 cases. *Child's Nervous System, 24*(1), 79–85.

EBP Reference: American College of Obstetricians and Gynecologists (ACOG). (2006). Mode of term singleton breech delivery. *ACOG Committee Opinion*, No. 3340, Washington, DC: Author.

362. A nurse is caring for two maternity clients who are in labor, one with a cephalic presentation and another with a breech presentation. The nurse determines that head entrapment is most likely to occur with which delivery presentation? Place an X on the correct illustration.

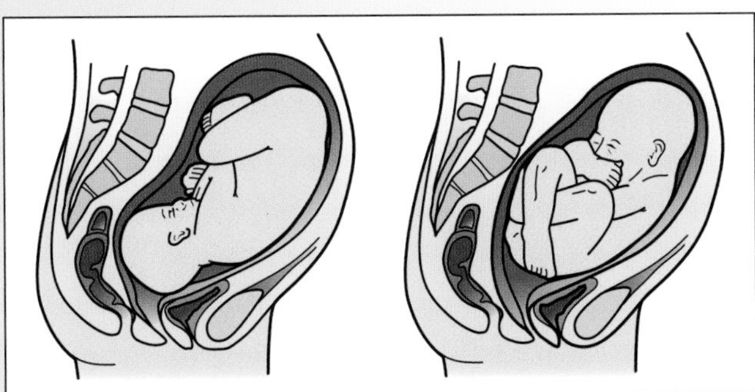

ANSWER:

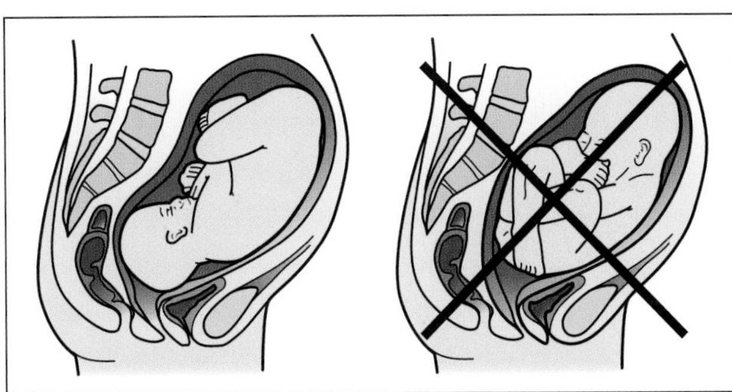

A breech delivery is most likely to be associated with head entrapment because the head is the largest part of the fetal body and it is delivered last in a breech delivery.

▶ ***Test-taking Tip:*** *View each delivery mentally and predict which image is most likely to result in head entrapment.*

Content Area: Childbearing Families; *Category of Health Alteration:* Intrapartal Management; *Integrated Processes:* Nursing Process Analysis; *Client Need:* Physiological Integrity/Reduction of Risk Potential/Potential for Complications from Surgical Procedures and Health Alterations; *Cognitive Level:* Analysis

Reference: Blackburn, S. (2007). *Maternal, Fetal, & Neonatal Physiology,* (3rd ed., p. 768). St. Louis, MO: Saunders/Elsevier.

---

363. EBP A pregnant client is concerned because she is now 14 days over her due date. A nurse should monitor the client for which most concerning problem for a post-term fetus?

1. Meconium-stained amniotic fluid
2. Macrosomia
3. Birth trauma
4. Fetal demise

ANSWER: 4

The most concerning problem is fetal demise or stillbirth. The mortality rate is double in post-term fetuses when compared to fetuses that are delivered before 42 gestational weeks. Meconium-stained fluid is increased in post-term pregnancies as is macrosomia and birth trauma; however, fetal death is the most concerning in this scenario.

➧ ***Test-taking Tip:*** *The key words are "most concerning." In this situation where all of the options are correct, select the worst problem, which is option 4.*

Content Area: Childbearing Families; *Category of Health Alteration:* Intrapartal Management; *Integrated Processes:* Nursing Process Implementation; *Client Need:* Physiological Integrity/Reduction of Risk Potential/Potential for Complications from Surgical Procedures and Health Alterations; *Cognitive Level:* Analysis

Reference: Davidson, M., London, M., & Ladewig, P. (2008). *Olds' Maternal-Newborn Nursing & Women's Health Across the Lifespan* (8th ed., p. 941). Upper Saddle River, NJ: Prentice Hall Health.

EBP Reference: American College of Obstetricians and Gynecologists (ACOG). (2004). Management of postterm pregnancy. *ACOG Practice Bulletin,* No. 55.

---

364. EBP A nurse is caring for a 30-weeks-pregnant client who is having contractions every 1½ to 2 minutes with spontaneous rupture of membranes 2 hours ago. The client's cervix is 8 cm dilated, and her cervix is 100% effaced. The nurse determines that delivery is imminent. Which nursing action is the most important at this time?

1. Administering a tocolytic agent
2. Providing teaching information on premature infant care
3. Notifying neonatology of the impending birth
4. Preparing for a cesarean birth

ANSWER: 3

The most important component of the client's care at this time is to notify the neonatal team of the delivery because they will be needed for respiratory support and possible resuscitation. It is too late to administer a tocolytic agent. A cesarean birth is indicated if there are other obstetrical needs. Teaching is important but is not appropriate at this time.

➧ ***Test-taking Tip:*** *Focus on the gestational age and the most important client needs at this time.*

Content Area: Childbearing Families; *Category of Health Alteration:* Intrapartal Management; *Integrated Processes:* Nursing Process Implementation; *Client Need:* Safe and Effective Care Environment/ Management of Care/Collaboration with Interdisciplinary Team; *Cognitive Level:* Analysis

Reference: Davidson, M., London, M., & Ladewig, P. (2008). *Olds' Maternal-Newborn Nursing & Women's Health Across the Lifespan* (8th ed., p. 493). Upper Saddle River, NJ: Prentice Hall Health.

EBP Reference: American College of Obstetricians and Gynecologists (ACOG). (2003). Management of preterm labor. *ACOG Practice Bulletin,* No. 43.

365. EBP A nurse is caring for a client who is in early labor and has been ambulating for the past 15 minutes when she states that her "water broke." Upon returning the client to her room, the nurse places the fetal monitor and obtains a fetal heart rate ranging from 82 to 87. A vaginal exam reveals that the cervix is 90% effaced and 1 to 2 cm dilated with the vertex presenting at a –2 station. There is a flesh-feeling, pulsating cord noted in the anterior portion of the cervical exam. Which critical intervention should be performed immediately?

1. Adjust the fetal monitor
2. Compare the maternal pulse to the FHR
3. Apply pressure to the presenting part to prevent pressure on the umbilical cord
4. Call for assistance

ANSWER: 3

The most critical intervention is to leave the examining hand in place and apply upward pressure to the presenting part because the umbilical cord is being compressed. The nurse should call for assistance as soon as possible. Readjusting the fetal monitor and comparing the FHR with the maternal pulse is not indicated because the nurse has identified the reason for the heart rate being low.

➧ ***Test-taking Tip:*** *First consider which of the options should be performed. Next, prioritize and determine which option is the most important in preventing further fetal decline.*

Content Area: Childbearing Families; *Category of Health Alteration:* Intrapartal Management; *Integrated Processes:* Nursing Process Implementation; *Client Need:* Safe and Effective Care Environment/Management of Care/Establishing Priorities; *Cognitive Level:* Application

Reference: Davidson, M., London, M., & Ladewig, P. (2008). *Olds' Maternal-Newborn Nursing & Women's Health Across the Lifespan* (8th ed., p. 749). Upper Saddle River, NJ: Prentice Hall Health.

EBP Reference: National Institute of Child Health and Human Development Maternal-Fetal Medicine Units Network. (2006). Decision-to-incision times and maternal and infant outcomes. *Obstetrics & Gynecology, 108*(1), 6–11.

366. A nurse is evaluating a client, who is 39 weeks pregnant, in triage. The client states that she thinks she has been leaking "stuff" from her vagina for about a week. The client reports a greenish, foul-smelling discharge and feels feverish. The client's oral temperature is 101.6°F (38.7°C), and the fetal heart rate is 120 with minimal variability and no accelerations. The client's group beta streptococcus (GBS) culture is positive. Which interventions should the nurse anticipate when planning for the client's care? SELECT ALL THAT APPLY.

1. Preparing for a cesarean birth because of chorioamnionitis
2. Starting oxytocin (Pitocin®) for an induction
3. Starting antibiotics for the GBS infection
4. Preparing for epidural anesthesia
5. Notifying the pediatrician or neonatologist of the status
6. Administering a cervical ripening agent for induction

ANSWER: 1, 3, 4, 5

When chorioamnionitis is suspected, immediate delivery is indicated. Because this woman is not in labor, a cesarean birth is indicated. The woman should be given antibiotics as ordered by her physician to treat the infection. Because epidural anesthesia offers the least risk to the fetus, preparation for epidural anesthesia should begin. The pediatrician or neonatologist should be notified of the impending delivery so he or she can be available as needed. Starting oxytocin or administering a cervical ripening agent would prolong the time to delivery.

➧ ***Test-taking Tip:*** *In this scenario, the woman needs to deliver as soon as possible. Identify which interventions would result in the quickest and safest delivery method.*

Content Area: Childbearing Families; *Category of Health Alteration:* Intrapartal Management; *Integrated Processes:* Nursing Process Planning; *Client Need:* Physiological Integrity/Reduction of Risk Potential/Potential for Alterations in Body Systems; *Cognitive Level:* Application

References: Davidson, M., London, M., & Ladewig, P. (2008). *Olds' Maternal-Newborn Nursing & Women's Health Across the Lifespan* (8th ed., pp. 493–494). Upper Saddle River, NJ: Prentice Hall Health; Anderson, B., Simhan, H., Simons, K., & Wiesenfeld, H. (2007). Untreated asymptomatic group B streptococcal bacteriuria early in pregnancy and chorioamnionitis at delivery. *American Journal of Obstetrics & Gynecology, 196*(6), 524.e1–e5.

367. A nurse is caring for a client who is about to undergo an emergency cesarean birth for severe preeclampsia at 26.3 weeks gestation. The client is admitted after 3 days of a severe headache and a 10-pound weight gain. Her blood pressure is 180/110 mm Hg, and she has a moderate abruption. The woman states, "It's my fault! If I would have called earlier, they could have stopped it and I wouldn't be having my baby delivered now!" What is the nurse's best response?

1. "This is not your fault. You are here now, and we are going to take care of you."
2. "Earlier intervention might have deemed a better outcome, but you can't think of that now."
3. "Your baby is going to be fine."
4. "Your health and well-being are what is important, you need to think of yourself and not the baby right now."

ANSWER: 1

The nurse needs to provide reassurance to the woman that she is not to blame and that everything is being done for her and the baby. Suggesting that an earlier presentation would have produced a better outcome places blame on the woman. Telling the woman that the baby will be fine may be providing false reassurance to her. Statements that indicate the woman should not worry about her baby are insensitive and are likely to leave the woman feeling that the nurse does not understand or care about her infant.

➧ ***Test-taking Tip:*** *Select options that are based on the principles of therapeutic communication.*

Content Area: Childbearing Families; *Category of Health Alteration:* Intrapartal Management; *Integrated Processes:* Caring; *Client Need:* Psychological Integrity/Crisis Intervention: Psychological Integrity/ Therapeutic Communications; *Cognitive Level:* Analysis

Reference: Berman, A., Snyder, S., Kozier, B., & Erb, G. (2008). *Kozier & Erb's Fundamentals of Nursing: Concepts, Process, and Practice* (8th ed., pp. 469–471). Upper Saddle River, NJ: Pearson Education.

Test 10: **Childbearing Families: Postpartal Management**

368. A delivery nurse is giving a report to a postpartum nurse on a client being transferred to a postpartum care area who just delivered her first baby, a term newborn. Which number should the delivery nurse report for the client's parity?

1. 0
2. 1
3. 2
4. 3

ANSWER: 2

Parity refers to the number of births after 20 weeks gestation. Because the woman has given birth to her first child, her parity is 1. The other options are incorrect.

➧ ***Test-taking Tip:*** *Determine the best answer based on your knowledge of the definition of parity.*

Content Area: Childbearing Families; *Category of Health Alteration:* Postpartum Management; *Integrated Processes:* Communication and Documentation; *Client Need:* Health Promotion and Maintenance/ Ante/Intra/Postpartum and Newborn Care; *Cognitive Level:* Application

Reference: Davidson, M., London, M., & Ladewig, P. (2008). *Olds' Maternal-Newborn Nursing & Women's Health Across the Lifespan* (8th ed., p. 338). Upper Saddle River, NJ: Prentice Hall Health.

---

369. A nurse is assisting in the delivery of a term newborn. Immediately after delivery of the placenta, the nurse palpates the uterine fundus and finds that it is firm and located halfway between the client's umbilicus and symphysis pubis. Which action should the nurse take based on the assessment findings?

1. Immediately begin to massage the uterus
2. Document the findings
3. Assess for bladder distension
4. Monitor the client closely for increased vaginal bleeding

ANSWER: 2

Immediately after birth, the uterus should contract and the fundus should be located one-half to two-thirds of the way between the symphysis pubis and umbilicus. Thus the only intervention required is to document the assessment finding. There is no indication that the bladder is full. A full bladder will cause uterine displacement to either side of the abdomen. Uterine massage is indicated only if the uterus does not feel firm and contracted. Since the uterus is firm, there is no reason to suspect that increased vaginal discharge would occur.

➧ ***Test-taking Tip:*** *Recall the process of uterine involution to correctly answer this question.*

Content Area: Childbearing Families; *Category of Health Alteration:* Postpartum Management; *Integrated Processes:* Nursing Process Implementation; *Client Need:* Physiological Integrity/Reduction of Risk Potential/System Specific Assessments; *Cognitive Level:* Application

References: Davidson, M., London, M., & Ladewig, P. (2008). *Olds' Maternal-Newborn Nursing & Women's Health Across the Lifespan* (8th ed., pp. 1041–1042, 1056). Upper Saddle River, NJ: Prentice Hall Health; Pillitteri, A. (2007). *Maternal & Child Health Nursing: Care of the Childbearing Families & Childrearing Family* (5th ed., p. 628). Philadelphia: Lippincott Williams & Wilkins.

---

370. A nurse walks into the room of a postpartum client and observes her looking in the mirror at her abdomen. The client says, "My stomach still looks like I'm pregnant!" The nurse explains that the abdominal muscles, which separate during pregnancy, will do which of the following?

1. Regain tone within the first week after birth
2. Regain prepregnancy tone with exercise
3. Remain permanently separated giving the abdomen a slight bulge
4. Regain tone as the client loses the weight gained during the pregnancy

ANSWER: 2

When the postpartum woman stands during the first days after birth, her abdomen protrudes and gives her a "still-pregnant" appearance. This is caused by relaxation of the abdominal wall. For the majority of postpartum women, the muscles of the abdominal wall will return to the prepregnancy state within 6 weeks with appropriate exercise. If the woman delivers a very large infant, the abdominal muscles may separate but the separation will become less apparent over time.

➧ ***Test-taking Tip:*** *Examine similar options first and eliminate one or both of these. Eliminate unrealistic options.*

Content Area: Childbearing Families; *Category of Health Alteration:* Postpartum Management; *Integrated Processes:* Teaching and Learning; *Client Need:* Health Promotion and Maintenance/Ante/Intra/ Postpartum and Newborn Care; *Cognitive Level:* Application

Reference: Wong, D., Hockenberry, M., Wilson, D., Perry, S., & Lowdermilk, D. (2006). *Maternal Child Nursing Care* (3rd ed., p. 593). Philadelphia: Lippincott Williams & Wilkins.

371. EBP A clinic nurse reviews the following laboratory results from a postpartum client who is 5 days post-delivery. What should the nurse do in response to these results?

Laboratory Value	Result
Hematocrit	35%
Hemoglobin	11 g/dL
White blood cells	20,000/mm^3

1. Record the findings
2. Assess the client for increased lochia
3. Assess the client's temperature
4. Notify the health-care provider immediately

ANSWER: 1

The only action required is to document the findings. Nonpathological leukocytosis often occurs during labor and in the immediate postpartum period because labor produces a mild proinflammatory state. White blood cell (WBC) values should return to normal levels by the end of the first postpartum week. Hemoglobin and hematocrit levels will decrease close to the end of the first postpartum week due to the hemodilution, which begins on postpartum day 3 or 4. Thus, all of these laboratory values are within the expected parameters. Assessing the client's lochia and temperature and notifying the health-care provider are unnecessary with these results.

▶ ***Test-taking Tip:*** *The key to this question is that the client is 5 days postdelivery. WBCs are still elevated in the first week postpartum, and hemodilution occurs also near the end of the first postpartum week.*

Content Area: Childbearing Families; *Category of Health Alteration:* Postpartum Management; *Integrated Processes:* Nursing Process Analysis; *Client Need:* Physiological Integrity/Reduction of Risk Potential/Laboratory Values; *Cognitive Level:* Analysis

Reference: Davidson, M., London, M., & Ladewig, P. (2008). *Olds' Maternal-Newborn Nursing & Women's Health Across the Lifespan* (8th ed., p. 1046). Upper Saddle River, NJ: Prentice Hall Health.

EBP Reference: Lurie, S., Rahamim, E., Piper, I., Golan, A., & Sadan, O. (2008). Total and differential leukocyte counts percentiles in normal pregnancy. *European Journal of Obstetrics & Gynecology and Reproductive Biology*, *136*(1), 16–19S.

---

372. EBP A Caucasian postpartum client asks a nurse if the stretch marks (striae gravidarum) on her abdomen will ever go away. Which response by the nurse is most accurate?

1. "Your stretch marks should totally disappear over the next month."
2. "Your stretch marks will always appear raised and reddened."
3. "Your stretch marks may become lighter in color if you keep that area of your skin hydrated."
4. "Your stretch marks will fade to pale white over the next 3 to 6 months."

ANSWER: 4

In Caucasian women, stretch marks will fade to a pale white over 3 to 6 months. Stretch marks will never completely disappear. Treatment is nonspecific, and a limited evidence base for treatment exists. Numerous creams, emollients, and oils (e.g., vitamin E cream, cocoa butter, aloe vera lotion, and olive oil) are used to prevent striae; however, there is no evidence that these treatments are effective. Postpartum treatments may include topical tretinoin (Retin-A®) or oral tretinoin (Vesanoid®) therapy (U.S. Food and Drug Administration pregnancy categories C and D, respectively; unknown safety in breastfeeding women) and laser treatment. There is no evidence that keeping the skin hydrated will lighten the appearance of the stretch marks.

▶ ***Test-taking Tip:*** *Recall the expected physiological changes that occur to the skin during pregnancy and postpartum. Options 1 and 2 reflect opposite ends of the spectrum of possible changes in striae gravidarum. Eliminate both of these options as too extreme.*

Content Area: Childbearing Families; *Category of Health Alteration:* Postpartum Management; *Integrated Processes:* Teaching and Learning; *Client Need:* Health Promotion and Maintenance/Self-Care; *Cognitive Level:* Application

References: Pillitteri, A. (2007). *Maternal & Child Health Nursing: Care of the Childbearing Families & Childrearing Family* (5th ed., p. 631). Philadelphia: Lippincott Williams & Wilkins; Orshan, S. (2008). *Maternity, Newborn, and Women's Health Nursing* (p. 446). Philadelphia: Lippincott Williams & Wilkins.

EBP Reference: Tunzi, M., & Gray, G. (2007). Common skin conditions during pregnancy. *American Family Physician*. Available at: www.aafp.org/afp/20070115/211.html

373. Twenty-four hours post–vaginal delivery, a postpartum client tells a nurse that she is concerned because she has not had a bowel movement since before delivery. In response to this information, the nurse should intervene by doing which of the following?

1. Documenting the information in the client's health-care records
2. Notifying the health-care practitioner immediately
3. Administering a laxative that has been ordered on an as needed basis
4. Assessing the client's bowel sounds

ANSWER: 1

Because of decreased muscle tone in the intestines during labor and the immediate postpartum period, possible prelabor diarrhea, decreased food intake during labor, and dehydration during labor, a spontaneous bowel evacuation may not occur for 2 to 3 days after childbirth. Thus, the only action required by the nurse is to document the lack of a bowel movement in the client's records. There is no need to notify the health-care practitioner or to administer a laxative. Bowel sounds are not altered by a vaginal delivery, even though the passage of stool through the intestines is slowed.

▶ ***Test-taking Tip:*** *Immediate notification of the health-care practitioner implies that a health-threatening problem is occurring. Lack of a bowel movement would not meet this criterion.*

Content Area: Childbearing Families; *Category of Health Alteration:* Postpartum Management; *Integrated Processes:* Nursing Process Analysis; *Client Need:* Physiological Integrity/Basic Care and Comfort/Elimination; *Cognitive Level:* Application

References: Wong, D., Hockenberry, M., Wilson, D., Perry, S., & Lowdermilk, D. (2006). *Maternal Child Nursing Care* (3rd ed., p. 594). Philadelphia: Lippincott Williams & Wilkins; Pillitteri, A. (2007). *Maternal & Child Health Nursing: Care of the Childbearing Families & Childrearing Family* (5th ed., p. 631). Philadelphia: Lippincott Williams & Wilkins.

374. A registered nurse (RN) is caring for a postpartum client who is 16 hours postdelivery. A student nurse is assisting with the care. The RN evaluates that the student needs more education about uterine assessment when the student is observed doing which of the following?

1. Elevating the client's head 30 degrees before beginning the assessment
2. Supporting the lower uterine segment during the assessment
3. Gently palpating the uterine fundus
4. Observing the abdomen before beginning palpation

ANSWER: 1

For uterine assessment, the client should be positioned in a supine position so the height of the uterus is not influenced by an elevated position. The abdomen should be observed for contour to detect distention and for the appearance of striae or a diastasis. When beginning the assessment, one hand should be placed at the base of the uterus just above the symphysis pubis to support the lower uterine segment. This prevents the inadvertent inversion of the uterus during palpation. Once the lower hand is in place, the fundus of the uterus can be gently palpated.

▶ ***Test-taking Tip:*** *The statement "needs further education" is a false-response item. Select the incorrect statement.*

Content Area: Childbearing Families; *Category of Health Alteration:* Postpartum Management; *Integrated Processes:* Nursing Process Evaluation; *Client Need:* Health Promotion and Maintenance/Techniques of Physical Assessment; *Cognitive Level:* Application

Reference: Pillitteri, A. (2007). *Maternal & Child Health Nursing: Care of the Childbearing Families & Childrearing Family* (5th ed., pp. 635, 636). Philadelphia: Lippincott Williams & Wilkins.

375. A nurse begins the assessment of a postpartum client, who is 5 hours postdelivery. Initially, the nurse is unable to palpate the uterine fundus. Which actions should the nurse take to locate the client's fundus? Prioritize the nurse's actions by placing each step in the correct order.

______ Place the side of one hand just above the client's symphysis pubis
______ Press deeply into the abdomen
______ Place a hand at the level of the umbilicus
______ Massage in a circular motion
______ Position the client in supine position
______ If the fundus is not felt, move the upper hand lower on the abdomen and repeat the massage

ANSWER: 2, 4, 3, 5, 1, 6

For uterine assessment, the client should be positioned in a supine position so the height of the uterus is not influenced by an elevated position. When beginning the assessment, one hand should be placed at the base of the uterus just above the symphysis pubis to support the lower uterine segment. This prevents the inadvertent inversion of the uterus during palpation. The second hand should then be placed at the level of the umbilicus because this is the expected location of the uterine fundus on the day of delivery. A nurse should then press deeply into the abdomen and massage in a circular motion. This massage should stimulate the uterus to contract and allow location of the fundus to be determined. If the fundus is still unable to be located, the nurse should move the upper hand lower on the abdomen because involution could potentially be occurring more rapidly than expected if the client is breastfeeding and/or had an uncomplicated labor and birth. At this point, the nurse should repeat the circular motion.

▶ ***Test-taking Tip:*** *Think about the order of the steps involved in assessing the postpartum fundus and recall that the uterine muscle will respond to massage by contracting.*

Content Area: Childbearing Families; *Category of Health Alteration:* Postpartum Management; *Integrated Processes:* Nursing Process Assessment; *Client Need:* Health Promotion and Maintenance/ Techniques of Physical Assessment; *Cognitive Level:* Application

References: Pillitteri, A. (2007). *Maternal & Child Health Nursing: Care of the Childbearing Families & Childrearing Family* (5th ed., pp. 628, 635). Philadelphia: Lippincott Williams & Wilkins; Davidson, M., London, M., & Ladewig, P. (2008). *Olds' Maternal-Newborn Nursing & Women's Health Across the Lifespan* (8th ed., p. 1056). Upper Saddle River, NJ: Prentice Hall Health.

---

376. A postpartum client, who delivered a full-term infant 2 days previously, calls a nurse to her room and states that she is concerned because her breasts "seem to be growing." She reports that the bra she wore during pregnancy is too small. She asks the nurse what is wrong with her. The nurse's response should be based on which of the following statements?

1. Enlarging breasts are a symptom of infection.
2. Increasing breast tissue may be a sign of postpartum fluid retention.
3. Thrombi may form in veins of the breast and cause increased breast size.
4. Breast tissue increases in the early postpartum period as milk forms.

ANSWER: 4

Breast tissue increases as breast milk forms, so a bra that was adequate during pregnancy may no longer be adequate by the second or third postpartum day. Infection in the breast tissue results in flu-like symptoms and redness and tenderness of the breast. It is usually unilateral and does not cause bilateral breast enlargement. Fluid is not retained during the postpartum period; rather, clients experience diuresis of the excess fluid volume accumulated during pregnancy. Symptoms of thrombi formation include redness, pain, and increased skin temperature over the thrombi. Fullness in both breasts would not be the result of thrombi formation.

▸ ***Test-taking Tip:*** *Recall the generic signs of infection: inflammation and thrombosis. Eliminate options 1 and 3 as bilateral breast fullness would not be caused by these conditions.*

Content Area: Childbearing Families; *Category of Health Alteration:* Postpartum Management; *Integrated Processes:* Nursing Process Planning; *Client Need:* Health Promotion and Maintenance/ Developmental Stages and Transitions; *Cognitive Level:* Application

References: Pillitteri, A. (2007). *Maternal & Child Health Nursing: Care of the Childbearing Families & Childrearing Family* (5th ed., pp. 630, 635). Philadelphia: Lippincott Williams & Wilkins; Davidson, M., London, M., & Ladewig, P. (2008). *Olds' Maternal-Newborn Nursing & Women's Health Across the Lifespan* (8th ed., p. 1127). Upper Saddle River, NJ: Prentice Hall Health.

---

377. While assessing a postpartum client who is 10 hours post-vaginal delivery, a nurse notes a perineal pad that is totally saturated with lochia. To determine the significance of this finding, which question should the nurse ask the client *first*?

1. "Are you having uterine cramping?"
2. "When was the last time you changed your peri pad?"
3. "Are you having any difficulty emptying your bladder?"
4. "Have you passed any clots?"

ANSWER: 2

Lochia amount should never exceed a moderate amount (less than a 6-inch stain on a perineal pad); however, the amount of lochia on a perineal pad at any given time is influenced by the individual client's pad changing practices. Therefore, the nurse should ask about the length of time the current pad has been in place before making a clinical judgment about whether the amount is concerning. Once the nurse has determined the length of time the pad has been in place, the nurse could decide if the other questions would be needed for further assessment.

▸ ***Test-taking Tip:*** *Note the key word "first."*

Content Area: Childbearing Families; *Category of Health Alteration:* Postpartum Management; *Integrated Processes:* Nursing Process Assessment; *Client Need:* Safe and Effective Care Environment/ Management of Care/Establishing Priorities; *Cognitive Level:* Analysis

Reference: Davidson, M., London, M., & Ladewig, P. (2008). *Olds' Maternal-Newborn Nursing & Women's Health Across the Lifespan* (8th ed., pp. 1058–1059). Upper Saddle River, NJ: Prentice Hall Health.

378. At 0600 hours, a registered nurse (RN) assesses the fundus of a postpartum client who had a vaginal birth at 0030 and finds that it is firm. The RN then asks a certified nursing assistant (CNA) to assist the client out of bed for the first time. Blood begins to run down the client's leg when she gets up, and the CNA immediately calls the RN back into the room. Which response by the nurse to the client's bleeding is correct?

1. Explain to the client that this extra bleeding can occur with initial ambulation
2. Immediately assist the client back to bed
3. Push the emergency call light in the room
4. Call the health-care provider to report this increased bleeding

ANSWER: 1

Lochia normally pools in the vagina when the postpartum woman remains in a recumbent position for any length of time. When the woman then stands, gravity causes the blood to flow out. As long as the nurse knows the fundus is firm and therefore not bleeding, a simple explanation to the client is all that is required. There is no reason to return the client to bed, push the emergency call light, or call the health-care provider.

Test-taking Tip: *Options 2, 3, and 4 are all interventions for a uterine hemorrhage. All of these interventions would be appropriate if the client were experiencing abnormal bleeding. Since all three cannot be selected, it would follow that the client in this situation is not hemorrhaging, therefore, eliminating options 2, 3, and 4.*

Content Area: Childbearing Families; *Category of Health Alteration:* Postpartum Management; *Integrated Processes:* Nursing Process Implementation; *Client Need:* Health Promotion and Maintenance/Ante/Intra/Postpartum and Newborn Care; *Cognitive Level:* Analysis

Reference: Davidson, M., London, M., & Ladewig, P. (2008). *Olds' Maternal-Newborn Nursing & Women's Health Across the Lifespan* (8th ed., pp. 1043, 1052). Upper Saddle River, NJ: Prentice Hall Health.

379. A licensed practical nurse (LPN) asks a registered nurse (RN) to assist in assessing the location of the fundus of a client who is 8 hours post-vaginal delivery. Place an X on the abdomen where the RN should expect to locate the client's fundus.

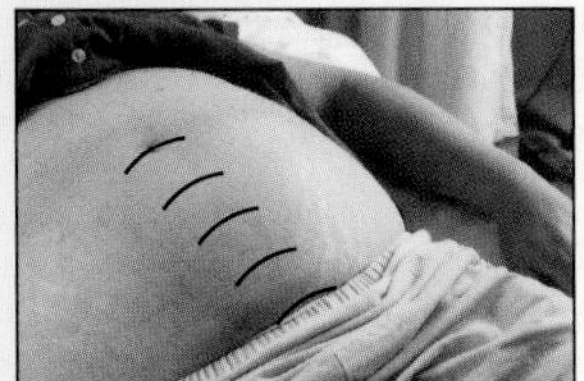

ANSWER:

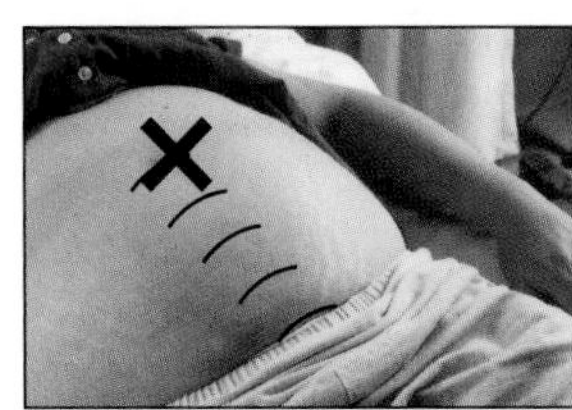

The nurse should expect to locate the client's fundus at the level of the umbilicus. Immediately after birth the uterus will contract and the fundus will be located one-half to two-thirds of the way between the symphysis pubis and umbilicus. However, within 6 to 12 hours after birth the fundus of the uterus rises to the level of the umbilicus because of blood and clots that remain within the uterus and changes in ligament support.

Test-taking Tip: *Use the process of elimination and review assessing postpartum clients.*

Content Area: Childbearing Families; *Category of Health Alteration:* Postpartum Management; *Integrated Processes:* Nursing Process Assessment; *Client Need:* Physiological Integrity Reduction of Risk Potential/System Specific Assessments; *Cognitive Level:* Application

Reference: Davidson, M., London, M., & Ladewig, P. (2008). *Olds' Maternal-Newborn Nursing & Women's Health Across the Lifespan* (8th ed., p. 1041). Upper Saddle River, NJ: Prentice Hall Health.

380. Which observation of a client should lead a nurse to be concerned about the client's attachment to her male infant?

1. Asking the licensed practical nurse (LPN) about how to change her infant's diaper
2. Comparing her baby's nose to her brother's nose
3. Calling the baby by name
4. Repeatedly telling her husband that she wanted a girl

ANSWER: 4

Attachment is demonstrated by expressing satisfaction with a baby's appearance and sex. Frequent expressions of dissatisfaction with the sex of the infant should be evaluated further. Seeking information about infant care, calling the infant by name, and pointing out family traits or characteristics seen in the newborn are all signs that the mother is developing attachment to her infant.

Test-taking Tip: *The statement "lead a nurse to be concerned" is a false-response item. Select the statement that describes incorrect attachment behaviors.*

Content Area: Childbearing Families; *Category of Health Alteration:* Postpartum Management; *Integrated Processes:* Nursing Process Evaluation; *Client Need:* Health Promotion and Maintenance/ Ante/Intra/Postpartum and Newborn Care; *Cognitive Level:* Application

Reference: Davidson, M., London, M., & Ladewig, P. (2008). *Olds' Maternal-Newborn Nursing & Women's Health Across the Lifespan* (8th ed., pp. 1065–1066). Upper Saddle River, NJ: Prentice Hall Health.

381. When caring for a postpartum family, a nurse determines that paternal engrossment is occurring when the newborn's father is observed:

1. talking to his newborn from across the room.
2. discussing the similarity between his ears and the newborn's ears.
3. expressing feelings of frustration when the infant cries.
4. being hesitant to touch his newborn.

ANSWER: 2

In North American culture, neonates have a powerful impact on their fathers, who become intensely involved with their babies. The term used for the father's absorption and interest in the infant is *engrossment.* Engrossment is demonstrated by touching the infant, making eye contact with the infant, and verbalizing awareness of features in the newborn that are similar to him and that validate his claim to that newborn. Not making face-to-face contact with the infant during communication and a hesitation to touch the infant demonstrate a lack of engrossment. Feelings of frustration are not uncommon to fathers and are characteristic of the second stage, or reality stage, of the transition to fatherhood but are not a sign of engrossment.

➧ ***Test-taking Tip:*** *Paternal engrossment like maternal attachment involves making close physical contact with the infant. Eliminate options 1 and 4 as these do not demonstrate that type of involvement.*

Content Area: Childbearing Families; *Category of Health Alteration:* Postpartum Management; *Integrated Processes:* Nursing Process Analysis; *Client Need:* Health Promotion and Maintenance/ Developmental Stages and Transitions; *Cognitive Level:* Application

Reference: Wong, D., Hockenberry, M., Wilson, D., Perry, S., & Lowdermilk, D. (2006). *Maternal Child Nursing Care* (3rd ed., pp. 640–641). Philadelphia: Lippincott Williams & Wilkins.

382. While caring for a postpartum primiparous client, who is 13 hours post-vaginal delivery, a nurse observes that the client is passive and hesitant about making decisions concerning her own care and the care of her newborn. In response to this observation, which interventions should be implemented by the nurse? SELECT ALL THAT APPLY.

1. Question her closely about the presence of pain
2. Ask her if she would like to talk about her birth experience
3. Encourage her to nap when her infant is napping
4. Encourage participation in any unit learning activities about infant care
5. Suggest that she begin to write her birth announcements

ANSWER: 1, 2, 3

Three phases are evident as the mother adjusts to her maternal role after birth. The initial phase is the dependent, or "taking-in," phase. This phase can last up to 48 hours after birth. During this phase, the mother's dependency needs predominate, and, if these needs are met by others, the mother is eventually able to divert her energy to her infant. The mother needs "mothering" herself to enable her to mother her child. Physical discomfort can be intense during this period and can interfere with rest. Many women may hesitate to ask for medication as they believe the pain they are experiencing is expected. Thus the nurse should ask the client about pain and assure her that there are methods to decrease her pain. During this period, the client may have a great need to talk about her birthing experience and ask questions for clarification as necessary. By encouraging this verbalization, the nurse helps the client to accept the experience and enables her to move to the next maternal phase. Sleep is a major need during this period and should be encouraged. Anxiety and preoccupation with her new role often narrow the client's perceptions, and information is not as easily assimilated at this time. Therefore, attending unit education sessions should be delayed if possible until the mother has completed this adjustment phase. Mothers also need to suspend their involvement in everyday responsibilities during this phase; so writing birth announcements should also be delayed until the mother has completed this adjustment phase.

➧ ***Test-taking Tip:*** *Select options which reflect nurturing and dependency.*

Content Area: Childbearing Families; *Category of Health Alteration:* Postpartum Management; *Integrated Processes:* Nursing Process Implementation; *Client Need:* Health Promotion and Maintenance/ Developmental Stages and Transitions; *Cognitive Level:* Analysis

References: Wong, D., Hockenberry, M., Wilson, D., Perry, S., & Lowdermilk, D. (2006). *Maternal Child Nursing Care* (3rd ed., pp. 636–637). Philadelphia: Lippincott Williams & Wilkins; Davidson, M., London, M., & Ladewig, P. (2008). *Olds' Maternal-Newborn Nursing & Women's Health Across the Lifespan* (8th ed., p. 1047). Upper Saddle River, NJ: Prentice Hall Health.

383. While assisting with the vaginal delivery of a full-term newborn, a nurse observes that, in spite of the fact that the client did not have an episiotomy or a perineal laceration, her perineum and labia are edematous. To promote comfort and decrease the edema, which intervention is most appropriate?

1. Applying an ice pack to the perineum
2. Teaching the client to relax her buttocks before sitting in a chair
3. Applying a warm pack
4. Providing the client with a plastic donut cushion to be used when sitting

ANSWER: 1

If perineal edema is present, ice packs should be applied for the first 24 hours. Ice reduces edema and vulvar irritation. After 24 hours, heat is recommended to increase circulation to the area. The client should be taught to tighten her buttocks when sitting because this compresses the buttocks and reduces pressure on the perineum. Donut cushions should be avoided because they promote separation of the buttocks and decrease venous blood flow to the area, thus increasing pain.

➧ ***Test-taking Tip:*** *Recall basic initial first aid for any acute injury that results in edema, and then select option 1.*

Content Area: Childbearing Families; *Category of Health Alteration:* Postpartum Management; *Integrated Processes:* Nursing Process Implementation; *Client Need:* Physiological Integrity/Basic Care and Comfort/Nonpharmacological Interventions; *Cognitive Level:* Application

References: Wong, D., Hockenberry, M., Wilson, D., Perry, S., & Lowdermilk, D. (2006). *Maternal Child Nursing Care* (3rd ed., pp. 610–611). Philadelphia: Lippincott Williams & Wilkins; Orshan, S. (2008). *Maternity, Newborn, and Women's Health Nursing* (p. 728). Philadelphia: Lippincott Williams & Wilkins.

384. A nurse enters the room of a postpartum, multiparous client and observes the client rubbing her abdomen. The nurse asks the client if she is having pain. The client says she feels like she is having menstrual cramps. In response to this information, which intervention should be implemented by the nurse?

1. Offer a warm blanket for her abdomen.
2. Encourage her to lie on her stomach until the cramping stops.
3. Instruct the client to avoid ambulation while having pain.
4. Check her lochia flow, as pain can sometimes precede hemorrhage.

ANSWER: 2

Multiparous women frequently experience intermittent uterine contractions called afterpains. Lying in a prone position will apply pressure to the uterus and therefore stimulate continuous uterine contraction. When the uterus maintains a state of contraction, the afterpains will cease. Heat application should be avoided as it may cause relaxation of the uterine muscle. Ambulation has been shown to decrease muscle pain. Afterpains are not a symptom of potential postpartum hemorrhage.

➧ ***Test-taking Tip:*** *Relate the uterine cramping to the fact that the client is multiparous. This should identify that the pain is most likely afterpains. Then select the most appropriate treatment for afterpains.*

Content Area: Childbearing Families; *Category of Health Alteration:* Postpartum Management; *Integrated Processes:* Nursing Process Implementation; *Client Need:* Physiological Integrity/Basic Care and Comfort/Nonpharmacological Interventions; *Cognitive Level:* Analysis

References: Davidson, M., London, M., & Ladewig, P. (2008). *Olds' Maternal-Newborn Nursing & Women's Health Across the Lifespan* (8th ed., pp. 1080–1081, 1159). Upper Saddle River, NJ: Prentice Hall Health; Pillitteri, A. (2007). *Maternal & Child Health Nursing: Care of the Childbearing Families & Childrearing Family* (5th ed., p. 637). Philadelphia: Lippincott Williams & Wilkins.

385. Two hours after delivery, a mother, who is bottle feeding, tells a nurse that she experienced "terrible pain when my milk came in with my last baby." The client asks if there is a way this can be prevented from happening after this birthing experience. Which response by the nurse is most appropriate?

1. "Once you have recovered from the birth I will help you bind your breasts."
2. "Development of engorgement is familial; if you had it with your last pregnancy there probably is no way to avoid it with this birth."
3. "You should put on a supportive bra as soon as possible and wear it continuously for the next 1 to 2 weeks."
4. "Engorgement usually occurs immediately after birth, so if you don't have it yet you probably won't develop it."

ANSWER: 3

Lactation can be suppressed by mechanical inhibition. This involves having the woman wear a supportive, well-fitting bra within 6 hours after birth. The bra should be worn continuously until lactation is suppressed (usually 7 to 14 days). It should be removed only for showers. In comparison studies between breast binders and bras, the mothers using binders experienced more engorgement and discomfort. Therefore, a supportive bra is a better choice for mechanical lactation suppression. Engorgement is not familial and not inevitable in bottle-feeding mothers. Signs of engorgement usually occur on the third to fifth postpartum day and engorgement will spontaneously resolve by the tenth day postpartum.

➧ ***Test-taking Tip:*** *Recall the physiological process of milk production. Breast emptying is required for continual milk production. Thus compressing the breast tissue would be the only way to suppress production. Eliminate options 2 and 4, as these do not address breast tissue compression.*

Content Area: Childbearing Families; *Category of Health Alteration:* Postpartum Management; *Integrated Processes:* Teaching and Learning; *Client Need:* Physiological Integrity/Reduction of Risk Potential/Potential for Complications from Surgical Procedures and Health Alterations; *Cognitive Level:* Analysis

References: Davidson, M., London, M., & Ladewig, P. (2008). *Olds' Maternal-Newborn Nursing & Women's Health Across the Lifespan* (8th ed., p. 1081). Upper Saddle River, NJ: Prentice Hall Health; Wong, D., Hockenberry, M., Wilson, D., Perry, S., & Lowdermilk, D. (2006). *Maternal Child Nursing Care* (3rd ed., p. 783). Philadelphia: Lippincott Williams & Wilkins.

---

386. EBP A postpartum client, who is 24 hours post-cesarean section, tells a nurse that she has had much less lochial discharge after this birth than she had with her vaginal birth 2 years ago. The client asks the nurse if this is a normal response to a cesarean birth. Which statement should be the basis for the nurse's response?

1. A decrease in lochia is not expected after cesarean section and further assessment is needed.
2. Women usually have increased lochial discharge after cesarean births.
3. Women normally have less lochia after cesarean births.
4. The amount of lochial discharge after cesarean section is related to method of placental delivery and whether the surgery was emergent or planned.

ANSWER: 3

Lochial discharge may be decreased in a woman after cesarean birth because the uterus is cleaned during surgery. Some lochia will always be present, and a total lack of lochia discharge should be reported to the health-care provider. The amount of lochia is not dependent on whether the surgery was emergent or planned or how the placenta was delivered.

➧ ***Test-taking Tip:*** *Knowledge of the cesarean surgical procedure is required to correctly answer this question.*

Content Area: Childbearing Families; *Category of Health Alteration:* Postpartum Management; *Integrated Processes:* Nursing Process Planning; *Client Need:* Physiological Integrity/Reduction of Risk Potential/System Specific Assessments; *Cognitive Level:* Application

Reference: Pillitteri, A. (2007). *Maternal & Child Health Nursing: Care of the Childbearing Families & Childrearing Family* (5th ed., p. 579). Philadelphia: Lippincott Williams & Wilkins.

EBP References: Bollapragada, S., & Edozien, L. (2002). Apparent absence of lochia after elective caesarean section. *Journal of Obstetrics and Gynecology, 22*(5), 558; Anorlu, R., Maholwana, B., & Hofmeyr, G. (2008). Methods of delivering the placenta at caesarean section. *Cochrane Database of Systematic Reviews,* Issue 3 Art. No. CD004737. DOI: 10.1002/14651858.CD004737.pub2. Available at: www.cochrane.org/reviews/en/ab004737.html.

---

387. In the process of preparing a client for discharge after cesarean section, a nurse addresses all of the following areas during discharge education. Which should be the priority advice for the client?

1. How to manage her incision
2. The need to plan for assistance at home
3. Infant care procedures
4. Increased need for rest

ANSWER: 2

Research suggests that women with cesarean births have several special needs following discharge. These include the increased need for rest, knowledge about incisional care, pain control, and infant care. However, because the client has had a surgical procedure, the priority consideration is for the mother to plan for additional assistance at home. Without this assistance, it is difficult for the mother to get the rest she needs for healing, pain control, and appropriate infant care.

➧ ***Test-taking Tip:*** *Think about which option if not accomplished would have a negative effect on the other options.*

Content Area: Childbearing Families; *Category of Health Alteration:* Postpartum Management; *Integrated Processes:* Nursing Process Implementation; *Client Need:* Physiological Integrity/Reduction of Risk Potential/Potential for Complications from Surgical Procedures and Health Alterations; *Cognitive Level:* Analysis

Reference: Davidson, M., London, M., & Ladewig, P. (2008). *Olds' Maternal-Newborn Nursing & Women's Health Across the Lifespan* (8th ed., p. 1092). Upper Saddle River, NJ: Prentice Hall Health.

388. A postpartum client, who is 24 hours post-vaginal birth and breastfeeding, asks a nurse when she can begin exercising to regain her prepregnancy body shape. Which response by the nurse is correct?

1. "Simple abdominal and pelvic exercises can begin right now."
2. "You will need to wait until after your 6-week postpartum checkup."
3. "Once your lochia has stopped you can begin exercising."
4. "You should not exercise while you are breastfeeding."

ANSWER: 1

On the first postpartum day, the client should be taught to start abdominal breathing and pelvic rocking. Kegel exercises, which should have been taught during pregnancy, should be continued. Simple exercises should be added daily until, by 2 to 3 weeks postpartum, the mother should be able to do sit-ups and leg raises. There is no reason that a breastfeeding mother should not follow this exercise schedule.

➧ ***Test-taking Tip:*** *Recall health education about resuming exercise after vaginal birth.*

Content Area: Childbearing Families; *Category of Health Alteration:* Postpartum Management; *Integrated Processes:* Teaching and Learning; *Client Need:* Health Promotion and Maintenance/Self-Care; *Cognitive Level:* Application

References: Davidson, M., London, M., & Ladewig, P. (2008). *Olds' Maternal-Newborn Nursing & Women's Health Across the Lifespan* (8th ed., pp. 1085–1086). Upper Saddle River, NJ: Prentice Hall Health; Wong, D., Hockenberry, M., Wilson, D., Perry, S., & Lowdermilk, D. (2006). *Maternal Child Nursing Care* (3rd ed., p. 781). Philadelphia: Lippincott Williams & Wilkins.

389. In the process of teaching a Muslim woman to breastfeed her infant, a nurse spends time with the mother attempting to help the baby correctly latch to the breast. During the teaching session, two student nurses are observing the instruction. Later that day, the client requests that the nurse who had given the breastfeeding instructions not be allowed to continue to provide her postpartum care. What most likely caused the client to be uncomfortable with the first nurse?

1. Muslim women do not want to breastfeed while in the hospital.
2. Muslim women prefer to wait for their milk to come in before they breastfeed.
3. Muslim women are uncomfortable breastfeeding in public situations.
4. Muslim women only breastfeed after the infant is given boiled water.

ANSWER: 3

Most Muslim women breastfeed because the Koran encourages it; however, they are uncomfortable about breastfeeding in public situations and prefer privacy. Having two students observing the feeding process most likely would make the client uncomfortable, as she would desire more privacy. Options 1, 2, and 4 are seen in other cultures. For example, Korean mothers resist breastfeeding in the hospital, and some Asian women believe colostrum is "bad" and therefore they do not feed until actual breast milk is present. Some Asian cultures also believe the newborn must be given boiled water until the milk is actually present.

➧ ***Test-taking Tip:*** *The key to this question is not only the culture of the client but also the fact that two students were present during the initial feeding process. Relate this most closely to a lack of privacy and select option 3.*

Content Area: Childbearing Families; *Category of Health Alteration:* Postpartum Management; *Integrated Processes:* Nursing Process Analysis; *Client Need:* Psychosocial Integrity/Cultural Diversity; *Cognitive Level:* Analysis

Reference: Davidson, M., London, M., & Ladewig, P. (2008). *Olds' Maternal-Newborn Nursing & Women's Health Across the Lifespan* (8th ed., pp. 919–920). Upper Saddle River, NJ: Prentice Hall Health.

390. While evaluating a breastfeeding session, a nurse determines that the infant has appropriately latched on to the mother's breast when which observations are made? SELECT ALL THAT APPLY.

1. The mother reports a firm tugging feeling on her nipple
2. A smacking sound is heard each time the baby sucks
3. The baby's mouth covers only the mother's nipple
4. The baby's nose, mouth, and chin are all touching the breast
5. The baby sucks with cheeks rounded
6. Swallowing is audible

ANSWER: 1, 4, 5, 6

When an infant is correctly latched to the breast, 2 to 3 centimeters (1/3 to 3/4 inch) of areola should be covered by the infant's mouth. If this occurs, it will result in the infant's nose, mouth, and chin touching the breast. The mother should not feel pain or pinching when the infant sucks if the latch is correct. Rather, she should feel only a firm tugging. When the infant is latched correctly, the cheeks will be rounded rather than dimpled, and swallowing will be audible. A smacking or clicking noise heard when the infant sucks is an indication that the latch is incorrect and that the infant's tongue may be inappropriately placed. Sucking only on the mother's nipple will cause sore nipples and also will not result in ejection of the milk from the milk ducts.

➧ ***Test-taking Tip:*** *Recall lactation physiology concerning the collection of breast milk in the milk ducts under the areola. This should enable elimination of option 3, as only sucking on the mother's nipple would not cause compression of these ducts and would therefore not promote optimum milk flow from the breast.*

Content Area: Childbearing Families; *Category of Health Alteration:* Postpartum Management; *Integrated Processes:* Nursing Process Evaluation; *Client Need:* Physiological Integrity/Basic Care and Comfort/Nutrition and Oral Hydration; *Cognitive Level:* Application

Reference: Wong, D., Hockenberry, M., Wilson, D., Perry, S., & Lowdermilk, D. (2006). *Maternal Child Nursing Care* (3rd ed., p. 776). Philadelphia: Lippincott Williams & Wilkins.

---

391. A primiparous client, who is bottle feeding her infant, asks a nurse when she can expect to start having her menstrual cycle again. Which response by the nurse is most accurate?

1. "Most women who bottle feed their infants can expect their periods to return within 6 to 10 weeks after birth."
2. "Your period should return a few days after your lochial discharge stops."
3. "You will notice a change in your vaginal discharge from pink to white; once that happens your period should return within a week."
4. "Bottle feeding will delay the return of a normal menstrual cycle until 6 months post-birth."

ANSWER: 1

In nonlactating women, the average time to first ovulation is 45 days and the return of menstruation usually happens within 6 to 10 weeks post birth. Most women can expect to have lochial discharge for up to 24 days. However, the cessation of discharge is not related to the return of menstruation. The return of ovulation and menstruation is associated with a rise in serum progesterone levels. Bottle feeding does not affect when this change occurs in the woman's body.

➧ ***Test-taking Tip:*** *Eliminate options that relate lochia to the return of menstruation.*

Content Area: Childbearing Families; *Category of Health Alteration:* Postpartum Management; *Integrated Processes:* Teaching and Learning; *Client Need:* Health Promotion and Maintenance/Ante/Intra/Postpartum and Newborn Care; *Cognitive Level:* Application

Reference: Davidson, M., London, M., & Ladewig, P. (2008). *Olds' Maternal-Newborn Nursing & Women's Health Across the Lifespan* (8th ed., p. 1043). Upper Saddle River, NJ: Prentice Hall Health.

---

392. While in the hospital after the birth of her first child, a 25-year-old single client tells a nurse that she has several different male sex partners and asks the nurse to recommend an appropriate birth control method for her. Considering her lifestyle, the nurse recognizes that which method of birth control would be contraindicated for this client?

1. An intrauterine device (IUD)
2. Depot-medroxyprogesterone acetate (Depo-Provera®) injections
3. A female condom
4. A diaphragm

ANSWER: 1

IUDs offer no protection against sexually transmitted diseases (STDs), and they are recommended for women who are in a stable, mutually monogamous relationship. A female condom does provide protection against some of the pathogens that cause STDs, and it would be readily available over the counter. A diaphragm would have to be fitted by a health-care practitioner, but, after that, it would be readily available to the client. Depo-Provera® is a long-acting progestin that is highly effective for birth control. A single injection will provide contraception for 3 months but does not offer protection against STDs.

➧ ***Test-taking Tip:*** *The phrase "a method of birth control that would be contraindicated for this client" is a false-response item. Select the incorrect statement.*

Content Area: Childbearing Families; *Category of Health Alteration:* Postpartum Management; *Integrated Processes:* Nursing Process Analysis; *Client Need:* Health Promotion and Maintenance/Developmental Stages and Transitions; *Cognitive Level:* Analysis

Reference: Davidson, M., London, M., & Ladewig, P. (2008). *Olds' Maternal-Newborn Nursing & Women's Health Across the Lifespan* (8th ed., pp. 93–94, 97). Upper Saddle River, NJ: Prentice Hall Health.

393. EBP After delivering a full-term infant, a breastfeeding mother, who is preparing for discharge, asks a nurse if there is any type of contraceptive method that should be avoided while she is breastfeeding. Which contraceptive should the nurse advise the client to avoid?

1. A diaphragm
2. An intrauterine device (IUD)
3. The combined oral contraceptive (COC) pill
4. The progesterone-only mini pill

ANSWER: 3

Birth control pills containing progesterone and estrogen (COC) can cause a decrease in milk volume and may affect the quality of the breast milk. The progesterone-only mini pill may be used by breastfeeding clients because it does not interfere with breast milk production. However, it is recommended that the mother wait 6 to 8 weeks before starting this method of contraception. After childbirth, the external cervical os is markedly irregular and closes slowly. Because a diaphragm must be fitted to the individual female cervix, the diaphragm must be rechecked for correct size after each childbirth; however, use of the diaphragm will not affect breast milk production. An IUD will not affect breast milk production unless the IUD is inserted within the first 48 hours postpartum; insertion should be delayed until 4 weeks postpartum.

▶ ***Test-taking Tip:*** *Eliminate option 1, as a diaphragm is a barrier device inserted over the cervix. It would be impossible for this device to affect the breastfeeding process.*

Content Area: Childbearing Families; *Category of Health Alteration:* Postpartum Management; *Integrated Processes:* Teaching and Learning; *Client Need:* Health Promotion and Maintenance/Developmental Stages and Transitions; *Cognitive Level:* Analysis

Reference: Davidson, M., London, M., & Ladewig, P. (2008). *Olds' Maternal-Newborn Nursing & Women's Health Across the Lifespan* (8th ed., 94, 99, 901, 1043). Upper Saddle River, NJ: Prentice Hall Health.

EBP Reference: Faculty of Family Planning and Reproductive Health Care Clinical Effectiveness Unit. (2004). Contraceptive choices for breastfeeding women. *Journal of Family Planning and Reproductive Health Care*, *30*(3), 181–189. Available at: www.guideline.gov/summary/summary.aspx?doc_id=7098&nbr=004270&string=IUD

394. While assessing a breastfeeding mother 24 hours postdelivery, a nurse notes that the client's breasts are hard and painful. In response to this assessment finding, which interventions should be implemented by the nurse? SELECT ALL THAT APPLY.

1. Instructing the mother to breastfeed the infant from both breasts at each feeding
2. Applying ice to the breasts at intervals between feedings
3. Giving supplemental formula at least one time in a 24-hour period
4. Administering anti-inflammatory medication
5. Applying warm, moist packs to the breast between feedings
6. Pumping the breasts as needed to ensure complete emptying

ANSWER: 2, 4, 6

Because engorgement is caused, in part, by swelling of the breast tissue surrounding the milk gland ducts, applying ice at intervals between feedings will help to decrease this swelling. Administering anti-inflammatory medication will also decrease breast pain and inflammation. Pumping the breasts may be necessary if the infant is unable to completely empty both breasts at each feeding. Pumping at this time will not cause a problematic increase in breast milk production. Moving the baby from the initial breast to the second breast during the feeding, before that breast is completely emptied, may result in neither breast being totally emptied and thus promote continued engorgement. Keeping the infant on the first breast until it is soft ensures that that breast has been emptied completely and allows the baby to receive the calorie-dense hind milk. The next feeding should then be initiated on the second breast. Giving supplemental formula and limiting the time the baby nurses at the breast also prevents total emptying of the breast and thus promotes increased engorgement. Because heat application increases blood flow, moist heat packs would exacerbate the engorgement.

▶ ***Test-taking Tip:*** *Giving supplemental formula to a healthy, breastfeeding baby is always contraindicated. Eliminate option 3. Since heat and cold applications cause opposite physiological body responses, do not select both options 2 and 5. Recall that engorgement is caused by increased blood flow to the breast and eliminate option 5 as counterproductive.*

Content Area: Childbearing Families; *Category of Health Alteration:* Postpartum Management; *Integrated Processes:* Nursing Process Implementation; *Client Need:* Health Promotion and Maintenance/Ante/Intra/Postpartum and Newborn Care; *Cognitive Level:* Application

References: Davidson, M., London, M., & Ladewig, P. (2008). *Olds' Maternal-Newborn Nursing & Women's Health Across the Lifespan* (8th ed., pp. 1126–1127). Upper Saddle River, NJ: Prentice Hall Health; Wong, D., Hockenberry, M., Wilson, D., Perry, S., & Lowdermilk, D. (2006). *Maternal Child Nursing Care* (3rd ed., pp. 777, 783). Philadelphia: Lippincott Williams & Wilkins.

395. A client who has been diagnosed with mastitis asks a nurse if she should stop breastfeeding since she has developed a breast infection. Which response by the nurse is best?

1. "Continuing to breastfeed will decrease the duration of the mastitis."
2. "Breastfeeding should only be continued if symptoms decrease."
3. "It is a good idea to discontinue feeding for 24 hours until antibiotic therapy begins to take effect."
4. "It is appropriate to discontinue breastfeeding because the infant may become infected."

ANSWER: 1

Improved outcomes, a decreased duration of symptoms, and decreased incidence of a breast abscess result if the breasts continue to be emptied by either breastfeeding or pumping. Thus continuing to breastfeed is recommended when the client has mastitis. The most common source of the organism that causes mastitis is the infant's nose and throat. Infants of women with mastitis generally remain well; therefore, concern that the mother will infect the infant if she continues breastfeeding is unwarranted.

▸ ***Test-taking Tip:*** *Recall that a major risk for mastitis development is poorly emptied breasts and plugged milk ducts. Discontinuing or decreasing breastfeeding would therefore be detrimental to the client with mastitis.*

Content Area: Childbearing Families; *Category of Health Alteration:* Postpartum Management; *Integrated Processes:* Nursing Process Implementation; *Client Need:* Physiological Integrity/Physiological Adaptation/Illness Management; *Cognitive Level:* Application

References: Davidson, M., London, M., & Ladewig, P. (2008). *Olds' Maternal-Newborn Nursing & Women's Health Across the Lifespan* (8th ed., pp. 1174–1175). Upper Saddle River, NJ: Prentice Hall Health; Wong, D., Hockenberry, M., Wilson, D., Perry, S., & Lowdermilk, D. (2006). *Maternal Child Nursing Care* (3rd ed., p. 785). Philadelphia: Lippincott Williams & Wilkins.

396. Before beginning an admission interview, a nurse reviews the health records of a 25-year-old postpartum client. After reading that the client is being admitted for mastitis, which interventions should the nurse anticipate including in the client's plan of care? SELECT ALL THAT APPLY.

1. Encouraging ambulation at least four times in 24 hours
2. Antibiotics
3. Local application of warm moist packs
4. Non steroidal anti-inflammatory agents
5. Decreasing oral fluid intake to 1,000 mL per day
6. Frequent emptying of the breasts

ANSWER: 2, 3, 4, 6

Treatment for mastitis includes administration of antibiotics to treat the infection and anti-inflammatory medications to treat fever and decrease breast inflammation. Improved outcomes, a decreased duration of symptoms, and decreased incidence of a breast abscess result if the breasts continue to be emptied by either breastfeeding or pumping. Application of warm packs decreases pain and promotes milk flow and breast emptying. Rest is extremely important to promote healing and bedrest may be ordered initially for 24 hours. Increasing fluid intake to at least 2 to 3 liters is recommended.

▸ ***Test-taking Tip:*** *Read the question carefully; it is asking for the recommended treatment plan for mastitis.*

Content Area: Childbearing Families; *Category of Health Alteration:* Postpartum Management; *Integrated Processes:* Nursing Process Planning; *Client Need:* Physiological Integrity/Physiological Adaptation/Illness Management; *Cognitive Level:* Application

References: Davidson, M., London, M., & Ladewig, P. (2008). *Olds' Maternal-Newborn Nursing & Women's Health Across the Lifespan* (8th ed., p. 1174). Upper Saddle River, NJ: Prentice Hall Health; Wong, D., Hockenberry, M., Wilson, D., Perry, S., & Lowdermilk, D. (2006). *Maternal Child Nursing Care* (3rd ed., p. 785). Philadelphia: Lippincott Williams & Wilkins.

397. EBP While assisting with the delivery of a term newborn, which intervention should a nurse anticipate to prevent postpartum hemorrhage during the third stage of labor?

1. Administration of intravenous oxytocin (Pitocin®)
2. Application of fundal pressure
3. Clamping the umbilical cord before pulsations stop
4. Administration of subcutaneous terbutaline sulfate (Brethine®)

ANSWER: 1

Active management of third-stage labor has been shown to decrease the risk of postpartum hemorrhage. Active management includes administration of oxytocin as the anterior shoulder of the infant is being delivered. Oxytocin causes uterine contraction. Fundal pressure in the third stage of labor will not prevent postpartum hemorrhage and is not routinely used because it may damage the uterine supports, invert the uterus, and is painful for the mother. Early clamping and cutting of the cord before pulsations have stopped has been deleted from the official definition of active management as it does not decrease the risk for postpartum hemorrhage. Terbutaline is a beta-mimetic agent that causes uterine relaxation. This would be contraindicated during the third stage of labor. The placenta cannot detach if the uterus is relaxed because the placental site is not reduced in size. The major cause of postpartum hemorrhage is uterine atony.

▸ ***Test-taking Tip:*** *Recall that uterine atony is the major cause of postpartum hemorrhage. Since terbutaline is a medication that relaxes the uterus, this drug would not be used to prevent hemorrhage. Eliminate option 4.*

Content Area: Childbearing Families; *Category of Health Alteration:* Postpartum Management; *Integrated Processes:* Nursing Process Planning; *Client Need:* Physiological Integrity/Reduction of Risk Potential/Potential for Alterations in Body Systems; *Cognitive Level:* Application

References: Davidson, M., London, M., & Ladewig, P. (2008). *Olds' Maternal-Newborn Nursing & Women's Health Across the Lifespan* (8th ed., pp. 674, 761, 1159). Upper Saddle River, NJ: Prentice Hall Health; Wong, D., Hockenberry, M., Wilson, D., Perry, S., & Lowdermilk, D. (2006). *Maternal Child Nursing Care* (3rd ed., p. 536). Philadelphia: Lippincott Williams & Wilkins.

EBP Reference: Anderson, J., & Etches, D. (2007). Prevention and management of postpartum hemorrhage. *American Family Physician, 75*(6), 875–882.

---

398. While working in a perinatal clinic, a nurse receives a phone call from a client who is 20 days postpartum. The client tells the nurse she has been having heavy, bright red bleeding since leaving the hospital 18 days ago. She is concerned and wonders what she should do. Which instruction to the client is correct?

1. Come to the clinic immediately
2. Decrease physical activity until the bleeding stops
3. Stop being concerned because this is expected after birth
4. Call again next week if the bleeding has not stopped by then

ANSWER: 1

Lochia rubra that persists for longer than 2 weeks is suggestive of subinvolution of the uterus, which is the most common cause of delayed postpartum hemorrhage. The client should be seen in the clinic immediately to determine what is causing her abnormal lochial discharge. Lochia rubra is expected to last for up to 3 days after birth and then the lochia becomes serosa and eventually alba. Increased physical activity can lead to increased lochial discharge; however, the client in the question is reporting continuous lochia rubra, which is abnormal.

➧ ***Test-taking Tip:*** *To answer this question correctly, recall that lochia rubra should last only 3 days postpartum.*

Content Area: Childbearing Families; *Category of Health Alteration:* Postpartum Management; *Integrated Processes:* Nursing Process Analysis; *Client Need:* Physiological Integrity/Reduction of Risk Potential/Potential for Alterations in Body Systems; *Cognitive Level:* Analysis

Reference: Davidson, M., London, M., & Ladewig, P. (2008). *Olds' Maternal-Newborn Nursing & Women's Health Across the Lifespan* (8th ed., pp. 1042, 1085, 1163). Upper Saddle River, NJ: Prentice Hall Health.

---

399. A nurse has been given a report on a postpartum client that includes the information that the client suffered a fourth-degree perineal laceration during her vaginal birth. In response to this information, which intervention should the nurse add to the client's plan of care?

1. Limit ambulation to bathroom privileges only.
2. Monitor the uterus for firmness every 2 hours.
3. Instruct the client on a high-fiber diet and administer stool softeners.
4. Decrease fluid intake to 1,000 mL every 24 hours.

ANSWER: 3

To help maintain bowel continence and decrease perineal trauma from constipation, the client with a third- or fourth-degree laceration should be instructed to increase dietary fiber and take stool softeners. Activity and fluids should also be increased, not decreased, to reduce the potential for constipation. A perineal laceration will not affect the condition of the uterus; therefore, there is no need to increase uterine monitoring over the unit standard of care.

➧ ***Test-taking Tip:*** *Eliminate any option that addresses the uterus as the question is concerning the perineum.*

Content Area: Childbearing Families; *Category of Health Alteration:* Postpartum Management; *Integrated Processes:* Nursing Process Planning; *Client Need:* Physiological Integrity/Reduction of Risk Potential/Potential for Complications from Surgical Procedures and Health Alterations; *Cognitive Level:* Application

References: Wong, D., Hockenberry, M., Wilson, D., Perry, S., & Lowdermilk, D. (2006). *Maternal Child Nursing Care* (3rd ed., p. 534). Philadelphia: Lippincott Williams & Wilkins; Pillitteri, A. (2007). *Maternal & Child Health Nursing: Care of the Childbearing Families & Childrearing Family* (5th ed., p. 661). Philadelphia: Lippincott Williams & Wilkins.

400. A postpartum client, who had a forceps-assisted vaginal birth 4 hours ago, calls a nurse to her room to report continuing perineal pain rated at 7 out of 10 on a numeric scale and rectal pressure, even though an oral analgesic was given and ice applied to the perineum. Considering this information, what should be the nurse's *next* intervention?

1. Call the health-care provider (HCP) to report the pain level
2. Closely reinspect the perineum
3. Encourage ambulation
4. Administer a stool softener

ANSWER: 2

Use of forceps for delivery places the client at risk for development of perineal hematomas. A symptom of a perineal hematoma is perineal pain, which is intense and disproportionate to initial objective findings. Also, if the hematoma is located in the posterior vaginal wall, the client may experience rectal pressure. If a hematoma is suspected, the nurse should closely examine the perineum and the vaginal introitus for ecchymosis and a bulging mass. Reexamination of the perineum should be completed before calling the HCP to report the pain level. A stool softener would be appropriate to avoid constipation but would not help the immediate problem. Ambulation also would not help the immediate pain concern.

➧ ***Test-taking Tip:*** *The key to this question is the nurse's "next intervention." Managing pain is always a priority; however, complete assessment should be the initial approach to allow the gathering of enough data to determine the appropriate course of action.*

Content Area: Childbearing Families; *Category of Health Alteration:* Postpartum Management; *Integrated Processes:* Nursing Process Analysis; *Client Need:* Physiological Integrity/Reduction of Risk Potential/Potential for Complications of Diagnostic Tests/Treatments/ Procedures; *Cognitive Level:* Analysis

Reference: Davidson, M., London, M., & Ladewig, P. (2008). *Olds' Maternal-Newborn Nursing & Women's Health Across the Lifespan* (8th ed., p. 1162). Upper Saddle River, NJ: Prentice Hall Health.

---

401. A postpartum client is being discharged to home with a streptococcal puerperal infection. The client is taking antibiotics but asks a nurse what precautions she should take at home to prevent spreading the infection to her husband, newborn, and toddler. Which is the best response by the nurse?

1. "You should wear a mask when caring for your newborn and toddler."
2. "You need to perform hand hygiene before caring for your children and after toileting and perineal care."
3. "Your husband should provide all of the care for both children until your infection is gone."
4. "No precautions are necessary since you are taking antibiotics."

ANSWER: 2

In addition to standard precautions, no additional precautions need to be taken by the client in her home. The course of an endometrial infection is approximately 7 to 10 days and thus standard precautions should be in place for that period of time even if the client has started antibiotics.

➧ ***Test-taking Tip:*** *Eliminate option 1, as puerperal infections are not spread by droplets and thus a mask would not be necessary.*

Content Area: Childbearing Families; *Category of Health Alteration:* Postpartum Management; *Integrated Processes:* Teaching and Learning; *Client Need:* Safe and Effective Care Environment/Safety and Infection Control/Standard/Transmission-based/Other Precautions; *Cognitive Level:* Application

References: Davidson, M., London, M., & Ladewig, P. (2008). *Olds' Maternal-Newborn Nursing & Women's Health Across the Lifespan* (8th ed., p. 1169). Upper Saddle River, NJ: Prentice Hall Health; Pillitteri, A. (2007). *Maternal & Child Health Nursing: Care of the Childbearing Families & Childrearing Family* (5th ed., p. 666). Philadelphia: Lippincott Williams & Wilkins.

402. EBP A student nurse is assisting a registered nurse (RN) in the care of a postpartum client who is 48 hours post–vaginal delivery. The student reports finding a warm, red, tender area on the client's left calf. The nurse assesses the client and explains to the student that postpartum clients are at increased risk for thrombophlebitis because of which of the following? SELECT ALL THAT APPLY.

1. The fibrinogen levels in the blood are elevated.
2. Fluids normally shift from the interstitial to the intravascular space.
3. Postpartum hormonal shifts irritate vascular basement membranes.
4. The legs are elevated in stirrups at the time of delivery.
5. Dilation of the veins in the lower extremities is present.
6. Compression of the common iliac vein occurs during pregnancy.

ANSWER: 1, 4, 5, 6

Major causes of thromboembolic disease are hypercoagulability of the blood and venous stasis. During pregnancy, fibrinogen levels increase, and this increase continues to be present in the postpartum period. Elevation of the legs in stirrups during delivery leads to pooling of blood and vascular stasis. Dilation of the veins in the lower extremities occurs during pregnancy as does compression of the common iliac vein. Both of these pregnancy changes increase the risk of venous stasis. There is not a shift of fluid from the interstitial to the vascular spaces in the postpartum period. Actual blood volume increases during pregnancy and is further increased immediately after delivery. This fluid volume is eventually lost through diuresis during the first postpartum week. Postpartum hormonal changes do occur but they do not affect the vascular basement membranes.

➧ ***Test-taking Tip:*** *Recall the physiological causes of thrombophlebitis, which are blood stasis and increased blood coagulability, to answer this question correctly.*

Content Area: Childbearing Families; *Category of Health Alteration:* Postpartum Management; *Integrated Processes:* Teaching and Learning; *Client Need:* Physiological Integrity/Physiological Adaptation/Pathophysiology; *Cognitive Level:* Application

References: Pillitteri, A. (2007). *Maternal & Child Health Nursing: Care of the Childbearing Families & Childrearing Family* (5th ed., p. 667). Philadelphia: Lippincott Williams & Wilkins; Davidson, M., London, M., & Ladewig, P. (2008). *Olds' Maternal-Newborn Nursing & Women's Health Across the Lifespan* (8th ed., pp. 317, 1046, 1176, 1179). Upper Saddle River, NJ: Prentice Hall Health.

EBP Reference: Finnish Medical Society Duodecim. (2006). *Deep Vein Thrombosis*. Hoboken, NJ: Wiley Interscience. John Wiley & Sons. Available at: www.guideline.gov/summary/summary.aspx?doc_id=9314&nbr=004983&string=postpartum+AND+thrombophlebitis

403. A nurse enters the room of a postpartum client who delivered a healthy newborn 36 hours previously. The nurse finds the client crying. When asked what is wrong, the client replies, "Nothing really. I'm not in pain or anything but I just seem to cry a lot for no reason." Based on this information, what should be the nurse's *first* intervention?

1. Call the client's support person to come and sit with her.
2. Remind the client that she has a healthy baby and there is nothing to cry about.
3. Call the health-care provider (HCP) immediately and report the incidence.
4. Ask the client to discuss her birth experience.

ANSWER: 4

A key feature of postpartum blues is episodic tearfulness without identifiable reason. Interventions for postpartum blues include allowing the client to relive her birth experience. The client's support person should be given information about postpartum blues before the client is discharged from the hospital. However, contacting that individual should not be the first intervention. There is no need to notify the HCP, as postpartum blues is a common self-limiting postpartum occurrence. Reminding the client that she has a healthy baby is a nontherapeutic communication technique that implies disapproval of the client's actions.

➧ ***Test-taking Tip:*** *Eliminate option 2, as this is a nontherapeutic response to the specific situation. Since this is not an emergent situation, eliminate option 3; there is no need to notify the HCP immediately.*

Content Area: Childbearing Families; *Category of Health Alteration:* Postpartum Management; *Integrated Processes:* Nursing Process Implementation; *Client Need:* Psychosocial Integrity/Therapeutic Communications; *Cognitive Level:* Application

References: Davidson, M., London, M., & Ladewig, P. (2008). *Olds' Maternal-Newborn Nursing & Women's Health Across the Lifespan* (8th ed., p. 1184). Upper Saddle River, NJ: Prentice Hall Health; Potter, P., & Perry, A. (2009). *Fundamentals of Nursing* (7th ed., pp. 355–356). St. Louis, MO: Mosby.

404. EBP As part of discharge education for a postpartum client, a nurse suggests prevention strategies for postpartum depression. Which prevention strategies should the nurse include when educating the client on postpartum depression? SELECT ALL THAT APPLY.

1. Attending a postpartum support group
2. Using the baby's nap time to complete household chores
3. Keeping a journal of feelings during the postpartum period
4. Notifying the health-care provider if feelings of being overwhelmed do not subside quickly.
5. Setting a daily schedule and following it
6. Completing major life changes within the first year after the birth

ANSWER: 1, 3, 4, 5

A postpartum support group can be a place where realistic information about postpartum depression can be discussed and symptoms recognized. Keeping a journal can be emotionally cathartic. Structuring activity with a schedule helps counteract inertia that comes with feeling sad or unsettled. Postpartum mothers should be encouraged to call their health-care providers if symptoms of postpartum depression, such as feelings of being overwhelmed, do not subside quickly or if the symptoms become severe. The presence of three symptoms on 1 day or one symptom for three days requires immediate attention. Fatigue is a major concern for all postpartum women. Clients should be encouraged to nap when their infant is napping rather than using that time for other activities. Other life stressors, such as major life changes, should be limited as much as possible until the infant is at least 1 year old.

➧ ***Test-taking Tip:*** *Think about activities that would decrease stress in general. Remember that problem-specific support groups are frequently utilized for psychological support no matter what the client's specific concern. Select option 1 for that reason.*

Content Area: Childbearing Families; *Category of Health Alteration:* Postpartum Management; *Integrated Processes:* Teaching and Learning; *Client Need:* Health Promotion and Maintenance/Disease Prevention; *Cognitive Level:* Application

Reference: Davidson, M., London, M., & Ladewig, P. (2008). *Olds' Maternal-Newborn Nursing & Women's Health Across the Lifespan* (8th ed., pp. 1185, 1188–1190). Upper Saddle River, NJ: Prentice Hall Health.

EBP Reference: Dennis, C., & Chung-Lee, L. (2006). Postpartum depression help-seeking barriers and maternal treatment preferences: A qualitative systematic review. *Birth*, *33*(4), 323–331.

---

405. The husband of a postpartum client, who has been diagnosed with postpartum depression (PPD), is concerned and asks a nurse what kind of treatment his wife will require. The nurse's response should be based on the knowledge that the collaborative plan of care for PPD includes which of the following?

1. Antidepressant medications and psychotherapy
2. Psychotherapy alone
3. Removal of the infant from the home
4. Hypnotic agents and psychotherapy

ANSWER: 1

Supportive treatment alone is not efficacious for PPD. Antidepressant medications and psychotherapy are required. If the client is displaying rejection of the infant or aggression toward the infant, she should not be left alone with the infant, but the infant does not need to be removed from the home. Hypnotic agents are medications that promote sleep and should not be used during the postpartum period.

➧ ***Test-taking Tip:*** *Recall that PPD is similar to depression, occurring at any time in an individual's life. Select the option that reflects best how depression is treated.*

Content Area: Childbearing Families; *Category of Health Alteration:* Postpartum Management; *Integrated Processes:* Nursing Process Planning; *Client Need:* Psychosocial Integrity/Crisis Intervention; *Cognitive Level:* Application

References: Wong, D., Hockenberry, M., Wilson, D., Perry, S., & Lowdermilk, D. (2006). *Maternal Child Nursing Care* (3rd ed., p. 675). Philadelphia: Lippincott Williams & Wilkins; Davidson, M., London, M., & Ladewig, P. (2008). *Olds' Maternal-Newborn Nursing & Women's Health Across the Lifespan* (8th ed., pp. 1185, 1189). Upper Saddle River, NJ: Prentice Hall Health; Lehne, R. (2007). *Pharmacology for Nursing Care* (6th ed., p. 363) St. Louis, MO: Saunders/Elsevier.

406. A nurse is caring for a postpartum client who is 15 years old. The nurse has concerns about this client's ability to parent a newborn because the nurse recognizes that developmentally the client is:

1. developing autonomy.
2. motivated to follow rules established by outside sources.
3. career oriented.
4. egocentric.

ANSWER: 4

Although it is biologically possible for the adolescent female to become a parent, her egocentricity and concrete thinking interfere with her ability to parent effectively. Because of this normal development, the adolescent may inadvertently neglect her child. The development of autonomy is a developmental task of toddlerhood. School-age children are motivated to follow rules established by others, and adult women are concerned about the effect of childbearing on careers.

➧ ***Test-taking Tip:*** *Read the question carefully. It is asking about developmental tasks of the adolescent.*

Content Area: Childbearing Families; *Category of Health Alteration:* Postpartum Management; *Integrated Processes:* Nursing Process Planning; *Client Need:* Health Promotion and Maintenance/Growth and Development; *Cognitive Level:* Application

Reference: Wong, D., Hockenberry, M., Wilson, D., Perry, S., & Lowdermilk, D. (2006). *Maternal Child Nursing Care* (3rd ed., pp. 643, 645, 1091, 1155). Philadelphia: Lippincott Williams & Wilkins.

Test 11: **Childbearing Families: Neonatal and High-Risk Neonatal Management**

407. A nurse meets a frantic father at an emergency department door who says he just delivered a full-term newborn baby in the car in the hospital parking lot. It is winter and the temperature outside is only 10°F (−12.2°C). In response to the cold environment, the nurse knows that the infant's body will immediately begin to produce heat by:

1. shivering.
2. metabolizing brown fat.
3. dilation of surface blood vessels.
4. decreasing flexion of the extremities.

ANSWER: 2

Brown adipose tissue first appears in the fetus at 26 to 30 weeks gestation. The ability to utilize brown adipose tissue (brown fat) to produce nonshivering thermogenesis is unique to full-term newborns. When skin receptors perceive a drop in environmental temperature, the sympathetic nervous system is stimulated. This in turn stimulates metabolism of brown fat, thus producing heat that is transferred to the peripheral circulation. Shivering is rarely seen in newborns, and it does little to produce heat. Newborns are able to conserve body heat by constricting blood vessels. Full-term newborns normally maintain a flexed posture, which decreases the skin surface area exposed to the environment and thus reduces heat loss. Decreasing flexion promotes heat loss in full-term newborns.

▶ ***Test-taking Tip:*** *Determine the best answer based on your knowledge of the physiological differences in adult and newborn metabolism.*

Content Area: Childbearing Families; *Category of Health Alteration:* Neonatal and High-Risk Neonatal Management; *Integrated Processes:* Nursing Process Analysis; *Client Need:* Physiological Integrity/Physiological Adaptation/Alterations in Body Systems; *Cognitive Level:* Application

References: Davidson, M., London, M., & Ladewig, P. (2008). *Olds' Maternal-Newborn Nursing & Women's Health Across the Lifespan* (8th ed., pp. 803–805). Upper Saddle River, NJ: Prentice Hall Health; Pillitteri, A. (2007). *Maternal & Child Health Nursing: Care of the Childbearing & Childrearing Family* (5th ed., p. 682). Philadelphia: Lippincott Williams & Wilkins; Wong, D., Hockenberry, M., Wilson, D., Perry, S., & Lowdermilk, D. (2006). *Maternal Child Nursing Care* (3rd ed., p. 707). Philadelphia: Lippincott Williams & Wilkins.

408. At a prenatal class, a nurse is discussing changes that occur in newborn circulation at birth. The nurse utilizes a picture of the fetal heart to explain that functional closure of the ductus arteriosus occurs within 15 hours after birth. Place an X on the fetal heart structure that the nurse would identify as the ductus arteriosus.

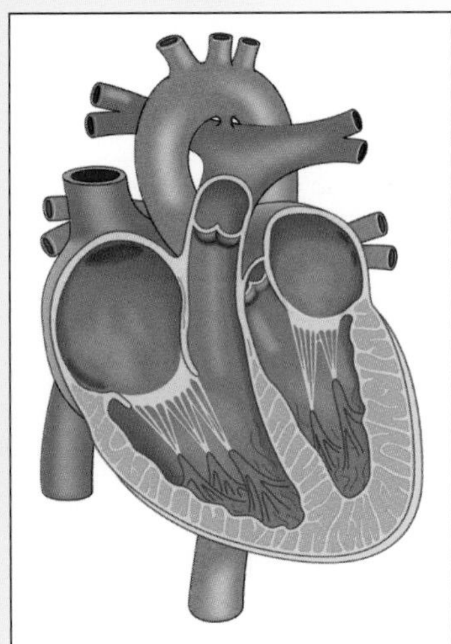

ANSWER:

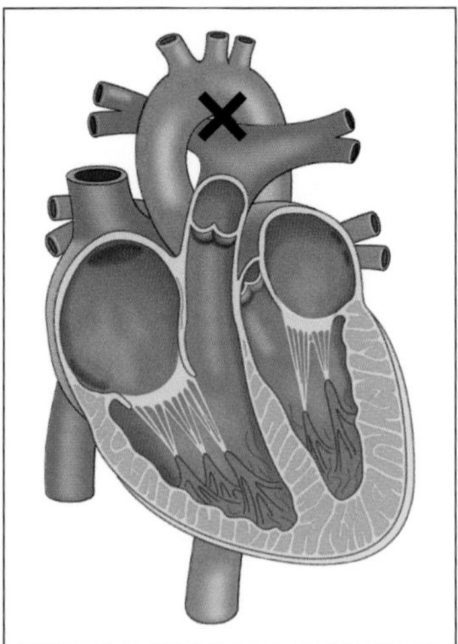

Oxygenation of the fetal blood is accomplished via diffusion from maternal circulation; therefore fetal lungs need limited amounts of blood. The ductus arteriosus connects the pulmonary artery to the descending aorta and acts as a shunt to carry blood directly from the right ventricle into the aorta.

▶ ***Test-taking Tip:*** *Focus on the differences between adult and fetal circulation to answer this question. Also note the term "ductus arteriosus," which indicates arterial connections.*

Content Area: Childbearing Families; *Category of Health Alteration:* Neonatal and High-Risk Neonatal Management; *Integrated Processes:* Teaching and Learning; *Client Need:* Physiological Integrity/ Physiological Adaptation/Hemodynamics; *Cognitive Level:* Application

Reference: Davidson, M., London, M., & Ladewig, P. (2008). *Olds' Maternal-Newborn Nursing & Women's Health Across the Lifespan* (8th ed., pp. 247–248, 799). Upper Saddle River, NJ: Prentice Hall Health.

---

409. While completing an assessment on a 4-hours-old newborn, a nurse notes the following documentation in the newborn's chart: "clamping of the umbilical cord was delayed until cord pulsations ceased." The nurse anticipates that this delayed cord clamping will result in:

1. more rapid expulsion of meconium from the newborn intestinal tract.
2. increased newborn alertness after birth.
3. an increase in initial newborn temperature.
4. an increase in the newborn's hemoglobin and hematocrit.

ANSWER: 4

Newborn hemoglobin and hematocrit values will be higher when placental transfusion, accomplished through delayed cord clamping, occurs at birth. Blood volume increases by up to 50% with delayed cord clamping. Full-term newborns normally pass meconium naturally within 8 to 24 hours after birth. In the later weeks of pregnancy, the intestinal peristalsis becomes active in preparation for meconium passage after birth. Delayed clamping of the umbilical cord will not affect this process. At birth, the newborn's temperature may fall due to evaporative heat loss. Delayed cord clamping will not affect this evaporation process. The healthy newborn is born awake and active. This period of alertness typically lasts for 30 minutes after birth and is known as the first period of reactivity. This will not be affected by delayed cord clamping.

► ***Test-taking Tip:*** *Recall that blood travels from the mother to the fetus via the umbilical cord. Option 4 is most related to circulation and therefore would be the best selection.*

Content Area: Childbearing Families; *Category of Health Alteration:* Neonatal and High-Risk Neonatal Management; *Integrated Processes:* Nursing Process Analysis; *Client Need:* Physiological Integrity/ Physiological Adaptation/Hemodynamics; *Cognitive Level:* Analysis

References: Pillitteri, A. (2007). *Maternal & Child Health Nursing: Care of the Childbearing & Childrearing Family* (5th ed., p. 537). Philadelphia: Lippincott Williams & Wilkins; Davidson, M., London, M., & Ladewig, P. (2008). *Olds' Maternal-Newborn Nursing & Women's Health Across the Lifespan* (8th ed., pp. 801–802, 810, 813). Upper Saddle River, NJ: Prentice Hall Health.

---

410. EBP A nurse is completing the 1-minute Apgar assessment on a full-term newborn. The heart rate is 80 beats per minute. In response to this assessment, the nurse should:

1. document a 2 for the heart rate parameter of the Apgar score.
2. document a 0 for the heart rate parameter of the Apgar score.
3. continue to evaluate the rest of the Apgar scoring parameters before determining a heart rate score.
4. begin immediate positive pressure ventilation.

ANSWER: 4

A newborn heart rate of less than 100 beats per minute equates to a 1 on the heart rate criterion and indicates a need to begin positive pressure ventilation by bag mask or Neopuff ventilation. To score a 2 on the heart rate criterion of the Apgar scoring, the newborn's heart rate must be above 100 beats per minute. An Apgar score of 0 on the heart rate criteria indicates that the heart rate is absent. Each Apgar parameter is evaluated and scored without regard to the other criteria.

► ***Test-taking Tip:*** *Apply parameters for Apgar scoring to answer this question.*

Content Area: Childbearing Families; *Category of Health Alteration:* Neonatal and High-Risk Neonatal Management; *Integrated Processes:* Nursing Process Assessment; *Client Need:* Health Promotion and Maintenance/Ante/Intra/Postpartum and Newborn Care; *Cognitive Level:* Application

References: Davidson, M., London, M., & Ladewig, P. (2008). *Olds' Maternal-Newborn Nursing & Women's Health Across the Lifespan* (8th ed., p. 670). Upper Saddle River, NJ: Prentice Hall Health; Pillitteri, A. (2007). *Maternal & Child Health Nursing: Care of the Childbearing & Childrearing Family* (5th ed., p. 701). Philadelphia: Lippincott Williams & Wilkins.

EBP Reference: Stringer, M., Brooks, P., King, K., & Biesecker, B. (2007). New guidelines for maternal and neonatal resuscitation. *Journal of Obstetric, Gynecologic, & Neonatal Nursing (JOGNN)*, 36(6), 624–635.

411. EBP A woman with oligohydraminos and suspected intrauterine growth restriction gives birth to an infant. The infant's 1-minute Apgar score was 6, and the 5-minute Apgar score is 7. Which conclusion should the nurse make from this information?

1. A low Apgar score at 1 minute correlates with infant mortality.
2. A 5-minute Apgar score of 7 to 10 is considered normal.
3. A 5-minute score greater than 9 indicates a decreased risk of neurological impairment.
4. Gestational age, resuscitation measures, and obstetrical medications did not affect the Apgar score.

ANSWER: 2

A 5-minute Apgar score above 7 is considered normal. Whereas a low 1-minute Apgar score does not, a low 5-minute Apgar score is associated with infant mortality. The Apgar score at 5 minutes in full-term infants is a poor predictor of neurological outcome. Variables such as gestational age, resuscitation measures, and medications can all affect the Apgar score.

➧ ***Test-taking Tip:*** *Read each option carefully, noting that the time of each Apgar score in the options is different from the infant's initial Apgar score. Consider the information that can be interpreted from an Apgar score.*

Content Area: Childbearing Families; *Category of Health Alteration:* Neonatal and High-Risk Neonatal Management; *Integrated Processes:* Nursing Process Analysis; *Client Need:* Physiological Integrity/ Reduction of Risk Potential/System Specific Assessments; *Cognitive Level:* Analysis

EBP Reference: American College of Obstetricians and Gynecologists (ACOG). (2006). The Apgar score. *ACOG Committee Opinion,* No. 333. Washington, DC: ACOG.

412. EBP A nurse knows that maintaining a newborn's axillary body temperature between 97.7°F (36.5°C) and 98.9°F (37.2°C) is an appropriate outcome. To accomplish this outcome the nurse should: SELECT ALL THAT APPLY.

1. dry the infant immediately after birth.
2. place the infant skin-to-skin with the mother.
3. apply leggings to the infant's legs.
4. cover the infant's head with a stocking cap.
5. place the infant in a crib close to the delivery room wall.
6. wrap the infant in warm blankets and place him under a radiant heat source.

ANSWER: 1, 2, 4

Drying the newborn immediately after birth prevents heat loss through evaporation. Skin-to-skin contact between mother and baby at birth assists to maintain newborn body temperature. The newborn's head is dried first after birth, and a stocking cap is placed on the head to conserve heat. A radiant heat source warms the outer surface of objects. A newborn placed under the radiant warmer will receive no extra warming benefit if it is wrapped in blankets. Placing the newborn's crib close to the delivery room wall will cause radiation heat loss because the wall is cooler in temperature than the infant. If other appropriate warming measures are taken, there is no need to wrap the infant's legs in leggings.

➧ ***Test-taking Tip:*** *Use the process of elimination to rule out option 5, as it is obvious that placing the newborn close to a cool surface such as a wall would be detrimental to body warming.*

Content Area: Childbearing Families; *Category of Health Alteration:* Neonatal and High-Risk Neonatal Management; *Integrated Processes:* Nursing Process Implementation; *Client Need:* Health Promotion and Maintenance/Ante/Intra/Postpartum and Newborn Care; *Cognitive Level:* Application

References: Davidson, M., London, M., & Ladewig, P. (2008). *Olds' Maternal-Newborn Nursing & Women's Health Across the Lifespan* (8th ed., pp. 670, 804). Upper Saddle River, NJ: Prentice Hall Health; Wong, D., Hockenberry, M., Wilson, D., Perry, S., & Lowdermilk, D. (2006). *Maternal Child Nursing Care* (3rd ed., p. 708). Philadelphia: Lippincott Williams & Wilkins.

EBP Reference: Moore, E., Anderson, G., & Bergman N. (2007). Early skin-to-skin contact for mothers and their healthy newborn infants. *Cochrane Database of Systematic Reviews*, Issue 3, Art. No. CD003519. DOI: 10.1002/14651858.CD003519.pub2. Available at: www.mrw.interscience.wiley.com.ezproxy.csbsju.edu/cochrane/clsysrev/articles/CD003519/frame.html

413. As a nurse prepares to administer prophylactic eye treatment to prevent gonorrheal conjunctivitis to a full-term newborn, the father of the newborn asks if it is really necessary to put something into his baby's eyes. The nurse's response is based on the knowledge that:

1. it is the law in the United States that newborns receive this treatment.
2. this treatment is recommended but may be omitted at the parent's verbal request.
3. the antibiotic used for the treatment can be given orally at the parent's request.
4. the eye prophylaxis can be given anytime up until the infant is 1 year old.

ANSWER: 1

Currently every U.S. state requires that newborns receive prophylactic eye treatment against gonorrheal conjunctivitis. If a parent objects to the procedure, he or she will be asked to sign formal documentation of informed refusal. The antibiotic can only be administered topically and it must be administered within 1 hour of birth to be effective. Administration may be delayed for a short period of time to allow for parent/infant bonding.

➧ ***Test-taking Tip:*** *Eliminate option 3 as a medication to specifically prevent eye conjunctivitis would be unlikely to be effective if administered orally.*

Content Area: Childbearing Families; *Category of Health Alteration:* Neonatal and High-Risk Neonatal Management; *Integrated Processes:* Teaching and Learning; *Client Need:* Safe and Effective Care Environment/Management of Care/Legal Rights and Responsibilities; *Cognitive Level:* Application

References: Pillitteri, A. (2007). *Maternal & Child Health Nursing: Care of the Childbearing & Childrearing Family* (5th ed., p. 712). Philadelphia: Lippincott Williams & Wilkins; Wong, D., Hockenberry, M., Wilson, D., Perry, S., & Lowdermilk, D. (2006). *Maternal Child Nursing Care* (3rd ed., p. 732). Philadelphia: Lippincott Williams & Wilkins.

414. EBP Immediately after assisting with the birth of a full-term infant, a nurse determines that promoting parent-infant attachment is an appropriate outcome. To accomplish this outcome, the nurse should: SELECT ALL THAT APPLY.

1. encourage the mother to take a short nap before interacting with her newborn.
2. dim the lights in the birthing room.
3. place the newly delivered infant on the mother's abdomen.
4. delay instillation of ophthalmic antibiotic 1 hour.
5. play loud music to keep the infant stimulated.
6. encourage the parents to delay phone calls for 1 hour after birth.

ANSWER: 2, 3, 4, 6

Dimming the lights in the birthing room encourages the newborn to open his or her eyes. This in turn encourages eye contact between the parent and the newborn. Instillation of ophthalmic antibiotic ointment may cause temporary blurred vision in the newborn, thereby decreasing the ability to engage in eye-to-eye contact with the parents. Skin-to-skin contact between mother and baby at birth improves mother-baby interaction. The newborn is alert for up to 1 hour after birth. Parents should be encouraged to use this time for attachment and delay phone calls. Avoiding loud noises encourages parent-infant communication. If the mother naps immediately after birth, the alert newborn period may be missed.

➧ ***Test-taking Tip:*** *Recall interventions that encourage parent-infant interactions.*

Content Area: Childbearing Families; *Category of Health Alteration:* Neonatal and High-Risk Neonatal Management; *Integrated Processes:* Nursing Process Planning; *Client Need:* Health Promotion and Maintenance/Ante/Intra/Postpartum and Newborn Care; *Cognitive Level:* Application

References: Davidson, M., London, M., & Ladewig, P. (2008). *Olds' Maternal-Newborn Nursing & Women's Health Across the Lifespan* (8th ed., pp. 673, 674). Upper Saddle River, NJ: Prentice Hall Health; Wong, D., Hockenberry, M., Wilson, D., Perry, S., & Lowdermilk, D. (2006). *Maternal Child Nursing Care* (3rd ed., p. 733). Philadelphia: Lippincott Williams & Wilkins.

EBP Reference: Moore, E., Anderson, G., & Bergman N. (2007). Early skin-to-skin contact for mothers and their healthy newborn infants. *Cochrane Database of Systematic Reviews*, Issue 3, Art. No. CD003519. DOI: 10.1002/14651858.CD003519.pub2. Available at: www.mrw.interscience.wiley.com.ezproxy.csbsju.edu/cochrane/clsysrev/articles/CD003519/frame.html

415. The father of a 12-hour-old newborn calls a nurse into his wife's hospital room. He is agitated and reports to the nurse that his baby's hands and feet are blue. The nurse confirms acrocyanosis and intervenes by:

1. immediately stimulating the infant to cry.
2. explaining to the father that this is an expected finding in a newborn.
3. assessing the newborn's temperature.
4. assessing the newborn's cardiac status.

ANSWER: 2

Acrocyanosis, which is blueness of hands and feet, is a normal newborn phenomenon in the first 24 to 48 hours after birth. The nurse should explain this to the father to relieve his anxiety. There is no need for any further action.

Test-taking Tip: *Recall that peripheral circulation in newborns is immature and may lead to acrocyanosis.*

Content Area: Childbearing Families; *Category of Health Alteration:* Neonatal and High-Risk Neonatal Management; *Integrated Processes:* Caring; *Client Need:* Physiological Integrity/Physiological Adaptation/ Alterations in Body Systems; *Cognitive Level:* Application

Reference: Pillitteri, A. (2007). *Maternal & Child Health Nursing: Care of the Childbearing & Childrearing Family* (5th ed., p. 690). Philadelphia: Lippincott Williams & Wilkins.

416. During the initial assessment of a full-term newborn, a nurse measures both the infant's chest and head circumference. The infant's father observes this assessment and asks the nurse why these measurements are necessary. Which explanation by the nurse is most accurate?

1. Comparing these measurements provides information about any head or chest growth abnormalities.
2. Measuring the head circumference provides information about future intellectual ability.
3. Measuring a newborn's chest provides data to assist with assessment of cardiac health.
4. Comparing head and chest circumference measurements provides information about future adult body size.

ANSWER: 1

The circumference of the normal newborn's head is approximately 2 centimeters greater than the circumference of the newborn's chest at birth. Any extreme difference in head size may indicate microcephalus, hydrocephalus, or increased intracranial pressure. Heredity, nutrition, and hormones are the major determinant of physical adult size. The relationship of the head and chest do not predict adult body size. Heredity and interpersonal relationships play critical roles in intellectual development of the child. Head size is not related to intelligence. Chest size does not provide information on cardiac status.

Test-taking Tip: *Eliminate options 2 and 4 as these relate to future data. These parameters will be affected by different outside influences as the child grows and could not be predicted by simple newborn head and chest measurements.*

Content Area: Childbearing Families; *Category of Health Alteration:* Neonatal and High-Risk Neonatal Management; *Integrated Processes:* Nursing Process Assessment; *Client Need:* Health Promotion and Maintenance/Techniques of Physical Assessment; *Cognitive Level:* Application

References: Davidson, M., London, M., & Ladewig, P. (2008). *Olds' Maternal-Newborn Nursing & Women's Health Across the Lifespan* (8th ed., pp. 830, 833). Upper Saddle River, NJ: Prentice Hall Health; Wong, D., Hockenberry, M., Wilson, D., Perry, S., & Lowdermilk, D. (2006). *Maternal Child Nursing Care* (3rd ed., pp. 710–711, 951, 952–953). Philadelphia: Lippincott Williams & Wilkins.

417. While assessing an 8-hour-old newborn, a nurse finds an axillary temperature of 97°F (36.1°C). In response to this finding, the nurse's first intervention should be to:

1. document the findings.
2. place the infant under a radiant warmer.
3. feed the infant warmed formula.
4. call the health-care provider to report the findings.

ANSWER: 2

The average temperature for a full-term newborn is 98.6°F (37°C) with a range of 98°F (36.6°C) to 99°F (37.2°C). If the infant's temperature drops below 97.7°F (36.5°C), the infant should be gradually rewarmed under a temperature-controlled radiant warmer. Following this intervention the nurse would then document the findings. There is no need to call the health-care provider unless the nurse is unable to warm the infant using appropriate interventions. Feeding warm formula is unnecessary.

Test-taking Tip: *The key word is "first." Consider that infants who become cold must increase their metabolic rate and thus their oxygen consumption to generate heat. This can lead to respiratory distress. Thus consider the ABCs (airway, breathing, circulation) of prioritization when selecting the correct option.*

Content Area: Childbearing Families; *Category of Health Alteration:* Neonatal and High-Risk Neonatal Management; *Integrated Processes:* Nursing Process Implementation; *Client Need:* Safe and Effective Care Environment/Management of Care/Establishing Priorities; *Cognitive Level:* Application

References: Davidson, M., London, M., & Ladewig, P. (2008). *Olds' Maternal-Newborn Nursing & Women's Health Across the Lifespan* (8th ed., p. 869). Upper Saddle River, NJ: Prentice Hall Health; Wong, D., Hockenberry, M., Wilson, D., Perry, S., & Lowdermilk, D. (2006). *Maternal Child Nursing Care* (3rd ed., p. 708). Philadelphia: Lippincott Williams & Wilkins.

418. EBP A nurse receives a call from the laboratory reporting a blood sugar of 46 mg/dL for a full-term newborn. In response to this information, the nurse should:

1. feed the infant formula.
2. immediately feed the infant water with 10% dextrose.
3. report the findings immediately to the health-care provider.
4. document the information in the newborn's health-care record.

ANSWER: 4

Standard blood sugar values for a full-term newborn are 45 to 65 mg/dL. Therefore the only intervention required is to document the findings. Early breastfeeding or formula feeding is a common practice that helps to prevent development of hypoglycemia in newborns; however, although not inappropriate, feeding is not necessary in response to a blood sugar of 46 mg/dL, which is within normal parameters. Oral glucose water can cause a rapid increase in glucose followed by an abrupt decrease and should not be given to treat hypoglycemia. Since the assessment finding was within normal parameters, there is no need to notify the health-care provider.

➧ ***Test-taking Tip:*** *Knowledge of normal blood sugar levels for a full-term newborn is necessary to correctly answer this question.*

Content Area: Childbearing Families; *Category of Health Alteration:* Neonatal and High-Risk Neonatal Management; *Integrated Processes:* Nursing Process Implementation; *Client Need:* Health Promotion and Maintenance/Ante/Intra/Postpartum and Newborn Care; *Cognitive Level:* Application

References: Davidson, M., London, M., & Ladewig, P. (2008). *Olds' Maternal-Newborn Nursing & Women's Health Across the Lifespan* (8th ed., p. 1006). Upper Saddle River, NJ: Prentice Hall Health; Wong, D., Hockenberry, M., Wilson, D., Perry, S., & Lowdermilk, D. (2006). *Maternal Child Nursing Care* (3rd ed., p. 741). Philadelphia: Lippincott Williams & Wilkins; Pillitteri, A. (2007). *Maternal & Child Health Nursing: Care of the Childbearing & Childrearing Family* (5th ed., p. 705). Philadelphia: Lippincott Williams & Wilkins.

EBP Reference: Newborn Nursery QI Committee. (2004). *Neonatal Hypoglycemia: Initial and Follow-up Management.* Portland, ME: The Barbara Bush Children's Hospital at Maine Medical Center. Available at: www.guideline.gov/summary/summary.aspx?doc_id=7180&nbr=004293&string=respiratory+AND+distress+AND+syndrome+AND+newborns

419. During the assessment of a full-term newborn infant who is 40 hours old, a nurse evaluates the infant for jaundice by:

1. removing the diaper and assessing the color of the genitalia.
2. applying pressure on the forehead for a few seconds and evaluating the skin color after the pressure is removed.
3. assessing the color of the palms of the hands and comparing that skin color to the color of the soles of the feet.
4. assessing the color of the infant's tongue and palate.

ANSWER: 2

To differentiate cutaneous jaundice from normal skin color, the nurse should apply pressure with a finger over a bony area such as the forehead. If jaundice is present, the blanched area will look yellow before the capillaries refill. Jaundice is generally first noticed in the head and then progresses gradually down the body; thus the change in skin color would not be evident as quickly in the extremities or the genitalia. Since the tongue and palate are naturally darker in color than the rest of the skin, it is more difficult to determine jaundice by assessing in these areas.

➧ ***Test-taking Tip:*** *Think carefully about the color of the body in the different areas described in the options. Select option 2 because the forehead would be the lightest skin selection and thus provide the easiest visualization of the change in skin color.*

Content Area: Childbearing Families; *Category of Health Alteration:* Neonatal and High-Risk Neonatal Management; *Integrated Processes:* Nursing Process Assessment; *Client Need:* Physiological Integrity/Reduction of Risk Potential/System Specific Assessments; *Cognitive Level:* Application

Reference: Wong, D., Hockenberry, M., Wilson, D., Perry, S., & Lowdermilk, D. (2006). *Maternal Child Nursing Care* (3rd ed., p. 737). Philadelphia: Lippincott Williams & Wilkins.

420. According to the date of the mother's last menstrual period (LMP), the nurse determines that the newborn just born has a gestational age of 40 weeks. Considering that data, the nurse anticipates that physical assessment of the newborn will demonstrate:
SELECT ALL THAT APPLY.

1. hypertonic flexion of all extremities.
2. sole creases on the anterior two-thirds of the sole.
3. well-defined incurving of the entire ear pinna.
4. a prominent clitoris.
5. the ability to touch the infant's heel to his or her ear in a supine position.
6. the ability of the infant to support his or her head momentarily when being pulled from a supine to a sitting position.

ANSWER: 1, 3, 6

As the newborn's muscular tone matures, the newborn posture becomes more flexed; thus the full-term newborn exhibits hypertonic flexion of all extremities. Cartilage gives the newborn ear its shape. At full term, the newborn ear has enough cartilage to produce a well-defined incurving of the entire pinna. The full-term infant has the muscle strength to momentarily support his or her head when pulled to a sitting position. Sole creases over the anterior two-thirds of the sole indicate a gestational age of approximately 37 weeks. A prominent clitoris is found in an infant whose gestational age is between 30 and 32 weeks. As the fetus matures, the labia majora become large enough to completely cover the clitoris and labia minora. With advancing gestational age, the infant demonstrates increasing resistance to having the heel pulled to the point of touching the ear. The ability to perform this maneuver indicates an immature infant.

➧ ***Test-taking Tip:*** *Muscle strength and resistance to positioning of arms and legs increases as gestational age increases. Eliminate any options suggesting a very immature infant.*

Content Area: Childbearing Families; *Category of Health Alteration:* Neonatal and High-Risk Neonatal Management; *Integrated Processes:* Nursing Process Assessment; *Client Need:* Health Promotion and Maintenance/Ante/Intra/Postpartum and Newborn Care; *Cognitive Level:* Application

Reference: Davidson, M., London, M., & Ladewig, P. (2008). *Olds' Maternal-Newborn Nursing & Women's Health Across the Lifespan* (8th ed., pp. 822–826). Upper Saddle River, NJ: Prentice Hall Health.

---

421. A new mother of a 2-hour-old full-term newborn calls a nurse into her room and very excitedly tells the nurse, "Something black is coming out of my baby." The nurse examines the diaper and finds that the infant has passed meconium stool. Which response by the nurse is most appropriate?

1. "Black stools often indicate bleeding in the gastrointestinal tract. I will notify your health-care provider immediately."
2. "Are you breastfeeding? If so, the stools will always have this dark color."
3. "All babies pass this type of stool initially."
4. "I'm going to check the baby's temperature. This happens when babies need to be warmed."

ANSWER: 3

At birth, the newborn intestine is filled with meconium, a substance formed during fetal life from amniotic fluid and intestinal secretions and cells. It is greenish-black in color and normally contains occult blood. The majority of full-term infants will normally pass the first meconium stool within 24 hours after birth. This stool is normal and does not indicate that a newborn has active gastrointestinal bleeding. Stools of breastfed babies are usually pale yellow once the meconium has passed. Exposure to cold will increase the infant's oxygen requirements, decrease glucose levels and surfactant production, and can eventually result in respiratory compromise; however, cold stress does not affect the passage of meconium.

➧ ***Test-taking Tip:*** *Base your answer on knowledge of normal newborn physiology*

Content Area: Childbearing Families; *Category of Health Alteration:* Neonatal and High-Risk Neonatal Management; *Integrated Processes:* Teaching and Learning; *Client Need:* Health Promotion and Maintenance/Ante/Intra/Postpartum and Newborn Care; *Cognitive Level:* Application

References: Wong, D., Hockenberry, M., Wilson, D., Perry, S., & Lowdermilk, D. (2006). *Maternal Child Nursing Care* (3rd ed., pp. 696–697). Philadelphia: Lippincott Williams & Wilkins; Davidson, M., London, M., & Ladewig, P. (2008). *Olds' Maternal-Newborn Nursing & Women's Health Across the Lifespan* (8th ed., pp. 810, 1004). Upper Saddle River, NJ: Prentice Hall Health.

422. While performing an initial assessment on a full-term female infant, a nurse notes the following skin discoloration. What should be the nurse's interpretation of this finding?

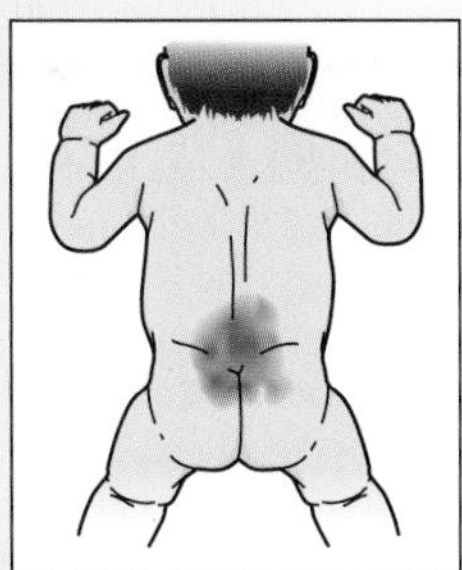

1. The infant was bruised during delivery.
2. This is a normally occurring skin variation in newborns.
3. The infant has been placed on her back inappropriately, and this has caused bruising.
4. Seepage of blood from the intestine occurred during the birth process.

ANSWER: 2

The image is illustrating Mongolian spots, a normal newborn skin variation. Mongolian spots are collections of pigmented cells that appear as slate-gray patches across the sacrum, buttocks, and, less commonly, arms and legs of newborns. Mongolian spots are more likely to occur in newborns of Asian, southern European, or African descent. They disappear by school age without treatment. They are not a result of injury or intestinal bleeding.

➧ ***Test-taking Tip:*** *Recall the cultural variations in newborn skin appearances.*

Content Area: Childbearing Families; *Category of Health Alteration:* Neonatal and High-Risk Neonatal Management; *Integrated Processes:* Nursing Process Assessment; *Client Need:* Physiological Integrity/Reduction of Risk Potential/System Specific Assessments; *Cognitive Level:* Application

Reference: Pillitteri, A. (2007). *Maternal & Child Health Nursing: Care of the Childbearing & Childrearing Family* (5th ed., p. 692). Philadelphia: Lippincott Williams & Wilkins.

---

423. While assessing a full-term newborn, a nurse notes molding on the infant's head. Considering this assessment finding, which information should the nurse expect to see on the mother's labor and delivery documentation?

1. Vaginal breech birth
2. Planned cesarean section, no labor
3. 16-hour labor
4. Precipitous delivery after a 30-minute labor

ANSWER: 3

Molding is a change in the shape of the fetal skull produced by the force of uterine contractions pressing the vertex of the head against the cervix during labor. The degree of molding varies with the amount and length of pressure exerted on the head. Thus a longer labor will increase molding. No molding occurs when the fetus is breech because the buttocks not the head are the presenting part. With planned cesarean section, the head is not pressed against the cervix because labor does not occur. A precipitous delivery following only 30 minutes of labor would mean limited time for the vertex to be pressing against the cervix.

➧ ***Test-taking Tip:*** *Recall what the term "molding" means and then use the process of elimination to eliminate options 1, 2, and 4, as there would be limited to no opportunity for the vertex to press against the cervix during these types of births.*

Content Area: Childbearing Families; *Category of Health Alteration:* Neonatal and High-Risk Neonatal Management; *Integrated Processes:* Nursing Process Analysis; *Client Need:* Health Promotion and Maintenance/Ante/Intra/Postpartum and Newborn Care; *Cognitive Level:* Analysis

References: Pillitteri, A. (2007). *Maternal & Child Health Nursing: Care of the Childbearing & Childrearing Family* (5th ed., pp. 493, 694). Philadelphia: Lippincott Williams & Wilkins; Davidson, M., London, M., & Ladewig, P. (2008). *Olds' Maternal-Newborn Nursing & Women's Health Across the Lifespan* (8th ed., p. 833). Upper Saddle River, NJ: Prentice Hall Health.

---

424. A nurse should prepare to assess the newborn's anterior fontanel by:

1. laying the infant on his or her back.
2. stimulating the infant to cry.
3. palpating over the infant's occipital bone.
4. placing the infant in a sitting position.

ANSWER: 4

When assessing the anterior fontanel, the infant should be in a sitting position (45° to 90°). The fontanel should not appear indented, which could indicate dehydration, or bulging, which could indicate increased intracranial pressure. Crying may cause a temporary bulging of the fontanel. Laying the infant supine may also cause bulging of the fontanel. The anterior fontanel is located at the juncture of the two parietal bones and the frontal bone.

➧ ***Test-taking Tip:*** *Recall anatomy of the newborn skull and eliminate option 3 as the fontanels are spaces between bones. Palpating over a bone would be an incorrect location.*

Content Area: Childbearing Families; *Category of Health Alteration:* Neonatal and High-Risk Neonatal Management; *Integrated Processes:* Nursing Process Assessment; *Client Need:* Health Promotion and Maintenance/Techniques of Physical Assessment; *Cognitive Level:* Application

References: Davidson, M., London, M., & Ladewig, P. (2008). *Olds' Maternal-Newborn Nursing & Women's Health Across the Lifespan* (8th ed., p. 834). Upper Saddle River, NJ: Prentice Hall Health; Pillitteri, A. (2007). *Maternal & Child Health Nursing: Care of the Childbearing & Childrearing Family* (5th ed., p. 694). Philadelphia: Lippincott Williams & Wilkins.

---

425. A nurse evaluates that a mother understands information provided about her newborn's milia when the mother says:

1. "I will put lotion on my infant's nose twice a day."
2. "I understand these raised white spots will clear up without treatment."
3. "I realize the baby will need surgery to remove these skin lesions."
4. "I will apply alcohol twice a day to the lesions until they disappear."

ANSWER: 2

Milia are exposed sebaceous glands that appear as raised white spots on the face, usually the nose, of the newborn. No treatment is necessary because they will clear up spontaneously within the first month. Treatment with lotion, alcohol, or surgery is not necessary.

➧ ***Test-taking Tip:*** *Read the question carefully; it is asking for the correct statement about milia.*

Content Area: Childbearing Families; *Category of Health Alteration:* Neonatal and High-Risk Neonatal Management; *Integrated Processes:* Nursing Process Evaluation; *Client Need:* Physiological Integrity/Basic Care and Comfort/Personal Hygiene; *Cognitive Level:* Application

Reference: Davidson, M., London, M., & Ladewig, P. (2008). *Olds' Maternal-Newborn Nursing & Women's Health Across the Lifespan* (8th ed., p. 832). Upper Saddle River, NJ: Prentice Hall Health.

---

426. While providing discharge education to the Native American parents of a 48-hour-old, full-term infant, a nurse recognizes the need for additional teaching about jaundice when the mother says:

1. "I know keeping my baby warm will help to decrease his jaundice."
2. "I know the jaundice should start to decrease after 5 days."
3. "The bilirubin causing the jaundice is eliminated in my baby's stools."
4. "Feeding my baby frequently will help to decrease the jaundice."

ANSWER: 2

Peak bilirubin levels are reached at 3 to 5 days of age for Caucasian infants. However, Native American babies have higher bilirubin levels than Caucasian babies, and the jaundice persists for longer periods with no apparent ill effects. The mother is correct to keep her baby warm as cold stress can result in acidosis, which will decrease available serum albumin binding sites. This in turn will result in a decrease in unconjugated bilirubin being transported via albumin to the liver. Bilirubin is eliminated in the newborn stools, therefore inadequate stooling may result in reabsorption of bilirubin. Frequent feeding promotes intestinal elimination and provides protein intake necessary for the formation of hepatic binding proteins.

➧ ***Test-taking Tip:*** *The phrase "the need for more teaching" indicates a false-response item. Look for the incorrect statement.*

Content Area: Childbearing Families; *Category of Health Alteration:* Neonatal and High-Risk Neonatal Management; *Integrated Processes:* Nursing Process Evaluation; *Client Need:* Health Promotion and Maintenance/Ante/Intra/Postpartum and Newborn Care; *Cognitive Level:* Analysis

Reference: Davidson, M., London, M., & Ladewig, P. (2008). *Olds' Maternal-Newborn Nursing & Women's Health Across the Lifespan* (8th ed., p. 808). Upper Saddle River, NJ: Prentice Hall Health.

427. In preparation to care for a primiparous client, who delivered a term newborn, a nurse reviews the client's history and notes that the client is a lesbian, achieved her pregnancy via artificial insemination, and is in a monogamous relationship with a female partner. In response to this information, which intervention should the nurse add to the newborn's care plan?

1. Avoid discussion of the lesbian relationship with the client.
2. Encourage the client's partner to participate in newborn cares.
3. Ask the partner to leave the room when the newborn is present.
4. Avoid telling the health-care staff who cares for the newborn about the client's situation.

ANSWER: 2

Acknowledgment of their partner has been reported as being clearly important to lesbian women. It is essential that caregivers afford partners of lesbian women the same respect, caring, and attention offered to the partners of heterosexual mothers. Including and integrating the nonchildbearing partner into the perinatal experience is a key component in the provision of caring and sensitive health care. Health-care providers who advocate for an inclusive, accepting environment will ensure that their clients feel respected and will ultimately achieve favorable health-care outcomes for the parents and their child. Health-care providers must ensure that the needs and desires of the couple are recognized and met by the entire health-care team. This can be accomplished by utilizing a process of anticipatory preparation for all health-care providers who will be present during the labor, birth, and postpartum experience.

➧ ***Test-taking Tip:*** *Select the option that represents a nonjudgmental inclusive approach to client care.*

Content Area: Childbearing Families; *Category of Health Alteration:* Neonatal and High-Risk Neonatal Management; *Integrated Processes:* Nursing Process Implementation; *Client Need:* Health Promotion and Maintenance/Developmental Stages and Transitions; *Cognitive Level:* Application

References: Wong, D., Hockenberry, M., Wilson, D., Perry, S., & Lowdermilk, D. (2006). *Maternal Child Nursing Care* (3rd ed., p. 640). Philadelphia: Lippincott Williams & Wilkins; McManus, A., Hunter, L., & Renn, H. (2006). Lesbian experiences and needs during childbirth: Guidance for health-care providers, *Journal of Obstetrics, Gynecology and Neonatal Nurses,* 35(1), 13–23.

428. **EBP** A nurse is preparing the parents of a full-term, 24-hour-old male newborn for discharge with their child. Which discharge criteria should be met before the infant leaves the hospital? SELECT ALL THAT APPLY.

1. Infant vital signs have been within normal range for the last 12 hours.
2. The infant has passed at least three meconium stools.
3. The infant has gained weight at the minimum 100 grams.
4. There has been no evidence of bleeding from the circumcision for the last 2 hours.
5. The infant has had 6 wet diapers.

ANSWER: 1, 4

The American Academy of Pediatrics has determined that newborn discharge criteria include stable vital signs for 12 hours and no bleeding from a circumcision for 2 hours. Successful urination and one meconium stool are also required for discharge. There is no weight gain requirement for discharge; newborns are expected to lose weight during the first 3 to 4 days after birth.

➧ ***Test-taking Tip:*** *Recall that newborns in the United States are usually discharged from the hospital within 48 hours after birth and then recall expected newborn physiology immediately after birth. This should allow elimination of options 2, 3, and 5.*

Content Area: Childbearing Families; *Category of Health Alteration:* Neonatal and High-Risk Neonatal Management; *Integrated Processes:* Nursing Process Evaluation; *Client Need:* Health Promotion and Maintenance/Ante/Intra/Postpartum and Newborn Care; *Cognitive Level:* Analysis

Reference: Davidson, M., London, M., & Ladewig, P. (2008). *Olds' Maternal-Newborn Nursing & Women's Health Across the Lifespan* (8th ed., pp. 810, 829). Upper Saddle River, NJ: Prentice Hall Health.

EBP References: American Academy of Pediatrics Committee on Fetus and Newborn. (2004). Hospital stays for healthy full-term newborns. *Pediatrics*, 113(5), 1434–1436. Available at: www.guideline.gov/summary/summary.aspx?doc_id=5088&nbr=003555&string=newborn+AND+care; Paul, I., Lehman, E., Hollenbeak, C., & Maisels, J. (2006). Preventable newborn readmissions since passage of the newborns' and mothers' health protection act. *Pediatrics*, 118, 2349–2358.

429. A nurse is caring for a full-term newborn male who is 24-hours-old and was circumcised with a Gomco® clamp 30 minutes ago. Which interventions should the nurse plan for care of the newborn's circumcision? SELECT ALL THAT APPLY.

1. Monitoring the penis hourly for 4 to 6 hours
2. Observing for and documenting the first voiding after circumcision
3. Using prepackaged commercial diaper wipes for perineal cleaning to prevent infection
4. Applying petroleum ointment around the penis after each diaper change
5. Applying the diaper tightly to provide hemostasis
6. Reporting penile swelling to the health-care provider

ANSWER: 1, 2, 4, 6

After circumcision, the penis should be closely monitored for bleeding. To evaluate for urinary obstruction, the infant should be monitored frequently for the first urination postcircumcision, and this finding should be documented. Petroleum and gauze should be applied to the circumcision site with each diaper change to prevent bleeding and to protect healing tissue. Penile swelling should be reported to the health-care provider. Prepackaged commercial diaper wipes should be avoided because they may contain alcohol, which could be irritating. When diapering the newborn the nurse ensures that the diaper is not too loose to cause rubbing with movement or too tight, which may cause pain.

➧ ***Test-taking Tip:*** *Recall care of the newly circumcised penis to correctly answer this question.*

Content Area: Childbearing Families; *Category of Health Alteration:* Neonatal and High-Risk Neonatal Management; *Integrated Processes:* Nursing Process Planning; *Client Need:* Physiological Integrity Reduction of Risk Potential/Potential for Complications from Surgical Procedures and Health Alterations; *Cognitive Level:* Application

References: Davidson, M., London, M., & Ladewig, P. (2008). *Olds' Maternal-Newborn Nursing & Women's Health Across the Lifespan* (8th ed., p. 876). Upper Saddle River, NJ: Prentice Hall Health; Wong, D., Hockenberry, M., Wilson, D., Perry, S., & Lowdermilk, D. (2006). *Maternal Child Nursing Care* (3rd ed., p. 755). Philadelphia: Lippincott Williams & Wilkins.

---

430. A nurse admits a term newborn who is at risk to develop neonatal abstinence syndrome (NAS) to the newborn nursery. The nurse correctly places this infant:

1. in the general nursery with 15 other infants.
2. in a small, well-lighted nursery with two other newborns.
3. alone in a small darkened nursery room.
4. right next to the charge nurse's desk.

ANSWER: 3

NAS is a term used to describe the set of behaviors exhibited by an infant who has been exposed to chemical substances in utero. Because some women are multidrug users, the newborn initially may exhibit a variety of withdrawal manifestations with varying times of onset. Nursing care of these infants includes reducing environmental stimuli by placing them in a small darkened nursery. Placing these infants where there are increased amounts of noise, activity, or light would be inappropriate.

➧ ***Test-taking Tip:*** *Select the option that describes the least stimulating environment for the newborn.*

Content Area: Childbearing Families; *Category of Health Alteration:* Neonatal and High-Risk Neonatal Management; *Integrated Processes:* Nursing Process Planning; *Client Need:* Physiological Integrity/ Physiological Adaptation/Illness Management; *Cognitive Level:* Application

References: Wong, D., Hockenberry, M., Wilson, D., Perry, S., & Lowdermilk, D. (2006). *Maternal Child Nursing Care* (3rd ed., pp. 848, 850–851). Philadelphia: Lippincott Williams & Wilkins; Pillitteri, A. (2007). *Maternal & Child Health Nursing: Care of the Childbearing & Childrearing Family* (5th ed., p. 792). Philadelphia: Lippincott Williams & Wilkins.

431. While reviewing discharge instructions with an African couple from Kenya who are being discharged to home with their 48-hour-old, full-term newborn, a nurse discovers that the parents have not named their newborn. Which action should the nurse take in response to this information?

1. Ask the parents to choose a name before discharge.
2. Encourage other appropriate attachment behaviors.
3. Document the finding.
4. Ask the health-care provider to delay discharge until the lack of appropriate parental attachment can be addressed.

ANSWER: 3

In Kenya, the naming of a child is an important event. In some areas, the name is given on the third day after birth and is marked by a celebration. Therefore, the only intervention needed is to document this information. It is always appropriate for the nurse to observe for and encourage attachment behaviors; however, in this situation, not naming the infant is not a sign of inappropriate attachment. There is no need to delay discharge. It would be culturally inappropriate to ask the parents to choose a name before discharge.

▶ ***Test-taking Tip:*** *Note that the stem of the question specifically addresses the ethnic origin of the parents. Consider cultural differences when answering the question.*

Content Area: Childbearing Families; *Category of Health Alteration:* Neonatal and High-Risk Neonatal Management; *Integrated Processes:* Nursing Process Analysis; *Client Need:* Psychosocial Integrity/Cultural Diversity; *Cognitive Level:* Application

Reference: Davidson, M., London, M., & Ladewig, P. (2008). *Olds' Maternal-Newborn Nursing & Women's Health Across the Lifespan* (8th ed., p. 878). Upper Saddle River, NJ: Prentice Hall Health.

---

432. EBP During a home-care visit to the parents of a 1-week-old newborn, a nurse correctly educates the parents about continuing care of the newborn's umbilical cord by instructing them to:

1. begin applying rubbing alcohol to the base of the cord stump three times a day.
2. attempt to gently dislodge the cord if it has not fallen off in the next week.
3. begin placing the infant in a tub of warm water that covers the cord twice a week until the cord falls off.
4. continue to place the diaper below the cord when diapering the infant.

ANSWER: 4

Keeping the cord dry and exposed to air promotes drying and eventual separation. Folding the diaper below the cord avoids cord contact with urine and stool, which could be detrimental because the wet, soiled environment slows drying and increases the risk of infection. There is no evidence that applying alcohol or any other sprays, creams, or powders to the cord are any better than keeping the baby's cord clean and dry. The cord should never be pulled and the parents should be instructed not to attempt to remove the cord because this could lead to bleeding and infection. Because placing the infant in a tub of water would moisten the cord and delay separation this practice should be avoided.

▶ ***Test-taking Tip:*** *Recall that the major outcome of umbilical cord care is prevention of infection and promotion of timely separation. Select the option that would most likely accomplish these outcomes.*

Content Area: Childbearing Families; *Category of Health Alteration:* Neonatal and High-Risk Neonatal Management; *Integrated Processes:* Teaching and Learning; *Client Need:* Health Promotion and Maintenance/Ante/Intra/Postpartum and Newborn Care; *Cognitive Level:* Application

Reference: Davidson, M., London, M., & Ladewig, P. (2008). *Olds' Maternal-Newborn Nursing & Women's Health Across the Lifespan* (8th ed., p. 881). Upper Saddle River, NJ: Prentice Hall Health.

EBP Reference: Zupan, J., Garner, P., & Omari, A. (2004). Topical umbilical cord care at birth. *Cochrane Database of Systematic Reviews,* Issue 3, Art. No. CD001057. DOI: 10.1002/14651858.CD001057.pub2. Available at www.cochrane.org/reviews/en/ab001057.html

---

433. A postpartum client (G2P2) is preparing for discharge with her term newborn. She is concerned about how her 3-year-old child will react to the infant and asks a nurse for suggestions to help facilitate sibling attachment and acceptance. Which action should the nurse suggest?

1. Providing a doll for the older child to care for and nurture
2. Avoiding bringing the older child to the hospital
3. Planning for dad to care for the older child while mom provides for the newborn
4. Encouraging the child to be "grown up," not tolerating regression developmentally

ANSWER: 1

Providing care to a doll encourages the older child to identify with the parents, which helps to decrease anger and the need to regress to get attention. Bringing the older child to the hospital and pointing out similarities to the older child's birth is encouraged and increases the bond between the two children. The older child needs individual attention from both parents to decrease jealousy, which may develop if the newborn is seen as taking all of the mother's time. Regression is a common occurrence even in well-prepared siblings, and parents should be counseled to expect this and not become concerned.

▶ ***Test-taking Tip:*** *Think about the developmental needs of the preschool child. Select the option that would best reflect adaptation to those needs.*

Content Area: Childbearing Families; *Category of Health Alteration:* Neonatal and High-Risk Neonatal Management; *Integrated Processes:* Nursing Process Implementation; *Client Need:* Health Promotion and Maintenance/Ante/Intra/Postpartum and Newborn Care; *Cognitive Level:* Application

References: Davidson, M., London, M., & Ladewig, P. (2008). *Olds' Maternal-Newborn Nursing & Women's Health Across the Lifespan* (8th ed., p. 1087). Upper Saddle River, NJ: Prentice Hall Health; Wong, D., Hockenberry, M., Wilson, D., Perry, S., & Lowdermilk, D. (2006). *Maternal Child Nursing Care* (3rd ed., p. 651). Philadelphia: Lippincott Williams & Wilkins.

---

434. While caring for a 30-year-old, single female who delivered a term newborn, a nurse determines that the best way to assess the impact of the newborn on the client's lifestyle would be to:

1. observe how the client interacts with her hospital visitors.
2. review the client's prenatal record.
3. ask the client what plans she has made for newborn care at home.
4. observe the relationship between the client and her newborn's father.

ANSWER: 3

Low income and lack of a reliable back-up person are common problems for the single parent. Open-ended questions such as, "What plans have you made for handling things when you get home?" will encourage sharing of feelings and examination of available lifestyle options. Reviewing the prenatal record will provide physical health information and information about attendance at prenatal visits. This may provide insight into the mother's commitment to the pregnancy and the newborn, but it will not provide information about the mother's postdelivery plans. Observing interaction with visitors and also who visits the mother will provide information about the mother's social support system. Since single mothers do not always have an involved father, this option would not always be available for the nurse.

➧ ***Test-taking Tip:*** *The key term is "best." Select the option which is most likely to provide the most information.*

Content Area: Childbearing Families; *Category of Health Alteration:* Neonatal and High-Risk Neonatal Management; *Integrated Processes:* Nursing Process Assessment; *Client Need:* Health Promotion and Maintenance/Family Systems; *Cognitive Level:* Analysis

References: Davidson, M., London, M., & Ladewig, P. (2008). *Olds' Maternal-Newborn Nursing & Women's Health Across the Lifespan* (8th ed., pp. 1073, 1083). Upper Saddle River, NJ: Prentice Hall Health; Pillitteri, A. (2007). *Maternal & Child Health Nursing: Care of the Childbearing & Childrearing Family* (5th ed., p. 29). Philadelphia: Lippincott Williams & Wilkins.

---

435. A new mother of a full-term newborn is concerned that her baby is not taking enough formula at each feeding. The baby weighs 7 pounds and the nurse explains that the infant needs approximately 3 ounces of fluid per pound of body weight per day. The mother then figures that her infant should be eating _______ ounces of formula every 4 hours.

ANSWER: 3.5

To meet the total fluid needs of a full-term infant, the baby needs to ingest 75 to 90 mL (2.5-3 ounces) per pound of body weight per 24-hour period. For an infant taking a commercial formula, this amount of formula will provide the appropriate number of calories (100-120 kcal/kg) needed per 24 hours. Each ounce of commercial formula provides 20 calories.

➧ ***Test-taking Tip:*** *Multiplying 3 ounces by 7 (the weight of the baby) = 21 ounces needed per day. Dividing 21 ounces by 6 (the number of feedings in 24 hours if the baby is fed every 4 hours) = 3.5 ounces per feeding.*

Content Area: Childbearing Families; *Category of Health Alteration:* Neonatal and High-Risk Neonatal Management; *Integrated Processes:* Nursing Process Evaluation; *Client Need:* Physiological Integrity/Basic Care and Comfort/Nutrition and Oral Hydration; *Cognitive Level:* Application

Reference: Pillitteri, A. (2007). *Maternal & Child Health Nursing: Care of the Childbearing & Childrearing Family* (5th ed., p. 743). Philadelphia: Lippincott Williams & Wilkins.

436. A healthy postpartum mother who is breastfeeding her term infant tells the nurse that she has noticed that her roommate is feeding iron-enriched formula to her newborn. The mother wonders if she should be giving her baby some supplemental iron also. The nurse replies:

1. "Your breast milk provides all the iron your baby needs."
2. "Once your breast milk comes in, you will need to take an iron supplement orally."
3. "In the next 2 weeks, your health-care practitioner will prescribe iron drops for your baby."
4. "If you give your baby one bottle of iron-fortified formula each day while you are breastfeeding, that will meet the infant's iron needs."

ANSWER: 1

Iron content in breast milk is much lower than iron-fortified formulas (0.5–1 mg compared to 12 mg); however, the iron in breast milk is much more completely absorbed. The infant receiving breast milk absorbs 50% to 80% of the iron in breast milk compared to only 12% absorption of the iron in formula. Therefore it is unnecessary to provide iron supplementation to a breastfeeding infant. The mineral content of breast milk is not influenced by maternal diet, therefore it would not increase breast milk iron if the mother took an oral iron supplement. Routine supplementation of breastfeeding babies with formula is not recommended as it decreases the amount of time the infant breastfeeds, thus decreasing breast milk supply. Using a bottle nipple for feeding also has the potential to produce nipple confusion in the newborn.

➧ ***Test-taking Tip:*** *Eliminate option 4 as healthy breastfeeding infants do not need and should not be given formula supplementation.*

Content Area: Childbearing Families; *Category of Health Alteration:* Neonatal and High-Risk Neonatal Management; *Integrated Processes:* Teaching and Learning; *Client Need:* Physiological Integrity/Basic Care and Comfort/Nutrition and Oral Hydration; *Cognitive Level:* Application

References: Davidson, M., London, M., & Ladewig, P. (2008). *Olds' Maternal-Newborn Nursing & Women's Health Across the Lifespan* (8th ed., p. 895). Upper Saddle River, NJ: Prentice Hall Health; Pillitteri, A. (2007). *Maternal & Child Health Nursing: Care of the Childbearing & Childrearing Family* (5th ed., p. 725). Philadelphia: Lippincott Williams & Wilkins.

437. A registered nurse (RN) is caring for a postpartum client who delivered a term newborn 24 hours previously. A student nurse is assisting the RN to care for this client. The nurse recognizes that the student needs more information on newborn nutrition when the nurse overhears the student telling the client that:

1. 50% of the infant's calorie needs are met by the fat contained in the breast milk or formula.
2. lactose is the primary source of carbohydrates in breast milk and formula.
3. calcium supplementation is not needed for the newborn regardless of the feeding method.
4. supplemental water should be given to all newborns every day, regardless of feeding method.

ANSWER: 4

Breast milk and formula contain almost 90% water, which meets the infant's water needs. Feeding supplemental water can cause hyponatremia and may result in seizures if water consumption is excessive. Full-term infants do receive about half of their required calories from the fat in breast milk (52%) or formula (49%). Lactose is the primary carbohydrate in both breast milk and formula, and its slow breakdown and absorption may increase calcium absorption. Therefore calcium levels are adequate in both types of milk for bone growth and prevention of tetany.

➧ ***Test-taking Tip:*** *The statement "nurse recognizes that the student needs more information" is a false-response item. Look for the incorrect statement.*

Content Area: Childbearing Families; *Category of Health Alteration:* Neonatal and High-Risk Neonatal Management; *Integrated Processes:* Nursing Process Evaluation; *Client Need:* Safe and Effective Care Environment/Management of Care/Supervision; *Cognitive Level:* Application

References: Davidson, M., London, M., & Ladewig, P. (2008). *Olds' Maternal-Newborn Nursing & Women's Health Across the Lifespan* (8th ed., p. 893). Upper Saddle River, NJ: Prentice Hall Health; Pillitteri, A. (2007). *Maternal & Child Health Nursing: Care of the Childbearing & Childrearing Family* (5th ed., p. 725). Philadelphia: Lippincott Williams & Wilkins; Wong, D., Hockenberry, M., Wilson, D., Perry, S., & Lowdermilk, D. (2006). *Maternal Child Nursing Care* (3rd ed., p. 770). Philadelphia: Lippincott Williams & Wilkins.

438. While preparing parents of a 2-day-old, bottle-feeding newborn for discharge, a nurse recognizes the need for additional teaching about formula feeding when one of the parents says:

1. "We will clean our baby's bottles in the dishwasher."
2. "I know we can warm the formula by placing it in a bowl of warm tap water."
3. "If there is formula left in the bottle after the baby finishes eating I know we should put it in the refrigerator."
4. "We live in the city, so I know we can use our tap water to mix the powdered formula."

ANSWER: 3

The formula remaining in the bottle after feeding has mixed with the infant's saliva and should be discarded. It should not be refrigerated. Bottles and nipples can be washed in the dishwasher with other family dishes. If the formula has been refrigerated, it can be warmed to room temperature by placing it in a bowl of warm water. It should never be warmed in the microwave. Infants may be fed cold formula; however, they most often prefer warm or room-temperature formula. Water from a municipal water supply is regulated by drinking water regulation and is safe for use with formula.

Test-taking Tip: *The statement "needs for additional teaching" in the stem is a false-response item. Look for the incorrect statement.*

Content Area: Childbearing Families; *Category of Health Alteration:* Neonatal and High-Risk Neonatal Management; *Integrated Processes:* Nursing Process Evaluation; *Client Need:* Physiological Integrity/Basic Care and Comfort/Nutrition and Oral Hydration; Safe and Effective Care Environment/Safety and Infection Control/Safe Use of Equipment; *Cognitive Level:* Analysis

References: Davidson, M., London, M., & Ladewig, P. (2008). *Olds' Maternal-Newborn Nursing & Women's Health Across the Lifespan* (8th ed., pp. 915–916). Upper Saddle River, NJ: Prentice Hall Health; Wong, D., Hockenberry, M., Wilson, D., Perry, S., & Lowdermilk, D. (2006). *Maternal Child Nursing Care* (3rd ed., p. 791). Philadelphia: Lippincott Williams & Wilkins.

439. A breastfeeding mother is being discharged with her 2-day-old, full-term newborn. A nurse recognizes that the mother understands how to determine if her newborn is getting enough breast milk when the mother says:

1. "I know he should have at least three wet diapers tomorrow."
2. "I am expecting him to have one stool per day during the next week."
3. "I know he should weigh at least 8 ounces more than his birth weight at his 1-week checkup."
4. "If he nurses for 5 minutes on each breast, I know he will be getting enough milk."

ANSWER: 1

The infant who is feeding well will have characteristic outputs. A 3-day-old infant should produce at least three wet diapers. After 5 days of age, the newborn should produce six well-saturated, wet diapers per day. Infants typically produce at least 3 to 4 stools per day, and it is not uncommon for a breastfed infant to have 10 stools per day for the first month of life. It is expected that newborns, especially breastfed newborns, will lose from 5% to 10% of their birth weight during the first week after birth; therefore, the mother should not expect an 8-ounce weight gain. The mother should be discouraged from watching the clock to determine appropriate intake. During a normal feeding session the infant will nurse 10 to 20 minutes on the first breast, with feeding time on the second breast varying.

Test-taking Tip: *Eliminate option 2 as this would obviously be abnormal stool production. Option 4 is incorrect because a time limit should not be placed on breastfeeding infants; however, common sense would dictate that 5 minutes on each breast would not be long enough for a feeding.*

Content Area: Childbearing Families; *Category of Health Alteration:* Neonatal and High-Risk Neonatal Management; *Integrated Processes:* Nursing Process Evaluation; *Client Need:* Health Promotion and Maintenance/Ante/Intra/Postpartum and Newborn Care; Physiological Integrity/Basic Care and Comfort/Nutrition and Oral Hydration; *Cognitive Level:* Analysis

Reference: Davidson, M., London, M., & Ladewig, P. (2008). *Olds' Maternal-Newborn Nursing & Women's Health Across the Lifespan* (8th ed., pp. 913–914). Upper Saddle River, NJ: Prentice Hall Health.

440. EBP A nurse is counseling an adoptive couple who is picking up their newborn from a facility. The newborn has some questionable facial characteristics, and a physician has advised the adoptive parents that the infant could have fetal alcohol syndrome (FAS). What information is needed to officially diagnose a baby with FAS? SELECT ALL THAT APPLY.

1. Documented presence of abnormal facial characteristics
2. Documented growth deficits
3. Documented central nervous system abnormalities
4. Documented statements of maternal alcohol consumption during pregnancy
5. Documented maternal treatment for alcohol abuse during pregnancy

ANSWER: 1, 2, 3

A diagnosis of FAS is made when there is documentation of abnormal facial characteristics, growth deficits, and nervous system abnormalities. Documentation of maternal alcohol consumption or treatment is not required because women may deny that they consumed alcohol during pregnancy or pregnant women who abuse alcohol may not seek treatment.

➧ ***Test-taking Tip:*** *Consider objective information about the infant. Eliminate information pertaining to the pregnant woman.*

Content Area: Childbearing Families; *Category of Health Alteration:* Neonatal and High-Risk Neonatal Management; *Integrated Processes:* Nursing Process Analysis; *Client Need:* Physiological Integrity/Physiological Adaptation/Alterations in Body Systems; *Cognitive Level:* Application

Reference: National Organization on Fetal Alcohol Syndrome (2007). *FASD Identification*. Available at: www.nofas.org/MediaFiles/PDFs/factsheets/identification.pdf

EBP Reference: Caley, L., Shipkey, N., Winkelman, T., Dunlap, C., Rivera, S. (2006). Evidence-based review of nursing interventions to prevent secondary disabilities in fetal alcohol spectrum disorder. *Pediatric Nursing*, 32(2), 155–162.

---

441. A nurse is caring for a woman on an intrapartum unit who has just given birth to a baby boy. The mother is O negative. The nurse should assess for ABO incompatibility and hyperbilirubinemia if the infants blood type is:

1. O positive.
2. O negative.
3. A negative.
4. any type, because all fetuses are equally affected.

ANSWER: 3

ABO incompatibility is limited to mothers with O blood type who have type A or B fetuses. The mother's O blood type has no red blood cell (RBC) antigens, and the plasma has A and B antibodies. The plasma of a fetus with A blood type will only have B antibodies, and the plasma of a fetus with B blood type will only have A antibodies. Group O fetuses are never affected, regardless of the mother's blood type, because the fetus does not have a RBC antigen and the plasma has A and B antibodies.

➧ ***Test-taking Tip:*** *If a mother is O negative, consider the absent RBC antigens and the presence of antibodies. Options 1 and 2 are opposites, so one or both of these can be eliminated as incorrect.*

Content Area: Childbearing Families; *Category of Health Alteration:* Neonatal and High-Risk Neonatal Management; *Integrated Processes:* Physiological Integrity/Physiological Adaptation/Pathophysiology; *Client Need:* Nursing Process Assessment; *Cognitive Level:* Application

References: Berman, A., Snyder, S., Kozier, B., & Erb, G. (2008). *Fundamentals of Nursing: Concepts, Process, and Practice* (8th ed., pp. 1472–1473). Upper Saddle River, NJ: Pearson Education; Pillitteri, A. (2007). *Maternal & Child Health Nursing: Care of the Childbearing & Childrearing Family* (5th ed., pp. 437–438). Philadelphia: Lippincott Williams & Wilkins.

---

442. Before beginning a newborn physical assessment, a nurse reviews the newborn's medical record and sees this notation: "31 weeks gestation." Considering this information, the nurse determines that a physical assessment of the infant should reveal:

1. flexion of all four extremities.
2. the ability to suck.
3. the absence of lanugo.
4. vernix covering the infant.

ANSWER: 4

The preterm infant, 24 to 36 weeks gestation, typically is covered with vernix caseosa—a waxy, white substance secreted by the fetus's sebaceous glands in utero. Lanugo is usually extensive in a 31-week infant, covering the back, forearms, forehead, and sides of the face. The sucking and swallowing reflexes are absent in an infant younger than 33 weeks gestation. The preterm infant's posture is characterized by very little, if any, flexion of extremities.

➧ ***Test-taking Tip:*** *Recall how the physical characteristics of infants change as their gestational age progresses.*

Content Area: Childbearing Families; *Category of Health Alteration:* Neonatal and High-Risk Neonatal Management; *Integrated Processes:* Nursing Process Analysis; *Client Need:* Health Promotion and Maintenance/Developmental Stages and Transitions; Physiological Integrity Reduction of Risk Potential/System Specific Assessments; *Cognitive Level:* Application

Reference: Pillitteri, A. (2007). *Maternal & Child Health Nursing: Care of the Childbearing & Childrearing Family* (5th ed., pp. 762–763). Philadelphia: Lippincott Williams & Wilkins.

443. At the end of a shift in the neonatal intensive care unit, a nurse is calculating the total output of a preterm infant. The infant had four wet diapers during the 8-hour shift. The weight of a dry diaper is 15 grams. The four wet diapers weighed 30 grams, 24 grams, 21 grams, and 25 grams. The calculation of total 8-hour urine output is______mL.

ANSWER: 40

Infant weight change is the most sensitive indicator of fluid balance in a neonate. However, weighing diapers is also important for accurate input and output measurement. One milliliter of urine output equals 1 gram of body weight.

Test-taking Tip: *If a dry diaper weighs 15 grams, subtract that weight from the weight of each of the infant's diapers: 30 − 15 = 15 grams, 24 − 15 = 9 grams, 21 − 15 = 6 grams, 25 − 15 = 10 grams. Then add all of the totals: 15 + 9 + 6 + 10 = 40 grams of fluid loss, which equals 40 mL of urine output.*

Content Area: Childbearing Families; *Category of Health Alteration:* Neonatal and High-Risk Neonatal Management; *Integrated Processes:* Nursing Process Assessment; *Client Need:* Physiological Integrity/Basic Care and Comfort/Elimination; *Cognitive Level:* Application

Reference: Davidson, M., London, M., & Ladewig, P. (2008). *Olds' Maternal-Newborn Nursing & Women's Health Across the Lifespan* (8th ed., p. 955). Upper Saddle River, NJ: Prentice Hall Health.

444. A nurse is caring for a preterm infant who must be fed via bolus gavage feeding. The infant has a 5 French feeding tube already secured in the left nare. The nurse has aspirated the infant's stomach contents, noting color, amount, and consistency, and reinserted the residual amount because it was less than a fourth of the previous feeding. Prioritize the remaining steps that the nurse should take to complete this feeding.

______ Separate the barrel of the syringe from the plunger and connect the syringe barrel to the feeding tube
______ Remove the syringe and clear the tubing with 2 to 3 mL of air.
______ Elevate the syringe 6 to 8 inches over the infant's head.
______ Position the infant on the right side.
______ Uncrimp the tubing and allow the feeding to flow by gravity at a slow rate.
______ Crimp the feeding tube and pour the specified amount of formula or breast milk into the barrel.
______ Cap the lavage feeding tube and tape or remove.

ANSWER: 2, 6, 4, 1, 5, 3, 7

First position the infant on the right side. This decreases the risk of aspiration should emesis occur. Next, the plunger is removed from the barrel of the syringe to allow the feeding to flow via gravity. Crimp the tube while pouring in the feeding to prevent inadvertent flow of the feeding before the total amount is in the syringe barrel. Elevate the syringe 6 to 8 inches to promote a slow gravity flow. When the syringe is at the correct height, uncrimp the tubing to allow the feeding to infuse. When the feeding is complete, instill 2 to 3 mL of air to clear the tube and make sure all the feeding is in the infant's stomach. Finally cap the tube. Capping it will prevent contamination if the tube is to be left in place, or fluid leakage and possible aspiration if the tube is to be removed.

Test-taking Tip: *Visualize the step-by-step process that would be needed to administer a bolus feeding through a feeding tube before placing items in the correct sequence.*

Content Area: Childbearing Families; *Category of Health Alteration:* Neonatal and High-Risk Neonatal Management; *Integrated Processes:* Nursing Process Implementation; *Client Need:* Physiological Integrity Reduction of Risk Potential/Therapeutic Procedures; *Cognitive Level:* Application

References: Davidson, M., London, M., & Ladewig, P. (2008). *Olds' Maternal-Newborn Nursing & Women's Health Across the Lifespan* (8th ed., pp. 950, 955). Upper Saddle River, NJ: Prentice Hall Health; Wong, D., Hockenberry, M., Wilson, D., Perry, S., & Lowdermilk, D. (2006). *Maternal Child Nursing Care* (3rd ed., pp. 808–809). Philadelphia: Lippincott Williams & Wilkins.

445. EBP A newborn who is 33-weeks gestation and 48 hours old has been diagnosed with respiratory distress syndrome (RDS). A health-care provider orders the administration of surfactant via endotracheal tube. The father asks a nurse to explain how this treatment will help his baby. The nurse explains that the preterm
infant is unable to produce adequate amounts of surfactant and giving it to his baby will:

1. increase $Paco_2$ levels in the bloodstream.
2. prevent alveoli collapse.
3. decrease Pao_2 levels in the bloodstream.
4. prevent pleural effusion.

ANSWER: 2

RDS is the result of a primary absence, deficiency, or alteration in the production of pulmonary surfactant. Lack of surfactant in the preterm infant causes decreased lung compliance, resulting in increased inspiratory pressure needed to expand the lungs with air. Surfactant replacement therapy decreases alveolar collapse and thus decreases the severity of RDS. Early surfactant replacement therapy is associated with a decreased need for mechanical ventilation and fewer complications. Preventing alveolar collapse allows the exchange of gases and thus will cause an increase in Pao_2 and a decrease in $Paco_2$. Pleural effusion does not occur in this disease.

➧ ***Test-taking Tip:*** *Recall that increasing $Paco_2$ and decreasing Pao_2 would indicate increasing respiratory distress and would not be a desired result. Eliminate options 1 and 3.*

Content Area: Childbearing Families; *Category of Health Alteration:* Neonatal and High-Risk Neonatal Management; *Integrated Processes:* Nursing Process Implementation; *Client Need:* Physiological Integrity/Physiological Adaptation/Pathophysiology; Physiological Integrity/Physiological Adaptation/Illness Management; *Cognitive Level:* Analysis

References: Davidson, M., London, M., & Ladewig, P. (2008). *Olds' Maternal-Newborn Nursing & Women's Health Across the Lifespan* (8th ed., pp. 943, 988, 990). Upper Saddle River, NJ: Prentice Hall Health; Pillitteri, A. (2007). *Maternal & Child Health Nursing: Care of the Childbearing & Childrearing Family* (5th ed., p. 767). Philadelphia: Lippincott Williams & Wilkins.

EBP Reference: Stevens, T., Blennow, M., Myers, E., & Soll, R. (2007). Early surfactant administration with brief ventilation vs. selective surfactant and continued mechanical ventilation for preterm infants with or at risk for respiratory distress syndrome. *Cochrane Database of Systematic Reviews,* Issue 4, Art. No. CD003063. DOI: 10.1002/14651858. CD003063.pub3. Available at: www.mrw.interscience.wiley.com.ezproxy. csbsju.edu/cochrane/clsysrev/articles/CD003645/frame.html

---

446. EBP A nurse is caring for a preterm infant with respiratory distress syndrome (RDS). To maximize the infant's respiratory status, the nurse should intervene by:

1. monitoring blood glucose levels every 4 hours.
2. cooling all inspired gases.
3. weighing the infant every other day.
4. positioning the infant in a prone position.

ANSWER: 4

The prone position is significantly superior to the supine position in terms of oxygenation in ventilated, preterm infants. Because this position is associated with sudden infant death, infants placed in this position should have continuous cardiorespiratory monitoring. All inspired gases should be warmed, as cold air/oxygen stimulates increased oxygen consumption by increasing the metabolic rate. Infants should be weighed daily to monitor for fluid imbalances, which may adversely affect respiratory status. While monitoring blood glucose levels is important, it will not assist in maximizing respiratory status.

➧ ***Test-taking Tip:*** *Eliminate option 3 as weights help monitor intake and output, not respiratory status. Similarly, eliminate option 1 as blood glucose is not linked with respiratory status.*

Content Area: Childbearing Families; *Category of Health Alteration:* Neonatal and High-Risk Neonatal Management; *Integrated Processes:* Nursing Process Implementation; *Client Need:* Physiological Integrity/ Physiological Adaptation/Illness Management; *Cognitive Level:* Application

Reference: Davidson, M., London, M., & Ladewig, P. (2008). *Olds' Maternal-Newborn Nursing & Women's Health Across the Lifespan* (8th ed., pp. 994–995). Upper Saddle River, NJ: Prentice Hall Health.

EBP Reference: Wells, D., Gillies, D., & Fitzgerald, D. (2005). Positioning for acute respiratory distress in hospitalized infants and children. *Cochrane Database of Systematic Reviews,* Issue 2, Art. No. CD003645. DOI: 10.1002/14651858.CD003645.pub2. Available at: www.mrw.interscience.wiley.com.ezproxy.csbsju.edu/cochrane/clsysrev/ articles/CD003645/frame.html

447. A nurse is reviewing the record of a 15-hour-old newborn before beginning a physical assessment. The nurse notes the following labor history: "Mother positive for group B streptococcal (GBS) infection at 37 weeks gestation. Membranes ruptured at home 14 hours before mother presented to the hospital at 40 weeks gestation. Precipitous labor, no antibiotic given." Considering this information, the nurse should observe the infant closely for:

1. temperature instability.
2. pink stains in the diaper.
3. meconium stools.
4. development of erythema toxicum.

ANSWER: 1

GBS is a bacterial infection found in the mother's urogenital tract. It can be transmitted to the fetus during childbirth if the mother has the infection. The risk of infection is increased if the membranes are ruptured for more than 12 hours before birth occurs and if the mother is not given antibiotics during labor. The infant infected with GBS may start to exhibit symptoms within the first 12 to 24 hours after birth. Temperature instability is one of the most common early symptoms. Erythema toxicum is a rash that is common to newborns and will disappear without treatment. Meconium stools are expected within the first 24 hours after birth. Pink stains in the diaper are caused by urates in the urine and are innocuous.

➧ ***Test-taking Tip:*** *Recall expected newborn characteristics. Options 2, 3, and 4 all describe expected physiological adaptations for newborns during the transition from fetal life.*

Content Area: Childbearing Families; *Category of Health Alteration:* Neonatal and High-Risk Neonatal Management; *Integrated Processes:* Nursing Process Planning; *Client Need:* Health Promotion and Maintenance/Ante/Intra/Postpartum and Newborn Care; *Cognitive Level:* Analysis

Reference: Davidson, M., London, M., & Ladewig, P. (2008). *Olds' Maternal-Newborn Nursing & Women's Health Across the Lifespan* (8th ed., pp. 533, 810–811, 832, 1026). Upper Saddle River, NJ: Prentice Hall Health.

448. EBP A nurse is caring for an infant in the neonatal intensive care unit who has an umbilical artery catheter (UAC) in place. To monitor for and prevent complications with this catheter, which interventions should be planned by the nurse? SELECT ALL THAT APPLY.

1. Assess the position of the catheter every shift.
2. Position the tubing close to the infant's lower limbs.
3. Assess for erythema or discoloration of the abdominal wall.
4. Palpate for femoral, pedal, and tibial pulses every 2 to 4 hours.
5. Reposition the tubing every hour.
6. Monitor blood glucose levels.

ANSWER: 1, 3, 4, 6

The nurse should verify that the catheter is secure and still at the prescribed, documented centimeter marking by examining the position of the centimeter marking on the catheter and comparing it to the mark recorded when the catheter was placed. After placement of a UAC, the nurse should perform abdominal assessments to monitor for intra-abdominal blood loss that may occur if an umbilical vessel becomes perforated. Alterations in circulation from UACs can lead to loss of digit(s) or an extremity. At least every 2 to 4 hours, the nurse should systematically evaluate perfusion to the distal extremities. This includes examining the legs for color, temperature, and capillary refill, as well as assessing the extremity pulses. Caregivers should monitor blood glucose levels and compare them to the amount of glucose the infant may be receiving. Abnormal values, especially hypoglycemia, may indicate that the catheter is out of position. The catheter should be positioned away from the infant's extremities to prevent the infant from accidentally dislocating or removing the catheter by toe or finger entrapment. Frequent manipulation of the catheter is a contributing factor in catheter-related bloodstream infection, therefore manipulation of the catheter should be avoided unless necessary for medical procedures and assessments.

➧ ***Test-taking Tip:*** *Knowledge of the care of umbilical arterial catheters is required to answer this question.*

Content Area: Childbearing Families; *Category of Health Alteration:* Neonatal and High-Risk Neonatal Management; *Integrated Processes:* Nursing Process Planning; *Client Need:* Physiological Integrity/Pharmacological and Parenteral Therapies/Parenteral/Intravenous Therapies; *Cognitive Level:* Application

Reference: Pillitteri, A. (2007). *Maternal & Child Health Nursing: Care of the Childbearing & Childrearing Family* (5th ed., p. 769). Philadelphia: Lippincott Williams & Wilkins.

EBP Reference: Furdon, S., Horgan, M., Bradshaw, T., & Clark, D. (2007). *Nurses' Guide to Early Detection of Umbilical Arterial Catheter Complications in Infants.* Available at: www.medscape.com/viewarticle/550544_1

449. While caring for a small for gestational age newborn (SGA), a nurse notes slight tremors of the extremities, a high-pitched cry, and an exaggerated Moro reflex. In response to these assessment findings, what should be the nurse's *first* action?

1. Assess the infant's blood sugar level
2. Document the findings in the infant's medical record
3. Immediately inform the health-care provider of the symptoms
4. Assess the infant's temperature.

ANSWER: 1

SGA infants are at risk for hypoglycemia because they have poor hepatic glycogen stores and inadequate supplies of enzymes to activate gluconeogenesis. Symptoms of hypoglycemia include tremors, high-pitched or weak cry, and exaggerated Moro reflex. The nurse should recognize that these symptoms in a SGA infant necessitate action rather than just documentation. The nurse should check the infant's blood glucose and notify the health-care provider if the level is abnormal. Assessing the infant's temperature should also be done, as a low temperature could contribute to hypoglycemia; however, this is not the first action in terms of priority.

➧ ***Test-taking Tip:*** *The key phase is "the nurse's first action," indicating a need for prioritization. Review the symptoms and then determine that more information is needed before calling the health-care provider. Eliminate option 3. Also recall that the symptoms are not normal/expected newborn adaptations; therefore, eliminate option 4.*

Content Area: Childbearing Families; *Category of Health Alteration:* Neonatal and High-Risk Neonatal Management; *Integrated Processes:* Nursing Process Analysis; *Client Need:* Physiological Integrity Reduction of Risk Potential/System Specific Assessments; *Cognitive Level:* Analysis

References: Davidson, M., London, M., & Ladewig, P. (2008). *Olds' Maternal-Newborn Nursing & Women's Health Across the Lifespan* (8th ed., pp. 932–933, 936, 1005). Upper Saddle River, NJ: Prentice Hall Health; Wong, D., Hockenberry, M., Wilson, D., Perry, S., & Lowdermilk, D. (2006). *Maternal Child Nursing Care* (3rd ed., p. 821). Philadelphia: Lippincott Williams & Wilkins.

450. A nurse is planning the care of a 2-hour-old infant at 38 weeks gestation whose mother has type 1 diabetes mellitus. The nurse writes the following NANDA diagnosis: "Altered Nutrition: less than body requirements" and appropriately adds which "related to" statement?

1. Decreased amounts of red blood cells secondary to low erythropoietin levels
2. Decreased amounts of total body fat secondary to decreased growth hormone
3. Increased glucose metabolism secondary to hyperinsulinemia
4. Increased amounts of body water

ANSWER: 3

While in utero, the fetus of a diabetic mother is exposed to high levels of maternal glucose. Hyperplasia of the fetal pancreas occurs resulting in hyperinsulinemia. When the fetus is born, the glucose supply from the mother is disrupted and the neonate's blood sugar falls rapidly in response to the corresponding high levels of circulating insulin. The infant of an insulin-dependent mother (IDM) has increased amounts of red blood cells (RBCs) because hemoglobin A1c binds to oxygen, decreasing the oxygen available to the fetal tissues. This tissue hypoxia stimulates increased erythropoietin production, which stimulates RBC production. The IDM has increased amounts of body fat as a result of hyperinsulinemia, which converts glucose to adipose tissue and stimulates production of pituitary growth hormone. IDMs have decreased total body water, particularly in the extracellular spaces.

➧ ***Test-taking Tip:*** *Recall the physiology of diabetes and the adaptations made by the IDM*

Content Area: Childbearing Families; *Category of Health Alteration:* Neonatal and High-Risk Neonatal Management; *Integrated Processes:* Nursing Process Analysis; *Client Need:* Physiological Integrity/Physiological Adaptation/Alterations in Body Systems; *Cognitive Level:* Analysis

References: Davidson, M., London, M., & Ladewig, P. (2008). *Olds' Maternal-Newborn Nursing & Women's Health Across the Lifespan* (8th ed., pp. 939–940). Upper Saddle River, NJ: Prentice Hall Health; Wong, D., Hockenberry, M., Wilson, D., Perry, S., & Lowdermilk, D. (2006). *Maternal Child Nursing Care* (3rd ed., p. 822). Philadelphia: Lippincott Williams & Wilkins.

451. While caring for a 6-hour-old, full-term newborn, a nurse notes that the newborn is showing signs of respiratory compromise. After reviewing the infant's labor and delivery record, the nurse suspects meconium aspiration syndrome (MAS) when which information is noted in the record?

1. 1-hour precipitous labor, small for gestational age infant
2. 40-hour labor, meconium-stained amniotic fluid
3. Forceps delivery, shoulder dystocia
4. Planned cesarean birth

ANSWER: 2

When fetal hypoxia occurs, the anal sphincter of the fetus relaxes and meconium is expelled into the amniotic fluid. Approximately 13% of live born, close-to-term, or full-term infants are born with meconium-stained amniotic fluid (MSAF). Any infant born with MSAF has the potential to aspirate the fluid and develop MAS. If the infant is not born with MSAF, then MAS will not occur.

➧ ***Test-taking Tip:*** *Think about the name of the syndrome: "Meconium aspiration." Eliminate options 1, 3, and 4 because there is no indication that meconium was present in the amniotic fluid.*

Content Area: Childbearing Families; *Category of Health Alteration:* Neonatal and High-Risk Neonatal Management; *Integrated Processes:* Nursing Process Analysis; *Client Need:* Physiological Integrity/ Physiological Adaptation/Alterations in Body Systems; *Cognitive Level:* Analysis

Reference: Davidson, M., London, M., & Ladewig, P. (2008). *Olds' Maternal-Newborn Nursing & Women's Health Across the Lifespan* (8th ed., pp. 997–998). Upper Saddle River, NJ: Prentice Hall Health.

---

452. When assessing an infant undergoing phototherapy for hyperbilirubinema, a nurse notes a maculopapular rash over the infant's buttocks and back. In response to this assessment finding, what action should the nurse take next?

1. Document the results in the newborn's medical record.
2. Call the health-care provider immediately to report this finding.
3. Discontinue the phototherapy immediately.
4. Assess the infant's temperature.

ANSWER: 1

As a side effect of phototherapy, some newborns develop a transient maculopapular rash that does not require treatment. The only action required is to document the findings. There is no need to call the health-care provider or discontinue phototherapy. Newborn temperatures should be monitored per institutional standards when an infant is being treated with phototherapy.

➧ ***Test-taking Tip:*** *Recall the side effects of phototherapy.*

Content Area: Childbearing Families; *Category of Health Alteration:* Neonatal and High-Risk Neonatal Management; *Integrated Processes:* Nursing Process Implementation; *Client Need:* Physiological Integrity Reduction of Risk Potential/Potential for Alterations in Body Systems; *Cognitive Level:* Application

References: Davidson, M., London, M., & Ladewig, P. (2008). *Olds' Maternal-Newborn Nursing & Women's Health Across the Lifespan* (8th ed., p. 1013). Upper Saddle River, NJ: Prentice Hall Health; Wong, D., Hockenberry, M., Wilson, D., Perry, S., & Lowdermilk, D. (2006). *Maternal Child Nursing Care* (3rd ed., p. 753). Philadelphia: Lippincott Williams & Wilkins.

---

453. EBP The parents of a healthy 15-hour-old term newborn are planning discharge from a hospital with their infant. The mother requests that the phenalketonuria (PKU) blood test be done before the infant leaves the hospital. The nurse's response to the mother is based on the knowledge that:

1. the PKU test must be done when the infant is at least 1 month of age.
2. the parents must sign a specific consent form if the PKU screening is done before the infant is 24 hours old.
3. the PKU screening is most accurate if performed after 24 hours of life but before the infant is 7 days old.
4. the PKU test is not needed as long as the infant is tolerating feedings without diarrhea or vomiting.

ANSWER: 3

Infants with PKU lack the ability to convert the amino acid phenylalanine to tyrosine. Phenylalanine accumulates in the blood and leads to progressive mental retardation. To allow sufficient intake of protein for accurate results, screening tests are most accurate if performed after 24 hours of life and before the infant is 7 days old. The PKU test is part of mandatory newborn screening. If parents leave the hospital before their infant is 24 hours old, they are required to obtain the test within the first week after discharge.

➧ ***Test-taking Tip:*** *PKU testing is mandatory, thus eliminating option 4.*

Content Area: Childbearing Families; *Category of Health Alteration:* Neonatal and High-Risk Neonatal Management; *Integrated Processes:* Nursing Process Planning; *Client Need:* Physiological Integrity Reduction of Risk Potential/Diagnostic Tests; *Cognitive Level:* Application

Reference: Davidson, M., London, M., & Ladewig, P. (2008). *Olds' Maternal-Newborn Nursing & Women's Health Across the Lifespan* (8th ed., pp. 975, 978). Upper Saddle River, NJ: Prentice Hall Health.

EBP Reference: U.S. Preventive Services Task Force. (2008). *Screening for Phenylketonuria (PKU)* (U.S. Preventive Services Task Force Reaffirmation Recommendation Statement). Available at: www.guideline.gov/summary/summary.aspx®view_id=1&doc_id=12270

454. If a nurse is concerned that a newborn may have congenital hydrocephalus, which assessment finding is noted?

1. Bulging anterior fontanel
2. Head circumference equal to the chest circumference
3. A narrowed posterior fontanel
4. Low-set ears

ANSWER: 1

A bulging anterior fontanel is an initial sign of congenital hydrocephalus. The posterior fontanel is normally smaller than the anterior fontanel, and molding may make it very narrow. The head and chest circumferences of a full-term newborn should be very close to the same size, within 2 to 3 cm. Low-set ears are a sign of trisomy 21.

▶ ***Test-taking Tip:*** *Recall that hydrocephalus is an enlargement in the ventricles of the brain. Thus, select option 1.*

Content Area: Childbearing Families; *Category of Health Alteration:* Neonatal and High-Risk Neonatal Management; *Integrated Processes:* Nursing Process Assessment; *Client Need:* Physiological Integrity/Physiological Adaptation/Alterations in Body Systems; *Cognitive Level:* Application

References: Davidson, M., London, M., & Ladewig, P. (2008). *Olds' Maternal-Newborn Nursing & Women's Health Across the Lifespan* (8th ed., pp. 281, 934, 960). Upper Saddle River, NJ: Prentice Hall Health; Wong, D., Hockenberry, M., Wilson, D., Perry, S., & Lowdermilk, D. (2006). *Maternal Child Nursing Care* (3rd ed., p. 855). Philadelphia: Lippincott Williams & Wilkins.

---

455. After assisting in the delivery of a full-term infant with anencephaly, the parents ask a nurse to explain treatments that might be available for their infant. The nurse's response is based on the knowledge that:

1. immediate surgery is necessary to repair the congenital defect.
2. anencephaly is incompatible with life, and only palliative care should be provided.
3. a shunting procedure will be necessary initially to relieve intracranial pressure.
4. antibiotics are needed initially before any treatment is started.

ANSWER: 2

Anencephaly is the absence of both cerebral hemispheres and of the overlying skull. It is a condition that is incompatible with life. Surgery, shunting, and/or antibiotics will not repair this defect.

▶ ***Test-taking Tip:*** *Focus on the definition of anencephaly.*

Content Area: Childbearing Families; *Category of Health Alteration:* Neonatal and High-Risk Neonatal Management; *Integrated Processes:* Nursing Process Planning; *Client Need:* Physiological Integrity/Physiological Adaptation/Alterations in Body Systems; *Cognitive Level:* Application

Reference: Wong, D., Hockenberry, M., Wilson, D., Perry, S., & Lowdermilk, D. (2006). *Maternal Child Nursing Care* (3rd ed., p. 854). Philadelphia: Lippincott Williams & Wilkins.

---

456. A nurse accompanies the parents of a newborn infant to the neonatal intensive care unit (NICU) to visit their newborn son who has been diagnosed with a terminal cardiac condition. The nurse understands that interventions to promote parental attachment should:

1. be delayed until it is certain that the newborn will live.
2. include encouraging the parents to provide as much care as possible for their newborn.
3. be limited to naming the baby only.
4. include reassurances that the condition is not a result of anything the mother did during her pregnancy.

ANSWER: 2

The parents should be encouraged to provide care for their infant, even if the baby is very sick and likely to die. If the infant should die, detachment is easier if attachment has been established because the parents will be comforted by the knowledge that they did all they could for their child while he or she was alive. Parents may be hesitant to bond with a sick infant; however, attachment should be encouraged. There is not enough information in the stem of the question to determine the cause of the cardiac condition, but feelings of guilt and failure often plague parents of sick newborns, and, rather than suppress or ignore these feelings, the nurse should acknowledge them as being expected.

▶ ***Test-taking Tip:*** *Read each option carefully and select options independently of the other options.*

Content Area: Childbearing; *Category of Health Alteration:* Neonatal and High-Risk Neonatal Management; *Integrated Processes:* Nursing Process Implementation; *Client Need:* Health Promotion and Maintenance/Developmental Stages and Transitions; *Cognitive Level:* Application

Reference: Davidson, M., London, M., & Ladewig, P. (2008). *Olds' Maternal-Newborn Nursing & Women's Health Across the Lifespan* (8th ed., p. 1032). Upper Saddle River, NJ: Prentice Hall Health.

Test 12: **Childbearing Families: Pharmacological and Parenteral Therapies**

457. EBP A client presents to a walk-in travel clinic to receive vaccinations. The client tells a nurse she thinks she may be pregnant. Which vaccines, if ordered by a physician, should the nurse prepare to administer to this client?

1. Rubella
2. Varicella
3. Hepatitis B
4. Mumps

ANSWER: 3

Hepatitis B vaccination can be safely administered during pregnancy. This vaccine is for the virus hepatitis B. The virus is transmitted through transfusions of contaminated blood or semen and can also be passed through contaminated syringes or needles through intravenous drug use. Hepatitis B may spread to the fetus if the mother is infected in the third trimester. Rubella, varicella, and mumps should not be administered to pregnant women because they are live viruses and are contraindicated during pregnancy.

➧ ***Test-taking Tip:** Identify which vaccinations are live. Live viruses should not be given in pregnancy. Use this information to make the best selection.*

Content Area: Childbearing Families; *Category of Health Alteration:* Pharmacological and Parenteral Therapies; *Integrated Processes:* Nursing Process Intervention; *Client Need:* Physiological Integrity/ Pharmacological and Parenteral Therapies/Parenteral/Intravenous Therapies; *Cognitive Level:* Application

Reference: Pillitteri, A. (2007). *Maternal & Child Health Nursing: Care of the Childbearing Families & Childrearing Family* (5th ed., pp. 1025, 1428). Philadelphia: Lippincott Williams & Wilkins.

EBP Reference: Kirkham, C., Harris, S., & Grzybowski, S. (2005). Evidence-based prenatal care: Part II. Third trimester care and prevention of infectious diseases. *American Family Physician,* 71(8), 1555–1560.

---

458. A pregnant woman presents to a clinic with a white, cottage-cheese like vaginal discharge, itching, and vulvar redness. A nurse should anticipate that a health-care provider will prescribe which medication?

1. Metronidazole (Flagyl®) 250 mg twice daily for 1 week
2. Butoconazole (Gynazole®) 2 g once
3. Imidazole vaginal cream daily for 1 week.
4. Fluconazole (Diflucan®) 150 mg by mouth once

ANSWER: 3

Imidazole vaginal cream for 1 week is indicated for the treatment of *Candida albicans*. This is also safe in pregnancy. Butoconazole should not be used in pregnancy. Metronidazole is used for the treatment of bacterial vaginosis. Fluconazole one-time treatment has not been well studied during pregnancy and therefore should not be used.

➧ ***Test-taking Tip:** Focus on the color of the discharge to recognize that this is caused by Candida albicans. Select the medication that would be most effective in treating a yeast infection.*

Content Area: Childbearing Families; *Category of Health Alteration:* Pharmacological and Parenteral Therapies; *Integrated Processes:* Nursing Process Intervention; *Client Need:* Physiological Integrity/ Pharmacological and Parenteral Therapies/Pharmacological Agents/ Actions; *Cognitive Level:* Analysis

Reference: Hockenberry, M., & Wilson, D. (2007). *Wong's Nursing Care of Infants and Children* (8th ed., p. 858). St. Louis, MO: Mosby/Elsevier.

---

459. EBP A hospital nurse is checking charts of second-trimester clients for health-care provider orders. Which order should be rewritten before the nurse can comply with the order?

1. Aldomet (Methyldopa®) 250 mg bid by mouth for elevated blood pressure
2. $MgSO_4$ 5 g intramuscular if BP > 160/90 mm Hg × 2 readings
3. Terbutaline (Brethine®) 5 mg q 6 hr by mouth for preterm labor
4. Prenatal vitamins one tablet daily by mouth

ANSWER: 2

According to the Joint Commission on Accreditation of Healthcare Organizations (JCAHO), certain abbreviations should not be used because of different meanings. $MgSO_4$ (magnesium sulfate) can be confused with MSO_4 (morphine sulfate) and should be written out as magnesium sulfate. The > and < symbols may be added to the list in the near future and should also be avoided when writing orders or other medical documentation. Terbutaline is a bronchodilator that is used off-label to treat preterm labor. The remaining orders are correctly written.

➧ ***Test-taking Tip:** Recall that abbreviations in medical orders have been demonstrated to contribute to medication errors. Select the option utilizing inappropriate abbreviations.*

Content Area: Childbearing Families; *Category of Health Alteration:* Pharmacological and Parenteral Therapies; *Integrated Processes:* Nursing Process Evaluation; *Client Need:* Physiological Integrity/ Pharmacological and Parenteral Therapies/Medication Administration; *Cognitive Level:* Application

Reference: Wilson, B., Shannon, M., Shields, K., & Stang, C. (2008). *Prentice Hall Nurse's Drug Guide 2008* (pp. 918–920, 1462). Upper Saddle River, NJ: Pearson Education.

EBP Reference: American College of Obstetricians and Gynecologists. (2006). *Do Not Use Abbreviations.* ACOG Committee Opinion No. 327. Washington, DC: Author.

---

460. EBP A nurse is caring for a 26-week-pregnant client who has been admitted twice in the past week for preterm labor. A physician orders corticosteroid therapy as a means to assist with fetal lung maturation. The nurse should anticipate that the medication and dosage to be ordered should be:

1. methylprednisolone (Medrol®) 40 mg IM weekly until 34 weeks.
2. betamethasone (Celestone®) 12 mg IM every 24 hours for 2 doses.
3. dexamethasone (Decadron®) 6 mg IM every 12 hours for 4 doses.
4. prednisone (Deltasone®) 12 mg IM every 24 hours for 2 doses.

ANSWER: 2

Betamethasone 12 mg IM every 24 hours for 2 doses is the recommended dosage for women between 24 and 34 weeks. Betamethasone is also associated with a decreased incidence of intraventricular brain hemorrhage in preterm infants. Betamethasone has been more widely studied and is preferred due to a reduced risk of fetal distress syndrome as compared with dexamethasone. Methylprednisolone has been shown to have altered placental transfer. It is a Category C medication, and may have teratogenic effects. It would not be prescribed.

➧ ***Test-taking Tip:*** *Look at the dosing and frequency of administration and examine options with duplicate information first. Use this information to choose the answer.*

Content Area: Childbearing Families; *Category of Health Alteration:* Pharmacological and Parenteral Therapies; *Integrated Processes:* Nursing Process Implementation; *Client Need:* Physiological Integrity/ Pharmacological and Parenteral Therapies/Pharmacological Agents/Actions; *Cognitive Level:* Application

Reference: Wilson, B., Shannon, M., Shields, K., & Stang, C. (2008). *Prentice Hall Nurse's Drug Guide 2008* (pp. 165–168). Upper Saddle River, NJ: Pearson Education.

EBP Reference: Roberts, D., & Dalziel, S. (2006). Antenatal corticosteroids for accelerating fetal lung maturation for women at risk of preterm birth. *Cochrane Database of Systematic Reviews*, Issue 3. Article. No.: CD004454. DOI: 10.1002/14651858.CD004454.pub2. Available at: www.cochrane.org/reviews/en/ab004454.html

---

461. A nurse is caring for a woman who was admitted at 25.2 weeks gestation in preterm labor. The woman received nifedipine (Procardia®) but continued having contractions. The nurse is now administering magnesium sulfate (Citro-Mag®). Which assessment findings indicate that the woman is experiencing an adverse effect from the magnesium sulfate? SELECT ALL THAT APPLY.

1. Shortness of breath
2. Nausea
3. Hypertension
4. Dizziness
5. Hypotension
6. Insomnia

ANSWER: 1, 2, 4, 5

Women receiving magnesium sulfate may encounter hypotension, shortness of breath, nausea, and dizziness. Hypertension and insomnia are not commonly associated with magnesium sulfate, and they also are not side effects of nifedipine. Hypotension is more common with nifedipine.

➧ ***Test-taking Tip:*** *The key words are "adverse effects." Think about the effect of magnesium on cells. Note that options 3 and 5 are opposites; eliminate one of these.*

Content Area: Childbearing Families; *Category of Health Alteration:* Pharmacological and Parenteral Therapies; *Integrated Processes:* Nursing Process Evaluation; *Client Need:* Physiological Integrity/ Pharmacological and Parenteral Therapies/Adverse Effects/ Contraindications; *Cognitive Level:* Analysis

References: Wilson, B., Shannon, M., Shields, K., & Stang, C. (2008). *Prentice Hall Nurse's Drug Guide 2008* (pp. 918–920, 1075). Upper Saddle River, NJ: Pearson Education; Lyell, D., Pullen, K., Campbell, L., Ching, S., Druzin, M., et al. (2007). Magnesium sulfate compared with nifedipine for acute tocolysis of preterm labor: A randomized controlled trial. *Obstetrics & Gynecology*, 110, 61–67.

462. EBP A nurse at an outpatient HIV Outreach Center is caring for a pregnant client diagnosed with HIV. The client is receiving highly active antiretroviral therapy (HAART). For which potential pregnancy-related risk factors associated with this therapy should a nurse monitor the client? SELECT ALL THAT APPLY.

1. Preterm labor
2. Preeclampsia
3. Low birth weight
4. Gestational diabetes
5. Birth defects

ANSWER: 1, 3, 4

Women receiving HAART during pregnancy are at higher risk for preterm labor, low birth weight babies, and gestational diabetes. There is no known association between HAART and preeclampsia or birth defects.

➧ ***Test-taking Tip:*** *HAART use in pregnancy is associated with pregnancy-related risk factors. Review these risk factors and eliminate incorrect options.*

Content Area: Childbearing Families; *Category of Health Alteration:* Pharmacological and Parenteral Therapies; *Integrated Processes:* Nursing Assessment Analysis

Client Need: Physiological Integrity/Pharmacological and Parenteral Therapies/Expected Outcomes; *Cognitive Level:* Application

Reference: Black, J., & Hokanson Hawks, J. (2009). *Medical-Surgical Nursing: Clinical Management for Positive Outcomes* (8th ed., p. 2094). St. Louis, MO: Saunders/Elsevier Inc.

EBP References: Martin, F., & Taylor, G. (2007). Increased rates of preterm delivery are associated with the initiation of highly active antiretroviral therapy during pregnancy: A single-center cohort study. *Journal of Infectious Disease*, 196(4), 558–561; Marti, C., Pena, J., Bates, I., Madero, R., de Jose, I., et al. (2007). Obstetric and perinatal complications in HIV-infected women. Analysis of a cohort of 167 pregnancies between 1997 and 2003. *Acta Obstetrics & Gynecology Scandanavia*, 86(4), 409–415.

---

463. EBP A client, who is 8 weeks pregnant, tells a nurse that she is experiencing nausea. The client also states that she does not like to take medication and asks if there are any herbal/natural remedies that she might try. Which herb should be safe for the nurse to suggest?

1. Ginger
2. Milk thistle
3. Black cohosh
4. Echinacea

ANSWER: 1

Ginger is a common remedy for nausea and vomiting in pregnancy. Ginger capsules of 250 mg taken four times a day have been demonstrated to be effective against nausea and vomiting associated with pregnancy, as well as hyperemesis, when compared with placebo. There is no evidence of significant side effects or adverse effects on pregnancy outcomes. The seeds of the milk thistle plant exert hepatoprotective and antihepatotoxic action over liver toxins. Milk thistle also activates the liver's regenerative capacity, making this herb beneficial in the treatment of hepatitis. Black cohosh is an herbal remedy used to treat menopausal and premenstrual syndrome symptoms. Echinacea is used to stimulate the immune system.

➧ ***Test-taking Tip:*** *Recall the action of herbal remedies to correctly answer this question.*

Content Area: Childbearing Families; *Category of Health Alteration:* Pharmacological and Parenteral Therapies; *Integrated Processes:* Teaching and Learning; *Client Need:* Physiological Integrity/Basic Care and Comfort/Nonpharmacological Comfort Interventions; *Cognitive Level:* Application

References: Lehne, R. (2007). *Pharmacology for Nursing Care* (6th ed., p. 1238). St. Louis, MO: Elsevier/Saunders; Monahan, F., Sands, J., Neighbors, M., Marek, J., & Green, C. (2007). *Phipps' Medical-Surgical Nursing: Health and Illness Perspectives* (8th ed., p. 1338). St. Louis, MO: Mosby.

EBP Reference: Wilcox, S. (2006). Pregnancy: Hyperemesis gravidarum, *E-Medicine from WebMD.* Available at: www.emedicine.com/emerg/topic479.htm

464. A health-care provider prescribes omeprazole (Prilosec®) to a client who is 28 weeks pregnant and experiencing heartburn. A nurse educates the client about this medication and explains that it reduces heartburn by:

1. blocking the action of the enzyme that generates gastric acid.
2. blocking the H_2 receptor located on the parietal cells of the stomach.
3. neutralizing the gastric acid.
4. coating the upper stomach and esophagus and decreasing the irritation from the stomach acid.

ANSWER: 1

Omeprazole is known as a proton pump inhibitor (PPI). This classification of medications causes irreversible inhibition of H^+, K^+-ATPase, which is the enzyme that actually produces gastric acid. Option 2 describes histamine blockers such as ranitidine. Option 3 describes the action of antacids, and option 4 describes sucralfate.

➧ ***Test-taking Tip:*** *Recall that the medication classification of omeprazole is a PPI. This should enable elimination of options 3 and 4.*

Content Area: Childbearing Families; *Category of Health Alteration:* Pharmacological and Parenteral Therapies; *Integrated Processes:* Teaching and Learning; *Client Need:* Physiological Integrity/Pharmacological and Parenteral Therapies/Pharmacological Agents/Actions; *Cognitive Level:* Application

Reference: Lehne, R. (2007). *Pharmacology for Nursing Care* (6th ed., pp. 895, 897–899). St. Louis, MO: Elsevier/Saunders.

---

465. A nurse admits a client who is 28 weeks pregnant and experiencing congestive heart failure. When initiating a health-care provider's admission orders for the client, which order should the nurse question?

1. Furosemide (Lasix®) 40 mg IV bid
2. Captopril (Capoten®) 25 mg PO daily
3. Digoxin (Lanoxin®) 0.125 mg IV daily
4. Metoprolol sustained release (Toprol XL®) 50 mg PO daily

ANSWER: 2

Captopril is an angiotensin-converting enzyme (ACE) inhibitor. ACE inhibitors are contraindicated in the second and third trimesters of pregnancy. They can cause oligohydramnios, intrauterine growth retardation (IUGR), congenital structural defects, and renal failure. Digoxin, furosemide, and metoprolol are all Category C medications, but they have not been shown to cause fetal harm. Digoxin exerts a positive inotropic action on the heart. Metoprolol, which is a beta blocker, can improve left ventricular ejection fraction and slow the progression of heart failure, and furosemide is a diuretic.

➧ ***Test-taking Tip:*** *Recall the medications used to treat heart failure in pregnant women and also those medications that are contraindicated for use during pregnancy.*

Content Area: Childbearing Families; *Category of Health Alteration:* Pharmacological and Parenteral Therapies; *Integrated Processes:* Nursing Process Implementation; *Client Need:* Safe and Effective Care Environment/Management of Care/Consultation; Physiological Integrity/Pharmacological and Parenteral Therapies/Medication Administration; *Cognitive Level:* Application

References: Lehne, R. (2007). *Pharmacology for Nursing Care* (6th ed., pp. 464, 467, 514, 520). St. Louis, MO: Elsevier/Saunders; Davidson, M., London, M., & Ladewig, P. (2008). *Olds' Maternal-Newborn Nursing & Women's Health Across the Lifespan* (8th ed., p. 472). Upper Saddle River, NJ: Prentice Hall Health.

---

466. A nurse is caring for a client who is diagnosed with severe preeclampsia and is receiving magnesium sulfate intraveneously (IV). When reviewing the client's laboratory results, which value should lead the nurse to conclude that the client's serum magnesium level is therapeutic?

1. 2 mg/dL
2. 10 mg/dL
3. 6 mg/dL
4. 0.5 mg/dL

ANSWER: 3

The normal magnesium level of an adult is 1.5–2.5 mg/dL. To assure prevention of seizure activity in a client with preeclampsia, the magnesium level should be between 4.8 to 9.6 mg/dL.

➧ ***Test-taking Tip:*** *Use the process of elimination and apply knowledge regarding the normal adult magnesium level, which is 1.5 to 2.5 mg/dL. Remember that a larger amount would be needed to prevent seizure activity.*

Content Area: Childbearing Families; *Category of Health Alteration:* Pharmacological and Parenteral Therapies; *Integrated Processes:* Nursing Process Evaluation; *Client Need:* Physiological Integrity/Pharmacological and Parenteral Therapies/Expected Effects/Outcomes; *Cognitive Level:* Application

References: Davidson, M., London, M., & Ladewig, P. (2008). *Olds' Maternal-Newborn Nursing & Women's Health Across the Lifespan* (8th ed., p. 513). Upper Saddle River, NJ: Prentice Hall Health; Kee, J. (2005). *Medical-Surgical Nursing: Assessment and Management of Clinical Problems* (7th ed., p. 298). St. Louis, MO: Mosby.

467. While caring for a client with severe preeclampsia who has been receiving intravenous magnesium sulfate for 24 hours, a nurse evaluates that the medication is effective when noting:

1. an increase in blood pressure.
2. an increase in urine output.
3. a decrease in platelet count.
4. an increase in hematocrit.

ANSWER: 2

Diuresis within 24 to 48 hours is an excellent prognostic sign. It is considered evidence that perfusion of the kidneys has improved as a result of the relaxation of arteriolar spasms. Women who develop preeclampsia become more sensitive to natural pressor agents. As the severity of the preeclampsia increases, the blood pressure also increases. An increase in blood pressure therefore would not be a positive sign. The preeclampsia syndrome also involves vasospasm. This vasospasm causes vascular damage that promotes platelet aggregation at the site of this damage. Decreasing platelet levels indicate more blood vessel damage, and it is not a positive sign. Vascular volume, which normally increases in pregnancy, may decrease as part of the preeclampsia syndrome. This decrease will cause a corresponding increase in hematocrit. Therefore, increasing hematocrit is a concerning sign related to preeclampsia.

Test-taking Tip: *Recall the pathophysiology of preeclampsia to correctly answer this question.*

Content Area: Childbearing Families; *Category of Health Alteration:* Pharmacological and Parenteral Therapies; *Integrated Processes:* Nursing Process Evaluation; *Client Need:* Physiological Integrity/ Pharmacological and Parenteral Therapies/Expected Effects/Outcomes; *Cognitive Level:* Analysis

Reference: Davidson, M., London, M., & Ladewig, P. (2008). *Olds' Maternal-Newborn Nursing & Women's Health Across the Lifespan* (8th ed., p. 504). Upper Saddle River, NJ: Prentice Hall Health.

468. A nurse is preparing to assist with an external cephalic version on a client who is 38 weeks pregnant. As part of the preparation, the nurse administers terbutaline sulfate subcutaneously and explains to the client that this medication will:

1. decrease uterine sensation.
2. relax her uterus.
3. cause her to feel sleepy.
4. stimulate labor contractions.

ANSWER: 2

Terbutaline is a beta-adrenergic agonist that, in pregnant women, causes uterine relaxation. This greatly enhances the comfort of the women during the version and facilitates the maneuver. It does not decrease the sensation in the uterus, stimulate contractions, or cause drowsiness.

Test-taking Tip: *Recall that an external cephalic version procedure is used to try and convert a breech presentation to a cephalic presentation. Eliminate option 4, as starting uterine contractions at the time of the version would be counterproductive to the procedure.*

Content Area: Childbearing Families; *Category of Health Alteration:* Pharmacological and Parenteral Therapies; *Integrated Processes:* Teaching and Learning; *Client Need:* Physiological Integrity/ Pharmacological and Parenteral Therapies/Expected Effects/Outcomes; *Cognitive Level:* Application

References: Davidson, M., London, M., & Ladewig, P. (2008). *Olds' Maternal-Newborn Nursing & Women's Health Across the Lifespan* (8th ed., pp. 759, 761). Upper Saddle River, NJ: Prentice Hall Health; Wilson, B., Shannon, M., Shields, K., & Stang, C. (2008). *Prentice Hall Nurse's Drug Guide 2008* (p. 1462). Upper Saddle River, NJ: Pearson Education.

469. A nurse is ordered to administer vaginal dinoprostone (Cervidil®) for cervical ripening. Place an X on the appropriate location for the medication.

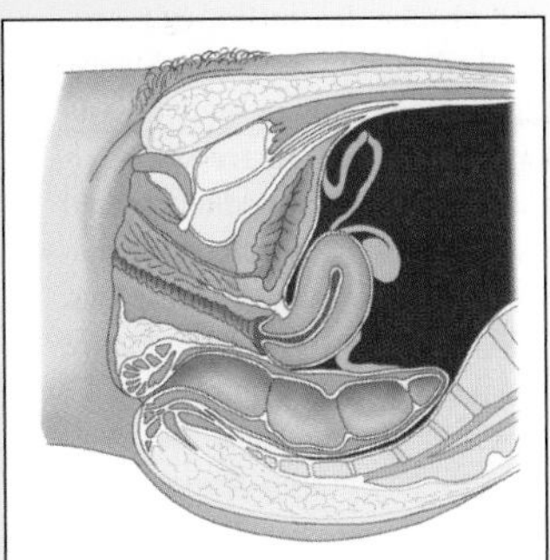

ANSWER:

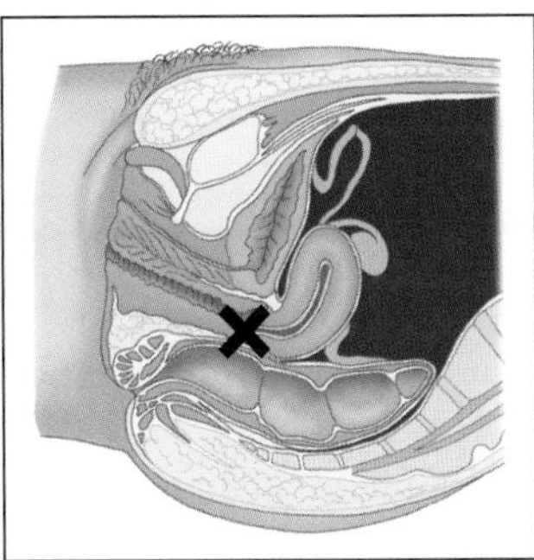

Dinoprostone is packaged as an intravaginal insert that resembles a 2 cm, square cardboard-like material. It should be placed transversely in the posterior fornix of the vagina and is left in place for 12 hours to provide a slow release of the medication. Cervical ripening may be necessary in a pregnant woman and in a nulliparous unpregnant woman before insertion of an intrauterine device.

▸ ***Test-taking Tip:*** *The key words are "vaginal" and "cervical ripening." The medication should be placed in the vagina, and since it is being used for cervical ripening, logically it should be placed close to the cervix.*

Content Area: Childbearing Families; *Category of Health Alteration:* Pharmacological and Parenteral Therapies; *Integrated Processes:* Nursing Process Implementation; *Client Need:* Physiological Integrity/Pharmacological and Parenteral Therapies/Medication Administration; *Cognitive Level:* Application

Reference: Davidson, M., London, M., & Ladewig, P. (2008). *Olds' Maternal-Newborn Nursing & Women's Health Across the Lifespan* (8th ed., p. 762). Upper Saddle River, NJ: Prentice Hall Health.

---

470. A nurse receives orders from a health-care provider for insertion of dinoprostone (Prepidil®) for cervical ripening for four inpatient clients. For which client should the nurse question this order?

1. Client A, who is G1P0000 and 41 weeks gestation
2. Client B, who is a G5P4004 at 40 and 4/7 weeks gestation
3. Client C, who is a G1P0000, type 1 diabetic at 38 weeks gestation, with evidence of fetal macrosomia
4. Client D, who is a G2P1001 at 40 weeks gestation attempting a vaginal birth after cesarean section with the client's other pregnancy

ANSWER: 4

A woman with a previous uterine incision from a cesarean section should not receive prostaglandin agents because the risk of uterine rupture is greatly increased. There is no contraindication to administering prostaglandins for cervical ripening to a primigravida client who is 41 weeks gestation. In fact, the use of cervical ripening agents has been shown to shorten labor and reduce the incidence of cesarean section for this population. Prostaglandins are not contraindicated in multiparous women until they have had six previous term vaginal births. Macrosomia in a pregnant diabetic woman may be an indication for early initiation of labor, and thus prostaglandins would be appropriate.

▸ ***Test-taking Tip:*** *Recall that dinoprostone is a synthetically prepared prostaglandin. Read the question carefully; it is asking for contraindications to the use of prostaglandins for cervical ripening or labor induction.*

Content Area: Childbearing Families; *Category of Health Alteration:* Pharmacological and Parenteral Therapies; *Integrated Processes:* Nursing Process Implementation; *Client Need:* Physiological Integrity/Pharmacological and Parenteral Therapies/Medication Administration; *Cognitive Level:* Analysis

Reference: Davidson, M., London, M., & Ladewig, P. (2008). *Olds' Maternal-Newborn Nursing & Women's Health Across the Lifespan* (8th ed., pp. 455, 763). Upper Saddle River, NJ: Prentice Hall Health.

471. A nurse is caring for a client receiving intravenous (IV) oxytocin (Pitocin®) for labor induction. Which manifestations would require the nurse to discontinue the IV infusion and notify the health-care provider? SELECT ALL THAT APPLY.

1. Consistent uterine resting tone of 18 mm Hg
2. Uterine contractions occurring every 4 minutes
3. Blood pressure increases from 100/60 to 130/85 mm Hg
4. Urine output of 60 mL in 2 hours
5. Fetal heart rate (FHR) of 90 beats/minute with decreased variability
6. Increasing client discomfort during uterine contractions

ANSWER: 1, 5

Intravenous oxytocin should be discontinued and the health-care provider notified if there is insufficient uterine relaxation (resting tone) between contractions. Expected resting uterine tone is 10 to 12 mm Hg. The IV infusion should also be discontinued if a nonreassuring fetal status develops. Fetal bradycardia is a FHR consistently below 90 beats per minute. When this is accompanied by decreased variability, it is considered an ominous sign of fetal distress. The goal of induction with IV oxytocin is a uterine contraction pattern of three 40- to 60-second contractions in 10 minutes. Therefore, uterine contractions occurring every 4 minutes would indicate a need for the administration of increased amounts of oxytocin. Blood pressure is expected to increase as much as 30% above baseline when oxytocin is administered. Larger doses of IV oxytocin will exert an antidiuretic effect and thus cause a marked decrease in urine output. While the client must be observed for water intoxication, a low normal urinary output is not a reason to stop the medication. A urine output of 60 mL/hr or more is considered to be within normal limits.

➧ ***Test-taking Tip:*** *Focus on concerning side effects of oxytocin. Eliminate options that describe expected responses to the use of oxytocin because these would be anticipated findings.*

Content Area: Childbearing Families; *Category of Health Alteration:* Pharmacological and Parenteral Therapies; *Integrated Processes:* Nursing Process Implementation; *Client Need:* Physiological Integrity/Physiological Adaptation/Unexpected Response to Therapies; *Cognitive Level:* Analysis

Reference: Davidson, M., London, M., & Ladewig, P. (2008). *Olds' Maternal-Newborn Nursing & Women's Health Across the Lifespan* (8th ed., pp. 584, 628, 766–768). Upper Saddle River, NJ: Prentice Hall Health.

---

472. While adding oxytocin (Pitocin®) to a 1,000-mL bag of intravenous solution, a 30-year-old, nonpregnant, female nurse inadvertently inserts the needle into her finger, and some of the oxytocin is injected into her body. The nurse goes immediately to the agency health service to report the incident. In addition to institutional treatment for a clean needlestick, the nurse should recognize that she will need:

1. subcutaneous terbutaline to relax her uterus.
2. ibuprofen for uterine cramping.
3. no further treatment.
4. to decrease her intake of free water for the next 24 hours.

ANSWER: 3

In the nonpregnant uterus, smooth muscle cells have low strength, demonstrate asynchronous contractions, and are fairly resistant to the effects of the oxytocin. Because the nurse in this question is not pregnant, the oxytocin should have little or no effect on the nurse's uterus, and, therefore, no additional treatment should be required. As gestation increases, the uterus becomes increasingly sensitive to oxytocin, and the number of oxytocin receptors increase. At the end of gestation, the number of receptors is about 200 times higher than that of a nonpregnant uterus, and excitability of the uterine cells is greatly increased. Oxytocin in larger doses does have an antidiuretic effect; however, since the dose received was relatively small, limiting water intake should not be necessary.

➧ ***Test-taking Tip:*** *Read the question carefully; it is asking about the action of oxytocin on the nonpregnant uterus. Note that two options include effects on the uterus, and two options are different. Use this information to eliminate the two options that include effects on the uterus.*

Content Area: Childbearing Families; *Category of Health Alteration:* Pharmacological and Parenteral Therapies; *Integrated Processes:* Nursing Process Planning; *Client Need:* Safe and Effective Care Environment/Management of Care/Continuity of Care; Physiological Integrity/Pharmacological and Parenteral Therapies/Expected Effects/Outcomes; *Cognitive Level:* Analysis

Reference: Davidson, M., London, M., & Ladewig, P. (2008). *Olds' Maternal-Newborn Nursing & Women's Health Across the Lifespan* (8th ed., p. 767). Upper Saddle River, NJ: Prentice Hall Health.

473. EBP A nurse is caring for multiple women in labor and notes a change in fetal heart rate (FHR) patterns following medication administration. Which medication, if used alone, should the nurse disregard as one that has an adverse effect on FHR patterns?

1. Magnesium sulfate
2. Meperidine hydrochloride (Demerol®)
3. Morphine sulfate (Avinza®)
4. Betamethasone (Diprolene AF®)

ANSWER: 2

Meperidine alone produces no characteristic changes in the FHR. However, meperidine used in combination with phenothiazines (a common method of administration due to the nauseating effects of meperidine) can produce significant FHR variability and accelerations. Magnesium sulfate, morphine sulfate (a narcotic analgesic), and betamethasone (a glucocorticosteroid) can affect the FHR.

Test-taking Tip: *Review the side effects associated with each of the medications and how they can affect the FHR.*

Content Area: Childbearing Families; *Category of Health Alteration:* Pharmacological and Parenteral Therapies; *Integrated Processes:* Nursing Process Evaluation; *Client Need:* Physiological Integrity/ Pharmacological and Parenteral Therapies/Adverse Effects/ Contraindications; *Cognitive Level:* Application

Reference: Wilson, B., Shannon, M., Shields, K., & Stang, C. (2008). *Prentice Hall Nurse's Drug Guide 2008* (pp. 942–945). Upper Saddle River, NJ: Pearson Education.

EBP Reference: American College of Obstetricians & Gynecologists (ACOG). (2005). Intrapartum fetal heart rate monitoring. *ACOG Practice Bulletin,* No. 70.

---

474. After admitting four clients to a labor and delivery suite, for which client should a nurse anticipate the administration of zolpidem tartrate (Ambien®)?

1. A 40-week G2P1001 client who is scheduled for a repeat cesarean section
2. A 39-week G3P1102 client who is 5 cm dilated, 80% effaced, and having contractions every 3 minutes
3. A 41-week G4P1112 client who is admitted for induction of labor
4. A 40-week G1P0000 client who is 1 cm dilated, 20% effaced, and having uncomfortable poor-quality uterine contractions

ANSWER: 4

The client who is at 40-weeks gestation, 1 cm dilated, and 20% effaced with poor-quality yet uncomfortable uterine contractions is experiencing hypertonic uterine dysfunction, a characteristic labor pattern that consists of poor-quality, ineffectual uterine contractions in the latent phase of labor. The treatment for this labor pattern is rest and sedation. Zolpidem tartrate (Ambien®) is a sedative-hypnotic barbiturate medication that will produce sleep and maternal relaxation. A barbiturate should not be administered to women in active labor or a woman whose delivery is imminent via cesarean section because it can cause fetal depression. The client admitted for induction of labor should be started on a medication to stimulate labor and should not be sedated.

Test-taking Tip: *Recall that zolpidem tartrate is a barbiturate medication. Eliminate option 2 because the client in this option is in active labor and does not need sedation. Also eliminate option 3 because sedation for a woman whose labor is to be induced would be counterproductive.*

Content Area: Childbearing Families; *Category of Health Alteration:* Pharmacological and Parenteral Therapies; *Integrated Processes:* Nursing Process Planning; *Client Need:* Physiological Integrity/ Pharmacological and Parenteral Therapies/Pharmacological Agents/Actions; *Cognitive Level:* Analysis

References: Davidson, M., London, M., & Ladewig, P. (2008). *Olds' Maternal-Newborn Nursing & Women's Health Across the Lifespan* (8th ed., p. 719). Upper Saddle River, NJ: Prentice Hall Health; Wilson, B., Shannon, M., Shields, K., & Stang, C. (2008). *Prentice Hall Nurse's Drug Guide 2008* (p. 1619). Upper Saddle River, NJ: Pearson Education.

475. A nurse is administering meperidine hydrochloride (Demerol®) intravenously (IV) to an actively laboring mother. The mother asks if the medication will affect her infant. Which statements should be the basis for the nurse's response? SELECT ALL THAT APPLY.

1. Meperidine hydrochloride crosses the placenta 90 seconds after IV administration to the mother.
2. When meperidine hydrochloride is given IV, the negative fetal effects can be avoided.
3. The fetal liver takes 2 to 3 hours to activate meperidine hydrochloride.
4. Newborns whose mothers have received meperidine hydrochloride have lower Apgar scores.
5. Meperidine hydrochloride has been associated with delay in initiation of successful breastfeeding.

ANSWER: 1, 3, 4, 5

Meperidine hydrochloride crosses the placenta 90 seconds after IV administration to the mother. However, it takes the fetus 2 to 3 hours to activate the medication. Therefore, if the newborn is born before activation of the medication or after the medication has been metabolized by the mother, the effect will be decreased. Meperidine has been associated with lower Apgar scores and delayed breastfeeding due to sucking problems. The negative fetal effects of meperidine are enhanced rather than avoided when it is administered IV.

▶ ***Test-taking Tip:*** *Recall the side effects of opioid medications. These will be manifested in all age populations. Select options 3 and 5 because they reflect these side effects. Of the remaining options, think about the adverse effects on the fetus.*

Content Area: Childbearing Families; *Category of Health Alteration:* Pharmacological and Parenteral Therapies; *Integrated Processes:* Nursing Process Analysis; *Client Need:* Physiological Integrity/ Pharmacological and Parenteral Therapies/Adverse Effects/Contradictions; *Cognitive Level:* Application

References: Davidson, M., London, M., & Ladewig, P. (2008). *Olds' Maternal-Newborn Nursing & Women's Health Across the Lifespan* (8th ed., p. 691). Upper Saddle River, NJ: Prentice Hall Health; Pillitteri, A. (2007). *Maternal & Child Health Nursing: Care of the Childbearing Families & Childrearing Family* (5th ed., p. 549). Philadelphia: Lippincott Williams & Wilkins.

476. A nurse administers butorphanol tartrate (Stadol®) to a laboring client who is 6 cm dilated. After 30 minutes, the client states that she feels the urge to bear down. The nurse assesses the client and finds the client's cervix completely dilated with the vertex at +2 station. The nurse determines delivery is imminent and is concerned that the fetus may be born during the time the butorphanol tartrate is peaking in the mother's body. In response to this concern, which medication should the nurse prepare for administration to the client?

1. Vitamin K
2. Oxytocin (Pitocin®)
3. Naloxone (Narcan®)
4. Erythromycin

ANSWER: 3

Naloxone is a narcotic antagonist that can be administered to the mother before birth or to the newborn after birth to prevent respiratory depression. Because the duration of action of naloxone may be less than the duration of the opioid medication, respiratory depression may return as the antagonistic effect of the naloxone wears off, and the dose may need to be repeated. Vitamin K is given to the newborn to decrease the risk of vitamin K–deficiency bleeding. Erythromycin eye ointment is given to the newborn as a prophylactic treatment for ophthalmia neonatorum. Oxytocin is not given to newborns.

▶ ***Test-taking Tip:*** *Focus on the medication classification of each of these medications and the effects on the newborn. Eliminate any medications that should not be given to newborns.*

Content Area: Childbearing Families; *Category of Health Alteration:* Pharmacological and Parenteral Therapies; *Integrated Processes:* Nursing Process Planning; *Client Need:* Physiological Integrity/ Pharmacological and Parenteral Therapies/Pharmacological Agents/Actions; *Cognitive Level:* Application

References: Davidson, M., London, M., & Ladewig, P. (2008). *Olds' Maternal-Newborn Nursing & Women's Health Across the Lifespan* (8th ed., pp. 693, 870–871). Upper Saddle River, NJ: Prentice Hall Health; Pillitteri, A. (2007). *Maternal & Child Health Nursing: Care of the Childbearing Families & Childrearing Family* (5th ed., p. 551). Philadelphia: Lippincott Williams & Wilkins.

477. EBP A nurse is caring for a laboring client who is receiving bupivacaine (Marcaine®) per epidural route for analgesia. For which adverse effects, specific to the local anesthetic agent, should the nurse closely monitor? SELECT ALL THAT APPLY.

1. Hypotension
2. Elevated temperature
3. Slowing of the second stage of labor
4. Nausea
5. Urinary retention
6. Sedation

ANSWER: 1, 2, 3, 5

Bupivacaine is a local anesthetic agent. The medication blocks sympathetic nerve fibers in the epidural space, which causes decreased peripheral resistance. This, in turn, causes hypotension. Maternal temperature may be elevated to 100°F (37.8°C) or higher due to sympathetic blockage that may decrease sweat production and diminish heat loss. The use of epidural analgesia has been demonstrated to slow the second stage of labor. The descent of the presenting part is slowed because the medication decreases the woman's ability to push effectively. Also, relaxation of the levator ani muscle impedes internal rotation. Bupivacaine alters transmission of impulses to the bladder, thus causing urinary retention. Nausea and sedation are not side effects of bupivacaine.

➧ *Test-taking Tip: Look at the suffix of the medication "-caine." This suffix is common for local anesthetic agents. Select options that would be related to this type of pain control.*

Content Area: Childbearing Families; *Category of Health Alteration:* Pharmacological and Parenteral Therapies; *Integrated Processes:* Nursing Process Implementation; *Client Need:* Physiological Integrity/Pharmacological and Parenteral Therapies/Adverse Effects/ Contradictions; *Cognitive Level:* Application

Reference: Davidson, M., London, M., & Ladewig, P. (2008). *Olds' Maternal-Newborn Nursing & Women's Health Across the Lifespan* (8th ed., p. 694). Upper Saddle River, NJ: Prentice Hall Health.

EBP Reference: Anim-Somuah, M., Smyth, R., & Howell, C. (2005). Epidural versus non-epidural or no analgesia in labour. *Cochrane Database of Systematic Reviews*, Issue 4, Art. No. CD000331. DOI: 10.1002/14651858.CD000331.pub2. Available at: www.cochrane.org/reviews/en/ab000331.html

478. A laboring client is to receive nalbuphine hydrochloride (Nubain®) 3 mg subcutaneously. The pharmacy supplies nalbuphine hydrochloride as 10 mg/mL. To provide the correct dose, the nurse should plan to administer _____ mL to the client.

ANSWER: 0.3

Use a proportion to determine the amount in milliliters. Multiply the extremes, then the means, and solve for X.

10 mg : 1 mL :: 3 mg : X mL

10 X = 3

X = 0.3.

➧ *Test-taking Tip: Since the ordered dose is less than 10 mg, the amount to give should be less than 1 mL. Use the formula dose needed/dose on hand or a proportion formula.*

Content Area: Childbearing Families; *Category of Health Alteration:* Pharmacological and Parenteral Therapies; *Integrated Processes:* Nursing Process Implementation; *Client Need:* Physiological Integrity/Pharmacological and Parenteral Therapies/Dosage Calculation; *Cognitive Level:* Application

References: Wilson, B., Shannon, M., Shields, K., & Stang, C. (2008). *Prentice Hall Nurse's Drug Guide 2008* (pp. 1039–1041). Upper Saddle River, NJ: Pearson Education; Craig, G. (2005). *Clinical Calculations Made Easy* (3rd ed., p. 63). Philadelphia: Lippincott Williams & Wilkins.

479. **EBP** A laboring client reports back pain, and a certified nurse midwife (CNM) suggests that sterile water injections may decrease the pain. A nurse prepares to position the client, recognizing that the CNM will administer these injections:

1. directly into the client's lactated Ringer's intravenous (IV) solution.
2. into the client's subcutaneous tissue on her abdomen.
3. intracutaneously into the client's lower back.
4. directly into the client's uterus.

ANSWER: 3

Sterile water injections for back pain during labor involve administering subcutaneous or intracutaneous injections of a small amount of sterile water in the lumbar-sacral region of the back. The intracutaneous route seems to give the best pain relief and is thought to work similarly to acupuncture. By introducing small amounts of sterile water into the intradermal layer of skin, a hyperstimulation of the large inhibitory nerve fibers occurs. The onset of pain relief is fast—usually within a few minutes—and can last 1 to 2 hours. The treatment can be repeated several times. There would be no benefit to adding sterile water to an existing IV maintenance solution. Administering the sterile water into the uterus or abdomen will not affect the back pain.

➧ *Test-taking Tip: Eliminate option 1 because there would be no benefit to adding sterile water to an existing IV maintenance solution. Of the other options, determine where the sterile water will have the most effect to minimize back pain.*

Content Area: Childbearing Families; *Category of Health Alteration:* Pharmacological and Parenteral Therapies; *Integrated Processes:* Nursing Process Implementation; *Client Need:* Physiological Integrity/Basic Care and Comfort/Nonpharmacological Comfort Interventions; *Cognitive Level:* Application

Reference: Ward, S., & Hisley, S. (2009). *Maternal-Child Nursing Care* (p. 410). Philadelphia: F. A. Davis.

EBP References: Märtensson, L., McSwiggin, M., & Mercer, S. (2008). US midwives' comprehension and use of sterile water injections for labor pain. *Journal of Midwifery & Women's Health,* 53(2), 115–122; Wiruchpongsanon, P. (2006). Relief of low back labor pain by using intracutaneous injections of sterile water: A randomized clinical trial. *Journal of the Medical Association of Thailand,* 89(5), 571–576. Available at: www.medassocthai.org/journal/index.php®command=preview&selvol=89&selno=5&selids=1162

480. A nurse is counseling a client who is 5 weeks pregnant and seeking information about pregnancy termination. The client asks for information about a medical abortion using mifepristone (Mifeprex®). Which information provided by the nurse about this medication is most accurate? SELECT ALL THAT APPLY.

1. It must be taken immediately after the last menstrual cycle to be effective.
2. It is a progesterone antagonist and will block the action of progesterone on the uterus.
3. To be certain that the abortion occurs, the mifepristone must be followed up with a vaginal douche of vinegar and water.
4. The success rate is 96% to 98% when taken within 42 days of conception.
5. The medication must be administered intravenously (IV) in the caregiver's office.
6. Most women will develop a transient temperature elevation when taking the medication.

ANSWER: 2, 4

Mifepristone blocks the uterine progesterone receptors in the uterus, thereby altering the endometrium and causing the detachment of the conceptus. The success rate for this medication is 96% to 98% when taken within 42 days of conception. The medication does not need to be taken immediately after the last menstrual cycle; however, to achieve a success rate at or above 91%, it should be taken within 49 days of conception. Douching is not required for abortion to occur. The medication is given orally. Temperature elevation is a sign of infection and should be reported immediately to the health-care provider.

➧ ***Test-taking Tip:*** *Douching is rarely recommended for any medical reason, thus eliminate option 3. Since most women do not realize they are pregnant until they have missed a menstrual period, it would be impossible to take the medication immediately after a menstrual cycle; thus eliminate option 1. Of the remaining options, think about the usual route of medication administration and signs of adverse effects to eliminate other options.*

Content Area: Childbearing Families; *Category of Health Alteration:* Pharmacological and Parenteral Therapies; *Integrated Processes:* Teaching and Learning; *Client Need:* Physiological Integrity/Pharmacological and Parenteral Therapies/Pharmacological Agents/Actions; *Cognitive Level:* Application

References: Davidson, M., London, M., & Ladewig, P. (2008). *Olds' Maternal-Newborn Nursing & Women's Health Across the Lifespan* (8th ed., p. 533). Upper Saddle River, NJ: Prentice Hall Health; Lehne, R. (2007). *Pharmacology for Nursing Care* (6th ed., p. 105). St. Louis, MO: Elsevier/Saunders.

481. A postpartum client, who just delivered a full-term infant, tells a nurse she is concerned about her Rh-negative status. She says that she received Rho(D) immune globulin (RhoGam®) during her pregnancy, and she wonders if she is going to need it again. The nurse correctly replies:

1. "To prevent you from building up antibodies against your next baby's blood you will need to have Rho(D) immune globulin within the next 72 hours."
2. "You will not need Rho(D) immune globulin again since you got it during your pregnancy."
3. "One dose of Rho(D) immune globulin will last for a lifetime."
4. "You will need Rho(D) immune globulin if your newborn is Rh positive."

ANSWER: 4

Rho(D) immune globulin is given in the postpartum period to Rh-negative women who have delivered Rh-positive newborns. Rho(D) immune globulin, when given at this time, prevents the mother from becoming sensitized from the fetomaternal transfusion of Rh-positive blood that occurred at delivery. When Rho(D) immune globulin is indicated, it should be given within 72 hours of the birth so the mother does not have time to produce antibodies to fetal cells. The mother will need rho(D) immune globulin with each subsequent pregnancy, pregnancy trauma, or pregnancy loss.

➧ ***Test-taking Tip:*** *Recall that Rho(D) immune globulin is an immune globulin that provides passive immunity to a foreign protein. Think of the Rh protein as a foreign protein for Rh-negative women and select the option that best demonstrates that concept.*

Content Area: Childbearing Families; *Category of Health Alteration:* Pharmacological and Parenteral Therapies; *Integrated Processes:* Teaching and Learning; *Client Need:* Physiological Integrity/Pharmacological and Parenteral Therapies/Pharmacological Agents/Actions; *Cognitive Level:* Application

Reference: Davidson, M., London, M., & Ladewig, P. (2008). *Olds' Maternal-Newborn Nursing & Women's Health Across the Lifespan* (8th ed., pp. 521, 523–524, 1082–1083). Upper Saddle River, NJ: Prentice Hall Health.

482. A breastfeeding, postpartum client is reporting afterpains. The client is requesting pain medication but does not want anything that will harm her breastfeeding infant. A nurse anticipates that a health-care provider will order which medication?

1. Meperidine (Demerol®)
2. Naproxen (Naprosyn®)
3. Ibuprofen (Motrin®)
4. Acetaminophen (Tylenol®)

ANSWER: 4

Acetaminophen is excreted in the breast milk in low concentrations and no adverse infant effects have been reported. Acetaminophen is the analgesic of choice for breastfeeding women. It has also been shown to decrease afterpains. Acetaminophen can be used in newborns for pain control. Medications that are safe for use directly in an infant of the nursing infant's age are generally also safe for the breastfeeding mother. Of the NSAIDs, ibuprofen is the preferred choice because it has poor transfer into milk and has been well studied in children. Therefore, occasional use of therapeutic doses is acceptable. Long half-life NSAIDs, such as naproxen, can accumulate in the infant with prolonged use. Meperidine is not the preferred analgesic for use in breastfeeding women because of the long half-life of its metabolite in infants.

➧ ***Test-taking Tip:*** *Evaluate each medication relative to its concentration in breast milk. Select option 4, recalling that acetaminophen is excreted in very low doses in breast milk.*

Content Area: Childbearing Families; *Category of Health Alteration:* Pharmacological and Parenteral Therapies; *Integrated Processes:* Nursing Process Planning; *Client Need:* Physiological Integrity/Pharmacological and Parenteral Therapies/Adverse Effects/Contradictions; *Cognitive Level:* Application

Reference: Pillitteri, A. (2007). *Maternal & Child Health Nursing: Care of the Childbearing Families & Childrearing Family* (5th ed., p. 1789). Philadelphia: Lippincott Williams & Wilkins.

---

483. **EBP** A health-care provider orders that carboprost tromethamine (Hemabate®) be given to a postpartum client who is experiencing uterine atony. Because of the side effects of this medication, a nurse should also prepare to give the client:

1. a sedative.
2. a stool softener.
3. an antiemetic.
4. extra oral fluids.

ANSWER: 3

Carboprost tromethamine is a synthetic analog of naturally occurring prostaglandin F_2 alpha, which stimulates myometrial contractions and is therefore used to treat postpartum hemorrhage caused by uterine atony. Because it is a synthetic prostaglandin, it also stimulates the smooth muscle of the gastrointestinal tract. Sixty percent of clients experience nausea and diarrhea. Thus, an antiemetic medication is often prescribed before and/or during carboprost tromethamine therapy. Carboprost tromethamine does not cause agitation; therefore, a sedative would not be required. Because carboprost tromethamine does cause diarrhea, a stool softener would be contraindicated. Oral fluids would be difficult to tolerate because the medication causes nausea and vomiting.

➧ ***Test-taking Tip:*** *Recall that carboprost tromethamine is a synthetic prostaglandin. Select the option that best describes a response to the common side effects of prostaglandins.*

Content Area: Childbearing Families; *Category of Health Alteration:* Pharmacological and Parenteral Therapies; *Integrated Processes:* Nursing Process Planning; *Client Need:* Physiological Integrity/Pharmacological and Parenteral Therapies/Adverse Effects/Contradictions; *Cognitive Level:* Application

Reference: Wilson, B., Shannon, M., Shields, K., & Stang, C. (2008). *Prentice Hall Nurse's Drug Guide 2008* (pp. 241–242). Upper Saddle River, NJ: Pearson Education.

EBP Reference: Briggs, G., & Wan, S. (2006). Drug therapy during labor and delivery: Part 2. *American Journal of Health-System Pharmacy*, 63(12), 1131–1139.

484. EBP While preparing to present women's health information at a college seminar, a nurse decides to include information on how combination oral contraceptives (COC) prevent conception. Which information should the nurse plan to include in the seminar? SELECT ALL THAT APPLY.

1. COCs inhibit ovulation.
2. COCs destroy the cell membrane of sperm.
3. COCs block uterine progesterone receptors.
4. COCs create an atrophic endometrium.
5. COCs promote the thickening of cervical mucous.
6. COCs have a reduced efficacy in obese individuals.

ANSWER: 1, 4, 5, 6

COCs are a combination of estrogen and progesterone. The estrogen acts to suppress follicle-stimulating hormone and luteinizing hormone, thereby suppressing ovulation. The progesterone action complements that of the estrogen by causing a decrease in the permeability of cervical mucus and endometrial proliferation. With a body mass index over 30, there is a greater risk of having an oral contraceptive failure resulting in an unintended pregnancy. Spermicides are chemical surfactants that kill sperm by destroying their cell membranes, and mifepristone blocks uterine progesterone receptors.

➧ ***Test-taking Tip:*** *Eliminate option 2 as COCs are taken orally by the female partner and do not come into contact with sperm. Think about another medication that blocks uterine progesterone receptors and then eliminate option 3.*

Content Area: Childbearing Families; *Category of Health Alteration:* Pharmacological and Parenteral Therapies; *Integrated Processes:* Teaching and Learning; *Client Need:* Physiological Integrity/Pharmacological and Parenteral Therapies/Pharmacological Agents/Actions; *Cognitive Level:* Application

Reference: Lehne, R. (2007). *Pharmacology for Nursing Care* (6th ed., p. 729). St. Louis, MO: Elsevier/Saunders.

EBP Reference: Brunner, H., & Toth, J. (2007). Obesity and oral contraceptive failure: Findings from the 2002 National Survey of Family Growth. *American Journal of Epidemiology,* 166(11), 1306–1311.

---

485. EBP A nurse is caring for an infant whose mother has tested positively for hepatitis B surface antigen. The nurse is preparing to administer the hepatitis B vaccine to the infant. To prevent infection, which medication should the nurse administer along with the hepatitis B vaccine?

1. Acyclovir (Zovirax®)
2. Ceftriaxone (Rocephin®)
3. Acetaminophen (Tylenol®)
4. Immune serum globulin (ISG)

ANSWER: 4

Those infants born to mothers who are hepatitis B surface antigen–positive should receive both the hepatitis B vaccine and 0.5 mL of hepatitis B immune globulin (HBIG) within 12 hours of birth. This combination has a greater effect in reducing the risk of developing hepatitis B than the vaccine alone. Hepatitis B is not treated with acyclovir at this age. Ceftriaxone is used to treat a bacterial infection. Acetaminophen could potentially be correct if the infant is uncomfortable or in pain, but it does not decrease the risk of an infection.

➧ ***Test-taking Tip:*** *Use the process of elimination of medications based on the disease causative agent and exposure of the infant to the disease. Eliminate a medication used to treat pain.*

Content Area: Childbearing Families; *Category of Health Alteration:* Pharmacological and Parenteral Therapies; *Integrated Processes:* Nursing Process Implementation; *Client Need:* Physiological Integrity/Pharmacological and Parenteral Therapies/Pharmacological Agents/Actions; *Cognitive Level:* Application

Reference: Pillitteri, A. (2007). *Maternal and Child Health Nursing* (5th ed. p. 790). Philadelphia: Lippincott Williams & Wilkins.

EBP Reference: Centers for Disease Control and Prevention. (2009). *Recommended Immunization Schedule for Persons Age 0–6 Years, United States.* Available at: www.cdc.gov/vaccines/recs/schedules/downloads/child/2009/09_0-6yrs_schedule_pr.pdf

---

486. EBP A nurse in a large urban hospital is admitting a 2-hour-old infant whose mother is positive for HIV. A neonatologist orders the infant to be started on zidovudine (Retrovir®). Which laboratory tests should the nurse analyze before administering the medication?

1. Complete blood count (CBC) with differential, prothrombin time (PT), and bleeding time
2. Cluster of differentiation 4 (CD4) count, CBC, and lactate
3. CBC with differential and alanine aminotransferase (ALT)
4. CBC, CD4 count, ALT, and serum protein

ANSWER: 3

A CBC with differential is indicated, along with an ALT to obtain baseline hemoglobin and liver function in the newborn and to identify if significant anemia or alteration in liver function is present before initiating therapy. Coagulation studies (PT and bleeding time) are unnecessary. Serum lactate is completed only if the infant develops severe clinical symptoms of unknown etiology. Zidovudine would be initiated regardless of the CD4 values. Serum protein values are unnecessary.

➧ ***Test-taking Tip:*** *Consider which laboratory tests would provide essential information before initiating an antiretroviral medication. Remember that ALT is a liver function test and CD4 cells are a type of lymphocyte.*

Content Area: Childbearing Families; *Category of Health Alteration:* Pharmacological and Parenteral Therapies; *Integrated Processes:* Nursing Process Implementation; *Client Need:* Physiological Integrity/ Reduction of Risk Potential/Laboratory Values; Physiological Integrity/ Pharmacological and Parenteral Therapies/Medication Administration; *Cognitive Level:* Analysis

Reference: Wilson, B., Shannon, M., Shields, K., & Stang, C. (2008). *Prentice Hall Nurse's Drug Guide 2008* (pp. 1611–1612). Upper Saddle River, NJ: Pearson Education.

EBP Reference: Public Health Service Task Force. (2006). *Recommendations For Use of Antiretroviral Medications in Pregnant HIV-1-Infected Women for Maternal Health and Interventions to Reduce HIV-1 Transmission in the United States.* Available at: http://aidsinfo.nih.gov/ContentFiles/ PerinatalGL.pdf

---

487. A nurse is preparing to administer indomethacin (Indocin®) to an infant diagnosed with patent ductus arteriosus (PDA). By which route should the nurse expect to administer the indomethacin for this infant?

1. Intravenously (IV)
2. Orally
3. Rectally
4. Intramuscularly (IM)

ANSWER: 1

The preferred administration route of indomethacin for treatment of a PDA is IV, so the medication can quickly enter the vascular system. Indomethacin is given to infants with PDA because it often stimulates closure of the defect. Although indomethacin can be administered orally and rectally, the onset of action is delayed. Indomethacin is not administered IM.

➧ ***Test-taking Tip:*** *Identify the point of impact for which the medication is being given.*

Content Area: Childbearing Families; *Category of Health Alteration:* Pharmacological and Parenteral Therapies; *Integrated Processes:* Nursing Process Planning; *Client Need:* Physiological Integrity/ Pharmacological and Parenteral Therapies/Medication Administration; *Cognitive Level:* Application

Reference: Hockenberry, M. (2007). *Wong's Essentials of Pediatric Nursing* (8th ed., pp. 767, 778, 1299). St. Louis, MO: Mosby/Elsevier.

---

488. A nurse is caring for a newborn infant of a diabetic mother. The infant requires intravenous (IV) D5/0.2 NS to manage blood glucose levels. When caring for the infant, which actions should be taken by the nurse? SELECT ALL THAT APPLY.

1. Assess for rebound hypoglycemia.
2. Maintain blood glucose levels between 45 mg/dL and 65 mg/dL.
3. Check blood glucose levels frequently in the first 2 to 4 days of life.
4. Titrate the IV solution rate to keep blood glucose levels within the ordered range.
5. Maintain blood glucose levels between 37 mg/dL and 40 mg/dL.

ANSWER: 2, 3, 4

An infant of a diabetic mother who requires IV therapy to maintain acceptable glucose levels requires close monitoring. Typically, blood glucose levels are maintained between 45 mg/dL and 65 mg/dL. The blood glucose should be frequently monitored, and the IV solution rate should be titrated based on glucose monitoring. Newborn hypoglycemia is a blood glucose level of less than 40 mg/dL. Maintaining glucose between 37 mg/dL and 40 mg/dL will cause the newborn to be hypoglycemic.

➧ ***Test-taking Tip:*** *Note that options 2 and 5 are similar. Either one or both of these must be incorrect.*

Content Area: Childbearing Families; *Category of Health Alteration:* Pharmacological and Parenteral Therapies; *Integrated Processes:* Nursing Process Assessment; *Client Need:* Physiological Integrity/ Pharmacological and Parenteral Therapies/Parenteral/Intravenous Therapies; *Cognitive Level:* Analysis

References: Pillitteri, A. (2007). *Maternal and Child Health Nursing* (5th ed., p. 791). Philadelphia: Lippincott Williams & Wilkins; Hockenberry, M. (2007). *Wong's Essentials of Pediatric Nursing* (8th ed., pp. 1724–1725). St. Louis, MO: Mosby/Elsevier.

489. A nurse is caring for a newborn infant of a diabetic mother. The infant is receiving D10/0.2 NS intravenously (IV) to manage blood glucose levels. After examining the infant, a primary care provider changes the order to D12.5/0.2 NS. Which action should the nurse take *first*?

1. Call pharmacy to get the newly ordered IV solution for the infant.
2. Obtain a blood glucose level prior to beginning the new infusion.
3. Contact the primary care provider to clarify the order.
4. Increase the current IV rate until the new bag is obtained from pharmacy.

ANSWER: 3

Neonates can have D10 in peripheral veins for short periods of time. Any solution that has higher concentrations of dextrose should be administered through a central line. The primary care provider should either place a central line or order the placement of a peripherally inserted central catheter (PICC). The nurse should not call the pharmacy for the solution because the solutions should not be administered as ordered. While obtaining blood glucose is acceptable, the infusion should not be started as ordered. The nurse should be concerned about fluid balance and should not adjust the rate to increase administration of dextrose. The nurse should not adjust the rate without an order.

➧ ***Test-taking Tip:*** *Recognize that there is a difference between what has been ordered and what has been infusing. Determine if the order change is appropriate.*

Content Area: Childbearing Families; *Category of Health Alteration:* Pharmacological and Parenteral Therapies; *Integrated Processes:* Nursing Process Implementation; *Client Need:* Physiological Integrity/Pharmacological and Parenteral Therapies/Parenteral/Intravenous Therapies; *Cognitive Level:* Analysis

References: Pillitteri, A. (2007). *Maternal and Child Health Nursing* (5th ed., p. 791). Philadelphia: Lippincott Williams & Wilkins; Hockenberry, M. (2007). *Wong's Essentials of Pediatric Nursing* (8th ed., pp. 1724–1725). St. Louis, MO: Mosby/Elsevier.

490. When completing an assessment on a 6-day-old infant, a nurse identifies white, adherent patches on the tongue, palate, and inner aspect of the checks. After consulting with a primary care provider, the nurse obtains an order for mycostatin (Nystatin®). Which is the most important information that the nurse should provide to the parent about this medication?

1. Monitor the infant's mouth for signs of improvement.
2. Monitor for signs of contact dermatitis.
3. Administer the medication and allow the infant to "swish and swallow."
4. Adverse effects of mycostatin can include nausea, vomiting, and diarrhea.

ANSWER: 1

The most important information for use of mycostatin is that the oral area is improving. Thrush is a disorder that can be self-limiting and can have a spontaneous resolution, although it could take up to 2 months. With the medication, the resolution should be much quicker. Monitoring for signs of contact dermatitis is correct for topical application, but contact dermatitis is an inflammation of the skin, not the mucous membranes. "Swish and swallow" administration is appropriate for an older person, but this is a 6-day-old infant. Adverse effects occur in less than 1% of the population and need not be stated at this time.

➧ ***Test-taking Tip:*** *Identify the option that is most consistent with the symptoms and treatment of the infection. Examine options with duplicate information first.*

Content Area: Childbearing Families; *Category of Health Alteration:* Pharmacological and Parenteral Therapies; *Integrated Processes:* Nursing Process Implementation; *Client Need:* Physiological Integrity/Pharmacological and Parenteral Therapies/Expected Actions/Outcomes; *Cognitive Level:* Application

References: Pillitteri, A. (2007). *Maternal and Child Health Nursing* (5th ed., p. 697). Philadelphia: Lippincott Williams & Wilkins; Wilson, B., Shannon, M., Shields, K., & Stang, C. (2008). *Nurse's Drug Guide* (pp. 1101–1102). Upper Saddle River, NJ: Pearson Education.

491. A nurse is caring for an infant who experienced asphyxiation at birth and is having seizure activity. The nurse has an order to administer phenobarbital 4 mg/kg/day in divided doses (q 8 hrs), with the infant weighing 4 kg. To provide the correct dose, the nurse should administer ____ mg to the infant.

ANSWER: 5.3

The nurse determines the dose by multiplying the dose (4 mg) by kilograms (4 kg) and dividing it by 3.

➧ ***Test-taking Tip:*** *Be sure to recognize that the 4 mg/kg/day is the total dose and that divided doses should be administered every 8 hours for a total of three doses.*

Content Area: Childbearing Families; *Category of Health Alteration:* Pharmacological and Parenteral Therapies; *Integrated Processes:* Nursing Process Planning; *Client Need:* Physiological Integrity/Pharmacological and Parenteral Therapies/Dosage Calculation; *Cognitive Level:* Application

References: Pillitteri, A. (2007). *Maternal and Child Health Nursing* (5th ed., pp. 1563–1564). Philadelphia: Lippincott Williams & Wilkins; Wilson, B., Shannon, M., Shields, K., & Stang, C. (2008). *Nurse's Drug Guide* (pp. 1200–1203). Upper Saddle River, NJ: Pearson Education.

Chapter Eight

Physiological Integrity: Care of Adults and Older Adults

Test 13: Adult Health: Developmental Needs

492. An unsteady 20-year-old surgical client persists in ambulating to the bathroom alone despite being reminded to call for assistance. A nurse concludes that, according to Havighurst's developmental tasks, this behavior reflects the client's need for:

1. adjusting to physiological changes.
2. independence.
3. industry.
4. integrity.

ANSWER: 2

The client is attempting to perform self-care and to demonstrate the ability to be self-sufficient and independent from other adults. Option 1 is a developmental task of middle age. Options 3 and 4 are Erikson's development tasks, not Havighurst's. Industry versus inferiority occurs from ages 6 to 12 years. Integrity versus despair occurs at 65 years and older.

➧ ***Test-taking Tip:*** *Apply knowledge of Havighurst's developmental tasks and use the process of elimination.*

Content Area: Adult Health; *Category of Health Alteration:* Developmental Needs; *Integrated Processes:* Nursing Process Analysis; *Client Need:* Health Promotion and Maintenance/Developmental Stages and Transitions; *Cognitive Level:* Application

Reference: Berman, A., Snyder, S., Kozier, B., & Erb, G. (2008). *Kozier & Erb's Fundamentals of Nursing: Concepts, Process, and Practice* (8th ed., p. 353). Upper Saddle River, NJ: Pearson Education.

---

493. A clinic nurse is planning to complete a physical examination on a 19-year-old female who has participated in strenuous physical activities while in high school. It would be most important for the nurse to plan to assess this client for:

1. lordosis.
2. an eating disorder.
3. an increase in muscle mass.
4. excessive bleeding with menses.

ANSWER: 2

Females who participate in strenuous physical activities are at risk for eating disorders, delayed menses, and osteoporosis. Lordosis is common in children before age 5. An increase in muscle mass is expected with physical activity. Delayed menses, not excessive bleeding, would be a concern.

➧ ***Test-taking Tip:*** *Note the key phrase "most important."*

Content Area: Adult Health; *Category of Health Alteration:* Developmental Needs; *Integrated Processes:* Nursing Process Planning; *Client Need:* Health Promotion and Maintenance/Growth and Development; *Cognitive Level:* Application

Reference: Berman, A., Snyder, S., Kozier, B., & Erb, G. (2008). *Kozier & Erb's Fundamentals of Nursing: Concepts, Process, and Practice* (8th ed., p. 642). Upper Saddle River, NJ: Pearson Education.

494. Place an X on the illustration that a nurse should expect to find when assessing the chest of a normal, healthy, young adult male client without chest abnormalities.

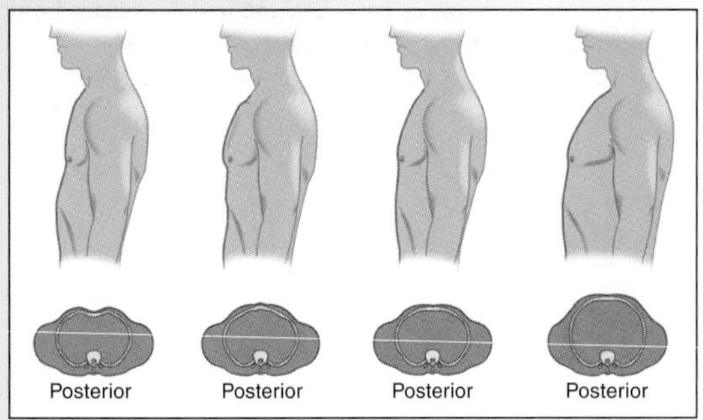

ANSWER:

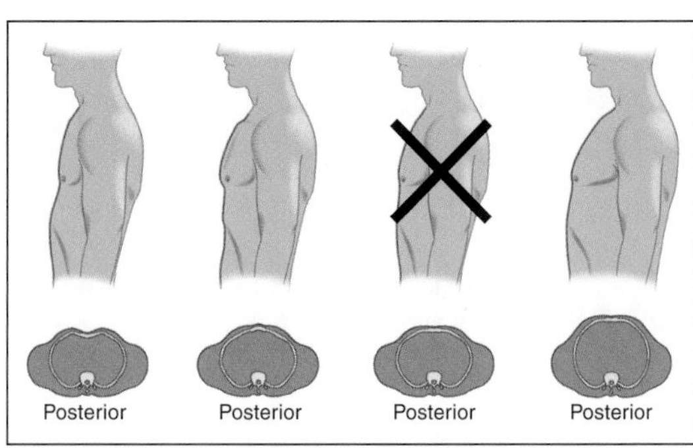

The normal adult chest has an anteroposterior-to-lateral ratio of approximately 1:2 and a costal angle less than 90 degrees. There should be no sternal or intercostal retractions or bulging at rest. Illustration 1 is pectus excavatum, or funnel chest, caused by sternal retraction. Illustration 2 is pectus carinatum, or pigeon breast, with sternal bulging. Illustration 4 is barrel chest with increased anteroposterior diameter of the chest, with near parallel rib sloping, and a costal angle greater than 90 degrees. Barrel chest occurs with chronic obstructive pulmonary disease.

➧ *Test-taking Tip: Note the key phrase, "normal, healthy . . . adult chest."*

Content Area: Adult Health; *Category of Health Alteration:* Developmental Needs; *Integrated Processes:* Nursing Process Assessment; *Client Need:* Health Promotion and Maintenance/Growth and Development; *Cognitive Level:* Application

Reference: Berman, A., Snyder, S., Kozier, B., & Erb, G. (2008). *Kozier & Erb's Fundamentals of Nursing: Concepts, Process, and Practice* (8th ed., p. 642). Upper Saddle River, NJ: Pearson Education.

---

495. EBP A nurse teaches an 18-year-old diabetic client to perform self-administration of insulin. The nurse notes that each time the client makes even a small mistake, the client constantly apologizes for getting it wrong. The nurse observes that the client also profusely apologizes when making a minimal mistake in other activities. The nurse concludes that, according to Erikson's development stages, the adult may have an unresolved development task of:

1. infancy.
2. early childhood.
3. school-age childhood.
4. adolescence.

ANSWER: 2

The behavior indicates an unresolved conflict of "autonomy versus shame and doubt" associated with the 18-month- to 3-year-old age group. When parents are overly critical and controlling, a child may develop an overly critical superego. As an adult it manifests in constantly apologizing for small mistakes. The central task of infancy is determining "trust versus mistrust." Unresolved conflict manifests itself in withdrawal, mistrust, or estrangement. The central task of the school age child is "industry versus inferiority." Unresolved conflict of this stage manifests itself in withdrawal from school and peers, loss of hope, or sense of being mediocre. The central task of adolescence is "identity versus role confusion." If unresolved, it manifests itself in indecisiveness, antisocial behavior, or feelings of confusion.

➧ *Test-taking Tip: Focus on the behaviors exhibited by the client and apply knowledge of Erikson's developmental stages.*

Content Area: Adult Health; *Category of Health Alteration:* Developmental Needs; *Integrated Processes:* Nursing Process Analysis; *Client Need:* Health Promotion and Maintenance/Developmental Stages and Transitions; *Cognitive Level:* Analysis

Reference: Berman, A., Snyder, S., Kozier, B., & Erb, G. (2008). *Kozier & Erb's Fundamentals of Nursing: Concepts, Process, and Practice* (8th ed., p. 353). Upper Saddle River, NJ: Pearson Education.

EBP Reference: Bowen, N. (2005). Histories of developmental task attainment in aggressive children and their relationship to behavior in middle childhood. *Journal of Emotional and Behavioral Disorders,* 13(2), 113–124.

496. A nurse is collecting information from a young adult client. Which psychosocial questions should the nurse ask during the admission assessment? SELECT ALL THAT APPLY.

1. "Do you have any pets?"
2. "How many hours of sleep do you get at night?"
3. "When was your last bowel movement?"
4. "How much alcohol do you consume and how frequently?"
5. "Can you describe your sexual activity?"

ANSWER: 1, 2, 4, 5

Pets can enhance mental well-being and promote responsibility. Insufficient amounts of sleep and rest can decrease coping and impair the immune system. Regular consumption of three or more alcoholic drinks a day increases risk of hypertension and decreases immune competence. Multiple sex partners and anal sex are risk factors for STDs and HIV. Asking for the date of the last bowel movement relates to physiological functions.

▶ ***Test-taking Tip:*** *Focus on the key word "psychosocial" and eliminate any options that relate to only physiological functioning.*

Content Area: Adult Health; *Category of Health Alteration:* Developmental Needs; *Integrated Processes:* Nursing Process Assessment; *Client Need:* Health Promotion and Maintenance/Growth and Development; *Cognitive Level:* Analysis

Reference: Dillon, P. (2007). *Nursing Health Assessment: A Critical Thinking, Case Studies Approach* (2nd ed., pp. 420–421). Philadelphia: F. A. Davis.

---

497. Which finding should a nurse expect when assessing a healthy, middle-aged adult?

1. Weight gain of 20 pounds in the past year
2. Tactile fremitus is absent at the apex of the lungs
3. Able to count backward from 100 subtracting 7 each time
4. Percussion indicates heart is larger then previous physical examination

ANSWER: 3

A middle-aged adult should be able to focus on a mental task such as subtraction. Tactile fremitus (the vibrations felt when the hand is held against the client's chest and the client is speaking) is a normal finding; it is decreased or absent with a pneumothorax. Although muscle is replaced by adipose tissue as a person ages, a weight gain of 20 pounds in a year is excessive. Percussion that indicates the heart is enlarged indicates that a medical problem has occurred since the last physical exam. If no disease is present, the heart stays the same size throughout life.

▶ ***Test-taking Tip:*** *Focus on the key words "healthy, middle-aged adult."*

Content Area: Adult Health; *Category of Health Alteration:* Developmental Needs; *Integrated Processes:* Nursing Process Assessment; *Client Need:* Health Promotion and Maintenance/Growth and Development; *Cognitive Level:* Application

Reference: Berman, A., Snyder, S., Kozier, B., & Erb, G. (2008). *Kozier & Erb's Fundamentals of Nursing: Concepts, Process, and Practice* (8th ed., pp. 615, 624, 638, 644). Upper Saddle River, NJ: Pearson Education.

---

498. A home health nurse is caring for a middle-aged client who is disabled due to a recent motor vehicle accident. The client has few interests, spends most days watching TV, and has become estranged from the family. Which of Erikson's developmental stages should the nurse conclude that the client is not meeting?

1. Industry versus inferiority
2. Initiative versus guilt
3. Generativity versus stagnation
4. Intimacy versus isolation

ANSWER: 3

The central task of adulthood is "generativity versus stagnation." The client has indicators of negative resolution of this developmental stage. "Industry versus inferiority" is the developmental stage for the school age child, 6 to 12 years. "Initiative versus guilt" is the developmental stage for late childhood, 3 to 5 years. "Intimacy versus isolation" is the developmental task for young adulthood, 18 to 25 years.

▶ ***Test-taking Tip:*** *Note that the client is middle-aged and focus on the client's behaviors. Then apply Erikson's developmental stages.*

Content Area: Adult Health; *Category of Health Alteration:* Developmental Needs; *Integrated Processes:* Nursing Process Analysis; *Client Need:* Health Promotion and Maintenance/Growth and Development; *Cognitive Level:* Analysis

Reference: Berman, A., Snyder, S., Kozier, B., & Erb, G. (2008). *Kozier & Erb's Fundamentals of Nursing: Concepts, Process, and Practice* (8th ed., p. 353). Upper Saddle River, NJ: Pearson Education.

499. A nurse is caring for a hospitalized 60-year-old Korean American client. Which statement, if made by the client, correctly reflects the Korean American culture and should alert the nurse that intervention is needed?

1. "Since 60 is considered old age, I retired as expected. I'm now worried about insurance."
2. "Value is on youth and beauty; so little attention is paid to problems of the elderly."
3. "Fathers are expected to continue to contribute financially even for their adult children."
4. "Grandchildren are raised by the grandparents until school age so we have a full house."

ANSWER: 1

In the Korean American culture, 60 is considered old age and elders are expected to retire. At a retirement age of 60, the client does not yet qualify for Medicare insurance coverage. A social worker consult may be needed to discuss insurance options. The European American culture focuses on youth and beauty. Option 3 is not an expectation of any one culture specifically. African American grandmothers often raise grandchildren and offer economic support.

▶ ***Test-taking Tip:*** *Focus on the key word "correctly" and apply knowledge of the Korean American culture to answer this question.*

Content Area: Adult Health; *Category of Health Alteration:* Developmental Needs; *Integrated Processes:* Nursing Process Analysis; *Client Need:* Health Promotion and Maintenance/Aging Process; Safe and Effective Care Environment/Management of Care/Referrals; *Cognitive Level:* Analysis

Reference: Dillon, P. (2007). *Nursing Health Assessment: Clinical Pocket Guide* (2nd ed., pp. 411–412). Philadelphia: F. A. Davis.

500. A 50-year-old client asks a nurse how to calculate the body mass index (BMI). The client weighs 134 pounds and is 5 feet 3 inches tall. Together, the client and nurse calculate the client's BMI to the nearest tenth. The client's BMI is ___.

ANSWER: 23.8

Formula: BMI = (705 times weight in pounds) ÷ (height in inches)^2
BMI = (705 × 134) ÷ 3,969 = 94,470 ÷ 3,969 = 23.8

▶ ***Test-taking Tip:*** *Use the formula and on-line calculator to calculate the BMI.*

Content Area: Adult Health; *Category of Health Alteration:* Developmental Needs; *Integrated Processes:* Nursing Process Analysis; *Client Need:* Health Promotion and Maintenance/Growth and Development; *Cognitive Level:* Analysis

Reference: Lutz, C., & Przytulski, K. (2006). *Nutrition & Diet Therapy: Evidence-Based Applications* (4th ed., p. 20). Philadelphia: F. A. Davis.

501. Which point should a nurse most specifically address when teaching a group of middle-aged female nurses about middle-aged moral development applicable only to women?

1. Gilligan's moral development theory includes responsibility and caring for self and others.
2. Kohlberg's moral development theory includes living according to universally agreed upon principles.
3. Westerhoff's stages of faith include putting faith into personal and social action and standing up for beliefs.
4. Fowler's stages of spiritual development include becoming aware of truth from a variety of viewpoints.

ANSWER: 1

Gilligan's theory is specific to women and proposes that women see morality in the integrity of relationships and caring. Women tend to consider what is right to be taking responsibility for others and caring, whereas men tend to consider what is right to be what is just. Kohlberg's theory is not specific to women. Option 2 describes Kohlberg's postconventional level of moral development for middle age or older adults. Westerhoff's stages of faith and Fowler's stages of spiritual development are both spiritual development theories and not moral development theories. These refer in part to the individual's perceptions about the direction and meaning of life.

▶ ***Test-taking Tip:*** *Focus on what the question is asking: moral development for women.*

Content Area: Adult Health; *Category of Health Alteration:* Developmental Needs; *Integrated Processes:* Teaching and Learning; *Client Need:* Health Promotion and Maintenance/Aging Process; Safe and Effective Care Environment/Management of Care/Staff Education; *Cognitive Level:* Analysis

Reference: Berman, A., Snyder, S., Kozier, B., & Erb, G. (2008). *Kozier & Erb's Fundamentals of Nursing: Concepts, Process, and Practice* (8th ed., pp. 359–362). Upper Saddle River, NJ: Pearson Education.

502. A 62-year-old client recently retired after working 30 years as a bank manager. Which statement to a nurse during a clinic visit best suggests that the client is achieving the developmental stage of "integrity versus despair"?

1. "Now that I have some free time, I want to treat my wife to a trip to Hawaii."
2. "I seem to be staying in bed longer and longer each day. There isn't a reason to get up now."
3. "I am noticing the little aches and pains more; before I was just too busy to notice them."
4. "I get calls a few times a week for advice; my coworkers still value my suggestions."

ANSWER: 4

"Integrity versus despair" is Erikson's stage of development from 65-years of age and older. Indicators of positive resolution include statements of acceptance of worth and uniqueness of one's own life. Option 1 is a statement reflecting positive resolution of generativity versus stagnation, showing concern for others. Option 2 indicates that the client is experiencing difficulty achieving the developmental stage. Option 3 is not reflective of any stage.

➧ ***Test-taking Tip:*** *Note the key word "best." Focus on the defining characteristics for a positive or negative resolution of the developmental stage integrity versus despair, that which occurs from 65 years to death.*

Content Area: Adult Health; *Category of Health Alteration:* Developmental Needs; *Integrated Processes:* Nursing Process Evaluation; Communication and Documentation; *Client Need:* Health Promotion and Maintenance/Growth and Development; Health Promotion and Maintenance/Aging Process; *Cognitive Level:* Analysis

Reference: Berman, A., Snyder, S., Kozier, B., & Erb, G. (2008). *Kozier & Erb's Fundamentals of Nursing: Concepts, Process, and Practice* (8th ed., p. 353). Upper Saddle River, NJ: Pearson Education.

---

503. EBP A 60-year-old client, admitted to a hospital with chest pain, has been functioning independently at home. During the night, the client is found wandering in the hallway and states, "I can't find my kitchen. I need a glass of milk." The nurse's best interpretation of the client's behavior is:

1. the client likely had a stroke.
2. the stress of being in unfamiliar surroundings has caused the client's confusion.
3. the decline in mental status, especially at night, is a normal part of aging.
4. this is an insidious change and it likely means the client has early dementia.

ANSWER: 2

Stress of unfamiliar situations or surroundings can cause confusion in an older adult. The client would be exhibiting other signs and symptoms if a stroke had occurred. Short-term memory is often less efficient, but a decline in mental status is not a normal part of aging. The confusion was an abrupt change in behavior, not insidious.

➧ ***Test-taking Tip:*** *Focus on the situation: an independent older adult who is now confused. Apply knowledge of age-related changes to answer this question.*

Content Area: Adult Health; *Category of Health Alteration:* Developmental Needs; *Integrated Processes:* Nursing Process Analysis; *Client Need:* Health Promotion and Maintenance/Aging Process; *Cognitive Level:* Application

Reference: Berman, A., Snyder, S., Kozier, B., & Erb, G. (2008). *Kozier & Erb's Fundamentals of Nursing: Concepts, Process, and Practice* (8th ed., p. 652). Upper Saddle River, NJ: Pearson Education.

EBP Reference: Park, M., Hsiao-Chen Tang, J., & Ledford, L. (2005). *Changing the Practice of Physical Restraint Use in Acute Care.* Iowa City: University of Iowa Gerontological Nursing Interventions Research Center, Research Translation and Dissemination Core. Available at: www.guideline.gov/summary/summary.aspx?doc_id=8626&nbr=004806&string=wandering

---

504. A nurse is caring for a 50-year-old client who reports having difficulty falling asleep. Which recommendations should a nurse make to this client? SELECT ALL THAT APPLY.

1. Drink a glass of wine or a beer before going to bed
2. Avoid exercising 3 to 4 hours before bedtime
3. Go to bed at the same time each night
4. Use the bed for sleeping or intimacy only
5. Eat later in the evening; people usually are sleepier after a large meal

ANSWER: 2, 3, 4

Avoidance of exercise near bedtime, going to bed at the same time, and using the bed for sleeping or intimacy only promote good sleep habits. Other actions that promote sleep include avoiding frequent napping during the day; sleeping in a cool, quiet environment; getting up upon awakening; and avoiding liquid intake after 6:00 p.m. Alcohol, nicotine, caffeine, large meals, and excitement should be avoided before bed.

➧ ***Test-taking Tip:*** *Apply knowledge of actions that promote sleep.*

Content Area: Adult Health; *Category of Health Alteration:* Developmental Needs; *Integrated Processes:* Nursing Process Intervention; *Client Need:* Health Promotion and Maintenance/Aging Process; *Cognitive Level:* Application

Reference: Craven, R., & Hirnle, C. (2007). *Fundamentals of Nursing: Human Health and Function* (5th ed., pp. 322–323). Philadelphia: Lippincott Williams & Wilkins.

505. A client states to a hospice nurse, "If I could live until my grandson's wedding in 2 months, then I would be ready to die." Based on this statement, the nurse should interpret that the client is in which stage of grief?

1. Denial
2. Depression
3. Bargaining
4. Acceptance

ANSWER: 3

Bargaining is one of the stages of grieving, noted by Kübler-Ross, which includes negotiating or making deals with God or fate. The client's statement is not representative of the other stages of grieving. In denial, a client may make a statement such as, "I don't need hospice care because I am not dying." The client would exhibit withdrawal, apathy, lack of appetite, or absence of interaction if experiencing depression. A statement of acceptance may include, for example, "I know that I might die before my grandson's wedding, but if I am still alive I plan to be present for awhile."

➧ ***Test-taking Tip:*** *Focus on the key phrase, "If I could live until," which suggests bargaining.*

Content Area: Adult Health; *Category of Health Alteration:* Developmental Needs; *Integrated Processes:* Communication and Documentation; *Client Need:* Psychosocial Integrity/Grief and Loss; *Cognitive Level:* Analysis

Reference: Lewis, S., Heitkemper, M., Dirksen, S., O'Brien, P., & Bucher, L. (2007). *Medical-Surgical Nursing: Assessment and Management of Clinical Problems* (7th ed., p. 153). St. Louis, MO: Mosby.

---

506. A client, who is experiencing mouth soreness precipitated by stress from completing multiple school examinations, visits a college health nurse. The nurse's priority nursing diagnosis at this time should be:

1. acute pain.
2. impaired tissue integrity.
3. potential fluid volume deficit.
4. imbalanced nutrition.

ANSWER: 1

The client is complaining of mouth soreness, thus acute pain is priority. The situation does not provide sufficient information to determine whether the pain is from impaired tissue integrity. It could be an infection. The data does not address the client's fluid or nutritional intake.

➧ ***Test-taking Tip:*** *Use the process of elimination, noting soreness in the situation and pain in the options. Avoid reading into the situation.*

Content Area: Adult Health; *Category of Health Alteration:* Developmental Needs; *Integrated Processes:* Nursing Process Analysis; *Client Need:* Physiological Integrity/Physiological Adaptation/Illness Management; *Cognitive Level:* Application

Reference: Lewis, S., Heitkemper, M., Dirksen, S., O'Brien, P., & Bucher, L. (2007). *Medical-Surgical Nursing: Assessment and Management of Clinical Problems* (7th ed., p. 1000). St. Louis, MO: Mosby.

---

507. EBP A 32-year-old client has been trying to get pregnant for the past 10 years. The client consults a family planning clinic after being unsuccessful with the calendar and basal body temperature methods to determine the time of ovulation. Which statement by a nurse would be most appropriate?

1. "Let me review the methods with you; maybe you have not been using them correctly."
2. "Have you considered that you might not be ovulating and that adoption is an option?"
3. "Test kits are available that will detect an enzyme in cervical mucus that signals ovulation."
4. "If you douche or your spouse wears restrictive underwear, these can reduce your chances of conception."

ANSWER: 3

An ovulation test kit, such as Ovulindex, is available over the counter, is easy to use, and is considered reliable. The kit can detect the presence of the enzyme, guaiacol peroxidase, in cervical mucus that signals ovulation 6 days beforehand. Option 1 is not the most appropriate response because the client has been unsuccessful for 10 years. Option 2 is premature since other options to test ovulation are still untried. Option 4 does not address the problem of determining the time of ovulation. Douching increases, not decreases, the chance of conception.

➧ ***Test-taking Tip:*** *Focus on the issue, determining time of ovulation. Only options 1 and 3 address the issue and option 1 has already been tried.*

Content Area: Adult Health; *Category of Health Alteration:* Developmental Needs; *Integrated Processes:* Teaching and Learning; *Client Need:* Health Promotion and Maintenance/Developmental Stages and Transitions; *Cognitive Level:* Analysis

Reference: Smeltzer, S., Bare, B., Hinkle, J., & Cheever, K. (2008). *Brunner & Suddarth's Textbook of Medical-Surgical Nursing* (11th ed., p. 1646). Philadelphia: Lippincott Williams & Wilkins.

EBP Reference: Institute for Clinical Systems Improvement. (2004). *Diagnosis and Management of Basic Infertility*. Bloomington, MN: Institute for Clinical Systems Improvement (ICSI). Available at: www.guideline.gov/summary/summary.aspx?doc_id=5567&nbr=003764&string=ovulation+AND+test+AND+kit

508. A nursing unit educator is planning teaching for other nurses after noting that some nurses are unfamiliar with insulin types and how to use the new insulin injection pens. When planning teaching, which question by the educator best reflects consideration that the nurses are adult learners?

1. "Does anyone want to volunteer to prepare a poster board?"
2. "What specifically regarding insulin and its administration do you need to learn?"
3. "Can you attend a presentation if I post various times during the day and evening shift?"
4. "What don't you understand about the information in the policy and procedure manual?"

ANSWER: 2

Adults are independent learners. Before deciding what nurses do not know, the nurses themselves should identify their specific learning needs and the methodology for learning. Adults learn best by demonstration and hands-on practice. Neither a poster board nor a presentation support adult learning styles. Asking staff what they don't understand about the policy and procedure is threatening.

➧ ***Test-taking Tip:*** *Note the key words "best reflects."*

Content Area: Adult Health; *Category of Health Alteration:* Developmental Needs; *Integrated Processes:* Teaching and Learning; *Client Need:* Health Promotion and Maintenance/Principles of Teaching and Learning; *Cognitive Level:* Application

Reference: Lewis, S., Heitkemper, M., Dirksen, S., O'Brien, P., & Bucher, L. (2007). *Medical-Surgical Nursing: Assessment and Management of Clinical Problems* (7th ed., pp. 54–55). St. Louis, MO: Mosby.

---

509. EBP A nurse has limited time to teach an adult postoperative client. The nurse should initially plan to:

1. provide brochures and handouts that the client can discuss with family members.
2. make a referral to outpatient resources for the client to receive the needed teaching.
3. establish learning needs that have the highest priority at this time and teach with each contact.
4. answer the client's questions and leave the extensive teaching for the nurse on the next shift.

ANSWER: 3

To make the most of limited time, the nurse and client should set priorities of the client's learning needs so that important teaching can be done during any contact with the client or family. Printed educational materials should be used with other teaching strategies. These must be appropriate for the reading level of the client. A referral might be an option if extensive teaching is needed, but it would not be an initial approach. Depending on the referral, there may be additional costs. The nurse has a professional responsibility to include client teaching. Teaching and practice can be broken into small time periods.

➧ ***Test-taking Tip:*** *Note the key word "initially" and use the process of elimination. Avoid reading into the responses.*

Content Area: Adult Health; *Category of Health Alteration:* Developmental Needs; *Integrated Processes:* Teaching and Learning; *Client Need:* Health Promotion and Maintenance/Principles of Teaching and Learning; *Cognitive Level:* Application

Reference: Lewis, S., Heitkemper, M., Dirksen, S., O'Brien, P., & Bucher, L. (2007). *Medical-Surgical Nursing: Assessment and Management of Clinical Problems* (7th ed., p. 56). St. Louis, MO: Mosby.

EBP Reference: Johnson, A., Sandford, J., & Tyndall, J. (2005). Written and verbal information versus verbal information only for patients being discharged from acute hospital settings to home. *Cochrane Database of Systematic Reviews*, Issue 3, Art. No. CD003716. DOI: 10.1002/14651858.CD003716. Available at: www.cochrane.org/reviews/en/ab003716.html

---

510. EBP An 18-year-old client has a college physical completed at a clinic. No problems are evident but the client tells a nurse, "I am getting stressed worrying about the demands of college. I am used to getting "As and Bs." Which statement should the nurse reserve until a follow-up visit with the client?

1. "Expressing your feelings of anxiety to a friend or nurse helps you cope emotionally."
2. "I will check with the physician about prescribing paroxetine hydrochloride (Paxil®)."
3. "Exercise increases the release of endorphins and can enhance your sense of well-being."
4. "If you like drawing or painting, register for an art class during your first semester in college."

ANSWER: 2

Other interventions should be tried before prescribing a medication. Paroxetine hydrochloride inhibits neuronal reuptake of serotonin in the central nervous system, thus potentiating the activity of serotonin. It has an antidepressant action and decreases the frequency of panic attacks or anxiety. Expressing feelings, physical activity, and art therapy all promote emotion-focused coping.

➧ ***Test-taking Tip:*** *Note the key word "reserve." Apply knowledge of coping strategies and use the process of elimination to eliminate options addressing emotion-focused coping strategies.*

Content Area: Adult Health; *Category of Health Alteration:* Developmental Needs; *Integrated Processes:* Communication and Documentation; *Client Need:* Health Promotion and Maintenance/Health and Wellness; Psychosocial Integrity/Stress Management; *Cognitive Level:* Application

Reference: Lewis, S., Heitkemper, M., Dirksen, S., O'Brien, P., & Bucher, L. (2007). *Medical-Surgical Nursing: Assessment and Management of Clinical Problems* (7th ed., p. 116). St. Louis, MO: Mosby.

EBP Reference: Ekeland, E., Heian, F., Hagen, K., Abbott, J., & Nordheim, L. (2004). Exercise to improve self-esteem in children and young people. *Cochrane Database of Systematic Reviews*, Issue 1, Art. No. CD003683. DOI: 10.1002/14651858.CD003683.pub2. Available at: www.mrw.interscience.wiley.com/cochrane/clsysrev/articles/CD003683/frame.html

511. A nurse is caring for a client diagnosed with hypertension. The nurse plans to teach the client progressive muscle relaxation to reduce stress and decrease the client's blood pressure. Which steps should the nurse take when teaching the client to perform progressive muscle relaxation? Prioritize the nurse's actions by placing each step in the correct order.

______ Relax the feet, imagining the tension flowing out with each exhalation.
______ Lie down in a quiet place where you are undisturbed.
______ Contract the muscles of your feet first as you inhale and hold the contraction briefly.
______ Relax your body, allowing it to feel heavy.
______ Lie still for a few minutes after the contraction and relaxation of all muscles.
______ Imagine the tension flowing out with each breath you take.
______ Move up the body, contracting then relaxing each muscle.

ANSWER: 5, 1, 4, 2, 7, 3, 6

The nurse should first instruct the client to lie down in a quiet place where the client will be undisturbed. Then the nurse should instruct the client to relax the body, allowing it to feel heavy. The nurse then tells the client to imagine the tension flowing out with each breath. The client is then instructed to contract the muscles of the feet first as the client inhales and to hold the contraction briefly. The client is then instructed to relax the feet, imagining the tension flowing out with each exhalation. The nurse then tells the client to move up the body, contracting then relaxing each muscle. Finally, the nurse instructs the client to lie still for a few minutes after experiencing the contraction and relaxation of all muscles. Another option is to start with the face first and moving down the body.

➧ ***Test-taking Tip:*** *Visualize the steps prior to placing the items in the correct order. Read all options first.*

Content Area: Adult Health; *Category of Health Alteration:* Developmental Needs; *Integrated Processes:* Teaching and Learning; *Client Need:* Health Promotion and Maintenance/Health and Wellness; Psychosocial Integrity/Stress Management; *Cognitive Level:* Analysis

Reference: Lewis, S., Heitkemper, M., Dirksen, S., O'Brien, P., & Bucher, L. (2007). *Medical-Surgical Nursing: Assessment and Management of Clinical Problems* (7th ed., p. 119). St. Louis, MO: Mosby.

512. A nurse is positioning a female client in the dorsal recumbent position for a routine examination. Which picture illustrates that the nurse has correctly positioned this client?

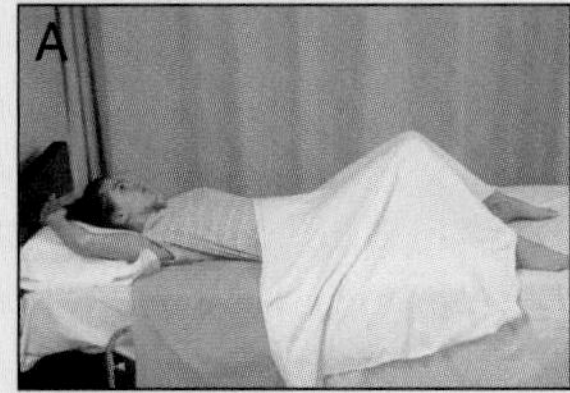

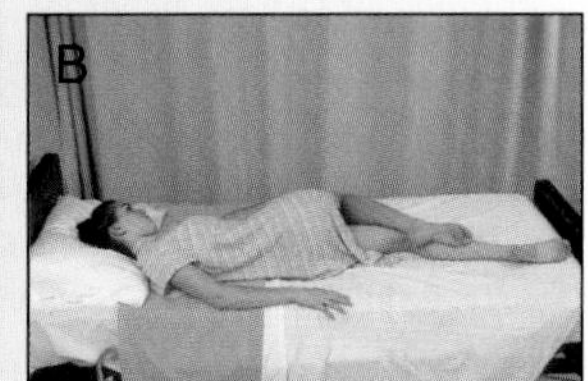

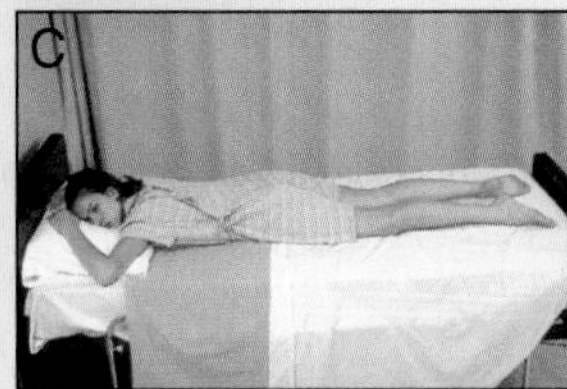

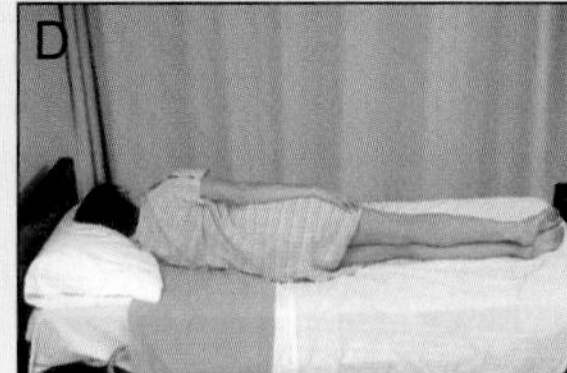

1. A
2. B
3. C
4. D

ANSWER: 1

The dorsal recumbent position involves lying supine with the knees slightly flexed to relax the abdominal muscles. It is used to assess the female pelvic area if the client is unable to assume the lithotomy, or Sims', position. Option 2 is Sims' position for examining the female pelvic and rectal areas. Option 3 is the prone position, often used to assess the back. Option 4 is the left lateral recumbent position used for cardiac auscultation.

➧ ***Test-taking Tip:*** *Apply knowledge of medical terminology; dorsum refers to back.*

Content Area: Adult Health; *Category of Health Alteration:* Developmental Needs; *Integrated Processes:* Nursing Process Application; *Client Need:* Health Promotion and Maintenance/Techniques of Physical Assessment; *Cognitive Level:* Application

Reference: Dillon, P. (2007). *Nursing Health Assessment: A Critical Thinking, Case Studies Approach* (2nd ed., pp. 75–76). Philadelphia: F. A. Davis.

513. A hospital nurse is teaching coworkers how to prevent varicose veins. Which recommendation by the nurse is most accurate?

1. Wear low-heeled comfortable shoes
2. Move your legs back and forth often
3. Wear support hose or thromboembolic deterrent stockings (TEDS).
4. Wear clean, white cotton socks with tennis shoes

ANSWER: 3

Support or compression hose help decrease edema and increase circulation back to the heart, thereby preventing varicose veins. Low-heeled shoes and clean white cotton socks with tennis shoes will decrease foot discomfort but will not prevent varicose veins. Leg movement helps prevent deep vein thrombosis, but not varicose veins.

***Test-taking Tip:** Use the process of elimination, ruling out options 1 and 4 because they address the feet. Eliminate option 2 after noting that back-and-forth movement of the legs is not the same as dorsiflexion and plantar flexion and will not promote return of blood to the heart.*

Content Area: Adult Health; *Category of Health Alteration:* Developmental Needs; *Integrated Processes:* Teaching and Learning; *Client Need:* Health Promotion and Maintenance/Disease Prevention; *Cognitive Level:* Analysis

Reference: Lewis, S., Heitkemper, M., Dirksen, S., O'Brien, P., & Bucher, L. (2007). *Medical-Surgical Nursing: Assessment and Management of Clinical Problems* (7th ed., p. 919). St. Louis, MO: Mosby.

514. EBP A nurse evaluates that a client correctly understands information regarding breast cancer screening when the client states:

1. "Women at average risk for breast cancer should begin having mammography at age 40."
2. "Women with fibrocystic breast disease should eliminate chocolate and caffeine from the diet."
3. "Women should perform monthly breast self-examination (BSE)."
4. "Only women with fibrocystic breast disease should have the addition of breast ultrasound or MRI."

ANSWER: 1

Mammography for cancer screening should be completed annually beginning at age 40 or younger for high-risk women. Some health-care providers suggest eliminating caffeine and chocolate from the diet if the breasts become tender, but there is no research that supports this to be effective in controlling the discomfort associated with fibrocystic breasts. The American Cancer Society states that it is acceptable for women to choose not to do BSE or to perform it only occasionally. Women should report any breast change promptly to their health-care provider. Beginning in their 20s, women should be told about the benefits and limitations of BSE. It still is advisable that women with known breast conditions perform BSE monthly to detect potential cancer. Women known to be at increased risk should have earlier screening and/or the addition of breast ultrasound or MRI.

***Test-taking Tip:** Eliminate option 4 because "only" is an absolute. Eliminate option 2 because it does not involve screening. Then eliminate option 3 applying knowledge of guideline changes.*

Content Area: Adult Health; *Category of Health Alteration:* Developmental Needs; *Integrated Processes:* Nursing Process Evaluation; *Client Need:* Health Promotion and Maintenance/Health Screening; *Cognitive Level:* Application

Reference: Lewis, S., Heitkemper, M., Dirksen, S., O'Brien, P., & Bucher, L. (2007). *Medical-Surgical Nursing: Assessment and Management of Clinical Problems* (7th ed., p. 282). St. Louis, MO: Mosby.

EBP Reference: Saslow, D., Boetes, C., Burke, W., Harms, S., Leach, M., et al. (American Cancer Society Breast Cancer Advisory Group). (2007). American Cancer Society guidelines for breast screening with MRI as an adjunct to mammography. *CA: A Cancer Journal for Clinicians*, 57(2), 75–89.

515. A 25-year-old client, who had a hysterectomy due to bleeding complications from a broken intrauterine device (IUD), tells a nurse, "My husband will probably leave me now because I won't be able to have any more children. I am so glad I have one child already." Which response by the nurse is most appropriate?

1. "That probably won't happen. He'll likely be thankful that you already have one child."
2. "Are you afraid your husband will leave you because he wants more children?"
3. "There are support groups you and your husband could attend to help cope with your loss."
4. "Your husband should be thankful that you are alive and didn't bleed to death!"

ANSWER: 2

This is a therapeutic response, restating and clarifying the client's feelings. Option 1 is unwarranted reassurance, ignoring the client's feelings and offering an opinion. The statement is a barrier to communication. Option 3 is problem solving and presenting options for coping, but the immediate response should be one that encourages the client to talk about her concerns. Option 4 is passing judgment and is a barrier to therapeutic communication.

***Test-taking Tip:** Use therapeutic communication techniques that encourage the client to discuss her feelings.*

Content Area: Adult Health; *Category of Health Alteration:* Developmental Needs; *Integrated Processes:* Communication and Documentation; *Client Need:* Psychosocial Integrity/Therapeutic Communications; *Cognitive Level:* Application

Reference: Berman, A., Snyder, S., Kozier, B., & Erb, G. (2008). *Kozier & Erb's Fundamentals of Nursing: Concepts, Process, and Practice* (8th ed., pp. 467–471). Upper Saddle River, NJ: Pearson Education.

516. A nurse assesses the coping-stress tolerance in the functional health assessment of a client diagnosed with anemia. The nurse notes that the client has a coping-stress tolerance problem. Which nursing diagnoses, pertaining to the client's coping-stress tolerance pattern, should the nurse document in the client's plan of care? SELECT ALL THAT APPLY.

1. Caregiver role strain
2. Defensive coping
3. Relocation stress syndrome
4. Stress overload
5. Ineffective coping
6. Readiness for enhanced coping

ANSWER: 1, 2, 3, 4, 5

Caregiver role strain, defensive coping, relocation stress syndrome, stress overload, and ineffective coping are all applicable to the coping-stress tolerance pattern. Each has different defining characteristics and variable interventions. Thus, the nurse should collect additional data. Readiness for enhanced coping indicates that the client is showing signs of resolution of a problem.

***Test-taking Tip:** Focus on what the question is asking, nursing diagnoses pertaining to coping-stress tolerance pattern.*

Content Area: Adult Health; *Category of Health Alteration:* Developmental Needs; *Integrated Processes:* Nursing Process Analysis; Communication and Documentation; *Client Need:* Psychosocial Integrity/Coping Mechanisms; *Cognitive Level:* Application

Reference: Lewis, S., Heitkemper, M., Dirksen, S., O'Brien, P., & Bucher, L. (2007). *Medical-Surgical Nursing: Assessment and Management of Clinical Problems* (7th ed., p. 121). St. Louis, MO: Mosby.

Test 14: **Adult Health: Older Client Needs**

517. A health-care provider documents, in the medical record of an 87-year-old hospitalized client, normal elder skin changes of senile purpura. The elder has no other skin changes. When assessing the client, which skin change, illustrated below, should the nurse expect to find?

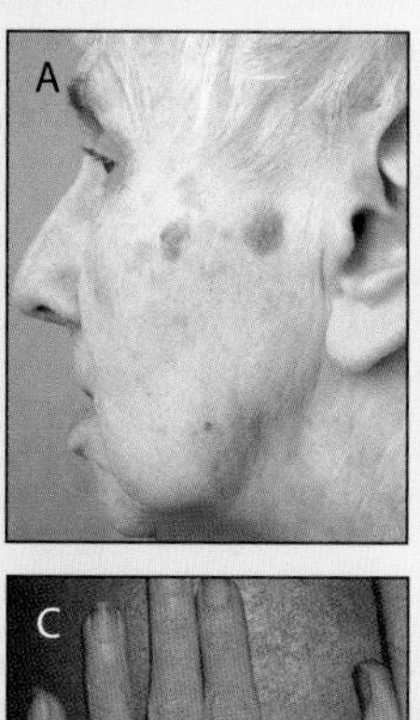

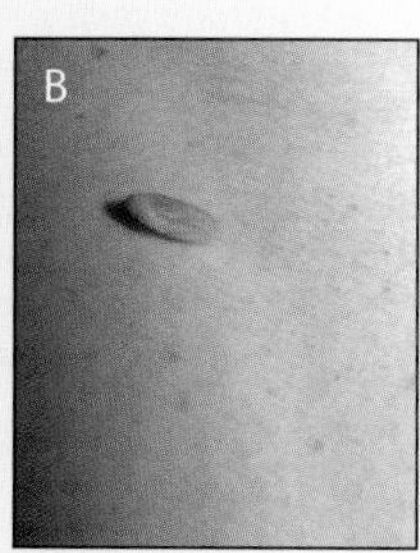

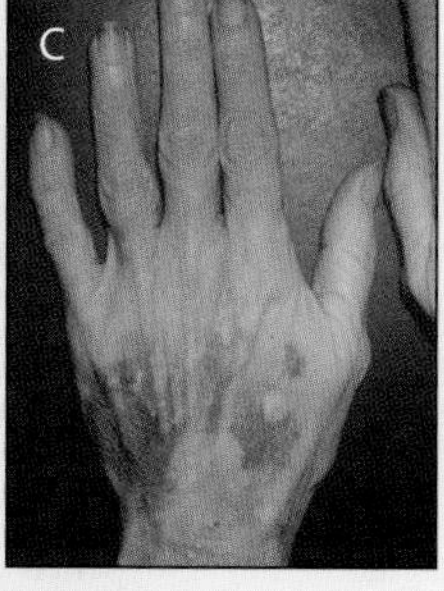

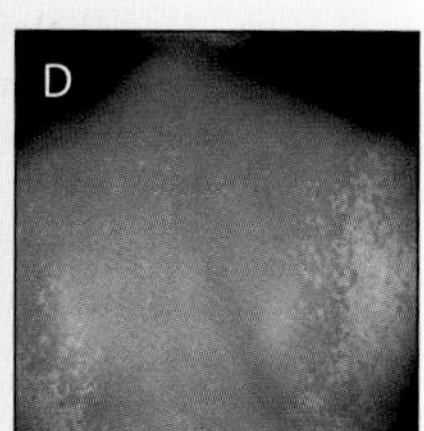

1. A
2. B
3. C
4. D

ANSWER: 3

Senile purpura is characterized by areas of ecchymosis and petechiae found on the hands, arms, and legs caused by the frail capillaries and decreased collagen support. It is a common skin lesion associated with aging. Seborrheic keratosis, option 1 (illustration A), is a benign pigmented lesion with a waxy surface on the face and trunk. Acrochordon, option 2 (illustration B), is a small, benign polyp-growth, also known as skin tags. Urticaria, option 4 (illustration D), is an abnormal lesion that can occur anywhere on the body from allergic reactions.

➧ ***Test-taking Tip:*** *Apply knowledge of medical terminology and age-related changes to eliminate options. Eliminate option 4 because it is an abnormal finding. Recalling that "purpura" relates to vascular, eliminate options 1 and 2.*

Content Area: Adult Health; *Category of Health Alteration:* Older Client Needs; *Integrated Processes:* Nursing Process Assessment; *Client Need:* Health Promotion and Maintenance/Aging Process; Health Promotion and Maintenance/Techniques of Physical Assessment; *Cognitive Level:* Application

Reference: Dillon, P. (2007). *Nursing Health Assessment: Clinical Pocket Guide* (2nd ed., pp. 47, 428). Philadelphia: F. A. Davis.

---

518. A nurse overhears a person say: "I'm having a senior moment because I forgot...." How should the nurse interpret this statement?

1. A comical statement without age bias
2. A stereotypical reference to older adults that can be termed ageism
3. Reflects age-related knowledge since memory decreases with age
4. A derogatory remark, but one that reflects a truism

ANSWER: 2

This statement is a form of ageism, comprises the prejudices and stereotypes that are applied to older people, and perpetuate negativism against them. The statement is biased against older adults. Research indicates that aging is blamed for many memory problems, but very few changes occur solely because of aging. In older adulthood, the processes of learning new information and recalling old information slow down somewhat, but the overall ability to learn and remember is not significantly affected in healthy older people. Inevitable decline in intellectual abilities in old age is a myth.

➧ ***Test-taking Tip:*** *Focus on "interpret." Look for a nonbiased interpretative statement.*

Content Area: Adult Health; *Category of Health Alteration:* Older Client Needs; *Integrated Processes:* Nursing Process Planning; *Client Need:* Health Promotion and Maintenance/Aging Process; *Cognitive Level:* Analysis

Reference: Miller, C. (2009). *Nursing for Wellness in Older Adults* (5th ed., pp. 5–9, 194). Philadelphia: Lippincott Williams & Wilkins.

519. When assessing the cardiovascular system of a 75-year-old male, a nurse auscultates a systolic heart murmur. This is the only abnormality noted. Which analysis by the nurse is correct?

1. Usually representative of some kind of underlying heart disease
2. Indication for valve replacement
3. Indication that the client has congestive heart failure (CHF)
4. Common due to age-related calcification and stiffening of the heart valves

ANSWER: 4

Age-related cardiovascular changes include calcification and stiffening of the heart valves (aortic and mitral), causing incomplete closure (systolic murmur). Approximately 60% of older adults have murmurs. Murmurs are abnormal, vibratory heart sounds. Other causes, including rheumatic fever and congenital defects of the valves, should not be the first consideration. More cardiac symptoms would need to be present to consider valve replacement. Following valve replacement, a murmur usually is auscultated.

➧ ***Test-taking Tip:*** *Focus on the cardiovascular physiological changes with aging. Option 3 is incorrect because an S_4 heart sound (or atrial diastolic gallop) would be heard with congestive heart failure.*

Content Area: Adult Health; *Category of Health Alteration:* Older Client Needs; *Integrated Processes:* Nursing Process Analysis; *Client Need:* Health Promotion and Maintenance/Techniques of Physical Assessment; Physiological Integrity/Physiological Adaptation/Pathophysiology; *Cognitive Level:* Analysis

Reference: Estes, M. (2006). *Health Assessment & Physical Examination* (3rd. ed., pp. 516–518). Clifton Park, NY: Thompson Delmar Learning.

---

520. In assessing a 75-year-old African American client, a nurse notes a blood pressure (BP) of 158/90 mm Hg. In planning care for this client, which interpretation by the nurse is correct?

1. Blood pressure tends to increase with age, so this elevation is considered acceptable and confers no special risk.
2. This reading indicates stage 1 hypertension, so health-promoting lifestyle modifications and medications are needed.
3. This reading indicates prehypertension, so only health-promoting lifestyle modifications are needed.
4. This reading indicates stage 2 hypertension, which is treatable only with thiazide-type diuretics, regardless of diet or exercise.

ANSWER: 2

The Joint National Committee on Prevention, Detection, Evaluation, and Treatment of High Blood Pressure's recommended BP levels list stage 1 hypertension as a systolic blood pressure of 140 to 159 mm Hg or a diastolic blood pressure of 90 to 99 mm Hg. Although BP increases with age, hypertension is a risk factor for cardiovascular disease and thus not an acceptable BP. Most clients with hypertension will require antihypertensive medications to achieve goal BP of less than 140/90 mm Hg. The client's BP is higher than the prehypertension stage (120–139/80–89). Stage 2 hypertension is a systolic BP of 160 or higher or a diastolic BP of 100 or higher. Lifestyle modifications are needed in all hypertensive states.

➧ ***Test-taking Tip:*** *Knowledge of blood pressure guidelines is needed to select the answer.*

Content Area: Adult Health; *Category of Health Alteration:* Older Client Needs; *Integrated Processes:* Nursing Process Assessment; *Client Need:* Health Promotion and Maintenance/Health Screening; *Cognitive Level:* Analysis

Reference: Tabloski, P. (2006). *Gerontological Nursing* (pp. 432–435). Upper Saddle River, NJ: Pearson/Prentice Hall.

---

521. When an office nurse completes height measurement for a 62-year-old female client, the woman says that she has lost half an inch. Which explanation by the nurse is most accurate?

1. "As we age, we lose muscle mass."
2. "Bone loss is due to lack of exercise."
3. "Aging changes in the cartilage of the knees and hips result in shortening stature."
4. "The vertebral column shortens due to compression and thinning of the vertebrae with aging."

ANSWER: 4

With aging, there is shortening and thinning of the vertebral column due to loss of water and bone density, causing compression resulting in decreased height. Loss of muscle mass does not affect height. Option 2 is a true statement but an incomplete statement, as bone loss also results from aging. Although there is loss of cartilage in joints, this does not affect height.

➧ ***Test-taking Tip:*** *Focus on the issue "loss of height in a 62-year-old." Knowledge of age-related changes in the musculoskeletal system is necessary to answer this question.*

Content Area: Adult Health; *Category of Health Alteration:* Older Client Needs; *Integrated Processes:* Teaching and Learning; *Client Need:* Health Promotion and Maintenance/Aging Process; *Cognitive Level:* Application

Reference: Tabloski, P. (2006). *Gerontological Nursing* (pp. 552–554). Upper Saddle River, NJ: Pearson/Prentice Hall.

522. An older adult client tells a clinic nurse that her hearing loss seems to have gotten worse in the last few days. A nurse asks if the client is experiencing any pain, has sustained any injuries, or has started taking any new medications. After performing an assessment, the nurse concludes that the recent hearing loss may be a result of a collection of cerumen. Which age-related change contributed to the collection of cerumen?

1. A diminution in sweat glands, longer and thicker hair growth, and thinning and drying of the skin lining the ear canal
2. Ossicular bone calcification and longer and thicker hair growth
3. Degenerative structural changes of the ear drum and drying of the skin lining the ear canal preventing cerumen passage
4. Prebycusis and reduction in sweat gland activity

ANSWER: 1

Since the hearing loss is recent, without any other suspected causes ear wax (cerumen) should be the first consideration. Cerumen collection is caused by these age-related changes: increased concentration of keratin, the growth of longer and thicker hair (especially in men), thinning and drying of the skin lining the canal, reduction in sweat gland activity causing drying of the wax, and prolapsed or collapsed ear canal. The buildup of wax affects the perception of sounds. Ossicular bone calcification, degenerative structural changes, and presbycusis are misnomers.

➧ ***Test-taking Tip:*** *Focus on the issue of the question and the client's signs and symptoms.*

Content Area: Adult Health; *Category of Health Alteration:* Older Client Needs; *Integrated Processes:* Nursing Process Analysis; Teaching and Learning; *Client Need:* Health Promotion and Maintenance/Aging Process; *Cognitive Level:* Analysis

Reference: Lewis, S., Heitkemper, M., Dirksen, S., O'Brien, P., & Bucher, L. (2007). *Medical-Surgical Nursing: Assessment and Management of Clinical Problems* (7th ed., pp. 438–439). St. Louis, MO: Mosby.

523. Which interventions should a nurse implement when teaching an 86-year-old client about glaucoma and demonstrating how to administer eye drops? SELECT ALL THAT APPLY.

1. Tell the client when the teaching session to be held so that the client may ask a relative to attend if needed or preferred.
2. Provide an environment that is private, quiet, and well lit.
3. Show the client how to administer eye drops in lying, sitting, and standing positions and be detailed with the explanations to ensure understanding.
4. Engage as many of the five senses as possible during the instruction linking the information with the client's life experience.
5. Give extensive written materials for each eye drop medication with a schedule to follow.

ANSWER: 1, 2, 4

The client's decreased vision may be a barrier to learning, so the presence of a relative may be needed. The client may also prefer to have the relative for support or for assistance. A private, quiet, and well-lit environment is needed so that the client can focus on the content and procedure. Engaging the five senses is important for retention of information through use of graphics, videos, or other teaching strategies. Too much information can overwhelm or fatigue the client. Follow the KISS principle—keep it short and simple; no longer than 15 minutes. Written materials should be concise, providing needed information and serving as a reference if questions or problems should arise.

➧ ***Test-taking Tip:*** *Focus on principles of teaching correlated with sensory age-related changes.*

Content Area: Adult Health; *Category of Health Alteration:* Older Client Needs; *Integrated Processes:* Nursing Process Intervention; *Client Need:* Health Promotion and Maintenance/Principles of Teaching and Learning; *Cognitive Level:* Application

Reference: Lewis, S., Heitkemper, M., Dirksen, S., O'Brien, P., & Bucher, L. (2007). *Medical-Surgical Nursing: Assessment and Management of Clinical Problems* (7th ed., pp. 434–436). St. Louis, MO: Mosby.

524. A nurse is caring for a 79-year-old client who was widowed last year and complains of being lonely. The nurse invites and encourages the client to attend local church services and activities. Which benefits are associated with participation in religious activities? SELECT ALL THAT APPLY.

1. Greater well-being and life satisfaction
2. Higher level of participation in health promotion activities
3. Coping mechanism for bereavement
4. Higher levels of hope and optimism
5. The services of a parish nurse who can provide medical care

ANSWER: 1, 2, 3, 4

Physical and mental health benefits have been associated with older adults' participation in religious activities by several research studies. Gerontologists have studied the various aspects of the role of religion in the psychosocial functioning of older adults and identified benefits including decreased anxiety and depression, better adaptation to medical illness, better immune system function, better adaptation to caregiving burden, faster recovery from depression, fewer hospitalizations, shorter hospital stays, lower rates of substance abuse, and lower rates of suicide.

➧ ***Test-taking Tip:*** *Focus on religious benefits and activities correlated with the psychosocial needs of older adults.*

Content Area: Adult Health; *Category of Health Alteration:* Older Client Needs; *Integrated Processes:* Nursing Process Implementation; Caring; *Client Need:* Health Promotion and Maintenance/Health and Wellness/Coping Mechanisms; *Cognitive Level:* Analysis

Reference: Miller, C. (2009). *Nursing for Wellness in Older Adults* (5th ed., p. 108). Philadelphia: Lippincott Williams & Wilkins.

525. A 62-year-old female client is attending a community health fair. A health fair nurse recommends that the client make an appointment with a physician and ask that a DEXA (dual-energy x-ray absorptiometry) scan be done to evaluate for osteoporosis because the client has many risk factors. Which risk factor likely influenced the health fair nurse's decision to recommend a DEXA scan?

1. Diabetes mellitus
2. Postmenopausal
3. Overweight
4. African American

ANSWER: 2

Major risk factors for osteoporosis include increased age, female sex, White or Asian race, family history of osteoporosis, and a thin body structure. Since osteoporosis is the most common metabolic disease, affecting 50% of women during their lifetime, it is important for women to be screened and begin appropriate treatment, if needed. Diabetes mellitus and being overweight are not risk factors for osteoporosis. Being overweight can contribute to the development of osteoarthritis.

➧ ***Test-taking Tip:*** *Focus on what the question is asking: risk factors of osteoporosis.*

Content Area: Adult Health; *Category of Health Alteration:* Older Client Needs; *Integrated Processes:* Nursing Process Evaluation; *Client Need:* Health Promotion and Maintenance/Health Screening; *Cognitive Level:* Application

Reference: Tabloski, P. (2006). *Gerontological Nursing* (p. 557). Upper Saddle River, NJ: Pearson/Prentice Hall.

---

526. EBP On the first postoperative day for a 74-year-old client who had a transurethral resection of the prostrate (TURP), a nurse assists the client to ambulate several times to maintain muscle strength. The nurse's action is based on knowing that:

1. passive exercises are not effective on aging muscles.
2. immobile gerontological clients can lose as much as 5% of muscle strength per day.
3. active exercise is the only type of exercise that aids in healing of the incision.
4. the weight-bearing exercise of walking increases deconditioning by 10%.

ANSWER: 2

Deconditioning and loss of muscle mass of hospitalized older adults can occur in brief periods of immobility. Passive exercise is effective with all age groups, and both passive and active exercise aids in the healing process by increasing circulation. Walking, a weight-bearing exercise increases "conditioning," not "deconditioning." Deconditioning describes the decrease in muscle mass and other physiological changes resulting in overall weakness.

➧ ***Test-taking Tip:*** *Focus on functional decline in older adults and the value of exercise.*

Content Area: Adult Health; *Category of Health Alteration:* Older Client Needs; *Integrated Processes:* Nursing Process Implementation; *Client Need:* Health Promotion and Maintenance/Aging Process; Physiological Integrity/Reduction of Risk Potential/Potential for Alterations in Body Systems; *Cognitive Level:* Application

Reference: Smeltzer, S., Bare, B., Hinkle, J., & Cheever, K. (2008). *Brunner & Suddarth's Textbook of Medical-Surgical Nursing* (11th ed., p. 246). Philadelphia: Lippincott, Williams & Wilkins.

EBP Reference: Graf, C. (2006). Functional decline in hospitalized older adults. *American Journal of Nursing,* 10, 58–68.

---

527. EBP A nurse should evaluate the hydration status of an older adult client by assessing: SELECT ALL THAT APPLY.

1. urine color.
2. serum blood urea nitrogen (BUN) and creatinine.
3. serum white blood cell (WBC) and differential count.
4. urine specific gravity.
5. 24-hour fluid intake and urine output.

ANSWER: 1, 2, 4, 5

Urine color indicates the concentration of the urine and varies with specific gravity. With overhydration, the urine will be dilute and light in color with a low specific gravity. With dehydration, the urine will be concentrated and dark in color with a high specific gravity. The BUN and creatinine tests are interpreted together and are directly proportional to renal excretory function; thus, overhydration tends to dilute the urine, resulting in lower levels, and dehydration tends to concentrate the urine, resulting in higher levels. Comparing intake and output measurements of the client's fluids for 24 hours assesses actual or potential imbalances. WBC and differential count evaluate infection, neoplasm, allergy, or immunosuppression, not hydration.

➧ ***Test-taking Tip:*** *Look for the correct indicators of fluid status and avoid reading into the question. Although the causes of elevated WBC and differential may result in fluid loss, this laboratory value is not used to evaluate hydration status.*

Content Area: Adult Health; *Category of Health Alteration:* Older Client Needs; *Integrated Processes:* Nursing Process Assessment; *Client Need:* Health Promotion and Maintenance/Aging Process; Physiological Integrity/Reduction of Risk Potential/Laboratory Values; *Cognitive Level:* Analysis

Reference: Pagana, K., & Pagana, T. (2007). *Mosby's Diagnostic and Laboratory Tests* (8th ed., pp. 322–323, 961–963, 969–971). St. Louis, MO: Mosby/Elsevier.

EBP Reference: GeronurseOnline.org. (2005). *Hydration Management.* Available at: www.geronurseonline.org

528. When assessing a 68-year-old client's laboratory test results, a nurse should anticipate common age-related changes. In the following box, place an X in the column for the laboratory values expected to be decreased due to age-related changes.

Lab Component	Age-Related Change
RBC	
WBC	
Platelets	
Hgb	
Hct	
BUN	

ANSWER:

Lab Component	Age-Related Change
RBC	X
WBC	X
Hgb	X
Hct	X
BUN	X

Due to the physiological changes of aging, red blood cell (RBC) values tend to decrease; white blood cell (WBC) counts tend to decrease slightly, platelet (thrombocytes) range does not vary, hemoglobin (Hgb) values slightly decrease, hematocrit (Hct) values slightly decrease; and blood urea nitrogen (BUN) may slightly increase.

▶ ***Test-taking Tip:*** *Knowledge of laboratory test normal values and age-related physiological changes is needed to complete the chart.*

Content Area: Adult Health; *Category of Health Alteration:* Older Client Needs; *Integrated Processes:* Nursing Process Assessment; *Client Need:* Health Promotion and Maintenance/Aging Process; *Cognitive Level:* Analysis

Reference: Pagana, K., & Pagana, T. (2007). *Mosby's Diagnostic and Laboratory Tests* (8th ed., pp. 518–519, 521–532, 732–733, 797–799, 961–962, 1003–1008). St. Louis, MO: Mosby/Elsevier.

529. For which age-related skin changes should a nurse assess an 81-year-old hospitalized client to best protect the client from developing ducubiti?

1. Increased tissue vascularity
2. Increase in subcutaneous tissue
3. Increased rate of cellular replacement
4. Loss of skin thickness and elasticity

ANSWER: 4

The replacement rate of the stratum corneum, which is the first layer of epidermis, declines by 50% as individuals age. A thinner epidermis allows more moisture to escape, decreasing strength and increasing the risk of skin tears. The dermis decreases in thickness by 20% with aging. Blood vessels decrease, not increase, from aging because of decreased skin thickness. A decrease in subcutaneous tissue (not an increase), causes diminished thermoregulatory function and inflammatory response. Loss of skin thickness and a decreased vascularity decrease the rate of cellular replacement.

▶ ***Test-taking Tip:*** *Note the key words "skin changes." Select the only option that is plural.*

Content Area: Adult Health; *Category of Health Alteration:* Older Client Needs; *Integrated Processes:* Nursing Process Assessment; *Client Need:* Health Promotion and Maintenance/Aging Process; Safe and Effective Care Environment/Safety and Infection Control/Injury Prevention; *Cognitive Level:* Application

Reference: Meiner, S., & Lueckenotte, A. (2006). *Gerontologic Nursing* (3rd ed., pp. 693–694). St. Louis, MO: Mosby/Elsevier.

530. A nurse reports to a health-care provider that a client has decreased peripheral vision. An ophthalmologist consult is ordered and the client is diagnosed with chronic open-angle glaucoma. The client cries when told the diagnosis. A nurse identifies the following nursing diagnoses. In which priority order should the nurse plan to address the nursing diagnoses?

____ Deficient knowledge related to glaucoma causes and treatment
____ Anxiety related to fear of vision loss and changes in quality of life
____ Sensory/perceptual alterations (visual) related to decreased peripheral vision
____ Dressing and grooming self-care deficit related to visual impairment

ANSWER: 3, 2, 1, 4

Implementing environmental precautions to accommodate loss of peripheral vision should be the first priority to protect the client from injury. Next, alleviate the client's anxiety by increasing the client's knowledge of the disease process and the use of medication to delay vision loss. Finally, assist the client in learning self-care adjustments needed because of the vision loss.

▶ ***Test-taking Tip:*** *Use Maslow's Hierarchy of Needs theory. Client safety and physiological needs are priority.*

Content Area: Adult Health; *Category of Health Alteration:* Older Client Needs; *Integrated Processes:* Nursing Process Planning; *Client Need:* Health Promotion and Maintenance/Aging Process; *Cognitive Level:* Analysis

Reference: Meiner, S., & Lueckenotte, A. (2006). *Gerontologic Nursing* (3rd ed., pp. 731–732). St. Louis, MO: Mosby/Elsevier.

531. EBP An older adult client tells a clinic nurse of a fear of falling due to improperly fitting shoes and sore feet. When assessing the client's feet, the nurse notes a bunion and refers the client to a podiatrist. Place an X on the illustration where the nurse noted the bunion.

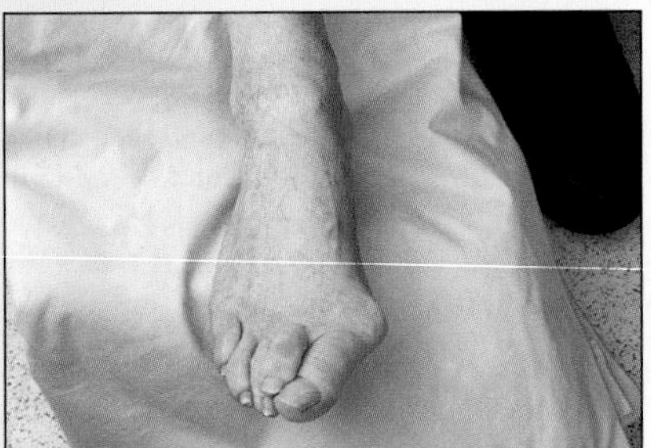

ANSWER:

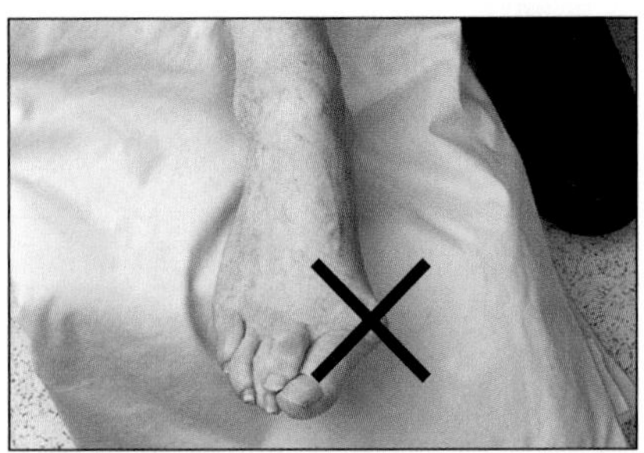

A bunion is caused from inflammation and thickening of the first metatarsal joint of the great toe, usually with marked enlargement of the joint and lateral displacement of the toe.

➧ *Test-taking Tip: Apply knowledge of medical terminology to answer this question.*

Content Area: Adult Health; *Category of Health Alteration:* Older Client Needs; *Integrated Processes:* Nursing Process Assessment; *Client Need:* Physiological Integrity/Basic Care and Comfort/Mobility/Immobility; *Cognitive Level:* Application

Reference: Black, J., & Hokanson Hawks, J. (2009). *Medical-Surgical Nursing: Clinical Management for Positive Outcomes* (8th ed., p. 503). St. Louis, MO: Saunders/Elsevier.

EBP Reference: Mann, W. (2005). A comparison of fallers and non-fallers in the frail elderly. *Technology & Disability*, 17(1), 25–32.

532. A client has a DEXA (dual-energy x-ray absorptiometry) scan that reveals osteoporosis. Which medication, if taken by the 62-year-old client, should a nurse identify as posing a secondary risk factor for the client's osteoporosis?

1. Baby aspirin daily for past 4 years
2. Escitalopram (Lexapro®) 5 mg daily for past 7 months
3. Multivitamin for many years
4. Budesonide (Pulmicort®) two sprays to each nostril two times a day for 9 to 10 years

ANSWER: 4

Long-term use of corticosteroids, such as Pulmicort, should be identified as a risk factor for osteoporosis. Baby aspirin, Lexapro®, and multivitamins have not been identified to cause bone loss (osteoporosis).

➧ *Test-taking Tip: Focus on the issue: osteoporosis. Knowledge of aspirin, Lexapro®, Pulmicort®, and multivitamins is needed to answer this question.*

Content Area: Adult Health; *Category of Health Alteration:* Older Client Needs; *Integrated Processes:* Nursing Process Analysis; *Client Need:* Health Promotion and Maintenance/Disease Prevention; Physiological Integrity/Pharmacological and Parenteral Therapies/Adverse Effects/Contradictions and Side Effects; *Cognitive Level:* Analysis

Reference: Tabloski, P. (2006). *Gerontological Nursing* (p. 557). Upper Saddle River, NJ: Pearson/Prentice Hall.

533. When assessing an older adult, which tools should a nurse select to identify the client's needs and care deficits?

1. Katz Index of Activities of Daily Living
2. Maslow's Hierarchy of Needs
3. Mini Mental State Exam (MMSE)
4. Erikson's Developmental Task Theory

ANSWER: 1

Katz Index of Activities of Daily Living is a widely used functional assessment tool for evaluating the client's ability to perform daily personal care activities. Maslow's is a human needs theory that is pertinent to everyone. Erikson's theory is a developmental theory differentiating needs of each age group. The MMSE only assesses cognition.

➧ *Test-taking Tip: Knowledge of these tools, and their assessment purposes, is needed to select the correct option.*

Content Area: Adult Health; *Category of Health Alteration:* Older Client Needs; *Integrated Processes:* Nursing Process Assessment; *Client Need:* Safe and Effective Care Environment/Safety and Infection Control/Injury Prevention; *Cognitive Level:* Application

Reference: Meiner, S., & Lueckenotte, A. (2006). *Gerontologic Nursing* (3rd ed., pp. 82–87). St. Louis, MO: Mosby/Elsevier.

534. A 74-year-old client is admitted from the emergency department after sustaining a knife cut to the left hand. The client has a dry and intact dressing on the left hand and has IV D5LR infusing at 100 mL/minute in the right hand. A nurse, performing the health assessment, writes a nursing diagnosis: *Disturbed thought processes due to inability to focus and memory deficits.* In analyzing the assessment data, the nurse determines that the signs supporting this nursing diagnosis may be a result of the client: SELECT ALL THAT APPLY

1. receiving pain medication in the ER.
2. having possible early dementia.
3. not eating dinner.
4. experiencing a strange environment.
5. feeling anxious about hospitalization.

ANSWER: 1, 2, 4, 5

Medication and dementia can affect the central nervous system, thus decreasing one's ability to focus and think. Age-related changes affect the pharmacokinetics and pharmacodynamics of the drugs, often causing exaggerated effects as well as adverse effects. Some memory deficits are often the first signs of dementia. Experiencing a strange environment and hospitalization cause threats to sense of security influencing the older adult client's ability to focus and think clearly. Although not having eaten dinner can precipitate nutrient losses, leading to electrolyte imbalances, the client is receiving D5LR to replace nutrients and electrolytes.

➧ ***Test-taking Tip:*** *Read the situation carefully and focus on the causes of confusion.*

Content Area: Adult Health; *Category of Health Alteration:* Older Client Needs; *Integrated Processes:* Nursing Process Analysis; *Client Need:* Physiological Integrity/Reduction of Risk Potential/Potential for Alterations in Body Systems; *Cognitive Level:* Analysis

Reference: Miller, C. (2009). *Nursing for Wellness in Older Adults* (5th ed., pp. 112–114, 190–191, 260–261, 273–274). Philadelphia: Lippincott Williams & Wilkins.

---

535. A 76-year-old client is admitted to a surgical unit following a right colectomy for a small tumor. The client has lactated Ringer's solution infusing intravenously at 125 mL/hr, O_2 per nasal cannula at 3 L, and a right abdominal dressing. A nurse analyzes the client's assessment information and identifies the nursing diagnosis: *Risk for infection (pneumonia) due to age-related functional changes in the respiratory system.* Which age-related assessment most likely prompted the nurse to establish the nursing diagnosis?

1. Decreased residual volume
2. Increased vital capacity
3. Increased PaO_2
4. Decreased cough reflex

ANSWER: 4

A decreased cough reflex is caused by blunting of the cough and laryngeal reflexes that occur with aging and increases the risk for aspiration. Age-related, decreased elastic recoil of the lungs produces increased, not decreased, residual volume (the amount of air remaining in the lungs at the end of exhalation) and decreased, not increased, vital capacity (the amount of air that moves in and out with inspiration and expiration). PaO_2 (arterial oxygen pressure) decreases, not increases, due to age-related changes in alveoli resulting in less surface area for gas exchange to take place. All of these factors interfere with oxygenation and the ability to clear secretions, predisposing the older adult client to pneumonia. The decreased mobility due to hospitalization and abdominal pain, which often prevents clients from taking deep breaths, is also a risk factor for pneumonia.

➧ ***Test-taking Tip:*** *Focus on what the question is asking: "age-related functional change in the respiratory system."*

Content Area: Adult Health; *Category of Health Alteration:* Older Client Needs; *Integrated Processes:* Nursing Process Analysis; *Client Need:* Health Promotion and Maintenance/Aging Process; Safe and Effective Care Environment/Safety and Infection Control/Injury Prevention; *Cognitive Level:* Application

References: Meiner, S., & Lueckenotte, A. (2006). *Gerontologic Nursing* (3rd ed., pp. 504–507). St. Louis, MO: Mosby/Elsevier; Miller, C. (2009). *Nursing for Wellness in Older Adults* (5th ed., pp. 442–448). Philadelphia: Lippincott Williams & Wilkins.

---

536. An 84-year-old client, hospitalized for repair of a fractured hip, is incontinent of urine, is sometimes confused, and is not eating well. A nurse notes nonblanchable erythema of the intact skin over the client's coccyx. The nurse's interventions to prevent further skin breakdown should include: SELECT ALL THAT APPLY

1. relieving pressure under the coccyx with an inflatable "donut."
2. repositioning the client at least every 2 hours.
3. keeping the head-of-bed raised above 30 degrees.
4. careful skin hygiene and reduction of pressure over the coccyx.
5. offering foods the client likes to eat.

ANSWER: 2, 4

Careful skin hygiene and reduction of pressure over the coccyx should be implemented to keep the client's skin dry and intact since moisture softens the skin and pressure reduces the blood supply, thereby weakening the skin. Clients should be repositioned at least every 2 hours so that ischemic areas can recover. An inflatable donut is contraindicated because it reduces blood supply to the affected area leading to even more ischemia. Keeping the head of the bed raised at 30 degrees would put additional pressure on the coccyx. Offering preferred foods would likely increase the client's intake and nutritional status but will not prevent further breakdown.

➧ ***Test-taking Tip:*** *Focus on interventions to prevent further skin breakdown and use the process of elimination to rule out incorrect options.*

Content Area: Adult Health; *Category of Health Alteration:* Older Client Needs; *Integrated Processes:* Nursing Process Implementation; *Client Need:* Physiological Integrity/Reduction of Risk Potential/Potential for Complications from Surgical Procedures and Health Alterations; *Cognitive Level:* Application

Reference: Black, J., & Hokanson Hawks, J. (2009). *Medical-Surgical Nursing: Clinical Management for Positive Outcomes* (8th ed., pp. 1210–1213). St. Louis, MO: Saunders/Elsevier.

537. EBP A nurse obtains information for a 75-year-old client and concludes that some findings are not age-related and require further follow-up because the client is at risk for falls. Which report by the client represents a non-age-related finding that requires additional investigation?

1. Reports experiencing a decreased ability to see at night
2. Reports seeing halos around lights
3. Reports having difficulty distinguishing some colors
4. Reports diminished visual acuity

ANSWER: 2

Seeing halos is not a normal age-related vision change. Halos are classic symptoms of glaucoma. Age-related changes include a decrease in the size of the pupil, limiting the amount of light entering the eye. The lens increases in density and rigidity, which cause the older adult client's night vision to decrease and reduce the client's ability to distinguish some colors.

➧ ***Test-taking Tip:*** *Knowledge of physiological changes of the eye due to aging is necessary to answer this question.*

Content Area: Adult Health; *Category of Health Alteration:* Older Client Needs; *Integrated Processes:* Nursing Process Assessment; *Client Need:* Safe and Effective Care Environment/Safety and Infection Control/Injury Prevention; Health Promotion and Maintenance/Aging Process; *Cognitive Level:* Analysis

Reference: Meiner, S., & Lueckenotte, A. (2006). *Gerontologic Nursing* (3rd ed., pp. 729–733). St. Louis, MO: Mosby/Elsevier.

EBP Reference: Gray-Micelli, D. (2008). Preventing falls in acute care. In: Capezuti, E., Zwicker, D., Mezey, M., & Fulmer, T., eds. *Evidence-Based Geriatric Nursing Protocols for Best Practice* (3rd ed., pp. 161–198). New York, NY: Springer Publishing Company.

538. A nurse is admitting an older adult client to a hospital medical unit. The nurse's assessment findings include: blood pressure (BP) 96/64 mm Hg, pulse 118/minute, respirations 20/minute, weight 110 pounds with an 8-pound weight loss in the last 3 months due to severe loss of appetite from chemotherapy for breast cancer, and body mass index (BMI) of 19. The client reports fatigue and decreased mobility (able to get around the house, but does not go out). Though tired, the client responds appropriately and clearly to questions and denies psychological problems. Which score should the nurse assign to the client when completing the Geriatric Mini Nutrition Assessment?

Geriatric Mini Nutrition Assessment	Score
Has food intake declined over the past 3 months due to loss of appetite, digestive problems, or chewing or swallowing difficulties? 0 = severe loss of appetite 1 = moderate 2 = no loss	
Weight loss during past 3 months 0 = more than 3 kg 1 = unknown 2 = 1–3 kg 3 = no weight loss	
Mobility 0 = bed or chair bound 1 = able to get out of bed/chair but does not go out 2 = goes out	
Psychological stress or acute disease in past 3 months 0 = yes 2 = no	
Neuropsychological problems 0 = severe dementia or depression 1 = mild dementia 2 = no psychological problems	
BMI 0 = less than 19 1 = 19–20.9 2 = 21–22.9 3 = 23 or more	
Score (max. 14): 12 or more = normal; 11 or less = possible malnutrition, continue assessing	

Source: Lutz, C., & Przytulski, K. (2006). *Nutrition & Diet Therapy: Evidence-Based Applications* (4th ed., p. 277). Philadelphia: F. A. Davis.

1. Score of 3
2. Score of 4
3. Score of 5
4. Score of 6

ANSWER: 2

Severe loss of appetite = 0; 8-lb (3.6 kg) weight loss during last 3 months is more than 3 kg = 0; able to get out of bed/chair but does not go out = 1; acute disease (cancer) in past 3 months = 0; no psychological problems = 2; and BMI 19 = 1.

Test-taking Tip: *Carefully read the client's information in the situation. Remember to convert pounds to kilograms for weight loss (2.2 pounds = 1 kilogram).*

Content Area: Adult Health; *Category of Health Alteration:* Older Client Needs; *Integrated Processes:* Nursing Process Analysis; *Client Need:* Physiological Integrity/Basic Care and Comfort/Nutrition and Oral Hydration; *Cognitive Level:* Analysis

Reference: Lutz, C., & Przytulski, K. (2006). *Nutrition & Diet Therapy: Evidence-Based Applications* (4th ed., p. 277). Philadelphia: F. A. Davis.

539. For which reason should a nurse plan to teach an older, hospitalized client about newly prescribed medications?

1. Most older adult clients are unable to read the unit-developed printed teaching materials.
2. Hospital admissions and readmissions of older adult clients occur from misuse of medications.
3. Most older adult clients are unable to retain information from printed teaching materials.
4. The client needs understanding of medications before prescriptions can be filled.

ANSWER: 2

Research findings, from hospital admission data, indicate that intentional or accidental misuse of medications among older clients contributes to frequent hospital admissions and readmissions. Medication teaching is an important intervention to enhance adherence and decrease the chances of readmissions and grave consequences. Although some older adult clients have limited education, teaching materials should be prepared at the fifth-grade reading level, a level at which most people can read and understand. Prescriptions are often filled by older adult clients without knowledge of the purpose, action, side effects, and administration instructions.

➧ ***Test-taking Tip:*** *Knowledge of misuse of medications by older people is necessary to answer this question.*

Content Area: Adult Health; *Category of Health Alteration:* Older Client Needs; *Integrated Processes:* Nursing Process Planning; *Client Need:* Health Promotion and Maintenance/Teaching and Learning; *Cognitive Level:* Application

Reference: Miller, C. (2009). *Nursing for Wellness in Older Adults* (5th ed., p. 124). Philadelphia: Lippincott Williams & Wilkins.

---

540. A client's family approaches a nurse with a complaint about a nursing assistant's inappropriate communication with their 89-year-old father. When evaluating the nursing assistant's communication, which statement most likely caused the family's complaint?

1. "Are you ready for the nurse to give you your medicine?"
2. "Grandpa, would you like to go to breakfast now?"
3. "Would you prefer to wear the brown socks today?"
4. "Your family will be visiting today. Isn't that nice?"

ANSWER: 2.

"Honey" and "grandpa" are diminutives (inappropriate intimate terms of endearment, implying a parent-child relationship). Asking the client questions is appropriate communication. Although the statement "Isn't that nice" uses a cliché that can block the feelings and thoughts of the client, it is not diminutive.

➧ ***Test-taking Tip:*** *Note the key words "inappropriate communication."*

Content Area: Adult Health; *Category of Health Alteration:* Older Client Needs; *Integrated Processes:* Nursing Process Evaluation; Communication and Documentation; *Client Need:* Psychosocial Integrity/Therapeutic Communications; Safe and Effective Care Environment/Management of Care/Supervision; *Cognitive Level:* Application

Reference: Berman, A., Snyder, S., Kozier, B., & Erb, G. (2008). *Kozier & Erb's Fundamentals of Nursing: Concepts, Process, and Practice* (8th ed., pp. 461–462). Upper Saddle River, NJ: Pearson Education.

---

541. At a community senior meal program, a nurse inquires about the health of an 80-year-old female attendee. The woman states that she is not taking her medication because it is too expensive and not needed. Based on knowledge of gerontological nursing, the nurse should recognize that the client is most likely refusing her medication because she:

1. has insufficient knowledge to realize that the medication is good for her.
2. is in a bad mood today and is being obstinate.
3. fears she will live longer than her resources will last.
4. prefers the sick role because it allows her to be "waited on."

ANSWER: 3

Fear of future lack of resources is a common concern of many older adults, resulting in the failure to seek or comply with medical treatments. While the other options are plausible, they are not major findings in medication assessments of the older adult.

➧ ***Test-taking Tip:*** *Note the key phrase "most likely" and the client's age.*

Content Area: Adult Health; *Category of Health Alteration:* Older Client Needs; *Integrated Processes:* Caring; Nursing Process Analysis; *Client Need:* Psychosocial Integrity/Coping Mechanisms; *Cognitive Level:* Application

Reference: Miller, C. (2009). *Nursing for Wellness in Older Adults* (5th ed., pp. 139–140). Philadelphia: Lippincott Williams & Wilkins.

542. An 87-year-old client, recovering from hip surgery, is ordered oxycodone (OxyContin®) as needed for pain. After giving this medication, for which side effects should a nurse assess the client?

1. Blood glucose elevation
2. Respiratory alkalosis
3. Urinary retention
4. Loss of appetite

ANSWER: 3

Oxycodone is a mild to moderate analgesic medication that should be used with caution in older adult clients because age-related changes in the renal system predispose these clients to urinary retention. Age-related decline in glomerular filtration decreases the clearance of this medication, thereby increasing its effects on urinary muscles, which are weakened due to age-related changes. Respiratory depression would result in respiratory acidosis, not alkalosis, from retention of carbonic acid. Blood glucose may decrease, but other factors may cause this change, and it is not considered a direct side effect of oxycodone. Loss of appetite may occur due to limited mobility and pain, but is not a side effect of oxycodone.

➧ ***Test-taking Tip:*** *Think of the effects of oxycodone and the effects of age-related changes.*

Content Area: Adult Health; *Category of Health Alteration:* Older Client Needs; *Integrated Processes:* Nursing Process Assessment; *Client Need:* Physiological Integrity/Pharmacological and Parenteral Therapies/Adverse Effects/Contradictions and Side Effects; *Cognitive Level:* Analysis

Reference: Wilson, B., Shannon, M., Shields, K., & Stang, C. (2008). *Prentice Hall Nurse's Drug Guide 2008* (pp. 1133–1135). Upper Saddle River, NJ: Pearson Education.

---

543. An 85-year-old client is hospitalized for diverticulitis. The client's 83-year-old girlfriend spends most of the day and evening with him. Several nurses have made comments about the couple's relationship. Which nurse's comment represents a myth about the intimacy needs of older adults in general?

1. Older adults require less physical contact than younger adults.
2. Sexual expression may enhance the quality of life of older adults.
3. Sexual expression may be difficult or impossible for some older adults.
4. Sexual interest tends to persist throughout one's life span.

ANSWER: 1

"Older adults require less physical contact than younger adults" is a myth. Options 2, 3, and 4 are true statements.

➧ ***Test-taking Tip:*** *Focus on the word "myth" and select the option that is a false statement.*

Content Area: Adult Health; *Category of Health Alteration:* Older Client Needs; *Integrated Processes:* Nursing Process Evaluation; *Client Need:* Health Promotion and Maintenance/Human Sexuality; *Cognitive Level:* Analysis

Reference: Ebersole, P., Hess, P., Touchy, T., Jett, K., & Luggen, A. (2008). *Toward Healthy Aging* (7th ed., pp. 460–466). St. Louis, MO: Mosby/Elsevier.

---

544. A nurse is caring for an 80-year-old hospitalized client of the Muslim belief who is near death. Which nursing action is most inappropriate?

1. Perfuming the room
2. Positioning the client supine facing Mecca
3. Offering grief counseling to family members
4. Reviewing the medical records to determine if the client wishes organ donation

ANSWER: 3

Discussion of death and grief counseling are discouraged in the Muslim faith. Perfuming the room and positioning the client supine facing Mecca are end-of-life care rituals in the Muslim faith. Organ donation is allowed.

➧ ***Test-taking Tip:*** *Note the key word "inappropriate." This is a false-response item so select the option that would not be correct.*

Content Area: Adult Health; *Category of Health Alteration:* Older Client Needs; *Integrated Processes:* Nursing Process Implementation; *Client Need:* Psychosocial Integrity/End of Life Care; Psychosocial Integrity/Cultural Diversity; *Cognitive Level:* Analysis

Reference: Tabloski, P. (2006). *Gerontological Nursing* (p. 319). Upper Saddle River, NJ: Pearson Education.

545. A 72-year-old male client with terminal cancer is receiving palliative care services in his home. He comments to the nurse, "I am such a feeble old man. My life is such a waste, and I hate having my wife see me like this. I just wish I could die now." The nurse's best interpretation of these comments is that the client is:

1. ashamed and ready to die.
2. expressing anxiety due to the diagnosis of terminal cancer.
3. experiencing Havighurst's developmental tasks of later maturity.
4. experiencing Erikson's developmental state of integrity versus despair.

ANSWER: 4

Indicators of a negative resolution (despair) include contempt for self or others and a sense of loss. Indicators of positive resolution (integrity) include acceptance of worth and acceptance of death. Shame would be from a sense of guilt. The client's comments do not reflect shame or anxiety. Havighurst's developmental tasks of later maturity include positive behaviors and adjustments, such as adjusting to decreasing physical strength and health. The client's comments indicate lack of adjustment.

▶ ***Test-taking Tip:*** *Note the key word "best" and use the process of elimination.*

Content Area: Adult Health; *Category of Health Alteration:* Older Client Needs; *Integrated Processes:* Nursing Process Analysis; *Client Need:* Psychosocial Integrity/End of Life Care; *Cognitive Level:* Analysis

Reference: Berman, A., Snyder, S., Kozier, B., & Erb, G. (2008). *Kozier & Erb's Fundamentals of Nursing: Concepts, Process, and Practice* (8th ed., pp. 353–355). Upper Saddle River, NJ: Pearson Education.

546. A client's plan of care includes a nursing diagnosis of *Anticipatory grieving/death anxiety related to anticipated loss of physiological well-being*. A nurse evaluates that the client has achieved one desired outcome pertinent to the diagnosis when the client:

1. dies with family members present.
2. continues normal life activities within abilities and verbalizes taking 1 day at a time.
3. verbalizes experiencing negative death images and unpleasant thoughts.
4. states worries about causing grief and suffering in others.

ANSWER: 2

Criteria to indicate that the client's grief is resolving include looking toward the future, taking 1 day at a time, and continuing with normal life activities. Option 1 should be a planned intervention so the client does not die alone. Options 3 and 4 are signs supporting the nursing diagnosis.

▶ ***Test-taking Tip:*** *Use the process of elimination, eliminating options 1, 3, and 4 because these are not outcome statements.*

Content Area: Adult Health; *Category of Health Alteration:* Older Client Needs; *Integrated Processes:* Nursing Process Evaluation; *Client Need:* Psychosocial Integrity/End of Life Care; *Cognitive Level:* Analysis

Reference: Doenges, M., Moorhouse, M., & Murr, A. (2005). *Nursing Care Plans* (7th ed., p. 884). Philadelphia: F. A. Davis.

547. A physician notifies the family of the death of their 90-year-old mother who died on admission to the emergency room. A nurse is meeting the family for the first time to escort them to the client's room. Which initial statement by the nurse would be best?

1. "I'm very sorry for the loss of your mother."
2. "This must be very hard for you. You have my sympathy."
3. "I am the nurse who was with your mother when she died."
4. "Let me take you to your mother's room where we can talk and you can be alone with her."

ANSWER: 1

Stating sorrow for the family's loss is a simple and direct statement that demonstrates caring. Telling the family that this must be very hard for them is a nontherapeutic statement because it makes an assumption (option 2). In option 3 the focus is on the nurse and not the family. Option 4 is too impersonal and doesn't demonstrate caring.

▶ ***Test-taking Tip:*** *Use techniques of therapeutic communication to identify the best response.*

Content Area: Adult Health; *Category of Health Alteration:* Older Client Needs; *Integrated Processes:* Communication and Documentation; Caring; *Client Need:* Psychosocial Integrity/Grief and Loss; *Cognitive Level:* Application

Reference: Berman, A., Snyder, S., Kozier, B., & Erb, G. (2008). *Kozier & Erb's Fundamentals of Nursing: Concepts, Process, and Practice* (8th ed., pp. 467–471, 1095–1096). Upper Saddle River, NJ: Pearson Education.

548. An 89-year-old client has recently been widowed. A nurse counseling the client explains that the client may experience grief for many years and may likely go through the phases of grief. Place each phase of the grief process in the correct order.

______ Full effects of widowhood set along with regret, self-doubt, and at times despair
______ Numb shock where the widow cannot believe that the spouse's death occurred
______ Reorganization with positive outlook on life and positive coping strategies
______ Emotional turmoil with alarm or panic-type reactions and anger, guilt, or longing

ANSWER: 3, 1, 4, 2

First the client experiences numb shock. Restless behavior, which includes stupor and withdrawal, are hallmarks of this phase. Next, the client experiences emotional turmoil and then the full effects of grief. Life's purpose becomes confusing, and the client can experience mood swings. Eventually, the client reaches reorganization where coping strategies and positive outlooks emerge.

▶ ***Test-taking Tip:*** *Visualize how one might respond if faced with the death of a spouse.*

Content Area: Adult Health; *Category of Health Alteration:* Older Client Needs; *Integrated Processes:* Teaching and Learning; *Client Need:* Psychosocial Integrity/Grief and Loss; *Cognitive Level:* Analysis

Reference: Tabloski, P. (2006). *Gerontological Nursing* (p. 318). Upper Saddle River, NJ: Pearson Education.

549. An 89-year-old female widow, who has been a resident of a long-term care facility for 2 years, is now incapacitated due to recurrent multiple strokes. A new nurse asks the client's only daughter to identify the goal for her mother's care and decide what interventions should be instituted should the resident develop acute problems. Which statement made by the new nurse should prompt an experienced nurse to intervene?

1. "If your mother should experience a cardiac arrest, should an attempt be made to resuscitate her?"
2. "If your mother should develop an acute illness, such as pneumonia, how aggressively should she be treated, and should she be transferred to an acute care facility?"
3. "If your mother should stop eating, should she be force fed, supplied artificial nutrition, or receive gentle spoon-feeding?"
4. "If your mother has another stroke, should she receive her regular hygienic and activity care, prescribed medications, and have regular visitors?"

ANSWER: 4

A client's hygiene, activity, and social needs must be met to promote well-being, comfort, and body integrity; thus, these basic nursing care interventions are never withdrawn. In addition, the medications that the client is prescribed for medical maintenance of chronic illnesses are not considered "extraordinary means." When a client is deteriorating and may be dying, it is important to determine which interventions the client and family wish to promote toward the client's comfort and quality at the end of life. These include resuscitation, additional care, and nutrition among others.

▶ *Test-taking Tip: Focus on ethical nursing practice and the rights of the client/family.*

Content Area: Adult Health; *Category of Health Alteration:* Older Client Needs; *Integrated Processes:* Caring/Communication and Documentation; *Client Need:* Safe and Effective Care Environment/Management of Care/Ethical Practice; *Cognitive Level:* Application

Reference: Meiner, S., & Lueckenotte, A. (2006). *Gerontologic Nursing* (3rd ed., pp. 41–46). St. Louis, MO: Mosby/Elsevier.

---

550. An 87-year-old client has severe coronary artery disease and has been advised to complete a living will and a durable power of attorney for health care. The client asks, "Why do I need both?" A nurse explains that a living will differs from a durable power of attorney in that a living will:

1. is an example of an advanced health-care directive.
2. allows the client to designate a person to make decisions should the client become unable to provide informed consent for health-care decisions.
3. provides a legal document for the client to specify what type of medical treatment is desired should the client becomes incapacitated and terminally ill.
4. is not a legal document, but makes it easier and quicker for medical personnel to care for the client if the client becomes terminally ill.

ANSWER: 3

A living will is a legal document allowing the person to specify what type of medical treatment is desired if the person becomes incapacitated or terminally ill. Both the living will and the health-care power of attorney are advance health-care directives and legal documents.

▶ *Test-taking Tip: Note the key words "differs from," and use the process of elimination to rule out incorrect options. Knowledge of advance health-care directive documents is needed to answer the question.*

Content Area: Adult Health; *Category of Health Alteration:* Older Client Needs; *Integrated Processes:* Teaching and Learning; *Client Need:* Safe and Effective Care Environment/Management of Care/Legal Rights and Responsibilities; *Cognitive Level:* Application

Reference: Lewis, S., Heitkemper, M., Dirksen, S., O'Brien, P., & Bucher, L. (2007). *Medical-Surgical Nursing: Assessment and Management of Clinical Problems* (7th ed., pp. 155–156). St. Louis, MO: Mosby.

---

551. An 82-year-old client is hospitalized for the fifth time within a year. The client's problems include urinary track infection, myocardial infarction, stroke, and gastrointestinal bleeding. The client's physician recommends discharge to a nursing home, but the client refuses, stating, "As long as I can take care of myself, I'm not going into a home!" Assuming that the client is mentally competent, which ethical principle should be the primary guide for making decisions about supporting or rejecting the client's desire to return to home?

1. Autonomy
2. Beneficence
3. Nonmalfeasance
4. Justice

ANSWER: 1

Autonomy is one's personal freedom to direct his or her own life as long as it does not infringe on the rights of others, thus letting the client decide. The principle of beneficence means attempting to do good for others, while nonmalfeasance is the principle of avoiding or preventing harm. Justice is a term meaning "giving to each what is their due" and, in health care, is the principle of fair distribution of health care in accordance to need and benefits it can provide.

▶ *Test-taking Tip: Select option 1, after noting the key phrase "mentally competent."*

Content Area: Adult Health; *Category of Health Alteration:* Older Client Needs; *Integrated Processes:* Caring; *Client Need:* Safe and Effective Care Environment/Management of Care/Client Rights; Safe and Effective Care Environment/Management of Care/Ethical Practice; *Cognitive Level:* Analysis

Reference: Miller, C. (2009). *Nursing for Wellness in Older Adults* (5th ed., pp. 147–148). Philadelphia: Lippincott Williams & Wilkins.

Test 15: **Adult Health: Cardiac Management**

552. A nurse is evaluating the blood pressure (BP) results for multiple clients with cardiac problems on a telemetry unit. Which BP reading suggests to the nurse that the client's mean arterial pressure (MAP) is abnormal and warrants notifying the physician?

1. 94/60 mm Hg
2. 98/36 mm Hg
3. 110/50 mm Hg
4. 140/78 mm Hg

ANSWER: 2

A MAP of less than 60 mm Hg indicates that there is inadequate perfusion to organs. The mean arterial pressure is calculated by the sum of the SBP + 2DBP and then divided by 3 [MAP = (SBP + 2DBP)/3]. Thus the MAP of 98/36 mm Hg is (98 + 72)/3 = 170/3 = 56.7. The mean arterial pressure of 94/60 is 71.3. The mean arterial pressure of 110/50 is 70. The mean arterial pressure of 140/78 is 98.7.

➧ ***Test-taking Tip:*** *Focus on the issue of the question, a BP reading with a MAP of less than 60. Though a BP of 94/60 mm Hg and 140/78 mm Hg may warrant notifying the physician, the question is asking for a BP with an abnormal MAP (less than 70). Normal MAP is 70 to 100.*

Content Area: Adult Health; *Category of Health Alteration:* Cardiac Management; *Integrated Processes:* Nursing Process Analysis; *Client Need:* Physiological Integrity/Physiological Adaptation/Hemodynamics; *Cognitive Level:* Analysis

Reference: Lewis, S., Heitkemper, M., Dirksen, S., O'Brien, P., & Bucher, L. (2007). *Medical-Surgical Nursing: Assessment and Management of Clinical Problems* (7th ed., pp. 743–744). St. Louis, MO: Mosby.

553. A nurse is assessing an older adult admitted with a diagnosis of left-sided heart failure and mitral regurgitation. Identify the area with an X where the nurse should place the stethoscope to best auscultate the murmur associated with mitral regurgitation.

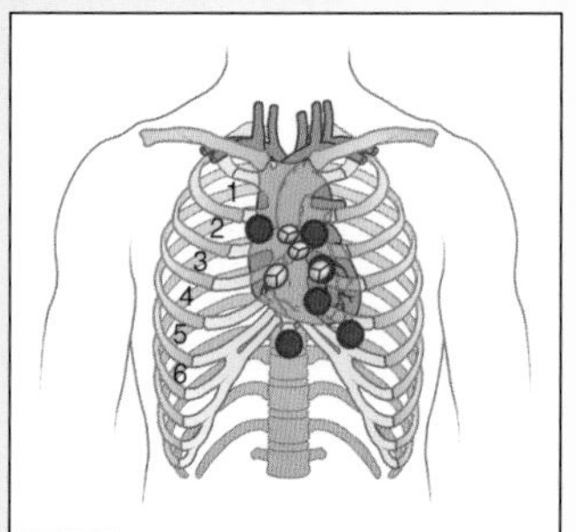

ANSWER:

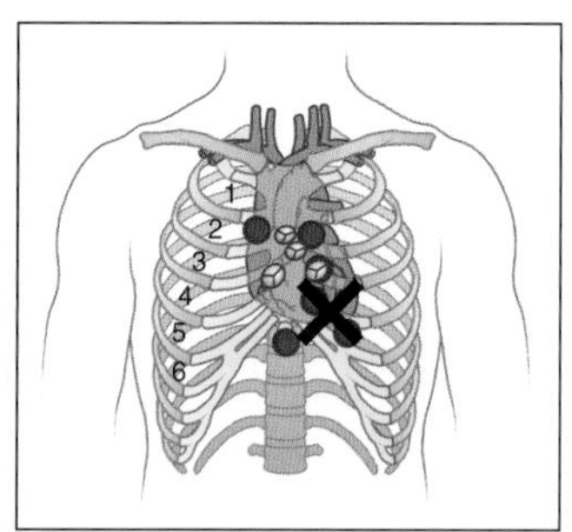

The mitral valve is best heard with the bell of the stethoscope at the fifth intercostal space, left midclavicular line. The bell is used to auscultate low-pitched sounds. Abnormalities, such as S_3 or S_4, are best heard with the bell of the stethoscope.

➧ ***Test-taking Tip:*** *The words "best" and "mitral" are key words in the stem. A mnemonic for remembering the auscultation points and the location of the heart valves is: "All Points To Monitor." The first letter of each word represents the auscultation point: Aortic valve, Pulmonic valve, Tricuspid valve, and Mitral valve.*

Content Area: Adult Health; *Category of Health Alteration:* Cardiac Management; *Integrated Processes:* Nursing Process Assessment; *Client Need:* Health Promotion and Maintenance/Techniques of Physical Assessment; *Cognitive Level:* Application.

Reference: Lewis, S., Heitkemper, M., Dirksen, S., O'Brien, P., & Bucher, L. (2007). *Medical-Surgical Nursing: Assessment and Management of Clinical Problems* (7th ed., pp. 748–750). St. Louis, MO: Mosby.

554. At 0730 hours, a nurse receives a verbal order for a cardiac catheterization to be completed on a client at 1400 hours. Which action should the nurse initiate first?

1. Initiate NPO (nothing per mouth) status for the client.
2. Teach the client about the procedure.
3. Start an intravenous (IV) infusion of 0.9% NaCl.
4. Ask the client to sign a consent form.

ANSWER: 1

A cardiac catheterization is an invasive procedure requiring the client to lie still in a supine position. The client is usually sedated with medication, such as midazolam (Versed®), during the procedure. To avoid aspiration, the client should be NPO 6 to 12 hours prior to the procedure. Because of the time element, NPO status should be initiated first and then teaching should occur. A consent form should be signed after the cardiologist has spoken with the client, and then an IV infusion order would be received.

➧ ***Test-taking Tip:*** *The term "cardiac catheterization" in the stem indicates that this is an invasive procedure that has the potential to cause aspiration from sedation. Use the ABCs (airway, breathing, circulation) to determine which action should be first. Any action that pertains to maintaining a patent airway should be first.*

Content Area: Adult Health; *Category of Health Alteration:* Cardiac Management; *Integrated Processes:* Nursing Process Implementation; *Client Need:* Safe and Effective Care Environment/Management of Care/Establishing Priorities; *Cognitive Level:* Analysis

Reference: Lewis, S., Heitkemper, M., Dirksen, S., O'Brien, P., & Bucher, L. (2007). *Medical-Surgical Nursing: Assessment and Management of Clinical Problems* (7th ed., pp. 755, 759). St. Louis, MO: Mosby.

555. Blood for cardiac enzymes and serum laboratory tests are drawn on a diabetic client admitted to an emergency department (ED) 5 hours after beginning to experience chest pressure. A nurse reviews the following laboratory results. Which serum laboratory findings should the nurse report to a primary healthcare provider (HCP) immediately due to the possibility that the client may be experiencing a myocardial infarction (MI)? SELECT ALL THAT APPLY.

Laboratory Tests	Client's Results
BUN (10–20 mg/dL)	30
SCr (0.4–1.4 mg/dL)	1.8
Ca (8.5–10.5 mg/dL)	9.0
Cl (100–108 mEq/L)	105
CO_2 (25–29 mEq/L)	24
Glucose (70–110 mg/dL)	160
Na (136–146 mEq/L)	135
K (3.8–5.3 mEq/L)	5.8
Mag (1.7–2.2 mg/dL)	1.6
CK (0–160 u/L)	320
CK-MB (0–16 u/L)	32
Troponin T (cTnT) (0.0–0.4 NG/mL)	34
WBC (3.9–11.9 K/μL)	14
RBC (4.08–5.79 m/μL)	5.0
Hgb (13.1–17.1%)	15
Hct (38.7–51 g/dL)	48
Platelets (PLT) (179–450 K/μL)	175
PT (9.2–11.9 sec)/INR (0.9–1.1 sec)	22/2.2
APTT (24–33 sec)	66

1. SCr
2. PT/INR
3. CK
4. CK-MB
5. Platelets
6. Troponin T

ANSWER: 3, 4, 6

A diabetic client may not experience the typical chest pain of a MI. Three to 12 hours after an MI the CK levels begin to rise, then peak in 24 hours, and return to normal within 2 to 3 days. The CK-MB band is specific to myocardial cells. Cardio-specific troponins (troponin T, cTnT, and troponin I, cTnI) are released into circulation after myocardial injury, are highly specific indicators of MI, and have greater sensitivity and specificity than CK-MB. SCr means serum creatinine, which is used to determine renal function and the kidneys' abilities to excrete creatinine. PT/INR (prothrombin time/international normalized ratio) is used to measure blood coagulation, especially with the use of warfarin (Coumadin®). Platelets are necessary for blood coagulation.

➧ ***Test-taking Tip:*** *Though all abnormal values should be reported to the HCP, the issue of the question is laboratory values specific for MI. Only select the options that pertain to MI.*

Content Area: Adult Health; *Category of Health Alteration:* Cardiac Management; *Integrated Processes:* Nursing Process Implementation; *Client Need:* Safe and Effective Care Environment/Management of Care/Collaboration with Interdisciplinary Team; *Cognitive Level:* Analysis

Reference: Lewis, S., Heitkemper, M., Dirksen, S., O'Brien, P., & Bucher, L. (2007). *Medical-Surgical Nursing: Assessment and Management of Clinical Problems* (7th ed., p. 806). St. Louis, MO: Mosby.

556. A nurse assesses a client who has just returned to a telemetry unit after having a coronary angiogram using the left femoral artery approach. The client's baseline blood pressure (BP) during the procedure was 130/72 mm Hg and the cardiac rhythm was a normal sinus throughout. Which assessment finding should indicate to the nurse that the client may be experiencing a complication?

1. BP 144/78 mm Hg
2. Pedal pulses palpable at +1
3. Left groin soft with 1 cm ecchymotic area
4. Apical pulse 132 beats per minute (bpm) with an irregular-irregular rhythm

ANSWER: 4

An apical pulse of 132 (bpm) with an irregular-irregular rhythm could indicate atrial fibrillation or a rhythm with premature beats. Dysrhythmias are a complication that can occur following coronary angiogram. The client should be placed on a cardiac monitor to determine the rhythm. A slight elevation of blood pressure could be related to pain at the incision site. It is not indicative of a complication without additional data. Usually pulses are palpable at +2, but without additional baseline data on the clients' pulses, this warrants monitoring but is not indicative in itself of a complication. A soft groin area where the puncture site is located is a normal finding. Ecchymosis (bruising) does not indicate a complication.

▸ ***Test-taking Tip:*** *Think about the potential complications that can occur after a coronary angiogram. Review each option to determine if the findings suggest a complication. Select the option that would be the most abnormal finding.*

Content Area: Adult Health; *Category of Health Alteration:* Cardiac Management; *Integrated Processes:* Nursing Process Evaluation; *Client Need:* Physiological Integrity/Physiological Adaptation/Unexpected Response to Therapies; *Cognitive Level:* Application

Reference: Lewis, S., Heitkemper, M., Dirksen, S., O'Brien, P., & Bucher, L. (2007). *Medical-Surgical Nursing: Assessment and Management of Clinical Problems* (7th ed., p. 759). St. Louis, MO: Mosby.

557. A nurse admits a client to a telemetry unit and obtains the following electrocardiogram (ECG) strip of the client's heart rhythm. What should be the nurse's interpretation of this rhythm strip?

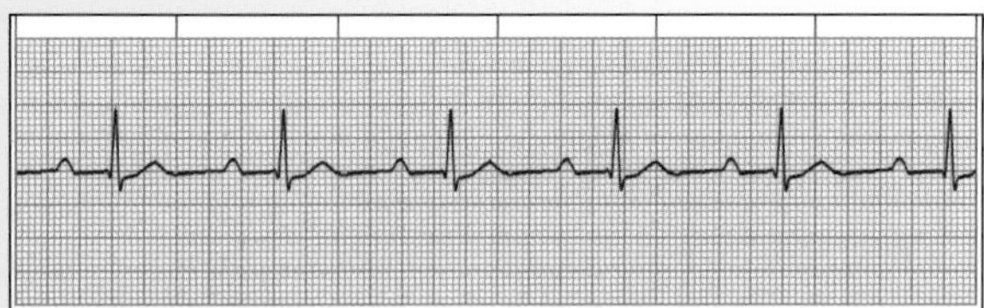

1. Atrial flutter
2. Atrial fibrillation
3. Sinus bradycardia
4. Sinus rhythm with premature atrial contractions (PACs)

ANSWER: 3

Sinus bradycardia is a regular rhythm with a ventricular rate less than 60 beats per minute (bpm), and one discernable P wave prior to each QRS. Atrial flutter is either a regular or an irregular rhythm with multiple discernable P waves prior to each QRS complex and no measurable PR interval. Atrial fibrillation is an irregular rhythm with multiple nondiscernable, fibrillatory P waves prior to each QRS and no measurable PR interval. Sinus rhythm with PACs is an irregular rhythm with a ventricular rate between 60 and 100 bpm, one discernable P wave prior to each QRS, and a PR interval between 0.12 and 0.20 seconds, with the presence of premature atrial beats that occur early in the cardiac cycle. The PACs also have one discernable P wave prior to each QRS and a PR interval between 0.08 and 0.20 seconds.

▸ ***Test-taking Tip:*** *Use the steps in interpreting an ECG rhythm to select the correct option. Note that the rhythm is regular, so eliminate option 4, which is an irregular rhythm. Recall that atrial fibrillation and atrial flutter do not have a measurable PR interval, so eliminate options 1 and 2.*

Content Area: Adult Health; *Category of Health Alteration:* Cardiac Management; *Integrated Processes:* Nursing Process Analysis; *Client Need:* Physiological Integrity/Physiological Adaptation/Hemodynamics; *Cognitive Level:* Application

Reference: Lewis, S., Heitkemper, M., Dirksen, S., O'Brien, P., & Bucher, L. (2007). *Medical-Surgical Nursing: Assessment and Management of Clinical Problems* (7th ed., p. 852). St. Louis, MO: Mosby.

558. EBP A nurse is planning care for a client admitted with a new diagnosis of persistent atrial fibrillation with rapid ventricular response. Although the client has had no previous cardiac problems, the client has been in atrial fibrillation for more than 2 days. The nurse should anticipate that the health-care provider is likely to initially order: SELECT ALL THAT APPLY.

1. oxygen.
2. immediate cardioversion.
3. administration of amiodarone (Cordarone®).
4. initiation of a IV heparin infusion.
5. immediate catheter-directed ablation of the AV node.
6. administration of a calcium channel antagonist such as diltiazem (Cardizem®).

ANSWER: 1, 3, 4, 6

The ineffective atrial contractions or loss of atrial kick with atrial fibrillation can decrease cardiac output. Administering oxygen enhances tissue oxygenation. Amiodarone is used for pharmacological cardioversion of the atrial fibrillation rhythm. The client is at risk for thrombi in the atria from stasis. Anticoagulant therapy is used to prevent thromboembolism. Diltiazem, a calcium channel antagonist, is prescribed to slow the ventricular response to atrial fibrillation. An alternative to a calcium channel antagonist would be the use of a beta blocker, such as esmolol, metoprolol, or propranolol. Cardioversion would only be considered if medications were ineffective in converting the client's rhythm and only after the presence of an atrial clot has been ruled out. Ablation of the AV node would only be considered if medications were ineffective in controlling the client's heart rate.

▶ ***Test-taking Tip:*** *Carefully read the information provided in the stem. The key phrase is "initially order." The nurse should direct interventions at the client's potential complications from the arrhythmia. Note that both options 2 and 5 contain the words "immediate." Eliminate one or both of those options, because both procedures cannot be immediate.*

Content Area: Adult Health; *Category of Health Alteration:* Cardiac Management; *Integrated Processes:* Nursing Process Planning; *Client Need:* Physiological Integrity/Physiological Adaptation/Illness Management; *Cognitive Level:* Application

Reference: Lewis, S., Heitkemper, M., Dirksen, S., O'Brien, P., & Bucher, L. (2007). *Medical-Surgical Nursing: Assessment and Management of Clinical Problems* (7th ed., p. 852). St. Louis, MO: Mosby.

EBP Reference: Institute for Clinical Systems Improvement. (2007). *Atrial Fibrillation.* Available at: www.guideline.gov/summary/summary.aspx?doc_id=10723&nbr=005585&string=heart

---

559. A nurse is caring for a client immediately following insertion of a permanent pacemaker via the right subclavian vein approach. The nurse best prevents pacemaker lead dislodgement by:

1. inspecting the incision site dressing for bleeding and the incision for approximation.
2. limiting the client's right arm activity and preventing the client reaching above shoulder level.
3. assisting the client with getting out of bed and ambulating with a walker.
4. ordering a stat chest x-ray following return from the implant procedure.

ANSWER: 2

Limiting arm and shoulder activity initially and up to 24 hours after the pacing leads are implanted helps prevent lead dislodgement. Often an arm sling is used as a reminder to the client to limit arm activity. The dressing should not be removed to check the incision immediately after insertion but should be checked for bleeding to monitor for potential complications. The nurse should assist the client the first time out of bed following a pacemaker implant, but the client should not use a walker for 24 hours after the procedure, and out of bed activity would not resume until the client is stable. A postinsertion chest x-ray is done to check lead placement and to rule out a pneumothorax. It does not promote the intactness of pacing leads.

▶ ***Test-taking Tip:*** *Focus on the issue of the question: measures to promote intactness of the pacing leads. Analyze the options to determine which would impact the desired result, maintaining intactness of the pacing leads.*

Content Area: Adult Health; *Category of Health Alteration:* Cardiac Management; *Integrated Processes:* Nursing Process Implementation; *Client Need:* Physiological Integrity/Reduction of Risk Potential/Therapeutic Procedures; *Cognitive Level:* Application

References: Lewis, S., Heitkemper, M., Dirksen, S., O'Brien, P., & Bucher, L. (2007). *Medical-Surgical Nursing: Assessment and Management of Clinical Problems* (7th ed., pp. 858–860). St. Louis, MO: Mosby; Smeltzer, S., Bare, B., Hinkle, J., & Cheever, K. (2008). *Brunner & Suddarth's Textbook of Medical-Surgical Nursing* (11th ed., pp. 844–849). Philadelphia: Lippincott Williams & Wilkins.

560. EBP A client experiences cardiac arrest at home and is successfully resuscitated. Following placement of an implantable cardioverter-defibrillator (ICD), a nurse is evaluating the effectiveness of teaching for the client. Which statement, if made by the client, indicates that further teaching is needed?

1. "The ICD will monitor my heart activity and provide a shock to my heart if my heart goes into ventricular fibrillation again."
2. "When I feel the first shock I should tell my family to start cardiopulmonary resuscitation (CPR) and call 911."
3. "I am fearful of my first shock since my friend stated his shock felt like a blow to the chest."
4. "I will need to ask my physician when I can resume driving because some states disallow driving until there is a 6-month discharge-free period."

ANSWER: 2

If the first shock is unsuccessful, the device will recycle and continue to deliver shocks. If the device fires more than once, the emergency medical services (EMS) system should be activated. The ICD continues to deliver shocks if indicated; CPR should only be initiated after the shocks have been delivered and only if the client is unresponsive and pulseless. The ICD monitors the client's heart rate and rhythm, identifies ventricular tachycardia or ventricular fibrillation, and delivers a 25-joule or less shock if a lethal rhythm is detected. Various sensations have been described when the device delivers a shock, including a blow to or kick in the chest. State laws vary regarding drivers with ICDs. The decision regarding driving is also based on whether dysrhythmias are present, the frequency of firing, and the client's overall health.

Test-taking Tip: *The key phrase "further teaching is needed" indicate a false-response item. Select the client's statement that is not correct.*

Content Area: Adult Health; *Category of Health Alteration:* Cardiac Management; *Integrated Processes:* Teaching and Learning; *Client Need:* Health Promotion and Maintenance/Principles of Teaching and Learning; *Cognitive Level:* Analysis

Reference: Smeltzer, S., Bare, B., Hinkle, J., & Cheever, K. (2008). *Brunner & Suddarth's Textbook of Medical-Surgical Nursing* (11th ed., pp. 834–849). Philadelphia: Lippincott Williams & Wilkins.

EBP Reference: Scottish Intercollegiate Guidelines Network (SIGN). (2007). *Cardiac Arrhythmias in Coronary Heart Disease. A National Clinical Guideline.* Edinburgh, Scotland: SIGN. Available at: www.guideline.gov/summary/summary.aspx®doc_id=10586&nbr=005528&string=heart

561. A nurse is teaching a client newly diagnosed with chronic stable angina. Which instructions should the nurse incorporate in the teaching session on measures to prevent future angina? SELECT ALL THAT APPLY.

1. Increase isometric arm exercises to build endurance.
2. Wear a face mask when outdoors in cold weather.
3. Take nitroglycerin before a stressful situation even though pain is not present.
4. Perform most exertional activities in the morning.
5. Avoid straining at stool.
6. Eliminate tobacco use.

ANSWER: 2, 3, 5, 6

Blood vessels constrict in response to cold and increase the workload of the heart. Sexual activity and straining at stool increases sympathetic stimulation and cardiac workload. Nitroglycerin produces vasodilation and improves blood flow to the coronary arteries; it can be used prophylactically to prevent angina. Nicotine stimulates catecholamine release, producing vasoconstriction and an increased heart rate. Isometric exercise of the arms can cause exertional angina. Exertional activity increases the heart rate, thus reducing the time the heart is in diastole, when blood flow to the coronary arteries is the greatest. A period of rest should occur between activities and activities should be spaced.

Test-taking Tip: *The key phrase is "measures to prevent future angina." Consider if each option could potentially increase myocardial oxygen demand or decrease available oxygen, either of which could precipitate angina.*

Content Area: Adult Health; *Category of Health Alteration:* Cardiac Management; *Integrated Processes:* Teaching and Learning; *Client Need:* Physiological Integrity/Physiological Adaptation/Illness Management; *Cognitive Level:* Application

Reference: Lewis, S., Heitkemper, M., Dirksen, S., O'Brien, P., & Bucher, L. (2007). *Medical-Surgical Nursing: Assessment and Management of Clinical Problems* (7th ed., pp. 797, 810–813). St. Louis, MO: Mosby.

562. EBP A nurse collects the following assessment data on a client who has no known health problems: blood pressure (BP) 135/89 mm Hg; body mass index (BMI) 23; waist circumference 34 inches; serum creatinine 0.9 mg/dL; serum K 4.0 mEq/L; low-density lipoprotein (LDL) cholesterol 200 mg/dL; high-density lipoprotein (HDL) cholesterol 25 mg/dL; and triglycerides 180 mg/dL. Which order from the client's health-care provider should the nurse anticipate?

1. 1,500-calorie regular diet.
2. No added salt, low saturated fat, low-potassium diet.
3. Hydrochlorothiazide (HydroDIURIL®) 25 mg twice daily.
4. Atorvastatin (Lipitor®) 20 mg daily.

ANSWER: 4

Atorvastatin is used to manage hypercholesterolemia. It lowers the total serum LDL cholesterol and triglycerides and slightly increases HDL cholesterol by inhibiting 3-hydroxy-3-methylglutaryl-coenzyme A (HMG-CoA) reductase, an enzyme that is responsible for catalyzing an early step in the synthesis of cholesterol. For persons with 0–1 risk factors, the goal for LDL is less than 160 mg/dL (4.14 mmol/L), and drug therapy is considered when LDL is greater than or equal to 190 mg/dL (4.91 mmol/L). Normal triglycerides are 40 to 150 mg/dL (0.45–1.69 mmol/L). A low-calorie diet is not indicated. The normal BMI is 18.5 to 24.9. While a low-saturated-fat diet in option 2 is indicated, a low-potassium diet is not because the serum K of 4.0 mEq/L is normal. The client's BP is slightly elevated but would be initially treated with lifestyle changes, not a diuretic.

▶ ***Test-taking Tip:*** *Focus on the data provided in the situation and identify the abnormal findings. If unable to identify the abnormal data because of lack of knowledge of normal lab values, note that the client's serum cholesterol level analysis includes more data than other problems. Conclude that these are abnormal data and then use "lipids" as a key to identifying the correct option. Review laboratory values and cardiac medications if you had difficulty with this question.*

Content Area: Adult Health; *Category of Health Alteration:* Cardiac Management; *Integrated Processes:* Nursing Process Planning; *Client Need:* Physiological Integrity/Reduction of Risk Potential/Laboratory Values; Health Promotion and Maintenance/Disease Prevention; *Cognitive Level:* Analysis

Reference: Smeltzer, S., Bare, B., Hinkle, J., & Cheever, K. (2008). *Brunner & Suddarth's Textbook of Medical-Surgical Nursing* (11th ed., pp. 863–865). Philadelphia: Lippincott Williams & Wilkins.

EBP Reference: Smith, S., Allen, J., Blair, S., et al. (2006). American Heart Association/American College of Cardiology guidelines for secondary prevention for patients with coronary and other atherosclerotic vascular disease: 2006 update. *Circulation*, 113, 2363.

563. A nurse is instructing a client diagnosed with coronary artery disease about care at home. The nurse determines that teaching is effective when the client states: SELECT ALL THAT APPLY.

1. "If I have chest pain, I should contact my physician immediately."
2. "I should carry my nitroglycerin in my front pants pocket so it is handy."
3. "If I have chest pain, I stop activity and place one nitroglycerin tablet under my tongue."
4. "I should always take three nitroglycerin tablets, 5 minutes apart."
5. "I plan to avoid being around people when they are smoking."
6. "I plan on walking on most days of the week for at least 30 minutes."

ANSWER: 3, 5, 6

Stopping activity decreases the body's demand for oxygen. One nitroglycerin tablet, taken sublingually, dilates the coronary arteries and increases oxygen to the myocardium. If pain is unrelieved, a second tablet should be taken 5 minutes later. Passive smoke can cause vasoconstriction and decrease blood flow velocity even in healthy young adults. The American Heart Association recommends exercising for 30 minutes on most days of the week. Medical attention is required only if pain persists and then the client should call 911 rather than the physician because emergency treatment may be necessary. Nitroglycerin loses its potency if stored in warm, moist areas, making the client's pants pocket an undesirable location for storage. If pain is relieved after one tablet, another tablet is not required. The standard dose for nitroglycerin is one tablet or spray 5 minutes apart until pain is relieved, to a maximum of three tablets.

▶ ***Test-taking Tip:*** *The key words are "teaching is effective." Select the client statements that are correct.*

Content Area: Adult Health; *Category of Health Alteration:* Cardiac Management; *Integrated Processes:* Nursing Process Evaluation; *Client Need:* Physiological Integrity/Physiological Adaptation/Illness Management; *Cognitive Level:* Analysis

References: Lewis, S., Heitkemper, M., Dirksen, S., O'Brien, P., & Bucher, L. (2007). *Medical-Surgical Nursing: Assessment and Management of Clinical Problems* (7th ed., pp. 790–795, 812). St. Louis, MO: Mosby; Smeltzer, S., Bare, B., Hinkle, J., & Cheever, K. (2008). *Brunner & Suddarth's Textbook of Medical-Surgical Nursing* (11th ed., pp. 862–874). Philadelphia: Lippincott Williams & Wilkins.

564. EBP A client admitted with a diagnosis of acute coronary syndrome calls for a nurse after experiencing sharp chest pains that radiate to the left shoulder. The nurse notes, prior to entering the client's room, that the client's rhythm is sinus tachycardia with a 10-beat run of premature ventricular contractions (PVCs). Admitting orders included all of the following interventions for treating chest pain. Which should the nurse implement *first*?

1. Obtain a stat 12-lead electrocardiogram (ECG).
2. Administer oxygen by nasal cannula.
3. Administer sublingual nitroglycerin.
4. Administer morphine sulfate intravenously.

ANSWER: 2

Oxygen should be available in the room and should be initiated first to enhance oxygen flow to the myocardium. Though a stat 12-lead ECG is needed to identify ischemia or infarct location, the first action is to treat the client. Sublingual nitroglycerin dilates coronary arteries and will enhance blood flow to the myocardium. Once oxygen is in place and the vital signs known, nitroglycerin should be administered. Morphine sulfate is a narcotic analgesic used for pain control and anxiety reduction. Because it is a controlled substance, extra steps are needed to retrieve the medication from a secure source, so this is not the first action.

▶ ***Test-taking Tip:*** *Use the ABCs (airway, breathing, circulation) to establish the priority action. Improving oxygen flow to the myocardium is priority.*

Content Area: Adult Health; *Category of Health Alteration:* Cardiac Management; *Integrated Processes:* Nursing Process Implementation; *Client Need:* Safe and Effective Care Environment/Management of Care/Establishing Priorities; Physiological Integrity/Physiological Adaptation/Medical Emergencies; *Cognitive Level:* Application

Reference: Smeltzer, S., Bare, B., Hinkle, J., & Cheever, K. (2008). *Brunner & Suddarth's Textbook of Medical-Surgical Nursing* (11th ed., pp. 880–883). Philadelphia: Lippincott Williams & Wilkins.

EBP Reference: Canadian Cardiovascular Society, American Academy of Family Physicians, American College of Cardiology, American Heart Association, Antman, E., Hand, M., Armstrong, P., et al. (2008). 2007 focused update of the ACC/AHA 2004 guidelines for the management of patients with ST-elevation myocardial infarction: a report of the American College of Cardiology/American Heart Association Task Force on Practice Guidelines. *Journal of the American College of Cardiology,* 51(2), 210–247.

---

565. A nurse is assessing a client diagnosed with an anterior-lateral myocardial infarction (MI). The nurse adds a nursing diagnosis to the client's plan of care of *decreased cardiac output* when which finding is noted on assessment?

1. One-sided weakness
2. Presence of an S_4 heart sound
3. Crackles auscultated in bilateral lung bases
4. Vesicular breath sounds over lung lobes

ANSWER: 3

An anterior-lateral MI can produce left ventricular dysfunction and low cardiac output. With low cardiac output, blood accumulates in the heart and backs up into the pulmonary system. The increased pulmonary pressure causes fluid to move into interstitial spaces and then into the alveoli. One-sided weakness suggests complications of a cerebrovascular accident, which can be caused from a clot or plaque embolus secondary to the MI. An S_4 heart sound is produced when blood flows forcefully from the atrium to a resistant ventricle during late ventricular diastole. Vesicular breath sounds are normal over lesser bronchi, bronchioles, and lobes of the lung.

▶ ***Test-taking Tip:*** *Recall that an anterior MI can produce left ventricular dysfunction. Focus on the issue of an assessment finding indicative of low cardiac output. Eliminate option 1 because it relates to tissue perfusion. If unsure of option 2, move to option 3. Note that options 3 and 4 relate to the lungs, so one or both of these must be wrong. Recall that crackles are always abnormal, whereas the presence of S_4 can be normal in an older adult, and vesicular lung sounds located over lung lobes is a normal finding.*

Content Area: Adult Health; *Category of Health Alteration:* Cardiac Management; *Integrated Processes:* Nursing Process Analysis; *Client Need:* Nursing Process Analysis; *Cognitive Level:* Analysis

Reference: Lewis, S., Heitkemper, M., Dirksen, S., O'Brien, P., & Bucher, L. (2007). *Medical-Surgical Nursing: Assessment and Management of Clinical Problems* (7th ed., pp. 523, 823–824). St. Louis, MO: Mosby.

566. A nurse increases activity for a client with an admitting diagnosis of acute coronary syndrome. Which symptoms experienced by the client best support a nursing diagnosis of activity intolerance?

1. Pulse rate increased by 15 beats per minute during activity
2. Blood pressure (BP) 130/86 mm Hg before activity; BP 108/66 mm Hg during activity
3. Increased dyspnea and diaphoresis relieved when sitting in a chair
4. A mean arterial pressure (MAP) of 80 following activity

ANSWER: 2

A drop in BP of 20 mm Hg from the baseline indicates that the client's heart is unable to adapt to the increased energy and oxygen demands of the activity. An increased heart rate during activity and the relief of dyspnea and diaphoresis with rest indicates the heart is able to adapt. A MAP of 80 is normal.

▶ ***Test-taking Tip:*** *The key words are "best supports." Select the option that is an abnormal finding.*

Content Area: Adult Health; *Category of Health Alteration:* Cardiac Management; *Integrated Processes:* Nursing Process Analysis; *Client Need:* Physiological Integrity/Physiological Adaptation/Alterations in Body Systems; *Cognitive Level:* Analysis

References: Newfield, S., Hinz, M., Tilley, D., Sridaromont, K., & Maramba, P. (2007). *Cox's Clinical Applications of Nursing Diagnosis* (5th ed., pp. 283–284). Philadelphia: F. A. Davis; Smeltzer, S., Bare, B., Hinkle, J., & Cheever, K. (2008). *Brunner & Suddarth's Textbook of Medical-Surgical Nursing* (11th ed., pp. 877–878). Philadelphia: Lippincott Williams & Wilkins.

---

567. After an inferior-septal wall myocardial infarction, which complication should a nurse suspect when noting jugular venous distention (JVD) and ascites?

1. Left-sided heart failure
2. Pulmonic valve malfunction
3. Right-sided heart failure
4. Ruptured septum

ANSWER: 3

Right-sided heart failure produces venous congestion in the systemic circulation resulting in JVD and ascites (from vascular congestion in the gastrointestinal tract). Additional signs include hepatomegaly, splenomegaly, and peripheral edema. Left-sided heart failure produces signs of pulmonary congestion, including crackles, S_3 and S_4 heart sounds, and pleural effusion. A characteristic finding of pulmonic valve malfunction would be a murmur. A murmur would also be auscultated with a ruptured septum, and the client would experience signs of cardiogenic shock.

▶ ***Test-taking Tip:*** *Note that options 1 and 3 focus on different types of heart failure. Either one or both of these must be wrong. Focus on the client's signs of JVD and ascites and the cardiac anatomy to eliminate all but option 3.*

Content Area: Adult Health; *Category of Health Alteration:* Cardiac Management; *Integrated Processes:* Nursing Process Analysis; *Client Need:* Physiological Integrity/Reduction of Risk Potential/Potential for Complications from Surgical Procedures and Health Alterations; *Cognitive Level:* Analysis

Reference: Lewis, S., Heitkemper, M., Dirksen, S., O'Brien, P., & Bucher, L. (2007). *Medical-Surgical Nursing: Assessment and Management of Clinical Problems* (7th ed., pp. 824–826). St. Louis, MO: Mosby.

---

568. EBP Which nursing actions should a nurse plan when caring for a client experiencing dyspnea due to heart failure and chronic obstructive pulmonary disease (COPD)? SELECT ALL THAT APPLY.

1. Apply oxygen 6 liters per nasal cannula
2. Elevate the head of the bed 30 to 40 degrees
3. Weigh client daily in the morning
4. Teach client pursed-lip breathing techniques
5. Turn and reposition the client every 1 to 2 hours

ANSWER: 2, 3, 4

Elevating the head of the bed will promote lung expansion. Daily weights will assess fluid retention. Fluid volume excess can increase dyspnea and cause pulmonary edema. Pursed-lip breathing techniques allow the client to conserve energy and slow the breathing rate. Applying greater than 4 liters of oxygen per nasal cannula is contraindicated for COPD. High flow rates can depress the hypoxic drive. Because the client with COPD suffers from chronically high CO_2 levels, the stimulus to breathe is the low O_2 level (a hypoxic drive). The situation does not warrant turning the client every 1 to 2 hours. This activity could increase the client's energy expenditure and dyspnea.

▶ ***Test-taking Tip:*** *Focus on the key words "dyspnea," "heart failure," and "COPD." Recall that dyspnea from heart failure is caused by fluid volume overload whereas dyspnea from COPD is caused from airway noncompliance. Combine actions for both of these problems in selecting the correct options.*

Content Area: Adult Health; *Category of Health Alteration:* Cardiac Management; *Integrated Processes:* Nursing Process Planning; *Client Need:* Physiological Integrity/Physiological Adaptation/Illness Management; *Cognitive Level:* Application

EBP Reference: Registered Nurses Association of Ontario (RNAO). (2005). *Nursing Care of Dyspnea: The 6th Vital Sign in Individuals with Chronic Obstructive Pulmonary Disease (COPD).* Available at: www.guideline.gov/summary/summary.aspx?doc_id=7008&nbr=004217&string=copd

569. A nurse notes that a client, who experienced a myocardial infarction (MI) 3 days ago, seems unusually fatigued. Upon assessment, the nurse finds that the client is dyspneic with activity, has a heart rate (HR) of 110 beats per minute (bpm), and has generalized edema. Which action by the nurse is most appropriate?

1. Administer high-flow oxygen
2. Encourage the client to rest more
3. Continue to monitor the client's heart rhythm
4. Compare the client's admission weight with the client's current weight

ANSWER: 4

A complication of MI is heart failure. Signs of heart failure include fatigue, dyspnea, tachycardia, edema, and weight gain. Other signs include nocturia, skin changes, behavioral changes, and chest pain. There is no indication that the client is hypoxic and in need of high-flow oxygen. To treat the dyspnea, oxygen by nasal cannula would be appropriate. The fatigue is caused by decreased cardiac output, impaired perfusion to vital organs, decreased tissue oxygenation, and anemia. Rest alone will not relieve the fatigue. Interventions are needed to improve cardiac output and tissue oxygenation. A heart rate of 110 bpm suggests tachycardia; the symptoms together imply heart failure. Further data collection is needed to confirm the findings. Continuing to monitor the client's heart rhythm, without further assessment, will delay an appropriate intervention.

➧ ***Test-taking Tip:*** *Use the nursing process to determine the next action. Before a conclusion can be reached, additional data are needed. The nurse should complete the assessment process. Eliminate options 1 and 2 because these are interventions. Of options 3 and 4 determine which option would provide the most immediate information to make a conclusion about the data.*

Content Area: Adult Health; *Category of Health Alteration:* Cardiac Management; *Integrated Processes:* Nursing Process Assessment; *Client Need:* Physiological Integrity/Reduction of Risk Potential/System Specific Assessments; *Cognitive Level:* Analysis

Reference: Lewis, S., Heitkemper, M., Dirksen, S., O'Brien, P., & Bucher, L. (2007). *Medical-Surgical Nursing: Assessment and Management of Clinical Problems* (7th ed., pp. 825–826). St. Louis, MO: Mosby.

570. A client is hospitalized for heart failure secondary to alcohol-induced cardiomyopathy. The client is started on milrinone (Primacor®) and placed on a transplant waiting list. The client has been curt and verbally aggressive in expressing dissatisfaction with the medication orders, overall care, and the need for energy conservation. A nurse should interpret that the client's behavior is likely related to the client's:

1. denial of the illness.
2. reaction to milrinone (Primacor®).
3. fear of the diagnosis.
4. response to cerebral anoxia.

ANSWER: 3

A threatening situation (need for heart transplant) can produce fear. Fear and helplessness may cause a client to verbally attack health team members to maintain control. There is no supporting evidence that the client denies the existence of a health problem. Minimizing symptoms or noncompliant behaviors would indicate denial. Milrinone is used in short-term treatment of congestive heart failure unresponsive to conventional therapy with digoxin, diuretics, and vasodilators. It increases myocardial contractility and decreases preload and afterload by direct dilating effect on the vascular smooth muscle. It does not cause behavior changes. Although a low cardiac output may lead to cerebral anoxia, there is insufficient evidence in this situation to support the conclusion of cerebral anoxia causing the client's reaction.

➧ ***Test-taking Tip:*** *Focus on the issue, the client's reaction to the illness and hospitalization.*

Content Area: Adult Health; *Category of Health Alteration:* Cardiac Management; *Integrated Processes:* Nursing Process Analysis; *Client Need:* Psychosocial Integrity/Coping Mechanisms; *Cognitive Level:* Analysis

Reference: Newfield, S., Hinz, M., Tilley, D., Sridaromont, K., & Maramba, P. (2007). *Cox's Clinical Applications of Nursing Diagnosis* (5th ed., pp. 553–555, 771–772). Philadelphia: F. A. Davis.

571. EBP A client diagnosed with class II heart failure according to the New York Heart Association Functional Classification has been taught about the initial treatment plan for this disease. A nurse determines that the client needs additional teaching if the client states that the treatment plan includes:

1. diuretics.
2. a low-sodium diet.
3. home oxygen therapy.
4. angiotensin-converting enzyme (ACE) inhibitors.

ANSWER: 3

In class II heart failure, normal physical activity results in fatigue, dyspnea, palpitations, or anginal pain. The symptoms are absent at rest. Home oxygen therapy is unnecessary unless there are other comorbid conditions. Diuretics mobilize edematous fluid, act on the kidneys to promote excretion of sodium and water, and reduce preload and pulmonary venous pressure. Dietary restriction of sodium aids in reducing edema. ACE inhibitors block the conversion of angiotensin I to the vasoconstrictor angiotensin II, prevent the degradation of bradykinin and other vasodilatory prostaglandins, and increase plasma renin levels and reduce aldosterone levels. The net result is systemic vasodilation, reduced systemic vascular resistance, and improved cardiac output.

➧ ***Test-taking Tip:*** *The key phrase "needs additional teaching" indicates that this is a false-response item. Select the option that is incorrect for treating class II heart failure.*

Content Area: Adult Health; *Category of Health Alteration:* Cardiac Management; *Integrated Processes:* Teaching and Learning; *Client Need:* Health Promotion and Maintenance/Principles of Teaching and Learning; *Cognitive Level:* Analysis

Reference: Lewis, S., Heitkemper, M., Dirksen, S., O'Brien, P., & Bucher, L. (2007). *Medical-Surgical Nursing: Assessment and Management of Clinical Problems* (7th ed., pp. 824–837). St. Louis, MO: Mosby.

EBP Reference: Heart Failure Society of America. (2006). Evaluation and therapy for heart failure in the setting of ischemic heart disease. *Journal of Cardiac Failure*, 12(1), e104–e111. Available at: www.guideline.gov/summary/summary.aspx?doc_id=9329&nbr=004998&string=heart

572. A client is admitted with a diagnosis of acute infective endocarditis (IE). Which findings during a nursing assessment support this diagnosis? SELECT ALL THAT APPLY.

1. Skin petechiae
2. Crackles in lung bases
3. Peripheral edema
4. Murmur
5. Arthralgia
6. Decreased erythrocyte sedimentation rate (ESR)

ANSWER: 1, 2, 3, 4, 5

Vegetations that adhere to the heart valves can break off into the circulation, causing embolism, valve incompetence, and a murmur. A vascular sign of microembolism is skin petechiae. Crackles and peripheral edema occur due to heart failure secondary to IE. Arthralgia (joint pain) can occur from microembolism and inadequate perfusion. The ESR (rate at which red blood cells settle) should increase, not decrease, during an inflammatory process.

➧ ***Test-taking Tip:*** *The issue of the question is signs and symptoms of infective endocarditis. Recall that the endocardium is the inner surface and cavities of the heart and that in IE microorganisms and debris from the inflammatory process can adhere to heart valves. Select signs and symptoms indicating the heart valves are affected and also those that can occur if portions of the vegetation should break off into the circulation.*

Content Area: Adult Health; *Category of Health Alteration:* Cardiac Management; *Integrated Processes:* Nursing Process Assessment; *Client Need:* Physiological Integrity/Reduction of Risk Potential/System Specific Assessments; *Cognitive Level:* Application

Reference: Lewis, S., Heitkemper, M., Dirksen, S., O'Brien, P., & Bucher, L. (2007). *Medical-Surgical Nursing: Assessment and Management of Clinical Problems* (7th ed., pp. 678–679, 866–869). St. Louis, MO: Mosby.

573. EBP A nurse evaluates that a client understands discharge teaching, following aortic valve replacement surgery with a synthetic valve, when the client states that he/she plans to: SELECT ALL THAT APPLY.

1. use a soft toothbrush for dental hygiene.
2. floss teeth daily to prevent plaque formation.
3. wear loose-fitting clothing to avoid friction on the sternal incision.
4. use an electric razor for shaving.
5. report black, tarry stools.
6. consume foods high in vitamin K, such as broccoli.

ANSWER: 1, 3, 4, 5

A synthetic heart valve requires long-term anticoagulation because of the risk of thromboembolism. Because low-dose aspirin, which prevents platelet aggregation, and oral anticoagulation together are more effective than just oral anticoagulation to reduce the risk of thromboembolism after valve replacement, both are prescribed, which increases the risk for bleeding. Bleeding precautions while on anticoagulation include using a soft toothbrush, avoiding injury (such as can occur with flossing), and using an electric razor. The client will have a sternal incision. Care must be taken to avoid tissue trauma. Black, tarry stools are a sign of bleeding. Flossing should be avoided because it causes tissue trauma, increases the risk of bleeding, and increases the risk of infective endocarditis. The diet should contain normal amounts of vitamin K; excessive amounts antagonize the effects of the anticoagulant.

Test-taking Tip: Focus on the issue: self-care following a synthetic valve replacement. Recall that anticoagulation will be required. Select options that include bleeding precautions and signs of bleeding.

Content Area: Adult Health; *Category of Health Alteration:* Cardiac Management; *Integrated Processes:* Teaching and Learning; Nursing Process Evaluation; *Client Need:* Physiological Integrity/Reduction of Risk Potential/Therapeutic Procedures; *Cognitive Level:* Analysis

Reference: Lewis, S., Heitkemper, M., Dirksen, S., O'Brien, P., & Bucher, L. (2007). *Medical-Surgical Nursing: Assessment and Management of Clinical Problems* (7th ed., pp. 882–885, 917). St. Louis, MO: Mosby.

EBP Reference: Little, S., & Massel, D. (2003). Antiplatelet and anticoagulation for patients with prosthetic heart valves. *Cochrane Database of Systematic Reviews*, Issue 4, Art. No. CD003464. DOI: 10.1002/14651858.CD003464. Available at: www.cochrane.org/reviews/en/ab003464.html

574. A male client confides to a clinic nurse that he is no longer dyspneic after receiving his new St. Jude's heart valve. He wants to have a vasectomy so that he can enjoy sexual intercourse again without the fear of his wife becoming pregnant. What is the nurse's best response?

1. "That's probably a good idea. The life expectancy after heart valve replacement is 10 to 15 years."
2. "You seem relieved that the heart valve replacement was successful and that you can enjoy a normal life again."
3. "If you have cardiac symptoms such as dyspnea during sexual intercourse, you can take a nitroglycerin tablet before sexual activity to prevent symptoms."
4. "Be sure to inform the physician that you have an artificial heart valve so you are given antibiotics as a preventive measure before the procedure."

ANSWER: 4

A St. Jude's valve is an artificial heart valve. Antibiotics are required prior to invasive procedures to prevent complications such as endocarditis. The physician also needs to know that the client has an artificial heart valve because the client should be receiving anticoagulants and there is the risk of increased bleeding. As long as the person receives regular follow-up with a health-care provider, the person can expect a normal life expectancy. Although mechanical valves are durable, they may need replacement in 10 to 15 years. Although responding that the client seems relieved is a therapeutic response, it is not the best response, because the client needs teaching. Nitroglycerin is not prescribed for persons with valvular heart disease unless the person also has coronary artery disease; thus he would not have nitroglycerin available.

Test-taking Tip: The key terms in the stem are "vasectomy" and "heart valve." Recall that antibiotics are prescribed prophylactically prior to invasive procedures.

Content Area: Adult Health; *Category of Health Alteration:* Cardiac Management; *Integrated Processes:* Communication and Documentation; *Client Need:* Physiological Integrity/Reduction of Risk Potential/Potential for Complications of Diagnostic Tests/Treatments/Procedures; *Cognitive Level:* Application

Reference: Lewis, S., Heitkemper, M., Dirksen, S., O'Brien, P., & Bucher, L. (2007). *Medical-Surgical Nursing: Assessment and Management of Clinical Problems* (7th ed., pp. 882–885). St. Louis, MO: Mosby.

575. EBP A client admitted with unstable angina is started on intravenous heparin and nitroglycerin. The client's chest pain resolves, and the client is weaned from the nitroglycerin. Noting that the client had a synthetic valve replacement for aortic stenosis 2 years ago, a physician writes an order to restart the oral warfarin (Coumadin®) 5 mg at 1900 hours. Which is the nurse's best action?

1. Administer the warfarin as prescribed.
2. Call the physician to question the warfarin order.
3. Discontinue the heparin drip and then administer the warfarin.
4. Hold the dose of warfarin until the heparin has been discontinued.

ANSWER: 1

Both heparin and warfarin are anticoagulants, but their actions are different. Oral warfarin requires 3 to 5 days to reach effective levels. It is usually begun while the client is still on heparin. Calling the physician is unnecessary. The nurse's scope of practice does not permit altering medication orders. The nurse should neither discontinue the heparin nor hold the warfarin without a written order.

➧ ***Test-taking Tip:*** *Use the process of elimination to eliminate options 3 and 4, which alter medication orders, because these are not within the nurse's scope of practice. Of the two remaining options, focus on the action of heparin and warfarin. Recall that warfarin takes 3 to 5 days to reach therapeutic effectiveness, during which time the client will continue to require anticoagulation.*

Content Area: Adult Health; *Category of Health Alteration:* Cardiac Management; *Integrated Processes:* Nursing Process Implementation; *Client Need:* Physiological Integrity/Pharmacological and Parenteral Therapies/Expected Outcomes/Effects; *Cognitive Level:* Application

Reference: Lewis, S., Heitkemper, M., Dirksen, S., O'Brien, P., & Bucher, L. (2007). *Medical-Surgical Nursing: Assessment and Management of Clinical Problems* (7th ed., pp. 882–883). St. Louis, MO: Mosby.

EBP Reference: Vahanian, A., Baumgartner, H., Bax, J., Butchart, E., Dion, R., et al. (2007). Guidelines on the management of valvular heart disease: The Task Force on the Management of Valvular Heart Disease of the European Society of Cardiology. *European Heart Journal,* 28(2), 230–268. Available at: www.guideline.gov/summary/summary.aspx?doc_id=10592&nbr=005534&string=aortic+AND+valve+AND+replacement

---

576. EBP A nurse is caring for a client following a coronary artery bypass graft. Which assessment finding in the immediate postoperative period should be most concerning to the nurse?

1. No chest tube output for 1 hour when previously it was copious
2. Client temperature of 99.1°F (37.2°C)
3. Arterial blood gas (ABG) results show pH 7.32; Pco_2 48; HCO_3 28; Po_2 80
4. Urine output of 160 mL in the last 4 hours

ANSWER: 1

A copiously draining chest tube that is no longer draining indicates an obstruction. There is an increased risk for cardiac tamponade or pleural effusion. A slight elevation in temperature could be the effects of rewarming after surgery. This should continue to be monitored, but is not immediately concerning. The ABG results show compensated respiratory acidosis. Though the pH is low and the Pco_2 is high, the kidneys are compensating by conserving bicarbonate (HCO_3). Normal pH is 7.35–7.45, Pco_2 32–42 mm Hg, HCO_3 20–24 mmol/L, and Po_2 75–100 mm Hg. A urine output of 160 mL/4 hr is equivalent to 40 mL/hr; adequate, but it warrants continued monitoring. Less than 30 mL/hr indicates decreased renal function.

➧ ***Test-taking Tip:*** *The key phrase in the question is "most concerning." Use the process of elimination and eliminate options 3 and 4 because these are normal findings. Of options 1 and 2, determine which option is most concerning.*

Content Area: Adult Health; *Category of Health Alteration:* Cardiac Management; *Integrated Processes:* Nursing Process Evaluation; *Client Need:* Physiological Integrity/Reduction of Risk Potential/Therapeutic Procedures; *Cognitive Level:* Analysis

Reference: Smeltzer, S., Bare, B., Hinkle, J., & Cheever, K. (2008). *Brunner & Suddarth's Textbook of Medical-Surgical Nursing* (11th ed., pp. 888–911). Philadelphia: Lippincott Williams & Wilkins.

EBP Reference: Eagle, K., Guyton, R., Davidoff, R., Edwards, F., Ewy, G., et al. (2004). ACC/AHA 2004 guideline update for coronary artery bypass graft surgery: Summary article. (A report of the American College of Cardiology/American Heart Association Task Force on Practice Guidelines [Committee to Update the 1999 Guidelines for Coronary Artery Bypass Graft Surgery]). *Circulation,* 110(9), 1168–1176.

577. EBP A nurse should anticipate instructing a client scheduled for a coronary artery bypass graft to: SELECT ALL THAT APPLY.

1. discontinue taking aspirin prior to surgery.
2. perform postoperative cardiac rehabilitation exercises and stress management strategies.
3. wash with an antimicrobial soap the evening prior to surgery.
4. shave the chest and legs and then shower to remove the hair.
5. resume normal activities when discharged from the hospital.
6. expect close monitoring after surgery, several intravenous (IV) lines, a urinary catheter, endotracheal tube, and chest tubes.

ANSWER: 1, 2, 3, 6

Aspirin decreases platelet aggregation and increases the risk of bleeding. It is usually discontinued a few days prior to surgery. A postoperative cardiac rehabilitation program is begun usually on the second postoperative day and includes exercises and stress management. The client should use an antimicrobial soap when showering or bathing the evening before and the day of surgery to decrease the risk of infection. Teaching about expectations of close monitoring, IV lines, a urinary catheter, endotracheal tube, and chest tubes can reduce client and family anxiety. The client may be offered a tour of the critical care unit prior to surgery or be given videos to view. Although the client's skin will be shaved, this will be completed just prior to surgery to avoid nicks and decrease the risk of infection. Activities that stress the sternum, such as lifting, driving, and overhead reaching, will be restricted after surgery.

➧ ***Test-taking Tip:*** *Use the process of elimination to eliminate options 4 and 5 because these increase surgical risk and the risk of complications after surgery.*

Content Area: Adult Health; *Category of Health Alteration:* Cardiac Management; *Integrated Processes:* Nursing Process Planning; *Client Need:* Physiological Integrity/Reduction of Risk Potential/Potential for Complications from Surgical Procedures and Health Alterations; *Cognitive Level:* Analysis

Reference: Smeltzer, S., Bare, B., Hinkle, J., & Cheever, K. (2008). *Brunner & Suddarth's Textbook of Medical-Surgical Nursing* (11th ed., pp. 888–911). Philadelphia: Lippincott Williams & Wilkins.

EBP Reference: Rees, K., Bennett, P., West, R., Smith, G., & Ebrahim, S. (2004). Psychological interventions for coronary heart disease. *Cochrane Database of Systematic Reviews*, Issue 2, Art. No. CD002902. DOI: 10.1002/14651858.CD002902.pub2. Available at: www.cochrane.org/reviews/en/ab002902.html

578. Because a step-down cardiac unit is unusually busy, a nurse fails to obtain vital signs at 0200 hours for a client 2 days postoperative for a mitral valve replacement. The client was stable when assessed at 0600 hours, so the nurse documents the electrocardiogram monitor's heart rate in the client's medical record for both the 0400 and 0600 vital signs. The charge nurse supervising the nurse determines that the nurse's behavior was: SELECT ALL THAT APPLY.

1. the correct action because neither complications nor harmful effects occurred.
2. a legal issue because the nurse has fraudulently falsified documentation.
3. demonstrating beneficence because the nurse decided what was best for the client.
4. an ethical issue of veracity because the nurse has been untruthful regarding the client's care.
5. an ethical legal issue of confidentiality because the nurse disclosed incorrect information.
6. demonstrating distributive justice because the nurse decided other clients' needs were priority.

ANSWER: 2, 4

Documenting vital signs that the nurse did not obtain is both a legal and ethical concern because documents were falsified and the nurse was untruthful regarding obtaining the vital signs. Veracity is telling the truth and not lying or deceiving others. Even if harm had not occurred, the nurse's behavior of falsifying documentation poses an ethical-legal concern and is never the correct action. Beneficence is doing good. There is no information to indicate the nurse did what was best for the client. Confidentiality relates to privacy and not disclosing private information about another. Documenting incorrect vital signs is not disclosing confidential information. Distributive justice is the distribution of resources to clients. There is no information about the resources available to the nurse.

➧ ***Test-taking Tip:*** *Focus on the nurse's behavior of falsifying documentation. Avoid reading into the question. Despite the unit being unusually busy, there is no information as to what the nurse was doing during the shift. Eliminate the options that are suggestive of nurse actions other than the behaviors presented.*

Content Area: Adult Health; *Category of Health Alteration:* Cardiac Management; *Integrated Processes:* Nursing Process Evaluation; *Client Need:* Safe and Effective Care Environment/Management of Care/Supervision; Safe and Effective Care Environment/Management of Care/Ethical Practice; *Cognitive Level:* Analysis

Reference: Smeltzer, S., Bare, B., Hinkle, J., & Cheever, K. (2008). *Brunner & Suddarth's Textbook of Medical-Surgical Nursing* (11th ed., p. 28). Philadelphia: Lippincott Williams & Wilkins.

579. A nurse, assessing a client hospitalized following a myocardial infarction (MI), obtains the following vital signs: blood pressure (BP) 78/38 mm Hg, heart rate (HR) 128, respiratory rate (RR) 32. For which life-threatening complication should the nurse carefully monitor the client?

1. Pulonary embolism
2. Cardiac tamponade
3. Cardiomyopathy
4. Cardiogenic shock

ANSWER: 4

The symptoms are indicative of cardiogenic shock (decreased cardiac output leading to inadequate tissue perfusion and initiation of the shock syndrome). Pulmonary embolism, cardiac tamponade, and cardiomyopathy are causes of cardiogenic shock. The cause of this client's cardiogenic shock is a myocardial infarction.

➧ ***Test-taking Tip:*** *Focus on the issue: life-threatening complications following MI.*

Content Area: Adult Health; *Category of Health Alteration:* Cardiac Management; *Integrated Processes:* Nursing Process Assessment; *Client Need:* Physiological Integrity/Physiological Adaptation/ Hemodynamics; *Cognitive Level:* Analysis

Reference: Smeltzer, S., Bare, B., Hinkle, J., & Cheever, K. (2008). *Brunner & Suddarth's Textbook of Medical-Surgical Nursing* (11th ed., pp. 965–966). Philadelphia: Lippincott Williams & Wilkins.

580. A client is admitted to a coronary care unit following an anterior myocardial infarction (MI). A nurse, caring for the client, obtains the following assessment findings. Based on these findings, the nurse should immediately notify the physician and plan which intervention?

TIME	7:00	8:00	8:30	9:00
Temp				
Tm=Tympanic O=Oral , R=Rectal Ax=Axillary		98.6 (0)		
Pulse		96	104	118
Resp		22	28	32
BP mm Hg		116/80	102/56	85/48
POx				
O_2 L/M/NC		2		4
Pain Rating: Numeric 0-10		0		4

INTAKE AND OUTPUT

	7:00	8:00	8:30	9:00	9:30
IVPB					
Oral Intake					
Urine Output		30 mL		20 mL	

1. Administering an IV fluid bolus of 0.9% NaCl because the client is in right heart failure
2. Initiating an IV infusion of dopamine (Intropin®) because the client is in cardiogenic shock
3. Preparing the client for pericardiocentesis since cardiac tamponade is suspected
4. Calling for a stat chest x-ray to rule out pulmonary embolism (PE)

ANSWER: 2

A complication of a anterior MI is left ventricular failure because a large portion of the left ventricle may have been damaged. Damage to the left ventricle leads to reduced cardiac output and cardiogenic shock. Hypotension, tachycardia, tachypnea, and decreasing urine output are classic signs of cardiogenic shock. A client with a systolic blood pressure (SBP) 85 mm Hg and a diastolic blood pressure (DBP) of 40 mm Hg has a mean arterial pressure (MAP) of 55. (MAP = [(SBP) + (2DBP)]/3 or 85 + 40 + 40 = 165/3 = 55). A MAP of less than 60 indicates impaired perfusion to organs. Vasopressors and positive inotropes are administered in cardiogenic shock to increase cardiac output. IV fluids may be administered if the client is showing signs of dehydration. However, the client is not experiencing right-sided heart failure (RHF). RHF produces signs of venous congestion, including jugular venous distention, hepatomegaly, splenomegaly, and ascites. Although symptoms of cardiac tamponade do include hypotension, tachycardia, and tachypnea, other signs include muffled heart sounds. Appropriate treatment for cardiac tamponade is pericardiocentesis. A chest x-ray is used to diagnose PE, but the data do not suggest PE. The signs of PE can be subtle and nonspecific but most commonly present with dyspnea, tachycardia, tachypnea, and/or chest pain.

➧ ***Test-taking Tip:*** *Focus on the client vital sign changes and decreased urine output. Complications of an anterior MI include left ventricular failure, reduced cardiac output, and cardiogenic shock.*

Content Area: Adult Health; *Category of Health Alteration:* Cardiac Management; *Integrated Processes:* Nursing Process Analysis; *Client Need:* Physiological Integrity/Reduction of Risk Potential/Potential for Complications from Surgical Procedures and Health Alterations; *Cognitive Level:* Application

Reference: Lewis, S., Heitkemper, M., Dirksen, S., O'Brien, P., & Bucher, L. (2007). *Medical-Surgical Nursing: Assessment and Management of Clinical Problems* (7th ed., pp. 598, 743–744, 1773–1774). St. Louis, MO: Mosby.

581. A client admitted to a telemetry unit with a diagnosis of Prinzmetal's angina, has the following medications ordered. Upon interpretation of the client's electrocardiogram (ECG) rhythm, the nurse notes a prolonged PR interval of 0.32 second. Based on this information, which medication order should the nurse question administering to the client?

1. Isosorbide mononitrate (Imdur®) 20 mg oral daily upon awakening
2. Amlodipine (Norvasc®) 10 mg oral daily
3. Nitroglycerin (Nitrostat®) 0.4 mg sublingual prn for chest pain
4. Atenolol (Tenormin®) 50 mg oral daily.

ANSWER: 4

Atenolol, a beta-blocker, blocks stimulation of $beta_1$ (myocardial)-adrenergic receptors, causing a reduction in blood pressure and heart rate. A side effect of the medication is a prolongation of the PR interval (normal PR interval is 0.12 to 0.20 second). Continued use of the drug can result in heart block. Nitrates and calcium channel blockers (CCBs) are the mainstays of medical therapy for variant angina rather than beta blockers. Isosorbide mononitrate, a nitrate, causes vasodilatation of the large coronary arteries. Nitrates act as an exogenous source of nitric oxide, which causes vascular smooth muscle relaxation resulting in a decrease in myocardial oxygen consumption and may have a modest effect on platelet aggregation and thrombosis. Amlodipine, a CCB, relaxes coronary smooth muscle and produces coronary vasodilation, which in turn improves myocardial oxygen delivery. Nitroglycerin sublingual effectively treats episodes of angina and myocardial ischemia within minutes of administration, and the long-acting nitrate preparation (Imdur®) reduces the frequency of recurrent events.

➧ ***Test-taking Tip:*** *The focus of the question is a medication contraindicated with a prolonged PR interval. Think about the action of the medications prescribed. Recall that Prinzmetal's angina is caused from coronary artery vasospasm and that nitrates and CCBs are the medications of choice for treatment. Both the prolonged PR interval and the diagnosis of Prinzmetal's angina are clues to selecting the correct option.*

Content Area: Adult Health; *Category of Health Alteration:* Cardiac Management; *Integrated Processes:* Nursing Process Analysis; *Client Need:* Physiological Integrity/Pharmacological and Parenteral Therapies/Medication Administration; *Cognitive Level:* Analysis

References: Lewis, S., Heitkemper, M., Dirksen, S., O'Brien, P., & Bucher, L. (2007). *Medical-Surgical Nursing: Assessment and Management of Clinical Problems* (7th ed., pp. 798–800, 853). St. Louis, MO: Mosby; Smeltzer, S., Bare, B., Hinkle, J., & Cheever, K. (2008). *Brunner & Suddarth's Textbook of Medical-Surgical Nursing* (11th ed., pp. 838, 869–874). Philadelphia: Lippincott Williams & Wilkins; Selwyn, A., & Orford, J. (2005). Coronary artery vasospasm. *E-Medicine from WebMD.* Available at: www.emedicine.com/med/topic447.htm

582. A nurse is to administer 40 mg of furosemide (Lasix®) to a client in heart failure. The prefilled syringe reads 100 mg/mL. In order to give the correct dose, the nurse should administer ____mL to the client.

ANSWER: 0.4

100 mg: 1 mL :: 40 mg : X mL
100 X = 40
X = 0.4
0.4 mL should be administered to the client.

➧ ***Test-taking Tip:*** *In this medication calculation problem, first determine the dose on hand, then determine the dose needed. Calculate the amount that should be administered. Recheck your answer using a calculator. With all calculation problems, the answer should make sense. The nurse should question unusually large amounts.*

Content Area: Adult Health; *Category of Health Alteration:* Cardiac Management; *Integrated Processes:* Nursing Process Implementation; *Client Need:* Physiological Integrity/Pharmacological and Parenteral Therapies/Dosage Calculation; *Cognitive Level:* Application

Reference: Pickar, G. (2007). *Dosage Calculations: A Ratio-Proportion Approach* (2nd ed.). Clifton Park, New York: Thomson Delmar Learning.

583. EBP A nurse receives a serum laboratory report for six different clients with admitting diagnoses of chest pain. After reviewing all of the lab reports, in which order should the nurse address each lab value? Prioritize the order in which the nurse should address each of the clients' results.

_____ Troponin T 42 ng/mL (0.0–0.4 ng/mL)
_____ WBC 11,000 K/μL
_____ Hgb 7.2 g/dL
_____ SCr 2.2 mg/dL
_____ K 2.2 mEq/L
_____ Total cholesterol 430 mg/dL

ANSWER: 1, 6, 3, 4, 2, 5

The nurse should address the elevated troponin level first. Cardio-specific troponins (troponin T, cTnT, and troponin I, cTnI) are released into circulation after myocardial injury and are highly specific indicators of myocardial infarction. Since "time is muscle," the client needs to be treated immediately to prevent extension of the infarct and possible death. The nurse should address the decreased serum potassium level (K) second. The normal serum K level is 3.5 to 5.8 mEq/L. A low serum K level can cause life-threatening dysrhythmias. The normal hemoglobin (Hgb) is 13.1 to 17.1 g/dL. A low Hgb can contribute to inadequate tissue perfusion and contribute to myocardial ischemia. The normal serum creatinine (SCr) is 0.4 to 1.4 mg/dL. Impaired circulation may be causing this alteration and further client assessment is needed. Medication doses may need to be adjusted with impaired renal perfusion. The normal total serum cholesterol should be less than 200 mg/dL. This is a risk factor for development of coronary artery disease. The client needs teaching. The normal white blood cell (WBC) count is 3.9 to 11.9 K/μL. Because the finding is normal, it can be addressed last.

▸ ***Test-taking Tip:*** *Knowledge of the normal ranges and the significance for critical laboratory values is expected on the NCLEX-RN®. Use the ABCs (airway, breathing, circulation) to determine priority. Of the laboratory values, determine those that are related to tissue perfusion (circulation), and then determine which value is most life threatening.*

Content Area: Adult Health; *Category of Health Alteration:* Cardiac Management; *Integrated Processes:* Nursing Process Implementation; *Client Need:* Safe and Effective Care Environment/Management of Care/Continuity of Care; Safe and Effective Care Environment/Management of Care/Establishing Priorities; *Cognitive Level:* Analysis

Reference: Lewis, S., Heitkemper, M., Dirksen, S., O'Brien, P., & Bucher, L. (2007). *Medical-Surgical Nursing: Assessment and Management of Clinical Problems* (7th ed., pp. 667–668, 752, 805–806, 1146–1147). St. Louis, MO: Mosby.

EBP Reference: Institute for Clinical Systems Improvement (ICSI). (2008). *Diagnosis and Treatment of Chest Pain and Acute Coronary Syndrome.* Bloomington, MN: ICSI. Available at: www.guideline.gov/summary/summary.aspx?doc_id=13480&nbr=006889&string=chest+AND+pain

584. EBP Following a normal chest x-ray for a client who had cardiac surgery, a nurse receives an order to remove the chest tubes. Which intervention should the nurse plan to implement *first*?

1. Auscultate the client's lung sounds
2. Administer 4 mg morphine sulfate intravenously
3. Turn off the suction to the chest drainage system
4. Prepare the dressing supplies at the client's bedside

ANSWER: 2

Because the peak action of morphine sulfate is 10 to 15 minutes, this should be administered first. Auscultating the client's lungs before and after the procedure, turning off the suction, and assembling the dressing supplies are all necessary, but administering the analgesic should be first.

▸ ***Test-taking Tip:*** *Recall that focusing on the client should be the priority.*

Content Area: Adult Health; *Category of Health Alteration:* Cardiac Management; *Integrated Processes:* Nursing Process Planning; *Client Need:* Physiological Integrity/Pharmacological and Parenteral Therapies/Pharmacological Pain Management; *Cognitive Level:* Application

Reference: Monahan, F., Sands, J., Neighbors, M., Marek, J., & Green, C. (2007). *Phipps' Medical-Surgical Nursing: Health and Illness Perspectives* (8th ed., pp. 848–850). St. Louis, MO: Mosby/Elsevier.

EBP Reference: Puntilo, K., & Ley, S. (2004). Appropriately timed analgesics control pain due to chest tube removal. *American Journal of Critical Care,* 13(4), 292–301.

585. A nurse who is beginning a shift on a cardiac step-down unit receives shift report for four clients. In which order should the nurse assess the clients? Prioritize the nurse's actions by placing each client in order from most urgent (1) to least urgent (4).

______ A 56-year-old client who was admitted 1 day ago with chest pain receiving intravenous (IV) heparin and has a partial thromboplastin time (PTT) due back in 30 minutes

______ A 62-year-old client with end-stage cardiomyopathy, blood pressure (BP) of 78/50 mm Hg, 20 mL/hr urine output, and a "Do Not Resuscitate" order and whose family has just arrived

______ A 72-year-old client who was transferred 2 hours ago from the intensive care unit (ICU) following a coronary artery bypass graft and has new onset atrial fibrillation with rapid ventricular response

______ A 38-year-old postoperative client who had an aortic valve replacement 2 days ago, BP 114/72 mm Hg, heart rate (HR) 100 beats/min, respiratory rate (RR) 28 breaths/min, and temperature 101.2°F (38.4°C)

ANSWER: 3, 4, 1, 2

The client with new onset atrial fibrillation should be assessed first because it is the most life threatening. The postoperative client with the elevated temperature should be assessed next because the elevated temperature, RR, and HR increase the demands on the heart and could be a sign of pulmonary complications. Third, the nurse should assess the client with the heparin infusion. PTT results should be back, and the dose may require adjustment. Last, the client with end-stage cardiomyopathy should be assessed. The family will have had time alone with the client, and the client and family may need emotional support.

➧ ***Test-taking Tip:*** *When establishing priorities, first determine life-threatening situations and then prioritize remaining clients by using the ABCs (airway, breathing, and circulation). Recall from Maslow's Hierarchy of Needs that physiological problems are priority over psychosocial issues, thus the client with end-stage cardiomyopathy should be assessed last.*

Content Area: Adult Health; *Category of Health Alteration:* Cardiac Management; *Integrated Processes:* Nursing Process Planning; *Client Need:* Safe and Effective Care Environment/Management of Care/Establishing Priorities; *Cognitive Level:* Analysis

Reference: Berman, A., Snyder, S., Kozier, B., & Erb, G. (2008). *Kozier & Erb's Fundamentals of Nursing: Concepts, Process, and Practice* (8th ed., pp. 217–218). Upper Saddle River, NJ: Pearson Education.

586. A nurse is working with a certified nursing assistant (CNA) providing care for four clients on a busy telemetry unit. All four clients are in need of immediate attention. The CNA is a senior nursing student who has been administering medications and performing procedures during clinical experiences as a student nurse. The charge nurse supervising care on the telemetry unit determines that care is appropriate when the registered nurse (RN) working with the CNA delegates: SELECT ALL THAT APPLY.

1. administering acetaminophen (Tylenol®) to the client with an elevated temperature.
2. taking vital signs on the client newly admitted with a diagnosis of heart failure.
3. finishing the discharge instructions so the client with a new pacemaker implant can go home.
4. changing a client's chest tube dressing because it got wet when the water pitcher overturned.
5. providing a sponge bath for the client with the elevated temperature.
6. checking the lung sounds of the client whose chest tube drainage system was tipped over and then righted

ANSWER: 2, 5

Legally a student nurse employed as a nursing assistant in a facility is only allowed to perform tasks listed in the job description of a nursing assistant even though the student nurse has received instruction and acquired competence in administering medications and performing sterile procedures. The tasks of a nursing assistant include taking vital signs and bathing clients. Medication administration, teaching, sterile procedures, and assessments are not within the nursing assistant's scope of practice.

➧ ***Test-taking Tip:*** *Read the information given in the question carefully. The issue of the question is tasks that the RN can legally delegate to a CNA who is also a student nurse. Delegated tasks must be within the job description of the nursing assistant.*

Content Area: Adult Health; *Category of Health Alteration:* Cardiac Management; *Integrated Processes:* Nursing Process Evaluation; *Client Need:* Safe and Effective Care Environment/Management of Care/Delegation; *Cognitive Level:* Analysis

Reference: Berman, A., Snyder, S., Kozier, B., & Erb, G. (2008). *Kozier & Erb's Fundamentals of Nursing: Concepts, Process, and Practice* (8th ed., pp. 74–75). Upper Saddle River, NJ: Pearson Education.

Test 16: **Adult Health: Endocrine Management**

587. EBP A nurse is reviewing serum laboratory data for four female clients. Which client would require the most immediate assessment?

Client	Lab Test	Result	Normal Ranges
A	Thyroid-stimulating hormone (TSH) level	5.2 mIU/L	0.4–4.2 mIU/L
B	Growth hormone	23 μg/L	8–18 μg/L
C	Free T_4 (thyroxin)	7.0 ng/dL	0.8–2.7 ng/dL
D	Glucose	140 mg/dL	70–110 mg/dL

1. Client A
2. Client B
3. Client C
4. Client D

ANSWER: 3

An excess of thyroid hormone is the most life threatening of the findings listed due to its effects on the cardiovascular system of hypertension and tachycardia. The client should be assessed for impending thyroid storm. An elevated thyroid-stimulating hormone (TSH) level occurs in hypothyroidism. TSH is needed to ensure proper synthesis and secretion of the thyroid hormones, which are essential for life. An elevated growth hormone produces acromegaly with resulting bone and soft tissue deformities and enlarged viscera. Though the glucose level is elevated, a level of 140 mg/dL does not require immediate assessment or intervention.

➧ ***Test-taking Tip:** Focus on the laboratory values and the normal ranges. Think about the functions of the hormones and the values that would be most life threatening to establish priority.*

Content Area: Adult Health; *Category of Health Alteration:* Endocrine Management; *Integrated Processes:* Nursing Process Analysis; *Client Needs:* Safe and Effective Care Environment/Management of Care/Establishing Priorities; *Cognitive Level:* Analysis

Reference: Smeltzer, S., Bare, B., Hinkle, J., & Cheever, K. (2008). *Brunner & Suddarth's Textbook of Medical-Surgical Nursing* (11th ed., pp. 1446, 1452, 1460–1461, 2586, 2591–2592). Philadelphia: Lippincott Williams & Wilkins.

EBP Reference: U. S. Preventive Services Task Force. (2004). *Screening for Thyroid Disease: Recommendation Statement.* Available at: www.ahrg.gov/clinic

588. A clinic nurse is evaluating a client with type 1 diabetes who intends to enroll in a tennis class. Which statement made by the client indicates that the client understands the effects of exercise on insulin demand?

1. "I will carry a high-fat, high-calorie food, such as a cookie."
2. "I will administer 1 unit of lispro insulin prior to playing tennis."
3. "I will eat a 15-gram carbohydrate snack before playing tennis."
4. "I will decrease the meal prior to the class by 15-grams of carbohydrates."

ANSWER: 3

Excessive exercise without sufficient carbohydrates can result in unexpected hypoglycemia. The food should be a simple sugar food because the fat content of a high-fat food will delay the absorption of the glucose in the food. Taking insulin or decreasing the carbohydrate intake prior to activity will lower the blood glucose level such that hypoglycemia can occur.

➧ ***Test-taking Tip:** Recall that type 1 diabetes mellitus requires daily insulin administration and that activity increases energy expenditure and the demand for glucose.*

Content Area: Adult Health; *Category of Health Alteration:* Endocrine Management; *Integrated Processes:* Nursing Process Evaluation; *Client Needs:* Physiological Adaptation/Illness Management; *Cognitive Level:* Application

Reference: Smeltzer, S., Bare, B., Hinkle, J., & Cheever, K. (2008). *Brunner & Suddarth's Textbook of Medical-Surgical Nursing* (11th ed., pp. 1388, 1411). Philadelphia: Lippincott Williams & Wilkins.

589. Two hours after taking a regular morning dose of Insulin Regular (Humulin R®), a client presents to a clinic with diaphoresis, tremors, palpitations, and tachycardia. Which nursing action is most appropriate for this client?

1. Check pulse oximetry and administer oxygen at 2 L per nasal cannula.
2. Administer a baby aspirin, one sublingual nitroglycerin tablet, and obtain an electrocardiogram (ECG).
3. Check blood glucose level and provide carbohydrates if less than 70 mg/dL (3.8 mmol/L).
4. Check vital signs and administer atenolol (Tenormin®) 25 mg orally if heart rate is greater than 120 beats per minute.

ANSWER: 3

Humulin R is regular insulin that peaks in 2 to 4 hours after administration. The client's symptoms suggest hypoglycemia, so a blood glucose level should be checked. The symptoms do not suggest a respiratory problem (option 1). Though diaphoresis, palpitations, and tachycardia are symptoms of both hypoglycemia and cardiac problems, the client had taken insulin 2 hours earlier. Treating the low blood sugar first will likely resolve the client's symptoms.

➧ ***Test-taking Tip:** Focus on the effects of Humulin R and the client's symptoms.*

Content Area: Adult Health; *Category of Health Alteration:* Endocrine Management; *Integrated Processes:* Nursing Process Implementation; *Client Needs:* Physiological Integrity/Physiological Adaptation/Unexpected Response to Therapies; *Cognitive Level:* Analysis

References: Smeltzer, S., Bare, B., Hinkle, J., & Cheever, K. (2008). *Brunner & Suddarth's Textbook of Medical-Surgical Nursing* (11th ed., pp. 1410–1411). Philadelphia: Lippincott Williams & Wilkins; Wilson, B., Shannon, M., Shields, K., & Stang, C. (2008). *Prentice Hall Nurse's Drug Guide 2008* (pp. 795–797). Upper Saddle River, NJ: Pearson Education.

590. A nurse working on a telemetry unit is planning to complete noon assessments for four assigned clients with type 1 diabetes mellitus. All of the clients received subcutaneous insulin aspart (NovoLog®) at 0800 hours. In which order should the nurse assess the clients? Place each answer option into the correct order.

_____ A 60-year-old client who is nauseous and has just vomited for the second time
_____ A 45-year-old client who is dyspneic and has chest pressure and new onset atrial fibrillation
_____ A 75-year-old client with a fingerstick blood glucose level of 300 mg/dL
_____ A 50-year-old client with a fingerstick blood glucose level of 70 mg/dL

ANSWER: 2, 1, 3, 4

First, the nurse should assess the client with new onset atrial fibrillation and dyspnea. Diabetes increases the risk of coronary artery disease and myocardial infarction. Next, assess the client who just vomited. The client with a 300 mg/dL blood glucose level should then be assessed. This blood glucose level is not immediately life-threatening, but needs to be lowered as soon as possible. The client with the blood glucose level of 70 mg/dL can be assessed last because this is a normal blood glucose level.

Test-taking Tip: *Use the ABC's (airway, breathing, circulation) to establish the priority client. Then, look at the information provided for each client to determine the next priority. Consider that all clients received insulin at 0800 hours.*

Content Area: Adult Health; *Category of Health Alteration:* Endocrine Management; *Integrated Processes:* Nursing Process Assessment; *Client Needs:* Safe and Effective Care Environment/Management of Care/Establishing Priorities; *Cognitive Level:* Analysis

Reference: Lewis, S., Heitkemper, M., Dirksen, S., O'Brien, P., & Bucher, L. (2007). *Medical-Surgical Nursing: Assessment and Management of Clinical Problems* (7th ed., pp. 1278–1281). St. Louis, MO: Mosby.

591. A client has eaten 45 grams of carbohydrate (carb) with the dinner meal. The client is ordered to receive 2 units of aspart insulin subcutaneously for each carb choice (CHO) eaten at a meal (1 carb choice = 15 grams). Place an X on the syringe that correctly identifies the amount of insulin the client should receive.

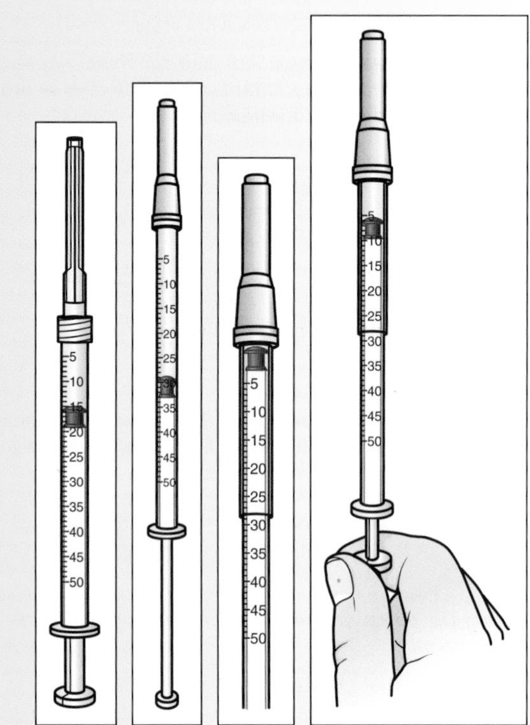

ANSWER:

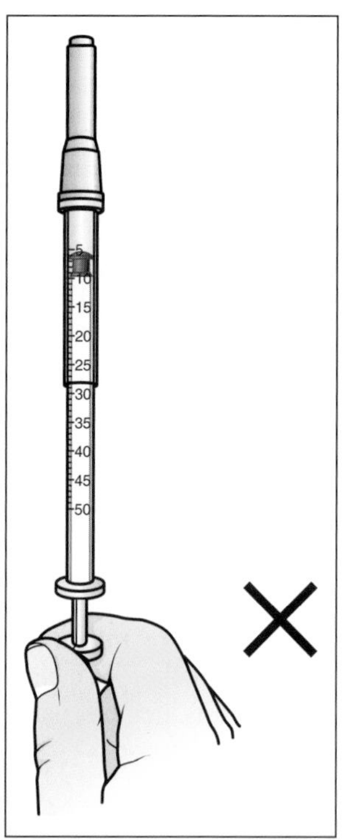

Eating 45 grams equals 3 CHOs. If the client is to receive 2 units of insulin for each CHO, the total amount of aspart insulin is 3 CHO times 2 units per CHO = 6 units.

Test-taking Tip: *Read the information in the question carefully. Calculate the amount of insulin the client should receive prior to making the selection.*

Content Area: Adult Health; *Category of Health Alteration:* Endocrine Management; *Integrated Processes:* Nursing Process Implementation; *Client Needs:* Physiological Integrity/Pharmacological and Parenteral Therapies/Dosage Calculation; *Cognitive Level:* Analysis

Reference: American Diabetes Association. (n.d.). *Carb Counting.* Available at: www.diabetes.org/for-parents-and-kids/diabetes-care/carb-count.jsp

592. A nurse is caring for a client with type 2 diabetes on a telemetry unit. The client is scheduled for cardiac rehabilitation exercises (cardiac rehab). The nurse notes that the client's blood glucose level is 300 mg/dL and the urine is positive for ketones. Which nursing action should be included in the nurse's plan of care?

1. Send the client to cardiac rehab because exercise will lower the client's blood glucose level.
2. Administer insulin and then send the client to cardiac rehab with a 15-gram carbohydrate snack.
3. Delay the cardiac rehab because blood glucose levels will decrease too much with exercise.
4. Cancel the cardiac rehab because blood glucose levels will increase further with exercise.

ANSWER: 4

Exercising with blood glucose levels exceeding 250 mg/dL and ketonuria increases the secretion of glucagon, growth hormone, and catecholamines, causing the liver to release more glucose. Exercise in the presence of hyperglycemia does not lower the blood glucose level (options 1 and 3). Administering insulin may be an option, but the blood glucose level should be known before sending the client to cardiac rehab (option 2).

▶ ***Test-taking Tip:*** *Think about the physiological effects of stress on blood glucose levels. Then eliminate options 1 and 3 because these are incorrect. Of the remaining two options, decide which action is safest for the client.*

Content Area: Adult Health; *Category of Health Alteration:* Endocrine Management; *Integrated Processes:* Nursing Process Planning; *Client Needs:* Physiological Integrity/Physiological Adaptation/Illness Management; *Cognitive Level:* Analysis

Reference: Smeltzer, S., Bare, B., Hinkle, J., & Cheever, K. (2008). *Brunner & Suddarth's Textbook of Medical-Surgical Nursing* (11th ed., p. 1388). Philadelphia: Lippincott Williams & Wilkins.

593. **EBP** A nurse administers 15 units of glargine (Lantus®) insulin at 2100 hours to a Hispanic client when the client's fingerstick blood glucose reading was 110 mg/dL. At 2300 hours, a nursing assistant reports to the nurse that an evening snack was not given because the client was sleeping. Which instruction by the nurse is most appropriate?

1. "You will need to wake the client to check the blood glucose and then give a snack. All diabetics get a snack at bedtime."
2. "It is not necessary for this client to have a snack because glargine insulin is absorbed very slowly over 24 hours and doesn't have a peak."
3. "The next time the client wakes up, check a blood glucose level and then give a snack."
4. "I will need to notify the physician because a snack at this time will affect the client's blood glucose level and the next dose of glargine insulin."

ANSWER: 2

The onset of glargine is 1 hour, it has no peak, and it lasts for 24 hours. Glargine lowers the blood glucose by increasing transport into cells and promoting the conversion of glucose to glycogen. Because it is peakless, a bedtime snack is unnecessary. Options 1 and 3 are unnecessary and option 4 is incorrect. Glargine is administered once daily, the same time each day, to maintain relatively constant concentrations over 24 hours.

▶ ***Test-taking Tip:*** *Apply knowledge of the action of glargine insulin.*

Content Area: Adult Health; *Category of Health Alteration:* Endocrine Management; *Integrated Processes:* Nursing Process Evaluation; *Client Needs:* Physiological Integrity/Pharmacological and Parenteral Therapies/Expected Effects/Outcomes; *Cognitive Level:* Application

Reference: Smeltzer, S., Bare, B., Hinkle, J., & Cheever, K. (2008). *Brunner & Suddarth's Textbook of Medical-Surgical Nursing* (11th ed., pp. 1392–1393). Philadelphia: Lippincott Williams & Wilkins.

EBP Reference: Philis-Tsimikas, A., Zhang, Q., & Walker, C. (2006). Glycemic control with insulin glargine as part of an ethnically diverse, community-based diabetes management program. *American Journal of Therapeutics*, 13, 466–472.

594. A client diagnosed with diabetes mellitus is on an insulin infusion drip. The insulin bag indicates there are 100 units of insulin in 1,000 milliliters (mL) of normal saline. Based on the client's blood glucose reading, the client should receive 1.5 units per hour. To ensure that the client receives 1.5 units per hour, the nurse should set the pump at ______ mL/hr.

ANSWER: 15

100 units : 1,000 mL :: 1.5 units : X mL
100X = 1,500
X = 15

▶ ***Test-taking Tip:*** *Use a drug calculation formula and the on-screen calculator and double-check the answer if it seems unusually large.*

Content Area: Adult Health; *Category of Health Alteration:* Endocrine Management; *Integrated Processes:* Nursing Process Analysis; *Client Needs:* Physiological Integrity/Pharmacological and Parenteral Therapies/Dosage Calculation; *Cognitive Level:* Analysis

Reference: Pickar, G. (2007). *Dosage Calculations: A Ratio-Proportion Approach* (2nd ed., pp. 46, 344). Clifton Park, NY: Thomson Delmar Learning.

595. EBP A nurse is teaching a client who has been newly diagnosed with type 2 diabetes mellitus (DM). Which teaching point should the nurse emphasize?

1. Use the arm when self-administering NPH insulin.
2. Exercise for 30 minutes daily, preferably after a meal.
3. Consume 30% of the daily calorie intake from protein foods.
4. Eat a 30-gram carbohydrate snack prior to strenuous activity.

ANSWER: 2

Exercise increases insulin receptor sites in the tissue and can have a direct effect on lowering blood glucose levels. Exercise also contributes to weight loss, which also decreases insulin resistance. Usually type 2 DM is controlled with oral hypoglycemic agents. If insulin is needed, sites should be rotated. For those with DM, protein should contribute less than 10% of the total energy consumed. Strenuous activity can be perceived by the body as a stressor, causing a release of counterregulatory hormones that subsequently increases blood glucose. Hyperglycemia can result from the combination of strenuous activity and extra carbohydrates.

Test-taking Tip: *The key terms are "type 2" and "emphasize." Apply knowledge of type 2 DM and eliminate options 1, 3, and 4 because type 2 diabetics will produce some insulin, and often weight reduction, calorie reduction, and exercise will help to normalize glucose levels.*

Content Area: Adult Health; *Category of Health Alteration:* Endocrine Management; *Integrated Processes:* Teaching and Learning; *Client Needs:* Health Promotion and Maintenance/Self-Care; *Cognitive Level:* Analysis

Reference: Lewis, S., Heitkemper, M., Dirksen, S., O'Brien, P., & Bucher, L. (2007). *Medical-Surgical Nursing: Assessment and Management of Clinical Problems* (7th ed., pp. 1268–1269). St. Louis, MO: Mosby.

EBP Reference: Thomas, D., Elliott, E., & Naughton, G. (2006). Exercise for type 2 diabetes mellitus. *Cochrane Database of Systematic Reviews*, Issue 3, Art. No. CD002968. DOI: 10.1002/14651858.CD002968.pub2. Available at: www.cochrane.org/reviews/en/ab002968.html

---

596. A nurse is evaluating a client's outcome. The client's nursing care plan includes the nursing diagnosis of fluid volume deficit related to hyperosmolar hyperglycemic nonketotic syndrome (HHNS) secondary to severe hyperglycemia. The nurse knows that the client has a positive outcome when which serum laboratory value has decreased to a normal range?

1. Glucose
2. Sodium
3. Osmolality
4. Potassium

ANSWER: 3

Extreme hyperglycemia produces severe osmotic diuresis; loss of sodium, potassium, and phosphorous; and profound dehydration. Consequently, hyperosmolality occurs. A normalizing of the serum osmolality indicates that the fluid volume deficit is resolving. A decrease in serum glucose indicates that the hyperglycemia is resolving, but not the fluid volume deficit. Serum sodium and potassium values should increase, not decrease, with treatment.

Test-taking Tip: *Focus on the issue: deficient fluid volume.*

Content Area: Adult Health; *Category of Health Alteration:* Endocrine Management; *Integrated Processes:* Nursing Process Evaluation; *Client Needs:* Physiological Integrity/Reduction of Risk Potential/Laboratory Values; *Cognitive Level:* Application

Reference: Lewis, S., Heitkemper, M., Dirksen, S., O'Brien, P., & Bucher, L. (2007). *Medical-Surgical Nursing: Assessment and Management of Clinical Problems* (7th ed., pp. 1280–1281). St. Louis, MO: Mosby.

---

597. A client with type 1 diabetes mellitus is scheduled for a total hip replacement. In reviewing the client's orders the evening prior to surgery, a nurse notes that the physician did not write an order to change the client's daily insulin dose. Which nursing action is most appropriate?

1. Notify the physician who wrote the insulin order in the client's medical record.
2. Write an order to decrease the morning insulin dose by one-half of the prescribed morning dose.
3. Do nothing because the physician would want the client to receive the usual insulin dose prior to surgery.
4. Inform the day shift nurse to check the client's fingerstick glucose before surgery and hold the morning dose of insulin.

ANSWER: 1

Because the client will be NPO (nothing per mouth) for surgery, the nurse must ensure that the usual insulin dosage has been changed to prevent hypoglycemia. The change may include eliminating the rapid-acting insulin and giving a decreased amount of intermediate-acting NPH or Lente insulin. A registered nurse is unable to prescribe medications. The nurse could write the order based on standing orders, but this is not noted in the option. Doing nothing could cause a hypoglycemic reaction because the client will be NPO for surgery. Holding the morning dose of insulin can cause hyperglycemia leading to diabetic ketoacidosis. Even without food, glucose levels increase from hepatic glucose production. Clients with type 1 diabetes require insulin 24 hours a day.

Test-taking Tip: *Note the key words "most appropriate." Eliminate options 2 and 4 knowing that the nurse should neither write an order to change the dose nor hold the dose. Both require a physician order. Next, look at options 1 and 3. Eliminate option 3, recalling the effects of insulin when the client is NPO.*

Content Area: Adult Health; *Category of Health Alteration:* Endocrine Management; *Integrated Processes:* Nursing Process Implementation; *Client Needs:* Safe and Effective Care Environment/Safety and Infection Control/Error Prevention; *Cognitive Level:* Application

Reference: Smeltzer, S., Bare, B., Hinkle, J., & Cheever, K. (2008). *Brunner & Suddarth's Textbook of Medical-Surgical Nursing* (11th ed., p. 1431). Philadelphia: Lippincott Williams & Wilkins.

598. A nurse administers a usual morning dose of 4 units of regular insulin and 8 units of NPH insulin at 7:30 a.m. to a client with a blood glucose level of 110 mg/dL. Which statements regarding the client's insulin are correct?

1. The onset of the regular insulin will be at 7:45 a.m. and the peak at 1:00 p.m.
2. The onset of the regular insulin will be at 8:00 a.m. and the peak at 10:00 a.m.
3. The onset of the NPH insulin will be at 8:00 a.m. and the peak at 10:00 a.m.
4. The onset of the NPH insulin will be at 12:30 p.m. and the peak at 11:30 p.m.

ANSWER: 2

The onset of regular insulin (short-acting) is one-half to 1 hour, and the peak is 2 to 3 hours. The onset of NPH insulin (intermediate acting) is 2 to 4 hours, and the peak is 4 to 12 hours. All other options have incorrect medication onset and peak times.

Test-taking Tip: *Apply knowledge of insulin onset and peak times.*

Content Area: Adult Health; *Category of Health Alteration:* Endocrine Management; *Integrated Processes:* Nursing Process Evaluation; *Client Needs:* Physiological Integrity/Pharmacological and Parenteral Therapies/Pharmacological Agents/Actions; *Cognitive Level:* Application

Reference: Smeltzer, S., Bare, B., Hinkle, J., & Cheever, K. (2008). *Brunner & Suddarth's Textbook of Medical-Surgical Nursing* (11th ed., p. 1392). Philadelphia: Lippincott Williams & Wilkins.

599. EBP A home-health nurse is planning the first home visit for a 60-year-old Hispanic client newly diagnosed with type 2 diabetes mellitus. The client has been instructed to take 70/30 combination insulin in the morning and at suppertime. Which interventions should be included in the client's plan of care? SELECT ALL THAT APPLY.

1. Instruct the client to inspect the feet daily.
2. Ensure that the client eats a bedtime snack.
3. Assess the client's ability to read small print.
4. Teach the client how to perform a hemoglobin A1c test.
5. Instruct the client on storing prefilled syringes in the refrigerator.
6. Teach the client to take one unit of 70/30 insulin after eating a snack.

ANSWER: 1, 2, 3, 5

Diabetes, diabetic complications, and increased mortality have been reported to occur at a higher rate in Hispanics compared with non-Hispanic whites of the same age. Therefore, careful daily skin assessment is necessary. Neuropathy, peripheral vascular disease, and immunocompromise can result in diabetic foot ulcer and complications. The 70/30 insulin is a combination of NPH and regular insulin. The NPH insulin will peak 4 to 12 hours after administration. A bedtime snack will cover the insulin peak to prevent hypoglycemia. Magnifying devices are available if the client is unable to read small print to prevent dosing errors. Syringes may be prefilled but should be stored in the refrigerator with the needle up. Blood is drawn in the laboratory to check the A1c. Only short-acting (regular) or rapid-acting insulin (aspart or lispro), not 70/30 insulin, would be administered to cover for additional carbohydrates if the client were on a carbohydrate-counting regimen with insulin coverage. This would be prescribed by the physician.

Test-taking Tip: *Focus on the situation, an older adult client with type 2 diabetes taking 70/30 insulin. Apply knowledge of care of the diabetic client and insulin types to select the correct options.*

Content Area: Adult Health; *Category of Health Alteration:* Endocrine Management; *Integrated Processes:* Nursing Process Planning; *Client Needs:* Physiological Integrity/Physiological Adaptation/Illness Management; *Cognitive Level:* Application

Reference: Smeltzer, S., Bare, B., Hinkle, J., & Cheever, K. (2008). *Brunner & Suddarth's Textbook of Medical-Surgical Nursing* (11th ed., pp. 1392–1429). Philadelphia: Lippincott Williams & Wilkins.

EBP Reference: Carlos, C. (2007). Addressing cultural barriers to the successful use of insulin in Hispanics with type 2 diabetes. *Southern Medical Journal,* 100(8), 812–820. Available at: http://web.ebscohost.com/ehost/pdf?vid=2&hid=114&sid=59059245-bbad-43cb-aefd-23ca9a35ae2f%40sessionmgr109

600. A friend brings an older adult homeless client to a free health-screening clinic because the friend is unable to continue administering the client's morning and evening insulin for type 1 diabetes mellitus. When advocating for this client, which action by the nurse is most appropriate?

1. Notify Adult Protective Services about the client's condition and living situation.
2. Ask where the client lives and if someone else can administer the insulin.
3. Contact the unit social worker to arrange for someone to give the client's insulin at a local homeless shelter.
4. Have the client return to the screening clinic mornings and evenings to receive the insulin injections.

ANSWER: 3

Advocacy focuses on the client's rights to make choices and decisions. The client has the right to receive and choose to receive treatment (autonomy). It is the nurse's responsibility to ensure that the client has access to health-care services to meet health needs. Adult Protective Services is an agency that investigates actual or potential abuse. Option 2 is data gathering and not advocacy. A screening clinic is not a permanent clinic where health-care services are provided.

➧ ***Test-taking Tip:** Note the key word "advocate."*

Content Area: Adult Health; *Category of Health Alteration:* Endocrine Management; *Integrated Processes:* Nursing Process Implementation; *Client Needs:* Safe and Effective Care Environment/Management of Care/Advocacy; *Cognitive Level:* Application

Reference: Berman, A., Snyder, S., Kozier, B., & Erb, G. (2008). *Kozier & Erb's Fundamentals of Nursing: Concepts, Process, and Practice* (8th ed., pp. 93–95). Upper Saddle River, NJ: Pearson Education.

---

601. EBP Which physician's order should the nurse question for a newly admitted client diagnosed with diabetic ketoacidosis (DKA)?

1. D5W at 125 mL per hour
2. KCL 10 mEq in 100 mL NaCl IV now
3. Stat arterial blood gases. Administer sodium bicarbonate if pH is less than 7.0.
4. Regular insulin infusion per protocol adjusting dose based on hourly glucose levels

ANSWER: 1

In DKA, the blood glucose level is above 300 mg/dL. Additional glucose will only increase the glucose level. Initially 0.45% or 0.9% sodium chloride (NaCl) is administered for fluid resuscitation. Glucose may be added when blood glucose levels approach 250 mg/dL. Insulin will drive potassium into the cells, so potassium chloride (KCL) is administered to prevent life-threatening hypokalemia. Normal pH is 7.35 to 7.45. Sodium bicarbonate will reverse the severe acidosis. Intravenous (IV) insulin will correct the hyperglycemia and hyperketonemia. Tight glucose control can be maintained by hourly glucose checks and adjusting the insulin infusion dose.

➧ ***Test-taking Tip:** Note the key word "question." Select the option that would not be included in the treatment of the client with DKA.*

Content Area: Adult Health; *Category of Health Alteration:* Endocrine Management; *Integrated Processes:* Nursing Process Analysis; *Client Needs:* Safe and Effective Care Environment/Safety and Infection Control/Error Prevention; *Cognitive Level:* Application

Reference: Lewis, S., Heitkemper, M., Dirksen, S., O'Brien, P., & Bucher, L. (2007). *Medical-Surgical Nursing: Assessment and Management of Clinical Problems* (7th ed., p. 1280). St. Louis, MO: Mosby.

EBP Reference: Egi, M., Bellomo, R., Stachowski, E., et al. (2006). Variability of blood glucose concentration and short-term mortality in critically ill patients. *Anesthesiology,* 105, 244–252.

---

602. EBP Which instructions should the nurse provide to a client regarding diabetes management during stress or illness? SELECT ALL THAT APPLY.

1. Notify the health-care provider if unable to keep fluids or foods down.
2. Test fingerstick glucose levels and urine ketones daily and keep a record.
3. Continue to take oral hypoglycemic medications and/or insulin as prescribed.
4. Supplement food intake with carbohydrate-containing fluids, such as juices or soups.
5. When on an oral agent, administer insulin in addition to the oral agent during the illness.
6. A minor illness, such as the flu, usually does not affect the blood glucose and insulin needs.

ANSWER: 1, 3

An acute or minor illness can evoke a counterregulatory hormone response resulting in hyperglycemia, thus the client should continue medications as prescribed. If the client is unable to eat due to nausea and vomiting, dehydration can occur from hyperglycemia and the lack of fluid intake. Blood glucose should be checked every 4 hours when ill and the ketones tested every 3 to 4 hours if the glucose is greater than 240 mg/dL. The client should supplement the diet with carbohydrate-containing fluids only if eating less than normal due to the illness. Insulin may or may not be necessary; it is based on the client's blood glucose level.

➧ ***Test-taking Tip:** Focus on the counterregulatory hormone response during an illness that causes hyperglycemia.*

Content Area: Adult Health; *Category of Health Alteration:* Endocrine Management; *Integrated Processes:* Teaching and Learning; *Client Needs:* Physiological Integrity/Physiological Adaptation/Illness Management; *Cognitive Level:* Application

Reference: Lewis, S., Heitkemper, M., Dirksen, S., O'Brien, P., & Bucher, L. (2007). *Medical-Surgical Nursing: Assessment and Management of Clinical Problems* (7th ed., pp. 1272–1273). St. Louis, MO: Mosby.

EBP Reference: Nield, L., Moore, H., Hooper, L., Cruickshank, J., Vyas, A., et al. (2004). Dietary advice for treatment of type 2 diabetes mellitus in adults. *Cochrane Database of Systematic Reviews*, Issue 2, Art. No. CD004097. DOI: 10.1002/14651858.CD004097.pub4. Available at: www.cochrane.org/reviews/en/ab004097.html

603. A nurse evaluates a client who is being treated for diabetic ketoacidosis (DKA). Which finding indicates that the client is responding to the treatment plan?

1. Eyes sunken, skin flushed
2. Skin moist with rapid elastic recoil
3. Serum potassium level is 3.3 mEq/L
4. ABG results are pH 7.25, $Paco_2$ 30, HCO_3 17

ANSWER: 2

Moist skin and good skin turgor indicate that dehydration secondary to hyperglycemia is resolving. Sunken eyes and flushing are signs of dehydration. Normal serum potassium levels are 3.5 to 5.8 mEq/L. The abnormal ABGs indicate compensating metabolic acidosis.

➧ ***Test-taking Tip:*** *Note the key phrase "responding to treatment." Select the option that is a normal finding.*

Content Area: Adult Health; *Category of Health Alteration:* Endocrine Management; *Integrated Processes:* Nursing Process Evaluation; *Client Needs:* Health Promotion and Maintenance/ Physiological Adaptation/Illness Management; *Cognitive Level:* Analysis

Reference: Lewis, S., Heitkemper, M., Dirksen, S., O'Brien, P., & Bucher, L. (2007). *Medical-Surgical Nursing: Assessment and Management of Clinical Problems* (7th ed., p. 1280). St. Louis, MO: Mosby.

604. A nurse is documenting nursing diagnoses for a client with elevated growth hormone (GH) levels. Which nursing diagnosis is *least* likely to be included in the client's plan of care?

1. Fluid volume deficit related to polyuria
2. Insomnia related to soft tissue swelling
3. Impaired communication related to speech difficulties
4. Disturbed body image related to undersized hands, feet, jaw, and soft body tissue

ANSWER: 4

GH excess causes overgrowth of the bones and soft tissues, resulting in a disturbance in body image. GH excess antagonizes the action of insulin causing hyperglycemia. Thus manifestations of diabetes mellitus occur: polyuria, polydipsia, and polyphagia. Sleep apnea occurs from upper airway narrowing and obstruction from increased amounts of pharyngeal tissue. Enlargement of the tongue may also result in speech difficulties.

➧ ***Test-taking Tip:*** *Focus on the issue, problems the client experiences with GH excess. The key phrase is "least likely." Select the nursing diagnoses that would be incorrect for the client with a GH excess.*

Content Area: Adult Health; *Category of Health Alteration:* Endocrine Management; *Integrated Processes:* Communication and Documentation; *Client Needs:* Physiological Integrity/Physiological Adaptation/Alterations in Body Systems; *Cognitive Level:* Application

Reference: Lewis, S., Heitkemper, M., Dirksen, S., O'Brien, P., & Bucher, L. (2007). *Medical-Surgical Nursing: Assessment and Management of Clinical Problems* (7th ed., pp. 1291–1292). St. Louis, MO: Mosby.

605. Which nursing actions are most appropriate when caring for a client diagnosed with diabetes insipidus (DI)? SELECT ALL THAT APPLY.

1. Monitoring fingerstick blood glucose before meals and at bedtime
2. Monitoring urine output hourly
3. Checking urine ketones
4. Administering desmopressin acetate (DDAVP)
5. Monitoring for signs of hyperkalemia
6. Monitoring daily weights

ANSWER: 2, 4, 6

DI is associated with decreased production and secretion of antidiuretic hormone (ADH). This causes increased urine output and increased plasma osmolality. Thus, urine output should be monitored hourly. DDAVP, administered orally, intravenously, or nasally, is an analog of ADH for ADH replacement. The client should be monitored for weight gain, hyponatremia, and water intoxication when taking DDAVP. Weight loss and hypernatremia are associated with DI. Elevated blood glucose levels are associated with diabetes mellitus, not DI. Checking urine ketones is unnecessary. Hypernatremia, not hyperkalemia, is associated with DI.

➧ ***Test-taking Tip:*** *Focus on the issue: management of DI.*

Content Area: Adult Health; *Category of Health Alteration:* Endocrine Management; *Integrated Processes:* Nursing Process Implementation; *Client Needs:* Physiological Integrity/Physiological Adaptation/Fluid and Electrolyte Imbalances; *Cognitive Level:* Application

Reference: Lewis, S., Heitkemper, M., Dirksen, S., O'Brien, P., & Bucher, L. (2007). *Medical-Surgical Nursing: Assessment and Management of Clinical Problems* (7th ed., pp. 1296–1297). St. Louis, MO: Mosby.

606. EBP A client has developed syndrome of inappropriate antidiuretic hormone (SIADH) secondary to a pituitary tumor. The client's symptoms include thirst, weight gain, and fatigue. The client's serum sodium is 127 mEq/L. Which physician order should the nurse anticipate when treating SIADH?

1. Elevate the head of the bed
2. Administer vasopressin intravenously (IV)
3. Fluid restriction of 800 to 1,000 mL per day
4. 0.3% sodium chloride IV infusion

ANSWER: 3

If symptoms are mild and serum sodium is greater than 125 mEq/L (125 mmol/L), treatment includes the restriction of fluid to 800 to 1,000 mL per day and discontinuation of medications that stimulate the release of antidiuretic hormone (ADH). The fluid restriction should result in a progressive rise in serum sodium concentration and osmolality and symptomatic improvement. Normal serum sodium levels are 136 to 146 mEq/L. The bed should be positioned flat or with no more than 10 degrees of elevation to enhance venous return to the heart and increase left atrial filling pressure, reducing ADH release. Vasopressin is an antidiuretic hormone, thus it will aggravate the client's problem. Hypertonic saline (3% to 5%) should be administered if the hyponatremia is severe (less than 120 mEq/L). Hypertonic solutions cause fluid to be drawn into the vascular system.

▸ ***Test-taking Tip:*** *Note that the client's symptoms are mild, but the serum sodium is low. Treatment is initially conservative.*

Content Area: Adult Health; *Category of Health Alteration:* Endocrine Management; *Integrated Processes:* Nursing Process Planning; *Client Needs:* Physiological Integrity/Physiological Adaptation/Alterations in Body Systems; *Cognitive Level:* Application

Reference: Lewis, S., Heitkemper, M., Dirksen, S., O'Brien, P., & Bucher, L. (2007). *Medical-Surgical Nursing: Assessment and Management of Clinical Problems* (7th ed., pp. 1295–1297). St. Louis, MO: Mosby.

EBP Reference: Johnson, A., & Criddle, L. (2005). Pass the salt: Indications for and implications of using hypertonic saline. *Critical Care Nurse*, 24, 36–48.

607. Which finding should the nurse anticipate when assessing a client newly diagnosed with diabetes insipidus (DI)?

1. Polyuria
2. Weight gain
3. Hyperglycemia
4. Profuse sweating and flushed skin

ANSWER: 1

DI is associated with decreased production or secretion of antidiuretic hormone (ADH). This causes increased urine output and increased plasma osmolality. Weight loss is secondary to polyuria. Hyperglycemia is associated with diabetes mellitus, not DI. Profuse sweating and flushed skin are associated with hyperthyroidism.

▸ ***Test-taking Tip:*** *The key word is "anticipate." Apply knowledge of signs and symptoms of DI to select the correct option.*

Content Area: Adult Health; *Category of Health Alteration:* Endocrine Management; *Integrated Processes:* Nursing Process Assessment; *Client Needs:* Physiological Integrity/Physiological Adaptation/Alterations in Body Systems; *Cognitive Level:* Application

Reference: Lewis, S., Heitkemper, M., Dirksen, S., O'Brien, P., & Bucher, L. (2007). *Medical-Surgical Nursing: Assessment and Management of Clinical Problems* (7th ed., p. 1296). St. Louis, MO: Mosby.

608. A client taking thyroid replacement hormone was involved in an automobile accident in another state and was hospitalized for a femur fracture. The physician did not prescribe replacement hormone because the client's medication history was unknown and the client was a poor historian at the time of the accident due to pain. A week after being hospitalized, a nurse notes that the client is becoming increasingly lethargic. Vital signs show a decreased blood pressure, respiratory rate, temperature, and pulse. Which actions should be taken by the nurse? Place each nursing action in the order of priority.

____ Warm the client
____ Administer intravenous fluids
____ Assist in ventilatory support
____ Administer the prescribed thyroxine

ANSWER: 3, 2, 1, 4

The client is experiencing myxedema coma. The initial action is to maintain a patent airway and administer oxygen. Fluid would be replaced next because of hypotension. The client should be warmed to prevent an increase in metabolic demand. Finally, thyroxine would be administered cautiously because the decreased metabolic rate and atherosclerosis of myxedema may result in angina.

Test-taking Tip: *Use the ABCs (airway, breathing, circulation) to establish priority and then the remaining actions.*

Content Area: Adult Health; *Category of Health Alteration:* Endocrine Management; *Integrated Processes:* Nursing Process Implementation; *Client Needs:* Physiological Integrity/Physiological Adaptation/Medical Emergencies; Safe and Effective Care Environment/Management of Care/Establishing Priorities; *Cognitive Level:* Analysis

Reference: Smeltzer, S., Bare, B., Hinkle, J., & Cheever, K. (2008). *Brunner & Suddarth's Textbook of Medical-Surgical Nursing* (11th ed., p. 1457). Philadelphia: Lippincott Williams & Wilkins.

609. A nurse is assessing a client following a total thyroidectomy. The client has a positive Trousseau's sign. Place an X on the illustration that supports the nurse's assessment finding.

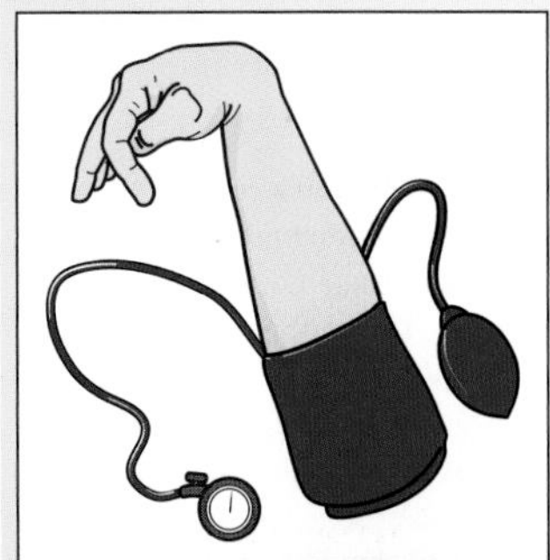

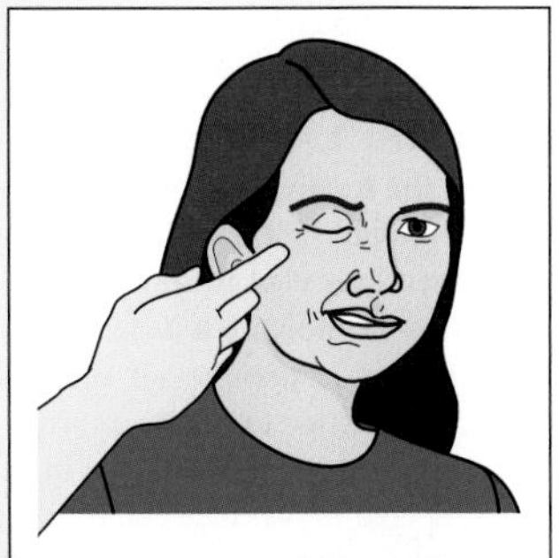

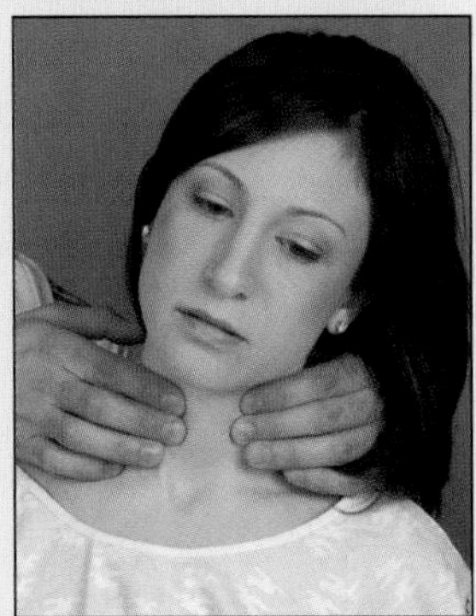

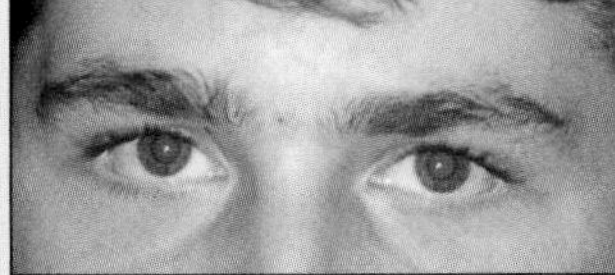

ANSWER:

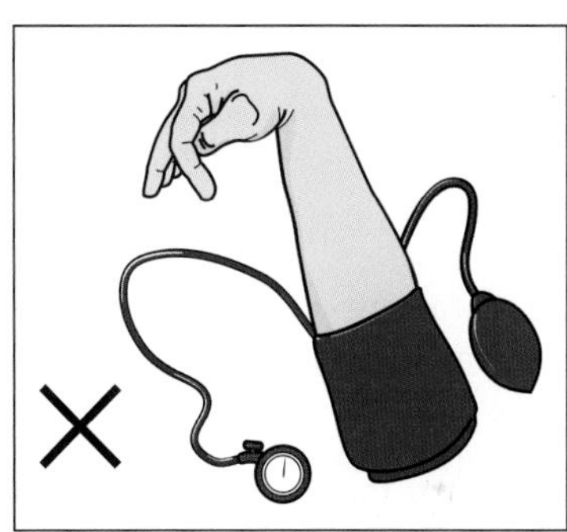

Trousseau's sign is carpal spasm as a result of hypocalcemia. During thyroid surgery, the parathyroid glands can be injured or removed affecting calcium metabolism resulting in hypocalcemia, nerve hyperirritability, and spasms. Chvostek's sign (illustration 2) is muscle twitching of the client's cheek when the facial nerve in front of the ear is tapped. Illustration 3 shows the method to palpate the thyroid gland using the posterior approach. Illustration 4 shows the red reflex over the pupil when performing an ophthalmic examination.

Test-taking Tip: *Apply knowledge of medical terminology to answer this question. Remember that Trousseau's sign involves spasms of the thumb and Chvostek's sign involves spasms of the cheek.*

Content Area: Adult Health; *Category of Health Alteration:* Endocrine Management; *Integrated Processes:* Nursing Process Assessment; *Client Needs:* Physiological Integrity/Physiological Adaptation/Fluid and Electrolyte Imbalances; *Cognitive Level:* Application

References: Lewis, S., Heitkemper, M., Dirksen, S., O'Brien, P., & Bucher, L. (2007). *Medical-Surgical Nursing: Assessment and Management of Clinical Problems* (7th ed., pp. 331, 1304). St. Louis, MO: Mosby; Dillon, P. (2007). *Nursing Health Assessment: A Critical Thinking, Case Studies Approach* (2nd ed., pp. 311, 357). Philadelphia: F. A. Davis.

610. EBP An agitated client is admitted to the emergency department (ED) with tachycardia, dyspnea, and intermittent chest palpitations. The client has a blood pressure of 170/110 mm Hg and heart rate of 130 beats per minute. The client's health history reveals thinning hair, recent 10-lb. weight loss, increased appetite, fine hand and tongue tremors, hyperreflexic tendon reflexes, and smooth moist skin. A physician writes orders for the client. Which order should the nurse implement first?

1. Obtain 12-lead electrocardiogram (ECG).
2. Administer propranolol (Inderal®) 2 mg intravenously q10–15min or until symptoms are controlled.
3. Administer propylthiouracil (PTU) 600 mg oral loading dose followed by 200 mg orally q4h.
4. Obtain thyroid-stimulating hormone (TSH), free T_4, and cardiac enzyme levels.

ANSWER: 2

The nurse should first administer propranolol as ordered by the physician. Propranolol is a beta-adrenergic blocker for symptomatic relief of thyrotoxicosis and decreasing peripheral conversion of T_4 to T_3. It controls cardiac and psychomotor manifestations within minutes. A beta blocker is also a first-line treatment for a client with acute coronary syndrome. Dysrhythmias can occur from beta-adrenergic receptor stimulation caused by excess thyroid hormone or following an acute coronary syndrome. PTU will inhibit the synthesis of thyroid hormone. Clinical effects may be seen as soon as 1 hour after administration. Decreased TSH and elevated free T_4 confirm the diagnosis of hyperthyroidism. Elevated cardiac enzymes confirm the diagnosis of acute coronary syndrome.

► ***Test-taking Tip:*** *Use the ABCs (airway, breathing, circulation) to establish priority. Controlling the client's blood pressure and heart rate is priority.*

Content Area: Adult Health; *Category of Health Alteration:* Endocrine Management; *Integrated Processes:* Nursing Process Implementation; *Client Needs:* Safe and Effective Care Environment/Management of Care/Establishing Priorities; *Cognitive Level:* Analysis

Reference: Lewis, S., Heitkemper, M., Dirksen, S., O'Brien, P., & Bucher, L. (2007). *Medical-Surgical Nursing: Assessment and Management of Clinical Problems* (7th ed., pp. 1300–1301). St. Louis, MO: Mosby.

EBP Reference: Schraga, E., & Manifold, C. (2006). Hyperthyroidism, thyroid storm, and Graves' disease. *E-Medicine*. Available at: www.emedicine.com/emerg/topic269.htm

611. A clinic nurse is teaching a client who has been diagnosed with hypothyroidism. Which instructions should the nurse provide regarding the use of levothyroxine sodium (Synthroid®)? SELECT ALL THAT APPLY.

1. Take the medication 1 hour before or 2 hours after breakfast.
2. Obtain a pulse rate before taking the medication, and call the clinic if the pulse rate is greater than 100 beats per minute.
3. Report adverse effects of the medication, including weight gain, cold intolerance, and alopecia.
4. Use levothyroxine sodium (Synthroid®) as a replacement hormone for diminished or absent thyroid function.
5. Have frequent laboratory monitoring to be sure your levels of T_3 and T_4 decrease.

ANSWER: 1, 2, 4

Taking the medication on an empty stomach promotes regular absorption. It should be taken in the morning to mimic normal hormone release and prevent insomnia. During initial dosage adjustment, tachycardia could indicate a dose that is too high. The replacement hormone is used in primary or secondary atrophy of the gland, after thyroidectomy, after excessive thyroid radiation, after the administration of antithyroid medications, or in congenital thyroid defects. Weight gain and cold intolerance could indicate that the dose is too low. Alopecia may indicate that the dose is too high. T_3 and T_4 should rise with treatment.

► ***Test-taking Tip:*** *Read each option carefully before selecting the correct options.*

Content Area: Adult Health; *Category of Health Alteration:* Endocrine Management; *Integrated Processes:* Teaching and Learning; *Client Needs:* Physiological Integrity/Pharmacological and Parenteral Therapies/Medication Administration; *Cognitive Level:* Application

Reference: Wilson, B., Shannon, M., Shields, K., & Stang, C. (2008). *Prentice Hall Nurse's Drug Guide 2008* (pp. 877–879). Upper Saddle River, NJ: Pearson Education.

612. A nurse is caring for a client who had a thyroidectomy 2 days ago. Based on the findings of the client's serum laboratory report, which medication should the nurse plan to administer first?

Serum Lab Test	Client's Value	Normal
BUN	24 mg/dL	5–25 mg/dL
Creatinine	1.2 mg/dL	0.5–1.5 mg/dL
Na	138 mEq/L	135–145 mEq/L
K	3.4 mEq/L	3.5–5.3 mEq/L
Calcium	6 mg/dL	9–11 mg/dL
Hgb	10.0 g/dL	13.5–17 g/dL
Hct	38%	40%–54%

1. K-dur® 20 mEq oral (PO) bid
2. Calcium gluconate 4.5 mEq intravenously (IV)
3. Dolasetron (Anzemet®) 12.5 mg IV as needed
4. Levothyroxine (Synthroid®) 50 mcg PO daily

ANSWER: 2

The nurse should administer calcium gluconate first. The serum calcium is critically low. Damage or removal of the parathyroid glands during surgery leads to hypocalcemia and tetany. Although the serum potassium is low, it is not as critically low as the serum calcium level. Dolasetron is an antiemetic. There is no indication from the laboratory analysis that the medication is needed at this time. The administration of levothyroxine, a thyroid hormone, is usually avoided immediately after surgery because the remaining thyroid tissue hypertrophies, recovering the capacity to produce sufficient hormone. Exogenous hormone inhibits pituitary production of thyroid-stimulating hormone and delays or prevents the restoration of thyroid tissue regeneration and function.

➧ ***Test-taking Tip:*** *The key word is "first." Analyze the laboratory report for critically low test values and use the process of elimination.*

Content Area: Adult Health; *Category of Health Alteration:* Endocrine Management; *Integrated Processes:* Nursing Process Planning; *Client Needs:* Safe and Effective Care Environment/Management of Care/Establishing Priorities; *Cognitive Level:* Synthesis

Reference: Lewis, S., Heitkemper, M., Dirksen, S., O'Brien, P., & Bucher, L. (2007). *Medical-Surgical Nursing: Assessment and Management of Clinical Problems* (7th ed., p. 1304). St. Louis, MO: Mosby.

613. A clinic nurse evaluates that a client's levothyroxine (Synthroid®) dose is too low when which findings are noted? SELECT ALL THAT APPLY.

1. Increased appetite
2. Decreased sweating
3. Apathy and fatigue
4. Paresthesias
5. Fine tremor of fingers and tongue
6. Slowed mental processes

ANSWER: 2, 3, 4, 6

Levothyroxine is used in treating hypothyroidism. Symptoms of hypothyroidism appear if the dose is too low and include decreased sweating, apathy and fatigue, paresthesias, and slowed mental processes. Increased appetite and fine tremors are signs of hyperthyroidism and can indicate the dose is too high.

➧ ***Test-taking Tip:*** *Recall that hypothyroidism is characterized by a slowing of body processes. Eliminate options 1 and 5 because these reflect increased sympathetic stimulation.*

Content Area: Adult Health; *Category of Health Alteration:* Endocrine Management; *Integrated Processes:* Nursing Process Evaluation; *Client Needs:* Physiological Integrity/Pharmacological and Parenteral Therapies/Expected Effects/Outcomes; *Cognitive Level:* Analysis

Reference: Lewis, S., Heitkemper, M., Dirksen, S., O'Brien, P., & Bucher, L. (2007). *Medical-Surgical Nursing: Assessment and Management of Clinical Problems* (7th ed., p. 1350). St. Louis, MO: Mosby.

614. Which nursing diagnosis should a nurse include when developing a plan of care for a client with hypothyroidism?

1. Diarrhea related to gastrointestinal hypermotility
2. Imbalance nutrition: less than body requirements related to calorie intake insufficient for metabolic rate
3. Activity intolerance related to increased metabolic rate
4. Anxiety related to forgetfulness, slowed speech, and impaired memory loss

ANSWER: 4

Disturbed thought processes can cause the client to be anxious. Diarrhea, imbalance nutrition related to insufficient calories, and activity intolerance related to increased metabolic rate are nursing diagnoses appropriate for hyperthyroidism.

➧ ***Test-taking Tip:*** *Focus on the issue: nursing diagnoses for hypothyroidism. Look for key words in each option. Eliminate option 1 because of the key word "hypermotility." Eliminate option 2 because of the key phrase "calorie intake insufficient." Eliminate option 3 because of the key phrase "increased metabolic rate."*

Content Area: Adult Health; *Category of Health Alteration:* Endocrine Management; *Integrated Processes:* Nursing Process Planning; *Client Needs:* Physiological Integrity/Physiological Adaptation/Alterations in Body Systems; *Cognitive Level:* Application

Reference: Lewis, S., Heitkemper, M., Dirksen, S., O'Brien, P., & Bucher, L. (2007). *Medical-Surgical Nursing: Assessment and Management of Clinical Problems* (7th ed., pp. 1307–1308). St. Louis, MO: Mosby.

615. A female client is being treated with radioactive iodine (RAI) therapy for an enlarged thyroid gland. The client asks if there are any precautions that are needed during RAI therapy. Which is the nurse's best response?

1. "No precautions are necessary. You receive radiation in the form of a capsule that will target and destroy the thyroid tissue only."
2. "Though a pregnancy test has confirmed that you are not pregnant, use contraceptives or abstain from sexual intercourse to avoid conceiving during treatment."
3. "Because maximum effects may not be seen for 6 months, you will need to continue taking the antithyroid medication and propranolol until the effects of radiation become apparent."
4. "Although RAI is usually effective, a few individuals will need life-long thyroid hormone replacement due to posttreatment hypothyroidism."

ANSWER: 2

Pregnancy should be postponed for at least 6 months after treatment. RAI is contraindicated during pregnancy because it crosses the placenta. Approximately 5% of individuals require more than one dose to destroy overactive thyroid cells. Precautions about avoiding pregnancy should be advised. Almost all of the radioactive iodine that enters and is retained by the body is concentrated in the thyroid gland and destroys thyroid tissue without jeopardizing other radiosensitive tissues. Symptoms of hyperthyroidism may subside in 3 to 4 weeks, but the maximum effects may not be seen for 3 to 4 months. Clients should continue with the antithyroid medication and propranolol. Almost 80% of individuals experience posttreatment hypothyroidism.

***Test-taking Tip:** The key word is "precaution." Eliminate option 4. Though correct, it does not address a precaution during RAI therapy.*

Content Area: Adult Health; *Category of Health Alteration:* Endocrine Management; *Integrated Processes:* Communication and Documentation; *Client Needs:* Physiological Integrity/Reduction of Risk Potential/Therapeutic Procedures; *Cognitive Level:* Analysis

References: Lewis, S., Heitkemper, M., Dirksen, S., O'Brien, P., & Bucher, L. (2007). *Medical-Surgical Nursing: Assessment and Management of Clinical Problems* (7th ed., p. 1301). St. Louis, MO: Mosby; Smeltzer, S., Bare, B., Hinkle, J., & Cheever, K. (2008). *Brunner & Suddarth's Textbook of Medical-Surgical Nursing* (11th ed., p. 1460). Philadelphia: Lippincott Williams & Wilkins.

616. A nurse is teaching a client experiencing hypoparathyroidism resulting from a lack of parathyroid hormone (PTH) about foods to consume. Which should be included on a list of appropriate foods for a client experiencing hypoparathyroidism?

1. Dark green vegetables, soybeans, and tofu
2. Spinach, strawberries, and yogurt
3. Whole grain bread, milk, and liver
4. Rhubarb, yellow vegetables, and fish

ANSWER: 1

Hypoparathyroidism from lack of PTH produces chronic hypocalcemia. Foods consumed should be high in calcium. Foods containing oxalic acid (spinach, rhubarb), and phytic acid (whole grains) reduce calcium absorption.

***Test-taking Tip:** Recall that hypoparathyroidism produces hypocalcemia.*

Content Area: Adult Health; *Category of Health Alteration:* Endocrine Management; *Integrated Processes:* Teaching and Learning; *Client Needs:* Physiological Integrity/Basic Care and Comfort/Nutrition and Oral Hydration; *Cognitive Level:* Application

Reference: Lewis, S., Heitkemper, M., Dirksen, S., O'Brien, P., & Bucher, L. (2007). *Medical-Surgical Nursing: Assessment and Management of Clinical Problems* (7th ed., p. 1311). St. Louis, MO: Mosby.

617. EBP Which nursing diagnoses should the nurse document in the plan of care for a client diagnosed with Cushing's syndrome? SELECT ALL THAT APPLY.

1. Fluid and electrolyte imbalance related to hyperkalemia and hypernatremia
2. Body image disturbance related to weight gain and facial hair
3. Risk for infection related to a decreased inflammatory response
4. Risk for injury related to weakness and fatigue
5. Disturbed thought processes related to mood swings and irritability

ANSWER: 2, 3, 4, 5

All nursing diagnoses should be included except fluid and electrolyte imbalance related to hyperkalemia and hypernatremia. The electrolyte imbalance seen in Cushing's syndrome is hypokalemia, not hyperkalemia.

***Test-taking Tip:** Focus on the manifestations of Cushing's syndrome to select the correct options.*

Content Area: Adult Health; *Category of Health Alteration:* Endocrine Management; *Integrated Processes:* Nursing Process Planning; *Client Needs:* Physiological Integrity/Physiological Adaptation/Illness Management; *Cognitive Level:* Analysis

Reference: Smeltzer, S., Bare, B., Hinkle, J., & Cheever, K. (2008). *Brunner & Suddarth's Textbook of Medical-Surgical Nursing* (11th ed., p. 1481). Philadelphia: Lippincott Williams & Wilkins.

EBP Reference: Ilias, I., Torpy, D., Pacak, K., Mullen, N., Wesley, R., et al. (2005). Cushing's syndrome due to ectopic corticotropin secretion: Twenty years' experience at the National Institutes of Health. *Journal of Clinical Endocrinology & Metabolism*, 90(8), 4955–4962.

618. EBP A client is admitted to the hospital with a diagnosis of Cushing's disease. A nurse reviews the client's laboratory results. Which findings would support a diagnosis of Cushing's syndrome? SELECT ALL THAT APPLY.

1. Hypokalemia
2. Eosinophilia
3. Hypocalcemia
4. Hyperglycemia
5. Thrombocytopenia
6. Elevated serum plasma cortisol

ANSWER: 1, 4, 6

Cushing's disease results from excessive adrenocortical activity producing hyperglycemia, hypokalemia, elevated plasma cortisol, and elevated adrenocorticotropic hormone levels. A decrease of eosinophils, rather than an increase, and hypercalcemia (high serum calcium levels), rather than hypocalcemia, are associated with Cushing's disease. Thrombocytopenia (low platelets) is not associated with the disorder.

➧ ***Test-taking Tip:*** *Focus on the effects of excess glucocorticoids and mineralocorticoids on the body.*

Content Area: Adult Health; *Category of Health Alteration:* Endocrine Management; *Integrated Processes:* Nursing Process Analysis; *Client Needs:* Physiological Integrity/Reduction of Risk Potential/Laboratory Values; *Cognitive Level:* Analysis

Reference: Smeltzer, S., Bare, B., Hinkle, J., & Cheever, K. (2008). *Brunner & Suddarth's Textbook of Medical-Surgical Nursing* (11th ed., p. 1480). Philadelphia: Lippincott Williams & Wilkins.

EBP Reference: Findling, J., & Raff, H. (2005). Screening and diagnosis of Cushing's syndrome. *Endocrinology and Metabolism Clinics of North America*, 34, 385.

619. A nurse's assessment of a client diagnosed with Cushing's syndrome includes the following findings: 4+ pitting leg edema, blood glucose 140 mg/dL, irregular heart rate, and ecchymosis on the right arm. Which action should be taken by the nurse first?

1. Weigh the client.
2. Administer insulin.
3. Notify the physician.
4. Measure the client's abdominal girth.

ANSWER: 3

Cushing's syndrome causes overproduction of aldosterone, retention of sodium and water, and excretion of potassium. An irregular heart rate can occur from hypokalemia. The physician should be notified immediately to obtain serum laboratory studies and to treat the irregular heart rate and hypokalemia if present. The other actions are appropriate for the client with Cushing's syndrome, but the first action addresses the major problem.

➧ ***Test-taking Tip:*** *The key word is "first." The best action should address the client's major problem to prevent complications. Use the ABCs (airway, breathing, circulation) to determine the client's major problem.*

Content Area: Adult Health; *Category of Health Alteration:* Endocrine Management; *Integrated Processes:* Nursing Process Implementation; *Client Needs:* Physiological Integrity/Physiological Adaptation/Medical Emergencies; *Cognitive Level:* Analysis

Reference: Lewis, S., Heitkemper, M., Dirksen, S., O'Brien, P., & Bucher, L. (2007). *Medical-Surgical Nursing: Assessment and Management of Clinical Problems* (7th ed., pp. 1312–1314). St. Louis, MO: Mosby.

620. A client diagnosed with Cushing's syndrome is admitted with fluid volume overload. The client weighed 190 pounds on admission to the hospital. After treatment, the client weighs 179 pounds. The nurse estimated that the amount of fluid the client lost was _______ mL.

ANSWER: 5,000

One liter of fluid (1,000 mL) weighs approximately 2.2 lb. An 11-lb weight loss equals 5,000 mL (11 lb/2.2 lb = 5.5 L × 1,000 mL per L = 5,000 mL). Use a proportion formula:
2.2 lb : 1,000 mL :: 11 lb : X mL
2.2X = 11,000
X = 11,000/2.2
X = 5,000

➧ ***Test-taking Tip:*** *Recall that 1 L of fluid is approximately equal to 2.2 lb.*

Content Area: Adult Health; *Category of Health Alteration:* Endocrine Management; *Integrated Processes:* Nursing Process Analysis; *Client Needs:* Physiological Integrity/Physiological Adaptation/Fluid and Electrolyte Imbalances; *Cognitive Level:* Analysis

Reference: Lewis, S., Heitkemper, M., Dirksen, S., O'Brien, P., & Bucher, L. (2007). *Medical-Surgical Nursing: Assessment and Management of Clinical Problems* (7th ed., p. 323). St. Louis, MO: Mosby.

621. Which medication should a nurse plan to administer to a client admitted in Addisonian crisis?

1. Regular insulin
2. Ketoconazole (Nizoral®)
3. Sodium nitroprusside (Nipride®)
4. Hydrocortisone (Solu-Cortef®)

ANSWER: 4

Addisonian crisis results from insufficient secretion of glucocorticoids and mineralocorticoids from the adrenal cortex. Hydrocortisone is a corticosteroid used in the absence of sufficient glucocorticoid production. Hypoglycemia, not hyperglycemia, is associated with Addisonian crisis. Ketoconazole is a systemic antifungal that has an unlabeled use in treating Cushing's syndrome as an adrenal enzyme inhibitor. Addisonian crisis produces severe hypotension; sodium nitroprusside is used to treat severe hypertension.

***Test-taking Tip:** Focus on the hormones secreted by the adrenal cortex to answer this question.*

Content Area: Adult Health; *Category of Health Alteration:* Endocrine Management; *Integrated Processes:* Nursing Process Planning; *Client Needs:* Physiological Integrity/Physiological Adaptation/Medical Emergencies; *Cognitive Level:* Application

Reference: Smeltzer, S., Bare, B., Hinkle, J., & Cheever, K. (2008). *Brunner & Suddarth's Textbook of Medical-Surgical Nursing* (11th ed., pp. 1476–1478). Philadelphia: Lippincott Williams & Wilkins.

---

622. A nurse is caring for a client who is hospitalized with adrenocortical insufficiency. The nurse reviews the client's serum laboratory values and immediately notifies the physician. Which serum laboratory value most likely prompted the nurse to notify the physician?

1. WBC 11.0 K/μL
2. Glucose 138 mg/dL
3. Sodium 148 mEq/L
4. Potassium 6.2 mEq/L

ANSWER: 4

The normal range for serum potassium is 3.8 to 5.0 mEq/L. Adrenocortical insufficiency causes excessive potassium reabsorption producing hyperkalemia. Hyperkalemia can result in dysrhythmias and cardiac arrest if not treated promptly. An acute infection can precipitate Addisonian crisis, but the white blood cell (WBC) count is on the high side of normal. Hypoglycemia and hyponatremia, not hyperglycemia nor hypernatremia, are associated with adrenocortical insufficiency. Both values are elevated, but not alarmingly. Normal serum glucose is 70–110 mg/dL and serum sodium is 136–146 mEq/L.

***Test-taking Tip:** Focus on the lab value that would be most life threatening.*

Content Area: Adult Health; *Category of Health Alteration:* Endocrine Management; *Integrated Processes:* Nursing Process Implementation; *Client Needs:* Physiological Integrity/Physiological Adaptation/Fluid and Electrolyte Imbalances; *Cognitive Level:* Application

Reference: Smeltzer, S., Bare, B., Hinkle, J., & Cheever, K. (2008). *Brunner & Suddarth's Textbook of Medical-Surgical Nursing* (11th ed., p. 1477). Philadelphia: Lippincott Williams & Wilkins.

---

623. Which clinical change should indicate to a nurse that the therapy for a client with Addisonian crisis is effective?

1. An increase of 25 mm Hg in the client's systolic blood pressure
2. A decrease of 25 mm Hg in the client's systolic blood pressure
3. An increase in the client's serum potassium level from 3.4 to 4.8 mEq/dL
4. An increase in the client's total serum calcium level from 8.6 to 10.0 mg/dL

ANSWER: 1

An increase in blood pressure is indicative of effective therapy. Addisonian crisis is caused by adrenocortical insufficiency with disturbances of sodium and potassium metabolism resulting in hyponatremia and hyperkalemia. Option 2 indicates therapy is not effective. The depletion of sodium and water causes severe dehydration and hypotension. Effective therapy would lower potassium levels. A serum potassium level of 3.4 to 4.8 mEq/dL is within the normal range. The normal serum calcium level is 8.6 to 10.2 mg/dL.

***Test-taking Tip:** The key word is "effective." Select the option that would show improvement for the client in Addisonian crisis. Use the ABCs (airway, breathing, circulation) to select an answer.*

Content Area: Adult Health; *Category of Health Alteration:* Endocrine Management; *Integrated Processes:* Nursing Process Evaluation; *Client Needs:* Physiological Integrity/Physiological Adaptation/Illness Management; *Cognitive Level:* Application

Reference: Smeltzer, S., Bare, B., Hinkle, J., & Cheever, K. (2008). *Brunner & Suddarth's Textbook of Medical-Surgical Nursing* (11th ed., pp. 1477–1478, 2583). Philadelphia: Lippincott Williams & Wilkins.

624. What should be a nurse's priority when admitting a client with suspected hyperaldosteronism?

1. Preparing the client for a computed tomography (CT) scan
2. Administering medications to treat headache
3. Obtaining an electrocardiogram (ECG) to assess for cardiac dysrhythmias
4. Protecting the client from falls due to muscle weakness

ANSWER: 3

The excessive aldosterone secretion of hyperaldosteronism causes sodium retention and potassium and hydrogen ion excretion. The potassium-wasting produces hypokalemia, which can cause life-threatening dysrhythmias. Assessing for life-threatening conditions is priority. Adenomas can be localized by a CT scan, but this is not priority. Headache occurs from hypertension, but this is not priority. Hypokalemia also produces generalized muscle weakness and fatigue which can predispose the client to falls.

*▶ **Test-taking Tip:** The key word is "priority." Use the ABCs (airway, breathing, circulation) and nursing process to establish the priority.*

Content Area: Adult Health; *Category of Health Alteration:* Endocrine Management; *Integrated Processes:* Nursing Process Implementation; *Client Needs:* Safe and Effective Care Environment/Management of Care/Establishing Priorities; *Cognitive Level:* Analysis

Reference: Lewis, S., Heitkemper, M., Dirksen, S., O'Brien, P., & Bucher, L. (2007). *Medical-Surgical Nursing: Assessment and Management of Clinical Problems* (7th ed., p. 1319). St. Louis, MO: Mosby.

---

625. A nurse is preparing to discharge a client following a unilateral adrenalectomy to treat hyperaldosteronism caused by an adenoma. Which instruction should be included in this client's discharge teaching?

1. Avoid foods high in potassium.
2. Self-monitor the blood pressure.
3. Discontinue medications taken prior to the adrenalectomy.
4. Carry an emergency kit that includes epinephrine.

ANSWER: 2

The hallmark of hyperaldosteronism is hypertension. Unilateral adrenalectomy is successful in controlling hypertension in only 80% of clients with adenoma, so the client should continue to self-monitor the blood pressure. There are no dietary potassium restrictions. Maintenance therapy for hypertension may include the administration of spironolactone, a potassium-sparing diuretic. However, hyperaldosteronism causes excretion of potassium. The client may still need medications to treat hyperaldosteronism after adrenalectomy. Clients with Addison's disease are instructed to carry an emergency kit with hydrocortisone.

*▶ **Test-taking Tip:** Focus on the problem, hyperaldosteronism, and the hypertension associated with the condition.*

Content Area: Adult Health; *Category of Health Alteration:* Endocrine Management; *Integrated Processes:* Teaching and Learning; *Client Needs:* Health Promotion and Maintenance/Self-Care; *Cognitive Level:* Application

Reference: Lewis, S., Heitkemper, M., Dirksen, S., O'Brien, P., & Bucher, L. (2007). *Medical-Surgical Nursing: Assessment and Management of Clinical Problems* (7th ed., pp. 1317, 1319–1320). St. Louis, MO: Mosby.

---

626. A nurse is caring for a client who is experiencing symptoms associated with pheochromocytoma. Which intervention should be included in the care of this client?

1. Offer distractions such as television or music.
2. Encourage frequent intake of oral fluids.
3. Assist with ambulation at least three times a day.
4. Administer nicardipine (Cardene®) to control hypertension.

ANSWER: 4

Pheochromocytoma is characterized by a tumor of the adrenal medulla that produces excessive catecholamines (epinephrine and norepinephrine). The increased catecholamines result in hypertension. Until the tumor can be surgically removed, calcium channel blockers are used to control blood pressure and other excess catecholamine symptoms. Noise can increase sympathetic nervous system stimulation and provoke a hypertensive and anxiety attack. A calm environment and reduced activity is needed to prevent hypertensive crisis prior to surgery.

*▶ **Test-taking Tip:** Knowledge of pheochromocytoma is needed to answer this question. Use medical terminology to decipher the meaning of the term. Recall that "oma" refers to tumor.*

Content Area: Adult Health; *Category of Health Alteration:* Endocrine Management; *Integrated Processes:* Nursing Process Planning; *Client Needs:* Physiological Integrity/Physiological Adaptation/Illness Management; *Cognitive Level:* Application

Reference: Lewis, S., Heitkemper, M., Dirksen, S., O'Brien, P., & Bucher, L. (2007). *Medical-Surgical Nursing: Assessment and Management of Clinical Problems* (7th ed., p. 1320). St. Louis, MO: Mosby.

Test 17: **Adult Health: Gastrointestinal Management**

627. EBP A nurse is assigned to four clients who have been diagnosed with gastric ulcers. Which one of these clients should the nurse conclude is most at risk to develop gastrointestinal (GI) bleeding?

1. A 40-year-old client who is positive for *Helicobacter pylori (H. pylori)*
2. A 45-year-old client who drinks 4 ounces of alcohol a day
3. A 70-year-old client who takes aspirin (Ecotrin®) 81 mg daily to prevent coronary artery disease
4. A 30-year-old pregnant client who uses acetaminophen (Tylenol®) as needed for headaches

ANSWER: 3

Aging is the most critical risk factor for GI bleeding. Aspirin use is one of the most common predisposing factors. The presence of *H. pylori* has not been proven to predispose to GI bleeding, and although alcohol is associated with gastric mucosal injury, its causative role in bleeding is unclear. Pregnancy and acetaminophen usage do not predispose to GI bleeding.

➧ ***Test-taking Tip:*** *Eliminate the obviously wrong answer option 4; note that aspirin, like NSAIDs, increases the risk of gastric damage.*

Content Area: Adult Health; *Category of Health Alteration:* Gastrointestinal Management; *Integrated Processes:* Nursing Process Analysis; *Client Need:* Safe and Effective Care Environment/ Management of Care/Establishing Priorities; *Cognitive Level:* Analysis

Reference: Monahan, F., Sands, J., Neighbors, M., Marek, J., & Green, C. (2007). *Phipps' Medical-Surgical Nursing: Health and Illness Perspectives* (8th ed., p. 1210). St. Louis, MO: Mosby.

EBP Reference: Antman, E., Bennett, J., Daugherty, A., Furberg, C., Roberts, H., et al. American Heart Association. (2007). Use of nonsteroidal anti-inflammatory drugs: An update for clinicians: a scientific statement from the American Heart Association. *Circulation,* 115(12), 1634–1642.

---

628. A nurse is assessing a client who is 24 hours postgastrointestinal (GI) hemorrhage. The assessment findings include blood urea nitrogen (BUN) of 40 mg/dL and serum creatinine of 0.8 mg/dL. After reviewing the assessment findings, the nurse should:

1. immediately call the physician to report these results.
2. monitor urine output as this may be a sign of kidney failure.
3. document the findings and continue monitoring the client.
4. encourage the client to limit his dietary protein intake.

ANSWER: 3

The BUN can be elevated after a significant GI hemorrhage related to the breakdown of blood proteins, which release nitrogen that is then converted to urea. No treatment is required. If acute kidney failure is present, both the BUN and creatinine would be elevated. Limiting protein intake in the presence of healthy kidneys is unnecessary.

➧ ***Test-taking Tip:*** *Focus on the situation: 24 hours post–GI hemorrhage. Knowledge of laboratory values and what causes increases in the BUN is the key to correctly answering this question.*

Content Area: Adult Health; *Category of Health Alteration:* Gastrointestinal Management; *Integrated Processes:* Nursing Process Implementation; *Client Need:* Physiological Integrity/Physiologic Adaptation/Illness Management; *Cognitive Level:* Analysis

Reference: Lewis, S., Heitkemper, M., Dirksen, S., O'Brien, P., & Bucher, L. (2007). *Medical-Surgical Nursing: Assessment and Management of Clinical Problems* (7th ed., pp. 1027, 1213). St. Louis, MO: Mosby.

---

629. An experienced nurse explains to a new nurse that the definitive diagnosis of peptic ulcer disease (PUD) involves:

1. a urea breath test.
2. upper gastrointestinal endoscopy with biopsy.
3. barium contrast studies.
4. the string test.

ANSWER: 2

The gastric mucosa can be visualized with an endoscope. A biopsy is possible to differentiate PUD from gastric cancer and to obtain tissue specimens to identify *Helicobacter pylori.* A urea breath test and a string test only test for the presence of *H. pylori.* Barium studies do not provide an opportunity for biopsy and *H. pylori* testing.

➧ ***Test-taking Tip:*** *The key words are "definitive diagnosis." This positive diagnosis usually involves actually viewing the tissue or taking biopsies.*

Content Area: Adult Health; *Category of Health Alteration:* Gastrointestinal Management; *Integrated Processes:* Teaching and Learning; *Client Need:* Health Promotion and Maintenance/Health Screening; *Cognitive Level:* Comprehension

References: Lewis, S., Heitkemper, M., Dirksen, S., O'Brien, P., & Bucher, L. (2007). *Medical-Surgical Nursing: Assessment and Management of Clinical Problems* (7th ed., p. 1018). St. Louis, MO: Mosby; Monahan, F., Sands, J., Neighbors, M., Marek, J., & Green, C. (2007). *Phipps' Medical-Surgical Nursing: Health and Illness Perspectives* (8th ed., p. 1212). St. Louis, MO: Mosby.

630. EBP During a hospital admission history, a nurse suspects gastrointestinal reflux disease (GERD) when the client says:

1. "I have been experiencing headaches immediately after eating."
2. "I have been waking up at night lately with a burning feeling in my chest."
3. "I have been waking up at night sweating."
4. "Immediately after eating I feel sleepy."

ANSWER: 2

Heartburn, which is described as a burning, tight sensation in the lower sternum, is the most common symptom of GERD. If will often wake a client from sleep. Headaches, night sweats, and postprandial sleepiness are symptoms not related to GERD.

Test-taking Tip: *Focus on what the question is actually asking: "symptoms of GERD."*

Content Area: Adult Health; *Category of Health Alteration:* Gastrointestinal Management; *Integrated Processes:* Nursing Process Assessment; *Client Need:* Physiological Integrity/Reduction of Risk Potential/System Specific Assessments; *Cognitive Level:* Analysis

Reference: Lewis, S., Heitkemper, M., Dirksen, S., O'Brien, P., & Bucher, L. (2007). *Medical-Surgical Nursing: Assessment and Management of Clinical Problems* (7th ed., p. 1004). St. Louis, MO: Mosby.

EBP Reference: University of Michigan Health System. (2007). *Gastroesophageal Reflux Disease (GERD)*. Available at: www.guideline.gov/summary/summary.aspx?doc_id=10631&nbr=005568&string=gastroesophageal+AND+reflux+AND+disease

---

631. EBP To assist a client to manage and decrease the sensation of nausea, which nonpharmacological intervention should a nurse recommend?

1. Drinking tea made from ginger root
2. Changing positions quickly when moving
3. Decreasing food intake
4. Playing loud rock music

ANSWER: 1

Ginger has demonstrated antiemetic properties, and it also has analgesic and sedative effects on gastrointestinal motility. Avoidance of sudden changes in position and decreasing activity are recommended to control nausea. All food should be stopped when nausea is present to prevent stomach stretching and stimulation of the afferent nerve fibers. A quiet, calm environment is recommended to decrease nausea.

Test-taking Tip: *Focus on the physiological causes of nausea, then eliminate options 2 and 3.*

Content Area: Adult Health; *Category of Health Alteration:* Gastrointestinal Management; *Integrated Processes:* Nursing Process Implementation; *Client Need:* Physiological Integrity/Basic Care and Comfort/Nonpharmacological Comfort Interventions; *Cognitive Level:* Application

Reference: Lewis, S., Heitkemper, M., Dirksen, S., O'Brien, P., & Bucher, L. (2007). *Medical-Surgical Nursing: Assessment and Management of Clinical Problems* (7th ed., pp. 991, 993). St. Louis, MO: Mosby.

EBP Reference: Ulbricht, C., & Basch, E. (2005). *Natural Standard Herb and Supplement Reference: Evidence-Based Clinical Reviews.* St. Louis, MO: Mosby.

---

632. A nurse, writing a nursing diagnosis in the care plan for a female client after bariatric surgery, should write, "Risk for nausea related to:

1. overfilling of the stomach pouch."
2. being female."
3. the lower half of the stomach becoming spastic."
4. handling of the duodenum with resulting inflammatory response."

ANSWER: 1

Bariatric surgery results in the construction of a small pouch (10–30 mL) in the upper part of the stomach. Overfilling of this pouch stimulates afferent nerve fibers, which relay information to the chemoreceptor trigger zone in the brain. Bariatric surgery is performed on both men and women. The function of the lower half of the stomach is not affected by this surgery, and the duodenum is not handled during this surgery.

Test-taking Tip: *Since the second half of a nursing diagnosis (the related to part) should focus on signs and symptoms for nursing interventions, select option 1, since the nurse can intervene with this situation. Understanding the causes of nausea and knowledge of the generic bariatric surgical procedure is required to answer correctly.*

Content Area: Adult Health; *Category of Health Alteration:* Gastrointestinal Management; *Integrated Processes:* Nursing Process Analysis; Communication and Documentation; *Client Need:* Physiological Integrity/Reduction of Risk Potential/Potential for Complications from Surgical Procedures and Health Alterations; *Cognitive Level:* Application

References: Lehne, R. (2007). *Pharmacology for Nursing Care* (6th ed., p. 911). St. Louis, MO: Saunders; Smeltzer, S., Bare, B., Hinkle, J., & Cheever, K. (2008). *Brunner & Suddarth's Textbook of Medical-Surgical Nursing* (11th ed., p. 1220). Philadelphia: Lippincott Williams & Wilkins.

633. A nurse is discharging a client after Billroth II surgery (gastrojejunostomy). To assist the client to control dumping syndrome, the client's discharge instructions should include:

1. drinking fluids with meals.
2. eating a high-carbohydrate, low-protein diet.
3. waiting at least 5 hours between meals.
4. lying down for 20 to 30 minutes after meals.

ANSWER: 4

Lying down after meals slows the passage of the food bolus into the intestine. To control dumping syndrome, the meal size must be reduced. Drinking fluids at meal time increases the size of the food bolus that enters the stomach. Carbohydrates are more rapidly digested than fats and proteins and would cause the food bolus to pass quickly into the intestine, increasing the likelihood that dumping syndrome would occur. Meals high in carbohydrates result in postprandial hypoglycemia, which is considered a variant of dumping syndrome. Small frequent meals are recommended to decrease dumping syndrome.

Test-taking Tip: *Focus on the anatomical changes that cause dumping syndrome.*

Content Area: Adult Health; *Category of Health Alteration:* Gastrointestinal Management; *Integrated Processes:* Nursing Process Implementation; Teaching and Learning; *Client Need:* Physiological Integrity/Reduction of Risk Potential/Therapeutic Procedures; *Cognitive Level:* Application

Reference: Lewis, S., Heitkemper, M., Dirksen, S., O'Brien, P., & Bucher, L. (2007). *Medical-Surgical Nursing: Assessment and Management of Clinical Problems* (7th ed., p. 1027). St. Louis, MO: Mosby.

---

634. After Billroth II surgery (gastrojejunostomy), a client experiences weakness, diaphoresis, anxiety, and palpations 2 hours after a high carbohydrate meal. A nurse should interpret that these symptoms indicate the development of:

1. steatorrhea.
2. duodenal reflux.
3. hypervolemic fluid overload.
4. postprandial hypoglycemia.

ANSWER: 4

When a client eats a large amount of carbohydrates at a meal, the rapid absorption of glucose from the chime results in hyperglycemia. This elevated glucose stimulates insulin production, which, in turn, causes an abrupt lowering of the blood glucose level, resulting in hypoglycemic symptoms. Although steatorrhea may occur after gastric resection, the symptoms are fatty stools with a foul odor. The symptoms of duodenal reflux are abdominal pain and vomiting, and they are not related to food intake. Symptoms of fluid overload would include increased blood pressure, edema, and weight gain.

Test-taking Tip: *Focus on the symptoms that are characteristic of hypoglycemia.*

Content Area: Adult Health; *Category of Health Alteration:* Gastrointestinal Management; *Integrated Processes:* Nursing Process Analysis; *Client Need:* Physiologic Integrity/Reduction of Risk Potential/Potential for Complications from Health Alterations; *Cognitive Level:* Nursing Process Analysis

References: Lewis, S., Heitkemper, M., Dirksen, S., O'Brien, P., & Bucher, L. (2007). *Medical-Surgical Nursing: Assessment and Management of Clinical Problems* (7th ed., p. 1026). St. Louis, MO: Mosby; Monahan, F., Sands, J., Neighbors, M., Marek, J., & Green, C. (2007). *Phipps' Medical-Surgical Nursing: Health and Illness Perspectives* (8th ed., p. 1224). St. Louis, MO: Mosby.

---

635. A nurse is performing an initial postoperative assessment on a client following upper gastrointestinal surgery. The client has a nasogastric tube to low, intermittent suction. To best assess the client for the presence of bowel sounds, the nurse should:

1. place the stethoscope to the left of the umbilicus.
2. turn off the nasogastric suction.
3. use the bell of the stethoscope.
4. turn the suction on the nasogastric tube to continuous.

ANSWER: 2

When listening for bowel sounds on a client who has a nasogastric tube to suction, the nurse should turn off the suction during auscultation to prevent mistaking the suction sound for bowel sounds. The diaphragm of the stethoscope should be utilized for bowel sounds and the bell for abdominal vascular sounds, such as bruits. When the client has hypoactive bowel sounds, which would be expected in a postsurgical client, the nurse should begin listening over the ileocecal valve in the right lower abdominal quadrant, as this normally is a very active area.

Test-taking Tip: *Focus on the presence of the nasogastric tube attached to suction, as this will alter the assessment procedure.*

Content Area: Adult Health; *Category of Health Alteration:* Gastrointestinal Management; *Integrated Processes:* Nursing Process Assessment; *Client Need:* Health Promotion and Maintenance/Techniques of Physical Assessment; *Cognitive Level:* Application

Reference: Dillon, P. (2007). *Nursing Health Assessment: A Critical Thinking, Case Studies Approach* (2nd ed., pp. 585–586). Philadelphia: F. A. Davis.

636. An experienced nurse is most likely to teach a new nurse that surgery to repair a hiatal hernia is becoming more common to prevent the emergency complication of:

1. severe dysphagia.
2. esophageal edema.
3. hernia strangulation.
4. aspiration.

ANSWER: 3

Like an abdominal hernia, a hiatal hernia can become strangulated. Although dysphagia and aspiration are complications of hiatal hernia, they are not emergency conditions. Esophageal edema is not a complication of hiatal hernia.

➧ ***Test-taking Tip:*** *Note the key phrase "most likely." Focus on general complications related to hernias.*

Content Area: Adult Health; *Category of Health Alteration:* Gastrointestinal Management; *Integrated Processes:* Teaching and Learning; *Client Need:* Physiological Integrity/Reduction of Risk Potential/Potential for Complications from Health Alterations; *Cognitive Level:* Application

Reference: Monahan, F., Sands, J., Neighbors, M., Marek, J., & Green, C. (2007). *Phipps' Medical-Surgical Nursing: Health and Illness Perspectives* (8th ed., p. 1193). St. Louis, MO: Mosby.

---

637. A nurse, caring for a client with a Zenker's diverticulum, knows that the priority nursing diagnosis for this client should be:

1. Pain related to gastric reflux.
2. Risk for aspiration related to regurgitation of food accumulated in the diverticula.
3. Constipation related to anatomical changes of the sigmoid colon.
4. Altered nutrition, less than body requirements related to dysphagia.

ANSWER: 2

Zenker's diverticulum is an outpouching of the esophagus near the hypopharyngeal sphincter. Food can become trapped in the diverticula and cause aspiration. The client may have difficulty with heartburn and weight loss, but these do not take priority over aspiration. Constipation is not a concern with this disorder.

➧ ***Test-taking Tip:*** *Note the key word "priority." Focus on the term "Zenker's diverticulum" and how this alters client anatomy. Use the ABCs (airway, breathing, circulation) to identify the priority.*

Content Area: Adult Health; *Category of Health Alteration:* Gastrointestinal Management; *Integrated Processes:* Nursing Process Analysis; *Client Need:* Safe and Effective Care Environment/Management of Care/Establishing Priorities; *Cognitive Level:* Comprehension

Reference: Sommers, M., Johnson, S., & Beery, T. (2007). *Diseases and Disorders: A Nursing Therapeutics Manual* (3rd ed., p. 338). Philadelphia: F. A. Davis.

---

638. A client returns to a surgical unit following a radical neck dissection for oral cancer. The nursing plan of care for this client should include:

1. positioning the client in a supine position.
2. monitoring the wound drainage tubes around the neck incision for amount and color of drainage and patency.
3. maintaining bed rest for 48 hours postsurgery.
4. offering ice chips orally 2 hours postsurgery.

ANSWER: 2

Wound suction, using portable surgical drains, should be placed around the surgical site to remove tissue fluid and, therefore, prevent edema, which could compress the airway. Positioning the client flat in bed would increase edema formation around the surgical site. The client can breathe best in a semi-Fowler's position. The client should be up in a chair on the first postoperative day (POD) and should begin to ambulate on the second POD. Edema at the surgical site prohibits oral intake. The client will return from surgery with a nasogastric tube in place, which should be used for feeding initially.

➧ ***Test-taking Tip:*** *Eliminate options 1 and 3 as these are contraindicated in the majority of postoperative clients.*

Content Area: Adult Health; *Category of Health Alteration:* Gastrointestinal Management; *Integrated Processes:* Nursing Process Planning; *Client Need:* Physiological Integrity/Reduction of Risk Potential/Potential for Complications from Surgical Procedures and Health Alterations; *Cognitive Level:* Application

References: Monahan, F., Sands, J., Neighbors, M., Marek, J., & Green, C. (2007). *Phipps' Medical-Surgical Nursing: Health and Illness Perspectives* (8th ed., pp. 608, 611–612). St. Louis, MO: Mosby; Lewis, S., Heitkemper, M., Dirksen, S., O'Brien, P., & Bucher, L. (2007). *Medical-Surgical Nursing: Assessment and Management of Clinical Problems* (7th ed., p. 556). St. Louis, MO: Mosby.

639. A nurse is caring for a client immediately after radical neck surgery. In which order should the nurse address the established nursing diagnoses? Prioritize the nurse's actions by placing each diagnosis in the correct order.

_____ Impaired swallowing related to tissue edema
_____ Risk for ineffective breathing pattern related to tissue edema
_____ Anxiety related to the surgical procedure
_____ Risk for infection related to altered tissue integrity

ANSWER: 1, 3, 2, 4

Actual problems are priority and then potential problems. The first priority is impaired swallowing related to tissue edema. Secretions can accumulate that could obstruct the airway. Next is anxiety, because it can also affect the breathing pattern and increase risk. Third, risk for ineffective breathing pattern. After radical neck surgery, inflammation and edema in the surgical areas may compress the trachea, so the client should be closely monitored. The last nursing diagnosis would be risk for infection.

➧ ***Test-taking Tip:*** *Keep in mind the ABCs (airway, breathing, circulation) to answer this question and addressing actual problems before potential problems.*

Content Area: Adult Health; *Category of Health Alteration:* Gastrointestinal Management; *Integrated Processes:* Nursing Process Analysis; *Client Need:* Safe and Effective Care Environment/Management of Care/Establishing Priorities; *Cognitive Level:* Application

Reference: Lewis, S., Heitkemper, M., Dirksen, S., O'Brien, P., & Bucher, L. (2007). *Medical-Surgical Nursing: Assessment and Management of Clinical Problems* (7th ed., p. 556). St. Louis, MO: Mosby.

---

640. A nurse is performing a health history on a client during a clinic visit. The client provides all of the following information. Which client statement should be most concerning to the nurse because it could be a symptom of esophageal cancer?

1. "I have been having a lot of indigestion lately."
2. "When I eat meat it seems to get stuck halfway down."
3. "I have been waking up at night lately with chest pain."
4. "I have been gaining weight, even though I have not changed my diet."

ANSWER: 2

Progressive dysphagia is the most common symptom, and it is initially experienced when eating meat. It is often described as a feeling that food is not passing. Indigestion and chest pain are not symptoms of this disease. Weight loss rather than gain is a symptom.

➧ ***Test-taking Tip:*** *Eliminate option 4 as weight gain is rarely a cancer symptom then think about how a cancerous tumor growing in the esophagus would manifest itself.*

Content Area: Adult Health; *Category of Health Alteration:* Gastrointestinal Management; *Integrated Processes:* Nursing Process Assessment; *Client Need:* Health Promotion and Maintenance/Health Screening; *Cognitive Level:* Application

References: Lewis, S., Heitkemper, M., Dirksen, S., O'Brien, P., & Bucher, L. (2007). *Medical-Surgical Nursing: Assessment and Management of Clinical Problems* (7th ed., p. 1009). St. Louis, MO: Mosby; Monahan, F., Sands, J., Neighbors, M., Marek, J., & Green, C. (2007). *Phipps' Medical-Surgical Nursing: Health and Illness Perspectives* (8th ed., p. 1199). St. Louis, MO: Mosby.

---

641. Following an esophagectomy with colon interposition (esophagoenterostomy) for esophageal cancer, a client is beginning to eat oral foods. A nurse is concerned about the risk of aspiration because the client no longer has a:

1. stomach.
2. pyloric sphincter.
3. pharynx.
4. lower esophageal sphincter.

ANSWER: 4

An esophagectomy for cancer involves removal of the lower esophageal sphincter, which normally functions to keep food from refluxing back into the esophagus. All or part of the stomach will remain intact as will the pharynx and pyloric sphincter.

➧ ***Test-taking Tip:*** *Focus on the esophagectomy with colon interposition surgical procedure, specifically what organs and tissues that are removed to treat the cancer.*

Content Area: Adult Health; *Category of Health Alteration:* Gastrointestinal Management; *Integrated Processes:* Nursing Process Analysis; *Client Need:* Physiological Integrity/Physiologic Adaptation/Pathophysiology; *Cognitive Level:* Analysis

Reference: Monahan, F., Sands, J., Neighbors, M., Marek, J., & Green, C. (2007). *Phipps' Medical-Surgical Nursing: Health and Illness Perspectives* (8th ed., p. 1202). St. Louis, MO: Mosby.

642. During a health promotion seminar for senior citizens, a seminar participant asks a nurse to discuss symptoms of gastric cancer. A nurse's response should be based on the knowledge that:

1. cancers that do not penetrate the gastric muscular layer are asymptomatic in the majority of clients.
2. pain from early gastric cancer lesions cannot be reduced by over-the-counter (OTC) histamine receptor antagonists.
3. unexplained weight gain and increased body mass index are early symptoms of gastric cancer.
4. anemia is uncommon in gastric cancer, but if it occurs it is likely due to the effects of aging.

ANSWER: 1

Eighty percent of clients with early gastric cancer do not have symptoms. Pain caused by gastric cancer can be alleviated by OTC histamine receptor antagonists. Weight loss and anemia are common symptoms. Anemia occurs from malabsorption and nutritional deficiencies.

➧ ***Test-taking Tip:*** *Read the question carefully noting that it is actually asking for symptoms of gastric cancer.*

Content Area: Adult Health; *Category of Health Alteration:* Gastrointestinal Management; *Integrated Processes:* Teaching and Learning; *Client Need:* Health Promotion and Maintenance/Health & Wellness; *Cognitive Level:* Application

References: Monahan, F., Sands, J., Neighbors, M., Marek, J., & Green, C. (2007). *Phipps' Medical-Surgical Nursing: Health and Illness Perspectives* (8th ed., p. 1221). St. Louis, MO: Mosby; Lewis, S., Heitkemper, M., Dirksen, S., O'Brien, P., & Bucher, L. (2007). *Medical-Surgical Nursing: Assessment and Management of Clinical Problems* (7th ed., p. 1028). St. Louis, MO: Mosby.

643. A nurse has just received report on a 55-year-old client who had Billroth II surgery 24 hours ago. The client's wife is listed as the designated contact person. Immediately after report, the client's son approaches the nurse in the hallway and asks for information regarding his father's condition. The nurse's best response would be:

1. "What has the surgeon told you about your father?"
2. "Let's go into your father's room together and ask him how he feels."
3. "Let's go to a more private place to discuss your father's condition."
4. "Let's review his medical record together."

ANSWER: 2

A nurse should not share confidential information about a client with anyone unless the client has specifically given permission. Going into the client's room allows the client to determine if he wants to disclose information and how much information he wants to disclose. Sharing information in a hospital hallway is inappropriate because individuals passing by could overhear confidential client information.

➧ ***Test-taking Tip:*** *The focus of this question is the provision of client confidentiality.*

Content Area: Adult Health; *Category of Health Alteration:* Gastrointestinal Management; *Integrated Processes:* Nursing Process Implementation; *Client Need:* Safe and Effective Care Environment/Management of Care/Confidentiality; *Cognitive Level:* Application

Reference: Harkreader, H., Hogan, M., & Thobaben, M. (2007). *Fundamentals of Nursing* (3rd ed., pp. 38–39). St. Louis, MO: Saunders/Elsevier.

644. A nurse is admitting a client with gastric cancer to an oncology unit for treatment. The nurse knows that the cancer has metastasized to the peritoneal cavity when which item of assessment data is collected?

1. The client is reporting nausea.
2. A nurse observes Grey Turner's sign.
3. The client is reporting rapid weight loss.
4. A nurse observes ascites.

ANSWER: 4

The presence of ascites indicates seeding of the tumor in the peritoneal cavity. Nausea is a sign of gastric outlet obstruction or impending hemorrhage. Grey Turner's sign is a symptom of pancreatitis. Weight loss is an initial sign of the disease.

➧ ***Test-taking Tip:*** *Read the question carefully; this question is asking for symptoms of gastric cancer metastasis.*

Content Area: Adult Health; *Category of Health Alteration:* Gastrointestinal Management; *Integrated Processes:* Nursing Process Assessment; *Client Need:* Physiological Integrity/Physiological Adaptation/Alterations in Body Systems; *Cognitive Level:* Application

Reference: Lewis, S., Heitkemper, M., Dirksen, S., O'Brien, P., & Bucher, L. (2007). *Medical-Surgical Nursing: Assessment and Management of Clinical Problems* (7th ed., pp. 1028, 1119). St. Louis, MO: Mosby.

645. A nurse is reviewing the health history of a client admitted to a hospital with a diagnosis of nonalcoholic fatty liver disease (NAFLD). When conducting the client's health history, which finding is consistent with this disease process?

1. 70 years old
2. Obese
3. History of recent antibiotic use
4. Living in colder climates

ANSWER: 2

The risk for developing NAFLD is directly related to body weight and is a major complication of obesity. Adults in their forties are most at risk for NAFLD. Antibiotic use and climate have no influence on disease development.

➧ ***Test-taking Tip:*** *The focus of the question is risk factors associated with NAFLD. If uncertain, note the stem addresses "fatty liver" and that option 2 is "obese."*

Content Area: Adult Health; *Category of Health Alteration:* Gastrointestinal Management; *Integrated Processes:* Nursing Process Assessment; *Client Need:* Health Promotion and Maintenance/Lifestyle Choices; *Cognitive Level:* Application

Reference: Lewis, S., Heitkemper, M., Dirksen, S., O'Brien, P., & Bucher, L. (2007). *Medical-Surgical Nursing: Assessment and Management of Clinical Problems* (7th ed., p. 1101). St. Louis, MO: Mosby.

---

646. The serum ammonia level of a client with cirrhosis is elevated. As a priority, a nurse should plan to:

1. monitor the client's temperature every 4 hours.
2. observe for increasing confusion.
3. measure the urine specific gravity.
4. restrict the client's oral fluid intake.

ANSWER: 2

Elevated serum ammonia levels may cause neurological changes, such as confusion. The client's temperature or urine specific gravity will not be affected. Oral fluid intake should be encouraged if tolerated by the client.

➧ ***Test-taking Tip:*** *Focus on the symptoms of hepatic encephalopathy, which is caused by increased circulating ammonia levels. If uncertain of the answer, use Maslow's Hierarchy of Needs theory to establish priority. Option 2 is a safety need.*

Content Area: Adult Health; *Category of Health Alteration:* Gastrointestinal Management; *Integrated Processes:* Nursing Process Planning; *Client Need:* Physiological Integrity/Reduction of Risk Potential/Potential for Complications from Surgical Procedures and Health Alterations; *Cognitive Level:* Analysis

Reference: Lewis, S., Heitkemper, M., Dirksen, S., O'Brien, P., & Bucher, L. (2007). *Medical-Surgical Nursing: Assessment and Management of Clinical Problems* (7th ed., pp. 1106, 1114). St. Louis, MO: Mosby.

---

647. EBP A client is hospitalized for conservative treatment of cirrhosis. As part of the collaborative plan of care, a nurse would anticipate:

1. monitoring the client's blood sugar.
2. maintaining NPO (nothing by mouth) status.
3. administering antibiotics.
4. encouraging frequent ambulation.

ANSWER: 1

Clients with cirrhosis may develop insulin resistance. Impaired glucose tolerance is common, and about 20% to 40% of clients with cirrhosis also have diabetes. For some clients with cirrhosis, however, hypoglycemia may occur during fasting because of decreased hepatic glycogen reserves and decreased gluconeogenesis. Clients with cirrhosis should receive a high-protein diet unless hepatic encephalopathy is present. Antibiotics are not part of the treatment plan of cirrhosis because it is not caused by microorganisms. The client with cirrhosis requires rest, thus activity should not be encouraged.

➧ ***Test-taking Tip:*** *Focus on the pathophysiology of cirrhosis to eliminate the incorrect options.*

Content Area: Adult Health; *Category of Health Alteration:* Gastrointestinal Management; *Integrated Processes:* Nursing Process Planning; *Client Need:* Physiological Integrity/Physiological Adaptation/Illness Management; *Cognitive Level:* Analysis

Reference: Smeltzer, S., Bare, B., Hinkle, J., & Cheever, K. (2008). *Brunner & Suddarth's Textbook of Medical-Surgical Nursing* (11th ed., pp. 1307–1308, 1321). Philadelphia: Lippincott Williams & Wilkins.

EBP Reference: McNeely, M. (2004). Case study: Diabetes in a patient with cirrhosis. *Clinical Diabetes*, 22(1), 42–43.

---

648. While caring for a male client with cirrhosis, a nurse adds the nursing diagnosis *Disturbed body image related to physical manifestations of illness* when the client is overheard telling his brother:

1. "I don't think I can handle this disease."
2. "I know the doctors say I have liver failure, but I don't really believe them."
3. "I know I should rest more, but I'm just not that type of person."
4. "I don't like the fact that I seem to have breasts now."

ANSWER: 4

One of the defining characteristics of the diagnosis *disturbed body image* is verbalization of feelings that reflect an altered view of one's body. Option 1 is an example of the client evaluating himself as unable to deal with the situation and would support the diagnosis *situational low self-esteem*. Option 2 is an example of the client denying the problem and would support the diagnosis *defensive coping*. Option 3 is an example of the client failing to take actions that would prevent further health problems and would support the diagnosis *impaired adjustment*.

➧ ***Test-taking Tip:*** *Recall that defining characteristics of disturbed body image involve the mental picture of one's physical self. This should allow elimination of options 1, 2, and 3.*

Content Area: Adult Health; *Category of Health Alteration:* Gastrointestinal Management; *Integrated Processes:* Communication and Documentation; *Client Need:* Psychosocial Integrity/Psychosocial Adaptation/Unexpected Body Image Changes; *Cognitive Level:* Analysis

Reference: NANDA International. (2005). *Nursing Diagnoses: Definitions and Classifications 2005–2006* (6th ed., pp. 5, 18, 46, 166). Philadelphia: NANDA International.

---

649. A client diagnosed with cirrhosis is scheduled for a transjugular intrahepatic portosystemic shunt (TIPS) placement. A nurse realizes the client does not understand the procedure when the client says:

1. "I hope my abdominal incision heals better after this procedure then it did when I had my appendix out."
2. "This procedure should decrease the risk that I might have another episode of bleeding from my esophagus."
3. "I know the shunt they are placing could become occluded in the future."
4. "This procedure should keep me from getting so much fluid buildup in my abdomen."

ANSWER: 1

The TIPS is placed through the jugular vein and threaded down to the hepatic vein. There is no need for an abdominal incision. The procedure will decrease pressure in the portal vein and thus decrease the risk of bleeding from esophageal varices. There is a risk that the stent that is placed will become occluded. The shunt will decrease ascites formation.

➧ ***Test-taking Tip:*** *The statement "does not understand the procedure" indicates a false-response item. Select the incorrect statement.*

Content Area: Adult Health; *Category of Health Alteration:* Gastrointestinal Management; *Integrated Processes:* Nursing Process Evaluation; *Client Need:* Physiological Integrity/Basic Care and Comfort/Nonpharmacological Interventions; Physiological Integrity/Physiological Adaptation/Illness Management; *Cognitive Level:* Application

References: Lewis, S., Heitkemper, M., Dirksen, S., O'Brien, P., & Bucher, L. (2007). *Medical-Surgical Nursing: Assessment and Management of Clinical Problems* (7th ed., p. 1108). St. Louis, MO: Mosby; Smeltzer, S., Bare, B., Hinkle, J., & Cheever, K. (2008). *Brunner & Suddarth's Textbook of Medical-Surgical Nursing* (11th ed., p. 1288). Philadelphia: Lippincott Williams & Wilkins.

---

650. After completing discharge education, a nurse recognizes the need for further teaching when a client, diagnosed with cirrhosis, says:

1. "I know propranolol (Inderal®) has been ordered to decrease my blood pressure."
2. "I plan to stop drinking alcohol."
3. "I am going to work only part-time."
4. "I know furosemide (Lasix®) will help to keep me from developing abdominal swelling."

ANSWER: 1

Prophylactic treatment with a nonselective beta blocker such as propranolol has been shown to reduce the risk of bleeding from esophageal varices and reduce bleeding-related deaths. Though it does decrease blood pressure, it is not ordered for this purpose. Alcohol intake is a major cause of cirrhosis and must be eliminated from the client's diet. Rest may enable the liver to restore itself and should be encouraged. Furosemide is used in combination with potassium-sparing diuretics to decrease ascites.

➧ ***Test-taking Tip:*** *The statement "need for further teaching" indicates a false-response item. Select the incorrect statement.*

Content Area: Adult Health; *Category of Health Alteration:* Gastrointestinal Management; *Integrated Processes:* Nursing Process Evaluation; Teaching and Learning; *Client Need:* Physiological Integrity/Physiological Adaptation/Illness Management; Physiological Integrity/Pharmacological and Parenteral Therapies/Expected Outcomes/Effects; *Cognitive Level:* Application

Reference: Lewis, S., Heitkemper, M., Dirksen, S., O'Brien, P., & Bucher, L. (2007). *Medical-Surgical Nursing: Assessment and Management of Clinical Problems* (7th ed., pp. 1102, 1107, 1111). St. Louis, MO: Mosby.

651. A client preparing for a liver transplantation, asks a nurse to show him where his new liver will be located. Which area should the nurse identify as the location of the client's liver transplant?

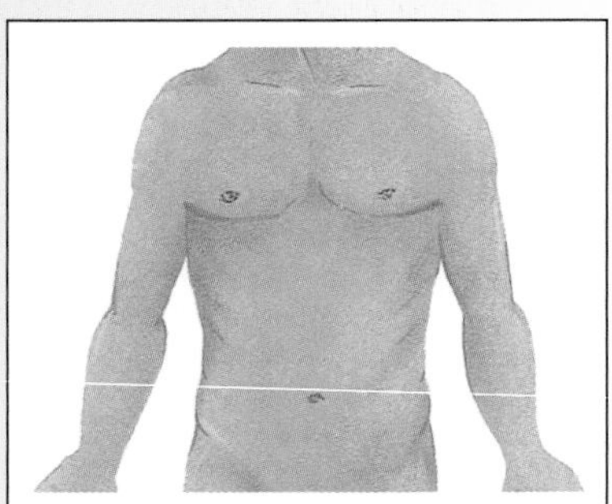

ANSWER:

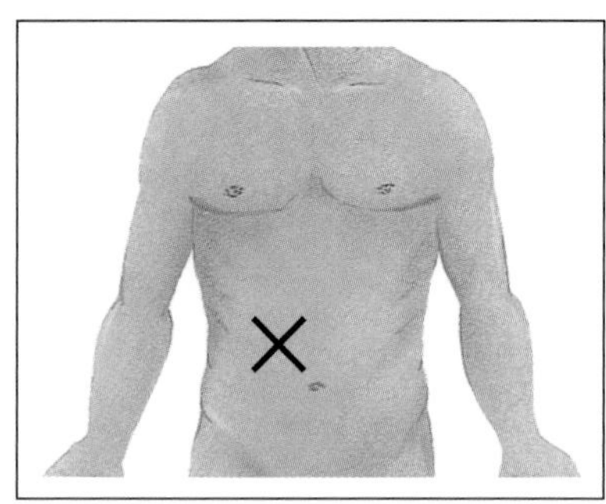

The liver transplantation procedure involves total removal of the diseased liver and replacement with a healthy liver in the same anatomical location.

▶ ***Test-taking Tip:*** *Think about the anatomical connection between the liver and the gallbladder and gastrointestinal tract. This makes it evident that the liver would need to be replaced in the approximate location from which the diseased liver was removed.*

Content Area: Adult Health; *Category of Health Alteration:* Gastrointestinal Management; *Integrated Processes:* Teaching and Learning; *Client Need:* Health Promotion and Maintenance/Principles of Teaching and Learning; Physiological Integrity/Reduction of Risk Potential/Potential for Complications from Surgical Procedures and Health Alterations; *Cognitive Level:* Application

Reference: Smeltzer, S., Bare, B., Hinkle, J., & Cheever, K. (2008). *Brunner & Suddarth's Textbook of Medical-Surgical Nursing* (11th ed., p. 1336). Philadelphia: Lippincott Williams & Wilkins.

---

652. A nurse suspects that a client, admitted with upper right-sided abdominal pain, may have liver cancer when which serum laboratory test result is noted to be elevated?

1. Creatinine
2. Serum α-fetoprotein (AFP) levels
3. Serum phosphorus levels
4. CA-125

ANSWER: 2

Serum α-fetoprotein is a major serum protein synthesized by fetal liver cells, by yolk track cells, and in small amounts the fetal gastrointestinal system. Reappearance of AFP in adults signals pathological problems. In 50% to 75% of clients with liver cancer, serum AFP levels are elevated. Elevated creatinine and phosphorus are symptoms of kidney failure. CA-125 is a tumor marker for ovarian cancer.

▶ ***Test-taking Tip:*** *Recall that cancer tumor markers are usually proteins, which are not normally present in the adult body. With this knowledge eliminate options 1 and 3.*

Content Area: Adult Health; *Category of Health Alteration:* Gastrointestinal Management; *Integrated Processes:* Nursing Process Analysis; *Client Need:* Physiological Integrity/Reduction of Risk Potential/Laboratory Values; *Cognitive Level:* Application

Reference: Lewis, S., Heitkemper, M., Dirksen, S., O'Brien, P., & Bucher, L. (2007). *Medical-Surgical Nursing: Assessment and Management of Clinical Problems* (7th ed., pp. 1116, 1200, 1403). St. Louis, MO: Mosby.

---

653. EBP A client tells a nurse that she has been diagnosed with a 2-cm cancerous tumor in the liver. The client wants to know what type of treatment should be anticipated. The nurse's response should reflect the knowledge that:

1. chemotherapy is the first-line treatment for liver cancer.
2. because of the vascularity of the liver, it is not possible to excise the cancerous tumor using an open surgical approach.
3. liver transplantation is not an option for clients with liver cancer.
4. radiofrequency ablation has been successful in treating tumors of that size.

ANSWER: 4

Radiofrequency ablation is a treatment technique that uses high-frequency, alternating electrical current that heats tissue cells to destroy them. It can be used to treat tumors less than 5 cm in size because these tumors tend to be slow-growing and encapsulated. Chemotherapy is only used for clients who are not likely to benefit from other therapies. Surgical resection of the tumor or liver transplantation is used when the tumor is large or localized.

▶ ***Test-taking Tip:*** *The key words are "a 2-cm tumor." Recall that cancer is treated with the most effective and least invasive therapy.*

Content Area: Adult Health; *Category of Health Alteration:* Gastrointestinal Management; *Integrated Processes:* Nursing Process Planning; *Client Need:* Physiological Integrity/Physiological Adaptation/Illness Management; *Cognitive Level:* Application

Reference: Lewis, S., Heitkemper, M., Dirksen, S., O'Brien, P., & Bucher, L. (2007). *Medical-Surgical Nursing: Assessment and Management of Clinical Problems* (7th ed., p. 1117). St. Louis, MO: Mosby.

EBP Reference: Bruix, J., & Sherman, M. (2005). Management of hepatocellular carcinoma. *Hepatology*, 42(5), 1208–1236. Available at: www.guideline.gov/summary/summary.aspx?doc_id=9401&nbr=005036&string=liver+AND+cancer+AND+treatment

---

654. A registered nurse (RN) is caring for a client following a liver biopsy with the assistance of a student nurse. The RN evaluates that the student understands the postprocedure care when the student nurse:

1. plans to monitor vital signs every hour.
2. promotes ambulation 1 hour after the procedure.
3. positions the client on the right side.
4. encourages the client to cough and deep breathe immediately following the procedure.

ANSWER: 3

Positioning the client on the right side after a liver biopsy splints the puncture site to prevent and decrease bleeding. Vital signs should be assessed every 15 minutes times two, every 30 minutes times four, and then every hour times four after a liver biopsy to monitor for shock, peritonitis, and pneumothorax. The client should be kept flat in bed for 12 to 14 hours following the procedure to prevent the risk of bleeding. The client should be cautioned to avoid coughing, which could precipitate bleeding.

➧ ***Test-taking Tip:*** *Recall that the liver is very vascular. Select the option that would decrease bleeding after the biopsy procedure.*

Content Area: Adult Health; *Category of Health Alteration:* Gastrointestinal Management; *Integrated Processes:* Nursing Process Evaluation; *Client Need:* Safe and Effective Care Environment/Management of Care/Supervision; Physiological Integrity/Reduction of Risk Potential/Diagnostic Tests; *Cognitive Level:* Application

References: Smeltzer, S., Bare, B., Hinkle, J., & Cheever, K. (2008). *Brunner & Suddarth's Textbook of Medical-Surgical Nursing* (11th ed., p. 1293). Philadelphia: Lippincott Williams & Wilkins; Lewis, S., Heitkemper, M., Dirksen, S., O'Brien, P., & Bucher, L. (2007). *Medical-Surgical Nursing: Assessment and Management of Clinical Problems* (7th ed., p. 944). St. Louis, MO: Mosby.

---

655. EBP During a hospital admission history, a nurse suspects acute pancreatitis when a 40-year-old client reports:

1. the sudden onset of intense pain in the upper left abdominal quadrant that radiates to the back.
2. persistent abdominal pain in the lower abdomen that has shifted to the lower right quadrant.
3. bloody diarrhea and colicky abdominal pain.
4. mild upper abdominal pain and projectile vomiting.

ANSWER: 1

The predominant symptom of acute pancreatitis is severe, deep or piercing, continuous or steady abdominal pain in the upper left quadrant. The pain may radiate to the back because of the retroperitoneal location of the pancreas. Middle-age individuals are at increased risk for developing acute pancreatitis. Abdominal pain, located mainly in the right lower quadrant, is a symptom of appendicitis, which is more common in younger adults. Bloody diarrhea and colicky abdominal pain are symptoms of inflammatory bowel disease, also more common in young adults. Upper abdominal pain and projectile vomiting are symptoms of gastric outlet obstruction.

➧ ***Test-taking Tip:*** *Think of the location of the pancreas. Look for key words in the location of each option and use the process of elimination. Only option 1 clearly describes the location of the pancreas.*

Content Area: Adult Health; *Category of Health Alteration:* Gastrointestinal Management; *Integrated Processes:* Nursing Process Analysis; *Client Need:* Physiological Integrity/Reduction of Risk Potential/System Specific Assessments; *Cognitive Level:* Application

Reference: Lewis, S., Heitkemper, M., Dirksen, S., O'Brien, P., & Bucher, L. (2007). *Medical-Surgical Nursing: Assessment and Management of Clinical Problems* (7th ed., pp. 1018, 1048, 1052, 1119). St. Louis, MO: Mosby.

EBP Reference: AGA Institute on Management of Acute Pancreatitis, Clinical Practice and Economics Committee, AGA Institute Governing Board (2007). AGA Institute medical position statement on acute pancreatitis. *Gastroenterology,* 132(5), 2019–2021.

656. While performing an assessment of a client with acute pancreatitis, a nurse notes the following skin appearance. What should be the nurse's interpretation of this finding?

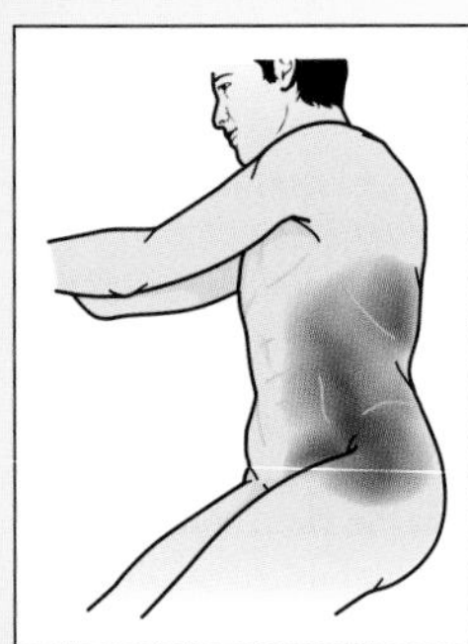

1. Seepage of blood-stained exudates from the pancreas has occurred.
2. The pancreatitis has caused the stomach to bleed and the blood is now in the interstitial tissue.
3. An intestinal obstruction that has increased vascular pressure has developed due to the pancreatic inflammation.
4. Portal hypertension has developed.

ANSWER: 1

Grey Turner's sign is a bluish flank discoloration. It is caused by the seepage of blood-stained exudates from the pancreas and indicates a severe disease process. Pancreatitis will not cause stomach bleeding or intestinal obstruction. Portal hypertension is related to cirrhosis.

➧ ***Test-taking Tip:*** *Eliminate options 2, 3, and 4 because these are describing related organs and not the pancreas. Only option 1 addresses the pancreas.*

Content Area: Adult Health; *Category of Health Alteration:* Gastrointestinal Management; *Integrated Processes:* Nursing Process Analysis; *Client Need:* Physiological Integrity/Reduction of Risk Potential/System Specific Assessments; *Cognitive Level:* Analysis

Reference: Lewis, S., Heitkemper, M., Dirksen, S., O'Brien, P., & Bucher, L. (2007). *Medical-Surgical Nursing: Assessment and Management of Clinical Problems* (7th ed., pp. 1104, 1118–1119). St. Louis, MO: Mosby.

657. EBP Which activities should a nurse, caring for a client with acute necrotizing pancreatitis, implement as part of a collaborative plan of care for this client? SELECT ALL THAT APPLY.

1. Administering 1,000 mL intravenous (IV) fluid bolus over 1 hour followed by IV fluids at 250 mL/hour
2. Initiating nasojejunal enteral feedings
3. Administering IV imipenem-cilastatin (Primaxin®) 500 mg every 6 hours
4. Ambulating four times daily
5. Positioning on left side with head of bed elevated
6. Inserting a Foley catheter

ANSWER: 1, 2, 3, 6

In the early phase of the illness, aggressive fluid resuscitation is critically important to prevent hypovolemia. Resuscitation should be enough to maintain hemodynamic stability, which is usually an initial fluid bolus of several liters followed by a 250 to 500 mL/hr continuous infusion. Early initiation of enteral nutritional supplementation and maintenance of a positive nitrogen balance is important in treating severe pancreatitis. Antibiotics, usually medications of the imipenem class, are used when pancreatitis is complicated by infected pancreatic necrosis. Urine output should be monitored closely to obtain data on circulating fluid volume. The client should be maintained on bedrest to decrease the metabolic rate and therefore reduce pancreatic secretions. Discomfort frequently improves with the client in the supine position rather than on the side.

➧ ***Test-taking Tip:*** *Use knowledge of generic treatment of inflammatory body conditions, which requires resting of the inflamed body part to eliminate option 4. Thinking about the location of the pancreas should allow elimination of option 5.*

Content Area: Adult Health; *Category of Health Alteration:* Gastrointestinal Management; *Integrated Processes:* Nursing Process Implementation; *Client Need:* Physiological Integrity/Physiological Adaptation/Illness Management; *Cognitive Level:* Analysis

Reference: Smeltzer, S., Bare, B., Hinkle, J., & Cheever, K. (2008). *Brunner & Suddarth's Textbook of Medical-Surgical Nursing* (11th ed., pp. 1361, 1362). Philadelphia: Lippincott Williams & Wilkins.

EBP Reference: Gardner, T., Berk, B., & Yakshe, P. (2006). Pancreatitis, acute. *E-Medicine from WebMD*. Available at: www.emedicine.com/med/topic1720.htm

658. EBP A client recovering from acute pancreatitis that has been NPO (nothing per mouth) asks a nurse when he can begin eating again. Which response by the nurse is most accurate?

1. "As soon as you start to feel hungry you can begin eating."
2. "When you have active bowel sounds and you are passing flatus."
3. "When your pain is controlled and your serum lipase level has decreased."
4. "Oral intake stimulates the pancreas so you will need to be NPO for at least 2 weeks from the day your disease was diagnosed to allow the pancreas to heal."

ANSWER: 3

Once pain is controlled and the serum enzyme levels begin to decrease, the client can begin oral intake. These are signs that the pancreas is healing. Intestinal peristalsis may be slowed due to the inflammation associated with acute pancreatitis, but return of bowel sounds and flatus are not used to determine when to begin oral intake. Regaining appetite is a positive sign, but it must be accompanied by a decrease in pain before the client is allowed to take food orally. There is no specific time limit for being NPO.

Test-taking Tip: *Recall that severe pain and elevated serum amylase and lipase are the main symptoms of pancreatitis. A decrease in these symptoms indicates healing. Do not be deceived by the length of time in option 4. The longest option is not always the correct option.*

Content Area: Adult Health; *Category of Health Alteration:* Gastrointestinal Management; *Integrated Processes:* Nursing Process Evaluation; Communication and Documentation; *Client Need:* Physiological Integrity/Physiological Adaptation/Illness Management; *Cognitive Level:* Application

References: Smeltzer, S., Bare, B., Hinkle, J., & Cheever, K. (2008). *Brunner & Suddarth's Textbook of Medical-Surgical Nursing* (11th ed., pp. 1359, 1362). Philadelphia: Lippincott Williams & Wilkins; Cresci, G. (2005). *Nutrition Support for the Critically Ill Patient: A Guide to Practice* (1st ed., p. 547). Boca Raton, FL: CRC Press.

EBP Reference: Gardner, T., Berk, B., & Yakshe, P. (2006). Pancreatitis, acute, *E-Medicine from WebMD*. Available at: www.emedicine.com/med/topic1720.htm

---

659. A 40-year-old client is recovering from an exacerbation of chronic pancreatitis. As the client prepares for discharge, the client makes several statements to a nurse. Which statement should be concerning to the nurse because it could inhibit the client's ability to accomplish the developmental tasks of middle adulthood?

1. "I'm planning on continuing to be active in the local town service club."
2. "I should be able to return to work in 3 weeks."
3. "I've really missed my friends. I'm looking forward to having a glass a wine with them."
4. "My spouse has been very supportive."

ANSWER: 3

The developmental task for the middle adult years is generativity versus stagnation. The individual who is working toward generativity is creatively giving of oneself to the world. The individual is volunteering and also working creatively in his/her job. Continuing to consume alcohol will cause continued progression of the pancreatic disease and could eventually result in the inability to work or to participate in community service.

Test-taking Tip: *Focus on developmental tasks of the middle adult as well as a lifestyle that would enhance disease progression.*

Content Area: Adult Health; *Category of Health Alteration:* Gastrointestinal Management; *Integrated Processes:* Nursing Process Evaluation; *Client Need:* Health Promotion and Maintenance/Developmental Stages and Transitions; *Cognitive Level:* Analysis

References: Berman, A., Snyder, S., Kozier, B., & Erb, G. (2008). *Kozier & Erb's Fundamentals of Nursing: Concepts, Process, and Practice* (8th ed., pp. 351–356). Upper Saddle River, NJ: Pearson Education; Harkreader, H., Hogan, M., & Thobaben, M. (2007). *Fundamentals of Nursing* (3rd ed., pp. 370–377). St. Louis, MO: Saunders/Elsevier.

---

660. A client diagnosed with chronic pancreatitis, is concerned about pain control. A nurse explains to the client that the initial plan for controlling the pain of chronic pancreatitis involves the administration of:

1. opioid analgesic medications.
2. NSAIDs.
3. pancreatic enzymes with H_2 blocker medications.
4. acetaminophen (Tylenol®) and low-carbohydrate diet.

ANSWER: 3

A trial of high-dose pancreatic enzymes coupled with H_2-blockers should precede the continuous use of narcotics or any invasive treatment for chronic pancreatitis pain. Nonopioid analgesics may be used to treat chronic pancreatic pain, but they are not the initial treatment and are usually not sufficient to control the pain. The client should be on a high-carbohydrate diet.

Test-taking Tip: *The key word is "initial." Opioid medications may be needed but are used only if other alternatives fail.*

Content Area: Adult Health; *Category of Health Alteration:* Gastrointestinal Management; *Integrated Processes:* Nursing Process Implementation; *Client Need:* Physiological Integrity/Pharmacological and Parenteral Therapies/Pharmacological Pain Management; Physiological Integrity/Physiological Adaptation/Illness Management; *Cognitive Level:* Application

Reference: Monahan, F., Sands, J., Neighbors, M., Marek, J., & Green, C. (2007). *Phipps' Medical-Surgical Nursing: Health and Illness Perspectives* (8th ed., p. 1297). St. Louis, MO: Mosby.

661. In preparation for providing care to a client immediately after a Whipple procedure, a nurse should anticipate that the nursing care plan may include:

1. monitoring the blood glucose levels.
2. administering enteral feedings.
3. irrigating the nasogastric (NG) tube with 30 mL of saline every 4 hours.
4. assisting the client to the commode to promote bowel elimination within the first 8 hours postsurgery.

ANSWER: 1

The Whipple procedure entails resection of the proximal pancreas, the adjoining duodenum, the distal portion of the stomach, and the distal segment of the common bile duct. The pancreatic duct, common bile duct, and stomach are then anastomosed to the jejunum. The Whipple procedure induces insulin-dependent diabetes. Thus, the blood glucose levels should be monitored closely starting immediately after surgery. The NG tube is strategically placed during surgery and should not be irrigated without a surgeon's order. With an order, gentle irrigation with 10 to 20 mL of normal saline is appropriate. Since this surgery reshapes the gastrointestinal tract, the client will not have peristalsis and bowel movements for several days. Parenteral feedings are the method of choice for providing nutrition immediately after surgery.

Test-taking Tip: Recall what is involved in a Whipple procedure, then note that the key word is "immediately." Options 2, 3, and 4 relate directly to the gastrointestinal tract. Option 1 is different.

Content Area: Adult Health; *Category of Health Alteration:* Gastrointestinal Management; *Integrated Processes:* Nursing Process Implementation; *Client Need:* Physiological Integrity/Physiological Adaptation/Illness Management; *Cognitive Level:* Application

Reference: Sommers, M., Johnson, S., & Beery, T. (2007). *Diseases and Disorders: A Nursing Therapeutics Manual* (3rd ed., pp. 690–691). Philadelphia: F. A. Davis.

662. While reviewing a client's medical records, a nurse notes the diagnosis of biliary colic. Considering this diagnosis, which additional sign will the nurse most likely find in the client's medical record?

1. Bloody diarrhea
2. Heartburn and regurgitation
3. Abdominal distention
4. Severe abdominal pain

ANSWER: 4

Biliary colic is the term used for the severe pain that is caused by a gallstone lodged in the cystic or common bile duct and/or traveling through the ducts. The presence of the stone causes the duct to spasm. Diarrhea, heartburn and regurgitation, and abdominal distention are not related to biliary colic.

Test-taking Tip: Recall that the term "biliary" refers to the gallbladder, which should enable elimination of options 1 and 2.

Content Area: Adult Health; *Category of Health Alteration:* Gastrointestinal Management; *Integrated Processes:* Nursing Process Assessment; *Client Need:* Physiological Integrity/Physiological Adaptation/Pathophysiology; *Cognitive Level:* Application

Reference: Lewis, S., Heitkemper, M., Dirksen, S., O'Brien, P., & Bucher, L. (2007). *Medical-Surgical Nursing: Assessment and Management of Clinical Problems* (7th ed., p. 1127). St. Louis, MO: Mosby.

663. A nurse anticipates that the conservative treatment of a client with acute cholecystitis will include:

1. a bland diet.
2. the administration of anticholinergic medications.
3. placing the client in a supine position with the head of the bed flat.
4. administering laxatives to clear the bowel.

ANSWER: 2

Anticholinergic medications decrease secretion and counteract smooth muscle spasms. The client should be NPO (nothing per mouth) rather than on a bland diet to decrease gallbladder stimulation. Laxatives would increase, rather than decrease, gastrointestinal stimulation. Positioning the client with the head of the bed elevated decreases the pressure of the abdominal contents on the diaphragm and promotes improved ventilation.

Test-taking Tip: Recall the generic treatment of inflammation, which is to rest the involved body part. Knowing this, options 1 and 4 should be eliminated.

Content Area: Adult Health; *Category of Health Alteration:* Gastrointestinal Management; *Integrated Processes:* Nursing Process Planning; *Client Need:* Physiological Integrity/Physiological Adaptation/Illness Management; Physiological Integrity/Pharmacological and Parenteral Therapies/Pharmacological Agents/Actions; *Cognitive Level:* Application

Reference: Lewis, S., Heitkemper, M., Dirksen, S., O'Brien, P., & Bucher, L. (2007). *Medical-Surgical Nursing: Assessment and Management of Clinical Problems* (7th ed., p. 1128). St. Louis, MO: Mosby.

664. A nurse is beginning client care and has been assigned to the following four clients. Which client should the nurse plan to assess first?

1. A 50-year-old client who has chronic pancreatitis and is reporting a pain level of 6 out of 10 on a numeric scale
2. A 47-year-old client with esophageal varices who has influenza and has been coughing for the last 30 minutes
3. A 60-year-old client who had an open cholecystectomy 15 hours ago and has been stable through the night
4. A 54-year-old client with cirrhosis and jaundice who is reporting itching

ANSWER: 2

Bleeding esophageal varices are the most life-threatening complication of cirrhosis. Coughing can precipitate a bleeding episode. The client with a pain rating of 6 out of 10 on a numeric scale and the client reporting itching also need attention, but the pain and itching are not life-threatening concerns. The client who is postcholecystectomy is reported as being stable and could be assessed last.

➧ ***Test-taking Tip:*** *Use the prioritization criteria: life-threatening concerns must be addressed first; client safety concerns second; and concerns essential to the plan of care third. Use the ABCs (airway, breathing, circulation) to determine priority. Determine if any of the clients are in a life-threatening situation, and select that option.*

Content Area: Adult Health; *Category of Health Alteration:* Gastrointestinal Management; *Integrated Processes:* Nursing Process Planning; *Client Need:* Safe and Effective Care Environment/ Management of Care/Establishing Priorities; *Cognitive Level:* Analysis

References: Lewis, S., Heitkemper, M., Dirksen, S., O'Brien, P., & Bucher, L. (2007). *Medical-Surgical Nursing: Assessment and Management of Clinical Problems* (7th ed., pp. 1104, 1107). St. Louis, MO: Mosby; LaCharity, L., Kumagai, C., & Bartz, B. (2006). *Prioritization, Delegation, Assignment: Practice Exercises for Medical-Surgical Nursing* (1st ed., p. 4). St. Louis, MO: Mosby.

---

665. A nurse is caring for a client who is 6 hours post–open cholecystectomy. The client's T-tube drainage bag is empty, and the nurse notes slight jaundice of the sclera. Which action by the nurse is most important?

1. Repositioning the client to promote T-tube drainage
2. Notifying the surgeon about these findings
3. Checking the client's blood pressure immediately
4. Recording the findings and continuing to monitor the client

ANSWER: 2

The T-tube is placed in the common bile duct to ensure patency of the duct. Lack of bile draining into the T-tube and jaundiced sclera are signs of an obstruction to bile flow and should be reported to the surgeon. Repositioning the client might promote bile flow into the T-tube if the client were lying on the tube. However, the jaundice indicates that the problem is internal. The client's blood pressure would not be affected by this situation. Recording the findings and continuing to monitor the client is inappropriate because the client is experiencing signs of a complication.

➧ ***Test-taking Tip:*** *Recall the cause of jaundice and the purpose of the T-tube in biliary surgery.*

Content Area: Adult Health; *Category of Health Alteration:* Gastrointestinal Management; *Integrated Processes:* Nursing Process Implementation; *Client Need:* Safe and Effective Care Environment/ Safety and Infection Control/Injury Prevention; Physiological Integrity/ Reduction of Risk Potential/Potential for Complications from Surgical Procedures and Health Alterations; *Cognitive Level:* Analysis

References: Lewis, S., Heitkemper, M., Dirksen, S., O'Brien, P., & Bucher, L. (2007). *Medical-Surgical Nursing: Assessment and Management of Clinical Problems* (7th ed., pp. 1104, 1129). St. Louis, MO: Mosby; Smeltzer, S., Bare, B., Hinkle, J., & Cheever, K. (2008). *Brunner & Suddarth's Textbook of Medical-Surgical Nursing* (11th ed., p. 1356). Philadelphia: Lippincott Williams & Wilkins.

666. A Chinese client with diarrhea refuses to drink the prescribed oral hydration solution and insists on having chicken broth instead. A nurse's intervention in this situation should be based on the knowledge that Chinese clients:

1. know that chicken is a food with yang qualities.
2. believe foods high in sodium should be used to treat diarrhea.
3. believe extra protein is needed to treat diarrhea.
4. mistrust modern medicine and often use simple foods to treat disease.

ANSWER: 1

An underlying principle of Chinese medicine is balance between yin and yang. Loose stools are a yin symptom, which should be treated with foods that have yang qualities, one of which is chicken. There is no Chinese belief related to using high-sodium or high-protein foods. The Chinese utilize both modern Western and Chinese medicine and may combine Western medicine and Chinese herbal medicines to treat disease.

➧ ***Test-taking Tip:*** *Focus on the specific norms of the Chinese culture.*

Content Area: Adult Health; *Category of Health Alteration:* Gastrointestinal Management; *Integrated Processes:* Nursing Process Planning, Communication and Documentation; *Client Need:* Psychosocial Integrity/Coping and Adaption/Cultural Diversity; *Cognitive Level:* Application

Reference: Harkreader, H., Hogan, M., & Thobaben, M. (2007). *Fundamentals of Nursing* (3rd ed., pp. 55–56). St. Louis, MO: Saunders/Elsevier.

---

667. During a hospital admission history, a nurse suspects irritable bowel syndrome (IBS) when the client says:

1. "I am having a lot of bloody diarrhea."
2. "I have been vomiting for 2 days."
3. "I have lost 10 pounds in the last month."
4. "I have noticed mucus in my stools."

ANSWER: 4

Mucus in the stools is a sign of IBS. Clients with this syndrome may have diarrhea, but it is not bloody. Vomiting is not a symptom of this disease, and clients do not experience unintentional weight loss.

➧ ***Test-taking Tip:*** *Read the question carefully. It is asking for identification of symptoms of IBS*

Content Area: Adult Health; *Category of Health Alteration:* Gastrointestinal Management; *Integrated Processes:* Nursing Process Analysis; *Client Need:* Physiological Integrity/Physiological Adaptation/Illness Management; *Cognitive Level:* Application

Reference: Monahan, F., Sands, J., Neighbors, M., Marek, J., & Green, C. (2007). *Phipps' Medical-Surgical Nursing: Health and Illness Perspectives* (8th ed., p. 1244). St. Louis, MO: Mosby.

---

668. A health-care provider writes the following admission orders for a client with possible appendicitis. Which order should the nurse question?

1. Apply heat to abdomen to decrease pain
2. Withhold analgesic medications to avoid masking critical changes in symptoms
3. Keep client NPO (nothing per mouth)
4. Start lactated Ringer's solution intravenously (IV) at 125 mL/hr

ANSWER: 1

Applying heat to the abdomen when appendicitis is suspected is contraindicated because heat increases circulation, which, in turn, could cause the appendix to rupture. Analgesic medications are usually withheld until a definitive diagnosis is established to avoid masking symptoms. Clients are kept NPO in case surgery is needed, and isotonic IV fluids are initiated to replace lost body fluid and prevent dehydration.

➧ ***Test-taking Tip:*** *"Which order should the nurse question" is a false-response item. Look for the incorrect statement.*

Content Area: Adult Health; *Category of Health Alteration:* Gastrointestinal Management; *Integrated Processes:* Nursing Process Implementation; *Client Need:* Safe and Effective Care Environment/Safety and Infection Control/Error Prevention; *Cognitive Level:* Analysis

References: Monahan, F., Sands, J., Neighbors, M., Marek, J., & Green, C. (2007). *Phipps' Medical-Surgical Nursing: Health and Illness Perspectives* (8th ed., pp. 1244, 1245). St. Louis, MO: Mosby; Sommers, M., Johnson, S., & Beery, T. (2007). *Diseases and Disorders: A Nursing Therapeutics Manual* (3rd ed., p. 101). Philadelphia: F. A. Davis.

669. A 22-year-old college senior has just been diagnosed with acute appendicitis requiring surgery. The client has been nauseated for 2 days, rates the pain as 4 out of 10 on a numeric scale, and tells the nurse, "I can't believe this is happening. I have final exams starting in 3 days. What am I going to do?" A nurse develops the following preoperative diagnoses for this client. Which nursing diagnosis should be priority?

1. Anxiety related to situational crisis
2. Acute pain related to tissue injury
3. Risk deficient fluid volume related to nausea
4. Risk for delayed development related to illness and need for recovery

ANSWER: 1

While all of these diagnoses are important, the client has expressed that the major concern is anxiety about this school situation. The client is not in immediate physical danger. In this situation, feedback from the client is an important consideration when the nurse determines priorities.

➧ ***Test-taking Tip:*** *Maslow's Hierarchy of Needs theory can be used to prioritize from the most crucial survival needs to safety and security needs.*

Content Area: Adult Health; *Category of Health Alteration:* Gastrointestinal Management; *Integrated Processes:* Nursing Process Analysis; Caring; *Client Need:* Safe and Effective Care Environment/Management of Care/Establishing Priorities; Psychosocial Integrity/Coping and Adaptation/Crisis Interventions; *Cognitive Level:* Analysis

References: Craven, R., & Hirnle, C. (2007). *Fundamentals of Nursing, Human Health and Function* (5th ed., p. 209). Philadelphia: Lippincott Williams & Wilkins; LaCharity, L., Kumagai, C., & Bartz, V. (2006). *Prioritization, Delegation & Assignment: Practice Exercises of Medical-Surgical Nursing* (pp. 4–5). St. Louis, MO: Mosby.

---

670. A nurse is reviewing the history and physical of a teenager admitted to a hospital with a diagnosis of ulcerative colitis. Based on this diagnosis, which information should the nurse expect to see on this client's medical record?

1. Abdominal pain and bloody diarrhea
2. Weight gain and elevated blood glucose
3. Abdominal distension and hypoactive bowel sounds
4. Heartburn and regurgitation

ANSWER: 1

The primary symptoms of ulcerative colitis are bloody diarrhea and abdominal pain. Weight loss often occurs in severe cases. Bowel sounds are often hyperactive. Heartburn and regurgitation are not symptoms of this disease.

➧ ***Test-taking Tip:*** *Read the question carefully. It is asking for symptoms of ulcerative colitis, so select the option that best describes those symptoms.*

Content Area: Adult Health; *Category of Health Alteration:* Gastrointestinal Management; *Integrated Processes:* Nursing Process Assessment; *Client Need:* Physiological Integrity/Physiological Adaptation/Pathophysiology; *Cognitive Level:* Application

Reference: Lewis, S., Heitkemper, M., Dirksen, S., O'Brien, P., & Bucher, L. (2007). *Medical-Surgical Nursing: Assessment and Management of Clinical Problems* (7th ed., p. 1052). St. Louis, MO: Mosby.

---

671. A 20-year-old male client is admitted to a hospital with an exacerbation of ulcerative colitis. A female nurse goes into the client's room to complete an initial assessment, and the client yells, "Get out of here! I'm tired of nurses and doctors looking at my body all the time!" Which is the nurse's best action?

1. Leave the room and ask a male colleague to complete the assessment.
2. Verbally acknowledge the client's frustration and anger.
3. Call the health-care practitioner and ask for a sedative order.
4. Tell the client that gathering data about his current condition will promote effective timely treatment of his health concerns.

ANSWER: 2

Ulcerative colitis can be a frustrating disease that often develops before the client has developed adequate coping mechanisms. When responding to an angry client, the nurse must make a determination about the possible cause of the anger. Assessment of the cause will then lead to an appropriate intervention. In the case of the client who is genuinely frustrated and/or frightened, the first implementation strategy should be supportive listening. Once the client has been given the opportunity to express his specific concerns, the nurse can take whatever action is needed to help him regain control.

➧ ***Test-taking Tip:*** *The key term is "best." Do not read into the question. The client has not told the nurse why he is frustrated and angry.*

Content Area: Adult Health; *Category of Health Alteration:* Gastrointestinal Management; *Integrated Processes:* Nursing Process Implementation; Caring; *Client Need:* Psychosocial Integrity/Coping and Adaptation/Therapeutic Communications; *Cognitive Level:* Application

References: Lewis, S., Heitkemper, M., Dirksen, S., O'Brien, P., & Bucher, L. (2007). *Medical-Surgical Nursing: Assessment and Management of Clinical Problems* (7th ed., p. 1057). St. Louis, MO: Mosby; Craven, R., & Hirnle, C. (2007). *Fundamentals of Nursing, Human Health and Function* (5th ed., pp. 389, 390). Philadelphia: Lippincott Williams & Wilkins; Monahan, F., Sands, J., Neighbors, M., Marek, J., & Green, C. (2007). *Phipps' Medical-Surgical Nursing: Health and Illness Perspectives* (8th ed., p. 1259). St. Louis, MO: Mosby.

672. A 25-year-old client, admitted to the hospital with an exacerbation of ulcerative colitis, is placed on mesalamine (Asacol®), which is to be administered rectally via enema. The client finds this procedure distasteful and asks the nurse why the medication cannot be given orally. Which is the best response by the nurse?

1. "It can be given orally; I'll contact the doctor and see if the change can be made."
2. "Rectal administration delivers the medication directly to the affected area."
3. "Oral administration will not be as effective for the disease condition."
4. "It can be given orally, I'll make the change and we'll tell the doctor in the morning."

ANSWER: 2

Treatment of inflammatory bowel disease often involves topical application of medication directly to the tissue involved. Rectal application of mesalamine decreases the side effects of the medication. Initially, the nurse should explain this to the client. If the client still desires a change in medication route, the health-care practitioner must be consulted. Nurses cannot order medications and cannot change medication routes without specific approval by a health-care practitioner who is licensed to prescribe medications.

▶ ***Test-taking Tip:*** *Focus on the legal scope of nursing practice and the medical treatment regime for ulcerative colitis.*

Content Area: Adult Health; *Category of Health Alteration:* Gastrointestinal Management; *Integrated Processes:* Nursing Process Implementation; Communication and Documentation; *Client Need:* Safe and Effective Care Environment/Management of Care/Ethical Practice; Physiological Integrity/Pharmacological and Parenteral Therapies/ Medication Administration; *Cognitive Level:* Analysis

Reference: Lewis, S., Heitkemper, M., Dirksen, S., O'Brien, P., & Bucher, L. (2007). *Medical-Surgical Nursing: Assessment and Management of Clinical Problems* (7th ed., p. 1057). St. Louis, MO: Mosby.

---

673. A 30-year-old client is 6 days post–total proctocolectomy with ileostomy creation for ulcerative colitis. During morning report, a nurse is told that the ileostomy is draining large amounts of liquid stool and the client has been reporting dizziness with ambulation. Based on this information, which parameters should the nurse assess immediately? SELECT ALL THAT APPLY.

1. Pulse rate for the last 24 hours.
2. Urine output.
3. Weight over the last 3 days.
4. Ability to move the lower extremities.
5. Temperature readings for the last 24 hours.

ANSWER: 1, 2, 3, 5

The client with an ileostomy can become dehydrated easily. Dizziness with ambulation is a sign of dehydration, as is increasing pulse rate, decreasing urine output and weight, and a low-grade temperature. The ability to move the lower extremities is not related to dehydration.

▶ ***Test-taking Tip:*** *Concentrate on the symptoms presented in the stem of the question: large ileostomy output and dizziness with ambulation. These should be recognized as signs of dehydration. Choose options that would provide more data about the client's fluid balance status.*

Content Area: Adult Health; *Category of Health Alteration:* Gastrointestinal Management; *Integrated Processes:* Nursing Process Analysis; *Client Need:* Physiological Integrity/Physiological Adaptation/Fluid and Electrolyte Imbalances; *Cognitive Level:* Analysis

References: Monahan, F., Sands, J., Neighbors, M., Marek, J., & Green, C. (2007). *Phipps' Medical-Surgical Nursing: Health and Illness Perspectives* (8th ed., pp. 367, 1263). St. Louis, MO: Mosby; Lewis, S., Heitkemper, M., Dirksen, S., O'Brien, P., & Bucher, L. (2007). *Medical-Surgical Nursing: Assessment and Management of Clinical Problems* (7th ed., p. 322). St. Louis, MO: Mosby.

---

674. A registered nurse (RN) overhears a licensed practical nurse (LPN) talking with a client who is being prepared for a total colectomy with the creation of an ileoanal reservoir for ulcerative colitis. To decrease the client's anxiety, the RN should intervene to clarify the information given by the LPN when the LPN is heard saying:

1. "this surgery will prevent you from developing colon cancer."
2. "after this surgery you will no longer have ulcerative colitis."
3. "when you return from surgery you will not be able to eat solid food for several days."
4. "you will have an ileostomy when you return from this surgery."

ANSWER: 4

Total colectomy with the creation of an ileoanal reservoir for ulcerative colitis is a two-stage surgery. The client will initially have an ileostomy, and, after the reservoir has healed, the ileostomy will be closed. Knowing that the ileostomy will be temporary is important information for the client to decrease stress. Since this surgery removes the total colon, the client will not be at risk for colon cancer and the ulcerative colitis will be cured.

▶ ***Test-taking Tip:*** *In this question, all of the other options are correct. Focus on what additional information, if provided to the client, would decrease client stress about this major surgery.*

Content Area: Adult Health; *Category of Health Alteration:* Gastrointestinal Management; *Integrated Processes:* Nursing Process Evaluation; Communication and Documentation; *Client Need:* Safe and Effective Care Environment/Management of Care/Supervision; *Cognitive Level:* Analysis

References: Lewis, S., Heitkemper, M., Dirksen, S., O'Brien, P., & Bucher, L. (2007). *Medical-Surgical Nursing: Assessment and Management of Clinical Problems* (7th ed., p. 1055). St. Louis, MO: Mosby; Monahan, F., Sands, J., Neighbors, M., Marek, J., & Green, C. (2007). *Phipps' Medical-Surgical Nursing: Health and Illness Perspectives* (8th ed., p. 1257). St. Louis, MO: Mosby.

675. A nurse is caring for a client diagnosed with Crohn's disease, who has undergone a barium enema that demonstrated the presence of strictures in the ileum. Based on this finding, the nurse should monitor the client closely for signs of:

1. peritonitis.
2. obstruction.
3. malabsorption.
4. fluid imbalance.

ANSWER: 2

Bowel strictures are a common complication of Crohn's disease and can result in an acute bowel obstruction. Peritonitis would not be an expected sequel of a bowel stricture nor would malabsorption. Fluid balance would be affected once total obstruction develops.

Test-taking Tip: *Focus on what can be expected if the bowel is narrowed in a specific area. This would help to eliminate options 3 and 4.*

Content Area: Adult Health; *Category of Health Alteration:* Gastrointestinal Management; *Integrated Processes:* Nursing Process Assessment; *Client Need:* Physiological Integrity/Reduction of Risk Potential/System Specific Assessments; *Cognitive Level:* Analysis

Reference: Monahan, F., Sands, J., Neighbors, M., Marek, J., & Green, C. (2007). *Phipps' Medical-Surgical Nursing: Health and Illness Perspectives* (8th ed., p. 1256). St. Louis, MO: Mosby.

---

676. While discharging a 25-year-old female client after a small bowel resection for Crohn's disease, a nurse overhears the client talking to her husband and realizes that the client needs more education when the client says:

1. "I'm so glad I won't ever need any more surgeries."
2. "I'll need to continue to monitor my weight."
3. "If I have another exacerbation I know they will probably put me back on hydrocortisone."
4. "I will probably have to take vitamin supplements all of my life."

ANSWER: 1

Crohn's disease can occur throughout the gastrointestinal (GI) tract. Surgery in one area of the GI tract will not prevent the disease from reoccurring in another area. This reoccurrence can result in the need for further surgery. Clients with Crohn's disease will always need to monitor their weight and will need vitamins to maintain adequate nutrient levels, since inflamed areas of the GI tract do not absorb nutrients well. Most likely, the client will need some type of glucocorticoid medication to treat a future exacerbation.

Test-taking Tip: *"Needs more education" is a false-response item. Look for the incorrect statement.*

Content Area: Adult Health; *Category of Health Alteration:* Gastrointestinal Management; *Integrated Processes:* Nursing Process Evaluation; *Client Need:* Physiological Integrity/Physiological Adaptation/Illness Management; *Cognitive Level:* Analysis

Reference: Monahan, F., Sands, J., Neighbors, M., Marek, J., & Green, C. (2007). *Phipps' Medical-Surgical Nursing: Health and Illness Perspectives* (8th ed., p. 1256). St. Louis, MO: Mosby.

---

677. A charge nurse on a medical unit is determining where on the unit to place a client who is being admitted with exacerbation of Crohn's disease. The client is female, 20 years old, alert and oriented, and has been taking azathioprine (Imuran®) for disease control. Into which room should the nurse place the client?

1. Private room right across from the nurses' station to allow constant visualization.
2. Room with a 22-year-old female client who also has Crohn's disease.
3. Private room with a private bathroom.
4. Room with an older adult female client who is oriented and on bedrest.

ANSWER: 3

Azathioprine suppresses cell-mediated immune responses and may cause bone marrow suppression. Thus, the client is at increased risk for infection and should be in a private room with a private bathroom. Because the client is alert and oriented, there is no need for constant visualization.

Test-taking Tip: *Focus on the adverse effects of azathioprine.*

Content Area: Adult Health; *Category of Health Alteration:* Gastrointestinal Management; *Integrated Processes:* Nursing Process Planning; *Client Need:* Safe and Effective Care Environment/Management of Care/Continuity of Care; *Cognitive Level:* Application

References: Lehne, R. (2007). *Pharmacology for Nursing Care* (6th ed., p. 920). St. Louis, MO: Saunders; Monahan, F., Sands, J., Neighbors, M., Marek, J., & Green, C. (2007). *Phipps' Medical-Surgical Nursing: Health and Illness Perspectives* (8th ed., p. 1254). St. Louis, MO: Mosby.

---

678. While conducting a home visit with a client who had a partial resection of the ileum for Crohn's disease 4 weeks previously, a nurse becomes concerned when the client says:

1. "My stools float and seem to have fat in them."
2. "I have gained 5 pounds since I left the hospital."
3. "I am still avoiding milk products."
4. "I only have two formed stools per day."

ANSWER: 1

Bile salts are absorbed in the terminal ileum. Disease in this area or resection of the ileum can result in poor fat absorption and loss of fat in the stool. Weight gain is a positive sign after small bowel resection for Crohn's disease, as are formed stools. Many clients with Crohn's disease develop lactose intolerance and therefore should avoid milk products.

Test-taking Tip: *Focus on the digestive process, what actually happens in the ileum, and what problems might develop if the ileum were resected.*

Content Area: Adult Health; *Category of Health Alteration:* Gastrointestinal Management; *Integrated Processes:* Nursing Process Analysis; *Client Need:* Physiological Integrity/Basic Care and Comfort/Nutrition and Oral Hydration; *Cognitive Level:* Analysis

Reference: Lewis, S., Heitkemper, M., Dirksen, S., O'Brien, P., & Bucher, L. (2007). *Medical-Surgical Nursing: Assessment and Management of Clinical Problems* (7th ed., pp. 1057, 1079). St. Louis, MO: Mosby.

---

679. A nurse is assessing a client, with a diagnosed inguinal hernia, at a scheduled clinic visit. The nurse suspects that the client's hernia may be strangulated when which finding is noted on assessment?

1. Shortness of breath
2. Intense abdominal pain
3. Constipation
4. Hyperactive bowel sounds

ANSWER: 2

When a hernia is irreducible and intestinal flow and blood supply are obstructed, the hernia is strangulated. Lack of blood supply causes severe pain in the strangulated area.

▶ ***Test-taking Tip:*** *Focus on the body response when blood supply to intestinal tissue is reduced. This would help to eliminate options 1 and 3.*

Content Area: Adult Health; *Category of Health Alteration:* Gastrointestinal Management; *Integrated Processes:* Nursing Process Assessment; *Client Need:* Physiological Integrity/Reduction of Risk Potential/System Specific Assessments; *Cognitive Level:* Application

Reference: Lewis, S., Heitkemper, M., Dirksen, S., O'Brien, P., & Bucher, L. (2007). *Medical-Surgical Nursing: Assessment and Management of Clinical Problems* (7th ed., pp. 322, 1078). St. Louis, MO: Mosby.

---

680. A nurse is reviewing the health history of a client being evaluated for treatment of hemorrhoids. Which information related to the development of hemorrhoids should the nurse expect to find in the client's medical history?

1. Body mass index (BMI) of 18
2. Chronic constipation
3. Nulliparous
4. Occupation: Salesperson

ANSWER: 2

Prolonged constipation is a risk factor for development of hemorrhoids. Since pregnancy is a common cause, nulliparous women would have a decreased risk, as would clients who are thin (BMI = 18). Sedentary occupations increase risk.

▶ ***Test-taking Tip:*** *Read the question carefully. The question is asking for identification of factors that increase the client's risk for development of hemorrhoids.*

Content Area: Adult Health; *Category of Health Alteration:* Gastrointestinal Management; *Integrated Processes:* Nursing Process Assessment; *Client Need:* Physiological Integrity/Reduction of Risk Potential/Potential for Alterations in Body Systems; *Cognitive Level:* Application

Reference: Monahan, F., Sands, J., Neighbors, M., Marek, J., & Green, C. (2007). *Phipps' Medical-Surgical Nursing: Health and Illness Perspectives* (8th ed., p. 1280). St. Louis, MO: Mosby.

---

681. A client is being admitted to a postsurgical unit following anorectal surgery. A nurse reviews the following postoperative orders from the surgeon. Which order should the nurse question?

1. Administer morphine sulfate per intravenous bolus before the first defecation
2. Administer sitz bath after each defecation
3. Begin high-fiber diet as soon as client can tolerate oral intake
4. Position client in supine position with the head of the bed elevated to 30 degrees.

ANSWER: 4

After anorectal surgery, the client should be positioned in a side-lying position to decrease rectal edema and client discomfort. Pain medication is recommended before the first defecation, and a sitz bath is encouraged for rectal cleansing after defecation. Prevention of constipation with a high-fiber diet is also recommended.

▶ ***Test-taking Tip:*** *"Which order should the nurse question?" is a false-response item. Look for the incorrect statement.*

Content Area: Adult Health; *Category of Health Alteration:* Gastrointestinal Management; *Integrated Processes:* Communication and Documentation; *Client Need:* Safe and Effective Care Environment/Safety and Infection Control/Injury Prevention; *Cognitive Level:* Analysis

Reference: Monahan, F., Sands, J., Neighbors, M., Marek, J., & Green, C. (2007). *Phipps' Medical-Surgical Nursing: Health and Illness Perspectives* (8th ed., p. 1282). St. Louis, MO: Mosby.

682. A client is admitted to a hospital for medical treatment of acute diverticulitis. A nurse should anticipate that this client's treatment plan will include: SELECT ALL THAT APPLY.

1. NPO (nothing per mouth) status.
2. frequent ambulation.
3. antibiotics.
4. antiemetic medication.
5. deep breathing every 2 hours.

ANSWER: 1, 3

When diverticulitis is managed medically, the goal is to promote bowel rest. Decreasing oral intake will help to achieve that goal. Antibiotics are part of the treatment regimen. Ambulation is not encouraged because resting the body also promotes bowel rest. Nausea is not a concern with diverticulitis, and, since the client did not have surgery, there is no need for deep breathing every 2 hours.

➧ ***Test-taking Tip:*** *Focus on basic treatment for any inflamed body part. This would help to eliminate option 2. Thinking about the location of diverticuli should enable the elimination of option 4.*

Content Area: Adult Health; *Category of Health Alteration:* Gastrointestinal Management; *Integrated Processes:* Nursing Process Implementation; *Client Need:* Physiological Integrity/Physiological Adaptation/Illness Management; *Cognitive Level:* Application

References: Monahan, F., Sands, J., Neighbors, M., Marek, J., & Green, C. (2007). *Phipps' Medical-Surgical Nursing: Health and Illness Perspectives* (8th ed., p. 1248). St. Louis, MO: Mosby; Sommers, M., Johnson, S., & Beery, T. (2007). *Diseases and Disorders: A Nursing Therapeutics Manual* (3rd ed., p. 301). Philadelphia: F. A. Davis.

683. EBP A nurse is assessing a client diagnosed with acute diverticulitis. Which finding should make the nurse suspect that the client has an intestinal perforation?

1. Elevated white blood cells (WBCs)
2. Temperature of 101°F (38.3°C)
3. Absent bowel sounds
4. Abdominal pain

ANSWER: 3

Clients with intestinal perforation will develop paralytic ileus. Increased temperature, WBCs, and abdominal pain are all symptoms of acute diverticulitis.

➧ ***Test-taking Tip:*** *Focus on symptoms of peritonitis and eliminate these.*

Content Area: Adult Health; *Category of Health Alteration:* Gastrointestinal Management; *Integrated Processes:* Nursing Process Assessment; *Client Need:* Physiological Integrity/Reduction of Risk Potential/Potential for Complications from Surgical Procedures and Health Alterations; *Cognitive Level:* Analysis

Reference: Lewis, S., Heitkemper, M., Dirksen, S., O'Brien, P., & Bucher, L. (2007). *Medical-Surgical Nursing: Assessment and Management of Clinical Problems* (7th ed., pp. 1076–1077). St. Louis, MO: Mosby.

EBP Reference: Society for Surgery of the Alimentary Tract (SSAT). (2003). *Surgical Treatment of Diverticulitis.* Available at: www.guideline.gov/summary/summary.aspx?doc_id=5509&nbr=003752&string=diverticulitis#s24

684. A family member tells a nurse that her father, who was told 24 hours ago that he has terminal colon cancer, refuses to see the family priest. He has also asked that his phone be disconnected so that he does not need to interact with other family members and friends. He told his daughter that he has decided he was never going to pray again in spite of the fact that previously he has been a very religious person. Based on this information, which nursing diagnosis should the nurse develop for this client?

1. Decisional conflict about how to manage his cancer diagnosis related to lack of experience with terminal illness
2. Risk for spiritual distress related to diagnosis of terminal cancer
3. Spiritual distress related to anxiety about the diagnosis of terminal cancer
4. Noncompliance related to spiritual values

ANSWER: 3

The client is exhibiting the defining characteristics for the diagnosis of spiritual distress. These include refusing interactions with family, friends, and spiritual leaders and the unwillingness to pray. The other nursing diagnoses do not fit the findings.

➧ ***Test-taking Tip:*** *Closely read the clients symptoms. They are not related to making a decision or noncompliance with a therapeutic plan. Thus eliminate options 1 and 4.*

Content Area: Adult Health; *Category of Health Alteration:* Gastrointestinal Management; *Integrated Processes:* Nursing Process Analysis; *Client Need:* Psychosocial Integrity/Coping and Adaptation/Religious and Spiritual Influences on Health; *Cognitive Level:* Analysis

Reference: Craven, R., & Hirnle, C. (2007). *Fundamentals of Nursing, Human Health and Function* (5th ed., pp. 1401–1403). Philadelphia: Lippincott Williams & Wilkins.

685. After examining a client's laboratory results, a nurse suspects that a client's colon cancer has metastasized to the liver. Which laboratory values should lead the nurse to make this conclusion?

Lab-Serum	Client Value	Normal Values
BUN	30	5–25 mg
Creatinine	2.0	0.5–1.5 mg/dL
Na	133	135–145 mEq/L
K	4.5	3.5–5.3 mEq/L
Cl	92	95–105 mEq/L
CO_2	23	22–30 mEq/L
Hgb/Hct	10/32%	13.5–17 g/dL, 40%–54%
WBC	12,000	4,500–10,000/μL
Neutrophils	85%	50%–70%
Albumin	2.5	3.5–5.0 g/dL
Alkaline phosphatase (ALP)	500	42–136 unit/L
Aspartate aminotransferase (AST)	76	8–38 unit/L
Calcium	3.0	4.5–5.5 mEq/L
Phosphorus	3.5	1.7–2.6 mg/dL

1. Elevated aspartate aminotransferase (AST) and alkaline phosphatase (ALP)
2. Elevated BUN (blood urea nitrogen) and Cr (creatinine)
3. Decreased albumin and calcium
4. Elevated WBCs (white blood cells) and neutrophils

ANSWER: 1

A common site for metastasis of colorectal cancer is the liver. ALP is an enzyme produced in the bone and liver, and AST is an enzyme produced in the heart and liver. Both are elevated when liver cancer is present. Elevated BUN and Cr could indicate kidney involvement. Decreased albumin and calcium could be related to the kidney or to poor nutrition. Elevated WBCs and neutrophils would indicate an acute inflammatory/infectious process.

➧ ***Test-taking Tip:*** *BUN and Cr are most commonly associated with the kidney, thus option 2 could be eliminated. Recall WBCs and neutrophils are commonly associated with infection, thus option 4 could be eliminated.*

Content Area: Adult Health; *Category of Health Alteration:* Gastrointestinal Management; *Integrated Processes:* Nursing Process Analysis; *Client Need:* Physiological Integrity/Reduction of Risk Potential/Laboratory Values; *Cognitive Level:* Analysis

References: Monahan, F., Sands, J., Neighbors, M., Marek, J., & Green, C. (2007). *Phipps' Medical-Surgical Nursing: Health and Illness Perspectives* (8th ed., p. 1274). St. Louis, MO: Mosby; Kee, J. (2005). *Laboratory and Diagnostic Tests with Nursing Implications* (7th ed., pp. 18, 25, 72, 83, 93, 102, 119, 142, 220, 336, 347, 400, 455, 457). Upper Saddle River, NJ: Pearson/Prentice Hall.

---

686. A nurse is caring for a client who had surgery for colon cancer, which included the creation of a temporary colostomy. The client is 24 hours postsurgery. During an assessment of the client, a nurse notes no stool in the colostomy bag. A review of the client's medical records indicates that, since surgery, there has not been stool in the bag. Considering this information, the nurse should:

1. call the doctor immediately to report this finding.
2. reposition the client to the left side.
3. document the findings.
4. administer pain medication.

ANSWER: 3

There is no need for action other than documentation because the colostomy will begin to produce feces when bowel peristalsis returns. After abdominal surgery, peristalsis in the large intestine may not return for 3 to 5 days. Thus, it would be expected that 24 hours postsurgery there would not be stool in the appliance.

➧ ***Test-taking Tip:*** *Focus on expected intestinal physiological changes as a result of bowel surgery.*

Content Area: Adult Health; *Category of Health Alteration:* Gastrointestinal Management; *Integrated Processes:* Nursing Process Analysis; *Client Need:* Physiological Integrity/Reduction of Risk Potential/Potential for Complications from Surgical Procedures and Health Alterations; *Cognitive Level:* Analysis.

Reference: Lewis, S., Heitkemper, M., Dirksen, S., O'Brien, P., & Bucher, L. (2007). *Medical-Surgical Nursing: Assessment and Management of Clinical Problems* (7th ed., pp. 390, 1071). St. Louis, MO: Mosby.

---

687. EBP A client, who had a sigmoid colectomy for colon cancer is instructed at a follow-up clinic visit to take 325 mg of aspirin (Ecotrin®) per day. A nurse explains to the client that the aspirin will:

1. decrease the surgical pain.
2. promote healing of the surgical incision.
3. prevent the return of cancer in the colon.
4. prevent metastasis of the cancer to other areas of the body.

ANSWER: 3

Aspirin 325 mg taken daily has been shown to decrease the risk of reoccurrence of colon cancer. Although aspirin may relieve some pain, it has a low analgesic effect to relieve postoperative pain. Aspirin will not promote healing or prevent metastasis of the cancer.

➧ ***Test-taking Tip:*** *Focus on the anti-inflammatory properties of aspirin. This would help to eliminate option 2. Also recall that opioids are the medication of choice for surgical pain followed by NSAIDs. This would eliminate option 1.*

Content Area: Adult Health; *Category of Health Alteration:* Gastrointestinal Management; *Integrated Processes:* Teaching and Learning; *Client Need:* Physiological Integrity/Pharmacological and Parenteral Therapies/Pharmacological Agents/Actions; *Cognitive Level:* Application

Reference: Lewis, S., Heitkemper, M., Dirksen, S., O'Brien, P., & Bucher, L. (2007). *Medical-Surgical Nursing: Assessment and Management of Clinical Problems* (7th ed., p. 389). St. Louis, MO: Mosby.

EBP Reference: Calonge, N., Petitti, D., DeWitt, T., Gordis, L., Gregory, K., et al. (2007). Routine aspirin or nonsteroidal anti-inflammatory drugs for the primary prevention of colorectal cancer: U.S. Preventive Services Task Force recommendation statement. *Annals of Internal Medicine*, 146(5), 361–364.

---

688. While caring for a surgical client during the first 24 hours after an abdominal–perineal resection, a nurse should give the highest priority to:

1. providing a low-residue diet.
2. monitoring the amount and color of stool in the colostomy bag.
3. assessing perineal dressings and drainage.
4. encouraging observation and acceptance of the colostomy site.

ANSWER: 3

After an abdominal–perineal resection, the client will have two incisions—one in the abdomen and one in the perineal area. A colostomy stoma will also be present. The perineal incision must be examined frequently to assess for drainage and the need for dressing changes. After bowel surgery, a temporary ileus is expected; thus the client would be NPO (nothing per mouth) initially, and there would not be stool coming from the colostomy. The client's physiological needs in the early postoperative period take precedence over the integration of the body image change into the client's self-concept.

➧ ***Test-taking Tip:*** *Note the key time period: 24 hours after surgery. Focus on nursing care required for all clients in the first 24 hours postsurgery and the physiological changes that occur as a result of surgery. Apply Maslow's Hierarchy of Needs theory to eliminate option 4 (physiological needs are priority over psychosocial needs).*

Content Area: Adult Health; *Category of Health Alteration:* Gastrointestinal Management; *Integrated Processes:* Nursing Process Planning; *Client Need:* Safe and Effective Care Environment/Management of Care/Establishing Priorities; *Cognitive Level:* Application.

References: Monahan, F., Sands, J., Neighbors, M., Marek, J., & Green, C. (2007). *Phipps' Medical-Surgical Nursing: Health and Illness Perspectives* (8th ed., pp. 1263, 1278, 1279). St. Louis, MO: Mosby; Lewis, S., Heitkemper, M., Dirksen, S., O'Brien, P., & Bucher, L. (2007). *Medical-Surgical Nursing: Assessment and Management of Clinical Problems* (7th ed., p. 1068). St. Louis, MO: Mosby.

---

689. EBP A nurse is conducting a home visit with a client who had surgery 3 months ago that involved the creation of a colostomy. When the nurse arrives at the home, the client's wife reports that her husband has lost interest in golf, which used to be his passion. She also says he cries often for no reason, is only able to sleep for a few hours each night, and reports fatigue daily. The wife asks the nurse for advice. A nurse's response should be based on the knowledge that:

1. twenty-five percent of all clients develop clinically significant depression after ostomy surgery.
2. athletic activities like golf are not possible after ostomy surgery.
3. after 3 months the client should have accepted his new body image.
4. it is difficult to sleep well with an ostomy.

ANSWER: 1

The client is exhibiting signs of depression. At least 25% of clients develop clinically significant depression following colostomy. Poor adjustment to a stoma correlates to development of depression. The adjustment period for ostomy clients is unique for each individual. Clients can be encouraged to gradually resume all their usual activities. Only sports where direct trauma to the stoma is likely should be avoided.

➧ ***Test-taking Tip:*** *Focus on signs of depression.*

Content Area: Adult Health; *Category of Health Alteration:* Gastrointestinal Management; *Integrated Processes:* Nursing Process Implementation; *Client Need:* Psychosocial Integrity/Psychosocial Adaptation/Psychopathology; *Cognitive Level:* Analysis

Reference: Lewis, S., Heitkemper, M., Dirksen, S., O'Brien, P., & Bucher, L. (2007). *Medical-Surgical Nursing: Assessment and Management of Clinical Problems* (7th ed., p. 1073). St. Louis, MO: Mosby.

EBP Reference: Brown, H., & Randle, J. (2005). Living with a stoma: A review of the literature. *Journal of Clinical Nursing*, 14(1), 74–81.

690. For a client with a newly created colostomy, a nurse creates this diagnosis: *risk for sexual dysfunction related to body image change*. To promote satisfying sexual functioning after ostomy surgery, which recommendation should the nurse make to the client?

1. Participate in sexual activity only in a darkened room
2. Utilize self-gratification for the majority of sexual needs
3. Empty and clean the ostomy pouch immediately before sexual activity
4. Utilize only the female superior position for sexual activity

ANSWER: 3
Emptying the pouch before sexual activity is suggested to decrease the concern of pouch breakage or leakage. Self-gratification, if it involves emotional distancing, can be destructive to the client's sexual relationship. Various positions should be explored during sexual activity with the goal of minimizing stress and pressure on the pouch. Participating in sex only in a darkened room may be a way of coping with body image concerns, but it is not necessary.

Test-taking Tip: *Focus on an intervention that would assist the client to cope with the body image change. This would eliminate option 2.*

Content Area: Adult Health; *Category of Health Alteration:* Gastrointestinal Management; *Integrated Processes:* Nursing Process Planning; *Client Need:* Psychosocial Integrity/Coping Mechanisms; *Cognitive Level:* Application.

Reference: Monahan, F., Sands, J., Neighbors, M., Marek, J., & Green, C. (2007). *Phipps' Medical-Surgical Nursing: Health and Illness Perspectives* (8th ed., p. 1267). St. Louis, MO: Mosby.

691. A nurse anticipates that the care of a client newly admitted to a medical unit with a diagnosis of peritonitis should include: SELECT ALL THAT APPLY.

1. intravenous (IV) fluids.
2. antibiotics.
3. NPO (nothing per mouth) status.
4. analgesic therapy.
5. positioning in a supine position.
6. nasogastric (NG) tube to suction.

ANSWER: 1, 2, 3, 4, 6
Interventions are supportive and include IV fluid and electrolyte replacement and resting the gastrointestinal tract with NG suction. Appropriate antibiotics are given, and analgesics are utilized for pain control. The client can assume any position that promotes comfort; a supine position is not required.

Test-taking Tip: *Recall treatment for all types of inflammatory/infectious health deviations.*

Content Area: Adult Health; *Category of Health Alteration:* Gastrointestinal Management; *Integrated Processes:* Nursing Process Implementation; *Client Need:* Physiological Integrity/Physiological Adaptation/Illness Management; *Cognitive Level:* Application

References: Lewis, S., Heitkemper, M., Dirksen, S., O'Brien, P., & Bucher, L. (2007). *Medical-Surgical Nursing: Assessment and Management of Clinical Problems* (7th ed., p. 1050). St. Louis, MO: Mosby; Sommers, M., Johnson, S., & Beery, T. (2007). *Diseases and Disorders: A Nursing Therapeutics Manual* (3rd ed., p. 719). Philadelphia: F. A. Davis.

Test 18: **Adult Health: Hematological and Oncological Management**

692. A nurse is preparing a client for a bone marrow biopsy of the iliac crest. Which actions should be taken by the nurse when preparing the client? Prioritize the nurse's actions by placing each step in the correct order.

_____ Premedicate with lorazepam (Ativan®).
_____ Obtain a signed informed consent.
_____ Position the client in a prone position.
_____ Verify that the physician has explained the procedure.
_____ Check for signs of bleeding every 2 hours for 24 hours.
_____ Support the client by holding the client's hand or using guided imagery.
_____ Teach that pressure or discomfort may be experienced.

ANSWER: 4, 3, 5, 1, 7, 6, 2

First, verify that the physician has explained the procedure, including the purpose and potential complications. Next, teach the client what to expect during the procedure, including that pressure or discomfort may be experienced. Once teaching has been completed, obtain a signed informed consent. Premedicate with lorazepam or other prescribed medication before positioning the client in a prone position (less commonly, the side-lying position could also be used). Next, provide support to the client by holding the client's hand or encouraging guided imagery. Following the procedure, a pressure dressing is applied by the health-care provider. Check for signs of bleeding every 2 hours for 24 hours.

▶ ***Test-taking Tip:*** *Visualize how to prepare and monitor a client for a bone marrow biopsy before prioritizing the nurse's actions.*

Content Area: Adult Health; *Category of Health Alteration:* Hematological and Oncological Management; *Integrated Processes:* Nursing Process Implementation; *Client Need:* Physiological Integrity/Reduction of Risk Potential/Diagnostic Tests; Safe and Effective Care Environment/Management of Care/Establishing Priorities; *Cognitive Level:* Analysis

Reference: Ignatavicius, D., & Workman, M. (2006). *Medical-Surgical Nursing: Critical Thinking for Collaborative Care* (5th ed., p. 885). St. Louis, MO: Elsevier/Saunders.

---

693. A homeless client, visiting a health clinic, is noted to have a smooth and reddened tongue and ulcers at the corners of the mouth. The client was tentatively diagnosed with a hematological disorder, and laboratory tests were prescribed. Based on this information, a nurse should expect the client's laboratory results to reveal:

1. low hemoglobin.
2. elevated red blood cells (RBCs).
3. prolonged prothrombin time (PT).
4. low white blood cells (WBCs).

ANSWER: 1

A smooth red tongue, ulcers at the corners of the mouth (angular cheilosis), and a low hemoglobin are signs of iron-deficiency anemia. Excess RBCs is associated with polycythemia vera. Prolonged PT is seen with clients taking anticoagulants or experiencing a coagulation disorder. Ulcers, if infected, would elevate the WBCs.

▶ ***Test-taking Tip:*** *Think about the conditions that would produce the altered lab values in each option before answering the questions.*

Content Area: Adult Health; *Category of Health Alteration:* Hematological and Oncological Management; *Integrated Processes:* Nursing Process Analysis; *Client Need:* Physiological Integrity/Reduction of Risk Potential/Laboratory Values; *Cognitive Level:* Analysis

Reference: Smeltzer, S., Bare, B., Hinkle, J., & Cheever, K. (2008). *Brunner & Suddarth's Textbook of Medical-Surgical Nursing* (11th ed., p. 1047). Philadelphia: Lippincott Williams & Wilkins.

---

694. EBP A nurse teaches a 55-year-old strict vegetarian that, to decrease the risk of developing megaloblastic anemia, the client should:

1. undergo a Schilling test.
2. increase intake of foods high in iron.
3. supplement the diet with vitamin B_{12}.
4. have a monthly hemoglobin level drawn.

ANSWER: 3

Megaloblastic anemia is caused by deficiency of vitamin B_{12} or folic acid. A vegetarian can prevent a deficiency with oral vitamin supplements or fortified soy milk. The U.S. Department of Agriculture's Dietary Guidelines for Americans 2005 also recommend that people over age 50, whether or not they are vegetarian, consume vitamin B_{12} in its crystalline form (i.e., fortified foods or supplements). The Schilling test is used to diagnose vitamin B_{12} deficiency. Consuming foods high in iron will prevent iron-deficiency anemia. Monthly laboratory work is unnecessary and costly.

▶ ***Test-taking Tip:*** *Focus on the issue, decrease the risk, and use the process of elimination. Eliminate options 1 and 4 because these do not decrease risk. Differentiate between iron deficiency and megaloblastic anemia to select the correct answer, option 3.*

Content Area: Adult Health; *Category of Health Alteration:* Hematological and Oncological Management; *Integrated Processes:* Teaching and Learning; *Client Need:* Health Promotion and Maintenance/Self-Care; *Cognitive Level:* Application

Reference: Smeltzer, S., Bare, B., Hinkle, J., & Cheever, K. (2008). *Brunner & Suddarth's Textbook of Medical-Surgical Nursing* (11th ed., p. 1053). Philadelphia: Lippincott Williams & Wilkins.

EBP Reference: U.S. Department of Health and Human Services, U.S. Department of Agriculture. (2005). *Dietary Guidelines for Americans.* Available at: www.guideline.gov/summary/summary.aspx?doc_id=6417&nbr=004048&string=anemia

695. A nurse should assess a client with hemolytic anemia for weakness, fatigue, malaise, skin and mucous membrane pallor, and:

1. jaundice.
2. a smooth red tongue.
3. a craving for ice.
4. a poor intake of fresh vegetables.

ANSWER: 1

Jaundice occurs from the shortened life span of the red blood cell and the breakdown of hemoglobin. About 80% of heme is converted to bilirubin, conjugated in the liver, and excreted in the bile. The increased bilirubin in the blood causes the jaundice. A smooth, red tongue and a craving for ice are seen with iron-deficiency anemia. Folate deficiency occurs in people who rarely eat fresh vegetables.

➧ ***Test-taking Tip:*** *Use knowledge of medical terminology, recalling that "-lytic" is destruction of red blood cells.*

Content Area: Adult Health; *Category of Health Alteration:* Hematological and Oncological Management; *Integrated Processes:* Nursing Process Assessment; *Client Need:* Physiological Integrity/Reduction of Risk Potential/System Specific Assessments; *Cognitive Level:* Comprehension

Reference: Smeltzer, S., Bare, B., Hinkle, J., & Cheever, K. (2008). *Brunner & Suddarth's Textbook of Medical-Surgical Nursing* (11th ed., pp. 1047, 1052). Philadelphia: Lippincott Williams & Wilkins.

696. A nurse is caring for multiple 25-year-old female clients. For which clients should the nurse plan to obtain a referral for genetic counseling and family planning? SELECT ALL THAT APPLY.

1. Client diagnosed with thalassemia major
2. Client diagnosed with sickle cell disease
3. Client diagnosed with hemophilia A
4. Client diagnosed with autoimmune hemolytic anemia
5. Client diagnosed with hemophilia B

ANSWER: 1, 2, 3, 5

Thalassemia, sickle cell disease, and hemophilia A and B are hereditary disorders. Autoimmune hemolytic anemia is an acquired hemolytic anemia.

➧ ***Test-taking Tip:*** *The key term is "genetic counseling." Eliminate an acquired condition.*

Content Area: Adult Health; *Category of Health Alteration:* Hematological and Oncological Management; *Integrated Processes:* Nursing Process Planning; *Client Need:* Safe and Effective Care Environment/Management of Care/Referrals; *Cognitive Level:* Application

Reference: Smeltzer, S., Bare, B., Hinkle, J., & Cheever, K. (2008). *Brunner & Suddarth's Textbook of Medical-Surgical Nursing* (11th ed., p. 1046). Philadelphia: Lippincott Williams & Wilkins.

697. A client is hospitalized with a diagnosis of sickle cell crisis. Which findings should lead a nurse to conclude that outcomes have been achieved for this client? SELECT ALL THAT APPLY.

1. Leukocyte count 7,500/mm^3
2. Describes the importance of keeping warm
3. Acute pain controlled at less than 3 on a 0 to 10 scale with analgesics
4. Free of chest pain or dyspnea
5. Blood transfusions effective in diminishing cell sickling
6. Hydroxyurea (Hydrea®) effective in suppressing leukocyte formation

ANSWER: 1, 2, 3, 4

A leukocyte count of 7,500/mm^3 is within normal range (5,000 to 10,000/mm^3 indicates the absence of an infection). Keeping warm and avoiding chills will help to prevent infection. Also, cold causes vasoconstriction, slowing blood flow and aggravating the sickling process. Acute pain is due to tissue hypoxia from the agglutination of sickled cells within blood vessels. Acute chest syndrome and pulmonary hypertension are two of the many complications associated with sickle cell disease. Red blood cell transfusions may help to prevent complications, but transfusions do not alter the person's body from producing the deformed erythrocytes. Hydroxyurea can decrease the permanent formation of sickled cells. A side effect (not therapeutic effect) of Hydroxyurea is suppression of leukocyte formation.

➧ ***Test-taking Tip:*** *Remember that outcomes need to be measurable. Options 5 and 6 are not measurable.*

Content Area: Adult Health; *Category of Health Alteration:* Hematological and Oncological Management; *Integrated Processes:* Nursing Process Evaluation; *Client Need:* Physiological Integrity/Physiological Adaptation/Illness Management; *Cognitive Level:* Analysis

Reference: Smeltzer, S., Bare, B., Hinkle, J., & Cheever, K. (2008). *Brunner & Suddarth's Textbook of Medical-Surgical Nursing* (11th ed., pp. 1055–1061). Philadelphia: Lippincott Williams & Wilkins.

698. A client with a diagnosis of chronic obstructive pulmonary disease (COPD) has developed polycythemia vera, and a nurse has completed teaching on measures to prevent complications. During a home health visit, the nurse evaluates that the client is correctly following the teaching when the client: SELECT ALL THAT APPLY.

1. tells the nurse about discontinuing iron supplements.
2. relays increasing alcohol intake to decrease blood viscosity.
3. records the amount consumed after drinking a glass of water.
4. discusses yesterday's phlebotomy treatment to remove blood.
5. shows the nurse a menu plan for eating three large meals daily.
6. reclines in a recliner chair with legs uncrossed, wearing antiembolic stockings (TEDS®).

ANSWER: 1, 3, 4, 6

Iron supplements, including those in multivitamins, should be avoided because the iron stimulates red blood cell production. Increasing fluid intake to 3,000 mL daily will help decrease blood viscosity. Phlebotomy is performed on a routine or intermittent basis to diminish blood viscosity, deplete iron stores, and decrease the client's ability to manufacture excess erythrocytes. Elevating the legs, avoiding constriction or crossing the legs, and wearing antiembolic socks help prevent deep vein thrombosis. Alcohol increases the risk of bleeding. Frequent, small meals are better tolerated, especially if the liver is involved.

➧ ***Test-taking Tip:*** *Focus on the issue: measures to prevent complications of polycythemia vera.*

Content Area: Adult Health; *Category of Health Alteration:* Hematological and Oncological Management; *Integrated Processes:* Teaching and Learning; *Client Need:* Health Promotion and Maintenance/Self-Care; *Cognitive Level:* Analysis

Reference: Smeltzer, S., Bare, B., Hinkle, J., & Cheever, K. (2008). *Brunner & Suddarth's Textbook of Medical-Surgical Nursing* (11th ed., pp. 1065–1066). Philadelphia: Lippincott Williams & Wilkins.

699. A nurse explains to another nurse that chronic lymphocytic leukemia (CLL) is: SELECT ALL THAT APPLY.

1. a malignancy of activated B lymphocytes.
2. the most common malignancy of older adults.
3. unresponsive to chemotherapy treatment.
4. often not treated in its early stages but the client is monitored.
5. an excessive accumulation of immature lymphocytes in the bone marrow.
6. often asymptomatic and diagnosed incidentally during routine physical examination.

ANSWER: 1, 2, 4, 6

CLL derives from a malignant clone of B lymphocytes. T-lymphocytic CLL is rare. Two-thirds of all persons with CLL are older than 60 years at diagnosis. Treatment is initiated when symptoms are severe (night sweats, painful lymphadenopathy) or the disease progresses to later stages. Because many persons are asymptomatic, it is often diagnosed during a routine physical or treatment for another condition. Treatment for CLL includes chemotherapy with fludarabine (Fludara®), but a major side effect is prolonged bone marrow suppression. In CLL there is an accumulation of mature-appearing but functionally inactive lymphocytes. Excessive accumulation of immature lymphocytes occurs in acute lymphocytic leukemia (ALL). ALL after 15 years of age is relatively uncommon.

➧ ***Test-taking Tip:*** *Recall that ALL frequently occurs in children, whereas CLL frequently occurs in adults. Learn the mnemonic for differentiating CLL from ALL: "**Be** **o**lder **a**nd **m**ature" (B = B lymphocytes; o = older adult; a = asymptomatic; m = mature but inactive lymphocytes).*

Content Area: Adult Health; *Category of Health Alteration:* Hematological and Oncological Management; *Integrated Processes:* Teaching and Learning; *Client Need:* Safe and Effective Care Environment/Management of Care/Staff Education; Physiological Integrity/Physiological Adaptation/Pathophysiology; *Cognitive Level:* Comprehension

Reference: Smeltzer, S., Bare, B., Hinkle, J., & Cheever, K. (2008). *Brunner & Suddarth's Textbook of Medical-Surgical Nursing* (11th ed., pp. 1073–1075). Philadelphia: Lippincott Williams & Wilkins.

700. EBP A client is neutropenic following treatment for acute lymphocytic leukemia and is now experiencing hypotension, tachycardia, and an elevated temperature. Because an infection is suspected, a nurse notifies a physician. Which physician order should be the nurse's priority?

1. Portable chest x-ray
2. Urine and blood cultures
3. Vancomycin (Vancocin®) 1 gm intravenously (IV) every 12 hours
4. Filgrastim (Neupogen®) 10 mg/kg subcutaneously daily

ANSWER: 2

Urine and blood cultures should be obtained before antibiotics are administered. National recommendations are to administer broad-spectrum antibiotics within 1 hour of suspected infection diagnosis. The antibiotics may be changed after culture and sensitivity reports are available (usually 24 to 48 hours). The results of the portable chest x-ray will help determine if the cause is a respiratory infection. It will not change the treatment. It takes 4 days for filgrastim to return the neutrophil count to baseline, so this is not a priority, but it should be administered as soon as possible.

Test-taking Tip: *Note the key word "priority." In questions of this type, all options will be correct, but one must be first. Recall that cultures are given before antibiotics.*

Content Area: Adult Health; *Category of Health Alteration:* Hematological and Oncological Management; *Integrated Processes:* Nursing Process Implementation; *Client Need:* Physiological Integrity/Physiological Adaptation/Illness Management; Safe and Effective Care Environment/Management of Care/Establishing Priorities; *Cognitive Level:* Analysis

Reference: Smeltzer, S., Bare, B., Hinkle, J., & Cheever, K. (2008). *Brunner & Suddarth's Textbook of Medical-Surgical Nursing* (11th ed., pp. 1067, 1069–1070). Philadelphia: Lippincott Williams & Wilkins.

EBP Reference: Hughes, W., Armstrong, D., Bodey, G., Bow, E., Brown, A., et al. (2002). Guidelines for the use of antimicrobial agents in neutropenic patients with cancer. *Clinical Infectious Diseases,* 34(6), 730–751. Available at: www.guideline.gov/summary/summary.aspx?doc_id=3206&nbr=002432&string=neutropenia

701. EBP A nurse is analyzing the serum laboratory report below for a client with a diagnosis of acute myeloid leukemia. Based on the findings of the serum laboratory report, which nursing action is most appropriate?

Serum Laboratory Test	Client's Value	Normal
WBC	15.0	3.9–11.9 K/μL
Neutrophils	40%	40%–43%
Lymphocytes	47%	16%–49%
Monocytes	11%	2%–13%
EOS	2%	0%–2%
Basophils	0%	0%–2%
RBC	2.1 m/μL	4.08–5.79 m/μL
Hgb	10.5 g/dL	13.5–17 g/dL
Hct	38%	40%–54%
Platelets	98 K/μL	179–450 K/μL

1. Instruct the client on foods to eat that are high in iron.
2. Assess the client for an allergic reaction.
3. Place the client on neutropenic precautions.
4. Teach the client to use an electric razor when shaving.

ANSWER: 4

The client is at risk for bleeding due to the low platelet count. Thrombocytopenia is a platelet count of less than 100 K/μL. Other bleeding precautions include a soft toothbrush; avoiding dental flossing, rectal temperatures, suppositories, and enemas; using stool softeners; and holding pressure to venipuncture sites for 5 minutes. Though the hemoglobin is low, the anemia that occurs in leukemia is unrelated to iron-deficiency anemia, so foods high in iron will not treat the anemia. The eosinophils (EOS) are in the normal range, so the client is not experiencing an allergic reaction. The neutrophils are within the normal range, so it is unnecessary to place the client on neutropenic precautions.

Test-taking Tip: *First focus on the laboratory values that are abnormal. Eliminate options 2 and 3 because the laboratory values associated with these actions are normal. If unsure between options 1 and 4, note that the laboratory value associated with the intervention in option 4 is very abnormal.*

Content Area: Adult Health; *Category of Health Alteration:* Hematological and Oncological Management; *Integrated Processes:* Nursing Process Implementation; *Client Need:* Physiological Integrity/Reduction of Risk Potential/Laboratory Values; Physiological Integrity/Physiological Adaptation/Illness Management; *Cognitive Level:* Analysis

Reference: Smeltzer, S., Bare, B., Hinkle, J., & Cheever, K. (2008). *Brunner & Suddarth's Textbook of Medical-Surgical Nursing* (11th ed., pp. 1071–1076). Philadelphia: Lippincott Williams & Wilkins.

EBP Reference: Seiter, K. (2006). Acute myelogenous leukemia. *E-Medicine.* Available at: www.emedicine.com/med/topic34.htm

702. A nurse obtains the following assessment data for a client diagnosed with acute myeloid leukemia. For which finding should a nurse plan interventions *first*?

1. Pain from mucositis
2. Weakness and fatigue
3. T 99°, P100, R 20, and BP 132/64 mm Hg
4. Ecchymosis and petechiae noted on arms

ANSWER: 1

Pain control is priority. The altered vital signs (other than temperature) could be related to pain. Weakness and fatigue are due to anemia and also the disease process. The temperature warrants further monitoring because it could indicate a developing infection. Ecchymosis and petechiae are associated with low platelets counts. The nurse should check the laboratory report for the platelet level.

➧ *Test-taking Tip: Use the ABCs (airway, breathing, circulation) to determine priority. In the absence of life-threatening findings, pain control should be priority.*

Content Area: Adult Health; *Category of Health Alteration:* Hematological and Oncological Management; *Integrated Processes:* Nursing Process Planning; *Client Need:* Safe and Effective Care Environment/Management of Care/Establishing Priorities; Physiological Integrity/Physiological Adaptation/Alterations in Body Systems; *Cognitive Level:* Analysis

Reference: Smeltzer, S., Bare, B., Hinkle, J., & Cheever, K. (2008). *Brunner & Suddarth's Textbook of Medical-Surgical Nursing* (11th ed., p. 1071). Philadelphia: Lippincott Williams & Wilkins.

703. A client who is receiving doxorubicin (Adriamycin®) for the first time to treat multiple myeloma develops flushing, facial swelling, headache, chills, and back pain. Which statement made by the nurse is best?

1. "These symptoms are uncomfortable for you, and I can give more medication for symptom control; these usually resolve in 1 day and are limited to the first dose."
2. "These symptoms are concerning. You may want to consider terminating treatment because these are signs of unacceptable toxicity."
3. "Next time you can receive premedication with ondansetron (Zofran®), an antiemetic to prevent these symptoms."
4. "Side effects will occur with chemotherapy. Focus on the goal of curing your cancer, and then the side effects will be more tolerable."

ANSWER: 1

This response demonstrates both compassion and competence, two aspects of caring. The nurse acknowledges the symptoms, offers treatment, and informs the client correctly that the symptoms are limited to the first dose. Responses in options 2, 3, and 4 do not demonstrate compassion and competence. The nurse is providing unsolicited advice, "consider terminating treatment," in option 2. Option 3 suggests that the nurse did not premedicate with the first dose of chemotherapy. Option 4 is belittling the client's symptoms. There is no cure for multiple myeloma. Treatment will control the illness and maintain the client's level of functioning for several years or more.

➧ *Test-taking Tip: Note the key word "best." Consider the option that demonstrates caring.*

Content Area: Adult Health; *Category of Health Alteration:* Hematological and Oncological Management; *Integrated Processes:* Communication and Documentation; Caring; *Client Need:* Physiological Integrity/Pharmacological and Parenteral Therapies/Adverse Effects/Contradictions; *Cognitive Level:* Application

References: Deglin, J., & Vallerand, A. (2007). *Davis's Drug Guide for Nurses* (10th ed., pp. 428-431). Philadelphia: F. A. Davis; Berman, A., Snyder, S., Kozier, B., & Erb, G. (2008). *Kozier & Erb's Fundamentals of Nursing: Concepts, Process, and Practice* (8th ed., p. 451). Upper Saddle River, NJ: Pearson Education.

704. Following a shift report on an oncology unit, a nurse determines that which client should be assessed first?

1. A client with breast cancer who has an order for ondansetron (Zofran®) 8 mg intravenously (IV) 30 minutes prior to chemotherapy
2. A client just admitted with a temperature of 101°F (38.3°C), diaphoresis, and an absolute neutrophil count of 98/mm^3
3. A client with breast cancer who is scheduled for external beam radiation in 15 minutes
4. A client with stomatitis associated with tonsilar cancer who receives gastrostomy tube feedings

ANSWER: 2

The newly admitted client should be assessed first because the client is neutropenic, showing signs of infection, and microorganisms from other clients would be less likely to be transmitted to the client if seen first. The client should be placed on neutropenic precautions. The client is at risk for severe sepsis if the absolute neutrophils count is less than 100/mm^3. In option 1, no time is noted for the chemotherapy treatment. In option 3, if the shift report indicates that the client has been stable, assessment can wait until the client returns or the client can be seen after first assessing the neutropenic client. The tube feeding can be initiated after the most critical clients are assessed.

➧ *Test-taking Tip: Use the nursing process to establish priorities. The most critical patient should be assessed first.*

Content Area: Adult Health; *Category of Health Alteration:* Hematological and Oncological Management; *Integrated Processes:* Nursing Process Assessment; *Client Need:* Physiological Integrity/Physiological Adaptation/Illness Management; Safe and Effective Care Environment/Management of Care/Establishing Priorities; *Cognitive Level:* Analysis

Reference: Smeltzer, S., Bare, B., Hinkle, J., & Cheever, K. (2008). *Brunner & Suddarth's Textbook of Medical-Surgical Nursing* (11th ed., pp. 1067–1070). Philadelphia: Lippincott Williams & Wilkins.

705. A clinic nurse is planning to assess the lymph nodes for a client with suspected Hodgkin's lymphoma, starting at the location where the disease usually begins. On the illustration below, at which area should the nurse plan to begin the examination?

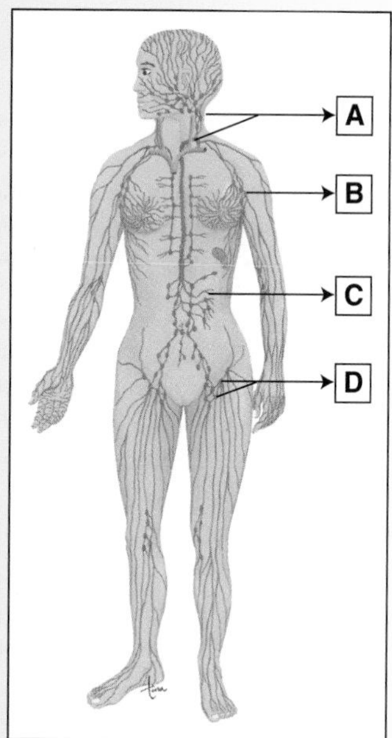

1. A
2. B
3. C
4. D

ANSWER: 1

Line A is pointing to the cervical lymph nodes. Hodgkin's lymphoma usually begins with a painless enlargement of one or more lymph nodes on one side of the neck (cervical or supraclavicular). Line B is pointing to the axillary nodes. Line C is pointing to the spleen. Line D is pointing to the inguinal nodes. The most common sites for lymphadenopathy are the cervical, supraclavicular, and mediastinal nodes; involvement of the iliac or inguinal nodes or spleen is much less common.

➧ ***Test-taking Tip:*** *Focus on the key phrase, "where the disease usually begins."*

Content Area: Adult Health; *Category of Health Alteration:* Hematological and Oncological Management; *Integrated Processes:* Nursing Process Planning; *Client Need:* Physiological Integrity/Reduction of Risk Potential/System Specific Assessments; Health Promotion and Maintenance/Techniques of Physical Assessment; *Cognitive Level:* Application

Reference: Smeltzer, S., Bare, B., Hinkle, J., & Cheever, K. (2008). *Brunner & Suddarth's Textbook of Medical-Surgical Nursing* (11th ed., pp. 94, 1080). Philadelphia: Lippincott Williams & Wilkins.

706. A female client is to receive chemotherapy and radiation for Hodgkin's lymphoma with cervical and axillary node involvement. A nurse evaluates that the client is coping positively when the client states:

1. "I selected a wig that matches my hair color, but I will miss my own hair."
2. "I am so glad that the chemotherapy and radiation treatments won't cause me to lose my hair."
3. "The chemotherapy-drug combination will prevent mucositis and immunosuppression."
4. "I have faith that my doctor will be able to cure me and I won't have any long-term effects."

ANSWER: 1

The client is expressing her feelings about her hair loss, but she has acted positively related to her feelings and selected a wig. Responses in options 2, 3, and 4 reflect either that the client is in denial or is uninformed regarding the effects of the chemotherapy and radiation treatments. Because chemotherapy and radiation will involve the cervical lymph nodes, side effects will include alopecia, mucositis, and immunosuppression. The risk for other cancers is increased after chemotherapy and radiation for Hodgkin's lymphoma so long-term surveillance is crucial.

➧ ***Test-taking Tip:*** *Note the key words "coping positively." Select the option that demonstrates either cognitive or behavioral effort to adapt to the stressful situation.*

Content Area: Adult Health; *Category of Health Alteration:* Hematological and Oncological Management; *Integrated Processes:* Nursing Process Evaluation; *Client Need:* Psychosocial Integrity/Coping Mechanisms; *Cognitive Level:* Analysis

Reference: Smeltzer, S., Bare, B., Hinkle, J., & Cheever, K. (2008). *Brunner & Suddarth's Textbook of Medical-Surgical Nursing* (11th ed., pp. 94, 1080–1081). Philadelphia: Lippincott Williams & Wilkins.

707. A physician documents that a client, diagnosed with stage III non-Hodgkin's lymphoma (NHL), is experiencing "B symptoms." A nurse interprets this to mean that the client has:

1. bleeding associated with low platelets counts.
2. a B lymphocyte malignancy and has progressed to an untreatable stage.
3. symptoms from exposure to a viral infection, such as Epstein-Barr virus.
4. recurrent fever, drenching night sweats, and an unintentional weight loss of 10% or more.

ANSWER: 4

Typically, NHL is not diagnosed until it progresses to stage III or IV because the client is asymptomatic. One-third of persons with NHL will have "B symptoms" at stage III or IV. Options 1, 2, and 3 do not describe "B symptoms." Most NHLs involve the B lymphocytes; only 5% involve the T lymphocytes. Treatment varies and depends on the actual classification of the disease, the stage, prior treatment (if any), and the person's ability to tolerate therapy. Although the cause of NHL is unknown, there is an increased incidence in people with viral infections.

▶ ***Test-taking Tip:*** *Select the option that focuses on symptoms (note plural).*

Content Area: Adult Health; *Category of Health Alteration:* Hematological and Oncological Management; *Integrated Processes:* Nursing Process Analysis; Communication and Documentation; *Client Need:* Physiological Integrity/Reduction of Risk Potential/Potential for Alterations in Body Systems; *Cognitive Level:* Application

Reference: Smeltzer, S., Bare, B., Hinkle, J., & Cheever, K. (2008). *Brunner & Suddarth's Textbook of Medical-Surgical Nursing* (11th ed., p. 1082). Philadelphia: Lippincott Williams & Wilkins.

708. A nurse is caring for a client hospitalized with idiopathic thrombocytopenic purpura (ITP). Which self-care measures should the nurse plan to include when teaching the client? SELECT ALL THAT APPLY.

1. "Use dental floss after brushing your teeth to prevent gum hyperplasia."
2. "Use only an electric razor when shaving."
3. "Remove throw rugs in your home, and avoid clutter."
4. "Increase fiber in your diet, and drink plenty of liquids to avoid constipation."
5. "Keep appointments for monthly platelet transfusions."

ANSWER: 2, 3, 4

Because the client is at risk for bleeding due to low platelets counts, measures to decrease the risk of bleeding should be implemented. Throw rugs and clutter increase the risk for falls with subsequent bleeding. Constipation can lead to hemorrhoids and increase the risk for bleeding. Dental floss can traumatize the gums and increase the risk for bleeding. Platelet transfusions are usually avoided because the person's antiplatelet antibodies bind with the transfused platelets, causing them to be destroyed.

▶ ***Test-taking Tip:*** *If unsure of ITP, recall that purpura is caused from bleeding into the tissues. Select the options that would prevent bleeding.*

Content Area: Adult Health; *Category of Health Alteration:* Hematological and Oncological Management; *Integrated Processes:* Nursing Process Planning; *Client Need:* Health Promotion and Maintenance/Self-Care; *Cognitive Level:* Application

Reference: Smeltzer, S., Bare, B., Hinkle, J., & Cheever, K. (2008). *Brunner & Suddarth's Textbook of Medical-Surgical Nursing* (11th ed., p. 1088). Philadelphia: Lippincott Williams & Wilkins.

709. A nurse teaches a coworker that the treatment for hemophilia will likely include periodic self-administration of:

1. platelets.
2. whole blood.
3. factor concentrates.
4. fresh frozen plasma.

ANSWER: 3

A person with hemophilia A is deficient in factor VIII; hemophilia B, factor IX; and von Willebrand's hemophilia, the von Willebrand's factor and factor VIII. Recombinant forms of the factors are available for the client to self-administer intravenously at home. Although whole blood and fresh frozen plasma contain the deficient factors, periodic administration of factor concentrates are safer. Platelets do not contain the deficient clotting factors.

▶ ***Test-taking Tip:*** *Apply knowledge of blood products and factor deficiencies in hemophilia.*

Content Area: Adult Health; *Category of Health Alteration:* Hematological and Oncological Management; *Integrated Processes:* Teaching and Learning; *Client Need:* Safe and Effective Care Environment/Management of Care/Staff Education; *Cognitive Level:* Comprehension

Reference: Smeltzer, S., Bare, B., Hinkle, J., & Cheever, K. (2008). *Brunner & Suddarth's Textbook of Medical-Surgical Nursing* (11th ed., pp. 1091, 1103). Philadelphia: Lippincott Williams & Wilkins.

710. A client diagnosed with von Willebrand's disease calls a clinic after experiencing hemarthrosis. Which treatment should a nurse recommend?

1. "Treat the pain with two 325-mg aspirin (Ecotrin®) tablets every 4 hours."
2. "Apply cold packs 2 hours on and 2 hours off of the affected site for 24 to 48 hours."
3. "Come to the clinic immediately so you can receive an infusion of fresh frozen plasma."
4. "If you are wearing a splint, remove it immediately to avoid compartment syndrome."

ANSWER: 2

Hemarthrosis is bleeding into the joint. The pressure of the ice pack and cold will reduce the bleeding and swelling. Aspirin and NSAIDs are contraindicated because they interfere with platelet aggregation. The client and family are usually taught how to administer factor concentrates at home at the first sign of bleeding. The splint should be left on initially to control bleeding. The client should be instructed on how to assess for adequate tissue perfusion.

➧ ***Test-taking Tip:*** *If unsure of the meaning of hemarthrosis, apply knowledge of medical terminology. "Heme-" refers to blood, and "arthrosis" refers to joints. Remember that cold reduces bleeding.*

Content Area: Adult Health; *Category of Health Alteration:* Hematological and Oncological Management; *Integrated Processes:* Nursing Process Implementation; *Client Need:* Physiological Integrity/Reduction of Risk Potential/Potential for Complications from Surgical Procedures and Health Alterations; *Cognitive Level:* Application

Reference: Smeltzer, S., Bare, B., Hinkle, J., & Cheever, K. (2008). *Brunner & Suddarth's Textbook of Medical-Surgical Nursing* (11th ed., p. 1091). Philadelphia: Lippincott Williams & Wilkins.

---

711. A client has a wound suction device for blood salvage following a left total knee replacement so that the blood can be reinfused into the client within the first 6 hours postoperatively. Which intervention should a nurse plan to implement to care for this wound suction device?

1. Discard the first 500 mL in the suction container and wait until the container is full again before beginning a reinfusion.
2. As soon as the prescribed amount is noted in the container, obtain the blood and prepare it for reinfusion into the client intravenously.
3. Separate the blood from the drainage, and reinfuse the blood back through the drainage system into the wound.
4. Remove the blood from the drainage system and send it to the blood bank to be prepared for an infusion.

ANSWER: 2

The blood salvage wound suction device drains blood from the surgical wound for reinfusion intravenously within 6 hours. The special device collects and filters the blood so it can be drained into a transfusion bag for infusion. The first 500 mL would be mostly blood and should not be discarded but reinfused. Usually all but 50 mL of the drainage in the collection device would be drained for infusion. There is no mechanism to separate the blood from other drainage. The blood is not reinfused into the wound but intravenously. There is no need to send the drainage to the blood bank. It will delay infusion, increase the risk of contamination, and increase the risk of administering mismatched blood.

➧ ***Test-taking Tip:*** *Note that option 2 is more complete than the other options.*

Content Area: Adult Health; *Category of Health Alteration:* Hematological and Oncological Management; *Integrated Processes:* Nursing Process Planning; *Client Need:* Physiological Integrity/Pharmacological and Parenteral Therapies/Blood and Blood Products; *Cognitive Level:* Application

Reference: Ignatavicius, D., & Workman, M. (2006). *Medical-Surgical Nursing: Critical Thinking for Collaborative Care* (5th ed., p. 917). St. Louis, MO: Elsevier/Saunders.

---

712. The family of a client who is scheduled for emergency surgery following an accident asks if they can donate blood for the client. The client's blood type is B negative. A nurse informs the family that packed red blood cells (PRBCs) could likely be used from family members whose blood type is:

1. type A positive.
2. type B positive.
3. type B negative.
4. type O positive.
5. type O negative.
6. type AB positive.

ANSWER: 3

The ABO system identifies the type of antigen present on the person's erythrocyte membrane, A, B, both A and B, or neither A or B (type O). The person with B negative blood type has B antigen on the erythrocyte and does not have an Rh (or D) antigen on the cell (whereas Rh positive does have a D antigen on the cell). The person can only receive PRBC of the same blood type (option 3) to prevent a significant PRBC reaction. Formerly in emergency situations, it was thought that O blood type was safe to administer when the client's blood type was not known. The American Red Cross now advises against this practice and recommends only administering blood of the same blood type.

➧ ***Test-taking Tip:*** *Focus on the issue: donating blood. Recall that blood typing and crossmatching is completed to assure that the client receives only blood of the same blood type.*

Content Area: Adult Health; *Category of Health Alteration:* Hematological and Oncological Management; *Integrated Processes:* Nursing Process Implementation; *Client Need:* Physiological Integrity/Pharmacological and Parenteral Therapies/Blood and Blood Products; *Cognitive Level:* Application

Reference: Smeltzer, S., Bare, B., Hinkle, J., & Cheever, K. (2008). *Brunner & Suddarth's Textbook of Medical-Surgical Nursing* (11th ed., p. 1106). Philadelphia: Lippincott Williams & Wilkins.

713. A nurse working in the blood mobile is screening clients to determine if they qualify for blood donation of whole blood. Which questions should the nurse ask during the screening interview? SELECT ALL THAT APPLY.

1. "What is your age?"
2. "If you have a tattoo, when did you receive it?"
3. "Have you had any close contact with anyone with HIV or hepatitis?"
4. "If you smoke, when was the last time you smoked tobacco products?"
5. "Have you been immunized for rubella, mumps, or varicella within the last month?"
6. "Did you receive a blood transfusion or blood product anywhere outside of the United States?"

ANSWER: 1, 2, 3, 5, 6

Persons ineligible to donate blood include those younger than 17 years of age; those immunized for rubella, mumps, or varicella within the last month; those with a history of a recent tattoo or close contact with a person with HIV or hepatitis; and those receiving transfusions in the United Kingdom, Gibraltar, or the Falkland Islands because of the increased likelihood of transmitting Creutzfeldt-Jakob disease. Persons who smoke tobacco products may donate blood unless they have a recent history of asthma.

▶ ***Test-taking Tip:*** *Focus on infectious disease transmission, noting that options 2, 3, 5, and 6 increase the risk of transmitting the diseases.*

Content Area: Adult Health; *Category of Health Alteration:* Hematological and Oncological Management; *Integrated Processes:* Nursing Process Assessment; *Client Need:* Health Promotion and Maintenance/Health Screening; Safe and Effective Care Environment/ Safety and Infection Control/Standard/Transmission-based/Other Precautions; *Cognitive Level:* Application

Reference: Smeltzer, S., Bare, B., Hinkle, J., & Cheever, K. (2008). *Brunner & Suddarth's Textbook of Medical-Surgical Nursing* (11th ed., pp. 1104–1105). Philadelphia: Lippincott Williams & Wilkins.

714. EBP A client with symptoms of anemia and a hemoglobin of 7.8 g/dL refuses blood and blood products transfusions for religious reasons. A nurse should anticipate that a health-care provider might prescribe: SELECT ALL THAT APPLY.

1. Epoetin alfa (Procrit®)
2. Folic acid
3. Albumin
4. Platelets
5. Fresh frozen plasma
6. Granulocytes

ANSWER: 1, 2

Epoetin alfa (erythropoietin growth factor) and folic acid promote erythropoiesis (production of red blood cells), thus decreasing the need for transfusions. Folic acid also stimulates production of white blood cells and platelets. According to the evidence base, for persons with hemoglobin less than 8 g/dL, the use of either transfusion or erythropoietic growth factor was rated "appropriate." Albumin, platelets, plasma, and granulocytes are all blood products.

▶ ***Test-taking Tip:*** *Focus on the issue: low hemoglobin and client refuses blood and blood products. Select options 1 and 2, because these are not blood products.*

Content Area: Adult Health; *Category of Health Alteration:* Hematological and Oncological Management; *Integrated Processes:* Nursing Process Planning; *Client Need:* Physiological Integrity/ Pharmacological and Parenteral Therapies/Pharmacological Agents/ Actions; *Cognitive Level:* Application

Reference: Smeltzer, S., Bare, B., Hinkle, J., & Cheever, K. (2008). *Brunner & Suddarth's Textbook of Medical-Surgical Nursing* (11th ed., p. 1103). Philadelphia: Lippincott Williams & Wilkins.

EBP Reference: Dubois, R., Goodnough, L., Ershler, W., Van Winkle, L., & Nissenson, A. (2006). Identification, diagnosis, and management of anemia in adult ambulatory patients treated by primary care physicians: Evidence-based and consensus recommendations. *Current Medical Research Opinion*, 22(2), 385–395. Available at: www.guideline.gov/summary/summary.aspx?doc_id=9925&nbr=005320&string=anemia

715. A client who has received 50 mL of a unit of whole blood complains of low back pain. In response to this client's symptom, a nurse should *first*:

1. reposition the client.
2. assess the pain further.
3. administer an analgesic.
4. stop the blood transfusion.

ANSWER: 4

Low back pain is a symptom of a potentially life-threatening acute hemolytic reaction. The pain is caused from agglutination of red blood cells in the kidneys and renal vasoconstriction. Hemolytic reactions occur most often within the first 50 mL of the infusion.

Test-taking Tip: When a question asks for the first action, all other actions may also be correct, but the answer is the option that should be first. Use the nursing process. Recall that this could be a life-threatening situation, thus an action follows the initial assessment, not further assessment. Eliminate option 2. Of the remaining options, think about which action is quickest, option 4.

Content Area: Adult Health; *Category of Health Alteration:* Hematological and Oncological Management; *Integrated Processes:* Nursing Process Implementation; *Client Need:* Physiological Integrity/Pharmacological and Parenteral Therapies/Blood and Blood Products; *Cognitive Level:* Application

Reference: Smeltzer, S., Bare, B., Hinkle, J., & Cheever, K. (2008). *Brunner & Suddarth's Textbook of Medical-Surgical Nursing* (11th ed., p. 1109). Philadelphia: Lippincott Williams & Wilkins.

---

716. At 1000 hours, a nurse is documenting after administering 275 mL of compatible platelets, unit number XR123, to a client. Which information should the nurse document? SELECT ALL THAT APPLY.

1. "One unit blood infused over 4 hours."
2. "Platelet number XR123 checked prior to administration."
3. "No transfusion reactions noted."
4. "D5W infused with platelets to prevent cell clumping."
5. "Infusion of 275 mL of platelets started at 0830 hours completed."

ANSWER: 2, 3, 5

Documentation should include the type of product infused (platelets), product number (compatible platelets were ordered), volume infused, time of infusion, and any adverse reactions. Platelets should be infused as fast as the client can tolerate the infusion to diminish clumping. Option 1 documents an incomplete blood type, and platelets are unlikely to be administered over 4 hours. Only 0.9% NaCl should be used when administering blood or blood products and usually only to purge the line before and after administration.

Test-taking Tip: Apply knowledge of information that should be documented in the client's chart when administering blood or blood products.

Content Area: Adult Health; *Category of Health Alteration:* Hematological and Oncological Management; *Integrated Processes:* Communication and Documentation; *Client Need:* Physiological Integrity/Pharmacological and Parenteral Therapies/Blood and Blood Products; *Cognitive Level:* Analysis

References: Ignatavicius, D., & Workman, M. (2006). *Medical-Surgical Nursing: Critical Thinking for Collaborative Care* (5th ed., p. 914). St. Louis, MO: Elsevier/Saunders; Smeltzer, S., Bare, B., Hinkle, J., & Cheever, K. (2008). *Brunner & Suddarth's Textbook of Medical-Surgical Nursing* (11th ed., p. 1108). Philadelphia: Lippincott Williams & Wilkins.

---

717. A young adult with a diagnosis of hemophilia A is receiving a monthly scheduled dose of factor VIII cryoprecipitate (Bioclate®). While a nurse is administering the Bioclate®, the client begins to cry. Which nursing response would be most appropriate?

1. "Why are you crying? You seem afraid when I am administering the Bioclate®."
2. "Is it painful when I administer the Bioclate® intravenous push? If it is, I can administer it by infusion."
3. "I know this is uncomfortable for you, but this will only take about 3 minutes to administer."
4. "If you want to talk to me about what you are feeling, I am here to listen."

ANSWER: 4

The nurse is offering self, which is a therapeutic communication technique. Option 1 challenges the client's feelings. Option 2 is seeking information, but is not most appropriate because the initial response from an adult would not be crying if it were painful. Option 3 ignores the client's feelings and presumes that the nurse knows what initiated the client's crying.

Test-taking Tip: Focus on the issue, the nurse's response to the client's crying and not on the nurse's administration of the Bioclate®. The client has been receiving this monthly, so there is likely another reason for the client's crying. Eliminate options 1, 2, and 3 because they focus on the nurse's procedure.

Content Area: Adult Health; *Category of Health Alteration:* Hematological and Oncological Management; *Integrated Processes:* Caring; *Client Need:* Psychosocial Integrity/Therapeutic Communication; *Cognitive Level:* Application

Reference: Berman, A., Snyder, S., Kozier, B., & Erb, G. (2008). *Kozier & Erb's Fundamentals of Nursing: Concepts, Process, and Practice* (8th ed., pp. 470–471). Upper Saddle River, NJ: Pearson Education.

718. EBP A client with leukemia asks a nurse to explain how donor cells are obtained for peripheral blood stem cell transplantation (PBSCT). Which statement by the nurse is correct?

1. "A large amount of bone marrow tissue is harvested from a donor's hip bone under general anesthesia in the operating room."
2. "Stem cells are collected from the donor's blood, which goes through a machine, removes the stem cells, and then returns the blood back to the donor."
3. "Stem cells are collected from a donor through a process called apheresis, which removes the stem cells from the blood. This typically takes 10 to 15 minutes."
4. "Stem cells are obtained similar to other blood donations, where the blood is collected and then administered to you immediately following collection."

ANSWER: 2

In PBSCT, stem cells are collected through apheresis via a machine that removes stem cells and returns the blood back to the donor. The cells that are collected can be frozen and stored until ready to be transplanted. Option 1 describes the process of obtaining donor cells by traditional harvesting, not PBSCT. Administering blood to the client immediately would be unsafe. While the process is called apheresis, the process takes from 4 to 6 hours and not 10 to 15 minutes. Too much blood would be removed to obtain the number of stem cells if whole blood were collected.

▶ ***Test-taking Tip:*** *Use the process of elimination and eliminate an option that refers to the bone marrow and not peripheral blood, an action that is unsafe and an option that addresses an insufficient amount of time for stem cell collection.*

Content Area: Adult Health; *Category of Health Alteration:* Hematological and Oncological Management; *Integrated Processes:* Teaching and Learning; *Client Need:* Physiological Integrity/Reduction of Risk Potential/Therapeutic Procedures; *Cognitive Level:* Application

Reference: Smeltzer, S., Bare, B., Hinkle, J., & Cheever, K. (2008). *Brunner & Suddarth's Textbook of Medical-Surgical Nursing* (11th ed., pp. 415, 1102, 1112–1113). Philadelphia: Lippincott Williams & Wilkins.

EBP Reference: National Cancer Institute (2004). *National Cancer Institute Fact Sheet: Bone Marrow Transplantation and Peripheral Blood Stem Cell Transplantation: Questions and Answers.* Available at: www.cancer.gov/cancertopics/factsheet/therapy/bone-marrow-transplant

---

719. A female nurse tells a coworker that she is confused because a physician stated that graft-versus-host disease (GVHD) symptoms were desirable for a particular client after a bone marrow transplant. In which type of malignancy is GVHD sometimes desirable?

1. Gastrointestinal
2. Reproductive
3. Neurological
4. Hematological

ANSWER: 4

The donor lymphocytes can mount a reaction against any lingering tumor cells and destroy them. Bone marrow transplant is not a treatment for gastrointestinal, reproductive, or neurological malignancies unless the primary source is hematological.

▶ ***Test-taking Tip:*** *Think about the purpose of a bone marrow transplant before attempting to answer this question. This should direct you to option 4.*

Content Area: Adult Health; *Category of Health Alteration:* Hematological and Oncological Management; *Integrated Processes:* Teaching and Learning; *Client Need:* Safe and Effective Care Environment/Management of Care/Staff Education; *Cognitive Level:* Application

Reference: Smeltzer, S., Bare, B., Hinkle, J., & Cheever, K. (2008). *Brunner & Suddarth's Textbook of Medical-Surgical Nursing* (11th ed., p. 1113). Philadelphia: Lippincott Williams & Wilkins.

---

720. EBP A client diagnosed with acute myeloid leukemia receives a bone marrow transplant. Which medication to prevent graft-versus-host disease (GVHD) should a nurse anticipate receiving an order to administer?

1. A cephalosporin antibiotic, such as ceftazidime (Fortaz®)
2. An immunosuppressant, such as cyclosporine (Neoral®)
3. A chemotherapeutic agent, such as cisplatin (Platinol A-Q®)
4. Peginterferon alfa-2a (Pegasys®) for prevention and treatment of hepatitis

ANSWER: 2

GVHD occurs when the T lymphocytes proliferate from the transplanted donor marrow and mount an immune response against the recipient's tissues. An immunosuppressant prevents the immune response. Antibiotics are administered to prevent infection. Cisplatin is administered mainly to treat metastatic testicular, ovarian, and cervical carcinoma; advanced bladder cancer; and head and neck cancer. Interferons have antiviral activity, which decrease the progression of hepatic damage associated with hepatitis A and B. This would only be administered if the transplanted cells transmitted the disease. The biological agent interferon is used to treat follicular low-grade lymphomas.

▶ ***Test-taking Tip:*** *Apply knowledge of medication effects to answer this question.*

Content Area: Adult Health; *Category of Health Alteration:* Hematological and Oncological Management; *Integrated Processes:* Nursing Process Planning; *Client Need:* Physiological Integrity/Pharmacological and Parenteral Therapies/Pharmacological Agents/Actions; *Cognitive Level:* Application

Reference: Smeltzer, S., Bare, B., Hinkle, J., & Cheever, K. (2008). *Brunner & Suddarth's Textbook of Medical-Surgical Nursing* (11th ed., p. 416). Philadelphia: Lippincott Williams & Wilkins.

EBP Reference: Milligan, D., Grimwade, D., Cullis, J., Bond, L., Swirsky, D., et al. (2005, May 23). *Guidelines on the Management of Acute Myeloid Leukemia in Adults*. London: British Society of Hematology. Available at: www.guideline.gov/summary/summary.aspx?doc_id=9557&nbr=005102&string=leukemia

---

721. EBP A nurse is evaluating a client's understanding of teaching about changes to expect following a bone marrow transplant (BMT). Which statement by the client indicates the client misunderstood the expected changes?

1. "You can have weight gain from the side effects of your steroid immunosuppressant medications."
2. "Sterility can occur from the destruction of your own stem cells with chemotherapy and radiation."
3. "Cataracts may develop after total body irradiation."
4. "Changes to the mouth include a white, patchy tongue."

ANSWER: 4

A white, patchy tongue is a sign of a fungal infection with *Candidiasis albicans* and would not be an expected change. Changes in weight, sexuality, and vision are common changes as a result of the total body irradiation after BMT.

▶ ***Test-taking Tip:*** *Note the key words "expected change" and "misunderstood." Look for the option that would not be an expected change.*

Content Area: Adult Health; *Category of Health Alteration:* Hematological and Oncological Management; *Integrated Processes:* Teaching and Learning; *Client Need:* Physiological Integrity/Physiological Adaptation/Unexpected Response to Therapies; *Cognitive Level:* Application

Reference: Smeltzer, S., Bare, B., Hinkle, J., & Cheever, K. (2008). *Brunner & Suddarth's Textbook of Medical-Surgical Nursing* (11th ed., pp. 416–417, 1112–1113). Philadelphia: Lippincott Williams & Wilkins.

EBP Reference: Tierney, D. (2004). Sexuality following hematopoietic cell transplantation. *Clinical Journal of Oncology Nursing*, 8(6), 43–47.

---

722. Which nursing diagnosis should have the highest priority for a client experiencing superior vena cava syndrome secondary to lung cancer?

1. Ineffective breathing pattern
2. Ineffective tissue perfusion
3. Risk for infection
4. Impaired skin integrity

ANSWER: 1

Ineffective breathing pattern occurs with superior vena cava syndrome because the superior vena cava is located next to the main stem bronchus and causes compression of the intrathoracic structures. Ineffective tissue perfusion occurs in lymphedema. Risk for infection occurs with chemotherapy treatment. Impaired skin integrity occurs with malignant skin conditions.

▶ ***Test-taking Tip:*** *Focus on the key term "superior vena cava syndrome" and think about the symptoms the client is likely to experience. Recall that the vena cava is located next to the main stem bronchus. Use the ABCs (airway, breathing, circulation) to establish priority.*

Content Area: Adult Health; *Category of Health Alteration:* Hematological and Oncological Management; *Integrated Processes:* Nursing Process Analysis; *Client Need:* Physiological Integrity/Physiological Adaptation/Medical Emergencies; *Cognitive Level:* Analysis

References: Black, J., & Hokanson Hawks, J. (2009). *Medical-Surgical Nursing: Clinical Management for Positive Outcomes* (8th ed., p. 297). St. Louis, MO: Saunders/Elsevier; Swearingen, P. (2007). *Manual of Medical-Surgical Nursing Care* (6th ed.). St. Louis, MO: Mosby.

723. A nurse explains "watchful waiting" (ongoing visits to a physician for observation of signs and symptoms without treatment) to a client with prostate cancer. Under which circumstance should the nurse recommend "watchful waiting"?

1. When bone cancer is diagnosed along with prostate cancer
2. When the client is older than age 70 with a life expectancy of less than 10 years with low-grade disease
3. When a client has extension of the tumor outside of the prostate
4. When a client has an elevated prostate specific antigen, has no symptoms, and is under the age of 60

ANSWER: 2

When a client is older than age 70 with a life expectancy of less than 10 years with low-grade disease, the nurse should recommend conservative management or "watchful waiting." The other three situations generally require aggressive therapy.

▶ ***Test-taking Tip:*** *Focus on the key phrases "watchful waiting" and "without treatment." Because options 1 and 3 indicate conditions requiring treatment, these would be eliminated, leaving no symptoms and under age 60 and the client older than age 70 years with less than 10 years to live with low-grade disease. Since clients under age 60 are more likely to receive treatment, that leaves the older client.*

Content Area: Adult Health; *Category of Health Alteration:* Hematological and Oncological Management; *Integrated Processes:* Nursing Process Implementation; *Client Need:* Physiological Integrity/Physiological Adaptation/Illness Management; *Cognitive Level:* Application

Reference: Langhorne, M., Fulton, J., & Otto, S. (2007). *Oncology Nursing* (5th ed., p. 168). St. Louis, MO: Mosby/Elsevier.

724. A nurse is teaching a client about self-breast examination and discusses where breast cancer commonly occurs. Identify with an X the area where the nurse should teach the client that breast cancer occurs most frequently.

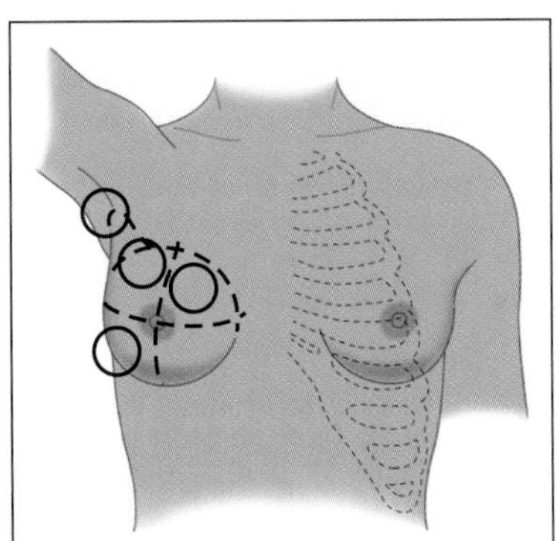

ANSWER:

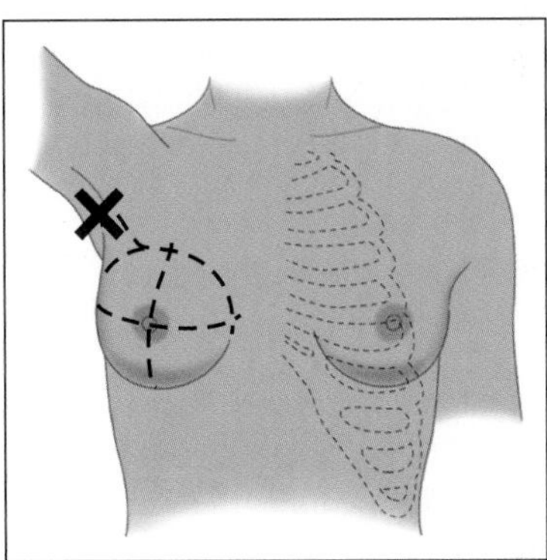

Breast cancer lesions are frequently found in the upper outer quadrant, near the axilla known as the tail of Spence (area A).

▶ ***Test-taking Tip:*** *The phrases "breast cancer" and "most frequently" are key phrases in the stem. Recall that lymph tissue from the breast empties into the lymph drainage system in the axilla.*

Content Area: Adult Health; *Category of Health Alteration:* Hematological and Oncological Management; *Integrated Processes:* Teaching and Learning; *Client Need:* Health Promotion and Maintenance/Health Screening; *Cognitive Level:* Application

References: Langhorne, M., Fulton, J., & Otto, S. (2007). *Oncology Nursing* (5th ed., p. 107). St. Louis, MO: Mosby/Elsevier; Dillon, P. (2007). *Nursing Health Assessment: A Critical Thinking, Case Studies Approach* (2nd ed., Fig. 16–1). Philadelphia: F. A. Davis.

725. Which actions should a nurse initiate for a client who had a left modified radical mastectomy (a total mastectomy with axillary node dissection and removal of the lining over the pectoralis major muscle)?

1. Elevate the left arm above the head.
2. Insert all intravenous (IV) access sites on the right side.
3. Have the client view the incision site as soon as possible.
4. Initiate strengthening exercises of the left arm within 24 hours of surgery.

ANSWER: 2

All IV access sites should be initiated on the nonoperative side to prevent circulatory impairment. The arm on the operative side should be elevated on a pillow, but not above the head. The nurse should assess the readiness of the client to look at the incision site, but at the readiness of the client and not as soon as possible. Only range of motion to the lower arm should be carried out for the first few days after surgery, with exercises and range of motion to the shoulder after the drains are removed.

Test-taking Tip: *Focus on the key word "actions," and think about the effects of the surgery on the body. Eliminate options 3 and 4 due to the time elements in the response. Since placing the arm above the head would be contraindicated due to the negative effect on the suture sites, option 2 is the only correct response.*

Content Area: Adult Health; *Category of Health Alteration:* Hematological and Oncological Management; *Integrated Processes:* Nursing Process Implementation; *Client Need:* Physiological Integrity Reduction of Risk Potential/Potential for Complications from Surgical Procedures and Health Alterations; *Cognitive Level:* Application

Reference: Langhorne, M., Fulton, J., & Otto, S. (2007). *Oncology Nursing* (5th ed., p. 114). St. Louis, MO: Mosby/Elsevier.

726. A nurse discusses the self-care guidelines to minimize the side effects of radiation on the skin. Which actions, to reduce radiation skin reactions, should the nurse explain to the client? SELECT ALL THAT APPLY.

1. Wear loose-fitting, soft clothing over the treated skin.
2. Use a straightedged razor to shave the hair in the treated area.
3. Swim only in swimming pools to avoid stagnant water.
4. Use only skin-care products suggested by the radiation staff.
5. Apply skin products immediately before radiation treatment.
6. Wash treated area gently with lukewarm water and mild soap.

ANSWER: 1, 4, 6

Wearing loose-fitting, soft clothing over the treated skin, using only skin-care products suggested by the radiation staff, and washing the treated area gently with lukewarm water and mild soap are recommended skin-care activities to reduce radiation skin reactions. The use of electric razors for shaving a treated area is recommended. Clients are advised to avoid swimming in chlorinated water and to delay the application of skin-care products within 4 hours of radiation treatment.

Test-taking Tip: *Focus on the "effects of radiation" and concentrate on the relationship between each of the options and protection of the skin. Options 2, 3, and 5 have negative effects on the skin and can be eliminated.*

Content Area: Adult Health; *Category of Health Alteration:* Hematological and Oncological Management; *Integrated Processes:* Teaching and Learning; *Client Need:* Physiological Integrity/Reduction of Risk Potential/Potential for Complications of Diagnostic Tests/Treatments/Procedures; *Cognitive Level:* Application

Reference: Langhorne, M., Fulton, J., & Otto, S. (2007). *Oncology Nursing* (5th ed., p. 349). St. Louis, MO: Mosby/Elsevier.

727. In discussing prevention of bladder cancer with a client, which factors that increase the client's risk for bladder cancer should the nurse emphasize? SELECT ALL THAT APPLY.

1. Consuming caffeine
2. Smoking tobacco
3. Consuming multivitamins
4. Being exposed to paint smells
5. Being exposed to the smell of tires in the rubber industry

ANSWER: 2, 4, 5

Smoking is the number one cause of bladder cancer in the world. Exposure to aromatic amines in the textile, paint, and rubber industries is clearly associated with bladder cancer. Consumption of caffeine is not associated with an increased risk for bladder cancer. Studies show a protective effect with an increased intake of vitamins A, B6, and E.

Test-taking Tip: *The key words are "risk factor" and "bladder cancer." Select options that pertain to inhalation.*

Content Area: Adult Health; *Category of Health Alteration:* Hematological and Oncological Management; *Integrated Processes:* Teaching and Learning; *Client Need:* Health Promotion and Maintenance/Disease Prevention; *Cognitive Level:* Application

Reference: Langhorne, M., Fulton, J., & Otto, S. (2007). *Oncology Nursing* (5th ed., p. 176). St. Louis, MO: Mosby/Elsevier.

728. A client diagnosed with Hodgkin's lymphoma develops radiation pneumonitis 3 months after radiation treatment. For which symptoms of radiation pneumonitis should a nurse observe the client?

1. Tachypnea, hypotension, and fever
2. Cough, fever, and dyspnea
3. Bradypnea, cough, and decreased urine output
4. Cough, tachycardia, and altered mental status

ANSWER: 2

Cough, fever, and dyspnea are classic symptoms in radiation pneumonitis due to a decrease in the surfactant in the lung. Hypotension, decreased urine output, and altered mental status are symptoms that are not common in radiation pneumonitis.

▶ ***Test-taking Tip:*** *Note the key words "radiation pneumonitis," and focus on the association with respiratory symptoms. Options 1, 3, and 4 can be eliminated because these options each contain a nonrespiratory response item.*

Content Area: Adult Health; *Category of Health Alteration:* Hematological and Oncological Management; *Integrated Processes:* Nursing Process Assessment; *Client Need:* Physiological Integrity/Reduction of Risk Potential/Potential for Complications of Diagnostic Tests/Treatments/Procedures; *Cognitive Level:* Analysis

Reference: Langhorne, M., Fulton, J., & Otto, S. (2007). *Oncology Nursing* (5th ed., p. 352). St. Louis, MO: Mosby/Elsevier.

729. EBP Which nursing actions should a nurse implement to prevent extravasation when administering vesicant chemotherapy medications such as doxorubicin hydrochloride (Adriamycin®)? SELECT ALL THAT APPLY.

1. Administer vesicant infusions through a peripheral intravenous (IV) device if it is to be infused in less than 60 minutes and check patency every 5 to 10 minutes.
2. Ask the client frequently about discomfort at the peripheral IV site during infusion.
3. Check the IV pump and alarm for indications of infiltration of the medication.
4. Check for blood return in a central venous catheter prior to administration of the vesicant medication.
5. Flush the peripheral and central venous catheters with 5 to 10 mL of normal saline between medications.
6. Use small-gauged syringes to flush all catheters.

ANSWER: 1, 2, 4, 5

National guidelines indicate the following actions contribute to the safe administration of vesicant medications: administering vesicant infusion through peripheral IV catheters under 60 minutes and checking patency of the IV catheter every 5 to 10 minutes, continuously asking the client if any discomfort exists at the IV insertion site, checking for blood return in the central venous catheter prior to administration of the vesicant medication, and flushing the venous access lines with 5 to 10 mL of normal saline between medications. IV pumps and alarms cannot be relied upon to detect extravasation because infiltration usually does not cause sufficient pressure to trigger an alarm. Small-gauge syringes produce high pressures and may cause injury to the blood vessel or damage a central line catheter.

▶ ***Test-taking Tip:*** *Visualizing the nursing actions and thinking about the procedures for safe administration of IV medication will assist in selecting the correct responses.*

Content Area: Adult Health; *Category of Health Alteration:* Hematological and Oncological Management; *Integrated Processes:* Nursing Process Implementation; *Client Need:* Safe and Effective Care Environment/Safety and Infection Control/Injury Prevention; *Cognitive Level:* Application

Reference: Black, J., & Hokanson Hawks, J. (2009). *Medical-Surgical Nursing: Clinical Management for Positive Outcomes* (8th ed., pp. 283–284). St. Louis, MO: Saunders/Elsevier.

EBP Reference: Oncology Nursing Society. (2005). *Chemotherapy and Biotherapy Guidelines and Recommendations for Practice* (2nd ed.). Pittsburgh, PA: Oncology Nursing Society. Available at: guidelines.gov/search/searchresults.aspx?Type=3&txtSearch=chemotherapy&num=20

730. A nurse cares for a client receiving combination chemotherapy of oxaliplatin (Eloxatin®), fluorouracil (5-FU), and leucovorin (Wellcovorin®). For which common side effects of this chemotherapy should the nurse assess the client?

1. Neurotoxicities and diarrhea
2. Cardiomyopathy and dysphagia
3. Renal insufficiency and gastritis
4. Photophobia and stomatitis

ANSWER: 1

Neurotoxicity and diarrhea occur frequently in clients receiving this medication regimen. Cardiomyopathy, dysphagia, renal insufficiency, gastritis, photophobia, and stomatitis are not common side effects of these chemotherapy agents.

▶ ***Test-taking Tip:*** *Focus on the key words "common side effects" and use the process of elimination to rule out incorrect options. Concentrate on the medication's effect on the body.*

Content Area: Adult Health; *Category of Health Alteration:* Hematological and Oncological Management; *Integrated Processes:* Nursing Process Analysis; *Client Need:* Physiological Integrity/Pharmacological and Parenteral Therapies/Pharmacological Agents/Actions; *Cognitive Level:* Analysis

Reference: Prescher-Hughes, D., & Alkhoudairy, C. (2007). *Clinical Practice Protocols in Oncology Nursing* (p. 167). Boston: Jones and Bartlett.

731. A nurse assesses that a client, who is receiving radiation for cervical cancer, continues to have diarrhea. Which nursing advice is most appropriate for this client?

1. Take sitz baths twice daily and eat a low-residue diet.
2. Drink fluids low in potassium and take frequent tub baths.
3. Increase your intake of milk products and take frequent showers.
4. Drink fluids high in sodium and apply hydrocolloid dressings to reddened areas.

ANSWER: 1

Clients are advised to take sitz (or tub) baths for comfort and to eat a low-residue diet to decrease roughage and bowel irritability. Intake of fluids that are high in potassium (not low) is recommended to replace electrolytes lost through diarrhea. Frequent tub bathing or showers can aggravate the skin and are not recommended. Milk products are discouraged because they increase bowel irritability. Intake of fluids high in sodium should be avoided because it contributes to water retention; but hydrocolloid dressings may be used on reddened areas to promote healing.

Test-taking Tip: Focus on the key word "diarrhea" and problems associated with diarrhea (skin breakdown, milk intolerance).

Content Area: Adult Health; *Category of Health Alteration:* Hematological and Oncological Management; *Integrated Processes:* Teaching and Learning; *Client Need:* Physiological Integrity/Basic Care and Comfort/Non-pharmacological Comfort Interventions; *Cognitive Level:* Application

Reference: Langhorne, M., Fulton, J., & Otto, S. (2007). *Oncology Nursing* (5th ed., p. 135). St. Louis, MO: Mosby/Elsevier.

---

732. When assessing a client who is recovering from a radical hysterectomy with vulvectomy, a nurse notes lymphedema of the lower extremities. Which intervention should be implemented by the nurse?

1. Elevate the head of the bed to a 45-degree angle.
2. Increase the client's intake of fluids high in sodium.
3. Encourage the client to exercise the lower extremities.
4. Apply lower-extremity splints.

ANSWER: 3

Leg exercises to improve drainage are a recommended treatment for lymphedema (the accumulation of lymph fluid in the tissues of the lower extremities). Head of the bed elevation to a 45-degree angle may increase lymphedema of the lower extremities. Intake of fluids high in sodium will cause fluid retention. Lower-extremity splints can cause skin breakdown of edematous tissue.

Test-taking Tip: Focus on the key word "lymphedema." Options 1 and 4 have no therapeutic effect on the lymphedema and thus can be eliminated. Intake of high sodium content would be contraindicated.

Content Area: Adult Health; *Category of Health Alteration:* Hematological and Oncological Management; *Integrated Processes:* Nursing Process Implementation; *Client Need:* Physiological Integrity/Basic Care and Comfort/Nonpharmacological Comfort Interventions; *Cognitive Level:* Analysis

Reference: Langhorne, M., Fulton, J., & Otto, S. (2007). *Oncology Nursing* (5th ed., p. 191). St. Louis, MO: Mosby/Elsevier.

---

733. A nurse is collecting data from a client with a suspected diagnosis of basal cell carcinoma (BCC). Which risk factors in the client's health history, identified by the nurse, support this diagnosis? SELECT ALL THAT APPLY.

1. Family history of BCC
2. Frequent use of indoor tanning devices (beds or lamps with artificial light)
3. Smoking history
4. Occupational exposure to carcinogens
5.

734. A client phones a nurse after having three basal cell carcinoma (BCC) lesions excised the day before and is concerned that the wounds are draining a small amount of serosanguineous fluid and that the small dressing is leaking. Which action should the nurse recommend?

1. Apply ice to the area.
2. Contact the physician.
3. Take medication for pain.
4. Change the dressings.

ANSWER: 4

The nurse should recommend changing the dressing because a small amount of serosanguineous drainage is a normal response to surgical removal of a lesion. Applying ice to the area is not necessary because the client did not mention swelling. Since the wounds do not drain purulent material, contacting the physician is not necessary. Because the client is not experiencing pain, pain medication is not needed.

➧ ***Test-taking Tip:*** *Note that "serosanguineous fluid" and "small dressing" indicate an expected finding, so options 1 and 2 should be eliminated. Option 3 does not address the concerns of the client and can also be eliminated.*

Content Area: Adult Health; *Category of Health Alteration:* Hematological and Oncological Management; *Integrated Processes:* Nursing Process Analysis; *Client Need:* Physiological Integrity/ Reduction of Risk Potential/Potential for Complications from Surgical Procedures and Health Alterations; *Cognitive Level:* Analysis

Reference: Langhorne, M., Fulton, J., & Otto, S. (2007). *Oncology Nursing* (5th ed., p. 482). St. Louis, MO: Mosby/Elsevier.

---

735. A client presents with a meningioma and symptoms of increased intracranial pressure. Which manifestations should a nurse *least expect* to find on assessment of this client?

1. Headache
2. Vomiting
3. Pyrexia
4. Papilledema

ANSWER: 3

Pyrexia (elevated temperature) is not a common symptom of increased intracranial pressure associated with meningioma (malignant brain tumor). Elevated temperature usually indicates an infection. Headache, nausea/vomiting, and papilledema are a common triad of symptoms for increased intracranial pressure often seen in persons presenting with a brain tumor. The symptoms are due to the pressure on surrounding structures.

➧ ***Test-taking Tip:*** *Focus on "increased intracranial pressure." Think about the brain structures and the location of the meninges. Eliminate options that are related to increased intracranial pressure.*

Content Area: Adult Health; *Category of Health Alteration:* Hematological and Oncological Management; *Integrated Processes:* Nursing Process Assessment; *Client Need:* Physiological Integrity/ Physiological Adaptation/Pathophysiology; *Cognitive Level:* Application

Reference: Langhorne, M., Fulton, J., & Otto, S. (2007). *Oncology Nursing* (5th ed., p. 87). St. Louis, MO: Mosby/Elsevier.

---

736. When caring for a client with epigastric pain and suspected gastric cancer, which diagnostic test should a nurse address with the client because it is the specific test used to diagnose the cancer?

1. Arthroscopy
2. Bronchoscopy
3. Colonoscopy
4. Esophagogastroduodenoscopy

ANSWER: 4

Esophagogastroduodenoscopy is an invasive procedure in which a lighted instrument (scope) is lowered into the stomach and duodenum to examine gastric tissues and obtain tissue to biopsy for cancer cell analysis. Thus it is the preferred test to diagnose gastric cancer. Arthroscopy is used to examine joints. Bronchoscopy is used to examine the lungs. Colonoscopy is used to inspect the large intestines.

➧ ***Test-taking Tip:*** *Focus on the key words "diagnostic test" and think about the organ (stomach) being examined. Since options 1, 2, and 3 do not involve the stomach, eliminate these as incorrect options.*

Content Area: Adult Health; *Category of Health Alteration:* Hematological and Oncological Management; *Integrated Processes:* Teaching and Learning; *Client Need:* Physiological Integrity/Reduction of Risk Potential/Potential for Complications of Diagnostic Tests/Treatments/ Procedures; *Cognitive Level:* Application

Reference: Langhorne, M., Fulton, J., & Otto, S. (2007). *Oncology Nursing* (5th ed., p. 146). St. Louis, MO: Mosby/Elsevier.

737. Which nursing diagnosis should a nurse plan to document for the client with gastric cancer experiencing hematemesis?

1. Impaired oral mucous membrane
2. Decreased cardiac output
3. Impaired gas exchange
4. Fluid volume deficit

ANSWER: 4

Fluid volume deficit occurs with hematemesis (blood in emesis) from both vomiting and the loss of blood. Impaired oral mucous membrane occurs with chemotherapy treatment. Decreased cardiac output may result from congestive heart failure. Impaired gas exchange happens with restrictive/obstructive lung disease.

▸ ***Test-taking Tip:*** *Note the key word "hematemesis," and focus on effects of losing blood.*

Content Area: Adult Health; *Category of Health Alteration:* Hematological and Oncological Management; *Integrated Processes:* Nursing Process Planning; Communication and Documentation; *Client Need:* Physiological Integrity/Physiological Adaptation/Alterations in Body Systems; *Cognitive Level:* Analysis

Reference: Doenges, M., & Moorhouse, M. (2006). *Nurses Pocket Guide: Diagnoses, Interventions, and Rationales* (10th ed.). Philadelphia: F.A. Davis.

738. A client diagnosed with esophageal cancer is having work-related problems. Which organization should a nurse advise the client to contact for assistance with these issues?

1. National Cancer Institute
2. Leukemia Society of America
3. Corporate Angel Network
4. Patient Advocate Foundation

ANSWER: 4

The Patient Advocate Foundation provides counseling to resolve job-related problems. The National Cancer Institute answers questions and has free information about cancer. The Leukemia Society of America provides education regarding leukemia. The Corporate Angel Network provides free plane transportation for cancer clients going to and from treatment centers.

▸ ***Test-taking Tip:*** *"Work-related problems" are key words in the stem and in understanding the role of each organization. By knowing the function of each organization, one can use the process of elimination to choose option 4 as the answer.*

Content Area: Adult Health; *Category of Health Alteration:* Hematological and Oncological Management; *Integrated Processes:* Caring; *Client Need:* Safe and Effective Care Environment/Management of Care/Consultation; *Cognitive Level:* Application

Reference: Langhorne, M., Fulton, J., & Otto, S. (2007). *Oncology Nursing* (5th ed., p. 542). St. Louis, MO: Mosby/Elsevier.

739. When caring for a client following a total laryngectomy, with which members of the multidisciplinary team should a nurse plan consultations? SELECT ALL THAT APPLY.

1. Physical therapist
2. Dietitian
3. Speech therapist
4. Dentist
5. Occupational therapist
6. Social worker

ANSWER: 1, 2, 3, 6

Total laryngectomy is removal of the entire larynx as well as the hyoid bone, the true vocal cords, the false vocal cords, the epiglottis, the cricoid cartilage, and two to three tracheal rings. The disciplines are needed for the following functions: the physical therapist for neck exercises, the dietitian for adequacy of oral intake, the speech therapist for other forms of communication and swallowing, and the social worker for contact with outside resources to assist the client in ongoing needs. The dentist and occupational therapist are not routinely used for care of the laryngectomy client.

▸ ***Test-taking Tip:*** *The words "laryngectomy" and "other members" are key words in the stem. Think about the roles of each of the disciplines. Knowing the voice box is removed, the neck muscles are excised, swallowing is affected, and outside resources may be needed would direct you to options 1, 2, 3, and 6. Since dentition and use of the upper extremities are not affected, options 4 and 5 can be eliminated.*

Content Area: Adult Health; *Category of Health Alteration:* Hematological and Oncological Management; *Integrated Processes:* Nursing Process Planning; *Client Need:* Safe and Effective Care Environment/Management of Care/Collaboration with Interdisciplinary Team; *Cognitive Level:* Analysis

Reference: Langhorne, M., Fulton, J., & Otto, S. (2007). *Oncology Nursing* (5th ed., p. 222). St. Louis, MO: Mosby/Elsevier.

740. A nurse assesses a client who has undergone a total laryngectomy. Which assessment findings should the nurse address first when caring for this client? Prioritize the nurse's actions by placing the nurse's findings on a scale of 1 to 4 in order of priority: 1 being the item requiring immediate attention by the nurse and 4 being the item requiring last consideration.

_____ Copious oral secretions and nasal mucus draining from the nose
_____ Restless and has a mucus plug in the tracheostomy
_____ Nasal gastric tube pulled halfway out and tube feeding continuing to infuse
_____ Oozing serosanguineous drainage around the tracheostomy tube and dressing saturated

ANSWER: 3, 1, 2, 4

Restlessness and mucus plugs from the tracheostomy require immediate attention due to the negative impact on air exchange. The nasal gastric tube coming part way out and the feeding running would have second highest priority. Although the esophagus does not communicate with the trachea, the nurse should turn off the tube feeding. The physician should be contacted to reinsert the nasal gastric tube because of the suture line in the esophagus. The third priority is to clear the copious oral secretions and nasal drainage. The mouth does not communicate with the trachea, so copious oral secretions and nasal drainage would not influence air exchange, but these create a source of discomfort for the client. The oozing of serosanguineous drainage around the tracheostomy is normal after surgery. A nurse would change the tracheostomy tube dressing last.

➧ ***Test-taking Tip:*** *The words "laryngectomy" and "immediate attention" are key words in the stem, and the nurse needs to think about the ABCs (airway, breathing, and circulation) to answer the question.*

Content Area: Adult Health; *Category of Health Alteration:* Hematological and Oncological Management; *Integrated Processes:* Nursing Process Implementation; *Client Need:* Safe and Effective Care Environment/Management of Care/Establishing Priorities; *Cognitive Level:* Application

Reference: Langhorne, M., Fulton, J., & Otto, S. (2007). *Oncology Nursing* (5th ed., p. 222). St. Louis, MO: Mosby/Elsevier.

---

741. EBP Which vaccine should a nurse recommend for prevention of liver cancer?

1. Varicella vaccine
2. Hepatitis A vaccine
3. Meningococcal vaccine
4. Hepatitis B vaccine

ANSWER: 4

Hepatitis B vaccine dramatically reduces the incidence of hepatitis B virus and, in turn, prevents liver cancer. The evidence does not support that the other vaccines have an effect on the incidence of liver cancer.

➧ ***Test-taking Tip:*** *Focus on the key words "liver cancer," and think about the effect of each vaccine. Eliminate options 1 and 3 because they have no association with the liver.*

Content Area: Adult Health; *Category of Health Alteration:* Hematological and Oncological Management; *Integrated Processes:* Teaching and Learning; *Client Need:* Health Promotion and Maintenance/Immunizations; *Cognitive Level:* Comprehension

Reference: Lewis, S., Heitkemper, M., Dirksen, S., O'Brien, P., & Bucher, L. (2007). *Medical-Surgical Nursing: Assessment and Management of Clinical Problems* (7th ed., p. 1117). St. Louis, MO: Mosby.

EBP Reference: United States Preventive Services Task Force. (2007). *Recommended Adult Health Immunization Schedule.* Rockville, MD: Agency for Healthcare Research and Quality. Available at: www.ahcpr.gov/clinic/uspstfix.htm#epss

---

742. A nurse is caring for a client diagnosed with hepatocellular carcinoma who is exhibiting a paraneoplastic syndrome. For which signs should the nurse assess?

1. Erythrocytosis and hypercalcemia
2. Hyperkalemia and hyperalbuminemia
3. Hypernatremia and hypomagnesemia
4. Hypocalcemia and hyperleukocytosis

ANSWER: 1

Erythrocytosis and hypercalcemia occur in hepatocellular carcinoma due to the cancer cells secreting parathyroid hormone and erythropoietin. The other laboratory abnormalities do not occur in liver cancer.

➧ ***Test-taking Tip:*** *Note the key words "paraneoplastic syndrome" and focus on what abnormalities are associated with this syndrome. Knowing that calcium levels are altered in many cancers can assist with the answer to the question by eliminating options 2 and 3. Since infection is not caused by tumors, option 4 can be eliminated (hyperleukocytosis or elevated white blood count).*

Content Area: Adult Health; *Category of Health Alteration:* Hematological and Oncological Management; *Integrated Processes:* Nursing Process Assessment; *Client Need:* Physiological Integrity/Physiological Adaptation/Pathophysiology; *Cognitive Level:* Comprehension

Reference: Langhorne, M., Fulton, J., & Otto, S. (2007). *Oncology Nursing* (5th ed., p. 150). St. Louis, MO: Mosby/Elsevier.

743. In the assessment of a client for endometrial cancer, a nurse would most likely find which symptoms at diagnosis of the disease?

1. Abnormal vaginal bleeding and pain in the pelvic region
2. Weight loss and profuse sweating
3. Anorexia and enlarged supraclavicular lymph node
4. Unexplained fevers and splenomegaly

ANSWER: 1

Abnormal vaginal bleeding and pain in the pelvic region appear as the most common presenting symptoms. Weight loss, anorexia, enlarged supraclavicular lymph nodes, unexplained fevers, and splenomegaly are not common presenting symptoms. Abnormal menstrual flow can occur as a presenting symptom but not in conjunction with weight loss.

➧ ***Test-taking Tip:*** *Note the key phrase "most likely" and focus on "presenting symptoms." Since options 2, 3, and 4 (profuse sweating, enlarged supraclavicular lymph node and unexplained fevers) are not associated with endometrial cancer, these options can be eliminated.*

Content Area: Adult Health; *Category of Health Alteration:* Hematological and Oncological Management; *Integrated Processes:* Nursing Process Assessment; *Client Need:* Physiological Integrity/Physiological Adaptation/Pathophysiology; *Cognitive Level:* Application

Reference: Langhorne, M., Fulton, J., & Otto, S. (2007). *Oncology Nursing* (5th ed., p. 194). St. Louis, MO: Mosby/Elsevier.

---

744. In discussing bad news with a client about a diagnosis of cancer, which actions are most appropriate for a nurse to use at this time of emotional impact? SELECT ALL THAT APPLY.

1. Advocate expression of feelings.
2. Avoid using the word *cancer*.
3. Give the client as much information as possible.
4. Maintain a professional detachment.
5. Promote a broad time frame by avoiding a definite time scale.
6. Provide for privacy and adequate time with family present.

ANSWER: 1, 5, 6

The current literature recommends advocating an expression of feelings, promoting a broad time frame, and providing privacy and adequate time with family present. The literature supports using the word *cancer* but advocates giving the client only as much information that he or she wants. Using a manner of professional detachment can offend the recipients of bad news. Using a gentle manner with a sense of reassurance is encouraged.

➧ ***Test-taking Tip:*** *Focus on the phrase "discussing bad news." Options 2, 3, and 4 can be eliminated because they are not appropriate behaviors under the circumstances.*

Content Area: Adult Health; *Category of Health Alteration:* Hematological and Oncological Management; *Integrated Processes:* Communication and Documentation; *Client Need:* Psychosocial Integrity/Therapeutic Communications; *Cognitive Level:* Application

Reference: Langhorne, M., Fulton, J., & Otto, S. (2007). *Oncology Nursing* (5th ed., p. 525). St. Louis, MO: Mosby/Elsevier.

---

745. A nurse counsels a family member of a cancer client about the caregiving role. Which self-care activity would help the family member cope with the caregiver role?

1. Being open to technologies and ideas that promote a loved one's dependence
2. Trusting that you are doing the right thing and staying focused on your loved one
3. Grieving over losing personal time for self or care of other family members
4. Self-education about a loved one's condition and how to communicate effectively with health-care providers

ANSWER: 4

Self-education about his or her loved one's condition and how to communicate effectively with health-care providers helps support the family member in the caregiver role. The family member needs to be open to technologies and ideas that promote his or her loved one's independence not dependence. The family member needs to trust his or her instincts and objectively make decisions about doing the right thing, which may or may not be focused on his or her loved one. It is healthy for the family member to grieve about his or her losses.

➧ ***Test-taking Tip:*** *Focus on the key words "care-giving role," and think about the meaning of "self-care activities." Since options 1, 2, and 3 focus on the ill person's role, these responses can be eliminated.*

Content Area: Adult Health; *Category of Health Alteration:* Hematological and Oncological Management; *Integrated Processes:* Nursing Process Analysis; *Client Need:* Psychosocial Integrity/Behavioral Interventions; *Cognitive Level:* Analysis

Reference: Langhorne, M., Fulton, J., & Otto, S. (2007). *Oncology Nursing* (5th ed., p. 538). St. Louis, MO: Mosby/Elsevier.

746. A nurse is counseling the family of a client who died from terminal cancer. Which interventions are effective in assisting the family through the grief process? SELECT ALL THAT APPLY.

1. Listening actively without judgment
2. Advising the family member to make change quickly to hasten the grieving process
3. Encouraging time with the body of the deceased at the time of death
4. Listening passively with minimal feedback to the family member
5. Advising the family member to move on with life and place no meaning on the death
6. Assisting the family member in further identifying the meaning of the loss in practical terms

ANSWER: 1, 3, 6

Interventions that assist the grieving family include, listening actively without judgments, encouraging time with the body of the deceased at the time of death, and assisting the family member in further identifying the meaning of the loss in practical terms. The family should be advised to minimize change. The nurse should listen actively and provide practical feedback as appropriate. The nurse should assist the family in grieving by allowing ample time to repeat the story of the death, come to an understanding of the meaning of the death, and then move to acceptance; the pace should be set by the grieving family.

Test-taking Tip: *Note the key phrase "work through the grief process" to determine which interventions connote a positive action. Options 2 and 5 are not appropriate interventions and can be eliminated. Passive listening is not a therapeutic communication technique and can be eliminated.*

Content Area: Adult Health; *Category of Health Alteration:* Hematological and Oncological Management; *Integrated Processes:* Nursing Process Analysis; *Client Need:* Psychosocial Integrity/Grief and Loss; *Cognitive Level:* Analysis

Reference: Langhorne, M., Fulton, J., & Otto, S. (2007). *Oncology Nursing* (5th ed., p. 615). St. Louis, MO: Mosby/Elsevier.

747. In discussing conditions important to the client at the terminal stages of cancer, which attributes should a nurse acknowledge as being important to the client at the end of life? SELECT ALL THAT APPLY.

1. Maintaining one's dignity
2. Being mentally sedated
3. Maintaining a sense of humor
4. Resolving unfinished business with family
5. Having others plan funeral arrangements
6. Saying goodbye to important people

ANSWER: 1, 3, 4, 6

Attributes considered important at the end of life by clients include maintaining one's dignity, maintaining a sense of humor, resolving unfinished business with family, and saying goodbye to important people. Clients want to be mentally alert, not sedated, and some clients want to plan their own funeral arrangements.

Test-taking Tip: *Note the key words "important" and "end of life." Since most clients want to be in control, options 2 and 5 are not attributes considered important at the end of life.*

Content Area: Adult Health; *Category of Health Alteration:* Hematological and Oncological Management; *Integrated Processes:* Caring; *Client Need:* Psychosocial Integrity/End of Life Care; *Cognitive Level:* Analysis

Reference: Langhorne, M., Fulton, J., & Otto, S. (2007). *Oncology Nursing* (5th ed., p. 604). St. Louis, MO: Mosby/Elsevier.

748. EBP For a client experiencing severe cancer pain (pain intensity of 7 to 10 on a scale of 0 to 10, where 0 equals no pain and 10 equals the worst possible pain), which medication should a nurse plan to administer?

1. Meperidine (Demerol®)
2. Propoxyphene (Darvon®)
3. Pentazocine (Talwin®)
4. Oxycodone (Oxycontin®)

ANSWER: 4

Opioids, such as oxycodone, remain the most frequently prescribed pain medication for severe pain in cancer. Meperidine and propoxyphene are not recommended because these medications cause central nervous system toxicity from metabolites. Pentazocine is used for moderate pain only, and it can cause confusion and hallucinations in older adults and clients with renal impairment.

Test-taking Tip: *Think about medications used for "severe pain" as opposed to mild or moderate pain. Option 1 is used for mild or moderate pain and can be eliminated. Knowing the side effects of options 2 and 3 would eliminate them as options.*

Content Area: Adult Health; *Category of Health Alteration:* Hematological and Oncological Management; *Integrated Processes:* Nursing Process Planning; *Client Need:* Physiological Integrity/Pharmacological and Parenteral Therapies/Pharmacological Pain Management; *Cognitive Level:* Analysis

Reference: Lewis, S., Heitkemper, M., Dirksen, S., O'Brien, P., & Bucher, L. (2007). *Medical-Surgical Nursing: Assessment and Management of Clinical Problems* (7th ed., pp. 136–138). St. Louis, MO: Mosby.

EBP Reference: Miaskowski, C., Cleary, J., Burney, R., Coyne, P., Finley, R., et al. (2005). *Guideline for the Management of Cancer Pain in Adults and Children*. Glenview, IL: American Pain Society. Available at: www.guideline.gov/summary/summary.aspx?doc_id=7297&nbr=004341&string=cancer+AND+pain

749. A nurse is caring for a client who is experiencing pain related to cancer treatment. The client tells the nurse, "Methadone (Dolophine®) has always worked well for me in the past." Which effects of methadone should the nurse consider before obtaining an order for the medication?

1. Long half-life and high potency
2. Central nervous system toxicity and potential to cause confusion
3. Frequent allergic reactions and therapeutic doses causing liver failure
4. Coagulation toxicity and short half-life

ANSWER: 1

Long half-life and high potency make methadone difficult to use in clients with cancer. Methadone administration is not usually associated with central nervous system toxicity, a potential to cause confusion, frequent allergic reactions, therapeutic doses causing liver failure, or coagulation toxicity. Methadone does not have a short half-life.

Test-taking Tip: *Focus on the actions of methadone. Options 2, 3, and 4 have items that are not actions of methadone and can be eliminated.*

Content Area: Adult Health; *Category of Health Alteration:* Hematological and Oncological Management; *Integrated Processes:* Nursing Process Assessment; *Client Need:* Physiological Integrity/ Pharmacological and Parenteral Therapies/Pharmacological Pain Management; *Cognitive Level:* Analysis

Reference: Langhorne, M., Fulton, J., & Otto, S. (2007). *Oncology Nursing* (5th ed., p. 687). St. Louis, MO: Mosby/Elsevier.

750. A cancer client is requesting nonpharmacological interventions for pain. Which research-supported interventions should the nurse implement to ease this client's pain? SELECT ALL THAT APPLY.

1. Acupuncture
2. Prayer
3. Dance therapy
4. Foot bracing
5. House cleaning
6. Music therapy

ANSWER: 1, 2, 6

Nonpharmacological interventions studied and found to be beneficial as adjuncts in pain include acupuncture, prayer, and music therapy. Dance therapy, foot bracing, and house cleaning have not been reported to be beneficial for the management of pain.

Test-taking Tip: *Focus on key words "research-supported interventions." Knowing options 3, 4, and 5 have no research basis should eliminate these as options.*

Content Area: Adult Health; *Category of Health Alteration:* Hematological and Oncological Management; *Integrated Processes:* Nursing Process Implementation; *Client Need:* Physiological Integrity/ Basic Care and Comfort/Complementary and Alternative Therapies/ Nonpharmacological Comfort Interventions; *Cognitive Level:* Application

Reference: Langhorne, M., Fulton, J., & Otto, S. (2007). *Oncology Nursing* (5th ed., p. 690). St. Louis, MO: Mosby/Elsevier

751. EBP A client with cancer pain may require treatment with coanalgesics or adjuvant medications to control pain. Which adjuvant medication gives the best response when given with opioids?

1. Promethazine (Phenergan®)
2. Gabapentin (Neurontin®)
3. Diphenhydramine (Benadryl®)
4. Droperidol (Inapsine®)

ANSWER: 2

Gabapentin is often administered with opioid pain medications because of its efficacy and limited adverse effects. Promethazine is given with pain medications, but its action is for nausea and vomiting, not pain. Diphenhydramine and droperidol are not coanalgesics, but hypnotic medications and can be given with other medications.

Test-taking Tip: *Focus on the key word "coanalgesics" (action is for pain along with the main medication). Since options 1, 3, and 4 do not have pain-relieving actions, these items can be eliminated.*

Content Area: Adult Health; *Category of Health Alteration:* Hematological and Oncological Management; *Integrated Processes:* Nursing Process Analysis; *Client Need:* Physiological Integrity/ Pharmacological and Parenteral Therapies/Pharmacological Pain Management; *Cognitive Level:* Analysis

Reference: Lewis, S., Heitkemper, M., Dirksen, S., O'Brien, P., & Bucher, L. (2007). *Medical-Surgical Nursing: Assessment and Management of Clinical Problems* (7th ed., p. 139). St. Louis, MO: Mosby.

EBP Reference: Institute for Clinical Systems Improvement (2007). *Assessment and Management of Chronic Pain.* Available at: www.guideline.gov/summary/summary.aspx?doc_id=10724&nbr=005586&string=brain+AND+tumor

Test 19: **Adult Health: Integumentary Management and Other Health Alterations**

752. A nurse is assessing the fluid status of a client with a second-degree burn who weighs 60 kg. The client is 5 hours postburn. The nurse determines that the client's fluid status is inadequate and immediately notifies a physician when the client exhibits:

1. blood pressure 92/60 mm Hg and pulse rate 100 beats per minute (bpm).
2. respiratory rate 18 breaths per minute and pulse rate 60 bpm.
3. pulse rate 130 bpm and urine output 25 mL/hr.
4. pulse rate 106 bpm and temperature 98.4°F (36.9°C).

ANSWER: 3

A client weighing 60 kilograms (kg) weighs 132 pounds (1 kg = 2.2 lbs). For an adult client, a pulse rate of 130 bpm (tachycardia) and a low urine output of 25 mL/hr are signs of inadequate circulating fluid volume. A pulse rate under 120 bpm and a urine output of greater than 50 mL/hr indicates adequate fluid intake in a burn client. A blood pressure of 92/60 mm Hg, a respiratory rate of 18 breaths per minute, and a temperature of 98.4°F (36.9°C) are considered normal or near normal.

➧ ***Test-taking Tip:*** *Note the key words "inadequate" and "immediately." Eliminate options with normal measurements.*

Content Area: Adult Health; *Category of Health Alteration:* Integumentary Management and Other Health Alterations; *Integrated Processes:* Nursing Process Assessment; *Client Need:* Physiological Integrity/Reduction of Risk Potential/System Specific Assessments; *Cognitive Level:* Analysis

Reference: Black, J., & Hokanson Hawks, J. (2009). *Medical-Surgical Nursing: Clinical Management for Positive Outcomes* (8th ed., pp. 1244–1246). St. Louis, MO: Saunders/Elsevier.

---

753. In planning the care for a client recovering from second- or third-degree burns, which psychosocial nursing diagnosis should have the highest priority?

1. Disturbed sensory perception
2. Disturbed thought processes
3. Disturbed body image
4. Disturbed personal identity

ANSWER: 3

Disturbed body image occurs during the recovering stages of the burn condition and should be a high priority. Disturbed sensory perception is a physiological nursing diagnosis. Disturbed thought processes and disturbed personal identity are less likely to occur than disturbed body image and are of a lesser priority.

➧ ***Test-taking Tip:*** *Focus on psychosocial nursing diagnoses and eliminate any option that is a physiological nursing diagnosis. Of the remaining options, determine which is most likely to occur.*

Content Area: Adult Health; *Category of Health Alteration:* Integumentary Management and Other Health Alterations; *Integrated Processes:* Nursing Process Analysis; *Client Need:* Psychosocial Integrity/Unexpected Body Image Changes; *Cognitive Level:* Analysis

References: Black, J., & Hokanson Hawks, J. (2009). *Medical-Surgical Nursing: Clinical Management for Positive Outcomes* (8th ed., pp. 1263–1264). St. Louis, MO: Saunders/Elsevier; Sommers, M., Johnson, S., & Beery, T. (2007). *Diseases and Disorders: A Nursing Therapeutics Manual* (3rd ed.). Philadelphia: F. A. Davis.

---

754. Which medication should a nurse apply topically in second- and third-degree burns to treat bacterial and yeast infections?

1. Bismuth subsalicylate (Kaopectate®)
2. Gold sodium thiomalate (Aurolate®)
3. Silver sulfadiazine (Silvadene®)
4. Arsenic trioxide (Trisenox®)

ANSWER: 3

Silver sulfadiazine is a topical anti-infective agent for prevention and treatment of wound sepsis in second- and third-degree burn clients. Gold sodium thiomalate is used to treat rheumatoid arthritis resistant to conventional therapy. Bismuth subsalicylate is an antidiarrheal medication. Arsenic trioxide is an antineoplastic.

➧ ***Test-taking Tip:*** *Note the key word "topically" in the stem. Options 1, 2, and 4 are not topical medications.*

Content Area: Adult Health; *Category of Health Alteration:* Integumentary Management and Other Health Alterations; *Integrated Processes:* Nursing Process Analysis; *Client Need:* Physiological Integrity/Pharmacological and Parenteral Therapies/Expected Effects/Outcomes; *Cognitive Level:* Application

Reference: Wilson, B., Shannon, M., Shields, K., & Stang, C. (2008). *Prentice Hall Nurse's Drug Guide 2008* (pp. 1387–1388). Upper Saddle River, NJ: Pearson Education.

755. EBP Which interventions should a nurse implement to assist a client with problems of anxiety and confusion in the critical phases of burn injury? SELECT ALL THAT APPLY.

1. Repeat statements of orientation to person, place, and time with the client.
2. Turn the client every 2 hours for reorientation.
3. Place familiar objects brought from home nearby so the client can touch them.
4. Implement a schedule for regular sleep/wake cycles.
5. Keep the door of the room closed so that distractions can be controlled.
6. Encourage the client to write notes to family members.

ANSWER: 1, 3, 4

Reiterating statements of orientation to the client decreases confusion. Employing a regular schedule for sleep-wake cycles assists in decreasing confusion and anxiety. Familiar objects reduce anxiety when clients are in unfamiliar surroundings. Repositioning the client improves circulation and aeration but does not affect confusion or anxiety. Closing the door of the room may increase anxiety. In the acute phase of burns, the client is too ill to write notes to family members.

▸ ***Test-taking Tip:*** *Note the key phrase "anxiety and confusion" and focus on what factors decrease these symptoms. The other options can be excluded by the process of elimination.*

Content Area: Adult Health; *Category of Health Alteration:* Integumentary Management and Other Health Alterations; *Integrated Processes:* Nursing Process Implementation; *Client Need:* Psychosocial Integrity/Behavioral Interventions; *Cognitive Level:* Application

Reference: Berman, A., Snyder, S., Kozier, B., & Erb, G. (2008). *Kozier & Erb's Fundamentals of Nursing: Concepts, Process, and Practice* (8th ed., p. 994). Upper Saddle River, NJ: Pearson Education.

EBP Reference: Blakeney, P., Rosenberg, L., Rosenberg, M., & Faber, A. (2007). Psychosocial care of persons with severe burns. *Burns,* 34(4), 433–440.

756. A nurse is caring for a client with a large, open sternal wound resulting from a burn injury. The client is receiving enteral feeding, Oxepa® (an anti-inflammatory, pulmonary 1.5 Cal/mL formula), at 25 mL/hour. Which abnormal laboratory value, reported in the exhibit below, indicates that the client is receiving inadequate nutrition?

Serum Lab Test	Client's Value	Normal Values
Phosphorus	2.0	3.0–4.5 mg/dL
Platelets	110,000	150,000–400,000/mm^3
Pre-albumin	10	15–36 mg/dL
Potassium	3.1	3.5–5.0 mEq/L

1. Phosphorus
2. Platelets
3. Pre-albumin
4. Potassium

ANSWER: 3

Pre-albumin has a half-life of 2 days and reflects changes in serum protein stores more rapidly than other indices. Phosphorus, platelets, and potassium do not measure protein stores. Phosphorus measures the serum level of phosphorus in the blood and has an inverse relationship to calcium; phosphorus levels decrease in malnutrition. The platelet count reflects platelet levels, which are essential to blood clotting. Potassium is the major cation within the cell and may be low due to renal failure or gastrointestinal disorders.

▸ ***Test-taking Tip:*** *Note the key words "inadequate nutrition" and focus on what this means. Eliminate options that do not measure protein stores.*

Content Area: Adult Health; *Category of Health Alteration:* Integumentary Management and Other Health Alterations; *Integrated Processes:* Nursing Process Analysis; *Client Need:* Physiological Integrity/Basic Care and Comfort/Nutrition and Oral Hydration; *Cognitive Level:* Analysis

Reference: Pagana, K., & Pagana, T. (2007). *Mosby's Diagnostic and Laboratory Test Reference* (8th ed., pp. 722, 732, 750, 755). St. Louis, MO: Mosby/Elsevier.

757. A nurse is assessing a client following a skin graft. The nurse should suspect infection in the grafted wound when observing that the client has:

1. a white blood cell count (WBC) of 9.9 K/μL.
2. serosanguineous drainage.
3. elevated temperature.
4. decreased urine output.

ANSWER: 3

Elevated temperature indicates the presence of an infection. Normal WBC is 3.9 to 11.9 K/μL. Clean wounds have serosanguineous drainage. Decreased urine output can indicate dehydration or renal failure.

▸ ***Test-taking Tip:*** *Note the key word "infection" and focus on what signs indicate an infection. The other options can be excluded by the process of elimination.*

Content Area: Adult Health; *Category of Health Alteration:* Integumentary Management and Other Health Alterations; *Integrated Processes:* Nursing Process Assessment; *Client Need:* Physiological Integrity/Reduction of Risk Potential/Vital Signs; *Cognitive Level:* Assessment

References: Bryant, R., & Nix, D. (2007). *Acute and Chronic Wounds* (3rd ed.). St. Louis, MO: Mosby/Elsevier; Lewis, S., Heitkemper, M., Dirksen, S., O'Brien, P., & Bucher, L. (2007). *Medical-Surgical Nursing: Assessment and Management of Clinical Problems* (7th ed., p. 1860). St. Louis, MO: Mosby/Elsevier.

758. EBP A nurse cares for a client with a venous leg ulcer who undergoes trilayer artificial skin grafting. The nurse understands that grafted skin heals best on venous leg ulcers when which intervention is implemented after grafting?

1. Applying a gauze dressing
2. Applying compression bandages
3. Applying Xeroform® dressing
4. Applying petrolatum bandages

ANSWER: 2

Research shows that bilayer artificial skin, used in conjunction with compression bandaging, speeds healing time for venous leg ulcers. Compression prevents fluid from accumulating between the grafting material and wound. Gauze or Xeroform® dressings are used to pack some open venous leg ulcers; gauze may be used to dress the wound, but compression aids healing. A petrolatum bandage is used for occlusion, such as over chest tube insertion site. There is no indication that it speeds healing time.

➧ ***Test-taking Tip:*** *Focus on the phrases "heals best" and "venous leg ulcers." Select the option that should best adhere the grafted skin to the wound.*

Content Area: Adult Health; *Category of Health Alteration:* Integumentary Management and Other Health Alterations; *Integrated Processes:* Nursing Process Analysis; *Client Need:* Physiological Integrity/Reduction of Risk Potential/Therapeutic Procedures; *Cognitive Level:* Application

Reference: Wilkinson, J., & Van Leuven, K. (2007). *Fundamentals of Nursing: Theory, Concepts & Applications* (Vol. 1, pp. 836–840). Philadelphia: F. A. Davis.

EBP Reference: Jones, J., & Nelson, E. (2008). Skin grafting for venous leg ulcers. *Cochrane Database of Systematic Reviews*, Issue 3. Available at: www.cochrane.org/reviews/en/ab001737.html

759. EBP A nurse is explaining facelift (rhytidectomy) surgery to a client. Place an X on the site where the incision most commonly used for rhytidectomy is made.

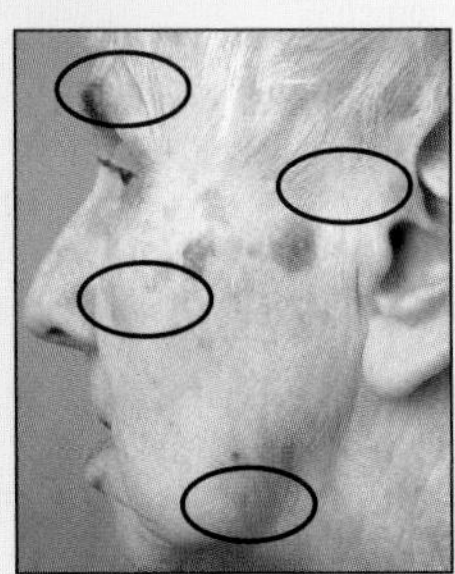

ANSWER:

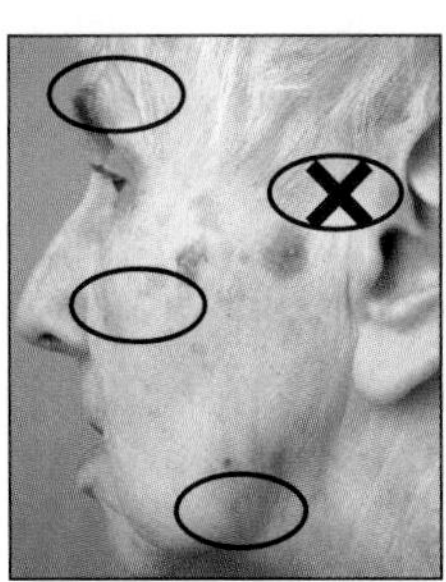

Excess skin and muscle laxity of the face are treated via rhytidectomy with an incision either in front or back of the ear. The forehead and periorbital areas are used for blepharoplasty and browlift. Head and neck reconstruction utilizes the chin site.

➧ ***Test-taking Tip:*** *Focus on the key word "rhytidectomy." Recall the physiology of the face to identify the appropriate site. Use the process of elimination to exclude the other sites.*

Content Area: Adult Health; *Category of Health Alteration:* Integumentary Management and Other Health Alterations; *Integrated Processes:* Teaching and Learning; *Client Need:* Physiological Integrity/Reduction of Risk Potential/Potential for Alterations in Body Systems; *Cognitive Level:* Application

EBP Reference: Kamer, F., & Nguyen D. (2007). Experience with fibrin glue in rhytidectomy. *Plastic and Reconstructive Surgery*, 120(4), 1045–1051.

760. Which home measures should a nurse discuss with a client who is diagnosed with a carbuncle? SELECT ALL THAT APPLY.

1. Leave the draining lesion open to the air.
2. Employ strict hand washing to prevent cross-contamination.
3. Cover mattress and pillows with plastic covers.
4. Apply ice to the affected area.
5. Wash all linens, towels, and clothing after each use.
6. Remove all throw rugs in the home.

ANSWER: 2, 3, 5

A carbuncle is an abscess of skin and subcutaneous tissue arising from a hair follicle. Treatments for an infected lesion should include strict hand washing to prevent cross-contamination, covering mattress and pillows with plastic covers, and washing all linens, towels, and clothing after each use. Leaving the draining lesion open to air is not advised as a dressing is needed to contain the drainage. Applying ice to the affected area and removing all throw rugs in the home do not pertain to the treatment of a carbuncle.

➧ ***Test-taking Tip:*** *Note the key word "carbuncle" in the stem and focus on treatments associated with carbuncles. Eliminate option 1 because it is contrary to care of a draining wound. Eliminate options 4 and 6 because they do not pertain to care of a carbuncle.*

Content Area: Adult Health; *Category of Health Alteration:* Integumentary Management and Other Health Alterations; *Integrated Processes:* Teaching and Learning; *Client Need:* Safe and Effective Care Environment/Safety and Infection Control/Standard/Transmission-based/Other Precautions; *Cognitive Level:* Application

Reference: Lewis, S., Heitkemper, M., Dirksen, S., O'Brien, P., & Bucher, L. (2007). *Medical-Surgical Nursing: Assessment and Management of Clinical Problems* (7th ed., p. 466). St. Louis, MO: Mosby/Elsevier.

---

761. During a physical assessment examination of the eyes, a nurse covers a client's right eye and then observes a shift in the client's gaze after the eye is uncovered. This finding suggests:

1. opacity of the lens.
2. absence of the blink reflex.
3. weakness in the extraocular muscles.
4. increased intraocular pressure.

ANSWER: 3

Covering and then uncovering the client's eye and then observing for a shift in the client's gaze is the cover-uncover test used to detect weakness in the extraocular muscles. Lens opacity is detected by direct observation. Stroking the eyelashes will evoke the blink reflex. The intraocular pressure is measured by tonometry.

➧ ***Test-taking Tip:*** *The issue of the question is the purpose of the cover-uncover test. The stem gives the result: a shift in the client's gaze. Shifting of the gaze involves movement. Select option 3 since the muscles are involved with movement. Eliminate the other options, which do not suggest movement.*

Content Area: Adult Health; *Category of Health Alteration:* Integumentary Management and Other Health Alterations; *Integrated Processes:* Nursing Process Assessment; *Client Need:* Physiological Integrity/Reduction of Risk Potential/System Specific Assessments; *Cognitive Level:* Application

Reference: Berman, A., Snyder, S., Kozier, B., & Erb, G. (2008). *Kozier & Erb's Fundamentals of Nursing: Concepts, Process, and Practice* (8th ed., p. 592). Upper Saddle River, NJ: Pearson Education.

---

762. EBP A nurse telephones a client who underwent cataract surgery the preceding day to assess the client's condition. Which client statement necessitates an evaluation by an ophthalmologist?

1. "My eye begins to hurt again about 4 hours after I take the pain pills the doctor ordered."
2. "The redness in my eye is much less than yesterday."
3. "I cannot see nearly as well as I could yesterday after the surgery."
4. "There is no swelling around my eye to speak of."

ANSWER: 3

A significant reduction in vision may indicate a complication such as infection or retinal detachment. Pain relieved by prescribed pain medication, decreasing redness, and no swelling are within normal assessment parameters.

➧ ***Test-taking Tip:*** *Read the stem carefully to determine the question is asking for a description of a complication. Evaluate each option and select the option that describes a decrease in vision, a complication.*

Content Area: Adult Health; *Category of Health Alteration:* Integumentary Management and Other Health Alterations; *Integrated Processes:* Nursing Process Evaluation; *Client Need:* Physiological Integrity/Reduction of Risk Potential/Potential for Complications from Surgical Procedures and Health Alterations; *Cognitive Level:* Analysis

Reference: Ignatavicius, D., & Workman, M. (2006). *Medical-Surgical Nursing: Critical Thinking for Collaborative Care* (5th ed., pp. 1092–1093). St. Louis, MO: Elsevier Saunders.

EBP Reference: American Academy of Ophthalmology (AAO). (2006). *Cataract in the Adult Eye: Preferred Practice Pattern.* San Francisco: AAO. Available at: www.guideline.gov/summary/summary.aspx?doc_id=10173&nbr5357

763. A client's eyes are tested with the use of a Snellen chart. The assessment is documented as 20/40 in the right eye and 20/30 in the left eye. How should a nurse interpret these results? SELECT ALL THAT APPLY.

1. The client has elevated intraocular pressure in both eyes.
2. The client needs eye pressure readings performed with a tonometer to determine if the client has glaucoma.
3. The vision in the left eye is closer to normal vision than the vision in the right eye.
4. The client has presbyopia.
5. The client has errors of refraction in both eyes consistent with myopia.

ANSWER: 3, 5

The Snellen chart is used to test distance vision. The numbers recorded indicate that at 20 feet (the first number) the client is able to read what a person with normal vision can read at another distance (second number). The eye's vision recorded as 20/30 has better vision that the eye with vision recorded as 20/40. The numbers indicate the client has myopia—that is, able to see near (nearsightedness)—and distant vision is not normal. The Snellen chart is not useful to diagnose glaucoma or measure intraocular pressure. Presbyopia is age-related inability to see close up.

➧ ***Test-taking Tip:*** *The issue of the test includes the purpose of Snellen chart testing and interpretation of the test results. Recall the Snellen chart is used to test distance vision, so eliminate options 1 and 2 that deal with glaucoma, a disease with increased pressure within the eye. Normal vision is often referred to as "20/20," so 20/30 is better than 20/40; include option 3 as a correct answer. Recall definitions of the terms myopia (near vision) and presbyopia (old-age vision: cannot focus close up). The Snellen chart is used to test distance vision, and results relate the client can see near, so select option 5.*

Content Area: Adult Health; *Category of Health Alteration:* Integumentary Management and Other Health Alterations; *Integrated Processes:* Nursing Process Analysis; *Client Need:* Physiological Integrity/Reduction of Risk Potential/System Specific Assessments; *Cognitive Level:* Analysis

Reference: Ignatavicius, D., & Workman, M. (2006). *Medical-Surgical Nursing: Critical Thinking for Collaborative Care* (5th ed., pp. 1074, 1078). St. Louis, MO: Elsevier/Saunders.

---

764. **EBP** A nurse speaks with a client who recently learned he has beginning cataracts in both eyes. Which statement made by the client should a nurse correct?

1. "It is important that I have surgery done as soon as possible to prevent permanent damage to my vision."
2. "Cataracts are corrected by surgery, with each eye done at different times."
3. "The surgical treatment of a cataract involves the removal of the client's own lens from the eye."
4. "An intraocular lens is placed in the eye at the time of surgery."

ANSWER: 1

The decrease in vision due to a cataract is caused by the opaque lens. The client's lens is removed, and an intraocular lens is implanted with surgery. No permanent damage occurs to other structures within the eye from the cataract. Surgery for cataracts involves removal of the client's lens and placement of an intraocular lens. If both eyes have cataracts, the eyes are treated in separate procedures

➧ ***Test-taking Tip:*** *Read the stem carefully and determine that the question calls for a false answer. Recall the definition of a cataract and what is done in surgical treatment. Cataract surgery is always elective and done when the vision and lifestyle of the client are affected. Select option 1 because it incorrectly describes urgency for cataract surgery.*

Content Area: Adult Health; *Category of Health Alteration:* Integumentary Management and Other Health Alterations; *Integrated Processes:* Nursing Process Evaluation; *Client Need:* Physiological Integrity/Physiological Adaptation/Illness Management; *Cognitive Level:* Analysis

Reference: Ignatavicius, D., & Workman, M. (2006). *Medical-Surgical Nursing: Critical Thinking for Collaborative Care* (5th ed., pp. 1092–1096). St. Louis, MO: Elsevier/Saunders.

EBP Reference: American Academy of Ophthalmology (AAO). (2006). *Cataract in the Adult Eye: Preferred Practice Pattern*, San Francisco: AAO. Available at: www.guideline.gov/summary/summary.aspx?doc_id=10173&nbr5357

765. EBP A family member of a client undergoing cataract surgery asks a nurse if there are ways to prevent cataracts. Which interventions decrease the risk for the development of cataracts? SELECT ALL THAT APPLY.

1. Wearing sunglasses that limit ultraviolet light penetration
2. Wearing sunscreen with a high number limiting ultraviolet light penetration
3. Wearing eye protection during activities that put the client at risk for eye injury
4. Avoiding activities such as reading in dimly lit environments
5. Eating foods high in vitamin C
6. Limiting saturated fat intake in the diet

ANSWER: 1, 3

Limiting eye exposure to ultraviolet light and avoiding trauma to the eye have been found to decrease the risk for cataracts. Sunscreen is applied to the skin, not the eyes. Straining the eyes to read does not lead to cataract formation. There is no evidence that nutrition prevents or delays progression of cataracts.

▶ ***Test-taking Tip:*** *The issue of the question is the cause of cataracts. Recall from pathophysiology that cataracts are associated with aging, trauma, and exposure to toxic agents. Eliminate option 2 since it pertains to skin exposure. Eliminate options 4 and 6 because these are deficiencies, not excessive toxic levels. Eliminate option 5 because vitamin C is water soluble and is usually excreted before toxicity is reached. Select options 1 and 3 that identify the risks of excessive ultraviolet light and trauma.*

Content Area: Adult Health; *Category of Health Alteration:* Integumentary Management and Other Health Alterations; *Integrated Processes:* Nursing Process Analysis; Teaching and Learning; *Client Need:* Physiological Integrity/Reduction of Risk Potential/Potential for Alterations in Body Systems; *Cognitive Level:* Application

Reference: Ignatavicius, D., & Workman, M. (2006). *Medical-Surgical Nursing: Critical Thinking for Collaborative Care* (5th ed., pp. 1092–1096). St. Louis, MO: Elsevier/Saunders.

EBP Reference: American Academy of Ophthalmology (AAO). (2006). *Cataract in the Adult Eye: Preferred Practice Pattern.* San Francisco: AAO. Available at: www.guideline.gov/summary/summary.aspx?doc_id=10173&nbr5357

766. EBP A nurse is discharging a client who underwent outpatient cataract surgery to home. Which intervention should be included in the discharge instructions to the client and family member? SELECT ALL THAT APPLY.

1. Observe the eye for increased redness, swelling, pain, and decrease in vision, and contact the surgeon if these problems develop.
2. Wear the eye shield at night.
3. Administer eye drops as directed.
4. Cough and deep breathe every 2 hours while awake.
5. Rest in bed with the head of the bed elevated at least 30 degrees.
6. Avoid getting water in the eye when washing the client's hair.

ANSWER: 1, 2, 3, 5, 6

The client should observe the eye for possible complications and contact the surgeon if symptoms occur. The client should avoid dependent positions and contact with water. The client should follow directions administering prescribed eye medications and wearing the eye shield. The client should not cough, because this will increase the pressure within the eye and risk for complications.

▶ ***Test-taking Tip:*** *The issue of the question is the selection of interventions for the client after cataract surgery. Postoperative complications include infection and damage from increased intraocular pressure or trauma. Select the options that prevent or detect the postoperative complications.*

Content Area: Adult Health; *Category of Health Alteration:* Integumentary Management and Other Health Alterations; *Integrated Processes:* Teaching and Learning; *Client Need:* Physiological Integrity/Reduction of Risk Potential/Potential for Complications from Surgical Procedures and Health Alterations; *Cognitive Level:* Analysis

Reference: Ignatavicius, D., & Workman, M. (2006). *Medical-Surgical Nursing: Critical Thinking for Collaborative Care* (5th ed., pp. 1092–1096). St. Louis, MO: Elsevier/Saunders.

EBP Reference: American Academy of Ophthalmology (AAO). (2006). *Cataract in the Adult Eye: Preferred Practice Pattern.* San Francisco: AAO. Available at: www.guideline.gov/summary/summary.aspx?doc_id=10173&nbr5357

767. A nurse at the family practice clinic routinely asks middle-aged and older clients if they have experienced any changes in their vision. Which are early symptoms that should alert the nurse to a client's onset of cataract formation? SELECT ALL THAT APPLY.

1. Blurring of vision
2. Difficulty seeing in the dark
3. Pain in the eye
4. Increased frequency of headaches
5. Floating dark spots in the vision field of the affected eye

ANSWER: 1, 2

A beginning cataract is a developing opacity of the lens that distorts the image reflected on the retina. This results in diminished vision, specifically blurriness and decreased night vision. Pain in the eye and headache are not associated with cataract formation. Floating dark spots in the vision field are associated with bleeding within the eye that occurs with detached retina.

➧ ***Test-taking Tip:*** *The issue of the question involves vision changes associated with early cataract formation. Recall by definition that a cataract is the opacity of the lens. A lens focuses vision. Select options 1 and 2, which describe minimal deficiencies in visual acuity. Eliminate options 3 and 4 because they deal with pain. Eliminate option 5 because it is a specific vision distortion, not a problem of the lens focusing.*

Content Area: Adult Health; *Category of Health Alteration:* Integumentary Management and Other Health Alterations; *Integrated Processes:* Nursing Process Assessment; *Client Need:* Physiological Integrity/Physiological Adaptation/Alterations in Body Systems; *Cognitive Level:* Analysis

Reference: Ignatavicius, D., & Workman, M. (2006). *Medical-Surgical Nursing: Critical Thinking for Collaborative Care* (5th ed., pp. 1092–1096). St. Louis, MO: Elsevier/Saunders.

768. Which symptoms should a nurse identify when a client asks about symptoms associated with retinal detachment? SELECT ALL THAT APPLY.

1. Redness in an eye
2. Seeing bright flashes of light
3. Eye pain
4. Severe headache
5. Diminished vision
6. Seeing floating dark spots in the vision field

ANSWER: 2, 5, 6

As the choroids and retina partially separate the client notices flashes of light, floating dark spots, or decreased vision often like "a curtain being drawn across." Eye redness or pain is not associated with retinal detachment. There are few pain fibers in the retina.

➧ ***Test-taking Tip:*** *Recall from anatomy and physiology that the retina is composed of cones and rods and transmits sensory impulses to the optic nerve. The retina is poorly innervated for pain. The condition "retinal detachment" by name implies the function of the retina has been insulted. Select the options listed that describe alternations in vision. Eliminate the options that describe the physical appearance of the eye or pain.*

Content Area: Adult Health; *Category of Health Alteration:* Integumentary Management and Other Health Alterations; *Integrated Processes:* Nursing Process Implementation; Teaching and Learning; *Client Need:* Physiological Integrity/Reduction of Risk Potential/ Potential for Alterations in Body Systems; *Cognitive Level:* Analysis

Reference: Ignatavicius, D., & Workman, M. (2006). *Medical-Surgical Nursing: Critical Thinking for Collaborative Care* (5th ed., pp. 1102–1103). St. Louis, MO: Elsevier/Saunders.

769. A nurse working in a long-term care facility suspects a client is experiencing detachment of the retina. A nurse should:

1. flush the eye thoroughly with saline solution and apply a pressure bandage.
2. apply an eye shield to the affected eye and administer the prescribed oral analgesic medication.
3. notify the primary care provider and have the client transported promptly to a facility for ophthalmologic referral and treatment.
4. patch both eyes and place the client in a prone position.

ANSWER: 3

The nurse should contact the primary care provider and secure ophthalmologic evaluation promptly. Early diagnosis and intervention for retinal detachment improve preservation of the client's vision. Other interventions to the eye are not substitutes for seeking medical attention for the client with suspected retinal detachment.

➧ ***Test-taking Tip:*** *The issue of the question is the treatment for a detached retina. Read the stem carefully and determine that the client is presently "experiencing the detached retina." This suggests a sense of urgency. Options 1, 2, and 4 are all similar in that the nurse eventually covers the eye and waits. Select option 3, which calls for the nurse to notify the primary care provider and obtain treatment for the client by an eye specialist.*

Content Area: Adult Health; *Category of Health Alteration:* Integumentary Management and Other Health Alterations; *Integrated Processes:* Nursing Process Implementation; *Client Need:* Physiological Integrity/Reduction of Risk Potential/Potential for Alterations in Body Systems; *Cognitive Level:* Analysis

Reference: Ignatavicius, D., & Workman, M. (2006). *Medical-Surgical Nursing: Critical Thinking for Collaborative Care* (5th ed., pp. 1102–1103). St. Louis, MO: Elsevier/Saunders.

---

770. A hospitalized client recently diagnosed with glaucoma tells a nurse that he finds it difficult to remember to administer the prescribed eye drops. The client states that he does not feel any pain or notice any vision changes if he forgets the drops. The best response by the nurse is:

1. "You should be diligent in administering those eye drops or you will need surgery or laser treatments."
2. "The medication controls the eye pressure. High pressure in the eye leads to gradual, painless nerve damage affecting sight. Tell me how it's been for you since your diagnosis of glaucoma."
3. "Tell me about your usual day so you can fit the eye drops into your schedule."
4. "I know this must be hard for you. Not everyone is able to remember everything."

ANSWER: 2

The client needs correct information about glaucoma, and the nurse should use open questioning to obtain further data to assist the client to follow the treatment plan. Current glaucoma treatment may include simultaneous pharmacological, laser, and surgical treatments. Dictating to or belittling the client does not include the client effectively into the treatment plan.

► ***Test-taking Tip:*** *Read the options carefully and select option 2, which addresses both the client's concern and knowledge deficit. Eliminate the options that are barriers to effective therapeutic communication.*

Content Area: Adult Health; *Category of Health Alteration:* Integumentary Management and Other Health Alterations; *Integrated Processes:* Nursing Process Implementation; Teaching and Learning; *Client Need:* Physiological Integrity/Reduction of Risk Potential/Potential for Alterations in Body Systems; Psychosocial Integrity/Therapeutic Communications; *Cognitive Level:* Analysis

Reference: Ignatavicius, D., & Workman, M. (2006). *Medical-Surgical Nursing: Critical Thinking for Collaborative Care* (5th ed., pp. 1096–1099). St. Louis, MO: Elsevier/Saunders.

---

771. A client diagnosed with glaucoma is prescribed pilocarpine hydrochloride 1% eye drops to both eyes four times per day. The expected action of this medication is to:

1. increase the outflow of aqueous humor in the eye.
2. improve vision in dimly lit environments.
3. increase production of aqueous humor.
4. increase pupillary dilation.

ANSWER: 1

Pilocarpine hydrochloride is a cholinergic agent used to treat glaucoma. It causes miosis (pupillary constriction), which then increases the angle of the channel in the anterior chamber of the eye. This improves the outflow of aqueous humor through the eye. The pupillary constriction from the pilocarpine also limits vision in dimly lit environments because when the pupil is constricted, less light reaches the retina to stimulate optic nerve function in sending impulses to the brain.

► ***Test-taking Tip:*** *Focus on the treatment aspect of glaucoma, a disease in which vision is slowly diminished due to increased intraocular pressure. Intraocular pressure will decrease if outflow of fluid is increased or production of fluid within the eyes is decreased. Constriction of the pupils improves the outflow of aqueous humor.*

Content Area: Adult Health; *Category of Health Alteration:* Integumentary Management and Other Health Alterations; *Integrated Processes:* Nursing Process Analysis; *Client Need:* Physiological Integrity/Pharmacological and Parenteral Therapies/Pharmacological Agents/Actions; *Cognitive Level:* Analysis

Reference: Wilson, B., Shannon, M., & Shields, K. (2009). *Prentice Hall Nurse's Drug Guide 2009* (pp. 1235–1237). Upper Saddle River, NJ: Pearson Education.

772. A client is seen in an emergency department and is diagnosed with closed-angle glaucoma. In a review of the client's medical record, which documented finding should the nurse question?

1. Eye pain
2. Sudden onset of symptoms
3. Normal intraocular pressure
4. Nausea and vomiting

ANSWER: 3

Closed-angle glaucoma causes an increased, not normal, intraocular pressure and this finding should be questioned. Symptoms of onset are acute, and the sudden rise in intraocular pressure causes eye pain, nausea, and vomiting. In closed-angle glaucoma the flow of aqueous is blocked when the iris moves against the cornea (closed angle).

➧ ***Test-taking Tip:*** *Note that three options are similar and one different. Often the option that is different is the answer.*

Content Area: Adult Health; *Category of Health Alteration:* Integumentary Management and Other Health Alterations; *Integrated Processes:* Communication and Documentation; *Client Need:* Physiological Integrity/Physiological Adaptation/Alterations in Body Systems; *Cognitive Level:* Application

Reference: Ignatavicius, D., & Workman, M. (2006). *Medical-Surgical Nursing: Critical Thinking for Collaborative Care* (5th ed., pp. 1096–1099). St. Louis, MO: Elsevier/Saunders.

---

773. A nurse, teaching a client with open-angle glaucoma, should instruct the client to:

1. restrict oral intake to lessen the need for glaucoma medications.
2. include foods high in omega 3 fatty acids in the diet.
3. remain under the care of and have regular eye examinations by an eye specialist physician.
4. administer prescribed eye drop medication when feeling pressure within the eyes.

ANSWER: 3

Glaucoma is a chronic progressive disease; clients with glaucoma should continue under the care of an eye specialist physician for life. Fluid restriction or dietary interventions are not effective treatment modalities. Clients should administer eye medications as prescribed. Elevated intraocular pressure cannot be felt.

➧ ***Test-taking Tip:*** *The issue of the question is treatment for glaucoma. Recall that glaucoma is a chronic progressive disease and that these diseases always require continued surveillance and treatment.*

Content Area: Adult Health; *Category of Health Alteration:* Integumentary Management and Other Health Alterations; *Integrated Processes:* Nursing Process Implementation, Teaching and Learning; *Client Need:* Physiological Integrity/Physiological Adaptation/Illness Management; *Cognitive Level:* Analysis

Reference: Ignatavicius, D., & Workman, M. (2006). *Medical-Surgical Nursing: Critical Thinking for Collaborative Care* (5th ed., p. 1096). St. Louis, MO: Elsevier/Saunders.

---

774. A client tells a nurse that he has been diagnosed with macular degeneration, "wet type." Based on the nurse's knowledge of this diagnosis, the nurse, examining this client's eyes using an ophthalmoscope, should expect to observe:

1. growth of abnormal blood vessels in the macula.
2. atrophy of structures in the macula.
3. clouding of the lens of the eye.
4. a thin, grayish-white area on the edge of the cornea.

ANSWER: 1

The "wet type" of macular degeneration results from the growth of abnormal blood vessels in the macula. The blood vessels often leak fluid and blood. The "dry type" of macular degeneration shows atrophy of structures in the macula. A cataract is the clouding of the lens. Corneal arcus is the thin grayish arc on the edge of the cornea, a normal finding in older clients.

➧ ***Test-taking Tip:*** *Read the stem and options carefully. Determine that the nurse will observe the macula using an ophthalmoscope. Eliminate options 3 and 4 since the macula is not observed. Eliminate option 2 because the term "atrophy" refers to the thinning or diminishment of structures viewed in the macula. Use the process of elimination to select option 1, which describes the growth of blood vessels, a source of blood, which is "wet."*

Content Area: Adult Health; *Category of Health Alteration:* Integumentary Management and Other Health Alterations; *Integrated Processes:* Nursing Process Assessment; *Client Need:* Physiological Integrity/Reduction of Risk Potential/System Specific Assessments; *Cognitive Level:* Application

Reference: Bouria, D., & Young, T. (2006). Age-related macular degeneration: A practical approach to a challenging disease. *Journal of American Geriatrics Society*, 54(7), 1130–1135.

775. A client diagnosed with macular degeneration is told the condition is progressing to an advanced stage. When completing the client's health assessment, which findings should the nurse expect the client to report? SELECT ALL THAT APPLY.

1. Curtain appearance over part of the visual field
2. Loss of peripheral vision
3. Difficulty seeing in dimly lit environments
4. Visual distortions in the central vision
5. Clouding of the lens

ANSWER: 3, 4

The macula is the area of central vision. Clients with macular degeneration experience loss or distortion of central vision and difficulty in lowly lit environments. A curtain appearance over the vision is associated with retinal detachment. Peripheral vision deficits result from progressive glaucoma. A cataract is the clouding of the lens.

➧ ***Test-taking Tip:*** *Recall from anatomy and physiology that the macula is the area near the fovea centralis, the area of most acute vision. Select options 3 and 4 because they identify visual defects associated with central vision. Eliminate options 1, 2, and 5 because they represent descriptions of other specific pathological conditions of the eye.*

Content Area: Adult Health; *Category of Health Alteration:* Integumentary Management and Other Health Alterations; *Integrated Processes:* Nursing Process Analysis; *Client Need:* Physiological Integrity/Physiological Adaptation/Illness Management; *Cognitive Level:* Application

Reference: Bouria, D., & Young, T. (2006). Age-related macular degeneration: A practical approach to a challenging disease. *Journal of American Geriatrics Society*, 54(7), 1130–1135.

---

776. A client with severely diminished vision has difficulty with visual discrimination. Which interventions should a nurse recommend to improve the client's sight in the home environment? SELECT ALL THAT APPLY.

1. Include contrasting colors in the environment but avoid the colors green and blue.
2. Write lists that will be used by the client with a black marker on a white background.
3. Keep light switches the same color as the wall, but place a Velcro® tab at the specific off/on switch.
4. Paint doorknobs on the doors a bright contrasting color.
5. Match the color of dishes with the color of tablecloths or placemats.

ANSWER: 1, 2, 4

Clients who have difficulty with vision discrimination are helped by interventions that emphasize color contrast in the environment. Similar colors within the environment worsen the client's ability for visual discrimination.

➧ ***Test-taking Tip:*** *The issue of the question is visual discrimination, the ability to discriminate different color tones. Read the options carefully and select those that emphasize the contrast of color tones within the home environment.*

Content Area: Adult Health; *Category of Health Alteration:* Integumentary Management and Other Health Alterations; *Integrated Processes:* Nursing Process Implementation; Teaching and Learning; *Client Need:* Physiological Integrity/Reduction of Risk Potential/Potential for Alterations in Body Systems; *Cognitive Level:* Analysis

Reference: Carpenito-Moyet, L. (2008). *Nursing Diagnosis Application to Clinical Practice* (12th ed., p. 365). Philadelphia: Wolters Kluwer/Lippincott Williams & Wilkins.

---

777. A client with diminished sight has problems secondary to glare with light. A nurse should advise the client to:

1. install fluorescent lighting throughout the home.
2. wear sunglasses and hats with brims when outdoors.
3. look directly at light sources.
4. utilize direct light from windows during the sunny times of the day.

ANSWER: 2

Wearing sunglasses and hats with brims while outdoors will block direct light from the client's eyes. Incandescent lighting produces fewer glares than fluorescent lighting. Glare problems are lessened when the client avoids looking at direct light, including sunlight.

➧ ***Test-taking Tip:*** *Read the stem carefully and determine the client's vision is harmed by the glare that occurs with light. Evaluate each option to determine whether it would decrease or increase the likelihood of glare. Picture yourself in each scenario to select the correct option.*

Content Area: Adult Health; *Category of Health Alteration:* Integumentary Management and Other Health Alterations; *Integrated Processes:* Nursing Process Implementation; *Client Need:* Physiological Integrity/Reduction of Risk Potential/Potential for Alterations in Body Systems; *Cognitive Level:* Application

Reference: Carpenito-Moyet, L. (2008). *Nursing Diagnosis Application to Clinical Practice* (12th ed., p. 365). Philadelphia: Wolters Kluwer/Lippincott Williams & Wilkins.

778. A nurse working in a hospital is assigned to care for a client who has a visual deficit. The nurse should plan to promote effective communication by:

1. announcing being present in the room and informing the client of the nurse's name.
2. standing directly in front of the client while speaking with the client.
3. using a loud, clear voice when talking with the client.
4. touching the client to get the client's attention before beginning to perform an assessment.

ANSWER: 1

Informing the client of the nurse's presence and name puts the client at ease and allows the client to participate in care. A nurse should stand in the client's field of vision, which may not be directly in front of the client. A nurse does not need to speak loudly since the client has a visual deficit but is able to hear. A nurse should explain what to expect before touching the client.

➧ ***Test-taking Tip:*** *Read the stem carefully to determine the question calls for interventions to enhance communication with a visually impaired person. Consider the effect of each option regarding whether it is effective or appropriate.*

Content Area: Adult Health; *Category of Health Alteration:* Integumentary Management and Other Health Alterations; *Integrated Processes:* Nursing Process Implementation; *Client Need:* Physiological Integrity/Reduction of Risk Potential/Potential for Alterations in Body Systems; *Cognitive Level:* Analysis

Reference: Berman, A., Snyder, S., Kozier, B., & Erb, G. (2008). *Kozier & Erb's Fundamentals of Nursing: Concepts, Process, and Practice* (8th ed., p. 990). Upper Saddle River, NJ: Pearson Education.

---

779. A client is seen in a primary care clinic because of a painful eye. The client is diagnosed with a hordeolum of the left eye. The client's treatment plan is likely to include:

1. wearing an eye patch on the left eye.
2. administering miotic eye drops twice daily.
3. applying warm compresses several times daily and applying antibiotic ointment.
4. avoiding reading and other close work.

ANSWER: 3

A hordeolum, or stye, is an infected sweat gland in the eyelid at the base of the eyelashes. Treatment includes warm compresses to promote drainage and antibiotic ointment to treat the infection, often due to a *Staphylococcus* or *Streptococcus* organism. Patching the eye is not indicated since the infection is in the outer eye. Miotic drops are ordered to treat glaucoma. Close work and reading are limited for clients who have undergone treatment for retinal detachment to limit rapid eye movement but would not be limited for clients diagnosed with a hordeolum.

➧ ***Test-taking Tip:*** *The issue of the question is treatment of a hordeolum or stye, which is an infection. Option 3 is the only response appropriate for treatment of an infection. If one cannot define hordeolum, option 2 can still be eliminated. The stem states the client is experiencing pain, and miotic drops are usually prescribed to treat open-angle glaucoma, a painless condition.*

Content Area: Adult Health; *Category of Health Alteration:* Integumentary Management and Other Health Alterations; *Integrated Processes:* Nursing Process Planning; *Client Need:* Physiological Integrity/Physiological Adaptation/Infectious Diseases; *Cognitive Level:* Application

Reference: Ignatavicius, D., & Workman, M. (2006). *Medical-Surgical Nursing: Critical Thinking for Collaborative Care* (5th ed., pp. 1086, 1088). St. Louis, MO: Elsevier/Saunders.

---

780. A hospitalized client tells a nurse that he feels as if he has something in his eye under the upper eyelid. The client does not recall any incident involving his eye. He has no eye pain or difficulty seeing. The eye is not reddened, and the client is able to open and shut his eye. The nurse should:

1. notify the client's primary care provider.
2. flush the eye with sterile saline.
3. don gloves, use a cotton-tipped applicator to evert the upper lid, and examine the eye and inner lid.
4. place a patch on the eye, taping the eye from the outside to the inside.

ANSWER: 3

Since the client is not experiencing pain or changes in vision, the nurse should further assess the client's eye by everting the upper eyelid safely with a cotton-tipped applicator to visualize the eye. Interventions such as contacting the primary care provider, irrigating the eye, or patching the eye should not be done until the assessment is complete.

➧ ***Test-taking Tip:*** *Read the stem carefully and determine that there are no specific signs or symptoms related to pathological condition. Use the nursing process to guide you to first perform a more complete assessment before proceeding with further interventions.*

Content Area: Adult Health; *Category of Health Alteration:* Integumentary Management and Other Health Alterations; *Integrated Processes:* Nursing Process Assessment; *Client Need:* Health Promotion and Maintenance/Techniques of Physical Assessment; *Cognitive Level:* Analysis

Reference: Berman, A., Snyder, S., Kozier, B., & Erb, G. (2008). *Kozier & Erb's Fundamentals of Nursing: Concepts, Process, and Practice* (8th ed., p. 589). Upper Saddle River, NJ: Pearson Education.

781. Which member of the interdisciplinary team should a nurse expect a consultation when planning the care of the client with Ménière's disease?

1. Rheumatologist
2. Otolaryngologist
3. Physiatrist
4. Oncologist

ANSWER: 2
Since Ménière's disease is a condition of the ear, the nurse would plan to include the otolaryngologist. The rheumatologist treats arthritic and immune conditions. The physiatrist cares for clients with musculoskeletal or rehabilitation conditions. The oncologist takes care of cancer clients.

▶ ***Test-taking Tip:*** *Focus on the key term "Ménière's disease," a condition involving the ear. Use knowledge of medical terminology to select the correct option. "Oto-" refers to ear.*

Content Area: Adult Health; *Category of Health Alteration:* Integumentary Management and Other Health Alterations; *Integrated Processes:* Nursing Process Planning; *Client Need:* Safe and Effective Care Environment/Management of Care/Consultation; *Cognitive Level:* Analysis

Reference: Lewis, S., Heitkemper, M., Dirksen, S., O'Brien, P., & Bucher, L. (2007). *Medical-Surgical Nursing: Assessment and Management of Clinical Problems* (7th ed., p. 441). St. Louis, MO: Mosby/Elsevier.

---

782. A client diagnosed with Ménière's disease tells a nurse that medication treatment for vertigo has been prescribed and provides the nurse with a list of medications recently received. Which medication is most likely prescribed for treating the vertigo?

1. Meclizine (Antivert®)
2. Megestrol (Megace®)
3. Meropenem (Merrem®)
4. Metoprolol (Lopressor®)

ANSWER: 1
The anticholinergic and antihistamine properties of meclizine treat the symptom of vertigo. Megestrol, an antineoplastic agent, is used to treat advanced breast cancer. The antibiotic, meropenem, treats intra-abdominal infections. The beta blocker, metopolol, controls hypertension and heart disease.

▶ ***Test-taking Tip:*** *Note the key word "vertigo." Remember what drugs treat this condition and eliminate options 2, 3, and 4.*

Content Area: Adult Health; *Category of Health Alteration:* Integumentary Management and Other Health Alterations; *Integrated Processes:* Nursing Process Implementation; *Client Need:* Physiological Integrity/Pharmacological and Parenteral Therapies/Pharmacological Agents/Actions; *Cognitive Level:* Application

Reference: Deglin, J., & Vallerand, A. (2009). *Davis's Drug Guide for Nurses* (11th ed.). Philadelphia: F. A. Davis.

---

783. EBP To reduce the risk of recurrent otitis media, which vaccine should a nurse recommend?

1. Varicella vaccine (Varivax®)
2. Pneumococcal vaccine (Prevnar®)
3. Typhoid vaccine (Typhim Vi®)
4. Zoster vaccine (Zostavax®)

ANSWER: 2
Pneumococcal vaccine can reduce the risk of ear infections. The evidence does not support the other vaccines having an effect on ear infections. Varicella vaccine is used to prevent chickenpox. Typhoid vaccine prevents typhoid fever. Zoster vaccine is used to prevent the development of herpes zoster.

▶ ***Test-taking Tip:*** *Focus on the key term of "otitis media," and think about the effect of each vaccine. Eliminate options with no association with ear infections.*

Content Area: Adult Health; *Category of Health Alteration:* Integumentary Management and Other Health Alterations; *Integrated Processes:* Teaching and Learning; *Client Need:* Health Promotion and Maintenance/Immunizations; *Cognitive Level:* Application

Reference: Youngkin, E., Sawin, K., Kissinger, K., & Israel, D. (2005). *Pharmacotherapeutics: A Primary Care Guide.* Upper Saddle River, NJ: Prentice Hall.

EBP Reference: University of Michigan Health System (UMHS). (2007). *Otitis Media.* Ann Arbor, MI: UMHS. Available at: www.guideline.gov/summary/summary.aspx?doc_id=11685&nbr=006032&string=Otitis+AND+Media

784. A client receives a prescription for sodium fluoride for otosclerosis and asks a nurse what the medication will do for his ears. Which response by the nurse is correct?

1. "The medication prevents the breakdown of bone cells and hardens the bone in the ear."
2. "The medication causes the breakdown of bone cells and softens the bone in the ear."
3. "The medication blocks the effect of histamine and dries the fluid in the ear."
4. "The medication causes the production of histamine and increases the fluid in the ear."

ANSWER: 1

The medication, sodium fluoride, retards bone reabsorption (prevents the breakdown of bone cells) and promotes calcification (hardening) of the bony lesions in the ear. No drug actions exist that reflect options 2 and 4. Antihistamine drugs treat the symptoms of allergic reaction but do not affect the fluid in the ear.

***Test-taking Tip:** Focus on the key words "sodium fluoride" and "otosclerosis." Recall the pathology that occurs in otosclerosis and the effect of the medication sodium fluoride. Use the process of elimination to exclude options 2, 3, and 4.*

Content Area: Adult Health; *Category of Health Alteration:* Integumentary Management and Other Health Alterations; *Integrated Processes:* Teaching and Learning; *Client Need:* Physiological Integrity/Pharmacological and Parenteral Therapies/Pharmacological Agents/Actions; *Cognitive Level:* Analysis

Reference: Lewis, S., Heitkemper, M., Dirksen, S., O'Brien, P., & Bucher, L. (2007). *Medical-Surgical Nursing: Assessment and Management of Clinical Problems* (7th ed., p. 441). St. Louis, MO: Mosby/Elsevier.

---

785. A client recovering from stapedectomy surgery for otosclerosis reports dizziness after surgery. To decrease symptoms, which interventions should a nurse advise the client to implement? SELECT ALL THAT APPLY.

1. Refrain from sudden movements.
2. Minimize chewing on the affected side.
3. Avoid lifting objects.
4. Minimize bending over.
5. Restrict fluid intake.
6. Avoid watching television.

ANSWER: 1, 3, 4

The eye, the inner ear, and kinesthetic senses are all responsible for maintaining balance. When one of these factors is affected, dizziness can result. The occurrence of dizziness can be decreased by refraining from sudden movements and avoiding lifting objects and bending at the waist. Dental conditions require the minimization of chewing on the affected side. Cardiac and renal conditions require restricting fluid intake. Television viewing may exacerbate symptoms in Ménière's disease.

***Test-taking Tip:** Focus on the key words "stapedectomy surgery" and "dizziness" and the physiological changes created by surgery. Use the process of elimination to exclude options 2, 5, and 6.*

Content Area: Adult Health; *Category of Health Alteration:* Integumentary Management and Other Health Alterations; *Integrated Processes:* Nursing Process Implementation; *Client Need:* Physiological Integrity/Reduction of Risk Potential/Therapeutic Procedures; *Cognitive Level:* Application

Reference: Lewis, S., Heitkemper, M., Dirksen, S., O'Brien, P., & Bucher, L. (2007). *Medical-Surgical Nursing: Assessment and Management of Clinical Problems* (7th ed., p. 441). St. Louis, MO: Mosby/Elsevier.

---

786. A client has a hearing loss from a suspected acoustic neuroma. Which diagnostic test should a nurse plan to prepare the client to confirm the presence of a tumor?

1. Tympanometry
2. Arteriogram of the cranial vessels
3. Magnetic resonance imaging (MRI)
4. Auditory canal biopsy

ANSWER: 3

MRI with gadolinium enhancement is the most reliable test in determining size and anatomic location of an acoustic neuroma. In tympanometry a probe is placed in the external ear canal and positive and negative pressures are then applied. It is used to diagnose middle ear effusions. Since the tumor arises from nerve cells, an arteriogram will not detect an acoustic neuroma. A biopsy is not possible in the inner ear.

***Test-taking Tip:** Note the key term "acoustic neuroma." Read each option carefully. Select an option in which the structures of the inner ear would be visible with the diagnostic test.*

Content Area: Adult Health; *Category of Health Alteration:* Integumentary Management and Other Health Alterations; *Integrated Processes:* Nursing Process Planning; *Client Need:* Physiological Integrity Reduction of Risk Potential/Diagnostic Tests; *Cognitive Level:* Application

Reference: Lewis, S., Heitkemper, M., Dirksen, S., O'Brien, P., & Bucher, L. (2007). *Medical-Surgical Nursing: Assessment and Management of Clinical Problems* (7th ed., pp. 414, 442). St. Louis, MO: Mosby/Elsevier.

787. A nurse assesses a postoperative client after surgical removal of a right-sided acoustic neuroma by a translabyrinthine approach and notes that the client is complaining of pain and has new onset of right-sided facial drooping and numbness. Determine which action the nurse should take next, and place the following items in order of priority, with 1 as the first activity carried out by the nurse and 4 the item requiring consideration last?

_____ Close the right eye and place a patch over it.
_____ Assess the operative incision site.
_____ Contact the physician to report facial drooping.
_____ Medicate the client for pain.

ANSWER: 4, 1, 2, 3

First, complete the client assessment by observing the operative incision site for bleeding or hematoma, as external problems, if any exist, this should be reported to the physician at once. Second, contact the physician, as facial drooping and numbness may indicate complications such as intracranial bleeding or nerve compression. Third, unless contraindicated by the physician, medicate the client for pain. Fourth, close the right eye and place a patch over it for corneal protection, because the client will be unable to close the eye due to nerve compression or damage.

Test-taking Tip: *Focus on the facial assessment. Visualize the process you would take in a real situation. Remember the urgent steps take priority (further assessment and contacting the physician).*

Content Area: Adult Health; *Category of Health Alteration:* Integumentary Management and Other Health Alterations; *Integrated Processes:* Nursing Process Analysis; *Client Need:* Safe and Effective Care Environment/Management of Care/Establishing Priorities; *Cognitive Level:* Analysis

References: Lewis, S., Heitkemper, M., Dirksen, S., O'Brien, P., & Bucher. L. (2007). *Medical-Surgical Nursing: Assessment and Management of Clinical Problems* (7th ed., p. 442). St. Louis, MO: Mosby/Elsevier; Roland, P. (2006). Skull base, acoustic neuroma (vestibular Schwannoma). *E-Medicine from WebMD.* Available at: www.emedicine.com/ent/TOPIC239.HTM

---

788. EBP A client's daughter tells a nurse of frustration while communicating with her elderly mother who wears hearing aides. A nurse suggests that the daughter should:

1. minimize oral communication to essential matters.
2. speak directly into the client's better ear.
3. use exaggerated mouth expressions while speaking.
4. attract the client's attention before speaking.

ANSWER: 4

Attracting the client's attention improves communication by including the client fully in the process from the start. Normal conversation, including a variety of topics, helps the client avoid social isolation. Speaking directly into the client's ear will amplify and perhaps distort the conversation. Additionally, the client will not be able to observe the speaker's mouth and receive visual cues. Exaggerated mouth expressions distort the visual cues and hinder communication.

Test-taking Tip: *Read the stem carefully and understand that the question calls for a true response. Consider each option and select the intervention that promotes communication and optimal functioning.*

Content Area: Adult Health; *Category of Health Alteration:* Integumentary Management and Other Health Alterations; *Integrated Processes:* Nursing Process Implementation; *Client Need:* Physiological Integrity/Reduction of Risk Potential/Potential for Alterations in Body Systems; *Cognitive Level:* Analysis

Reference: Berman, A., Snyder, S., Kozier, B., & Erb, G. (2008). *Kozier & Erb's Fundamentals of Nursing: Concepts, Process, and Practice* (8th ed., p. 597). Upper Saddle River, NJ: Pearson Education.

EBP Reference: Adams-Wendling, L., & Pimple, C. (2007). *Nursing Management of Hearing Impairment in Nursing Facility Residents.* Iowa City: University of Iowa Gerontological Nursing Interventions Research Center, Research Dissemination Core. Available at: www.guideline.gov/summary/summary.aspx?doc_id=11053&nbr=005832&string=hearing

789. EBP A resident of a long-term care facility tells the nurse that he is having increased difficulty hearing during conversations and while watching television. A nurse should:

1. teach the client to eliminate background noises.
2. assess the client's hearing and examine the client's ears using an otoscope.
3. contact the primary care provider and schedule the client for bilateral ear irrigations.
4. teach the client to look directly at the speaker's face in conversations or while watching a television program.

ANSWER: 2

A nurse assesses the client's hearing and performs an examination using an otoscope. A nurse performs the assessment to verify the client's symptoms and attempts to find the source of the client's problem. Interventions to improve communication are useful to the client, but a new hearing loss must be investigated. A nurse should obtain additional data before referring the client for medical evaluation.

Test-taking Tip: *Read the stem carefully and ascertain if further information is needed before planning an intervention. Utilize the steps of the nursing process and select option 2, which calls for the nurse to perform an assessment.*

Content Area: Adult Health; *Category of Health Alteration:* Integumentary Management and Other Health Alterations; *Integrated Processes:* Nursing Process Implementation; *Client Need:* Physiological Integrity/Reduction of Risk Potential/System Specific Assessments; *Cognitive Level:* Analysis

Reference: Berman, A., Snyder, S., Kozier, B., & Erb, G. (2008). *Kozier & Erb's Fundamentals of Nursing: Concepts, Process, and Practice* (8th ed., p. 597). Upper Saddle River, NJ: Pearson Education.

EBP Reference: Adams-Wendling, L., & Pimple, C. (2007). *Nursing Management of Hearing Impairment in Nursing Facility Residents.* Iowa City: University of Iowa Gerontological Nursing Interventions Research Center, Research Dissemination Core. Available at: www.guideline.gov/summary/summary.aspx?doc_id=11053&nbr=005832&string=hearing

790. EBP A client is admitted to a nursing care facility for rehabilitation after suffering a stroke. Observations by a nurse that should suggest the client has impaired hearing include: SELECT ALL THAT APPLY.

1. the client nods and agrees to all statements by the nurse.
2. the client asks for more information about the physical therapy schedule.
3. the client is slow to respond verbally but answers questions appropriately.
4. the client speaks in a loud tone of voice.
5. the client leans in toward the nurse when the nurse speaks.
6. the client asks the nurse to be careful before the nurse begins the otoscopic examination.

ANSWER: 1, 4, 5

Clients with hearing defects are sometimes overly agreeable in an effort to avoid dealing with the issue of not hearing what is being discussed. They often speak louder than normal to compensate and lean in toward the speaker to enhance their hearing. Asking details about a schedule, responding slowly, or expressing concern before a physical exam are not suggestive of deficient hearing.

Test-taking Tip: *Read the stem carefully and understand the question calls for negative findings. Consider each option and select the option describing behaviors a client utilizes to adapt to a hearing deficit.*

Content Area: Adult Health; *Category of Health Alteration:* Integumentary Management and Other Health Alterations; *Integrated Processes:* Nursing Process Assessment; *Client Need:* Physiological Integrity/Reduction of Risk Potential/System Specific Assessments; *Cognitive Level:* Analysis

Reference: Berman, A., Snyder, S., Kozier, B., & Erb, G. (2008). *Kozier & Erb's Fundamentals of Nursing: Concepts, Process, and Practice* (8th ed., p. 597). Upper Saddle River, NJ: Pearson Education.

EBP Reference: Adams-Wendling, L., & Pimple, C. (2007). *Nursing Management of Hearing Impairment in Nursing Facility Residents.* Iowa City: University of Iowa Gerontological Nursing Interventions Research Center, Research Dissemination Core. Available at: www.guideline.gov/summary/summary.aspx?doc_id=11053&nbr=005832&string=hearing

791. Which interventions should the nurse advise a client to implement for home treatment of acute sinusitis? SELECT ALL THAT APPLY.

1. Take over-the-counter antacids.
2. Apply warm compresses to the face.
3. Use saline nasal spray.
4. Take over-the-counter decongestants.
5. Drink plenty of fluids.
6. Spend time outdoors in the sunlight.

ANSWER: 2, 3, 4, 5

Implementing options 2, 3, 4, and 5 helps treat the symptoms of acute sinusitis. Over-the-counter antacids will not treat sinusitis but treat epigastric pain from dyspepsia. Spending time in the sunlight will treat psoriasis but not sinusitis.

***Test-taking Tip:** Note the key word "interventions," and use the process of elimination to exclude options 1 and 6.*

Content Area: Adult Health; *Category of Health Alteration:* Integumentary Management and Other Health Alterations; *Integrated Processes:* Teaching and Learning; *Client Need:* Physiological Integrity/Basic Care and Comfort/Nonpharmacological Comfort Interventions; *Cognitive Level:* Application

Reference: Lewis, S., Heitkemper, M., Dirksen, S., O'Brien, P., & Bucher, L. (2007). *Medical-Surgical Nursing: Assessment and Management of Clinical Problems* (7th ed., pp. 540–541). St. Louis, MO: Mosby/Elsevier.

Test 20: **Adult Health: Musculoskeletal Management**

792. A nurse should teach a client, following a diagnostic arthroscopy, to: SELECT ALL THAT APPLY.

1. elevate the involved extremity for 24 to 48 hours.
2. apply ice continually for 24 hours.
3. report severe joint pain immediately to the physician.
4. resume usual activities to help reduce swelling.
5. treat pain with a mild analgesic such as acetaminophen (Tylenol®).

ANSWER: 1, 3, 5

Elevation will help to decrease edema. Severe joint pain may indicate a possible complication and should be reported immediately. Usually, a mild analgesic is sufficient for pain control following a diagnostic arthroscopy. Ice should be applied intermittently (usually 20 to 30 minutes with a 10- to 15-minute warming period between applications). Hypothermia causes vasoconstriction; lower temperatures cause worsening of the condition and decrease circulation to the area. Activity is initially limited and slowly progressed.

➧ ***Test-taking Tip:*** *Note that this is a diagnostic arthroscopy.*

Content Area: Adult Health; *Category of Health Alteration:* Musculoskeletal Management; *Integrated Processes:* Teaching and Learning; *Client Need:* Health Promotion and Maintenance/Self-Care; *Cognitive Level:* Application

References: Berman, A., Snyder, S., Kozier, B., & Erb, G. (2008). *Kozier & Erb's Fundamentals of Nursing: Concepts, Process, and Practice* (8th ed., p. 932). Upper Saddle River, NJ: Pearson Education; Ignatavicius, D., & Workman, M. (2006). *Medical-Surgical Nursing: Critical Thinking for Collaborative Care* (5th ed., p. 1154). St. Louis, MO: Elsevier/Saunders.

---

793. EBP Which treatments should a nurse plan for a client being seen in the clinic for a second-degree ankle sprain?

1. Rest, elevate the extremity, apply ice, and apply a compression bandage.
2. Perform range of motion to determine the extent of injury, apply heat, check circulation and sensation, and examine the ankle.
3. Reduce pain with moist heat, then apply ice to reduce swelling; check circulation, motion, and sensation; and elevate the ankle.
4. Refer the client immediately to an orthopedic surgeon, administer analgesics, control swelling with ice, and encourage rest and elevation.

ANSWER: 1

A second-degree ankle sprain involves tearing of ligament fibers producing edema, tenderness, pain with motion, joint instability, and partial loss of normal joint function. Rest prevents further injury and promotes healing. However, encourage walking with a normal gate as soon as possible, allowing for some discomfort. Inversion should be avoided. Ice and elevation control swelling. Compression with an elastic bandage controls bleeding, reduces edema, and provides support for injured tissues. Performing range of motion would be contraindicated initially because it causes pain and possible further injury. Progressive passive and active exercises may begin as soon as tolerated without pain, usually in 2 to 5 days. Heat causes vasodilation, increasing edema, and should not be used if swelling is present. Immediate orthopedic referral is reserved for emergent, frequently open, injuries.

➧ ***Test-taking Tip:*** *Recall the acronym RICE: rest, ice, compression, and elevation.*

Content Area: Adult Health; *Category of Health Alteration:* Musculoskeletal Management; *Integrated Processes:* Nursing Process Planning; *Client Need:* Physiological Integrity/Reduction of Risk Potential/Therapeutic Procedures; *Cognitive Level:* Application

Reference: Smeltzer, S., Bare, B., Hinkle, J., & Cheever, K. (2008). *Brunner & Suddarth's Textbook of Medical-Surgical Nursing* (11th ed., p. 2426). Philadelphia: Lippincott Williams & Wilkins.

EBP Reference: Institute for Clinical Systems Improvement. (2006). *Ankle Sprain.* Available at: www.guideline.gov/summary/summary.aspx?doc_id=8948&nbr=004870&string=ankle+AND+fracture

794. A client involved in a work-related accident is scheduled for surgery to repair a comminuted femur fracture. Three days following surgery, the client asks a nurse to describe what is meant by "a comminuted femur fracture." In describing the fracture, which illustration should the nurse show the client?

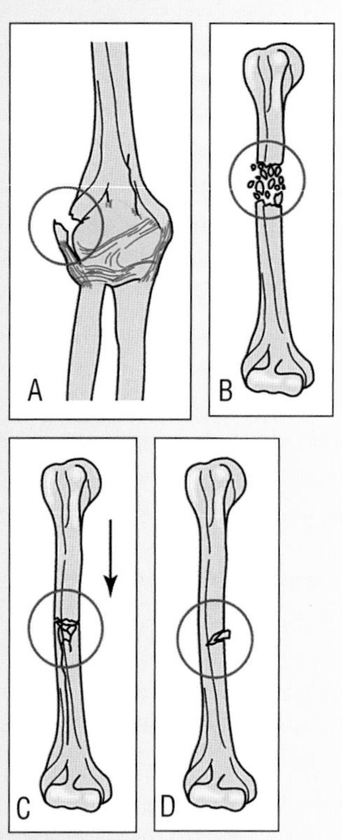

1. Illustration A
2. Illustration B
3. Illustration C
4. Illustration D

ANSWER: 2

A comminuted fracture has bone fragments that are splintered or shattered into numerous fragments. This often occurs following a crushing injury and is considered an unstable fracture. Option 1 (illustration A) shows an avulsion, where a piece of bone is torn away from the main bone while still attached to a ligament or tendon. Option 3 (illustration C) is an impacted bone where bone is pushed into bone. Option 4 (illustration D) is a greenstick fracture. Often seen in children, this is an incomplete fracture that occurs when the bone is bent and a fracture occurs on the outer arc of the bend.

▶ ***Test-taking Tip:*** *Apply knowledge of fracture types to answer this question.*

Content Area: Adult Health; *Category of Health Alteration:* Musculoskeletal Management; *Integrated Processes:* Teaching and Learning; *Client Need:* Health Promotion and Maintenance/Principles of Teaching and Learning; *Cognitive Level:* Application

Reference: Lewis, S., Heitkemper, M., Dirksen, S., O'Brien, P., & Bucher, L. (2007). *Medical-Surgical Nursing: Assessment and Management of Clinical Problems* (7th ed., p. 1636). St. Louis, MO: Mosby.

795. A college student walking with a stiff left leg visits a campus health service reporting knee pain and a click when walking. He is concerned because sometimes his knee either "locks" or "gives way." He thinks he twisted his knee wrong during a tennis match, but is not sure. A nurse suspects the client has:

1. an injury of the meniscus cartilage.
2. a fracture of the lateral tibial condyle.
3. a fractured patella.
4. a lateral collateral ligament injury.

ANSWER: 1

The cartilage of the knee (meniscus) can be torn or detached from the head of the tibia with twisting or repetitive squatting and impact. The loose cartilage can slip between the femur and tibia, preventing full leg extension and "locking." If the cartilage slips during walking, a clicking sound is heard, and during running the leg can "give way." Locking and clicking are not associated with a tibial or patella fracture. In a collateral ligament injury, the client experiences acute pain, joint instability, and inability to walk without assistance.

▶ ***Test-taking Tip:*** *Focus on the client's symptoms and the fact that he is walking; then use the process of elimination to rule out incorrect options.*

Content Area: Adult Health; *Category of Health Alteration:* Musculoskeletal Management; *Integrated Processes:* Nursing Process Analysis; *Client Need:* Physiological Integrity/Physiological Adaptation/Alterations in Body Systems; *Cognitive Level:* Analysis

Reference: Smeltzer, S., Bare, B., Hinkle, J., & Cheever, K. (2008). *Brunner & Suddarth's Textbook of Medical-Surgical Nursing* (11th ed., pp. 2429–2430). Philadelphia: Lippincott Williams & Wilkins.

796. A client is suspected of having a fat embolism following a pelvic fracture from a motor vehicle accident. A nurse should assess for which sign that is specific to a fat emboli?

1. Dyspnea
2. Chest pain
3. Delirium
4. Petechiae

ANSWER: 4

Petechiae (small purplish hemorrhagic spots on the skin) are thought to be due to transient thrombocytopenia. They can occur over the chest, anterior axillary folds, hard palate, buccal membranes, and conjunctival sacs. The other symptoms are not specific to fat emboli but are associated with blood emboli. Dyspnea and chest pain can occur when pulmonary or cardiac vessels are occluded. Cerebral disturbances, due to hypoxia and the lodging of emboli in the brain, vary from headache and mild agitation to delirium.

➧ *Test-taking Tip: Note the key word "specific." This should direct you to option 4.*

Content Area: Adult Health; *Category of Health Alteration:* Musculoskeletal Management; *Integrated Processes:* Nursing Process Assessment; *Client Need:* Physiological Integrity/Physiological Adaptation/ Alterations in Body Systems; *Cognitive Level:* Application

Reference: Smeltzer, S., Bare, B., Hinkle, J., & Cheever, K. (2008). *Brunner & Suddarth's Textbook of Medical-Surgical Nursing* (11th ed., pp. 2435–2436). Philadelphia: Lippincott Williams & Wilkins.

---

797. Which order written by a physician should be a priority for a nurse caring for a client who sustained an unstable pelvic fracture in a motor vehicle accident?

1. Urinalysis
2. Blood alcohol level
3. Computed tomography (CT) scan of the pelvis
4. Two units of cross-matched whole blood

ANSWER: 4

A type and cross-match needs to be completed prior to administering blood, which takes time. Significant blood loss occurs because the pelvis is a highly vascular area. Approximately 20% of persons with unstable pelvic fractures require more than 15 units of blood products within the first 24 hours of injury. The client is at risk for fat emboli. Free fat may show in the urine, but this is not priority. The administration of analgesics and anesthetics is affected by blood alcohol results, but this is not priority. CT of the pelvis will determine the extent of the fracture, but is not the priority.

➧ *Test-taking Tip: Use the ABCs (airway, breathing, and circulation). An intervention that promotes circulation is priority if airway or breathing interventions are not indicated.*

Content Area: Adult Health; *Category of Health Alteration:* Musculoskeletal Management; *Integrated Processes:* Nursing Process Analysis; *Client Need:* Safe and Effective Care Environment/Management of Care/Establishing Priorities; Physiological Integrity/Physiological Adaptation/Medical Emergencies; *Cognitive Level:* Analysis

Reference: Smeltzer, S., Bare, B., Hinkle, J., & Cheever, K. (2008). *Brunner & Suddarth's Textbook of Medical-Surgical Nursing* (11th ed., p. 2445). Philadelphia: Lippincott Williams & Wilkins.

---

798. A licensed practical nurse is reporting observations and cares to a registered nurse (RN). Based on the report, which client should the RN assess immediately?

1. The client, 2 hours following a total knee replacement, who has 100 mL bloody drainage in the suction container of an autotransfusion drainage system
2. The client with a crush injury to the arm who was given another analgesic and a skeletal muscle relaxant for throbbing, unrelenting pain
3. The client in a new body cast who was turned every 2 hours and supported with waterproof pillows
4. The client with an external fixator on the left leg, having serous drainage from the pin sites

ANSWER: 2

Throbbing, unrelenting pain could be the first sign of compartment syndrome. The neurovascular status of the extremity should be assessed. Unrelieved pressure can lead to compromised circulation and avascular necrosis. Postoperative drainage from a total knee replacement ranges from 200 to 400 mL during the first 24 hours. This amount is neither alarming nor sufficient enough to autotransfuse. The client in a body cast should be turned q2h to promote drying of the cast. To avoid cracking or denting of the cast, the client is supported with waterproof pillows that touch each other without open spaces. Some serous drainage, which is due to tissue trauma and edema, is expected from pin sites of an external fixator.

➧ *Test-taking Tip: Focus on the issue, the client that needs immediate assessment, and use the ABCs (airway, breathing, and circulation). Focus on the information in option 2 that suggests circulation is potentially compromised: throbbing, unrelenting pain.*

Content Area: Adult Health; *Category of Health Alteration:* Musculoskeletal Management; *Integrated Processes:* Nursing Process Analysis; *Client Need:* Physiological Integrity/Physiological Adaptation/Unexpected Response to Therapies; *Cognitive Level:* Analysis

Reference: Smeltzer, S., Bare, B., Hinkle, J., & Cheever, K. (2008). *Brunner & Suddarth's Textbook of Medical-Surgical Nursing* (11th ed., pp. 2363–2364, 2375, 2438). Philadelphia: Lippincott Williams & Wilkins.

799. A clinic nurse has completed teaching for a client with a rotator cuff tear who is being treated conservatively. Which client statement indicates that further teaching is needed?

1. "I received a corticosteroid injection in my shoulder to reduce the inflammation."
2. "I will be doing progressive stretching and strengthening exercises now that the pain is controlled."
3. "I should continue taking ibuprofen (Advil®) with food for pain control."
4. "I will need an open acromioplasty surgery to repair the torn cuff after the swelling is reduced."

ANSWER: 4

Surgery is not a conservative treatment. However, some rotator cuff tears do require arthroscopic débridement or an open acromioplasty with tendon repair. Initial conservative treatment includes rest with modified activities, corticosteroid injections, NSAIDs, and progressive exercises.

➧ ***Test-taking Tip:*** *Focus on the key words "conservative" and "further teaching is needed." This is a false-response item. Select the client statement that is incorrect.*

Content Area: Adult Health; *Category of Health Alteration:* Musculoskeletal Management; *Integrated Processes:* Teaching and Learning; Nursing Process Evaluation; *Client Need:* Physiological Integrity/Reduction of Risk Potential/Therapeutic Procedures; *Cognitive Level:* Analysis

Reference: Smeltzer, S., Bare, B., Hinkle, J., & Cheever, K. (2008). *Brunner & Suddarth's Textbook of Medical-Surgical Nursing* (11th ed., p. 2429). Philadelphia: Lippincott Williams & Wilkins.

800. Which findings should a nurse expect when assessing a client diagnosed with a left femoral neck fracture? SELECT ALL THAT APPLY.

1. Left leg is abducted.
2. Left leg is externally rotated.
3. Left leg is shorter than right leg.
4. Pain in the lateral side of the left knee.
5. Pain in the groin area.

ANSWER: 2, 3, 5

With a left femoral neck fracture, the leg is externally rotated and shortened and pain is experienced in the groin area. Additional findings include an adducted (not abducted) left leg and pain in the medial (not lateral) side of the knee and hip.

➧ ***Test-taking Tip:*** *Visualize the fracture before selecting the options.*

Content Area: Adult Health; *Category of Health Alteration:* Musculoskeletal Management; *Integrated Processes:* Nursing Process Assessment; *Client Need:* Physiological Integrity/Reduction of Risk Potential/System Specific Assessments; *Cognitive Level:* Application

Reference: Smeltzer, S., Bare, B., Hinkle, J., & Cheever, K. (2008). *Brunner & Suddarth's Textbook of Medical-Surgical Nursing* (11th ed., p. 2446). Philadelphia: Lippincott Williams & Wilkins.

801. A client with a lower left leg fracture and a cast is using crutches. A nurse is evaluating whether the client is able to correctly get into a chair. Prioritize the actions that the client should be taking to correctly get into the chair.

______ Grasp the arm of the chair with the right hand.
______ Stand with the back of the unaffected leg centered against the chair.
______ Lean forward and flex the knees and hips.
______ Lower the body into the chair.
______ Brace the chair against the wall.
______ Transfer the crutches to the left hand, holding the crutches by the hand bars.

ANSWER: 4, 2, 5, 6, 1, 3

The client should first brace the chair against the wall. Then, stand with the back of the unaffected leg centered against the chair. Next, transfer the crutches to the left hand, holding them by the hand bars, and grasp the arm of the chair with the right hand. The client should lean forward and flex the knees and hips, then lower the body into the chair.

➧ ***Test-taking Tip:*** *First visualize getting into a chair while keeping weight off the affected extremity and holding crutches. Then read each option and place each in the correct order.*

Content Area: Adult Health; *Category of Health Alteration:* Musculoskeletal Management; *Integrated Processes:* Nursing Process Evaluation; *Client Need:* Safe and Effective Care Environment/Management of Care/Establishing Priorities; *Cognitive Level:* Analysis

Reference: Berman, A., Snyder, S., Kozier, B., & Erb, G. (2008). *Kozier & Erb's Fundamentals of Nursing: Concepts, Process, and Practice* (8th ed., p. 1155). Upper Saddle River, NJ: Pearson Education.

802. A 28-year-old client and his spouse were involved in a motorcycle accident in which his spouse was killed. The client, being treated in the progressive care unit for multiple rib fractures and a broken leg, asks the nurse in which room his wife is located. Which response is most appropriate?

1. "Your wife is not in the hospital."
2. "I'm sorry, but your wife did not survive the accident."
3. "I need to get your family so that you can talk to them about your wife."
4. "The doctor will be talking to you about your wife and where she is located."

ANSWER: 2

Because a nurse-client relationship is built on trust, the nurse should not withhold information from the client. Though telling the client his wife is not in the hospital is correct, it is deceitful, and the client will likely want more information. Options 3 and 4 do not answer the client's question. Leaving the client or deferring the explanation to someone else without providing an answer could increase the client's anxiety.

▶ ***Test-taking Tip:** Think about the client's rights and building a trusting therapeutic relationship.*

Content Area: Adult Health; *Category of Health Alteration:* Musculoskeletal Management; *Integrated Processes:* Communication and Documentation; *Client Need:* Psychosocial Integrity/Therapeutic Communications; *Cognitive Level:* Application

Reference: Berman, A., Snyder, S., Kozier, B., & Erb, G. (2008). *Kozier & Erb's Fundamentals of Nursing: Concepts, Process, and Practice* (8th ed., pp. 460, 471). Upper Saddle River, NJ: Pearson Education.

803. An elderly client with Alzheimer's dementia is being admitted from a postanesthesia unit following a hip hemiarthroplasty to treat a hip fracture. Which intervention should a nurse *initially* plan for the client's pain control?

1. Apply a fentanyl (Duragesic®) transdermal patch.
2. Initiate morphine sulfate per patient-controlled analgesia (PCA) with a basal rate.
3. Administer intravenous morphine sulfate based on the client's report of pain.
4. Administer scheduled doses of morphine sulfate intravenously around the clock.

ANSWER: 4

In addition to scheduling pain medication around the clock, supplemental NSAIDs can be administered to reduce inflammation and enhance the effects of the analgesic. A transdermal analgesic patch is used to treat chronic, not acute, pain. Usually a PCA affords the client better control over the pain and avoids the peaks and valleys associated with intermittent analgesics. However, the client with dementia would be unable to adequately use PCA. The client with dementia typically cannot report the level of pain accurately.

▶ ***Test-taking Tip:** Note the client has Alzheimer's dementia. This influences the treatment choices.*

Content Area: Adult Health; *Category of Health Alteration:* Musculoskeletal Management; *Integrated Processes:* Nursing Process Planning; *Client Need:* Physiological Integrity/Pharmacological and Parenteral Therapies/Pharmacological Pain Management; *Cognitive Level:* Application

Reference: Monahan, F., Sands, J., Neighbors, M., Marek, J., & Green, C. (2007). *Phipps' Medical-Surgical Nursing: Health and Illness Perspectives* (8th ed., p. 1544). St. Louis, MO: Mosby/Elsevier.

804. A diabetic client is admitted with a tentative diagnosis of osteomyelitis secondary to a wound on the ankle. The client's ankle is painful, red, swollen, and warm, and the wound is persistently draining. The client's temperature is 102.2°F (39°C). Based on the client's status, which written physician's order should a nurse plan to defer until later?

1. Obtain wound culture.
2. Administer ceftriaxone (Rocephin®) 1 g IV (intravenously) q12 hours.
3. Apply splint to immobilize ankle.
4. Begin teaching on self-administration of home IV antibiotics.

ANSWER: 4

The nurse should defer teaching. Pain and an elevated temperature are barriers to learning. The wound culture should be obtained before antibiotics are started. Ceftriaxone is a third-generation cephalosporin used in treating bone infections. The usual dose ranges from 1 to 2 g every 12 or 24 hours. Immobilizing with a splint helps to decrease pain and muscle spasms.

▶ ***Test-taking Tip:** Focusing on the client's symptoms and the question should direct you to option 4.*

Content Area: Adult Health; *Category of Health Alteration:* Musculoskeletal Management; *Integrated Processes:* Nursing Process Analysis; *Client Need:* Physiological Integrity/Physiological Adaptation/Illness Management; Health Promotion and Maintenance/Principles of Teaching and Learning; *Cognitive Level:* Analysis

Reference: Smeltzer, S., Bare, B., Hinkle, J., & Cheever, K. (2008). *Brunner & Suddarth's Textbook of Medical-Surgical Nursing* (11th ed., p. 2414). Philadelphia: Lippincott Williams & Wilkins.

805. A nurse is assessing an elderly client in Buck's traction to temporally immobilize a fracture of the proximal femur prior to surgery. Which finding requires the nurse to intervene immediately?

1. Reddened area on the sacrum
2. Voiding concentrated urine, 50 mL/hr
3. Capillary refill 3 seconds, dorsiflexion and sensation intact, pedal pulses palpable
4. Lower leg secure in traction boot and ropes and pulleys and 5 lb weight hanging freely

ANSWER: 1

A reddened sacrum is the first sign of a pressure ulcer that is caused by pressure or friction and sheer. Sheer results from the weight of the skin traction pulling the client to the foot of the bed and then the client sliding back up in bed. Immediate interventions are required before it develops into a stage II ulcer. The 50 mL/hr output is adequate, though the nurse should evaluate the client's amount of intake. Option 3 findings are normal. Buck's traction is skeletal traction. Traction (usually 5 to 8 lbs) is applied either to a boot in which the client's lower extremity is secured or to traction tapes applied to the client's extremity.

➧ ***Test-taking Tip:*** *The key word is "immediately." Eliminate options 3 and 4 because they are normal findings.*

Content Area: Adult Health; *Category of Health Alteration:* Musculoskeletal Management; *Integrated Processes:* Nursing Process Analysis; *Client Need:* Physiological Integrity/Reduction of Risk Potential/Potential for Complications of Diagnostic Tests/Treatments/Procedures; *Cognitive Level:* Application

Reference: Smeltzer, S., Bare, B., Hinkle, J., & Cheever, K. (2008). *Brunner & Suddarth's Textbook of Medical-Surgical Nursing* (11th ed., pp. 208–211, 2366–2367). Philadelphia: Lippincott Williams & Wilkins.

---

806. A nurse is providing instructions to a client who has a plaster cast to attain adequate molding following a fracture to the right wrist. Which statement, if made by the nurse, is incorrect?

1. "Keep your cast uncovered while drying so that moisture can evaporate."
2. "Your cast will have a musty odor and dull gray appearance until it dries. But once fully dry, your cast should be odorless and shiny white."
3. "Your cast will feel sticky and very warm during the drying process, but it will dry very quickly in about 30 minutes."
4. "Support the cast by elevating it on pillows and avoid any sharp or hard surfaces, especially while your cast is drying, because it can cause denting and pressure areas."

ANSWER: 3

Although the cast will feel very warm for about 15 to 20 minutes, a plaster cast requires 24 to 72 hours to dry completely. The freshly applied cast should be exposed to circulating air and not covered by clothing or bed linens. A wet plaster cast is musty smelling and dull gray until it dries. The pillows used to elevate the casted extremity should not be plastic coated, to avoid burning and inadequate drying. Sharp objects, firm surfaces, and pressure from fingers can dent the cast during drying.

➧ ***Test-taking Tip:*** *The key word is "least likely." Select the nurse's statement that is incorrect. Recall that a fiberglass cast, not a plaster cast, dries quickly.*

Content Area: Adult Health; *Category of Health Alteration:* Musculoskeletal Management; *Integrated Processes:* Teaching and Learning; *Client Need:* Physiological Integrity/Reduction of Risk Potential/Therapeutic Procedures; *Cognitive Level:* Application

Reference: Smeltzer, S., Bare, B., Hinkle, J., & Cheever, K. (2008). *Brunner & Suddarth's Textbook of Medical-Surgical Nursing* (11th ed., p. 2356). Philadelphia: Lippincott Williams & Wilkins.

---

807. A client has an external fixator for reduction of a tibial fracture. A nurse is evaluating the client's effectiveness in ambulating with crutches. Place an X on the *three areas* where the client should be bearing weight when crutch walking.

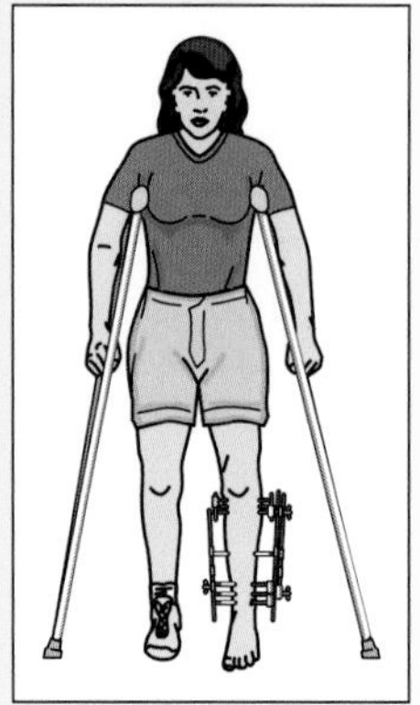

ANSWER:

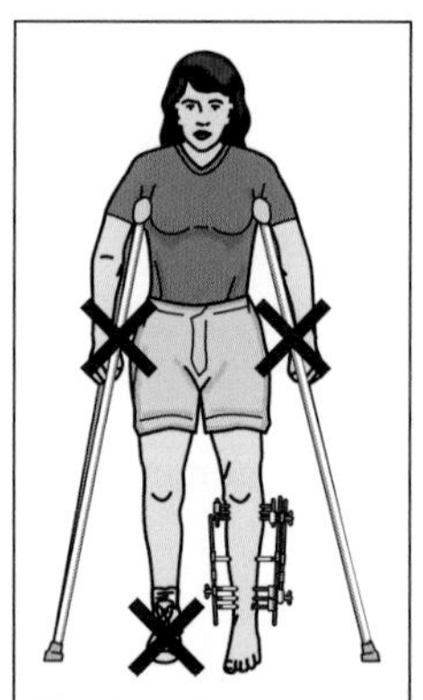

The client should be bearing weight on the hand grips when bringing legs forward. When moving crutches, the weight should be borne on the unaffected leg. If weight is borne on the axilla, the brachial plexus nerves can be damaged from the pressure of the crutch.

➧ ***Test-taking Tip:*** *Visualize crutch walking without bearing weight on the affected extremity.*

Content Area: Adult Health; *Category of Health Alteration:* Musculoskeletal Management; *Integrated Processes:* Nursing Process Evaluation; *Client Need:* Physiological Integrity/Basic Care and Comfort/Mobility/Immobility; *Cognitive Level:* Application

Reference: Smeltzer, S., Bare, B., Hinkle, J., & Cheever, K. (2008). *Brunner & Suddarth's Textbook of Medical-Surgical Nursing* (11th ed., p. 205). Philadelphia: Lippincott Williams & Wilkins.

808. A male client has been in a body cast for the past 2 days to treat numerous broken vertebrae from a fall. The client is reporting dyspnea, vomiting, epigastric pain, and abdominal distention. Which action demonstrates the best clinical judgment by a nurse?

1. Immediately notifies the client's physician of these findings
2. Initiates oxygen at 2 liters per nasal cannula to relieve the dyspnea
3. Places ice packs around the cast to reduce the abdominal distention
4. Administers ondansetron (Zofran®), the prescribed antiemetic on the client's MAR

ANSWER: 1

Vomiting, epigastric pain, and abdominal distention are classic symptoms of cast syndrome, with partial or complete upper intestinal obstruction from compression of the duodenum between the superior mesenteric artery and the aorta. A window in the abdominal portion of the cast or bivalving is needed to relieve the pressure. The actions in options 2, 3, and 4 should also be implemented, but option 1 demonstrates the nurse's best clinical judgment of suspecting cast syndrome.

► ***Test-taking Tip:*** *Note the key words "best clinical judgment." Select the action that interprets the data and the treatment correctly.*

Content Area: Adult Health; *Category of Health Alteration:* Musculoskeletal Management; *Integrated Processes:* Nursing Process Analysis; *Client Need:* Physiological Integrity/Physiological Adaptation/Unexpected Response to Therapies; *Cognitive Level:* Analysis

Reference: Ignatavicius, D., & Workman, M. (2006). *Medical-Surgical Nursing: Critical Thinking for Collaborative Care* (5th ed., p. 1199). St. Louis, MO: Elsevier/Saunders.

809. **EBP** An experienced nurse observes a new nurse caring for a client in skeletal traction to stabilize a fracture of the proximal femur prior to surgery. Which observation by the experienced nurse indicates the new nurse needs additional orientation?

1. Positions the client so the feet stay clear of the bottom of the bed
2. Checks ropes so that they are positioned in the wheel groves of the pulleys
3. Removes weights from the ropes until the weights hang freely off the bed frame
4. Performs pin site care with chlorhexidine solution twice daily

ANSWER: 3

Weights should be hanging freely, but weights should never be removed (unless a life-threatening situation occurs) because removal could result in injury and defeats the purpose of the traction. The lengths of the ropes need to be adjusted so the weights do not rest on the bed frame. The client slipping down in bed or ropes not in the pulleys result in ineffective traction. Chlorhexidine is recommended by some as the most effective cleansing solution. Water and saline are alternate choices. Hydrogen peroxide and povidone-iodine (Betadine®) solutions are believed to be cytotoxic to osteoblasts. However, systematic reviews of research found little evidence as to which pin site care regimen best reduces infection rates.

► ***Test-taking Tip:*** *Note the key words "needs additional orientation." Select the option that is incorrect.*

Content Area: Adult Health; *Category of Health Alteration:* Musculoskeletal Management; *Integrated Processes:* Nursing Process Evaluation; *Client Need:* Physiological Integrity/Reduction of Risk Potential/Potential for Complications of Diagnostic Tests/Treatments/Procedures; *Cognitive Level:* Application

Reference: Smeltzer, S., Bare, B., Hinkle, J., & Cheever, K. (2008). *Brunner & Suddarth's Textbook of Medical-Surgical Nursing* (11th ed., pp. 2368–2369). Philadelphia: Lippincott Williams & Wilkins.

EBP Reference: Parker, M., & Handoll, H. (2006). Pre-operative traction for fractures of the proximal femur in adults. *Cochrane Database of Systematic Reviews*, Issue 3, Art. No. CD000168. DOI: 10.1002/14651858.CD000168.pub2. Available at: www.cochrane.org/reviews/en/ab000168.html.

810. A client diagnosed with osteoarthritis, tells a clinic nurse about the inability to ambulate and staying on bedrest because of hip stiffness. In addition to teaching the client measures to reduce joint stiffness, which referral for the client should the nurse plan to discuss with the health-care provider?

1. Psychiatrist
2. Social worker
3. Physical therapist
4. Arthritis Foundation

ANSWER: 3

The physical therapist can assist the client in adopting self-management strategies and teach isometric, postural, and aerobic exercises that prevent joint overuse. A psychiatrist would assist the client in dealing with the mental health aspects related to the disease, such as ineffective coping, loss, or anger. There is no evidence that the client has mental health issues. The social worker would address issues such as finances, home assistance, placement, or acquiring assistive devices. The Arthritis Foundation provides a wealth of information to the client, but a referral is not necessary. The client can initiate the contact.

Test-taking Tip: *Focus on the issue, joint stiffness, and the health-care specialty that can best assist the client.*

Content Area: Adult Health; *Category of Health Alteration:* Musculoskeletal Management; *Integrated Processes:* Nursing Process Planning; *Client Need:* Safe and Effective Care Environment/ Management of Care/Referrals; *Cognitive Level:* Application

Reference: Smeltzer, S., Bare, B., Hinkle, J., & Cheever, K. (2008). *Brunner & Suddarth's Textbook of Medical-Surgical Nursing* (11th ed., p. 1915). Philadelphia: Lippincott Williams & Wilkins.

811. EBP A client is admitted for a total hip arthroplasty for chronic degenerative joint disease of the left hip. A nurse documents during the admission assessment that the client uses alternative therapies for osteoarthritis treatment. The evidence for this documentation would include the client stating: SELECT ALL THAT APPLY

1. taking ibuprofen (Advil®) every 4 to 6 hours for pain control.
2. wearing a copper bracelet continuously.
3. taking glucosamine sulfate 1,000 mg daily.
4. applying magnets to the hip joint and securing with an ace wrap.
5. sleeping on the unaffected hip with a pillow between the legs.

ANSWER: 2, 3, 4

Alternative therapies for arthritis treatment include those which have not been proven to be efficacious in the treatment of the disease, such as herbal and dietary supplements of glucosamine or wearing copper bracelets or magnets. Other alternative therapies include special diets, acupuncture, acupressure, and participation in Tai Chi. Although it has been suggested that glucosamine modifies cartilage structure, studies have shown it to be ineffective. Taking NSAIDs and sleeping on the unaffected side are proven interventions that reduce or minimize pain.

Test-taking Tip: *Focus on what the question is asking: what are the alternative therapies. Use the process of elimination, discard accepted treatment options 1 and 5.*

Content Area: Adult Health; *Category of Health Alteration:* Musculoskeletal Management; *Integrated Processes:* Communication and Documentation; Nursing Process Analysis; *Client Need:* Physiological Integrity/Basic Care and Comfort/Complementary and Alternative Therapies; *Cognitive Level:* Application

Reference: Smeltzer, S., Bare, B., Hinkle, J., & Cheever, K. (2008). *Brunner & Suddarth's Textbook of Medical-Surgical Nursing* (11th ed., p. 1915). Philadelphia: Lippincott Williams & Wilkins.

EBP Reference: Towheed, T., Maxwell, L., Anastassiades, T., Shea, B., Houpt, J., et al. (2005). Glucosamine therapy for treating osteoarthritis. *Cochrane Database of Systematic Reviews*, Issue 2, Art. No. CD002946. DOI: 10.1002/14651858.CD002946.pub2. Available at: www.cochrane.org/reviews/en/ab002946.html

812. EBP Which nursing action should be implemented on the second postoperative day for a client who received a right total hip replacement (THR) with a cemented prosthesis?

1. Assisting the client to the bathroom, which has an elevated toilet seat, using a walker and partial weight bearing of the right leg
2. Removing the Hodgkin's splint, which maintained leg alignment during the night, and positioning pillows to adduct the client's right leg
3. Reinfusing the returns from a Stryker® wound autotransfusion drainage system, which has collected 400 mL in the past 24 hours
4. Assisting the client to get out of bed on the left side so the client can stand to use the urinal

ANSWER: 1

On the second postoperative day following THR, the client should have weight-bearing restrictions but should be able to ambulate with the use of a walker. An elevated toilet seat is used to prevent hip flexion of greater than 90 degrees when the client sits. The client's legs should be abducted, not adducted. Drainage from a wound drain reinfusion system would not be used 6 hours postoperatively because the drainage would primarily be fluid and debris and not blood. Not every client may have a wound drainage system following a THR. The best side for the client to get out of bed is the affected side. This allows the client to shift position with the good leg and the trapeze to the edge of the bed, lower the affected leg over the edge of the bed, and, with the assistance of the nurse, turn to a sitting position without exceeding the 90-degree hip flexion.

Test-taking Tip: *Focus on the actions that would promote client safety.*

Content Area: Adult Health; *Category of Health Alteration:* Musculoskeletal Management; *Integrated Processes:* Nursing Process Implementation; *Client Need:* Physiological Integrity/Physiological Adaptation/Alterations in Body Systems; *Cognitive Level:* Analysis

Reference: Smeltzer, S., Bare, B., Hinkle, J., & Cheever, K. (2008). *Brunner & Suddarth's Textbook of Medical-Surgical Nursing* (11th ed., pp. 2373–2374). Philadelphia: Lippincott Williams & Wilkins.

EBP Reference: Parker, M., Livingstone, V., Clifton, R., & McKee, A. (2007). Closed suction surgical wound drainage after orthopedic surgery. *Cochrane Database of Systematic Reviews*, Issue 3, Art. No. CD001825. DOI: 10.1002/14651858.CD001825.pub2. Available at: www.cochrane.org/reviews/en/ab001825.html.

813. To prevent dislocation of the hip prosthesis following total hip replacement, a nurse should plan to: SELECT ALL THAT APPLY.

1. place pillows or a wedge pillow between the client's legs to keep them adducted.
2. use a fracture bedpan and instruct the client to flex the unaffected hip and use the trapeze to lift the pelvis while the nurse places the pan.
3. prevent hip flexion by not elevating the head of the bed more than 90 degrees.
4. place a pillow between the client's knees when initially assisting the client out of bed.
5. elevate both of the client's legs when sitting in the wheelchair to decrease swelling.

ANSWER: 2, 4

The client's hip should never be flexed more than 90 degrees. A regular bedpan is too large, so a fracture pan should be used. The client should be reminded not to flex the affected hip when using the bedpan. In initial transfers, a pillow is used to remind the client to maintain abduction and prevent internal and external hip rotation. A pillow should be used to maintain abduction (not adduction). The head of the bed should not be elevated more than 60 degrees. This allows the client no more than 30 degrees of hip flexion if lifting the leg. The hip should never be flexed more than 90 degrees. Elevating the affected leg when sitting increases the risk of flexing the client's hip beyond 90 degrees.

➧ ***Test-taking Tip:*** *Read each option carefully and apply total hip precautions of protecting the hip from adduction, flexion, internal or external rotation, and excessive weight bearing to select the correct options.*

Content Area: Adult Health; *Category of Health Alteration:* Musculoskeletal Management; *Integrated Processes:* Nursing Process Planning; *Client Need:* Physiological Integrity/Reduction of Risk Potential/Potential for Complications from Surgical Procedures and Health Alterations; *Cognitive Level:* Analysis

Reference: Smeltzer, S., Bare, B., Hinkle, J., & Cheever, K. (2008). *Brunner & Suddarth's Textbook of Medical-Surgical Nursing* (11th ed., pp. 2373–2374). Philadelphia: Lippincott Williams & Wilkins.

814. EBP One month after discharge, a client who had a left total hip replacement calls a clinic reporting acute constant pain in the left groin and hip area and feeling like the left leg is shorter than the right. A nurse advises the client to come to the clinic immediately suspecting:

1. wound infection.
2. deep vein thrombosis (DVT).
3. dislocation of the prosthesis.
4. aseptic loosening of the prosthesis.

ANSWER: 3

Indicators of a prosthesis dislocation include increased surgical site pain, acute groin pain, shortening of the leg, abnormal external or internal rotation, restricted ability or inability to move the leg, and reports of a popping sensation in the hip. Signs of a wound infection include swelling, purulent drainage, pain, and fever. Signs of DVT include calf pain and swelling. Aseptic loosening of the prosthesis causes pain that diminishes with rest.

➧ ***Test-taking Tip:*** *Focus on the key findings: pain and one leg is shorter than the other. Use the process of elimination.*

Content Area: Adult Health; *Category of Health Alteration:* Musculoskeletal Management; *Integrated Processes:* Nursing Process Analysis; *Client Need:* Physiological Integrity/Reduction of Risk Potential/Potential for Complications from Surgical Procedures and Health Alterations; *Cognitive Level:* Analysis

Reference: Smeltzer, S., Bare, B., Hinkle, J., & Cheever, K. (2008). *Brunner & Suddarth's Textbook of Medical-Surgical Nursing* (11th ed., p. 2376). Philadelphia: Lippincott Williams & Wilkins.

EBP Reference: Best, J. (2005). Revision total hip and total knee arthroplasty. *Orthopaedic Nursing*, 24(3), 174–182.

815. To prevent circulatory complications after a right total knee replacement, a nurse should ensure that the client is:

1. flexing both feet and exercising uninvolved joints every hour while awake.
2. using the continuous passive motion device (CPM) every 2 hours for 30 minutes.
3. assisted up to a chair as soon as the effects of anesthesia have worn off.
4. using the trapeze to lift the buttocks off the bed and then rotating each leg intermittently.

ANSWER: 1

Dorsiflexion of the foot promotes muscle contraction which compresses veins. This reduces venous stasis and risk of thrombus formation. It should be performed every hour while awake. The CPM device should be on and used most of the time. The client may be up the evening of surgery or the following day. Rotating the right knee could result in dislocation of the knee prosthesis. The knee should be kept in a neutral position.

➧ ***Test-taking Tip:** Visualize each of the activities and determine if they would be safe following a total knee replacement.*

Content Area: Adult Health; *Category of Health Alteration:* Musculoskeletal Management; *Integrated Processes:* Nursing Process Implementation; *Client Need:* Physiological Integrity/Reduction of Risk Potential/Therapeutic Procedures; *Cognitive Level:* Application

Reference: Smeltzer, S., Bare, B., Hinkle, J., & Cheever, K. (2008). *Brunner & Suddarth's Textbook of Medical-Surgical Nursing* (11th ed., pp. 2375–2376). Philadelphia: Lippincott Williams & Wilkins.

---

816. A nurse assesses a client 4 hours after a left total knee replacement. The client has a knee immobilizer in place with medial and lateral ice packs that have warmed. The surgical extremity's neurovascular status is intact and vital signs stable. A Stryker® wound drain, an autotransfusion drainage system, has 350 mL drainage collected. The client reports pain at a level 3, which is tolerable, and denies nausea. The client has not voided since before surgery. Which interventions should the nurse plan to implement at this time? SELECT ALL THAT APPLY.

1. Notify the client's physician.
2. Reinfuse the salvaged blood loss.
3. Remove the immobilizer and place a pillow behind the client's knee to create a 90-degree knee flexion.
4. Stand the client at the bedside to facilitate bladder emptying.
5. Place the affected extremity in a continuous passive motion device (CPM) to begin early motion.
6. Replace the ice packs in the knee immobilizer.

ANSWER: 2, 6

An autotransfusion drainage system should be used in the immediate postoperative period if extensive bleeding is anticipated. Collected drainage can be reinfused up to 6 hours postoperatively. Ice packs, used to reduce swelling and control bleeding, are replaced every 2 hours. If they have warmed, they need to be replaced. If the vital signs are stable, it is unnecessary to notify the physician. This amount of blood is expected and does not indicate excessive bleeding. Flexing the knee to 90 degrees staunches excessive bleeding. The client's bladder should be scanned using a bedside bladder ultrasound to determine the amount of urine in the bladder. Research indicates bladder scanning reduces the need for catheterization and is cost effective. Four hours after surgery may be too soon to stand the client at the bedside. The nurse assists the client to get out of bed in the evening or the day after surgery. The client's leg would not begin cycling in the CPM machine until the amount of drainage decreases.

➧ ***Test-taking Tip:** Focus on the situation and the information that would be expected following a total knee replacement.*

Content Area: Adult Health; *Category of Health Alteration:* Musculoskeletal Management; *Integrated Processes:* Nursing Process Planning; *Client Need:* Physiological Integrity/Physiological Adaptation/Alterations in Body Systems; *Cognitive Level:* Analysis

Reference: Smeltzer, S., Bare, B., Hinkle, J., & Cheever, K. (2008). *Brunner & Suddarth's Textbook of Medical-Surgical Nursing* (11th ed., pp. 2375–2376). Philadelphia: Lippincott Williams & Wilkins.

---

817. Which priority nursing diagnosis should a nurse document in the plan of care for a client following a C5–C6 anterior cervical discectomy?

1. Potential ineffective breathing pattern
2. Potential impaired tissue perfusion
3. Risk for infection
4. Impaired skin integrity

ANSWER: 1

Retractors used during surgery can injure the recurrent laryngeal nerve resulting in the inability to cough effectively to clear secretions. Edema and bleeding can also compromise the airway and compress the spinal cord. Risk for ineffective tissue perfusion, risk for infection, and impaired skin integrity should also be included in the plan of care but are not the priority.

➧ ***Test-taking Tip:** Focus on the ABCs (airway, breathing, and circulation). Assessment of the client's airway is the priority.*

Content Area: Adult Health; *Category of Health Alteration:* Musculoskeletal Management; *Integrated Processes:* Communication and Documentation; *Client Need:* Physiological Integrity/Reduction of Risk Potential/Potential for Complications from Surgical Procedures and Health Alterations; *Cognitive Level:* Application

Reference: Smeltzer, S., Bare, B., Hinkle, J., & Cheever, K. (2008). *Brunner & Suddarth's Textbook of Medical-Surgical Nursing* (11th ed., p. 2327). Philadelphia: Lippincott Williams & Wilkins.

818. A nurse receives an order to administer cyclobenzaprine (Flexeril®) 30 mg orally three times daily to a client hospitalized with acute cervical neck pain. The pharmacy has supplied 10-mg tablets. Which action by the nurse is best?

1. Administer three 10-mg tablets with food.
2. Call the physician to question the order.
3. Observe the client for drowsiness after administration.
4. Administer morphine sulfate intravenously for immediate pain control.

ANSWER: 2

Cyclobenzaprine is a centrally acting skeletal muscle relaxant. The total daily dose should not exceed 60 mg. The medication can be administered with food to decrease gastric distress; but 30 mg is too high a dose. If the correct dose were administered, the nurse should assess for drowsiness because it is a side effect. Also, the nurse should consider immediate pain control if the correct dose is ordered because the onset of action is 1 hour.

▶ ***Test-taking Tip:*** *The key word is "best." Apply knowledge of the usual daily dose of cyclobenzaprine to answer this question.*

Content Area: Adult Health; *Category of Health Alteration:* Musculoskeletal Management; *Integrated Processes:* Nursing Process Implementation; *Client Need:* Physiological Integrity/Pharmacological and Parenteral Therapies/Pharmacological Agents/Actions; *Cognitive Level:* Analysis

Reference: Wilson, B., Shannon, M., Shields, K., & Stang, C. (2008). *Prentice Hall Nurse's Drug Guide 2008* (pp. 390–391). Upper Saddle River, NJ: Pearson Education.

819. EBP A college student consults a clinic nurse and reports acute lower back pain of sudden onset. In addition to taking the prescribed medications, which instructions should the nurse include? SELECT ALL THAT APPLY.

1. Continue routine activity within your pain tolerance while paying attention to correct posture.
2. Temporarily avoid specific activities known to increase mechanical stress on the spine, such as lifting.
3. When sleeping on your side, flex your hips and knees and place a pillow between your knees.
4. Maintain bedrest for 1 week in a contour position and then begin leg flexion and hyperextension exercises.
5. Stand intermittently when attending classes and sit with a soft support at the small of the back.
6. When sleeping on your back, elevate your head and chest with pillows 30 degrees, flex your knees slightly, and support your knees with a pillow

ANSWER: 1, 2, 3, 5, 6

Remaining active is best. Prolonged bedrest is no longer recommended because it contributes to deconditioning. Mechanical stress can increase pain. Prolonged unsupported sitting, heavy lifting, and bending or twisting the back, especially while lifting, should be avoided. Using pillows and hip and knee flexion promotes lumbar flexion and back alignment (options 3 and 6). Prolonged standing, walking, or sitting should be avoided because fatigue contributes to spasm of the back muscles. Lordosis can be decreased by using a soft support at the small of the back. Heat or cold can be used for comfort.

▶ ***Test-taking Tip:*** *Note key words in the incorrect option: "bedrest for 1 week."*

Content Area: Adult Health; *Category of Health Alteration:* Musculoskeletal Management; *Integrated Processes:* Teaching and Learning; *Client Need:* Health Promotion and Maintenance/Self-Care; Physiological Integrity/Reduction of Risk Potential/Potential for Complications from Surgical Procedures and Health Alterations; *Cognitive Level:* Application

Reference: Smeltzer, S., Bare, B., Hinkle, J., & Cheever, K. (2008). *Brunner & Suddarth's Textbook of Medical-Surgical Nursing* (11th ed., pp. 2395–2396). Philadelphia: Lippincott Williams & Wilkins.

EBP Reference: Institute for Clinical Systems Improvement (ICSI). (2006). Adult low back pain. Available at: www.guideline.gov/summary/summary.aspx?doc_id=9863&nbr=005287&string=ankle+AND+fracture.

820. A nurse assesses a client 6 hours postoperatively following a lumbar spinal fusion. The client is experiencing a headache rated at 8 out of 10 but denies nausea. The neurovascular status of the lower extremities is intact, and the vital signs are within the normal range. The client log rolls with assistance. The lungs have fine crackles in the left base. The back dressing has a dime-sized bloody spot surrounded by a moderate amount of clear yellowish drainage. Which nursing action demonstrates the nurse's best clinical judgment?

1. Administering morphine sulfate intravenously
2. Encouraging coughing and deep breathing
3. Reinforcing the incisional dressing
4. Notifying the client's physician

ANSWER: 4

A bloody area surrounded by clear yellowish fluid on the dressing and the client's headache suggest a cerebral spinal fluid leak, a complication following spinal fusion. The client may need to be kept on bedrest for a few days while the dural tear heals or may need a blood patch to seal the leak because the client is at risk for a central nervous system infection. All other actions are correct and should also be implemented.

▶ ***Test-taking Tip:*** *Focus on the data and what the question is asking: "the best clinical judgment."*

Content Area: Adult Health; *Category of Health Alteration:* Musculoskeletal Management; *Integrated Processes:* Nursing Process Implementation; *Client Need:* Physiological Integrity/Physiological Adaptation/Unexpected Response to Therapies; Physiological Integrity/Reduction of Risk Potential/Potential for Complications from Surgical Procedures and Health Alterations; *Cognitive Level:* Analysis

Reference: Ignatavicius, D., & Workman, M. (2006). *Medical-Surgical Nursing: Critical Thinking for Collaborative Care* (5th ed., p. 981). St. Louis, MO: Elsevier/Saunders.

821. Which action should a nurse plan in the care of the client who had a surgical repair of a right Dupuytren's contracture?

1. Elevating the right lower extremity above the level of the heart
2. Assisting the client with bathing, dressing, grooming, and toileting
3. Instructing the client on obtaining proper fitting shoes
4. Frequent rewrapping of the elastic bandage on the right extremity to decrease edema

ANSWER: 2

A Dupuytren's contracture is a slowly progressive contracture of the palmar fascia, which severely impairs function of the fourth, fifth, and sometimes middle fingers. Independent self-care is impaired for a few days after surgery because the hand is bandaged. Interventions involving the lower extremities (options 1 and 3) are irrelevant. The elastic bandage should be kept clean and dry and removed only by the surgeon.

➧ ***Test-taking Tip:*** *Apply knowledge of a Dupuytren's contracture to answer this question.*

Content Area: Adult Health; *Category of Health Alteration:* Musculoskeletal Management; *Integrated Processes:* Nursing Process Planning; *Client Need:* Physiological Integrity/Basic Care and Comfort/Personal Hygiene; *Cognitive Level:* Application

Reference: Smeltzer, S., Bare, B., Hinkle, J., & Cheever, K. (2008). *Brunner & Suddarth's Textbook of Medical-Surgical Nursing* (11th ed., pp. 2399–2400). Philadelphia: Lippincott Williams & Wilkins.

---

822. A clinic nurse suspects that a client may have developed osteomyelitis 3 months following a left shoulder arthroplasty. Which findings on assessment prompted the nurse's conclusion? SELECT ALL THAT APPLY.

1. Sudden onset of chills
2. Temperature 103°F (39.4°C)
3. Bradycardia
4. Report by the client of a pulsating pain in the area that intensifies with movement
5. Painful, swollen area on the left shoulder

ANSWER: 1, 2, 4, 5

A sudden onset of chills and a high fever suggest the infection is bloodborne. The pulsating pain is caused from the pressure of the collecting pus. The infected area becomes swollen, painful, and extremely tender. Tachycardia, not bradycardia, would be present.

➧ ***Test-taking Tip:*** *Apply knowledge of medical terminology; osteomyelitis is an infection of the bone. Visualizing the client's signs and symptoms may help to eliminate option 3.*

Content Area: Adult Health; *Category of Health Alteration:* Musculoskeletal Management; *Integrated Processes:* Nursing Process Analysis; *Client Need:* Physiological Integrity/Reduction of Risk Potential/Potential for Complications from Surgical Procedures and Health Alterations; *Cognitive Level:* Analysis

Reference: Smeltzer, S., Bare, B., Hinkle, J., & Cheever, K. (2008). *Brunner & Suddarth's Textbook of Medical-Surgical Nursing* (11th ed., p. 2413). Philadelphia: Lippincott Williams & Wilkins.

---

823. To which client should a nurse plan to provide teaching about genetic resources?

1. Client who had an ankle fracture secondary to a boating accident
2. Client who had a ganglion removed from the dorsum of the wrist
3. Client who had a surgical repair of a fracture due to osteoporosis
4. Client who had a total knee replacement due to degenerative joint disease

ANSWER: 3

Genetic factors influence the development of osteoporosis. There is no known genetic link for a ganglion, degenerative joint disease, or accidental fractures (except those due to osteoporosis).

➧ ***Test-taking Tip:*** *Use the process of elimination to narrow the options to 3 and 4 because these options include secondary causes within the body. Of these two options, eliminate option 4, recalling that degenerative joint disease is caused by osteoarthritis.*

Content Area: Adult Health; *Category of Health Alteration:* Musculoskeletal Management; *Integrated Processes:* Teaching and Learning; *Client Need:* Safe and Effective Care Environment/Management of Care/Continuity of Care; *Cognitive Level:* Analysis

Reference: Smeltzer, S., Bare, B., Hinkle, J., & Cheever, K. (2008). *Brunner & Suddarth's Textbook of Medical-Surgical Nursing* (11th ed., p. 2345). Philadelphia: Lippincott Williams & Wilkins.

---

824. When analyzing the serum laboratory report for a client diagnosed with lung cancer that has metastasized to the pelvic bone, which finding should a nurse anticipate?

1. Elevated calcium
2. Decreased hemoglobin
3. Elevated creatinine (Scr)
4. Elevated creatine kinase (CK)

ANSWER: 1

Malignant tumors cause hypercalcemia through a variety of mechanisms, one being an increased release of calcium from the bones. A low hemoglobin is seen with bleeding, insufficient intake of iron, or with renal disease. An elevated Scr is seen with renal disease. An elevated CK would be seen with muscle damage.

➧ ***Test-taking Tip:*** *Apply knowledge of critical laboratory results. If unsure, use the process of elimination, eliminating those options known to be incorrect.*

Content Area: Adult Health; *Category of Health Alteration:* Musculoskeletal Management; *Integrated Processes:* Nursing Process Analysis; *Client Need:* Physiological Integrity/Reduction of Risk Potential/Laboratory Values; *Cognitive Level:* Application

Reference: Smeltzer, S., Bare, B., Hinkle, J., & Cheever, K. (2008). *Brunner & Suddarth's Textbook of Medical-Surgical Nursing* (11th ed., pp. 327, 2417–2419). Philadelphia: Lippincott Williams & Wilkins.

---

825. A nurse reads the chart of a 25-year-old male and notes that he has been diagnosed with an osteosarcoma of the distal femur. Which statement indicates the nurse's correct interpretation of the client's diagnosis?

1. The tumor originated elsewhere in the client's body and metastasized to the bone.
2. Osteosarcoma is the most common and most often fatal primary malignant bone tumor.
3. The only treatment for osteosarcoma is a leg amputation well above the tumor growth.
4. Osteosarcoma is a nonmalignant growth that can be excised and the bone replaced with a bone graft.

ANSWER: 2

Osteosarcoma is a malignant primary tumor of the bone, appearing most frequently in males between 10 and 25 years (when bones grow rapidly). Prognosis depends on whether the tumor has metastasized to the lungs, but it is often fatal. Options 1 and 4 are incorrect because osteosarcoma is a primary malignant tumor. Treatment includes combined chemotherapy that is started before and continued after surgery.

➧ ***Test-taking Tip:*** *Apply knowledge of medical terminology; "sarcoma" is cancer arising from underlying tissue and "osteo" is bone. Thus, eliminate options 1 and 4. If uncertain, the "only" in option 3 should lead to eliminating this option.*

Content Area: Adult Health; *Category of Health Alteration:* Musculoskeletal Management; *Integrated Processes:* Nursing Process Analysis; *Client Need:* Physiological Integrity/Physiological Adaptation/Pathophysiology; *Cognitive Level:* Application

Reference: Smeltzer, S., Bare, B., Hinkle, J., & Cheever, K. (2008). *Brunner & Suddarth's Textbook of Medical-Surgical Nursing* (11th ed., p. 2417). Philadelphia: Lippincott Williams & Wilkins.

---

826. A nurse reports to a physician that a 75-year-old client continues to experience phantom limb pain following an above-the-knee amputation (AKA) despite nursing interventions of distraction and administering the prescribed morphine sulfate. Which interventions to minimize the altered sensory perceptions should the nurse anticipate that the physician might prescribe? SELECT ALL THAT APPLY.

1. Local anesthetic to the residual limb
2. Transcutaneous electrical nerve stimulation (TENS)
3. A beta-blocker medication such as atenolol (Tenormin®)
4. An antiseizure medication such as oxcarbazepine (Trileptal®)
5. Reducing the client's activity level until the sensations resolve
6. A different analgesic, such as meperidine hydrochloride (Demerol®)

ANSWER: 1, 2, 3, 4

A local anesthetic or TENS provide pain relief for some. Beta-blockers may relieve dull, burning discomfort, and antiseizure medications control stabbing and cramping pain. Additional medications include tricyclic antidepressants to improve mood and coping ability. Increasing the client's activity, not decreasing it, helps to decrease the occurrence of phantom limb pain. A different analgesic could be prescribed, but meperidine is contraindicated in the elderly due to the increased incidence of confusion and seizures.

➧ ***Test-taking Tip:*** *Focus on the issue, controlling phantom limb pain. Note the client's age. Use the process of elimination to select the options that can assist with pain control for this client.*

Content Area: Adult Health; *Category of Health Alteration:* Musculoskeletal Management; *Integrated Processes:* Nursing Process Planning; *Client Need:* Physiological Integrity/Physiological Adaptation/Alterations in Body Systems; *Cognitive Level:* Application

Reference: Smeltzer, S., Bare, B., Hinkle, J., & Cheever, K. (2008). *Brunner & Suddarth's Textbook of Medical-Surgical Nursing* (11th ed., p. 2464). Philadelphia: Lippincott Williams & Wilkins.

827. A client, with a lower leg amputation, is experiencing edema, so a nursing assistant (NA) elevates the client's residual left limb on pillows. What is the most appropriate action by the nurse when observing that the client's leg has been elevated?

1. Thank the NA for being so observant and intervening appropriately.
2. Remove the pillows, raise the foot of the bed, and inform the NA that the limb should not be elevated on pillows because it could cause a flexion contracture.
3. Inform the NA that this was the correct action at this time in the client's recovery, but once the client's incision heals the leg should not be elevated.
4. Report the incident to the surgeon and tell the NA to complete a variance report because the client's leg should not have been elevated.

ANSWER: 2

Flexion, abduction, and external rotation of the residual lower limb are avoided to prevent hip contracture. All other options are incorrect. It is unnecessary for the nurse to report the incident to the surgeon and to complete a variance report unless the client was in the position for an extended period of time.

➧ ***Test-taking Tip:*** *Select the option that is most complete and yet addresses the issue with the nursing assistant.*

Content Area: Adult Health; *Category of Health Alteration:* Musculoskeletal Management; *Integrated Processes:* Nursing Process Evaluation; *Client Need:* Safe and Effective Care Environment/Management of Care/Supervision; *Cognitive Level:* Application

Reference: Smeltzer, S., Bare, B., Hinkle, J., & Cheever, K. (2008). *Brunner & Suddarth's Textbook of Medical-Surgical Nursing* (11th ed., pp. 2465–2466). Philadelphia: Lippincott Williams & Wilkins.

Test 21: **Adult Health: Neurological Management**

828. A client is scheduled for an outpatient electroencephalogram (EEG). A nurse instructs the client to prepare for the test by:

1. removing all hair pins.
2. avoiding eating or drinking at least 6 hours prior to the test.
3. being prepared to have some of the scalp shaved.
4. having blood drawn for a glucose level 2 hours before the test.

ANSWER: 1

In an EEG, electrodes are placed on the scalp over multiple areas of the brain to detect and record patterns of electrical activity. Preparation includes clean hair without any objects in the hair to prevent inaccurate test results. The client should not be NPO (nothing per mouth) since a usual glucose level is important for normal brain functioning. The scalp will not be shaved; the electrodes are applied with paste. There is no indication to have a serum glucose drawn before the test.

▶ ***Test-taking Tip:*** *The question calls for a true response. The prefix "cephalo-" refers to head, so the test involves the head. Consider each option separately and use the process of elimination.*

Content Area: Adult Health; *Category of Health Alteration:* Neurological Management; *Integrated Processes:* Nursing Process Analysis; *Client Need:* Physiological Integrity/Reduction of Risk Potential/Laboratory Values; *Cognitive Level:* Application

Reference: Ignatavicius, D., & Workman, M. (2006). *Medical-Surgical Nursing: Critical Thinking for Collaborative Care* (5th ed., pp. 942–944). St. Louis, MO: Elsevier/Saunders.

---

829. A client is seen by a primary care provider because of difficulty walking. A neurological assessment is done. A nurse informs the client that which assessment procedure was done to test the functioning of the cerebellum?

1. Ask the client to shut the eyes and distinguish whether the touch is with a sharp or dull object (either end of a cotton-tipped applicator).
2. Ask the client to hold hands with palms up perpendicular to the body with eyes closed.
3. Ask the client to grasp and squeeze 2 fingers of each of the examiner's hands.
4. Ask the client to alternate placing hands up and then hands down on thighs as fast as possible.

ANSWER: 4

Repetitive, alternating motion tests the client's coordination; an indicator of cerebella function. Detecting sharp or dull touch is a test for peripheral nerve function. Assessing for pronator drift is a test for muscle weakness due to cerebral or brainstem dysfunction. Assessment of hand grasps compares equality of muscle strength bilaterally.

▶ ***Test-taking Tip:*** *Key words in the stem are "difficulty walking" and "cerebella function." Consider each option separately. Note that the client's problem involves movement, as does the correct answer. The other options assess strength and sensation. Use the process of elimination.*

Content Area: Adult Health; *Category of Health Alteration:* Neurological Management; *Integrated Processes:* Teaching and Learning; *Client Need:* Health Promotion and Maintenance/Techniques of Physical Assessment; *Cognitive Level:* Analysis

Reference: Ignatavicius, D., & Workman, M. (2006). *Medical-Surgical Nursing: Critical Thinking for Collaborative Care* (5th ed., pp. 935–936). St. Louis, MO: Elsevier/Saunders.

---

830. A nurse is admitting a client with a diagnosis of meningitis. Which of the nurse's assessment findings support this diagnosis? SELECT ALL THAT APPLY.

1. Nuchal rigidity
2. Severe headache
3. Pill-rolling tremor
4. Photophobia
5. Fever
6. Micrographia

ANSWER: 1, 2, 4, 5

Meningitis is an inflammation affecting the arachnoid and pia mater that cover the brain and spinal cord. There is meningeal irritation that causes nuchal rigidity (stiff neck), severe headache, and photophobia (light irritates the eyes). The body responds with fever. Pill-rolling tremors and micrographia (small, cramped handwriting) are associated with Parkinson's disease.

▶ ***Test-taking Tip:*** *The suffix "-itis" suggests an inflammation or infection. Evaluate each option as it relates to the "meninges," three layers protecting the brain tissue called the dura mater, arachnoid mater, and the pia mater.*

Content Area: Adult Health; *Category of Health Alteration:* Neurological Management; *Integrated Processes:* Nursing Process Analysis; *Client Need:* Physiological Integrity/Physiological Adaptation/Alteration in Body Systems; *Cognitive Level:* Application

Reference: Ignatavicius, D., & Workman, M. (2006). *Medical-Surgical Nursing: Critical Thinking for Collaborative Care* (5th ed., pp. 955–956). St. Louis, MO: Elsevier/Saunders.

831. A client is hospitalized with a diagnosis of meningococcal meningitis. The client is at risk for the complication of septic emboli. Which intervention by a nurse directly addresses this risk?

1. Monitoring vital signs on an hourly basis
2. Administering meningitis polysaccharide vaccine (Menoune®)
3. Assessing neurological function with the Glasgow coma scale every 2 hours
4. Completing a vascular assessment of all extremities every 2 hours

ANSWER: 4

Frequent vascular assessments will detect vascular compromise secondary to septic emboli. Early detection allows for interventions that will prevent gangrene and possible loss of limb. Monitoring vital signs and frequent neurological assessments are indicated but do not address the complication of septic emboli. Immunization with the meningitis vaccine is a preventive measure against meningitis, not treatment.

▶ ***Test-taking Tip:*** *Key words in the stem are "meningococcal meningitis" and "septic emboli." The word emboli suggests a vascular concern. Eliminate options 2 and 3, and then decide which remaining option is best.*

Content Area: Adult Health; *Category of Health Alteration:* Neurological Management; *Integrated Processes:* Nursing Process Analysis; *Client Need:* Physiological Integrity/Reduction of Risk Potential/System Specific Assessments; *Cognitive Level:* Analysis

Reference: Ignatavicius, D., & Workman, M. (2006). *Medical-Surgical Nursing: Critical Thinking for Collaborative Care* (5th ed., pp. 956–958). St. Louis, MO: Elsevier/Saunders.

---

832. A client is admitted to an emergency department (ED). A nurse in the ED documents that the client is "postictal upon transfer" as evidenced by which observation?

1. Yellowing of the skin
2. Recently experienced a seizure and is in a drowsy or confused state
3. Severe itching of the eyes
4. Abnormal sensations including tingling of the skin

ANSWER: 2

The client has experienced a tonic-clonic seizure recently and is now in a state of deep relaxation and is breathing quietly. During this period the client may be unconscious, gradually awakens, but is often confused and disoriented. Often the client is amnesic regarding the seizure. Jaundice and icteric are terms for yellowing of the skin. Pruritus is a term for itching. Paresthesia is the term for abnormal sensations such as tingling and burning of the skin.

▶ ***Test-taking Tip:*** *Read the stem carefully. Consider that the client has a condition that was treated in an ED and is now being admitted to the hospital for further treatment. The correct answer describes a medical event that could merit a visit to an ED. The term "postictal" can be broken down into the prefix "post-," which means "after" and "-ictal," which means attack. Evaluate each option separately.*

Content Area: Adult Health; *Category of Health Alteration:* Neurological Management; *Integrated Processes:* Communication and Documentation; *Client Need:* Physiological Integrity/Reduction of Risk Potential/Potential for Alterations in Body Systems; *Cognitive Level:* Application

Reference: Johnson, K., & Hausman, K. (2006). Sensory perceptual disorders. In K. Wagner, K. Johnson, & P. Kidd (Eds.), *High-Acuity Nursing* (4th ed., pp. 459–483). Upper Saddle River, NJ: Pearson Education.

---

833. A client being admitted for surgery has a vagus nerve stimulation (VNS) device that was implanted several months earlier for seizure management. The nurse determines that the VNS is working properly when:

1. it stimulates the heart to beat when the client has bradycardia during a seizure.
2. the client activates the device to stop a seizure from occurring.
3. it defibrillates the client when the client experiences a lethal dysrhythmia during a seizure.
4. the client does not experience any airway obstruction from secretions during a seizure.

ANSWER: 2

A VNS is a medical device that is implanted in the chest and stimulates the vagus nerve to control seizures unresponsive to medical treatment. Clients who experience auras before a seizure use a magnet to activate the VNS to stop the seizure. It is a treatment option used for clients with seizures who do not respond to treatment with anticonvulsant medications. It does not stimulate the heart to beat as a pacemaker or defibrillate the heart as an implantable cardioverter/defibrillator (ICD) does. The device does not have an effect on the airway or secretions.

▶ ***Test-taking Tip:*** *The question is "What is vagus nerve stimulation?" Read the stem carefully. The question states that the client has a history of seizures, so consider the major aim of the device to deal with that focus and then eliminate nonrelevant options.*

Content Area: Adult Health; *Category of Health Alteration:* Neurological Management; *Integrated Processes:* Nursing Process Evaluation; *Client Need:* Physiological Integrity/Reduction of Risk Potential/Potential for Complications of Diagnostic Tests/Treatments/Procedures; *Cognitive Level:* Application

Reference: Ignatavicius, D., & Workman, M. (2006). *Medical-Surgical Nursing: Critical Thinking for Collaborative Care* (5th ed., pp. 954–955). St. Louis, MO: Elsevier/Saunders.

834. EBP A client with a history of epilepsy has consecutive seizures lasting more than 5 minutes and is in status epilepticus. Which interventions should be included in this client's immediate treatment? SELECT ALL THAT APPLY.

1. Administer dexamethasone (Decadron®) intravenously.
2. Administer oxygen and prepare for endotracheal intubation.
3. Prepare for immediate defibrillation.
4. Continue to protect the patient from injury.
5. Administer lorazepam (Ativan®) intravenously.
6. Transfer to a facility with expertise in treating status epilepticus.

ANSWER: 2, 4, 5

Status epilepticus is a medical emergency. The client is at risk for brain hypoxia and permanent brain damage. The client needs additional oxygen, and intubation will secure the airway. Care is taken to protect the client from injury during the seizure. Either lorazepam or diazepam is administered initially to terminate the seizure, because they can be administered more rapidly than phenytoin. Anticonvulsant medications such as phenytoin (Dilantin®), and not anti-inflammatory medications such as dexamethasone, are administered intravenously to control seizure activity. Defibrillation is treatment for ventricular fibrillation, a lethal heart dysrhythmia. Failure to terminate the seizures or need for critical care may be reasons for transfer to a facility with expertise in this area, which may be desirable after the client's condition has been stabilized.

Test-taking Tip: *Read the stem carefully: status epilepticus is defined. Consider the effect of continuous seizures. Control of the seizure will stop the medical problem. Use the ABCs (airway, breathing, circulation) to identify airway and oxygen as priority interventions. Use Maslow's Hierarchy of Needs to include protection from injury. Eliminate the options that do not apply to the problem or the immediate situation.*

Content Area: Adult Health; *Category of Health Alteration:* Neurological Management; *Integrated Processes:* Nursing Process Implementation; *Client Need:* Physiological Integrity/Physiological Adaptation/Medical Emergencies; *Cognitive Level:* Analysis

Reference: Ignatavicius, D., & Workman, M. (2006). *Medical-Surgical Nursing: Critical Thinking for Collaborative Care* (5th ed., pp. 953–954). St. Louis, MO: Elsevier/Saunders.

EBP Reference: Meierkord, H., Boon, P., Engelsen, B., Gocke, K., Shorvon, S., et al. (2006). EFNS guideline on the management of status epilepticus. *European Journal of Neurology*, 13(5), 445–450. Available at: www.guideline.gov/summary/summary.aspx?doc_id=10459&nbr=005482&string=status+AND+epilepticus

835. A client has undergone a lumbar laminectomy with spinal fusion 12 hours earlier. Which assessment finding should indicate to a nurse that the client has a leakage of cerebrospinal fluid?

1. Backache not relieved by analgesics
2. 100 mL of serosanguineous fluid measured from the Jackson-Pratt® drain since surgery
3. Clear fluid drainage noted on the surgical dressing
4. Temperature of 101.3°F (38.5°C)

ANSWER: 3

Cerebrospinal fluid (CSF) is clear; clear drainage on the surgical dressing is indicative of a CSF leak. Pain relieved by morphine sulfate and 100 mL of serosanguineous drainage in the Jackson-Pratt are normal findings. The temperature elevation could indicate an infection.

Test-taking Tip: *Consider the normal characteristics of CSF and normal surgical findings. Eliminate options 1 and 2 because these are normal findings.*

Content Area: Adult Health; *Category of Health Alteration:* Neurological Management; *Integrated Processes:* Nursing Process Analysis; *Client Need:* Physiological Integrity/Reduction of Risk Potential/Potential for Complications from Surgical Procedures and Health Alterations; *Cognitive Level:* Application

Reference: Ignatavicius, D., & Workman, M. (2006). *Medical-Surgical Nursing: Critical Thinking for Collaborative Care* (5th ed., pp. 980–981). St. Louis, MO: Elsevier/Saunders.

836. A client has had recurrent episodes of low back pain. Which statement indicates that the client has incorporated positive lifestyle changes to decrease the incidence of future back problems?

1. "I stoop and avoid twisting when I lift objects."
2. "I wear my old comfortable shoes whenever I go for a walk to avoid blisters."
3. "I walk 5 miles each day on the weekends."
4. "I sit as much as possible and elevate my legs."

ANSWER: 1

Stooping and avoiding twisting motions when lifting objects lessens the likelihood of injury. Clients should wear supportive shoes, include regular daily exercise as a program (not excessive walking over 2 days on the weekend), and avoid prolonged sitting or standing.

Test-taking Tip: *Focus on the issue: activities that prevent back injury. This should lead you to select option 1.*

Content Area: Adult Health; *Category of Health Alteration:* Neurological Management; *Integrated Processes:* Nursing Process Evaluation; *Client Need:* Health Promotion and Maintenance/Health and Wellness; *Cognitive Level:* Analysis

Reference: Ignatavicius, D., & Workman, M. (2006). *Medical-Surgical Nursing: Critical Thinking for Collaborative Care* (5th ed., pp. 978–979). St. Louis, MO: Elsevier/Saunders.

---

837. A nurse in an emergency department assesses a client injured in a diving accident 2 hours earlier. A computed tomography (CT) scan reveals a fracture of the C4 cervical vertebra. The client is breathing independently but has no movement or muscle tone from below the area of injury. The nurse understands that the client:

1. has suffered a complete spinal cord injury (SCI).
2. is experiencing spinal shock.
3. has sustained an upper motor neuron injury.
4. will be a quadriplegic.

ANSWER: 2

The client is experiencing spinal shock that manifests within a few hours after the injury. There is hypotension, flaccid paralysis, and absence of muscle contractions. Spinal shock lasts 7 to 20 days, and the SCI cannot be classified accurately until spinal shock resolves. There is insufficient evidence at this early time of the injury to support the other options. A complete spinal cord injury is a complete transection resulting in no reflexes or movement distal to the injury. An injury of the upper motor neuron results in spastic paralysis. Quadriplegia is paralysis involving all four extremities.

Test-taking Tip: *Focus on the client's symptoms, location of the fracture, and the time of the accident to select the answer. Recalling that SCI cannot be accurately classified at the time of the injury should direct you to option 2.*

Content Area: Adult Health; *Category of Health Alteration:* Neurological Management; *Integrated Processes:* Nursing Process Analysis; *Client Need:* Physiological Integrity/Reduction of Risk Potential/Potential for Alterations in Body Systems; *Cognitive Level:* Analysis

Reference: Johnson, K., & Hausman, K. (2006). Sensory perceptual disorders. In K. Wagner, K. Johnson, & P. Kidd (Eds.), *High-Acuity Nursing* (4th ed., pp. 459–483). Upper Saddle River, NJ: Pearson Education.

---

838. A nurse learns in report that a client admitted with a vertebral fracture has a halo external fixation device in place. Based on this information, for which intervention should the nurse plan?

1. Ensure the weight with the traction is hanging freely.
2. Remove the vest at bedtime.
3. Perform pin site care.
4. Progressively loosen the pins in the skull each day.

ANSWER: 3

A halo external fixation device is a static device that consists of a "halo" that is screwed into the skull by four pins. It is attached to a vest that the client wears. The device provides immobilization and stability to the spinal cord while healing occurs with or without surgical intervention. Care includes inspection of the pin sites and cleansing the pin sites. Traction or weights are not part of the halo device. The external fixation devices are worn continuously until the neurosurgeon discontinues the external fixation after sufficient healing has occurred and the injury has stabilized. Because the pins are secured in the skull to maintain alignment of the cervical vertebrae, the pins should be checked for loosening and, if loose, should be reported to the physician for tightening.

Test-taking Tip: *The key words are "external fixation" and "intervention." Recall that external fixation devices are attached to bones with pins. Eliminate option 1 because it pertains to assessment, not an intervention. Note that options 2 and 4 focus on the vest. Think about these options and the implications for client safety.*

Content Area: Adult Health; *Category of Health Alteration:* Neurological Management; *Integrated Processes:* Nursing Process Planning; *Client Need:* Physiological Integrity/Reduction of Risk Potential/Potential for Complications of Diagnostic Tests/Treatments/Procedures; *Cognitive Level:* Analysis

Reference: Johnson, K., & Hausman, K. (2006). Sensory perceptual disorders. In K. Wagner, K. Johnson, & P. Kidd (Eds.), *High-Acuity Nursing* (4th ed., pp. 459–483). Upper Saddle River, NJ: Pearson Education.

839. EBP A nurse is caring for a client with a spinal cord injury at the level of the sixth cervical vertebra. The client is at risk for the complication of autonomic dysreflexia. For which associated symptoms should a nurse monitor the client? SELECT ALL THAT APPLY.

1. Sweating
2. Headache
3. Hypotension
4. Blurred vision
5. Anxiety
6. Tachycardia

ANSWER: 1, 2, 4, 5

Autonomic dysreflexia results from uncontrolled sympathetic nervous system discharges causing vasoconstriction below the level of the injury and hypertension. Sweating, headache, blurred vision, and anxiety occur secondary to the hypertension. Hypertension (not hypotension) is a symptom of autonomic dysreflexia. Bradycardia (not tachycardia) is secondary to vagal parasympathetic stimulation.

Test-taking Tip: First, eliminate the cardiovascular symptoms listed in the options that are opposite symptoms associated with sympathetic nervous system stimulation. Then, select the options with the symptoms associated with severe hypertension. Finally, consider the symptoms associated with parasympathetic stimulation and select this option.

Content Area: Adult Health; *Category of Health Alteration:* Neurological Management; *Integrated Processes:* Nursing Process Analysis; *Client Need:* Physiological Integrity/Physiological Adaptation/Medical Emergencies; *Cognitive Level:* Synthesis

Reference: Johnson, K., & Hausman, K. (2006). Sensory perceptual disorders. In K. Wagner, K. Johnson, & P. Kidd (Eds.), *High-Acuity Nursing* (4th ed., pp. 459–483). Upper Saddle River, NJ: Pearson Education.

EBP Reference: Paralyzed Veterans of America/Consortium for Spinal Cord Medicine. (2006). *Acute Management of Autonomic Dysreflexia: Individuals with Spinal Cord Injury Presenting to Health-Care Facilities.* Available at: www.guideline.gov/summary/summary.aspx?doc_id=2964&nbr=002190&string=autonomic+AND+dysreflexia.

840. EBP A client with multiple sclerosis is seen in an office of a primary care provider. The client states that fatigue is the present concern. A nurse performs an assessment and reviews the client's current medications and blood laboratory results. Which findings by the nurse are most likely to contribute to the client's fatigue? SELECT ALL THAT APPLY.

1. Hemoglobin is 9.5 g/dL and hematocrit is 31.8%
2. Taking baclofen (Lioresal®) 15 mg 3 times per day
3. Working 4 to 8 hours per week in the family business
4. Stopped taking amytriptyline (Elavil®) 8 weeks earlier.
5. Presence of a cardiac murmur at the fifth intercostal space to the left of the sternum
6. Leans on cane and right leg weakness noted when walking in room

ANSWER: 1, 2, 4, 5, 6

The lower than normal hemoglobin and hematocrit reflect anemia, which stresses the body to provide adequate oxygen to the cells. Baclofen, a skeletal muscle relaxant has adverse effects of drowsiness and fatigue. The client has stopped amytriptyline, an antidepressant, and may be clinically depressed. Fatigue is a major symptom of depression. A tricuspid murmur indicates an incompetent cardiac valve, which will decrease the amount of oxygenated blood reaching the tissues. The increased energy expenditure with ambulation can increase fatigue. Limited hours working should not factor into the fatigue symptom.

Test-taking Tip: The issue of the question is "causes of fatigue." Consider that abnormal laboratory values, medication adverse effects, and the primary and other conditions can all contribute to fatigue. Thus, select all but option 3.

Content Area: Adult Health; *Category of Health Alteration:* Neurological Management; *Integrated Processes:* Nursing Process Analysis; *Client Need:* Physiological Integrity/Reduction of Risk Potential/Potential for Alterations in Body Systems; *Cognitive Level:* Synthesis

Reference: Springhouse Publishing Company Staff. (2007). *Springhouse Nurse's Drug Guide 2007* (8th ed., pp. 142–143, 204–206). Philadelphia: Lippincott Williams & Wilkins.

EBP Reference: O'Leary, S., & Phillips, J. (2007). Optimizing quality of life in multiple sclerosis patients. *Medscape Neurology & Neurosurgery.* Available at: www.medscape.com/viewarticle/558261

841. A client develops muscle weakness and seeks medical attention from a primary care provider. The client asks a nurse during the initial assessment if the symptoms suggest "Lou Gehrig's" disease. Which is the most appropriate response to the client?

1. "You may have been working too much and that is why you are tired. Let's not think the worst."
2. "Tell me what has you thinking that you might have Lou Gehrig's disease."
3. "Have you been having trouble remembering things along with this weakness?"
4. "Well, you are in the right place to figure out what is going on."

ANSWER: 2

The most appropriate response focuses on the client's concern, encourages verbalization of concerns, and solicits more information to assist with diagnosis of the client's problem. Responses that do not take the client seriously, give false reassurance, or cut off the client are not appropriate. Amyotrophic lateral sclerosis (Lou Gehrig's disease) is a degenerative disease that affects the motor system and does not have a dementia component; thus a question about memory is inappropriate.

▶ ***Test-taking Tip:*** *Evaluate each option according to principles of therapeutic communication and then eliminate options 1 and 4 because these are nontherapeutic and option 3 because it does not pertain to the disease.*

Content Area: Adult Health; *Category of Health Alteration:* Neurological Management; *Integrated Processes:* Communication and Documentation; *Client Need:* Psychosocial Integrity/Therapeutic Communications; *Cognitive Level:* Application

References: Berman, A., Snyder, S., Kozier, B., & Erb, G. (2008). *Kozier & Erb's Fundamentals of Nursing: Concepts, Process, and Practice* (8th ed., p. 470). Upper Saddle River, NJ: Pearson Education; Ignatavicius, D., & Workman, M. (2006). *Medical-Surgical Nursing: Critical Thinking for Collaborative Care* (5th ed., p. 1003). St. Louis, MO: Elsevier/Saunders.

---

842. A client with a diagnosis of Guillain-Barré syndrome is scheduled to receive plasmapheresis treatments. A nurse explains to the client's spouse that the purpose of plasmapheresis is to:

1. remove excess fluid from the bloodstream.
2. restore protein levels in the blood.
3. remove circulating antibodies from the bloodstream.
4. infuse lipoproteins to restore the myelin sheath.

ANSWER: 3

Plasmapheresis is a procedure in which the circulating antibodies are removed from the blood. During the procedure, blood is removed from the client, the plasma is separated, and blood cells without the plasma are returned to the client during the procedure. The purpose does not involve removing excess fluid, restoring protein, or infusing lipoproteins.

▶ ***Test-taking Tip:*** *Use the process of elimination. Eliminate option 4 because plasma is associated with the blood. Apheresis means separation, thus eliminate option 2. Of the remaining two options, think about the etiology of Guillain-Barré syndrome. Eliminate option 1 because research suggests that Guillain-Barré syndrome is a cell-mediated immunological reaction.*

Content Area: Adult Health; *Category of Health Alteration:* Neurological Management; *Integrated Processes:* Teaching and Learning; *Client Need:* Physiological Integrity/Reduction of Risk Potential/Potential for Complications of Diagnostic Tests/Treatments/Procedures; *Cognitive Level:* Application

Reference: Ignatavicius, D., & Workman, M. (2006). *Medical-Surgical Nursing: Critical Thinking for Collaborative Care* (5th ed., p. 1010). St. Louis, MO: Elsevier/Saunders.

---

843. For which associated complication should a nurse monitor the client experiencing Guillain-Barré syndrome?

1. Autonomic dysreflexia
2. Septic emboli
3. Increased intracranial pressure (ICP)
4. Respiratory failure

ANSWER: 4

Ascending paralysis that occurs in Guillain-Barré syndrome can affect the innervation of the muscles used in respiration, leading to respiratory failure. Clients with spinal cord injuries are at risk for autonomic dysreflexia. Clients who have bacterial meningitis are at risk for septic emboli. Clients with conditions involving brain pathology such as traumatic brain injury are at risk to develop ICP.

▶ ***Test-taking Tip:*** *Evaluate each option as it relates to the pathophysiology involved in Guillain-Barré syndrome. Recall that the syndrome can lead to muscular paralysis, so select the most serious complication.*

Content Area: Adult Health; *Category of Health Alteration:* Neurological Management; *Integrated Processes:* Nursing Process Analysis; *Client Need:* Physiological Integrity/Reduction of Risk Potential/Potential for Alterations in Body Systems; *Cognitive Level:* Application

Reference: Ignatavicius, D., & Workman, M. (2006). *Medical-Surgical Nursing: Critical Thinking for Collaborative Care* (5th ed., pp. 1007–1010). St. Louis, MO: Elsevier/Saunders.

844. A home health nurse evaluates the foot care of a client with peripheral neuropathy. Which client actions in providing foot care are appropriate? SELECT ALL THAT APPLY.

1. Visually inspects the feet on a daily basis including using a handled mirror to see the bottom of the foot
2. Applies a lubricating lotion to the feet and legs daily, but not in between the toes
3. Goes barefoot in the house to air out the feet
4. States wearing warm socks and boots when outside in cold weather
5. Tests bath water with a thermometer
6. Trims toenails weekly to a rounded contour

ANSWER: 1, 2, 4, 5

Clients with peripheral neuropathy experience altered sensation and are at increased risk for injury. Clients need to use other means to become aware of risks. These include visual inspection, testing water before bathing or soaking feet, and monitoring environmental extremes and wearing appropriate clothing to avoid sunburns or frostbite. Keeping the skin adequately lubricated prevents drying and cracking—a key risk for infection. Clients should avoid going barefoot because this increases the risk of injury from stepping on an object. Toenails should be trimmed straight across to avoid damaging the tissue, which is slow to heal.

▸ ***Test-taking Tip:*** *The key words are "client actions" and "peripheral neuropathy." Neuropathy pertains to diseases of the nerves. Focus on foot care that protects the client from injury and infection. All options are actions. Look for key words in each option that would eliminate that option. The key word in option 3 is "barefoot," and the key words in option 6 are "trims toenails . . . rounded."*

Content Area: Adult Health; *Category of Health Alteration:* Neurological Management; *Integrated Processes:* Nursing Process Evaluation; *Client Need:* Physiological Integrity/Basic Care and Comfort/Personal Hygiene; Physiological Integrity/Reduction of Risk Potential/Potential for Alterations in Body Systems; *Cognitive Level:* Analysis

Reference: Ignatavicius, D., & Workman, M. (2006). *Medical-Surgical Nursing: Critical Thinking for Collaborative Care* (5th ed., p. 1020). St. Louis, MO: Elsevier/Saunders.

845. A nurse is performing hourly neurological assessment checks on a client who is admitted with changes in mental status. The nurse understands that frequent assessments are used to determine if a client is developing increased intracranial pressure (ICP). Which option correctly describes the outcome if ICP is untreated and progresses?

1. Displacement of brain tissue
2. Increase in cerebral circulation and perfusion
3. Increase in serum pH
4. Improved brain tissue oxygenation

ANSWER: 1

The outcome of undetected and untreated ICP is displacement of brain tissue, also referred to as brain herniation. Unchecked ICP progresses to cause shifts in brain tissue, resulting in irreversible brain damage and possibly death. ICP compresses structures within the cranium and leads to a decrease in cerebral perfusion, hypoxia, and acidosis. In acidosis, the pH level is decreased.

▸ ***Test-taking Tip:*** *The issue of the question is "the complication of progressive ICP." The question asks for the result of progressive ICP—a negative outcome for the client. Evaluate each option according to the effect on the client. Eliminate options 2, 3, and 4 since these represent improvement in the client's condition.*

Content Area: Adult Health; *Category of Health Alteration:* Neurological Management; *Integrated Processes:* Nursing Process Analysis; *Client Need:* Physiological Integrity/Physiological Adaptation/Alterations in Body Systems; *Cognitive Level:* Application

References: Ignatavicius, D., & Workman, M. (2006). *Medical-Surgical Nursing: Critical Thinking for Collaborative Care* (5th ed., pp. 1045–1046). St. Louis, MO: Elsevier/Saunders; Johnson, K. (2006). Determinants and assessment of cerebral tissue perfusion. In K. Wagner, K. Johnson, & P. Kidd (Eds.), *High-Acuity Nursing* (4th ed., pp. 409–410). Upper Saddle River, NJ: Pearson Education.

846. EBP A client who receives a diagnosis of right-sided stroke should be assessed for risk factors of stroke during the initial hospitalization, and measures should be instituted to lessen the client's risk. A nurse should address these risk factors as a priority and institute measures because: SELECT ALL THAT APPLY.

1. one of every four strokes occurs as a recurrent stroke.
2. the time period of greatest risk for a second stroke is the first 30 days after ischemic symptoms occur.
3. the potential for recovery continues for at least 6 months after the initial stroke event.
4. controlling modifiable risk factors is too difficult for persons who have already experienced a stroke.
5. the resultant deficit will cause the client to deny or minimize that there is a problem.
6. most stroke victims develop depression and less interest in learning preventive measures as the recovery process lengthens.

ANSWER: 1, 2, 3

Clients who have had strokes should be assessed for risk of stroke and receive adequate treatment because the risk for a repeat stroke is high, especially in the initial 30 days after the stroke event. The capacity for rehabilitation continues at least 6 months, although clients often receive more intensive therapy for the first few months. Clients who have had strokes are capable of making the lifestyle changes needed to lower their risk of another stroke. A person with a stroke on the right side of the brain (left-sided stroke) tends to deny or minimize problems. Although depression can occur, it is variable and doesn't affect most stroke victims.

▶ ***Test-taking Tip:*** *Read the stem of the question carefully. The question asks "Why should clients who have already had a stroke be assessed and treated to decrease their risk factors for stroke?" Select options 1, 2, and 3 because these options support the fact that strokes are likely to reoccur, and clients benefit from prevention of another stroke.*

Content Area: Adult Health; *Category of Health Alteration:* Neurological Management; *Integrated Processes:* Nursing Process Analysis; *Client Need:* Health Promotion and Maintenance/Disease Prevention; *Cognitive Level:* Application

EBP Reference: Stokowski, L. (2007). Stroke and stroke nursing: Safeguarding the brain. *Medscape Nurses.* Available at: www.medscape.com/viewarticle/558615

847. A client who has had a stroke stares at a nurse but does not attempt to verbally respond to the nurse's questions. The client follows instructions without any problems. The nurse understands that the client is displaying symptoms consistent with:

1. receptive aphasia.
2. global aphasia.
3. expressive aphasia.
4. both receptive and expressive aphasia.

ANSWER: 3

The client is showing symptoms of expressive aphasia (Broca's aphasia). The client has difficulty and is nonfluent with speech. Clients are often aware of their speech errors and are reluctant to speak. The client is able to comprehend and responds appropriately. With receptive aphasia (Wernicke's aphasia) the client receives but is unable to comprehend auditory impulses. Global aphasia is a combination of receptive and expressive aphasia. The client is severely limited in both the comprehension and expression of speech.

▶ ***Test-taking Tip:*** *Read the stem of the question to determine the client's communication technique. Determine that the problem involves language and eliminate option 4. Determine whether the problem involves client response (expression), comprehension (receiving), or both. Use the process of elimination.*

Content Area: Adult Health; *Category of Health Alteration:* Neurological Management; *Integrated Processes:* Nursing Process Analysis; *Client Need:* Physiological Integrity/Physiological Adaptation/Alterations in Body Systems; *Cognitive Level:* Analysis

Reference: Johnson, K., & Tarbay, A. (2006). Alterations in cerebral tissue perfusion: Acute brain attack. In K. Wagner, K. Johnson, & P. Kidd (Eds.), *High-Acuity Nursing* (4th ed., pp. 426–447). Upper Saddle River, NJ: Pearson Education.

848. EBP A client is admitted to the intensive care unit with a severe stroke. The client is receiving a continuous intravenous insulin infusion titrated according to hourly blood glucose results to control hyperglycemia. The client's spouse asks the nurse why the client is receiving insulin when the client is not diabetic. Which explanations to the client's spouse should the nurse include? SELECT ALL THAT APPLY

1. "The body reacts to stress by producing various hormones, which results in elevated glucose levels."
2. "The body has less effective utilization of glucose during serious illness."
3. "Insulin lessens the likelihood of brain tissue becoming swollen."
4. "Use of insulin will decrease the likelihood of the client becoming diabetic in the future."
5. 'The stroke affected the part of the brain that controls the release of insulin."
6. "A side effect of the medications administered is the development of type 1 diabetes mellitus."

ANSWER: 1, 2, 3

During critical illness, the body responds by producing hormones such as epinephrine and glucagons. These hormones increase the glucose level in the blood. Peripheral muscle tissues utilize glucose less effectively during critical illness, and this also elevates glucose levels. Insulin lessens the likelihood of cerebral edema by improving cell membrane stability. Maintaining intensive control of hyperglycemia during critical illness will not prevent diabetes in the future. Insulin is produced in the pancreas. If the client were receiving steroids in treatment, these can increase blood glucose levels, but do not cause diabetes.

➧ ***Test-taking Tip:*** *The issue of the question is "the physiological changes that occur during critical illness that cause increased glucose levels necessitating intensive insulin therapy." Evaluate each option to determine if it addresses the issue of the question correctly. Select the options that refer to the issue of the question: physiological response to critical illness. Eliminate option 4 since it refers to the future.*

Content Area: Adult Health; *Category of Health Alteration:* Neurological Management; *Integrated Processes:* Nursing Process Analysis; *Client Need:* Physiological Integrity/Pharmacological and Parenteral Therapies/Expected Effects/Outcomes; *Cognitive Level:* Analysis

EBP Reference: Paolino, A., & Garner, K. (2005). Effects of hyperglycemia on neurologic outcome in stroke patients. *Journal of Neuroscience Nursing*, 37(3), 130–135.

---

849. EBP A client with a deteriorating mental status after suffering a stroke has a rectal temperature of 102.3°F (39.1°C). For which reason should a nurse initiate interventions to bring the temperature to a normal level?

1. A normal temperature will strengthen the client's immune system against infection.
2. Hyperthermia lowers the incidence of mortality.
3. A normal temperature will decrease the score on the Glasgow coma scale.
4. Hyperthermia increases the likelihood of a larger area of brain infarct.

ANSWER: 4

Temperature elevation in neurological cases is thought to be associated with dysfunction of the hypothalamus. Research has shown that temperature elevations in the client post stroke result in an increase in the size of the infarct. Hyperthermia was associated with higher mortality rates and lower scores on the Glasgow coma scale. A normal temperature does not strengthen the immune system.

➧ ***Test-taking Tip:*** *The issue of the question asks why hyperthermia is detrimental to clients with stroke. Read each option separately and evaluate whether it describes the outcomes of hyperthermia negatively. Eliminate option 1 due to incorrect data about temperature and immune system function. Eliminate option 2 because it describes hyperthermia with a positive outcome. Eliminate option 3 because it attributes a decline in neurological status with a normal temperature. Select option 4 since it describes a negative outcome with hyperthermia.*

Content Area: Adult Health; *Category of Health Alteration:* Neurological Management; *Integrated Processes:* Nursing Process Analysis; *Client Need:* Physiological Integrity/Reduction of Risk Potential/Vital Signs; *Cognitive Level:* Application

EBP Reference: Thompson, H., Kirkness, C., Mitchell, P., & Webb, D. (2007). Fever management practices of neuroscience nurses: National and regional perspectives. *Journal of Neuroscience Nursing*, 39(3), 151–162.

---

850. A client is diagnosed with a stroke that affects the right hemisphere of the brain. A nurse, receiving report prior to the care of this client, should expect the client to have which symptom?

1. Right hemiparesis
2. Expressive aphasia
3. Poor impulse control
4. Marked anxiety when learning new tasks

ANSWER: 3

The client with a stroke affecting the right side of the brain often exhibits impulsive behavior and is unaware of the neurological deficits. The client with a stroke affecting the left side of the brain will experience motor function deficits on the right side because motor fibers in the brain cross over in the medulla before entering the spinal column. This client is more likely to experience aphasia because the center for language is located on the left side of the brain in 75% to 80% of the population. This client is often cautious, depressed about the neurological deficits, and anxious when learning new tasks.

▶ ***Test-taking Tip:*** *Key words in the stem are "stroke affecting the right side of the brain." Consider that the nerves cross resulting in contralateral effect from the stroke. Determine the location of the areas controlling the behaviors listed. Eliminate options 1, 2, and 4 because they are all symptoms associated with strokes affecting the left hemisphere.*

Content Area: Adult Health; *Category of Health Alteration:* Neurological Management; *Integrated Processes:* Nursing Process Analysis; *Client Need:* Physiological Integrity/Physiological Adaptation/Alterations in Body Systems; Safe and Effective Care Environment/Management of Care/Continuity of Care; *Cognitive Level:* Analysis

References: Ignatavicius, D., & Workman, M. (2006). *Medical-Surgical Nursing: Critical Thinking for Collaborative Care* (5th ed., p. 1034). St. Louis, MO: Elsevier/Saunders; Smeltzer, S., Bare, B., Hinkle, J., & Cheever, K. (2008). *Brunner & Suddarth's Textbook of Medical-Surgical Nursing* (11th ed., p. 2209). Philadelphia: Lippincott Williams & Wilkins.

---

851. A client seeks medical attention at an emergency department after experiencing left-sided weakness and slurred speech. The client receives a diagnosis with an ischemic stroke and is evaluated for treatment with thrombolytic therapy. A definite contraindication for thrombolytic therapy is:

1. a normal computed tomography (CT) scan of the brain.
2. a serious head injury 4 weeks earlier.
3. a history of diabetes mellitus.
4. the onset of neurological deficits 2 hours earlier.

ANSWER: 2

Contraindications to thrombolytic therapy for a client with an ischemic stroke include a serious head injury within the previous 3 months. This would put the client at risk of developing serious bleeding problems, specifically cerebral hemorrhage. A negative CT scan and onset of neurological deficits within 3 hours are criteria for administering the thrombolytic therapy. History of diabetes is not a contraindication.

▶ ***Test-taking Tip:*** *The word "thrombolytic" means break down of a blood clot so a risk associated with the thrombolytic therapy is bleeding. Read each option carefully and select the option that relates to bleeding.*

Content Area: Adult Health; *Category of Health Alteration:* Neurological Management; *Integrated Processes:* Nursing Process Analysis; *Client Need:* Physiological Integrity/Reduction of Risk Potential/Potential for Complications of Diagnostic Tests/Treatments/ Procedures; *Cognitive Level:* Comprehension

Reference: Ignatavicius, D., & Workman, M. (2006). *Medical-Surgical Nursing: Critical Thinking for Collaborative Care* (5th ed., pp. 1038–1039). St. Louis, MO: Elsevier/Saunders.

---

852. A client is admitted to an intensive care unit because of a leaking cerebral aneurysm. A family member asks a nurse why the client is awakened and questioned about his orientation so frequently when he needs to rest. The nurse answers the family member based on the knowledge that the earliest sign of increased intracranial pressure (ICP) is:

1. pupillary changes.
2. drop in the blood pressure.
3. altered sensation.
4. changes in the level of consciousness.

ANSWER: 4

A change in the level of consciousness is the first sign of neurological deterioration and is often associated with development of ICP. Pupillary changes may occur with ICP as it progresses or with actual cranial nerve injury. A drop in blood pressure is not directly associated with neurological deterioration. A blood pressure with a wide pulse pressure is a late sign of ICP. Altered sensation may be associated with peripheral nerve pathology.

▶ ***Test-taking Tip:*** *The key words are "earliest sign of ICP." Consider that the earliest sign may be the most subtle. Evaluate each option separately. Eliminate options 2 and 3 because these are not subtle signs.*

Content Area: Adult Health; *Category of Health Alteration:* Neurological Management; *Integrated Processes:* Teaching and Learning; *Client Need:* Physiological Integrity/Reduction of Risk Potential/System Specific Assessments; *Cognitive Level:* Application

Reference: Johnson, K. (2006). Determinants and assessment of cerebral tissue perfusion. In K. Wagner, K. Johnson, & P. Kidd (Eds.), *High-Acuity Nursing* (4th ed., pp. 402–425). Upper Saddle River, NJ: Pearson Education.

853. A nurse is orienting a new nurse to a unit. The experienced nurse evaluates that the new nurse understands information related to a stroke resulting from a subarachnoid hemorrhage when which points are addressed by the new nurse? SELECT ALL THAT APPLY.

1. Subarachnoid hemorrhage is often associated with a rupture of a cerebral aneurysm.
2. Subarachnoid hemorrhage usually occurs while the client is sleeping and is noticed when the client awakens.
3. Subarachnoid hemorrhage is accompanied by complaints of an extremely severe headache.
4. Subarachnoid hemorrhage may be treated with thrombolytic therapy if no contraindications exist.
5. Subarachnoid hemorrhage often results in bloody cerebrospinal fluid (CSF).
6. Subarachnoid hemorrhage causes nuchal rigidity.

ANSWER: 1, 3, 5, 6

A subarachnoid hemorrhage is usually caused by rupture of a cerebral aneurysm. There is bleeding in the subarachnoid space causing bloody CSF and symptoms of meningeal irritation, such as nuchal rigidity (stiff neck) and a severe headache. Ischemic stroke in elderly clients often occurs during sleep when the blood pressure drops and the circulation is decreased. Thrombolytic therapy would not be used to treat the stroke because the etiology is bleeding, not a clot. A subarachnoid hemorrhage is a contraindication to thrombolytic therapy.

➧ ***Test-taking Tip:*** *Focus on the issue of the question, symptoms, diagnostic findings, and whether thrombolytic therapy is indicated for treatment of a subarachnoid hemorrhage stroke. Consider the location of the hemorrhage and associated symptoms and treatment. Consider the anatomy of the meninges, which contains the subarachnoid space. Recall that options 3 and 6 represent symptoms of meningeal irritation.*

Content Area: Adult Health; *Category of Health Alteration:* Neurological Management; *Integrated Processes:* Teaching and Learning; Nursing Process Evaluation; *Client Need:* Physiological Integrity/Physiological Adaptation/Pathophysiology; *Cognitive Level:* Synthesis

Reference: Johnson, K., & Tarbay, A. (2006). Alterations in cerebral tissue perfusion: Acute brain attack. In K. Wagner, K. Johnson, & P. Kidd (Eds.), *High-Acuity Nursing* (4th ed., pp. 426–447). Upper Saddle River, NJ: Pearson Education.

---

854. **EBP** A nurse should plan for which measure to treat an elderly client with normal pressure hydrocephalus (NPH)?

1. Carotid endarterectomy
2. Ventriculoperitoneal shunt
3. Lumbar drain
4. Anticonvulsant medications

ANSWER: 2

NPH is a reversible neurological condition in older adults. The clients have mild dementia, bladder and bowel incontinence, and a specific hypokinetic gait disorder. The clients have dilated ventricles in the brain despite normal cerebrospinal pressure. NPH is treated with a procedure that involves removal of excess cerebral spinal fluid (CSF): the placement of a shunt in a lateral ventricle of the brain that drains into the peritoneal cavity. Symptoms improve with removal of CSF. A carotid endarterectomy involves removal of plaque from the carotid artery. A lumbar drain can be used to remove CSF with disorders that increase CSF in the subarachnoid space in the lumbar area, such as a tumor. Anticonvulsant medications are used to treat seizures.

➧ ***Test-taking Tip:*** *The issue of the question is the procedure used to treat NPH. Evaluate each option to determine whether it is a method to remove excess CSF.*

Content Area: Adult Health; *Category of Health Alteration:* Neurological Management; *Integrated Processes:* Nursing Process Analysis; *Client Need:* Physiological Integrity/Reduction of Risk Potential/Potential for Complications of Diagnostic Tests/Treatments/Procedures; *Cognitive Level:* Comprehension

EBP Reference: Fraser, J., & Fraser, C. (2007). Gait disorder is the cardinal sign of normal pressure hydrocephalus: a case study. *Journal of Neuroscience Nursing,* 39(3), 132–134, 192.

---

855. Following an industrial accident in which a client sustained a severe craniocerebral trauma, the client develops the complication of diabetes insipidus (DI). A nurse suspects this complication is occurring when observing which symptom?

1. Hyperglycemia
2. Large amounts of urinary output
3. Elevated urine specific gravity
4. Decrease in level of consciousness

ANSWER: 2

DI occurs due to a lack of antidiuretic hormone (ADH), a hormone secreted by the posterior pituitary gland. With a head injury there may be compression of the pituitary gland and loss of ADH production. Improper water balance results and the client excretes large amounts of pale, dilute urine and becomes hypotensive. Elevated glucose levels are not associated with DI. The urine of clients with DI is very dilute and therefore has a very low specific gravity. Decrease in level of consciousness is not directly associated with DI but rather from craniocerebral swelling or bleeding from the trauma.

➧ *Test-taking Tip: Read the question carefully and note the condition is diabetes insipidus, not mellitus. Use the process of elimination. Note that large amounts of urinary output and a high specific gravity are not usually associated together, so one of these answers must be correct. Consider that the term diabetes insipidus means excessive urination.*

Content Area: Adult Health; *Category of Health Alteration:* Neurological Management; *Integrated Processes:* Nursing Process Analysis; *Client Need:* Physiological Integrity/Reduction of Risk Potential/ Potential for Alterations in Body Systems; *Cognitive Level:* Analysis

Reference: DaDeppo, A. (2006). Decreased adaptive capacity: Closed head injury. In K. Wagner, K. Johnson, & P. Kidd (Eds.), *High-Acuity Nursing* (4th ed., pp. 448–458). Upper Saddle River, NJ: Pearson Education.

856. EBP A client hits her head in a minor motor vehicle accident and refuses medical attention at the time of the accident. The client makes an appointment with a primary care provider 6 weeks later because of headaches. The primary care provider diagnoses the client with mild traumatic brain injury (TBI). Which details noted by a nurse in the client's history of the injury support this diagnosis? SELECT ALL THAT APPLY.

1. The client has had no episodes of vomiting after the accident.
2. The client remembers the events leading up to the accident and what occurred during the accident.
3. The client has experienced episodes of headache and dizziness on a daily basis since the accident.
4. The client has difficulty concentrating and focusing while at work.
5. The client reported a loss of consciousness for a few seconds at the time of the injury.
6. The client describes a funny taste in the mouth since the accident that is "disgusting."

ANSWER: 3, 4, 5, 6

Mild TBI results from damage to axonal injury or neuronal and glia cell injury. Recurrent problems with headache and dizziness are the most prominent symptoms of mild TBI. At the time of the accident, the person may experience a loss of consciousness for a few seconds or minutes. Cognitive difficulties, including inability to concentrate and forgetfulness, also occur with mild TBI. Other symptoms of mild TBI include confusion, lightheadedness, blurred vision or tired eyes, ringing in the ears, bad taste in the mouth, fatigue or lethargy, a change in sleep patterns, behavioral or mood changes, and trouble with memory, attention, or thinking. Clients with mild TBI usually experience symptoms commonly associated with mild concussion such as vomiting and amnesia regarding the accident or injury event.

➧ *Test-taking Tip: The key words are "supports the diagnosis." Focus on symptoms of mild TBI. Eliminate options that are normal findings and those that would occur with a more severe head injury.*

Content Area: Adult Health; *Category of Health Alteration:* Neurological Management; *Integrated Processes:* Nursing Process Analysis; *Client Need:* Physiological Integrity/Physiological Adaptation/Alterations in Body Systems; *Cognitive Level:* Analysis

Reference: Smeltzer, S., Bare, B., Hinkle, J., & Cheever, K. (2008). *Brunner & Suddarth's Textbook of Medical-Surgical Nursing* (11th ed., pp. 2233–2250). Philadelphia: Lippincott Williams & Wilkins.

EBP Reference: Bay, E., & McLean, S. (2007). Mild traumatic brain injury: An update for advanced practice nurses. *Journal of Neuroscience Nursing*, 39(1), 43–51.

857. An anxious client is seen in a clinic because the client suspects that he/she has a brain tumor. The client questions a nurse about treatment options if tests show the presence of a tumor. The nurse answers the client based on the knowledge that treatment of a brain tumor depends on: SELECT ALL THAT APPLY.

1. rate of growth of the tumor.
2. whether the tumor is malignant or benign.
3. cell type from which the tumor originates.
4. location within the brain.
5. whether the tumor will reoccur.
6. the client's age and type of insurance.

ANSWER: 1, 2, 3, 4, 5

Treatment of a brain tumor depends on the tumor type, including whether it is malignant, tendency to reoccur, and the rate of growth. The area within the brain or adjacent structure also is considered when planning treatment. Treatment is planned to remove or decrease tumor size without damaging the normal tissue. Comorbid conditions, not age, may be a determining factor in treatment options. The type of insurance is irrelevant to treatment unless treatment is experimental.

➧ *Test-taking Tip: The issue of the question is what factors determine the appropriate treatment of a brain tumor. Consider each option separately and evaluate how each factor affects the outcome.*

Content Area: Adult Health; *Category of Health Alteration:* Neurological Management; *Integrated Processes:* Nursing Process Analysis; *Client Need:* Physiological Integrity/Physiological Adaptation/Pathophysiology; *Cognitive Level:* Synthesis

References: Ignatavicius, D., & Workman, M. (2006). *Medical-Surgical Nursing: Critical Thinking for Collaborative Care* (5th ed., pp. 1055–1058). St. Louis, MO: Elsevier/Saunders; Smeltzer, S., Bare, B., Hinkle, J., & Cheever, K. (2008). *Brunner & Suddarth's Textbook of Medical-Surgical Nursing* (11th ed., pp. 2305–2311). Philadelphia: Lippincott Williams & Wilkins.

858. A nurse is caring for a group of clients on a medical unit in a rural hospital. Which client would the nurse be *least* likely to monitor for the potential complication of a brain abscess?

1. Client with endocarditis
2. Client with idiopathic epilepsy
3. Client who has had a liver transplant
4. Client with meningitis

ANSWER: 2

Brain abscess denotes a collection of pus in the brain that occurs from an infection. The client who has idiopathic epilepsy has the lowest risk of developing a brain abscess because epilepsy from an unknown cause does not have the risk factors of an active infectious process or an impaired immune system. The client with endocarditis has an infective process within the body's circulation and is at risk for septic emboli. The client with the liver transplant is at risk because of treatment with immunosuppressant medications. The client with meningitis has an infective process in close proximity to the brain.

Test-taking Tip: *The key words are "least likely" and "brain abscess." Evaluate each option and determine if it relates to an infective process or increased risk of infection. The question calls for the option with the weakest link to a brain abscess. Eliminate options 1 and 4 because these directly relate to an infection, thus the suffix "-itis." Eliminate option 3 because transplant clients are immunosuppressed and at increased risk of infection.*

Content Area: Adult Health; *Category of Health Alteration:* Neurological Management; *Integrated Processes:* Nursing Process Analysis; *Client Need:* Physiological Integrity/Reduction of Risk Potential/Potential for Complications from Surgical Procedures and Health Alterations; *Cognitive Level:* Application

Reference: Ignatavicius, D., & Workman, M. (2006). *Medical-Surgical Nursing: Critical Thinking for Collaborative Care* (5th ed., p. 1066). St. Louis, MO: Elsevier/Saunders.

---

859. A client who had a craniotomy 2 days earlier is receiving mannitol (Osmitrol®) intravenously to decrease intracranial pressure. Which diagnostic laboratory value should be monitored while the client is receiving this medication?

1. Serum osmolarity
2. White blood cell (WBC) count
3. Serum cholesterol
4. Erythrocyte sedimentation rate (ESR)

ANSWER: 1

Mannitol, an osmotic diuretic, increases the serum osmolarity and pulls fluid from the tissues, decreasing cerebral edema postoperatively. Serum osmolarity levels are assessed as a parameter to determine proper dosage. The WBC, serum cholesterol, and ESR are not affected by mannitol.

Test-taking Tip: *The question asks for the effect of mannitol and which laboratory value reflects that effect. The brand name Osmitrol suggests that the medication acts by regulation of osmosis. Consider each option separately and use the process of elimination.*

Content Area: Adult Health; *Category of Health Alteration:* Neurological Management; *Integrated Processes:* Nursing Process Analysis; *Client Need:* Physiological Integrity/Reduction of Risk Potential/Laboratory Values; *Cognitive Level:* Comprehension

Reference: Ignatavicius, D., & Workman, M. (2006). *Medical-Surgical Nursing: Critical Thinking for Collaborative Care* (5th ed., p. 1052). St. Louis, MO: Elsevier/Saunders.

---

860. A client with epilepsy is prescribed phenytoin sodium (Dilantin®) 100 mg 3 times per day orally as anticonvulsant therapy. The most precise method for a nurse to determine if this is the proper dose for the client is:

1. observation of the client for seizures.
2. observation of the client for adverse effects.
3. determining whether the client is able to participate in usual activities.
4. monitoring serum phenytoin levels.

ANSWER: 4

Dosages of anticonvulsant medications are individualized and monitored by measuring medication levels in the blood of the client. Observing client for symptoms and seizure activity is not as specific as monitoring drug levels for therapeutic range.

Test-taking Tip: *Key words in the stem are "most precise method" and "proper dose." Evaluate each option regarding how it specifically addresses whether the medication is prescribed at the proper dose.*

Content Area: Adult Health; *Category of Health Alteration:* Neurological Management; *Integrated Processes:* Nursing Process Evaluation; *Client Need:* Physiological Integrity/Pharmacological and Parenteral Therapies/Expected Effects/Outcomes; *Cognitive Level:* Analysis

Reference: Fagley, M. (2007). Taking charge of seizure activity. *Nursing 2007,* 37(9), 42–47.

861. An elderly client with Parkinson's disease is prescribed levodopa and carbidopa (Sinemet®). Which point should a nurse include in the teaching plan for the client and spouse?

1. The client is at increased risk for falls due to dizziness and orthostatic hypotension.
2. The client should stop taking multiple vitamins.
3. The medication should not be taken with food.
4. The medication has very few adverse effects.

ANSWER: 1

Sinemet® is an antiparkinsonian agent. Levodopa is converted to dopamine in the central nervous system, where it serves as a neurotransmitter, and carbidopa, a decarboxylase inhibitor, prevents peripheral destruction of levodopa. When first taking Sinemet®, clients are likely to experience dizziness and orthostatic hypotension due to the dopamine agonist properties. Clients must be alerted about the increased risk for falls. The medication can be taken with multiple vitamins and with food to decrease gastrointestinal upset. There are many, not few, adverse effects associated with Sinemet® including involuntary movements, anxiety, memory loss, blurred vision, and mydriasis.

▶ ***Test-taking Tip:*** *Focus on the main issue of the question: "what are key points to teach clients beginning Sinemet®?" Note that the most serious issue listed among the options is the answer.*

Content Area: Adult Health; *Category of Health Alteration:* Neurological Management; *Integrated Processes:* Teaching and Learning; *Client Need:* Physiological Integrity/Pharmacological and Parenteral Therapies/Adverse Effects/Contradictions; *Cognitive Level:* Application

Reference: Ignatavicius, D., & Workman, M. (2006). *Medical-Surgical Nursing: Critical Thinking for Collaborative Care* (5th ed., pp. 956–958). St. Louis, MO: Elsevier.

---

862. A home health nurse is making a home visit to a client with multiple sclerosis. The nurse reviews the home medications taken by the client. Which question should the nurse ask to determine the effectiveness of the client's medication, baclofen (Lioresal®)?

1. "How has your appetite been?"
2. "Are you having any difficulty with having regular bowel movements?"
3. "Are you having trouble with spasms?"
4. "Does your urine look clear and not infected?"

ANSWER: 3

Baclofen is a skeletal muscle relaxant used to control spasticity. The medication does not affect appetite, act as a stool softener, or treat a urinary tract infection.

▶ ***Test-taking Tip:*** *The key word is "effectiveness." Select option 3 recalling that the intended effect is to reduce spasms.*

Content Area: Adult Health; *Category of Health Alteration:* Neurological Management; *Integrated Processes:* Nursing Process Evaluation; *Client Need:* Physiological Integrity/Pharmacological and Parenteral Therapies/Expected Effects/Outcomes; *Cognitive Level:* Analysis

Reference: Springhouse Publishing Company Staff. (2007). *Springhouse Nurse's Drug Guide 2007* (8th ed., pp. 204–206). Philadelphia: Lippincott Williams & Wilkins.

Test 22: **Adult Health: Perioperative Management**

863. A nurse plans care for a client and notes that all of the following must be completed for a client being prepared for surgery. Which intervention should the nurse complete *first*?

1. Complete the preoperative checklist.
2. Assess the client's preoperative vital signs.
3. Remove the client's rings, gold chain, and wristwatch.
4. Administer 10 mEq KCL IV for a serum potassium level of 3.0 mEq/L.

ANSWER: 4

Intravenous potassium is ordered for low serum potassium levels. Low levels could induce cardiac dysrhythmias and delay surgery. Administering the potassium should be the nurse's priority because abnormalities must be corrected before surgery. Completing the preoperative checklist ensures that all requirements are completed. This would be the second priority. Although important, assessing the client's preoperative vital signs is not the first priority. Although important, removing the client's rings, gold chain, and wristwatch is not the first priority.

▶ ***Test-taking Tip:*** *Use the process of elimination and Maslow's Hierarchy of Needs. Physiological needs would take priority over safety needs, unless life threatening. Replacing serum potassium poses both a physiological and safety need and could be life threatening.*

Content Area: Adult Health; *Category of Health Alteration:* Perioperative Management; *Integrated Processes:* Nursing Process Planning; *Client Need:* Safe and Effective Care Environment/Management of Care/Establishing Priorities; *Cognitive Level:* Application

Reference: Ignatavicius, D., & Workman, M. (2006). *Medical-Surgical Nursing: Critical Thinking for Collaborative Care* (5th ed., p. 301). St. Louis, MO: Elsevier/Saunders.

---

864. Which client statement made during a presurgical admission assessment needs the most immediate follow-up?

1. "I haven't eaten foods or had any fluids for the past 12 hours."
2. "I donated my own blood in case I need a transfusion; the last donation was 4 days ago."
3. "I took my usual dose of warfarin (Coumadin®) and other cardiac meds this morning with a sip of water."
4. "I brought a copy of my Health Care Directives so others will know my wishes should my heart stop during surgery."

ANSWER: 3

Warfarin is an anticoagulant. Usually this is stopped a few days before surgery due to the increased risk of bleeding. The exact amount of time a client must be NPO before surgery is controversial. Older adults may have imbalances of fluids, electrolytes, and blood glucose levels from fasting longer. However, there is no indication in the question that this is a concern. Blood can be donated up to 72 hours before the scheduled surgery. Clients should be encouraged to bring a copy of the Health Care Directives so others are aware of the client's wishes. The surgeon, nurse, and other health-care providers should be aware of the client's wishes.

▶ ***Test-taking Tip:*** *Note the key words "most immediate." Knowledge of the anticoagulant effects of warfarin is needed to answer this question.*

Content Area: Adult Health; *Category of Health Alteration:* Perioperative Management; *Integrated Processes:* Nursing Process Implementation; *Client Need:* Physiological Integrity/Reduction of Risk Potential/Potential for Complications from Surgical Procedures and Health Alterations; *Cognitive Level:* Application

Reference: Ignatavicius, D., & Workman, M. (2006). *Medical-Surgical Nursing: Critical Thinking for Collaborative Care* (5th ed., pp. 299, 306). St. Louis, MO: Elsevier/Saunders.

---

865. A nurse is to witness the signature of a surgical consent for multiple clients scheduled for surgery the following day. In evaluating the health history of each client, the nurse should plan to obtain a signature from the next of kin for:

1. a 75-year-old client who is blind.
2. a 60-year-old client who does not understand English.
3. a 50-year-old client who is forgetful, but fully oriented.
4. a 16-year-old educated client who fully understands the surgery.

ANSWER: 4

The legal age for consent is 18 years unless the adolescent has emancipated status granted by a judge. The client may sign his or her signature with an "X" as long as the client understands the nature and reason for surgery, who will perform the surgery, available options, the benefits and risks of surgery, and the consent form that is read to the client. Another person besides the nurse should witness the client's "X" signature. An interpreter should be available to read the consent in the client's native language. The client can then provide written consent in the presence of two witnesses. A client is able to sign a consent form unless determined incompetent. If the client is fully oriented, a signed consent can be obtained from the client.

▶ ***Test-taking Tip:*** *Note the key words "next of kin." Focus on the ages of the clients, and use the process of elimination.*

Content Area: Adult Health; *Category of Health Alteration:* Perioperative Management; *Integrated Processes:* Nursing Process Planning; *Client Need:* Safe and Effective Care Environment/Management of Care/Informed Consent; *Cognitive Level:* Application

Reference: Ignatavicius, D., & Workman, M. (2006). *Medical-Surgical Nursing: Critical Thinking for Collaborative Care* (5th ed., pp. 304–306). St. Louis, MO: Elsevier/Saunders.

866. A nurse receives the written laboratory results of a positive pregnancy test for a client scheduled for an emergency appendectomy. The nurse should first:

1. call the lab to verify the results of the test.
2. inform the client of the positive results.
3. report the results immediately to the surgeon.
4. notify the client's primary physician of the results.

ANSWER: 3

The surgeon should be notified because a positive pregnancy test result could influence the choice of anesthetic agents, medications, and surgical approach. Verifying laboratory results is unnecessary. Some hospitals may require critical laboratory tests repeated. Discussing laboratory results with the client is the physician's responsibility.

As a courtesy, the primary physician should be notified. However, it is more important to notify the surgeon.

➧ ***Test-taking Tip:*** *Note the key word "first." Read each stem and determine what action would be most important.*

Content Area: Adult Health; *Category of Health Alteration:* Perioperative Management; *Integrated Processes:* Nursing Process Implementation; *Client Need:* Physiological Integrity/Reduction of Risk Potential/Potential for Complications from Surgical Procedures and Health Alterations; *Cognitive Level:* Application

Reference: Ignatavicius, D., & Workman, M. (2006). *Medical-Surgical Nursing: Critical Thinking for Collaborative Care* (5th ed., p. 301). St. Louis, MO: Elsevier/Saunders.

867. During a presurgical admission assessment, a client states, "I've told my surgeon that I am a Jehovah's Witness and I won't accept a blood transfusion." Which statement by the nurse would be most appropriate?

1. "Tell me about your fear of receiving a blood transfusion."
2. "Your request to not receive a transfusion would be honored. Your consent is needed to administer blood or blood products."
3. "You don't need to worry about getting a blood transfusion. We have newer equipment that causes less blood loss during surgery."
4. "Are you sure you wouldn't want a blood transfusion if one is needed during surgery? You can always change your mind after surgery."

ANSWER: 2

A client's consent is needed prior to administering blood or blood products. Even in a life-threatening situation, the client has the right to refuse blood and blood products for religious reasons. There is no indication the client is fearful. The client is refusing blood for religious reasons. Telling the client not to worry belittles the client and does not address the client's statement about not getting a blood transfusion. Response 4 is incorrect. Asking the client if he or she is sure he or she does not want a transfusion is requesting an explanation and questions the client's decision. The client has a right to his or her religious beliefs.

➧ ***Test-taking Tip:*** *Use therapeutic communication principles to answer this question. Eliminate a response that belittles the client's feelings, questions the client's decision, and misinterprets the client's feelings.*

Content Area: Adult Health; *Category of Health Alteration:* Perioperative Management; *Integrated Processes:* Communication and Documentation; *Client Need:* Psychosocial Integrity/Religious and Spiritual Influences on Health; *Cognitive Level:* Application

Reference: Ignatavicius, D., & Workman, M. (2006). *Medical-Surgical Nursing: Critical Thinking for Collaborative Care* (5th ed., p. 299). St. Louis, MO: Elsevier/Saunders.

868. A nurse is analyzing serum laboratory results for a 73-year-old female client scheduled for surgery in 2 hours. The nurse concludes that which result would warrant the most immediate notification of the physician?

1. Hemoglobin 10 g/dL
2. Creatinine 1.0 mg/dL
3. Potassium 4.5 mEq/dL
4. Prothrombin time 22 seconds

ANSWER: 4

The normal prothrombin time is 11 to 12.5 seconds. Because it is prolonged, the client is at risk for bleeding. Normal hemoglobin for a 73-year-old female is 11.7 to 16.1 g/dL. Although a little low, this does not warrant the most immediate notification. The normal creatinine level is 0.6 to 1.2 mg/dL for a 73-year-old female. The normal potassium level is 3.5 to 5.0 mEq/dL.

➧ ***Test-taking Tip:*** *The nurse would be expected to know ranges of these essential laboratory values. Analyze each laboratory value against the normal ranges to determine which value is incorrect.*

Content Area: Adult Health; *Category of Health Alteration:* Perioperative Management; *Integrated Processes:* Nursing Process Analysis; *Client Need:* Physiological Integrity/Reduction of Risk Potential/Laboratory Values; *Cognitive Level:* Analysis

Reference: Ignatavicius, D., & Workman, M. (2006). *Medical-Surgical Nursing: Critical Thinking for Collaborative Care* (5th ed., pp. 302–303). St. Louis, MO: Elsevier/Saunders.

869. A nurse is reviewing preoperative orders for a client who is to have surgery on the large intestine the next day. Which written orders should the nurse question? SELECT ALL THAT APPLY.

1. NPO after midnight
2. Erythromycin 500 mg bid
3. Tap water enemas until hard stool passed
4. Clear liquid diet the day before surgery
5. Begin incentive spirometer (IS) use prior to surgery

ANSWER: 2, 3

Tap water enemas would be administered until the returns are clear. Stool present in the colon could predispose the client to peritonitis and infection. Antibiotics are administered to sterilize the bowel prior to surgery but no route is prescribed. The client should be NPO after midnight to prevent aspiration of gastric contents during surgery. A clear liquid diet the day before surgery minimizes roughage in the bowel. IS use allows for presurgical evaluation of lung capacity.

▸ ***Test-taking Tip:*** *Note the type of surgery and the written orders that pose a risk to the client or are incomplete.*

Content Area: Adult Health; *Category of Health Alteration:* Perioperative Management; *Integrated Processes:* Nursing Process Analysis; *Client Need:* Physiological Integrity/Reduction of Risk Potential/Potential for Complications from Surgical Procedures and Health Alterations; *Cognitive Level:* Application

Reference: Ignatavicius, D., & Workman, M. (2006). *Medical-Surgical Nursing: Critical Thinking for Collaborative Care* (5th ed., p. 306). St. Louis, MO: Elsevier/Saunders.

870. A physician writes an order to hold all medications the morning of surgery for a client with a history of type 1 diabetes mellitus and hypertension. A nurse should call the physician to clarify the hold order for what medication?

1. Acetylsalicylic acid (aspirin)
2. Ducosate sodium (Colace®)
3. Regular and NPH insulin (Humulin®)
4. Clonidine (Catapres®)

ANSWER: 3

The diabetic client who takes insulin should be given a reduced dose of intermediate or long-acting insulin based on the blood glucose levels. Regular insulin in divided doses on the day of surgery or an insulin drip may be initiated for tight glucose control. Aspirin has anticoagulant properties and should be discontinued to avoid bleeding complications. Colace® is a stool softener. It is appropriate to hold this the morning of surgery. Antihypertensive medications are often held prior to surgery to prevent a hypotension crisis intraoperatively.

▸ ***Test-taking Tip:*** *Focus on the medication actions and use the process of elimination. Remember that stress increases blood glucose levels.*

Content Area: Adult Health; *Category of Health Alteration:* Perioperative Management; *Integrated Processes:* Nursing Process Implementation; *Client Need:* Safe and Effective Care Environment/ Management of Care/Legal Rights and Responsibilities; *Cognitive Level:* Analysis

Reference: Ignatavicius, D., & Workman, M. (2006). *Medical-Surgical Nursing: Critical Thinking for Collaborative Care* (5th ed., p. 306). St. Louis, MO: Elsevier/Saunders.

871. EBP Which client statement indicates that a client who is scheduled for a 3-hour surgery under general anesthesia needs further teaching?

1. "A breathing tube will be placed when I am in the operating room."
2. "I should shave the skin in the surgical area the evening prior to surgery."
3. "I should splint my incision with a pillow when coughing and deep breathing after surgery."
4. "I might need a urinary catheter inserted before surgery so my urine output can be monitored."

ANSWER: 2

If any shaving of the surgical area is to be done, it should be done immediately prior to surgery in a holding area, treatment room, operating suite, or the operating room by qualified personnel. The client should not shave the surgical area. Nicks increase the risk for infection. Either an endotracheal or nasotracheal tube would be placed for a client under general anesthesia. Postoperatively, the client should cough and deep breathe. The incision can be splinted with a pillow, towel, or folded blanket placed over the surgical incision. Because the surgery is prolonged (3 hours), a urinary catheter should be inserted and urine output monitored.

▸ ***Test-taking Tip:*** *Read the stem carefully and focus on the key words "needs further teaching." Select the client statement that indicates that the nurse needs to provide further instructions.*

Content Area: Adult Health; *Category of Health Alteration:* Perioperative Management; *Integrated Processes:* Nursing Process Implementation; Teaching and Learning; *Client Need:* Physiological Integrity/Reduction of Risk Potential/Potential for Complications from Surgical Procedures and Health Alterations; *Cognitive Level:* Application

Reference: Ignatavicius, D., & Workman, M. (2006). *Medical-Surgical Nursing: Critical Thinking for Collaborative Care* (5th ed., pp. 307–309). St. Louis, MO: Elsevier/Saunders.

EBP Reference: The Joanna Briggs Institute. (2003). The impact of preoperative hair removal on surgical site infection. *Best Practice*, 7(2). Available at: www.joannabriggs.edu.au/pubs/best_practice.php

---

872. EBP Which nursing action would be best when a preoperative client verbalizes fear of postoperative pain?

1. Providing diversional activities when client reports fear of pain
2. Encouraging the client to verbalize concerns regarding the fear of pain
3. Informing the client of experiences and the likelihood of pain pre- and postoperatively
4. Explaining the medications ordered for pain control, availability, and treatment goals

ANSWER: 4

The client should be reassured that there are medications available to prevent and treat pain. Diversional activities are used to enhance the pharmacological effect. Pharmacological management is the mainstay for acute pain. Although allowing the client to verbalize fears is a therapeutic communication technique, allaying the fear is best. Informing the client of experiences may heighten the client's fear. The client needs reassurance that the pain will be controlled.

➧ ***Test-taking Tip:*** *Note the key word "best." Look at the verbs provide, encourage, inform, explain. Providing diversional activities does not address the client's verbalization. Eliminate responses 2 and 3 because they are lower-level verbs.*

Content Area: Adult Health; *Category of Health Alteration:* Perioperative Management; *Integrated Processes:* Nursing Process Implementation; *Client Need:* Physiological Integrity/Pharmacological and Parenteral Therapies/Pharmacological Pain Management; *Cognitive Level:* Application

Reference: Lewis, S., Heitkemper, M., Dirksen, S., O'Brien, P., & Bucher, L. (2007). *Medical-Surgical Nursing: Assessment and Management of Clinical Problems* (7th ed., pp. 388–389). St. Louis, MO: Mosby.

EBP Reference: Institute for Clinical Systems Improvement (ICSI). (2008). *Assessment and Management of Acute Pain.* Available at: www.guideline.gov/summary/summary.aspx?doc_id=12302&nbr=006371&string=acute+AND+pain+AND+management+AND+perioperative+AND+setting.

---

873. Which statement by a nurse is most effective when collecting data about a preoperative client's recreational drug use?

1. "Describe the drugs you use and the frequency that you use these drugs."
2. "Do you use any over-the-counter medications or illegal substances?"
3. "Tell me about all medications and substances you take because complications can occur if you are taking something we do not know about."
4. "Because herbs, medications, and recreational drugs such as marijuana and cocaine affect the type and amount of anesthesia you need, list any of these you take and how often you use them."

ANSWER: 4

When clients are aware of the potential interactions of drugs with anesthetics, most clients respond honestly about their drug use. This statement is nonjudgmental and nonthreatening. Clients are less likely to respond honestly to drug use if they are unaware of potential drug interactions. Open-ended questions should be used because close-ended questions elicit only a "yes/no" response. Statements and questions made to a patient should be nonthreatening to elicit a more honest answer.

➧ ***Test-taking Tip:*** *Use therapeutic communication techniques to answer this question.*

Content Area: Adult Health; *Category of Health Alteration:* Perioperative Management; *Integrated Processes:* Nursing Process Implementation; Communication and Documentation; *Client Need:* Physiological Integrity/Reduction of Risk Potential/Potential for Complications from Surgical Procedures and Health Alterations; Psychosocial Integrity/Therapeutic Communications; *Cognitive Level:* Analysis

Reference: Lewis, S., Heitkemper, M., Dirksen, S., O'Brien, P., & Bucher, L. (2007). *Medical-Surgical Nursing: Assessment and Management of Clinical Problems* (7th ed., p. 354). St. Louis, MO: Mosby.

874. A nurse evaluates that a preoperative client can properly use a volume incentive spirometer when which client action is noted?

1. Sits upright, inserts the mouthpiece, and blows until the lungs are emptied of air
2. Sits upright, exhales, seals lips around the mouthpiece, inhales, and holds breath for 5 seconds
3. Sits at the edge of the bed, coughs, inserts the mouthpiece, and blows slowly for 10 seconds
4. Sits at the edge of the bed, breathes deeply five times, inserts the mouthpiece, and inhales quickly

ANSWER: 2

Sitting upright promotes lung expansion. With all types of incentive spirometers, the client must be able to seal the lips tightly around the mouthpiece and inhale slowly. The client then holds the breath for 3 to 5 seconds for effective lung expansion. The client should be inhaling, not blowing. Coughing will help expel secretions and allow for full lung aeration. The client should be inhaling slowly and holding the breath before exhalation to promote lung expansion.

➧ ***Test-taking Tip:** Visualize a client using an incentive spirometer before trying to answer this question.*

Content Area: Adult Health; *Category of Health Alteration:* Perioperative Management; *Integrated Processes:* Nursing Process Evaluation; *Client Need:* Physiological Integrity/Reduction of Risk Potential/Therapeutic Procedures; *Cognitive Level:* Analysis

Reference: Ignatavicius, D., & Workman, M. (2006). *Medical-Surgical Nursing: Critical Thinking for Collaborative Care* (5th ed., p. 309). St. Louis, MO: Elsevier/Saunders.

875. EBP A nurse is teaching a client prior to surgery about the device illustrated. The nurse teaches the client that the *primary purpose* of the device illustrated is to:

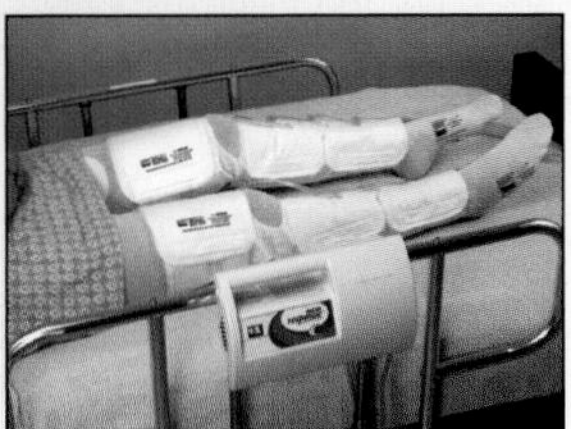

1. improve circulation prior to surgery.
2. prevent intra- and postoperative deep vein thrombosis.
3. assist in keeping the client warm during surgery.
4. promote dehiscence and wound healing postoperatively.

ANSWER: 2

Sequential compression devices (SCDs) are used postoperatively to prevent deep vein thrombosis. The device promotes fluid movement by simulating leg muscles contraction. The stocking compartments inflate to 35 to 55 mm Hg, inflating from the ankle, to the calf, and finally the thigh. Circulation may be improved, but this is not the primary purpose. SCDs have a cooling and warming option, but this is not the primary purpose. SCDs will have no effect on wound healing.

➧ ***Test-taking Tip:** Note the key words "primary purpose."*

Content Area: Adult Health; *Category of Health Alteration:* Perioperative Management; *Integrated Processes:* Teaching and Learning; *Client Need:* Physiological Integrity/Reduction of Risk Potential/Potential for Complications from Surgical Procedures and Health Alterations; *Cognitive Level:* Application

Reference: Lewis, S., Heitkemper, M., Dirksen, S., O'Brien, P., & Bucher, L. (2007). *Medical-Surgical Nursing: Assessment and Management of Clinical Problems* (7th ed., pp. 911–912). St. Louis, MO: Mosby.

EBP Reference: Blondin, M. (2006). *Prevention of Deep Vein Thrombosis.* Iowa City: University of Iowa Gerontological Nursing Research Center, Research Dissemination Core. Available at: www.guideline.gov/summary/summary.aspx?doc_id=9266&nbr=004960&string=graduated+AND+compression+AND+stockings.

876. A client in an operating room holding area, who is to receive general anesthesia, reports having a dry mouth because food and fluids have been withheld for 8 hours. Which action by a nurse is most appropriate?

1. Teach the client that the primary reason food and fluids have been withheld is to prevent vomiting and potential complications
2. Clarify that food and fluids should have been withheld only for 4 hours and offer a small sip of water
3. Explain to the client that a full stomach puts pressure on the diaphragm and prevents full lung expansion during surgery
4. Tell the client that the general anesthetic will soon make the client sleepy and unaware of the mouth dryness

ANSWER: 1

The client should have nothing by mouth (NPO) for 6 to 8 hours prior to general anesthesia to prevent vomiting and aspiration. The client may have ordered medications with a sip of water (about 20 mL). Prior to general anesthesia, the client should be NPO for 6 to 8 hours. A full stomach putting pressure on the diaphragm and preventing full lung expansion during surgery is not the primary reason for the NPO status. Telling the client that the anesthesia will soon cause unawareness of the dry mouth disregards the client's concerns.

➧ ***Test-taking Tip:** Note the key words "most appropriate." Client teaching is most appropriate in the preoperative period.*

Content Area: Adult Health; *Category of Health Alteration:* Perioperative Management; *Integrated Processes:* Nursing Process Implementation; *Client Need:* Physiological Integrity/Reduction of Risk Potential/Potential for Complications from Surgical Procedures and Health Alterations; *Cognitive Level:* Application

Reference: Ignatavicius, D., & Workman, M. (2006). *Medical-Surgical Nursing: Critical Thinking for Collaborative Care* (5th ed., p. 306). St. Louis, MO: Elsevier/Saunders.

877. A nurse is caring for a client who received conscious sedation during a surgical procedure. Which assessment of this client is most important for a nurse to make postoperatively?

1. Lung sounds
2. Amount of urine output
3. Ability to swallow liquids
4. Rate and depth of breathing

ANSWER: 4

The rate and depth of breathing should be assessed to determine the adequacy of air exchange. A respiratory rate of less than 10 breaths per minute indicates drug-induced respiratory depression. The primary concern with conscious sedation is the effect of the medications on the central nervous system (CNS). Lung sounds are assessed to determine the adequacy of ventilation of all lung lobes or the presence of fluid or secretions in the airways and lung tissue. Though assessing the lung sounds is important postoperatively, assessing the rate and depth of breathing is *most* important with conscious sedation. Though urine output should be at least 30 mL/hr and medications administered can potentially be nephrotoxic, it is more important to assess the rate and depth of respirations with conscious sedation. The client swallowing ability should be assessed prior to administering liquids. However, it is more important to assess the rate and depth of respirations with conscious sedation.

➧ ***Test-taking Tip:*** *Note the key words "most important." Use the ABCs (airway, breathing, circulation) to identify the correct response.*

Content Area: Adult Health; *Category of Health Alteration:* Perioperative Management; *Integrated Processes:* Nursing Process Assessment; *Client Need:* Physiological Integrity/Reduction of Risk Potential/System Specific Assessments; *Cognitive Level:* Application

Reference: Ignatavicius, D., & Workman, M. (2006). *Medical-Surgical Nursing: Critical Thinking for Collaborative Care* (5th ed., p. 332). St. Louis, MO: Elsevier/Saunders.

878. Upon arrival to an operating room holding area, a client who is scheduled for abdominal surgery is noted to have replaced a tongue ring that was removed when the operative checklist was completed. Which is the most appropriate initial action by a nurse?

1. Document the findings on the client's medical record
2. Request that the client once again remove the tongue ring
3. Complete a variance report, noting that the client has replaced the tongue ring
4. Notify the surgeon and the anesthesiologist of the replacement of the tongue ring

ANSWER: 2

Because anesthesia and surgery have not yet started, it is safe to ask the client to remove the tongue ring. If the client refuses, then the surgeon and anesthesiologist should be notified. Documentation regarding finding the tongue ring replaced should occur after the intervention. A variance report should be completed because the item should have been removed before the client arrived to the holding area. Tongue rings increase the risk of aspiration, burns, and injury during surgery. Notifying the surgeon and the anesthesiologist is not the first action. If the client removes the tongue ring, the surgeon and anesthesiologist would not need to be notified.

➧ ***Test-taking Tip:*** *Note the key word "first." Use the nursing process. The nurse has already assessed and analyzed. The next step is intervention. Decide the priority action.*

Content Area: Adult Health; *Category of Health Alteration:* Perioperative Management; *Integrated Processes:* Nursing Process Implementation; *Client Need:* Physiological Integrity/Reduction of Risk Potential/Potential from Surgical Procedures and Health Alterations; *Cognitive Level:* Application

Reference: Ignatavicius, D., & Workman, M. (2006). *Medical-Surgical Nursing: Critical Thinking for Collaborative Care* (5th ed., p. 333). St. Louis, MO: Elsevier/Saunders.

879. EBP A nurse is orienting a new nurse to a postanesthesia care unit (PACU). Which statement by the new nurse indicates further orientation is needed?

1. "Lactated Ringer's (LR) and 5% dextrose with LR are typical IV solutions administered in the PACU."
2. "If a client has an opioid overdose, I should expect to administer naloxone hydrochloride (Narcan®)."
3. "I should monitor vital signs and perform a pain assessment every 15 minutes or more often if necessary."
4. "Once a client responds verbally after a spinal anesthetic, the client can be transferred to the nursing unit."

ANSWER: 4

The client receiving a spinal anesthetic should remain in the PACU until feeling and voluntary motor movement of the lower extremities has begun to return. Because the client did not receive a general anesthetic that depressed the central nervous system, the client may be verbally responsive immediately after surgery. Both LR and dextrose with LR solutions are isotonic and are used for fluid replacement in the PACU. After returning to the medical-surgical unit, the type and amount of solution are based on client need. Naloxone hydrochloride (Narcan®) is an antagonist for opioids and is used for reversing the respiratory-depressive effects of opioid analgesics. Vital sign observations and pain assessment should be completed every 15 minutes or more frequently based on the client's condition.

▶ ***Test-taking Tip:*** *Note the key words "further orientation is needed." The correct answer is the wrong statement.*

Content Area: Adult Health; *Category of Health Alteration:* Perioperative Management; *Integrated Processes:* Teaching and Learning; *Client Need:* Safe and Effective Care Environment/Management of Care/Concepts of Management; *Cognitive Level:* Analysis

Reference: Ignatavicius, D., & Workman, M. (2006). *Medical-Surgical Nursing: Critical Thinking for Collaborative Care* (5th ed., pp. 344, 353). St. Louis, MO: Elsevier/Saunders.

EBP Reference: The Joanna Briggs Institute. (1999). Vital signs. *Best Practice,* 3(3). Available at: www.joannabriggs.edu.au/pubs/best_ practice.php

880. Which information is most important for a postanesthesia care unit nurse to include in a report on a postoperative client to a surgical unit nurse?

1. Location of the relatives
2. Review of the surgical consent
3. Placement of client belongings
4. Last dose and type of pain medication

ANSWER: 4

Pain is the fifth vital sign. Time and dose is the reference for implementing the pain protocol or developing a plan for the client's pain control. The hand-off of the client to another area is the ideal time to insure the continuation of care, as well as the transfer of responsibility. The nurse should check for the presence of family or significant others. However, this is not the most important. Reviewing the consent is unnecessary postoperatively. If the client needs a blood transfusion, the nurse may need to review the consent for a blood transfusion prior to administering blood or blood products. This may be a part of the surgical consent but varies by institution. The nurse should note where the client's belongings are placed if the client was not previously on the surgical unit. However, this is not the most important.

▶ ***Test-taking Tip:*** *Use Maslow's Hierarchy of Needs to identify the correct option. Note the physiological need.*

Content Area: Adult Health; *Category of Health Alteration:* Perioperative Management; *Integrated Processes:* Nursing Process Implementation; *Client Need:* Safe and Effective Care Environment/Management of Care/Continuity of Care; *Cognitive Level:* Application

Reference: Lewis, S., Heitkemper, M., Dirksen, S., O'Brien, P., & Bucher, L. (2007). *Medical-Surgical Nursing: Assessment and Management of Clinical Problems* (7th ed., pp. 378, 388). St. Louis, MO: Mosby.

881. A nurse evaluates that a client has achieved an expected outcome for the second postoperative day following abdominal surgery under general anesthesia. Which finding supports the nurse's conclusion?

1. Passing flatus
2. Urine output 680 mL in 24 hours
3. Crackles in bilateral lung bases
4. Rates incisional pain at 4 out of 10 on a 0 to 10 rating scale 60 minutes after analgesic given

ANSWER: 1

Passing flatus indicates increased gastrointestinal motility and the return of bowel function. The urine output should be at least 30 mL per hour or at least 720 mL in 24 hours. Crackles indicate atelectasis or fluid accumulation in the lungs. Incisional pain is the most intense in the first 48 hours. An expected outcome should be a pain level of 3 or less.

▶ ***Test-taking Tip:*** *Focus on the key words "achieved an expected outcome." Look for an indication that the client's status is improving.*

Content Area: Adult Health; *Category of Health Alteration:* Perioperative Management; *Integrated Processes:* Nursing Process Evaluation; *Client Need:* Physiological Integrity/Physiological Adaptation/Alterations in Body Systems; *Cognitive Level:* Analysis

Reference: Ignatavicius, D., & Workman, M. (2006). *Medical-Surgical Nursing: Critical Thinking for Collaborative Care* (5th ed., p. 345). St. Louis, MO: Elsevier/Saunders.

882. A nurse is planning the discharge of a client following recovery from an exploratory laparotomy. The client has a history of chronic back pain and limited ability to ambulate. The nurse plans for further discharge teaching when the client states:

1. "I can leave my elastic antiembolic (TEDS®) stockings off once I get home."
2. "I should be eating a diet high in protein, calories, and vitamin C now and when I get home."
3. "An alternative method to control pain and reduce swelling is applying ice to my incision."
4. "I use my incentive spirometer every 2 hours so I can reach my volume goal before discharge."

ANSWER: 1

Because the client has limited ability to ambulate, the client should continue to wear the TED stockings at home to prevent deep vein thrombosis until the client increases ambulation. The TEDS should be removed one to two times daily for skin care and inspection. Clients provided with preoperative teaching pamphlets learn proper exercise techniques or skills faster than those provided the information postadmission. A diet high in protein, calories, and vitamin C will promote wound healing. A nonpharmacological method to reduce postoperative pain and promote comfort includes ice application. Specific volume goals are usually set based on the client's ability and the type of incentive spirometer. Achievement of the volume goal is an expected postoperative outcome that should be met prior to discharge.

▸ ***Test-taking Tip:*** *Focus on the key words "limited ability to ambulate." Both TEDS and ambulation promote venous return.*

Content Area: Adult Health; *Category of Health Alteration:* Perioperative Management; *Integrated Processes:* Nursing Process Planning; *Client Need:* Physiological Integrity/Reduction of Risk Potential/Potential for Complications from Surgical Procedures and Health Alterations; *Cognitive Level:* Application

Reference: Ignatavicius, D., & Workman, M. (2006). *Medical-Surgical Nursing: Critical Thinking for Collaborative Care* (5th ed., p. 354). St. Louis, MO: Elsevier/Saunders.

---

883. A nurse is reviewing a plan of care for a postoperative client with a history of sickle cell disease. Which nursing diagnosis, documented on the client's care plan, should the nurse address *first*?

1. Anxiety
2. Impaired skin integrity
3. Deficient fluid volume
4. Ineffective airway clearance

ANSWER: 4

An open airway is a physiological need that is priority. Ineffective airway clearance in a postoperative client is often due to an ineffective or absent cough and the accumulation of secretions that compromise the airway. Anxiety is a psychosocial need and is not the priority. Impaired skin integrity is a physiological need, but of lower priority than an open airway. Deficient fluid volume is a physiological problem, but of lower priority than an open airway.

▸ ***Test-taking Tip:*** *Note the key word "first." Use Maslow's Hierarchy of Needs theory to identify that physiological needs are the first priority. Then use the ABCs (airway, breathing, circulation) to further prioritize the physiological needs.*

Content Area: Adult Health; *Category of Health Alteration:* Perioperative Management; *Integrated Processes:* Nursing Process Planning; *Client Need:* Physiological Integrity/Physiological Adaptation/Alterations in Body Systems; *Cognitive Level:* Application

Reference: Ignatavicius, D., & Workman, M. (2006). *Medical-Surgical Nursing: Critical Thinking for Collaborative Care* (5th ed., p. 348). St. Louis, MO: Elsevier/Saunders.

---

884. A nurse is caring for a postoperative client who reports an inability to void. Which initial action by the nurse is most appropriate?

1. Turning on running water
2. Inserting a urinary catheter
3. Palpating the client's bladder
4. Reviewing the client's chart for the time of the last voiding

ANSWER: 3

The bladder should be palpated for distention. The nurse should also observe for other signs of a full bladder such as restlessness or an elevated blood pressure. The nurse should first determine the underlying reason for the client's inability to void. Turning on running water assumes that the client has a full bladder. A urinary catheter should only be inserted if the client has a full bladder and other measures to initiate voiding have been unsuccessful. Though reviewing the chart for the time of the last voiding may assist in determining the underlying problem, client assessment should be the first action.

▸ ***Test-taking Tip:*** *Use the steps in the nursing process to identify the correct answer. Assessment should be completed before interventions are implemented.*

Content Area: Adult Health; *Category of Health Alteration:* Perioperative Management; *Integrated Processes:* Nursing Process Assessment; *Client Need:* Physiological Integrity/Basic Care and Comfort/Elimination; *Cognitive Level:* Application

Reference: Ignatavicius, D., & Workman, M. (2006). *Medical-Surgical Nursing: Critical Thinking for Collaborative Care* (5th ed., p. 344). St. Louis, MO: Elsevier/Saunders.

885. A postoperative client who received a spinal anesthetic is experiencing a headache, photophobia, and double vision. A nurse's initial intervention should be to:

1. immediately notify the surgeon.
2. position the client flat in bed.
3. limit the client's fluid intake.
4. administer steroid medications.

ANSWER: 2

The client is experiencing a postdural puncture headache caused by leakage of cerebrospinal fluid (CSF) from the needle insertion made in the dura for the spinal anesthetic. Placing the client in the flat position minimizes the leakage of CSF. The surgeon should be notified of the development as well as the anesthesiologist if the headache persists despite interventions or there is noticeable leakage of CSF. Fluids should be increased to hydrate the client and replace fluids lost from the CSF leakage. If the headache persists, steroids may be ordered to decrease inflammation, but this is not an initial intervention.

➧ ***Test-taking Tip:*** *Note the key word "initial." Also note that positioning the client flat in bed is an intervention that the nurse could accomplish quickly to reduce the client's headache.*

Content Area: Adult Health; *Category of Health Alteration:* Perioperative Management; *Integrated Processes:* Nursing Process Implementation; *Client Need:* Physiological Integrity/Physiological Adaptation/Unexpected Response to Therapies; *Cognitive Level:* Application

References: Ignatavicius, D., & Workman, M. (2006). *Medical-Surgical Nursing: Critical Thinking for Collaborative Care* (5th ed., p. 942). St. Louis, MO: Elsevier/Saunders; Williams, L., & Hopper, P. (2007). *Understanding Medical-Surgical Nursing* (3rd ed., p. 189). Philadelphia: F. A. Davis.

886. A physician documents in a client's postoperative progress notes that the client is experiencing a respiratory infection with a shift to the left in the white blood cell (WBC) differential count. Which finding by a nurse reviewing the client's laboratory report would support the physician's documentation?

1. Decreased WBC count
2. Increased band cells
3. Decreased hemoglobin
4. Increased C-reactive protein

ANSWER: 2

An early indication of infection is an increase in the band cells, which are immature neutrophils in the WBC differential count. The increase is termed a *shift to the left*. The total WBC count should be elevated, not decreased. However, this does not describe the shift to the left. Decreased hemoglobin in a postoperative client is usually due to blood loss. An increased C-reactive protein indicates nonspecific inflammation and is not part of the WBC differential count.

➧ ***Test-taking Tip:*** *Note the key words "shift to the left" and "WBC differential." Decreased hemoglobin and increased C-reactive protein do not pertain to the WBC. Increased C-reactive protein is opposite of what is expected with infection.*

Content Area: Adult Health; *Category of Health Alteration:* Perioperative Management; *Integrated Processes:* Nursing Process Evaluation; *Client Need:* Physiological Integrity/Reduction of Risk Potential/Laboratory Values; *Cognitive Level:* Analysis

Reference: Ignatavicius, D., & Workman, M. (2006). *Medical-Surgical Nursing: Critical Thinking for Collaborative Care* (5th ed., p. 347). St. Louis, MO: Elsevier/Saunders.

887. EBP In reviewing a physician's orders for a postoperative client who underwent gynecological surgery, which order should a nurse determine is specifically written with the intent to prevent postoperative thrombophlebitis and pulmonary embolism?

1. Have the client dangle the legs the evening of surgery
2. Administer enoxaparin (Lovenox®) 40 mg subcutaneously daily
3. Administer hydromorphone (Dilaudid®) 1 to 4 mg IV every 3 to 4 hours as needed (prn)
4. Encourage coughing and deep breathing (C&DB) every hour while awake

ANSWER: 2

Enoxaparin is an anticoagulant that potentiates the inhibitory effect of antithrombin on factor Xa and thrombin. Early postoperative ambulation instead of dangling is a major preventive technique for thrombophlebitis. Hydromorphone is a narcotic analgesic for pain control. Coughing and deep breathing promote lung expansion and prevent atelectasis and pneumonia.

➧ ***Test-taking Tip:*** *Note the key words "specifically written," and then eliminate options 1, 3, and 4 because they are not specific to preventing postoperative thrombophlebitis and pulmonary embolism. Knowledge of medications is needed to answer this question.*

Content Area: Adult Health; *Category of Health Alteration:* Perioperative Management; *Integrated Processes:* Nursing Process Analysis; *Client Need:* Physiological Integrity/Reduction of Risk Potential/Therapeutic Procedures; *Cognitive Level:* Analysis

Reference: Lewis, S., Heitkemper, M., Dirksen, S., O'Brien, P., & Bucher, L. (2007). *Medical-Surgical Nursing: Assessment and Management of Clinical Problems* (7th ed., pp. 911–912). St. Louis, MO: Mosby.

EBP Reference: American College of Obstetricians and Gynecologists. (2007). Prevention of deep vein thrombosis and pulmonary embolism. Available at: www.guideline.gov/summary/summary.aspx?doc_id=11429&nbr=005947&string=postoperative+AND+care

---

888. A nurse assesses that a client on the second postoperative day following abdominal surgery has diminished breath sounds in both lung bases, is taking shallow breaths, is able to achieve only 500 mL on an incentive spirometer, and has been smoking one pack of cigarettes per day prior to surgery. The nurse's best interpretation of these findings is that the client is experiencing:

1. atelectasis.
2. pneumonia.
3. a normal postoperative course.
4. chronic obstructive pulmonary disease (COPD).

ANSWER: 1

Atelectasis is a common finding in smokers after abdominal surgery due to the accumulation of secretions. It is caused from collapsed alveoli or mucus that prevents some alveoli from opening and manifests with diminished breath sounds, diminished vital capacity, and decreased oxygen saturation. There is no indication, such as elevated temperature or increased white blood cells, that the client has an infection. It should also be noted that the client is experiencing abnormal findings for the second postoperative day. Smoking can cause COPD, but the diminished lung bases suggest alveoli are not expanding.

➧ ***Test-taking Tip:*** *Note that the client is 2 days postabdominal surgery. Eliminate the options that occur over time.*

Content Area: Adult Health; *Category of Health Alteration:* Perioperative Management; *Integrated Processes:* Nursing Process Analysis; *Client Need:* Physiological Integrity/Physiological Adaptation/Alterations in Body Systems; *Cognitive Level:* Analysis

Reference: Lewis, S., Heitkemper, M., Dirksen, S., O'Brien, P., & Bucher, L. (2007). *Medical-Surgical Nursing: Assessment and Management of Clinical Problems* (7th ed., pp. 511–512, 597). St. Louis, MO: Mosby.

---

889. A nurse notes redness, swelling, and warmth of and around the incision when assessing a client's leg incision 48 hours after femoral popliteal bypass surgery. The nurse's best analysis should be that the incision is:

1. healing normally for the second postoperative day.
2. showing signs of rejection of the suture materials.
3. inflamed and could indicate the presence of an infection.
4. infected and showing signs of wound dehiscence.

ANSWER: 3

Redness, swelling, and warmth are signs of inflammation and could indicate the presence of an infection. Other signs of an infection include excessive pain or tenderness on palpation and purulent or odorous drainage. Slight crusting, a pink color to the incision line, and slight swelling under the sutures or staples are normal findings for the second postoperative day due to inflammation from the surgical procedure. Though these findings could indicate rejection of the sutures, rejection occurs less frequently than a wound infection. If the wound is dehiscing, bloody or serosanguineous drainage would also be present.

➧ ***Test-taking Tip:*** *Use the process of elimination and focus on the findings (redness, swelling, and warmth).*

Content Area: Adult Health; *Category of Health Alteration:* Perioperative Management; *Integrated Processes:* Nursing Process Analysis; *Client Need:* Physiological Integrity/Reduction of Risk Potential/Potential for Complications from Surgical Procedures and Health Alterations; *Cognitive Level:* Analysis

Reference: Ignatavicius, D., & Workman, M. (2006). *Medical-Surgical Nursing: Critical Thinking for Collaborative Care* (5th ed., p. 346). St. Louis, MO: Elsevier/Saunders.

890. Which outcome should indicate to a nurse that a post-surgical client's coughing and deep breathing (C&DB) is most effective?

1. Respirations are 16 per minute and unlabored.
2. Lung sounds are audible and clear on auscultation.
3. Coughs include small amount of clear secretions.
4. Cough effort is strong and productive.

ANSWER: 2

The purpose of postoperative C&DB is to expel secretions, keep the lungs clear, allow full aeration, and prevent pneumonia and atelectasis. Auscultating for clear and audible lung sounds is a definitive means for evaluating the effectiveness of C&DB. Secretions could still be present in the lungs with normal respirations and nonlabored breathing. Coughing clear secretions and a productive cough indicates that secretions are still present.

➧ ***Test-taking Tip:*** *Note the key words "most effective," and eliminate options that include abnormal data.*

Content Area: Adult Health; *Category of Health Alteration:* Perioperative Management; *Integrated Processes:* Nursing Process Evaluation; *Client Need:* Physiological Integrity/Physiological Adaptation/Illness Management; *Cognitive Level:* Application

Reference: Ignatavicius, D., & Workman, M. (2006). *Medical-Surgical Nursing: Critical Thinking for Collaborative Care* (5th ed., p. 309). St. Louis, MO: Elsevier/Saunders.

---

891. A client is to receive a second dose of oxycodone/acetaminophen (Percocet®) for postoperative incisional pain. When a nurse brings the medication to the client, the client says, "Why bring this medication again? It makes me feel sick." Which statement is the most appropriate initial nurse response?

1. "I can call the doctor to see what else can be ordered for your pain."
2. "Describe what you feel when you say that the medication makes you feel sick."
3. "The doctor has ordered an antacid. I can give you this along with the medication."
4. "Many people say the same thing. The aspirin in the medication is hard on your stomach."

ANSWER: 2

The nurse is using the therapeutic communication technique, known as clarifying, to determine the effects of the medication on the client. This focuses on the client's feelings. Simply offering new medication avoids the client's feelings. Also, without questioning the client, the nurse would have insufficient information to give to the physician regarding the client's reaction to the medication. Offering an antacid also avoids the client's concerns and assumes that the client has a gastrointestinal reaction to the medication. Even though option 4 focuses on the client's nausea, incorrect information is provided. Oxycodone/acetaminophen does not contain aspirin.

➧ ***Test-taking Tip:*** *Use therapeutic communication techniques and focus on the client's feelings, concerns, fears, or anxieties. Eliminate options that provide incorrect information.*

Content Area: Adult Health; *Category of Health Alteration:* Perioperative Management; *Integrated Processes:* Communication and Documentation; *Client Need:* Psychosocial Integrity/Therapeutic Communications; *Cognitive Level:* Application

References: Berman, A., Snyder, S., Kozier, B., & Erb, G. (2008). *Kozier & Erb's Fundamentals of Nursing: Concepts, Process, and Practice* (8th ed., pp. 469–471). Upper Saddle River, NJ: Pearson Education; Wilson, B., Shannon, M., Shields, K., & Stang, C. (2008). *Prentice Hall Nurse's Drug Guide 2008* (p. 1656). Upper Saddle River, NJ: Pearson Education.

---

892. A nurse evaluates that the drainage from a client's nasogastric (NG) tube, inserted for gastric decompression during emergency surgery, would be normal if it:

1. returns brown-liquid in color.
2. returns greenish-yellow in color.
3. has an alkalotic hydrogen level (pH).
4. measures less than 25 mL in volume.

ANSWER: 2

Normal NG drainage fluid is greenish yellow in color. Brown liquid or drainage with a "coffee-ground" appearance indicates old bleeding. The pH of gastric secretions would be acidic. In emergency surgery, large amounts of output would be expected because the client's stomach was unlikely to be empty.

➧ ***Test-taking Tip:*** *Note the key word "normal."*

Content Area: Adult Health; *Category of Health Alteration:* Perioperative Management; *Integrated Processes:* Nursing Process Evaluation; *Client Need:* Physiological Integrity/Physiological Adaptation/Fluid and Electrolyte Imbalances; *Cognitive Level:* Application

Reference: Ignatavicius, D., & Workman, M. (2006). *Medical-Surgical Nursing: Critical Thinking for Collaborative Care* (5th ed., p. 345). St. Louis, MO: Elsevier/Saunders.

893. A nurse notifies a physician after assessing a client 5 days after an exploratory laparotomy and noting a distended abdomen, abdominal pain, absence of flatus, and absent bowel sounds. Which *typical* complication of abdominal surgery should the nurse conclude may be occurring?

1. Paralytic ileus
2. Silent peritonitis
3. Fluid volume excess
4. Malabsorption syndrome

ANSWER: 1

Paralytic ileus results from a neuromuscular disturbance and does not involve a physical obstruction in or outside the intestine. Peristalsis is decreased or absent, resulting in a slowing of the movement or a backup of intestinal contents. In addition to the symptoms the client is experiencing, nausea and vomiting may be present. The client would not have any signs or symptoms with silent peritonitis. The distended abdomen could indicate that fluid may have shifted into the abdomen. However, fluid volume deficit would then occur and not excess. There is an interference with absorption of nutrients in malabsorption syndrome. Typical signs and symptoms include weight loss, bloating and flatus, edema, bone pain, anemia, easy bruising, and decreased libido.

▶ ***Test-taking Tip:*** *Note the key words "typical complication of abdominal surgery" and eliminate options that occur over a longer period of time.*

Content Area: Adult Health; *Category of Health Alteration:* Perioperative Management; *Integrated Processes:* Nursing Process Analysis; *Client Need:* Physiological Integrity/Reduction of Risk Potential/Potential for Complications from Surgical Procedures and Health Alterations; *Cognitive Level:* Analysis

Reference: Ignatavicius, D., & Workman, M. (2006). *Medical-Surgical Nursing: Critical Thinking for Collaborative Care* (5th ed., pp. 345, 1326–1327). St. Louis, MO: Elsevier/Saunders.

---

894. Which statement should a nurse include when teaching a client prior to discharge following abdominal surgery?

1. "Return to work in about 4 weeks because working increases your physical activity gradually."
2. "The ordered iron and vitamins tablets will promote wound healing and red blood cell growth."
3. "Daily walking carrying 10-pound weights will help to strengthen your incision."
4. "Home-care nursing service is usually paid by insurance if you need help around the house."

ANSWER: 2

In addition to vitamins and iron, supplemental vitamin C and a diet high in protein and calories will promote wound healing. Surgery stresses the body, and time and rest are needed for healing. The client should return to work only after consulting with the surgeon. If work involves a moderate amount of physical labor, up to 6 weeks time off may be needed for recovery. Daily walking should be encouraged, but carrying 10-pound weights or lifting heavy objects stresses the incision. Although the wound may appear to be healed in 2 to 3 weeks, it takes up to 2 years for complete wound healing and strengthening of the scar. A referral to a home-care agency should be made if skilled nursing care such as complex dressing changes is needed. Nursing service does not include household help.

▶ ***Test-taking Tip:*** *Note the key words "should . . . include." Read each option carefully noting key words that would make an option incorrect.*

Content Area: Adult Health; *Category of Health Alteration:* Perioperative Management; *Integrated Processes:* Teaching and Learning; *Client Need:* Health Promotion and Maintenance/Self-Care; *Cognitive Level:* Analysis

Reference: Ignatavicius, D., & Workman, M. (2006). *Medical-Surgical Nursing: Critical Thinking for Collaborative Care* (5th ed., pp. 354–355). St. Louis, MO: Elsevier/Saunders.

---

895. A nurse is calculating nasogastric (NG) tube drainage for a postoperative client. At 0700 hours, the client's drainage container was marked at 150 mL. At 1500 hours, there was 575 mL in the container. During the nursing shift, the nurse instilled 30 mL of saline irrigation into the tube four times as prescribed by the physician. The nurse calculates that the actual NG tube drainage for the client from 0700 to 1500 hours is _____ mL.

ANSWER: 305

575 mL – 150 mL = 425 mL of drainage in the container
30 mL × 4 = 120 mL of irrigation solution
425 mL – 120 mL = 305 mL of actual drainage

▶ ***Test-taking Tip:*** *Focus on the information in the question and use the on-screen calculator. Verify your response especially if it seems like an unusual amount.*

Content Area: Adult Health; *Category of Health Alteration:* Perioperative Management; *Integrated Processes:* Nursing Process Implementation; *Client Need:* Physiological Integrity/Physiological Adaptation/Alterations in Body Systems; *Cognitive Level:* Analysis

Reference: Ignatavicius, D., & Workman, M. (2006). *Medical-Surgical Nursing: Critical Thinking for Collaborative Care* (5th ed., p. 345). St. Louis, MO: Elsevier/Saunders.

896. A nurse assesses that two areas of a client's postoperative leg incision are not approximated. Place an X on the two areas in the illustration that correctly depict the nurse's wound assessment.

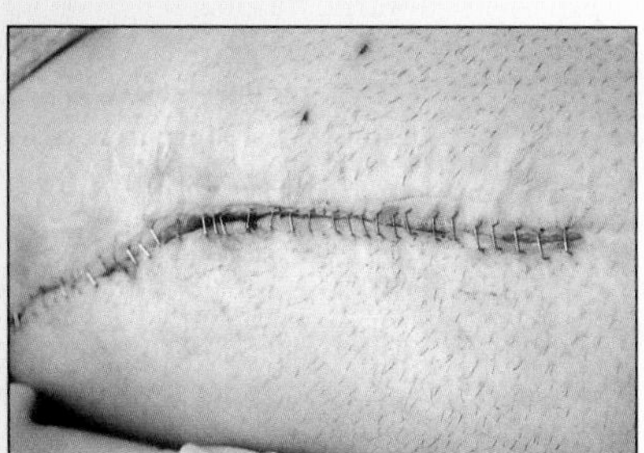

ANSWER:

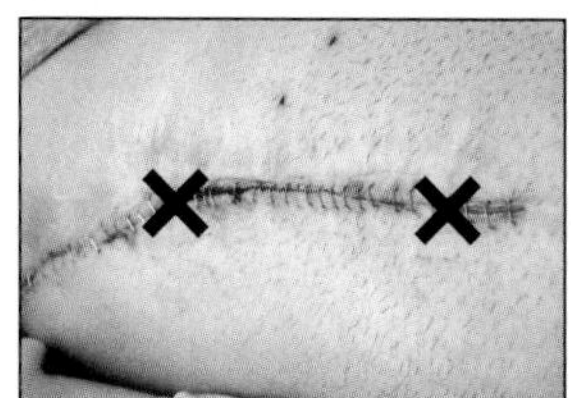

A nonapproximated incision is one in which wound edges are not closed. The wound will close by secondary intention healing.

➧ *Test-taking Tip: Read the stem carefully, noting the words "not approximated."*

Content Area: Adult Health; *Category of Health Alteration:* Perioperative Management; *Integrated Processes:* Nursing Process Assessment; *Client Need:* Health Promotion and Maintenance/Techniques of Physical Assessment; *Cognitive Level:* Application

Reference: Lewis, S., Heitkemper, M., Dirksen, S., O'Brien, P., & Bucher, L. (2007). *Medical-Surgical Nursing: Assessment and Management of Clinical Problems* (7th ed., p. 392). St. Louis, MO: Mosby.

897. A nurse is interpreting the serum laboratory report illustrated for a postoperative client. The nurse, notifying a physician of the laboratory results, should expect the physician to order which stat order?

Serum Laboratory Test	Client's Value	Normal Values
BUN	40	5–25 mg/dL
Creatinine	1.4	0.5–1.5 mg/dL
Na	140	135–145 mEq/L
K	3.2	3.5–5.3 mEq/L
Cl	99	95–105 mEq/L
CO_2	16	22–30 mEq/L
Phosphate	1.9	1.7–2.6 mEq/L
Calcium	9	9–11 mg/dL
Hgb	11	13.5–17 g/dL
Hct	38%	40%–54%

1. Administer 1 unit packed red blood cells (RBCs).
2. Administer potassium chloride 10 mEq in 100 mL 0.9% NaCl via intravenous piggyback (IVPB).
3. Hold the ACE inhibitor enalapril (Vasotec®).
4. Administer calcium gluconate 10 mEq in 100 mL 0.9% NaCl via IVPB.

ANSWER: 2

A low serum potassium (K) level can cause cardiac dysrhythmias. Potassium is lost through nasogastric (NG) suctioning and tissue destruction. The potassium needs to be replaced immediately. Unless the client is showing symptoms of inadequate tissue perfusion, blood would not be replaced with a hemoglobin (Hgb) level of 11.0. The nurse should be alert for the development of hyperkalemia, not hypokalemia, with angiotensin-converting enzyme (ACE) inhibitors such as enalapril (Vasotec®) especially with clients who have diabetes mellitus, impaired kidney function, or congestive heart failure (CHF). Calcium gluconate is administered in acute hypocalcemia to replace calcium. It is also administered when a client's serum potassium level is elevated to raise the threshold for cardiac muscle excitation, thereby preventing life-threatening dysrhythmias.

➧ *Test-taking Tip: Use the ABCs (airway, breathing, circulation) to determine the priority intervention. Both the serum K level and the hemoglobin/hematocrit (Hgb/Hct) affect oxygenation and circulation. However, the low serum K level is more critical than the low Hgb/Hct level because the serum K level affects cardiac muscle function.*

Content Area: Adult Health; *Category of Health Alteration:* Perioperative Management; *Integrated Processes:* Nursing Process Analysis; *Client Need:* Physiological Integrity/Physiological Adaptation/Fluid and Electrolyte Imbalances; *Cognitive Level:* Analysis

Reference: Wilson, B., Shannon, M., Shields, K., & Stang, C. (2008). *Prentice Hall Nurse's Drug Guide 2008* (pp. 221–223, 543–545, 1243–1245). Upper Saddle River, NJ: Pearson Education.

Test 23: **Adult Health: Renal and Urinary Management**

898. A nurse is planning care for a client who is scheduled for an intravenous pyelogram (IVP). Which intervention should the nurse include in the care of this client?

1. Teaching the client that a warm, flushing sensation may be experienced as the dye is injected
2. Preparing the client for a bladder catheterization before the procedure
3. Keeping the client NPO after the procedure until test results are obtained
4. Ambulating the client in the hall to promote excretion of the dye

ANSWER: 1

The client may experience a warm, flushing sensation up the arm or upper body and experience a strange taste when the dye is injected. Bladder catheterization is needed only if the client is unable to void. The client should increase intake of fluids to promote clearance of the dye. The client is usually allowed activity as tolerated. No activity is prescribed. Fluids, not ambulation, promote dye excretion.

▶ ***Test-taking Tip:*** *Use the process of elimination and focus on the issue of pre- and post-procedure care for an IVP.*

Content Area: Adult Health; *Category of Health Alteration:* Renal and Urinary Management; *Integrated Processes:* Nursing Process Planning; *Client Need:* Physiological Integrity/Reduction of Risk Potential/Diagnostic Tests; *Cognitive Level:* Analysis

Reference: Monahan, F., Sands, J., Neighbors, M., Marek, J., & Green, C. (2007). *Phipps' Medical-Surgical Nursing: Health and Illness Perspectives* (8th ed., p. 956). St. Louis, MO: Mosby/Elsevier.

---

899. A nurse assessing a client's right groin puncture site after a renal angiogram finds a saturated, bloody dressing and blood pooling on the sheets. What should be the nurse's *first* action?

1. Remove the dressing to further assess the puncture site
2. Reinforce the dressing with a compression dressing
3. Apply firm pressure directly over the puncture site dressing with a gloved hand
4. Have the client flex the right leg to help control the bleeding by constriction

ANSWER: 3

The assessment suggests arterial bleeding, so 5 minutes of direct pressure should be applied to the site first. A saturated dressing with blood pooling indicates the client is hemorrhaging. Direct pressure is required to control bleeding before removing the dressing to check the puncture site. A compression dressing is insufficient to control arterial bleeding, although it can be used to prevent further bleeding. Flexing the leg is contraindicated. It can dislodge an already partially formed clot and initiate further bleeding.

▶ ***Test-taking Tip:*** *Note the key word "first." Read the question carefully and focus on the stem of the question. Because this is an emergency situation, an intervention, not further assessment, is the first priority.*

Content Area: Adult Health; *Category of Health Alteration:* Renal and Urinary Management; *Integrated Processes:* Nursing Process Implementation; *Client Need:* Physiological Integrity/Reduction of Risk Potential/Potential for Complications of Diagnostic Tests/Treatments/Procedures; *Cognitive Level:* Application

References: Monahan, F., Sands, J., Neighbors, M., Marek, J., & Green, C. (2007). *Phipps' Medical-Surgical Nursing: Health and Illness Perspectives* (8th ed., p. 957). St. Louis, MO: Mosby/Elsevier; Smeltzer, S., Bare, B., Hinkle, J., & Cheever, K. (2008). *Brunner & Suddarth's Textbook of Medical-Surgical Nursing* (11th ed., pp. 2526–2527). Philadelphia: Lippincott Williams & Wilkins.

---

900. A nurse notes blood clots in a client's urine after a cystoscopy. Which is the most appropriate *initial* action by the nurse?

1. Perform bladder irrigation
2. Notify the health-care provider (HCP)
3. Apply heat to the client's bladder area
4. Administer the prescribed antispasmodic agent

ANSWER: 2

Blood-tinged urine is expected after a cystoscopy, but bright red bleeding and clots are abnormal and should be reported to the HCP. Hemorrhage is a complication of cystoscopy. Although the HCP may order bladder irrigation, this should not be the nurse's initial action. Heat may decrease the client's discomfort, but may increase bleeding. An antispasmodic medication will reduce the pain from spasms and contractions of the bladder and sphincter, but will not control bleeding.

▶ ***Test-taking Tip:*** *Note the key word "initial." Clots suggest a potential complication of hemorrhage; thus, the priority should be to notify the health-care provider.*

Content Area: Adult Health; *Category of Health Alteration:* Renal and Urinary Management; *Integrated Processes:* Nursing Process Implementation; *Client Need:* Safe and Effective Care Environment/ Management of Care/Establishing Priorities; Physiological Integrity/ Physiological Adaptation/Unexpected Response to Therapies; *Cognitive Level:* Analysis

Reference: Lewis, S., Heitkemper, M., Dirksen, S., O'Brien, P., & Bucher, L. (2007). *Medical-Surgical Nursing: Assessment and Management of Clinical Problems* (7th ed., p. 1149). St. Louis, MO: Mosby/Elsevier.

---

901. EBP Which nursing action should a nurse perform *first* for a client experiencing a suspected hospital-acquired bladder infection?

1. Obtain a clean-catch urine specimen for culture and sensitivity
2. Start antibiotic medications
3. Teach the client to wipe the perineum front to back after toileting
4. Prepare the client for bladder catheterization

ANSWER: 1

Urine should be cultured to identify the causative organism and the number of bacteria present. Urine should be collected before antibiotic treatment begins to avoid affecting results. Once the results of the urine culture are obtained (24 to 48 hours), the antibiotic may need to be changed to one to which the causative organism is sensitive. Using the appropriate antibiotic also prevents antibiotic resistance. A broad-spectrum antibiotic is usually ordered but should be started after a urine culture is obtained. Although the client should be taught to wipe the perineum from front to back, this is not the first action. Bladder catheterization is needed only if the client is unable to void.

Test-taking Tip: *Note the key word "first" in the stem.*

Content Area: Adult Health; *Category of Health Alteration:* Renal and Urinary Management; *Integrated Processes:* Nursing Process Implementation; *Client Need:* Safe and Effective Care Environment/ Management of Care/Establishing Priorities; Physiological Integrity/ Physiological Adaptation/Alterations in Body Systems; *Cognitive Level:* Application

Reference: Monahan, F., Sands, J., Neighbors, M., Marek, J., & Green, C. (2007). *Phipps' Medical-Surgical Nursing: Health and Illness Perspectives* (8th ed., p. 964). St. Louis, MO: Mosby/Elsevier.

EBP Reference: Larson, E., Quiros, D., Giblin, T., & Lin, S. (2007). Relationship of antimicrobial control policies and hospital and infection control characteristics to antimicrobial resistance rates. *American Journal of Critical Care*, 16(2), 110–119.

---

902. After completing a health history for a female client experiencing recurrent urinary tract infections (UTI), a nurse determines that the client should be taught to reduce her risk for a UTI by:

1. eliminating caffeine and tea from her diet.
2. taking tub baths rather than showers.
3. wearing good quality synthetic underwear.
4. abstaining from sexual intercourse.

ANSWER: 1

Caffeine-containing beverages, such as coffee, tea, and cocoa, and alcoholic beverages irritate the bladder and should be avoided. Showers, rather than tub baths, are recommended. Synthetic underwear and constricting clothing, such as tight jeans, should be avoided. Abstinence is unnecessary. The client should urinate after intercourse.

Test-taking Tip: *Note the key words "reduce her risk." Use the process of elimination to select option 1.*

Content Area: Adult Health; *Category of Health Alteration:* Renal and Urinary Management; *Integrated Processes:* Nursing Process Planning; Teaching and Learning; *Client Need:* Health Promotion and Maintenance/Self-Care; *Cognitive Level:* Analysis

Reference: Smeltzer, S., Bare, B., Hinkle, J., & Cheever, K. (2008). *Brunner & Suddarth's Textbook of Medical-Surgical Nursing* (11th ed., p. 1577). Philadelphia: Lippincott Williams & Wilkins.

903. A home health client verbalizes concerns about producing brown-colored urine after taking nitrofurantoin (Furadantin®) for a urinary tract infection. Which response by a nurse is most appropriate?

1. "Your urine is too concentrated. Take only one-half the dose of your medication."
2. "Discontinue taking the medication and make an appointment for a urine culture."
3. "Continue taking the medication because nitrofurantoin (Furadantin®) discolors the urine."
4. "Drink 500 mL of fluid every 3 hours to lighten your urine color."

ANSWER: 3

Nitrofurantoin (Furadantin®) produces a harmless, brown color to the urine. The medication should be discontinued only after the client's symptoms are alleviated or the prescribed dose is completed. Concentrated urine would be dark amber, not necessarily brown-colored. Medication dosages should not be changed without a physician's order. A urine culture should be performed before treatment is initiated, if treatment is ineffective, and during the follow-up appointment. A urine culture is not indicated at this time. Although increasing fluid intake will lighten the urine color, the urine will remain brown-colored.

➧ ***Test-taking Tip:*** *Use the process of elimination. Note the key word "most appropriate." Apply knowledge that nitrofurantoin (Furadantin®) turns the urine to a brownish color.*

Content Area: Adult Health; *Category of Health Alteration:* Renal and Urinary Management; *Integrated Processes:* Nursing Process Implementation; *Client Need:* Physiological Integrity/Pharmacological and Parenteral Therapies/Adverse Effects/Contraindications and Side Effects; *Cognitive Level:* Application

Reference: Deglin, J., & Vallerand, A. (2007). *Davis's Drug Guide for Nurses* (10th ed., pp. 867–868). Philadelphia: F. A. Davis.

904. EBP A client is admitted to a hospital with a diagnosis of acute pyelonephritis. Which symptom occurs most frequently and should be monitored by the nurse?

1. Low-grade fever
2. Bradycardia
3. Flank pain on the affected side
4. Rebound tenderness in left lower quadrant

ANSWER: 3

Typical manifestations of pyelonephritis include high fever, chills, tachycardia and tachypnea, nausea and vomiting, abdominal discomfort (often colicky), flank pain on the affected side with costovertebral angle tenderness, generalized weakness, nocturia, and urinary burning, urgency, or frequency. Fever is often present in acute pyelonephritis. Tachycardia, not bradycardia, occurs with fever. Rebound tenderness in the right lower quadrant could indicate appendicitis.

➧ ***Test-taking Tip:*** *Focus on the diagnosis of acute pyelonephritis. Note that "-itis" means inflammation or infection. Eliminate options 1 and 2 because these are not correct signs and symptoms of infection. Eliminate option 4 because it involves the lower abdomen and pyelonephritis involves the upper urinary tract.*

Content Area: Adult Health; *Category of Health Alteration:* Renal and Urinary Management; *Integrated Processes:* Nursing Process Assessment; *Client Need:* Physiological Integrity/Physiological Adaptation/Alterations in Body Systems; *Cognitive Level:* Application

Reference: Ignatavicius, D., & Workman, M. (2006). *Medical-Surgical Nursing: Critical Thinking for Collaborative Care* (5th ed., p. 1713). St. Louis, MO: Elsevier/Saunders.

EBP Reference: Institute for Clinical Systems Improvement (ICSI). (2006). *Uncomplicated Urinary Tract Infection in Women.* Available at: www.ngc.gov/summary/summary.aspx?doc_id=9657&nbr=005173&string=pyelonephritis

905. During a teaching session with a client, a nurse shows the client an illustration indicating the area of inflammation during a bout of pyelonephritis. Identify this area of inflammation with an X.

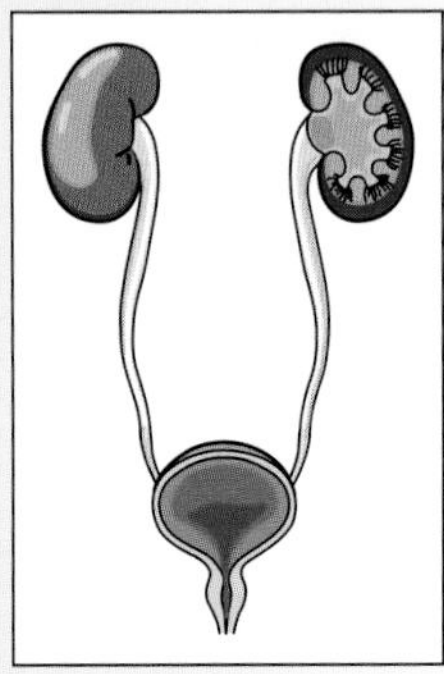

ANSWER:

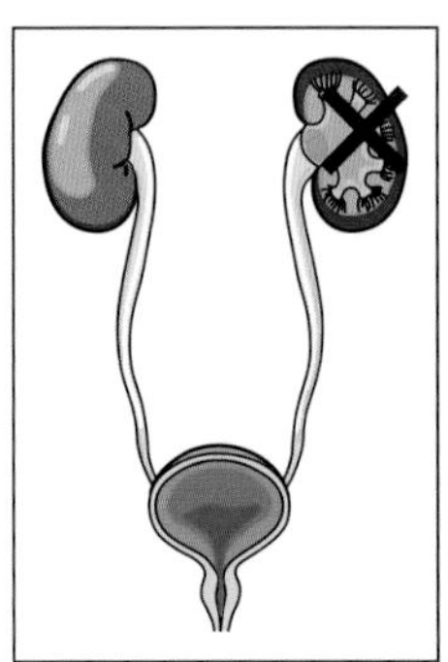

Pyelonephritis is an inflammation, usually from an infection, which occurs in the renal parenchyma and collecting system, including the renal pelvis.

Test-taking Tip: If pyelonephritis is unfamiliar, break the word down. "Pyelo" means pelvis and "nephro" means kidney (pelvis of the kidney).

Content Area: Adult Health; *Category of Health Alteration:* Renal and Urinary Management; *Integrated Processes:* Teaching and Learning; *Client Need:* Health Promotion and Maintenance/Principles of Teaching and Learning; *Cognitive Level:* Analysis

Reference: Lewis, S., Heitkemper, M., Dirksen, S., O'Brien, P., & Bucher, L. (2007). *Medical-Surgical Nursing: Assessment and Management of Clinical Problems* (7th ed., pp. 1161–1162). St. Louis, MO: Mosby/Elsevier.

---

906. A nurse evaluates that a client, diagnosed with obstructing left ureterolithiasis, may have passed the calculi in the urine when which outcome has been achieved?

1. Voiding clear amber urine greater than 30 mL per hour
2. No hematemesis or urinary tract infection (UTI)
3. Absence of epigastric pain, nausea, and vomiting
4. Absence of colicky pain in the left lateral flank and groin

ANSWER: 4

Symptoms of a urinary stone include abdominal or flank pain (usually severe), hematuria, and renal colic. As the stone moves along the ureter, it produces flank pain radiating to the genitalia and groin. The pain is from the spasm of the ureter and ureter wall anoxia from the pressure of the stone. The absence of the colicky pain indicates the stone may have been excreted. An ureterolithiasis is a calculus in the ureter. The kidneys will continue to produce urine and the client should be voiding at least 30 mL per hour even with the calculi. Hematemesis occurs with gastrointestinal problems. UTI may occur from the calculi's irritation to the ureter, but an absence of UTI does not mean the stone has been excreted in the urine. Option 3 would be an outcome for a client with cholecystitis because it describes the pain characteristics of cholecystitis.

Test-taking Tip: Focus on the issue of passing the calculi and the major symptoms of ureterolithiasis. Eliminate options 1, 2, and 3 because they are not characteristic of the major symptoms of ureterolithiasis, which is flank pain and renal colic.

Content Area: Adult Health; *Category of Health Alteration:* Renal and Urinary Management; *Integrated Processes:* Nursing Process Evaluation; *Client Need:* Physiological Integrity/Physiological Adaptation/Illness Management; *Cognitive Level:* Analysis

Reference: Lewis, S., Heitkemper, M., Dirksen, S., O'Brien, P., & Bucher, L. (2007). *Medical-Surgical Nursing: Assessment and Management of Clinical Problems* (7th ed., pp. 1169–1171). St. Louis, MO: Mosby/Elsevier.

---

907. A nurse is completing an admission assessment for a client suspected of having an obstructing struvite calculus of the right ureter. During the assessment, which is the *best* question for the nurse to ask the client?

1. "Are you experiencing any left flank pain?"
2. "Do you like to drink cranberry, prune, or tomato juice?"
3. "Have you had a history of chronic urinary tract infections (UTIs)?"
4. "How often do you eat organ meats, poultry, fish, and sardines?"

ANSWER: 3

A frequent UTI is a predisposing factor for struvite stones. These stones are commonly referred to as "infection stones" because they form in alkaline urine that is rich in ammonia. Though assessing pain is a priority, pain associated with a calculus in the right ureter would be in the right (not left) flank or costovertebral area. Asking a client about juice preferences is irrelevant. The client with a UTI would be instructed to increase intake of cranberries, prunes, plums, and tomatoes because they acidify the urine. This is a good question to ask the client when planning teaching but is not the best question during the admission assessment. Organ meats, poultry, fish, gravies, red wines, sardines, goose, and venison are high in purines. These can contribute to the development of uric acid stones not struvite stones.

Test-taking Tip: Use the process of elimination. Focus on the information provided in the question. Option 1 can be eliminated because the calculus involves the right ureter. Note that options 2 and 4 are similar, and these would not be important to ask during an admission assessment; thus, these can be eliminated.

Content Area: Adult Health; *Category of Health Alteration:* Renal and Urinary Management; *Integrated Processes:* Nursing Process Assessment; *Client Need:* Physiological Integrity/Reduction of Risk Potential/System Specific Assessments; *Cognitive Level:* Analysis

Reference: Lewis, S., Heitkemper, M., Dirksen, S., O'Brien, P., & Bucher, L. (2007). *Medical-Surgical Nursing: Assessment and Management of Clinical Problems* (7th ed., pp. 1168–1170). St. Louis, MO: Mosby/Elsevier.

908. EBP A nurse is admitting a client with a diagnosis of renal calculi to a hospital nursing unit. Which nursing action should be performed *first*?

1. Encourage the client to increase oral fluids
2. Obtain supplies to measure and strain all urine
3. Assess the severity and location of the client's pain
4. Obtain consent for an extracorporeal shock wave lithotripsy (ESWL)

ANSWER: 3

Assessment should be the priority and is the first step in the nursing process. Severe colic pain, which is most severe in the first 24 to 36 hours, can cause a vasovagal reaction with syncope and hypotension. Pain can also interfere with the client's admission process. A nurse should use a systematic, validated pain assessment tool to assess the parameters of pain. Increasing fluids will promote passage of the renal stone through the ureter and decrease pain, but it is not the first action. Urine should be measured and strained, but this is not priority. ESWL may be ordered after other measures to assist the client to pass the stone are ineffective.

▶ ***Test-taking Tip:*** *Assessment is the first step in the nursing process and should be implemented first (except in life-threatening situations, then an intervention might be first). When the question asks which is first, all four options may be appropriate for the client's diagnosis, but only one has priority.*

Content Area: Adult Health; *Category of Health Alteration:* Renal and Urinary Management; *Integrated Processes:* Nursing Process Implementation; *Client Need:* Physiological Integrity/Physiological Adaptation/Illness Management; Safe and Effective Care Environment/Management of Care/Establishing Priorities; *Cognitive Level:* Analysis

Reference: Ignatavicius, D., & Workman, M. (2006). *Medical-Surgical Nursing: Critical Thinking for Collaborative Care* (5th ed., pp. 1698–1699). St. Louis, MO: Elsevier/Saunders.

EBP Reference: Institute for Clinical Systems Improvement (ICSI). (2008). *Assessment and Management of Acute Pain.* Available at: www.guideline.gov/summary/summary.aspx?doc_id=12302&nbr=006371&string=pain.

909. Which nursing actions should a nurse plan in the care of a client immediately after extracorporeal shock wave lithotripsy (ESWL)? SELECT ALL THAT APPLY.

1. Measure and strain all urine
2. Keep the client NPO for 24 hours
3. Check for ecchymosis on the flank of the affected side
4. Assess the incision to see if it is clean, dry, and intact
5. Remove the stent if one has been placed before or during ESWL

ANSWER: 1, 3

Urine is strained to monitor the passage of stone fragments. Some bruising may occur on the flank of the affected side after ESWL because sound, laser, or dry shock wave energies are used to break the stone into small fragments. Once the client has recovered from the effects of the sedative, foods and fluids are given. Increasing fluids assists with passage of the stone fragments. There is no incision with ESWL. A small incision is made during percutaneous ultrasonic lithotripsy. A stent is occasionally placed in the ureter before ESWL to dilate the ureter and ease passage of the stone fragments. Stent placement prevents the stone from coming in contact with the ureteral mucosa, thereby reducing pain. The stent is not removed until stone fragments have passed.

▶ ***Test-taking Tip:*** *Recall that ESWL uses laser and does not involve an incision. Eliminate options pertaining to an open surgical procedure.*

Content Area: Adult Health; *Category of Health Alteration:* Renal and Urinary Management; *Integrated Processes:* Nursing Process Planning; *Client Need:* Physiological Integrity/Physiological Adaptation/Illness Management; Physiological Integrity/Reduction of Risk Potential/Therapeutic Procedures; *Cognitive Level:* Analysis

Reference: Ignatavicius, D., & Workman, M. (2006). *Medical-Surgical Nursing: Critical Thinking for Collaborative Care* (5th ed., p. 1699). St. Louis, MO: Elsevier/Saunders.

910. Which interventions should a nurse include when caring for a female client experiencing new onset urge urinary incontinence? SELECT ALL THAT APPLY.

1. Take the client to the bathroom every 4 hours
2. Administer diuretics at supper time so the bladder is empty at night
3. Turn on the water or flush the toilet to assist the client to void
4. Space fluids at regular intervals during the day and limit fluids after the dinner hour
5. Instruct the client on insertion of vaginal weights which are to be worn throughout the day

ANSWER: 3, 4

Turning on the water utilizes the power of suggestion to promote voiding. Spacing fluids helps avoid fluid overload on the bladder and allows urine to accumulate at a steady pace. An initial toileting schedule should be every 1 to 2 hours. Diuretics should be given early in the day, preferably at breakfast-time. Vaginal weights (vaginal cone therapy) are helpful in strengthening the pelvic muscles and decreasing stress (not urge) urinary incontinence.

▶ ***Test-taking Tip:*** *Focus on the situation urge urinary incontinence. Eliminate option 5 because it is associated with stress incontinence. Eliminate options 1 and 2 because these would result in a full bladder and could increase incontinence.*

Content Area: Adult Health; *Category of Health Alteration:* Renal and Urinary Management; *Integrated Processes:* Nursing Process Implementation; *Client Need:* Physiological Integrity/Reduction of Risk Potential/Therapeutic Procedures; Physiological Integrity/Physiological Adaptation/Illness Management; *Cognitive Level:* Application

Reference: Potter, P., & Perry, A. (2009). *Fundamentals of Nursing* (7th ed., pp. 1149–1150, 1152). St. Louis, MO: Mosby/Elsevier.

911. EBP A nurse admits a client diagnosed with polycystic kidney disease (PKD). The client is experiencing dull flank pain, nocturia, and diluted urine with a low urine specific gravity. A nurse is reviewing orders written by a health-care provider. Which orders should the nurse question? SELECT ALL THAT APPLY.

1. Increase fluid intake to 2 L daily
2. Restrict sodium intake to 500 mg daily
3. Initiate referral for genetic counseling
4. Lisinopril (Prinivil®) 2.5 mg daily for hypertension
5. Metoprolol (Lopressor®) 12.5 mg (oral) bid

ANSWER: 2, 4

A client with PKD can have salt wasting and should not be on a sodium-restricted diet (500 mg). A low-sodium (but not sodium-restricted) diet may be ordered to control hypertension. Antihypertensive agents include angiotensin-converting enzyme (ACE) inhibitors such as lisinopril (Prinivil®), calcium channel blockers, beta blockers, and vasodilators; but the route is not specified for lisinopril. When renal impairment results in decreased urine concentration with nocturia and low urine specific gravity, the client should drink at least 2 liters of fluid daily to prevent dehydration. Children of parents who have the autosomal dominant form of PKD (the most common form) have a 50% chance of inheriting the gene that causes the disease. Blood pressure control is necessary to slow the progression of the renal dysfunction and reduce cardiovascular complications.

▶ ***Test-taking Tip:*** *Read the stem and question carefully. Note that the question is asking which order should be questioned. Therefore, look for the wrong intervention for PKD.*

Content Area: Adult Health; *Category of Health Alteration:* Renal and Urinary Management; *Integrated Processes:* Nursing Process Analysis; Communication and Documentation; *Client Need:* Physiological Integrity/Physiological Adaptation/Illness Management; Safe and Effective Care Environment/Safety and Infection Control/Injury Prevention; *Cognitive Level:* Analysis

Reference: Ignatavicius, D., & Workman, M. (2006). *Medical-Surgical Nursing: Critical Thinking for Collaborative Care* (5th ed., pp. 1708–1709). St. Louis, MO: Elsevier/Saunders.

EBP Reference: Schiffrin, E., Lipman, M., & Mann, J. (2007). Chronic kidney disease: Effects on the cardiovascular system. *Circulation*, 116, 85–97.

912. When which assessment finding is noted, for a client with polycystic kidney disease (PKD), should a nurse suspect that a cyst has ruptured?

1. Reports a decrease in pain
2. Voids cola-colored urine
3. Passes bloody stools
4. Has decreased serum creatinine levels

ANSWER: 2

The client could have bright red or cola-colored urine if a cyst ruptures. Sharp, intermittent pain occurs when a cyst ruptures. Bloody stools would indicate a gastrointestinal problem, not a renal problem. Serum creatinine is a measure of renal function. As kidney function deteriorates, serum creatinine and blood urea nitrogen (BUN) levels rise.

▶ ***Test-taking Tip:*** *Focus on the information in the question. Note that it relates to PKD, so eliminate option 3. Eliminate option 1 because a ruptured cyst would cause increased pain. Eliminate option 4 because with altered renal function, the serum creatinine would increase.*

Content Area: Adult Health; *Category of Health Alteration:* Renal and Urinary Management; *Integrated Processes:* Nursing Process Assessment; *Client Need:* Physiological Integrity/Reduction of Risk Potential/System Specific Assessments; *Cognitive Level:* Application

Reference: Ignatavicius, D., & Workman, M. (2006). *Medical-Surgical Nursing: Critical Thinking for Collaborative Care* (5th ed., pp. 1708–1709). St. Louis, MO: Elsevier/Saunders.

---

913. A client is diagnosed with renal cell carcinoma. Which specific symptoms should a nurse expect when completing an assessment of the client?

1. Hematuria and nocturia
2. Abdominal pain and dysuria
3. Flank pain and hematuria
4. Suprapubic pain and foul-smelling urine

ANSWER: 3

Clients with renal cell cancer may report flank pain (not abdominal or suprapubic pain), gross hematuria, and a palpable renal mass. Hematuria and nocturia are nonspecific symptoms that could be associated with other renal problems, such as benign prostatic hypertrophy. Abdominal pain is not associated with renal cell carcinoma unless it has metastasized. Metastasis is not addressed in the question. Painful urination could indicate a lower urinary tract problem, such as cystitis or a bladder infection. Suprapubic pain and foul-smelling urine could indicate an infection.

➧ ***Test-taking Tip:*** *Note the key words "specific symptoms" and "renal." Eliminate options 2 and 4 because the location of the kidney is in the flank area. Eliminate option 1 because these are nonspecific symptoms. Avoid reading into the question.*

Content Area: Adult Health; *Category of Health Alteration:* Renal and Urinary Management; *Integrated Processes:* Nursing Process Analysis; *Client Need:* Physiological Integrity/Physiological Adaptation/Alterations in Body Systems; *Cognitive Level:* Application

Reference: Ignatavicius, D., & Workman, M. (2006). *Medical-Surgical Nursing: Critical Thinking for Collaborative Care* (5th ed., p. 1723). St. Louis, MO: Elsevier/Saunders.

---

914. A client asks a nurse to clarify a health-care provider's explanations about the client's scheduled cystectomy with an ileal conduit for urinary diversion. Regarding this procedure, a nurse should explain that:

1. no stoma is required with this surgery and the normal anatomic urinary flow is maintained.
2. a permanent external urinary collecting device will be required.
3. urinary continence is possible with muscle control and Kegel exercises.
4. bladder retraining will be taught later during the recovery.

ANSWER: 2

An ileal conduit collects urine in a portion of the intestine that opens onto the skin surface as a stoma. After the creation of a stoma, the client must wear a pouch to collect urine. A stoma will also be formed when the *ileal* conduit is created for the urinary diversion, so option 1 is incorrect. An *ileal* conduit creates a noncontinent stoma. Kegel exercises are used to control urinary incontinence. Kegel exercises and bladder retraining will have no effect on muscle strengthening and bladder control because the bladder is removed during cystectomy.

➧ ***Test-taking Tip:*** *Focus on the issue: cystectomy with an ileal conduit. Knowledge of the urinary diversion procedures used in the treatment of bladder cancer is needed to answer this question.*

Content Area: Adult Health; *Category of Health Alteration:* Renal and Urinary Management; *Integrated Processes:* Teaching and Learning; *Client Need:* Physiological Integrity/Physiological Adaptation/Illness Management; *Cognitive Level:* Application

Reference: Ignatavicius, D., & Workman, M. (2006). *Medical-Surgical Nursing: Critical Thinking for Collaborative Care* (5th ed., p. 1703). St. Louis, MO: Elsevier/Saunders.

---

915. EBP Which intervention should a nurse include in the care of a client who had continent urinary diversion surgery with creation of a Kock pouch?

1. Insert a catheter at 4- to 6-hour intervals to drain the urine
2. Cleanse the skin around the stoma with alcohol and water daily
3. Instruct the client to sleep on the side of the stoma to promote urine drainage
4. Apply the stoma pouch so that it fits snuggly around the stoma

ANSWER: 1

A Kock pouch is a continent internal ileal reservoir that should be catheterized every 4 to 6 hours. The stoma is sutured to the abdominal wall. Fluid pressure closes the valve inside the pouch to prevent outflow of urine. Alcohol is drying and can result in skin breakdown. Sleeping on the side of the stoma is unnecessary. Urine will flow from the ureters into the reservoir regardless of the client's position. The flange of the stoma pouch should be 1/16 to 1/8 inch larger than a stoma. However, a stoma pouch would not be required. The client may initially have a plastic catheter in the stoma until the suture line heals.

➧ ***Test-taking Tip:*** *Focus on the issue of a continent urinary diversion and use the process of elimination.*

Content Area: Adult Health; *Category of Health Alteration:* Renal and Urinary Management; *Integrated Processes:* Nursing Process Implementation; *Client Need:* Health Promotion and Maintenance/Self-Care; *Cognitive Level:* Application

Reference: Ignatavicius, D., & Workman, M. (2006). *Medical-Surgical Nursing: Critical Thinking for Collaborative Care* (5th ed., p. 1190). St. Louis, MO: Elsevier/Saunders.

EBP Reference: Brown, H., & Randle, J. (2005). Living with a stoma: A review of the literature. *Journal of Clinical Nursing,* 14(1), 74–81.

916. A nurse is reviewing the care plan for a client after a urinary diversion with an ileal conduit that includes all of the nursing diagnoses listed. Which nursing diagnosis should the nurse place as the *lowest* priority?

1. Altered skin integrity
2. Disturbed body image
3. Deficient fluid volume
4. Acute pain

ANSWER: 2

Disturbed body image is a psychosocial need. According to Maslow's Hierarchy of Needs theory, physiological needs are the priority, followed by safety needs, and then psychosocial needs. Altered skin integrity, deficient fluid volume, and acute pain are physiological needs and take priority over a psychosocial or safety need.

Test-taking Tip: *Read the stem, carefully noting the key words "lowest priority." Use Maslow's Hierarchy of Needs theory to answer the question.*

Content Area: Adult Health; *Category of Health Alteration:* Renal and Urinary Management; *Integrated Processes:* Nursing Process Analysis; *Client Need:* Physiological Integrity/Physiological Adaptation/Illness Management; *Cognitive Level:* Application

Reference: Lewis, S., Heitkemper, M., Dirksen, S., O'Brien, P., & Bucher, L. (2007). *Medical-Surgical Nursing: Assessment and Management of Clinical Problems* (7th ed., pp. 1191–1192). St. Louis, MO: Mosby/Elsevier.

917. A nurse teaches a client with a noncontinent urostomy created during urinary diversion that the stoma should be:

1. flush with the skin.
2. constrained with clothing.
3. intermittently catheterized.
4. red, moist, and protruding.

ANSWER: 4

The ideal urinary stoma is symmetrical; has no skin breakdown; protrudes about 1.5 cm, and has healthy, red, moist mucosa. A noncontinent urinary diversion stoma may be flush with the skin. The client should be taught to avoid restrictive clothing that could impair blood supply to the stoma and the flow of urine. A noncontinent urostomy drains urine continually, so there is no need for intermittent catheterization unless complications occur with the stoma such as a stricture.

Test-taking Tip: *Use the process of elimination to rule out incorrect options. Focusing on characteristics of a noncontinent urostomy, eliminate options 1 and 3. Recalling that clothing should be nonrestrictive leads to the elimination of option 2.*

Content Area: Adult Health; *Category of Health Alteration:* Renal and Urinary Management; *Integrated Processes:* Teaching and Learning; *Client Need:* Health Promotion and Maintenance/Self-Care; *Cognitive Level:* Application

Reference: Lewis, S., Heitkemper, M., Dirksen, S., O'Brien, P., & Bucher, L. (2007). *Medical-Surgical Nursing: Assessment and Management of Clinical Problems* (7th ed., p. 1190). St. Louis, MO: Mosby/Elsevier.

918. A client has a nephrostomy tube in place after a partial nephrectomy. When caring for a nephrostomy tube, a nurse should: SELECT ALL THAT APPLY.

1. clamp the tube periodically to allow the remaining nephrons to adapt.
2. irrigate only if ordered and then with less than 5 mL of sterile saline solution.
3. observe for signs of infection, such as cloudy foul-smelling urine draining from the tube.
4. maintain patency of the closed drainage system by keeping it below the level of the kidney.
5. add the amount of output from the nephrostomy tube to the output from the urinary drainage tube to calculate the hourly urine output.
6. record the amount of output from each tube separately.

ANSWER: 2, 3, 4, 5, 6

Irrigation should be performed only with an order. Using more than 5 mL of sterile solution may cause overdistention and renal damage. The output and surrounding tissue should be assessed for signs of infection. The nephrostomy tube is draining urine from the kidney, so the tube must be kept below the flank level to prevent backflow of urine. The nephrostomy tube drains urine from the affected kidney. The urinary drainage device drains urine from the bladder (collected from the other kidney). Hourly urine output should be monitored by adding the two amounts together. To determine kidney function, drainage from each tube should be recorded separately. Clamping, compressing, or kinking the tube can cause renal damage.

➧ ***Test-taking Tip:*** *"Nephro" means kidney. Although option 1 may sound plausible, it is unsafe.*

Content Area: Adult Health; *Category of Health Alteration:* Renal and Urinary Management; *Integrated Processes:* Nursing Process Implementation; *Client Need:* Physiological Integrity/Physiological Adaptation/Illness Management; *Cognitive Level:* Application

Reference: Lewis, S., Heitkemper, M., Dirksen, S., O'Brien, P., & Bucher, L. (2007). *Medical-Surgical Nursing: Assessment and Management of Clinical Problems* (7th ed., pp. 1178, 1187–1188). St. Louis, MO: Mosby/Elsevier.

919. A nurse reviews the laboratory report of a client with acute renal failure (ARF) and notes that the serum potassium level is 6.8 mEq/L. Which medication should the nurse plan to administer specifically to protect the heart from the high potassium levels?

1. Erythropoietin
2. Regular insulin
3. 50% dextrose
4. Calcium gluconate

ANSWER: 4

Calcium gluconate raises the threshold for cardiac muscle excitation, thereby reducing the incidence of life-threatening dysrhythmias that can occur with hyperkalemia. Erythropoietin triggers the production of red blood cells by bone marrow. It is used to treat anemia, which is common in renal failure. Regular insulin, along with 5% to 50% dextrose, forces the potassium into the cells; temporarily lowering serum potassium levels.

➧ ***Test-taking Tip:*** *Note the key word "specifically." Read the question carefully and use the process of elimination to find the medication that protects the heart.*

Content Area: Adult Health; *Category of Health Alteration:* Renal and Urinary Management; *Integrated Processes:* Nursing Process Planning; *Client Need:* Physiological Integrity/Pharmacological and Parenteral Therapies/Pharmacological Agents/Actions; *Cognitive Level:* Application

Reference: Lewis, S., Heitkemper, M., Dirksen, S., O'Brien, P., & Bucher, L. (2007). *Medical-Surgical Nursing: Assessment and Management of Clinical Problems* (7th ed., p. 1202). St. Louis, MO: Mosby/Elsevier.

920. A client with chronic renal failure receives a hemodialysis treatment. The client's weight before dialysis was 83 kilograms and after dialysis 80 kilograms. A nurse estimates that the amount of fluid that the client lost was ____ liters.

ANSWER: 3

Because 1 kilogram of weight is equivalent to 1 liter of fluid, a weight loss of 3 kilograms would be approximately 3 liters of fluid loss.

➧ ***Test-taking Tip:*** *Knowledge that 1 liter of fluid is equivalent to 1 kilogram is needed to answer this question.*

Content Area: Adult Health; *Category of Health Alteration:* Renal and Urinary Management; *Integrated Processes:* Nursing Process Analysis; *Client Need:* Physiological Integrity/Reduction of Risk Potential/Therapeutic Procedures; *Cognitive Level:* Analysis

Reference: Lewis, S., Heitkemper, M., Dirksen, S., O'Brien, P., & Bucher, L. (2007). *Medical-Surgical Nursing: Assessment and Management of Clinical Problems* (7th ed., p. 1205). St. Louis, MO: Mosby/Elsevier.

921. A nurse evaluates that a client is in the recovery phase of acute renal failure (ARF). Achievement of which outcomes supports the nurse's conclusion? SELECT ALL THAT APPLY.

1. Increased urine specific gravity
2. Increased serum creatinine level
3. Decreased serum potassium level
4. Absence of nausea and vomiting
5. Absence of muscle twitching

ANSWER: 1, 3, 4, 5

Urine specific gravity increases because of the kidneys' ability to concentrate urine and excrete electrolytes. Potassium is decreased because of the kidneys' ability to excrete potassium. Nausea, vomiting, and diarrhea are common in ARF because of accumulation of nitrogenous wastes. An absence of these indicates that the client is in the recovery phase of ARF. Neurologically, the client in renal failure may have muscle twitching, drowsiness, headache, and seizures because of the electrolyte imbalances and accumulation of metabolic wastes. In the recovery period, the client should not have muscle twitching. The client should have a decreased, not increased, serum creatinine level in the recovery period.

▶ *Test-taking Tip: Look for signs that show improvement, thus eliminating option 2. Avoid reading into the question. Muscle twitching could occur from other problems, but consider if it can also occur with ARF.*

Content Area: Adult Health; *Category of Health Alteration:* Renal and Urinary Management; *Integrated Processes:* Nursing Process Evaluation; *Client Need:* Physiological Integrity/Physiological Adaptation/Illness Management; *Cognitive Level:* Application

Reference: Ignatavicius, D., & Workman, M. (2006). *Medical-Surgical Nursing: Critical Thinking for Collaborative Care* (5th ed., pp. 1730–1731). St. Louis, MO: Elsevier/Saunders.

922. A nurse is interpreting the serum laboratory report below for a client with a diagnosis of acute renal failure (ARF) secondary to cardiac catheterization. Based on the findings of the serum laboratory report, which action should the nurse establish as the priority?

Serum Laboratory Test	Client's Value	Normal Values
BUN	40	5–25 mg/dL
Creatinine	4.2	0.5–1.5 mg/dL
Na	150	135–145 mEq/L
K	6.9	3.5–5.3 mEq/L
Cl	99	95–105 mEq/L
CO_2	16	22–30 mEq/L
Phosphate	5.0	1.7–2.6 mEq/L
Calcium	7	9–11 mg/dL
Hgb	10	13.5–17 g/dL
Hct	32%	40%–54%
PTH	88	11–54 μg/mL

1. Administer intravenous (IV) calcium gluconate
2. Administer IV furosemide
3. Begin cardiac monitoring
4. Restrict foods high in potassium.

ANSWER: 1

The client has severe hyperkalemia. Calcium gluconate raises the threshold for cardiac muscle excitation, thereby reducing the incidence of life-threatening dysrhythmias. The first action is to protect the heart. Furosemide is a loop diuretic that inhibits reabsorption of sodium and chloride and promotes the excretion of potassium. The amount of potassium excreted in the urine will be insufficient to quickly lower the severely elevated serum potassium levels to protect the heart from the hyperkalemic effects. Though it is important to place the client on cardiac monitoring, the heart needs to be protected from the hyperkalemic effects. Restricting foods high in potassium is not the priority.

▶ *Test-taking Tip: Focus on the situation in the stem ARF. Then read the information in the chart carefully, looking for abnormal information that pertains to the situation. Note the key word "priority" in the stem. The most life-threatening problem needs to be addressed first.*

Content Area: Adult Health; *Category of Health Alteration:* Renal and Urinary Management; *Integrated Processes:* Nursing Process Analysis; *Client Need:* Physiological Integrity/Physiological Adaptation/Medical Emergencies; *Cognitive Level:* Analysis

Reference: Lewis, S., Heitkemper, M., Dirksen, S., O'Brien, P., & Bucher, L. (2007). *Medical-Surgical Nursing: Assessment and Management of Clinical Problems* (7th ed., p. 1202). St. Louis, MO: Mosby/Elsevier.

923. After a diagnosis of chronic renal failure, a client was started on epoetin alfa (Epogen®). Which finding should a nurse expect when evaluating the desired therapeutic effectiveness of the medication?

1. Decrease in serum creatinine levels (SCr)
2. Increase in white blood cells (WBCs)
3. Increase in serum hematocrit (Hct)
4. Decrease in blood pressure (BP)

ANSWER: 3

Epoetin alfa (Epogen®) stimulates red blood cell production and increases Hct levels. Initial effects should be seen in 1 to 2 weeks, and normal Hct levels should be achieved within 2 to 3 months. Epoetin alfa (Epogen®) does not have a direct effect on SCr levels. Elevated WBCs could indicate the client has an infection. Epoetin alfa (Epogen®) does not affect WBCs. As the Hct rises, there can be a transient increase in BP.

Test-taking Tip: *Use the process of elimination, focusing on the desired effects of Epoetin alfa (Epogen®).*

Content Area: Adult Health; *Category of Health Alteration:* Renal and Urinary Management; *Integrated Processes:* Nursing Process Evaluation; *Client Need:* Physiological Integrity/Pharmacological and Parenteral Therapies/Expected Effects/Outcomes; *Cognitive Level:* Application

Reference: Deglin, J., & Vallerand, A. (2009). *Davis's Drug Guide for Nurses* (11th ed., pp. 487–490). Philadelphia: F. A. Davis.

924. A client hospitalized with a diagnosis of chronic renal failure (CRF) is experiencing hypotension, cold and clammy skin, and dysrhythmias. An arterial blood gas (ABG) is drawn with orders to notify the physician if abnormal. Based on the following results, a nurse should notify the physician to report that the client is experiencing:

ABG Laboratory Value	Client's Value	Normal Values
pH	7.20	7.35–7.45
$PaCO_2$	32	35–45 mm Hg
HCO_3	14	Bicarb 22–26 mEq/L
Base excess/deficit	–3	+ 2 mEq/L
PO_2	80	80–100 mm Hg

1. respiratory acidosis.
2. respiratory alkalosis.
3. metabolic acidosis.
4. metabolic alkalosis.

ANSWER: 3

In metabolic acidosis, the pH and HCO_3 (bicarbonate) are decreased, and the $Paco_2$ is normal (or decreased if compensation is occurring). In compensation, the client would be hyperventilating to decrease the $Paco_2$ and conserve the HCO_3. In CRF, metabolic acidosis occurs because the kidneys are unable to excrete the increased amounts of acids. The inability of the kidney tubules to excrete ammonia (NH_3) and to reabsorb sodium bicarbonate (HCO_3) causes the decreased acid secretion. The decreased excretion of phosphates and other organic acids contributes to the accumulation of acids. Respiratory acidosis would result in a decreased pH, an increased $Paco_2$, and a normal or decreased HCO_3. Respiratory alkalosis would result in an increased pH, a decreased $Paco_2$, and a normal or decreased HCO_3. Metabolic alkalosis would result in an increased pH, an increased HCO_3, and a normal or increased $Paco_2$.

Test-taking Tip: *Recall that the $Paco_2$ is the respiratory component and HCO_3 is the metabolic component. For abnormal values, visualize the pH, $Paco_2$, and HCO_3 each separately on an acid–base scale to determine whether the client's value is acidic, basic, or within a normal pH range. Write this down. The value that matches the pH as being either acidic or basic is the system (respiratory or metabolic) that initiated the imbalance.*

Content Area: Adult Health; *Category of Health Alteration:* Renal and Urinary Management; *Integrated Processes:* Nursing Process Analysis; *Client Need:* Physiological Integrity/Reduction of Risk Potential/Laboratory Values; Physiological Integrity/Physiological Adaptation/Medical Emergencies; *Cognitive Level:* Analysis

Reference: Smeltzer, S., Bare, B., Hinkle, J., & Cheever, K. (2008). *Brunner & Suddarth's Textbook of Medical-Surgical Nursing* (11th ed., pp. 335–340, 1529). Philadelphia: Lippincott Williams & Wilkins.

925. EBP A client with a diagnosis of end-stage renal disease states to a nurse, "I don't think I want to be on dialysis anymore; it's just too painful for me." What is the most appropriate response by the nurse?

1. "Why do you think you will be unable to stay on dialysis?"
2. "You feel that dialysis is painful for you. Tell me more about that."
3. "It really isn't hard to stay on dialysis. Remember you can sleep during the dialysis run."
4. "You need to stay on dialysis to avoid getting worse. You could die if you don't go to dialysis regularly."

ANSWER: 2

Paraphrasing the client's statement encourages the client to verbalize feelings and conveys that the message is understood by the nurse. An open-ended response allows for a more lengthy response from the client. The client could be experiencing emotional distress, something troublesome, or physical pain. According to research (Davison, 2007), chronic pain and depression are not adequately assessed and treated in clients with chronic renal failure. The World Health Organization's (WHO) stepwise progression of analgesics should be used for treating client pain. Asking a "why" question is asking for information that the client may not be able to express. Telling the client that dialysis treatment "isn't really hard" devaluates the client's feelings. Telling the client what to do, giving advice, and threatening the client block communication.

► ***Test-taking Tip:*** *Use therapeutic communication techniques, focusing on the client's statements in the stem. Response 2 is the only response that uses a therapeutic communication technique (paraphrasing).*

Content Area: Adult Health; *Category of Health Alteration:* Renal and Urinary Management; *Integrated Processes:* Caring; Communication and Documentation; *Client Need:* Psychosocial Integrity/Therapeutic Communications; *Cognitive Level:* Application

Reference: Ignatavicius, D., & Workman, M. (2006). *Medical-Surgical Nursing: Critical Thinking for Collaborative Care* (5th ed., p. 1744). St. Louis, MO: Elsevier/Saunders.

EBP Reference: Davison, S. (2007). Chronic kidney disease: Psychosocial impact of chronic pain. *Geriatrics*, 62(2), 17–18, 20–23.

926. Which notation should a nurse document as an appropriate outcome in the plan of care for a client with chronic renal failure?

1. Consumption of three large meals daily without nausea
2. Daily weight gain of no more than 3 pounds
3. Reduced serum albumin levels within 1 week
4. Absence of bleeding

ANSWER: 4

The client with chronic renal failure is at risk for bleeding because of impaired platelet function. The absence of bleeding is an appropriate client outcome. The client with chronic renal failure has the potential for imbalanced nutrition due to anorexia, nausea, and stomatitis secondary to the effects of urea excess on the gastrointestinal system. The client should consume small, frequent meals, not large meals. The client with chronic renal failure is at risk for fluid volume excess because of the kidneys' inability to excrete water. A weight gain indicates fluid retention. The client with chronic renal failure has the potential for imbalanced nutrition because of a protein-restricted diet. Serum albumin levels should be within normal limits.

► ***Test-taking Tip:*** *Use the ABCs (airway, breathing, circulation) to identify option 4 as the correct answer to the question.*

Content Area: Adult Health; *Category of Health Alteration:* Renal and Urinary Management; *Integrated Processes:* Communication and Documentation; *Client Need:* Physiological Integrity/Physiological Adaptation/Illness Management; *Cognitive Level:* Application

Reference: Monahan, F., Sands, J., Neighbors, M., Marek, J., & Green, C. (2007). *Phipps' Medical-Surgical Nursing: Health and Illness Perspectives* (8th ed., pp. 1014–1019). St. Louis, MO: Mosby/Elsevier.

927. A nursing assistant reports to a nurse that a client diagnosed with chronic renal failure has "white crystals" and dry, itchy skin. Based on this information, the nurse should instruct the nursing assistant to:

1. apply the prescribed antipruritic cream to the client's skin.
2. offer the client a glass of warm milk to drink.
3. bathe the client in tepid water.
4. assess the client's serum creatinine levels.

ANSWER: 3

Bathing the client in cool water will remove crystals, decrease itching, and promote client comfort. The crystals (uremic frost) and itching are from irritating toxins and deposits of calcium phosphate precipitates on the skin. Although an antipruritic cream could be applied to relieve itching, applying the medication would not be within the scope of practice of a nursing assistant. Fluid intake is usually restricted for the client with chronic renal failure. Assessment is not within the scope of practice of a nursing assistant. Knowing the serum creatinine levels will not address the problem of the uremic frost and itchy skin.

► ***Test-taking Tip:*** *Focus on the problem, the "white crystals" and dry, itchy skin and delegate appropriately. Knowing the scope of practice for a nursing assistant and interventions for uremic frost and pruritis will help answer this question.*

Content Area: Adult Health; *Category of Health Alteration:* Renal and Urinary Management; *Integrated Processes:* Nursing Process Analysis; *Client Need:* Physiological Integrity/Physiological Adaptation/Illness Management; Safe and Effective Care Environment/Management of Care/Delegation; *Cognitive Level:* Analysis

Reference: Lewis, S., Heitkemper, M., Dirksen, S., O'Brien, P., & Bucher, L. (2007). *Medical-Surgical Nursing: Assessment and Management of Clinical Problems* (7th ed., pp. 1214–1215). St. Louis, MO: Mosby/Elsevier.

---

928. EBP Which nursing assessment is most accurate in determining the patency of a client's newly placed left forearm internal arteriovenous (AV) fistula for hemodialysis?

1. Feeling for a bruit on the left forearm
2. Palpating for a thrill over the fistula
3. Aspirating blood from the fistula every 8 hours
4. Checking the client's distal pulses and circulation

ANSWER: 2

An AV fistula is created by the anastomosis of an artery to a vein. A thrill is the arterial blood rushing into the vein. Its presence indicates that the fistula is not occluded. Bruits are auscultated, not palpated. Aspirating for blood is unnecessary and can damage the fistula because it takes 4 to 6 weeks to mature. Although checking circulation, motion, and sensation (CMS) is important to assess circulation to the hand, it does not provide information about the patency of the fistula.

➧ ***Test-taking Tip:*** *Focus on the issue of patency of the fistula and the key words "most accurate" to answer this question.*

Content Area: Adult Health; *Category of Health Alteration:* Renal and Urinary Management; *Integrated Processes:* Nursing Process Assessment; *Client Need:* Physiological Integrity/Reduction of Risk Potential/Therapeutic Procedures; *Cognitive Level:* Application

Reference: Ignatavicius, D., & Workman, M. (2006). *Medical-Surgical Nursing: Critical Thinking for Collaborative Care* (5th ed., p. 1754). St. Louis, MO: Elsevier/Saunders.

EBP Reference: Clinical Practice Guidelines for Hemodialysis Adequacy. (2006). *American Journal of Kidney Disease,* 48(1), S13–S97. Available at: www.ajkd.org/issues/contents?issue_key=TOC@@JOURNALS@YAJKD@0048@9999s1

---

929. A nurse is initiating peritoneal dialysis for a client with renal failure. During the infusion of the dialysate, the client reports abdominal pain. Which intervention by the nurse is most appropriate?

1. Stopping the dialysis
2. Slowing the infusion
3. Asking if the client is constipated
4. Explaining that the pain will subside after a few exchanges

ANSWER: 4

Peritoneal irritation, from the inflow of the dialysate, commonly causes pain during the first few exchanges. The pain usually subsides within 1 to 2 weeks. Positioning the client supine in a low-Fowler's position reduces intra-abdominal pressure. The infusion should not be stopped or slowed, because it is peritoneal irritation causing the pain. The pain should be treated. Constipation may cause slowing and the client may feel pressure, but not pain, during inflow of the dialysate solution.

➧ ***Test-taking Tip:*** *Use the process of elimination, ruling out options 1 and 2 because these are similar actions.*

Content Area: Adult Health; *Category of Health Alteration:* Renal and Urinary Management; *Integrated Processes:* Nursing Process Implementation; *Client Need:* Physiological Integrity/Reduction of Risk Potential/Therapeutic Procedures; *Cognitive Level:* Application

Reference: Ignatavicius, D., & Workman, M. (2006). *Medical-Surgical Nursing: Critical Thinking for Collaborative Care* (5th ed., pp. 1758–1759). St. Louis, MO: Elsevier/Saunders.

930. The spouse of a client who has been on hemodialysis for the past 5 years, calls a clinic because the client has stopped eating, is taking long naps, and refuses to talk with the spouse. A nurse interprets that the client is most likely experiencing:

1. depression.
2. displacement.
3. noncompliance.
4. activity intolerance.

ANSWER: 1

In response to illness, persons on dialysis may demonstrate noncompliance, depression, and suicidal tendencies. Depression is an extreme feeling of sadness, despair, dejection, lack of worth, or emptiness. Emotional signs and symptoms include tiredness, sadness, emptiness, or numbness. Behavioral signs include irritability, inability to concentrate, difficulty making decisions, crying, sleep disturbance, social withdrawal, and loss of sexual desire. Physical signs include anorexia, weight loss, constipation, headache, and dizziness. Displacement is releasing pent-up feelings on persons less threatening than those who initially aroused the feelings. Noncompliance is behaviors or actions that would be contraindicated for a particular situation. For example, rather than stopping eating, the client might eat foods that are to be avoided and drink more fluids than allocated. The defining characteristics of activity intolerance, such as dyspnea, fatigue, or weakness, are not noted in the stem.

Test-taking Tip: *Focus on the information given in the stem. Based on the information, the only applicable interpretation is depression.*

Content Area: Adult Health; *Category of Health Alteration:* Renal and Urinary Management; *Integrated Processes:* Nursing Process Analysis; *Client Need:* Psychosocial Integrity/Mental Health Concepts; *Cognitive Level:* Analysis

References: Lewis, S., Heitkemper, M., Dirksen, S., O'Brien, P., & Bucher, L. (2007). *Medical-Surgical Nursing: Assessment and Management of Clinical Problems* (7th ed., p. 1224). St. Louis, MO: Mosby/Elsevier; Berman, A., Snyder, S., Kozier, B., & Erb, G. (2008). *Kozier & Erb's Fundamentals of Nursing: Concepts, Process, and Practice* (8th ed., pp. 1066–1067). Upper Saddle River, NJ: Pearson Education.

---

931. A nurse is concerned that a client receiving peritoneal dialysis may be experiencing peritonitis. Which finding noted on the nurse's assessment supported this concern?

1. Abdominal numbness
2. Cloudy dialysis output
3. Radiating sternal pain
4. Decreased white blood cells

ANSWER: 2

Manifestations of peritonitis include cloudy dialysate, fever, abdominal tenderness, abdominal pain, general malaise, nausea, and vomiting. The client would experience abdominal tenderness and pain, not numbness or sternal pain. White blood cells (WBCs) would increase in the presence of an infection.

Test-taking Tip: *Focus on the issue of peritonitis and use the process of elimination. Eliminate option 4 because WBCs should be elevated. Eliminate 1 and 3 because they are uncharacteristic of peritonitis.*

Content Area: Adult Health; *Category of Health Alteration:* Renal and Urinary Management; *Integrated Processes:* Nursing Process Assessment; *Client Need:* Physiological Integrity/Physiological Adaptation/Alterations in Body Systems; *Cognitive Level:* Application

Reference: Ignatavicius, D., & Workman, M. (2006). *Medical-Surgical Nursing: Critical Thinking for Collaborative Care* (5th ed., p. 1758). St. Louis, MO: Elsevier/Saunders.

932. A nurse is admitting a client with possible renal trauma after a motor vehicle accident. When caring for this client, which actions should be taken by the nurse? Prioritize the nurse's actions by numbering each action from the highest priority (1) to the lowest priority (5).

____ Teach the client signs of a urinary tract infection (UTI)
____ Palpate both flanks for asymmetry
____ Assess for pain in the flank area
____ Prepare the client for a CT scan
____ Inspect the abdomen and the urethra for gross bleeding

ANSWER: 5, 3, 1, 4, 2

First assess for pain. Unrelieved pain can prolong the stress response. A nurse should treat pain before the physical exam, sending the client for a test, or teaching. Next, the nurse would inspect the abdomen and urethra for gross bleeding. Third, the flanks should be palpated for asymmetry. If gross bleeding is present, the abdomen should not be palpated. Once the physical examination is completed, the client should be prepared for a computed tomography (CT) exam. The least priority would be to teach the client about signs of a UTI.

Test-taking Tip: *Use the nursing process and the physical assessment process to prioritize the nursing actions. Assessment is the first step in the nursing process. Look for the key word "assess." Inspection should occur before palpation because the findings could lead to deciding not to palpate because it could cause harm. Use the other steps of the nursing process to prioritize the remaining items.*

Content Area: Adult Health; *Category of Health Alteration:* Renal and Urinary Management; *Integrated Processes:* Nursing Process Analysis; *Client Need:* Safe and Effective Care Environment/Management of Care/Establishing Priorities; *Cognitive Level:* Analysis

Reference: Ignatavicius, D., & Workman, M. (2006). *Medical-Surgical Nursing: Critical Thinking for Collaborative Care* (5th ed., pp. 1662, 1724–1725). St. Louis, MO: Elsevier/Saunders.

Test 24: **Adult Health: Reproductive Management**

933. EBP A nurse is preparing to conduct a women's wellness seminar at a local civic center. What information should the nurse plan to include about risk factors for development of breast cancer? SELECT ALL THAT APPLY.

1. Breast cancer occurs most frequently in women younger than 30 years.
2. The longer the interval between menarche and menopause, the more the risk increases.
3. Nulliparous women are at increased risk.
4. Risk is increased in postmenopausal women with body mass indexes below 20.
5. Women whose sisters or mothers have had breast cancer are at increased risk.
6. The risk increases for women with fibrocystic breast disease.

ANSWER: 2, 3, 5

Early menarche and/or late menopause increase the risk of developing breast cancer. Childless women are at increased risk as are women with first-degree relatives, such as a mother or sister, who had breast cancer. Breast cancer is diagnosed most commonly in women older than 50 years. Postmenopausal women who are obese are at increased risk and fibrocystic breast disease is not related to breast cancer development.

➧ ***Test-taking Tip:*** *Recall the risk factors for the majority of cancers, which are age, diet (overeating), and heredity. Use the process of elimination then to eliminate options opposite of these risk factors.*

Content Area: Adult Health; *Category of Health Alteration:* Reproductive Management; *Integrated Processes:* Nursing Process Planning; *Client Need:* Health Promotion and Maintenance/Disease Prevention; *Cognitive Level:* Application

Reference: Monahan, F., Sands, J., Neighbors, M., Marek, J., & Green, C. (2007). *Phipps' Medical-Surgical Nursing: Health and Illness Perspectives* (8th ed., pp. 1750–1752). St. Louis, MO: Mosby/Elsevier.

EBP Reference: Qaseem, A., Snow, V., Sherif, K., Aronson, M., Weiss, K., et al. (2007). Screening mammography for women 40 to 49 years of age: A clinical practice guideline from the American College of Physicians. *Annals of Internal Medicine*, 146(7), 511–515. Available at: www.guideline.gov/summary/summary.aspx?doc_id=10715&nbr=005578&string=breast+AND+cancer+AND+risk

---

934. An oncologist tells a nurse that he has informed a client that her breast cancer is stage 1. After overhearing the client talking with her husband, the nurse determines that the client has not fully understood the diagnosis. Which statement was most likely made by the client to her husband?

1. "I guess I won't be here to see our daughter graduate this spring."
2. "I understand that I will need some type of chemotherapy."
3. "I will be starting radiation therapy soon."
4. "I think I have a good chance to be a 5-year survivor."

ANSWER: 1

Ninety percent of women with localized tumors (stage 1 and 2) can be expected to achieve long-term disease-free survival. Both chemotherapy and radiation are recommended for stage 1 and 2 breast cancer. Both are usually started after surgical removal of the tumor.

➧ ***Test-taking Tip:*** *The statement about the nurse's concern that the client has "not fully understood" indicates a false-response item. Look for the incorrect statement.*

Content Area: Adult Health; *Category of Health Alteration:* Reproductive Management; *Integrated Processes:* Nursing Process Evaluation; *Client Need:* Physiological Integrity/Physiological Adaptation/Illness Management; Safe and Effective Care Environment/Management of Care/Collaboration with Interdisciplinary Team; *Cognitive Level:* Application

Reference: Monahan, F., Sands, J., Neighbors, M., Marek, J., & Green, C. (2007). *Phipps' Medical-Surgical Nursing: Health and Illness Perspectives* (8th ed., p. 1759). St. Louis, MO: Mosby/Elsevier.

935. EBP A client with newly diagnosed breast cancer asks a nurse to explain the advantages of a sentinel lymph node biopsy (SLNB). Which explanation should the nurse state to the client?

1. "The sentinel node biopsy improves the potential that the total tumor will be removed."
2. "The sentinel node biopsy can decrease the number of axillary lymph nodes that must be removed during surgery."
3. "The sentinel node biopsy makes breast reconstruction easier to perform."
4. "The sentinel node biopsy, if performed, will make hormonal therapy unnecessary."

ANSWER: 2

An SLNB helps to identify axillary node involvement before axillary dissection has occurred. If the sentinel node is identified and is found to be negative for tumor cells, then further axillary lymph node dissection is unnecessary. Thus the lymph drainage of the involved arm can be preserved. The SLNB will not improve the ability of the surgeon to remove the total tumor, and it will not make breast reconstruction easier. The use of hormonal therapy for breast cancer treatment is determined by the receptor status of the tumor.

➧ ***Test-taking Tip:*** *Note that only one option mentions lymph nodes. Connect this to the SLNB and select that option.*

Content Area: Adult Health; *Category of Health Alteration:* Reproductive Management; *Integrated Processes:* Nursing Process Implementation; Teaching and Learning; *Client Need:* Physiological Integrity/Reduction of Risk Potential/Diagnostic Tests; *Cognitive Level:* Application

Reference: Monahan, F., Sands, J., Neighbors, M., Marek, J., & Green, C. (2007). *Phipps' Medical-Surgical Nursing: Health and Illness Perspectives* (8th ed., pp. 1762, 1763). St. Louis, MO: Mosby/Elsevier.

EBP Reference: Al-Shibli, K., Mohammed, H., & Mikalsen, K. (2005). Sentinel lymph nodes and breast carcinoma: Analysis of 70 cases by frozen section. *Annals of Saudi Medicine,* 25(2), 111–114. Available at: www.medscape.com/medline/abstract/15977687

---

936. EBP A nurse is conducting a breast cancer awareness seminar at a local church. After the seminar, a 40-year-old female tells the nurse that she is at high risk for developing breast cancer and her health-care provider suggests that she begin taking tamoxifen (Soltamox®). She asks the nurse to explain how this drug will help her avoid developing breast cancer. The nurse's response should be based on the knowledge that tamoxifen is:

1. a potent anti-inflammatory drug that prevents the body's inflammatory response to the tumor growth.
2. a type of chemotherapy agent that has minimal side effects if taken prophylactically.
3. a drug that will decrease the risk of endometrial cancer, which is related to breast cancer development.
4. a drug that blocks estrogen receptors on tumor cells and causes tumor regression.

ANSWER: 4

Tamoxifen is recommended as a primary prevention modality for women at high risk for breast cancer. It blocks estrogen receptors on tumor cells, and thus the cell growth declines and the tumor regresses. It does not have anti-inflammatory properties, and it is a hormonal rather than a chemotherapeutic agent. A major side effect is that is increases the risk of endometrial cancer.

➧ ***Test-taking Tip:*** *Focus on the information provided and note that the woman does not have cancer, but is at high risk. Eliminate options that would pertain to a diagnosis of cancer and a side effect of tamoxifen.*

Content Area: Adult Health; *Category of Health Alteration:* Reproductive Management; *Integrated Processes:* Nursing Process Planning; *Client Need:* Physiological Integrity/Pharmacological and Parenteral Therapies/Pharmacological Agents/Actions; Health Promotion and Maintenance/Prevention and Early Detection of Disease/Disease Prevention; *Cognitive Level:* Application

References: Smeltzer, S., Bare, B., Hinkle, J., & Cheever, K. (2008). *Brunner & Suddarth's Textbook of Medical-Surgical Nursing* (11th ed., p. 1714). Philadelphia: Lippincott Williams & Wilkins; Lehne, R. (2007). *Pharmacology for Nursing Care* (6th ed., pp. 1176–1177). St. Louis, MO: Elsevier/Saunders.

EBP Reference: Chustecka, Z. (2006). Tamoxifen continues to prevent breast cancer for years after therapy is stopped. *Medscape Medical News.* Available at: www.medscape.com/viewarticle/549550.

937. In preparation to provide care to a client after a TRAM (transrectus abdominis myocutaneous) flap breast reconstruction, which actions should a nurse anticipate including in the collaborative plan of care for the client?

1. Initiating passive range of motion to the affected side immediately after surgery and continue every 4 hours
2. Assessing capillary refill, color, and temperature of the flap every hour for 24 hours
3. Maintaining a pressure dressing on the reconstructed breast for 48 hours
4. Keeping the affected arm below the level of the reconstructed breast for 48 hours

ANSWER: 2

To monitor for viability and adequacy of blood supply to the TRAM flap, the flap must be assessed every hour for the first 24 hours. Upper extremity exercise is restricted to reduce strain on the incision site. Pressure over the flap is avoided until healing is complete. The affected arm should be elevated to promote venous return.

➧ ***Test-taking Tip:*** *Focus on the TRAM flap breast reconstruction procedure. Use the nursing process and ABCs (airway, breathing, circulation) to select the option that ensures that circulation is adequate.*

Content Area: Adult Health; *Category of Health Alteration:* Reproductive Management; *Integrated Processes:* Nursing Process Planning; *Client Need:* Physiological Integrity/Reduction of Risk Potential/Potential for Complications from Surgical Procedures and Health Alterations; *Cognitive Level:* Application

Reference: Monahan, F., Sands, J., Neighbors, M., Marek, J., & Green, C. (2007). *Phipps' Medical-Surgical Nursing: Health and Illness Perspectives* (8th ed., pp. 1774, 1775). St. Louis, MO: Mosby/Elsevier.

938. EBP A client who is 5 days post–abdominal surgery is discussing her general health with a nurse. In the process of the discussion, the client tells the nurse that she has been experiencing breast pain for which she has had several diagnostic procedures, all of which have been negative. The client asks if the nurse has any advice on how this breast pain can be controlled without using prescription medications. Which suggestions should the nurse make? SELECT ALL THAT APPLY.

1. Take evening primrose oil, 1,000 mg three times per day.
2. Go without a bra for at least 4 hours a day.
3. Reduce caffeine in the diet.
4. Supplement the diet with B complex vitamins.
5. Apply hot packs to the breast.

ANSWER: 1, 3, 4, 5

Breast pain can be cyclic related to the menstrual cycle or noncyclic. Once specific disease has been ruled out, few women will require treatment with more than reassurance and well-tolerated medications and nonpharmacological treatment. Taking evening primrose oil, reducing caffeine, supplementing with B complex vitamins, and applying hot packs can be used to help control breast pain. The women should also be told to wear a support bra, not to go without a bra.

➧ ***Test-taking Tip:*** *Focus on the treatment for noncancerous breast pain. Eliminate any option that potentially could increase pain through gravitational pull.*

Content Area: Adult Health; *Category of Health Alteration:* Reproductive Management; *Integrated Processes:* Nursing Process Implementation; Teaching and Learning; *Client Need:* Physiological Integrity/Basic Care and Comfort/Nonpharmacological Comfort Interventions; *Cognitive Level:* Application

Reference: Lewis, S., Heitkemper, M., Dirksen, S., O'Brien, P., & Bucher, L. (2007). *Medical-Surgical Nursing: Assessment and Management of Clinical Problems* (7th ed., p. 1345). St. Louis, MO: Mosby/Elsevier.

EBP Reference: Institute for Clinical Systems Improvement. (2008). *Diagnosis of Breast Disease.* Available at: www.guideline.gov/summary/summary.aspx?doc_id=12232&nbr=006317&string=diagnosis+AND+breast+AND+disease

939. EBP A nurse is conducting a health history interview with a 20-year-old college sophomore when the client starts crying and says, "I'm so worried. I found a lump in my breast last night and I'm scared I might have cancer!" Which fact should the nurse consider when formulating a response to the client?

1. Young women are at increased risk to develop breast cancer.
2. A nondiscrete possible mass or thickening has a high index of suspicion for breast cancer.
3. Benign fibroadenomas are the most frequent cause of breast masses in women under 25 years.
4. College students often develop infectious breast disorders due to the close personal contact required in dormitory living.

ANSWER: 3

Fibroadenomas are the most common benign breast neoplasm, and most often occur in women younger than 25 years. Breast cancer is diagnosed most commonly in women older than 50 years. A nondiscrete possible mass or thickening has a lower (not higher) index of suspicion for breast cancer. Mastitis is a bacterial infection of the breast tissue and is not contagious and therefore would not be spread by dormitory living. Most cancerous tumors are usually not tender.

➧ ***Test-taking Tip:*** *Review knowledge of breast cancer, which should allow elimination of options 1 and 2, as these are not true statements about breast cancer. The key word in option 4 is "often." Think about how many college students you know who develop infectious breast disorders; probably none.*

Content Area: Adult Health; *Category of Health Alteration:* Reproductive Management; *Integrated Processes:* Nursing Process Planning; *Client Need:* Psychosocial Integrity/Crisis Intervention; Physiological Integrity/Physiological Adaptation/Pathophysiology; *Cognitive Level:* Application

References: Monahan, F., Sands, J., Neighbors, M., Marek, J., & Green, C. (2007). *Phipps' Medical-Surgical Nursing: Health and Illness Perspectives* (8th ed., pp. 1750, 1755–1776). St. Louis, MO: Mosby/Elsevier; Lewis, S., Heitkemper, M., Dirksen, S., O'Brien, P., & Bucher, L. (2007). *Medical-Surgical Nursing: Assessment and Management of Clinical Problems* (7th ed., p. 1347). St. Louis, MO: Mosby/Elsevier.

EBP Reference: University of Michigan Health System. (2007). *Common Breast Problems*. Available at: www.guideline.gov/summary/summary.aspx?doc_id=12015&nbr=006199&string=herbal

940. At a 6-week postpartum visit, a client tells a nurse that she is considering breast reduction and wants to know if she could still breastfeed a baby after such a procedure. Which statement should be the basis for the nurse's response?

1. Breast reduction does not affect the ability to breastfeed.
2. If the nipples are left connected to breast tissue, lactation is possible.
3. Breast reduction makes lactation impossible due to the amount of breast tissue removed.
4. Breastfeeding is impossible due to the changes that take place in the nipple structure from the surgery.

ANSWER: 2

Lactation can usually be accomplished if the nipples are left connected to breast tissue. Breast reduction has the potential to negatively affect lactation if large amounts of breast tissue are removed. The nipple structure is not changed with breast reduction; however, some surgeries may necessitate relocation of the nipple.

► ***Test-taking Tip:*** *Recall breast anatomy. Acini cells, which produce milk, are connected to ducts that eventually empty into lactiferous sinuses under the nipple. These connections must be maintained for lactation to occur.*

Content Area: Adult Health; *Category of Health Alteration:* Reproductive Management; *Integrated Processes:* Nursing Process Implementation; *Client Need:* Physiological Integrity/Reduction of Risk Potential/Potential for Complications of Diagnostic Tests/Treatments/Procedures; *Cognitive Level:* Application

Reference: Lewis, S., Heitkemper, M., Dirksen, S., O'Brien, P., & Bucher, L. (2007). *Medical-Surgical Nursing: Assessment and Management of Clinical Problems* (7th ed., pp. 1327, 1361). St. Louis, MO: Mosby/Elsevier.

941. While working in a urology clinic, a nurse receives a phone call from a concerned client diagnosed with known benign prostatic hyperplasia (BPH). The client says he developed a cold a few days ago and since then his urinary frequency and urgency have increased. The nurse should immediately ask the client if he has:

1. been drinking large amounts of water.
2. been exercising more than usual.
3. been taking any over-the-counter cold remedies.
4. increased the amount of dairy products in his diet.

ANSWER: 3

Compounds found in common cough and cold remedies, such as pseudoephedrine and phenylephrine, are alpha-adrenergic agonists that cause contraction of smooth muscle. Since the bladder is smooth muscle, these medications could result in increased symptoms of urinary urgency and frequency. Clients with BPH should maintain fluid intake at normal levels to prevent dehydration. Drinking large amounts of water, however, could lead to bladder distention, which would result in abdominal discomfort. Increased exercise will not alter BPH symptoms. Increased amounts of alcohol and caffeine can increase BPH symptoms, but dairy products should not affect BPH symptoms.

► ***Test-taking Tip:*** *The key information in this question is that the client has a cold and his symptoms increased with the onset of the cold symptoms. Option 3 directly mentions cold remedies.*

Content Area: Adult Health; *Category of Health Alteration:* Reproductive Management; *Integrated Processes:* Nursing Process Analysis; *Client Need:* Physiological Integrity/Pharmacological and Parenteral Therapies/Adverse Effects/Contraindications; *Cognitive Level:* Application

Reference: Lewis, S., Heitkemper, M., Dirksen, S., O'Brien, P., & Bucher, L. (2007). *Medical-Surgical Nursing: Assessment and Management of Clinical Problems* (7th ed., p. 1421). St. Louis, MO: Mosby/Elsevier.

942. A client is admitted to a surgical unit following a transurethral prostatectomy. The client has a continuous bladder irrigation (CBI) running. A nurse assesses the client's urine and finds dark red urine containing several small clots. In response to this finding, which action should the nurse take?

1. Increase the flow of the bladder irrigation fluid.
2. Immediately turn off the bladder irrigation.
3. Irrigate the catheter manually.
4. Deflate the balloon on the catheter.

ANSWER: 1

The purpose of the CBI is to remove clots from the bladder and ensure drainage of urine through the catheter. The flow rate of the CBI fluid should be set so that the urine remains free from clots and remains light red to pink. If the urine is dark red, the flow rate of the CBI should be increased. Turning off the CBI would increase the risk that the catheter would become blocked and the flow of urine interrupted. There is no need to manually irrigate a catheter if a CBI is infusing unless the catheter becomes obstructed. Deflating the catheter balloon would be contraindicated because this could result in dislodging the catheter.

➧ ***Test-taking Tip:*** *Recall the purpose of a CBI is to maintain catheter patency. Eliminate option 2 as this would negate the functioning of the CBI.*

Content Area: Adult Health; *Category of Health Alteration:* Reproductive Management; *Integrated Processes:* Nursing Process Implementation; *Client Need:* Physiological Integrity/Reduction of Risk Potential/Therapeutic Procedures; *Cognitive Level:* Application

References: Monahan, F., Sands, J., Neighbors, M., Marek, J., & Green, C. (2007). *Phipps' Medical-Surgical Nursing: Health and Illness Perspectives* (8th ed., p. 1731). St. Louis, MO: Mosby/Elsevier; Lewis, S., Heitkemper, M., Dirksen, S., O'Brien, P., & Bucher, L. (2007). *Medical-Surgical Nursing: Assessment and Management of Clinical Problems* (7th ed., p. 1421). St. Louis, MO: Mosby/Elsevier.

943. During the last 8 hours, a nurse cared for a client who had a transurethral prostatectomy. The client has continuous bladder irrigation (CBI) infusing. At the end of the 8 hours, a nurse determines that the client received 3,050 mL of irrigation fluid and that 4,030 mL of fluid was emptied from the urinary drainage bag. The nurse calculates the actual urine output for 8 hours to be _______ mL.

ANSWER: 980

Subtract the amount of CBI solution from the total amount of fluid emptied from the urinary drainage device: 4,030 mL – 3,050 mL = 980 mL. The intake and output record should reflect the urinary output compared with the amount of irrigation solution infused.

➧ ***Test-taking Tip:*** *Carefully read the question to determine what is being asked. Be sure to subtract the amount of irrigation solution from the total amount in the urinary drainage bag to obtain the urine output. Use the onscreen calculator to ensure accuracy with calculations.*

Content Area: Adult Health; *Category of Health Alteration:* Reproductive Management; *Integrated Processes:* Nursing Process Assessment; *Client Need:* Physiological Integrity/Basic Care and Comfort/Elimination; *Cognitive Level:* Application

Reference: Monahan, F., Sands, J., Neighbors, M., Marek, J., & Green, C. (2007). *Phipps' Medical-Surgical Nursing: Health and Illness Perspectives* (8th ed., p. 1731). St. Louis, MO: Mosby/Elsevier.

944. A nurse is caring for a client who is 24-hours post–transurethral prostatectomy. The nurse suspects the client may be having bladder spasms when he describes abdominal pain rated as 5 on a 0 to 10 numeric scale. A nurse assesses the Foley catheter and finds it draining freely. Based on this information, what should be the most appropriate nursing intervention?

1. Administer morphine sulfate intravenously, which is ordered as needed (prn).
2. Administer a belladonna and opium suppository, which is ordered prn.
3. Ambulate the client.
4. Apply cold compresses to the client's abdomen.

ANSWER: 2

Belladonna and opium suppositories inhibit smooth muscle contraction, which will decrease bladder spasms and also reduce pain. Opioid medications will decrease the pain sensations but will not decrease the muscle spasms. Ambulation will not decrease the discomfort and heat, rather than cold, is the recommended nonpharmacological treatment for bladder spasms.

➧ ***Test-taking Tip:*** *Think about therapies to relieve muscle spasms. That should allow elimination of options 1 and 3. Then consider the effects of applying cold versus warmth to the skin.*

Content Area: Adult Health; *Category of Health Alteration:* Reproductive Management; *Integrated Processes:* Nursing Process Planning; *Client Need:* Physiological Integrity/Pharmacological and Parenteral Therapies/Expected Actions or Outcomes; *Cognitive Level:* Application

Reference: Smeltzer, S., Bare, B., Hinkle, J., & Cheever, K. (2008). *Brunner & Suddarth's Textbook of Medical-Surgical Nursing* (11th ed., p. 1766). Philadelphia: Lippincott Williams & Wilkins.

945. While obtaining a hospital admission history for a 35-year-old client, which statement made by the client should prompt a nurse to consider that the client has chronic prostatitis?

1. "I am having difficulty obtaining erection."
2. "When I ejaculate I have pain."
3. "I have been feeling pressure around my rectum."
4. "I don't think I am totally emptying my bladder."

ANSWER: 2
Both chronic bacterial prostatitis and chronic prostatitis/pelvic pain syndrome manifest with ejaculatory pain. Other symptoms include irritative voiding symptoms, backache, and perineal/pelvic pain. Chronic prostatitis does not cause erectile dysfunction or rectal pain. Obstructive bladder symptoms, such as incomplete bladder emptying, are uncommon unless the client also has benign prostatic hyperplasia.

➧ ***Test-taking Tip:*** *Recall the physiology of male sexual response: during ejaculation the prostate gland contracts. Thus, disease in the prostate gland would predispose to ejaculation pain.*

Content Area: Adult Health; *Category of Health Alteration:* Reproductive Management; *Integrated Processes:* Nursing Process Assessment; *Client Need:* Physiological Integrity/Physiological Adaptation/Alterations in Body Systems; *Cognitive Level:* Application

Reference: Lewis, S., Heitkemper, M., Dirksen, S., O'Brien, P., & Bucher, L. (2007). *Medical-Surgical Nursing: Assessment and Management of Clinical Problems* (7th ed., pp. 1429, 1434). St. Louis, MO: Mosby/Elsevier.

---

946. A nurse is reviewing hospital admission orders for a client diagnosed with acute prostatitis. Before initiating the orders, which order should the nurse question?

1. Begin intravenous trimethoprim/sulfamethoxazole (Bactrim®) 1 gram every 6 hours.
2. Give ibuprofen (Motrin®) 600 mg orally every 6 hours prn (as needed).
3. Maintain bedrest with bathroom privileges.
4. Insert a Foley urinary drainage catheter.

ANSWER: 4
Passage of a catheter through an inflamed urethra is contraindicated in acute prostatitis. If urinary retention is a concern, a suprapubic catheter should be used. Bactrim® is a common antibiotic used to treat acute prostatitis. Adequate hydration should be maintained. Analgesics, such as NSAIDs, should be used for pain control, and rest encouraged.

➧ ***Test-taking Tip:*** *Select the option that is unsafe for the client.*

Content Area: Adult Health; *Category of Health Alteration:* Reproductive Management; *Integrated Processes:* Nursing Process Evaluation; *Client Need:* Safe and Effective Care Environment/Safety and Infection Control/Injury Prevention; *Cognitive Level:* Application

References: Lehne, R. (2007). *Pharmacology for Nursing Care* (6th ed., p. 1007). St. Louis, MO: Elsevier/Saunders; Lewis, S., Heitkemper, M., Dirksen, S., O'Brien, P., & Bucher, L. (2007). *Medical-Surgical Nursing: Assessment and Management of Clinical Problems* (7th ed., pp. 1423, 1429). St. Louis, MO: Mosby/Elsevier.

---

947. A community health nurse is asked to prepare health education on testicular cancer. To obtain the maximal impact, the nurse should plan to present this education to which group?

1. High school males
2. Males over 30-years-old who have never fathered a child
3. Males over 21-years-old who have fathered at least one child
4. Males who are over the age of 50 years

ANSWER: 1
Testicular cancer is the most common type of cancer in young men between 15 and 34 years of age. Therefore, education should be directed at high-school-age males. Fathering a child does not change the risk for development of testicular cancer; all males in the high-risk age group should be educated. Increasing age decreases risk.

➧ ***Test-taking Tip:*** *Read the situation carefully. The focus of the question is the age group most at risk to develop testicular cancer. Select the option that best represents that group.*

Content Area: Adult Health; *Category of Health Alteration:* Reproductive Management; *Integrated Processes:* Nursing Process Planning; *Client Need:* Health Promotion and Maintenance/Health Promotion and Disease Prevention; *Cognitive Level:* Application

Reference: Lewis, S., Heitkemper, M., Dirksen, S., O'Brien, P., & Bucher, L. (2007). *Medical-Surgical Nursing: Assessment and Management of Clinical Problems* (7th ed., pp. 1423, 1432). St. Louis, MO: Mosby/Elsevier.

948. A client with testicular cancer is admitted to a hospital for treatment of the disease. A nurse reviews the client's laboratory values. After this review, the nurse concludes that the:

Laboratory-Serum	Client Value	Normal Values
BUN	20	5–25 mg
Creatinine	1.0	0.5–1.5 mg/dL
Na	137	135–145 mEq/L
K	3.4	3.5–5.3 mEq/L
Cl	99	95–105 mEq/L
CO_2	24	22–30 mEq/L
Glucose	132	70–110 mg/dL
Hgb/Hct	10/32%	13.5–17 g/dL, 40%–54%
WBC	9,000	4,500–10,000/μL
Neutrophils	65%	50%–70%
Aspartate aminotransferase (AST)	200 units/L	8–38 units/L
Alanine aminotransferase (ALT)	150 units/L	10–35 units/L

1. client may have developed an infection.
2. client's nutrient intake has been inadequate.
3. client's liver has been activated in an attempt to fight the disease.
4. client's disease may have metastasized.

ANSWER: 4

Anemia and elevated liver function tests are present when testicular cancer has metastasized. There is no indication of developing infection or inadequate nutrition, and laboratory results will not demonstrate the liver's attempt to fight cancer. The client's elevated glucose and lowered potassium could be related to the body's physiological and/or psychological response to stress.

▶ ***Test-taking Tip:*** *When reviewing the laboratory results, determine which are abnormal. Then use the process of elimination to eliminate options 1 and 2, as there is not information to support these options.*

Content Area: Adult Health; *Category of Health Alteration:* Reproductive Management; *Integrated Processes:* Nursing Process Assessment; *Client Need:* Physiological Integrity/Reduction of Risk Potential/Laboratory Values; Physiological Integrity/Physiological Adaptation/Alterations in Body Systems; *Cognitive Level:* Analysis

References: Lewis, S., Heitkemper, M., Dirksen, S., O'Brien, P., & Bucher, L. (2007). *Medical-Surgical Nursing: Assessment and Management of Clinical Problems* (7th ed., pp. 114, 328, 1432). St. Louis, MO: Mosby/Elsevier; Smeltzer, S., Bare, B., Hinkle, J., & Cheever, K. (2008). *Brunner & Suddarth's Textbook of Medical-Surgical Nursing* (11th ed., p. 95). Philadelphia: Lippincott Williams & Wilkins.

949. A client is told that he will require a right orchiectomy for treatment of testicular cancer. The client asks a nurse if he will be infertile after this procedure. Which response should be made by the nurse?

1. "This procedure will make you infertile."
2. "Has your surgeon discussed cryopreservation of your sperm?"
3. "Since only one testicle is being removed your fertility will not be affected."
4. "Don't be concerned about this now, at this point you need to be concerned about removal of the cancer."

ANSWER: 2

The impact of treatment for testicular cancer on fertility varies. The involvement of chemotherapy, lymph node removal, and/or radiation in the treatment plan may all impact a client's ability to procreate. Clients should be encouraged to consider cryopreservation of sperm in a sperm bank before beginning treatment for testicular cancer. The client's fertility can be affected to varying degrees, so it is inappropriate to say the client will absolutely be infertile or absolutely not be infertile. Telling the client not to be concerned is inappropriate communication because it is negating the client's feelings and changing the subject.

▶ ***Test-taking Tip:*** *Note that options 1 and 3 offer absolute yes and no answers to the question of infertility. Rarely is this the case in any aspect of health care. Eliminate both of these options for this reason.*

Content Area: Adult Health; *Category of Health Alteration:* Reproductive Management; *Integrated Processes:* Nursing Process Implementation; Communication and Documentation; *Client Need:* Health Promotion and Maintenance/Health and Wellness; *Cognitive Level:* Application

References: Lewis, S., Heitkemper, M., Dirksen, S., O'Brien, P., & Bucher, L. (2007). *Medical-Surgical Nursing: Assessment and Management of Clinical Problems* (7th ed., pp. 1432–1433). St. Louis, MO: Mosby/Elsevier; Craven, R., & Hirnle, C. (2007). *Fundamentals of Nursing: Human Health and Function* (5th ed., p. 380). Philadelphia: Lippincott Williams & Wilkins.

950. A male client who is considering a vasectomy for contraception asks a nurse where the incision for the procedure will be made. The nurse utilizes the picture below to educate the client. On which area of the body should the nurse inform the client that the incision will most likely be made?

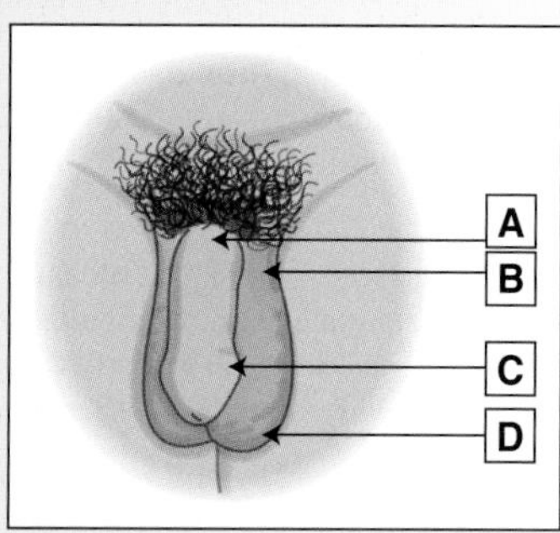

1. Location A
2. Location B
3. Location C
4. Location D

ANSWER: 2

A vasectomy is a resection of the vas deferens to prevent passage of sperm from the testes to the urethra during ejaculation. Because the vas deferens travels out of the scrotum and into the abdomen (gut cavity) through the inguinal canal, it cannot be seen from the outside of the body. A small incision is made in the upper portion of the scrotum to expose the vas deferens (location B). The vas deferens is then severed, and the severed ends are occluded with ligatures or by electrocautery. Neither the upper or lower portion of the penis, nor the lower portions of the scrotum are incised during a vasectomy.

➧ ***Test-taking Tip:*** *Think about the location of the vas deferens and then where anatomically it would be most accessible.*

Content Area: Adult Health; *Category of Health Alteration:* Reproductive Management; *Integrated Processes:* Nursing Process Implementation; Teaching and Learning; *Client Need:* Physiological Integrity/Physiological Adaptation/Alterations in Body Systems; *Cognitive Level:* Application

Reference: Smeltzer, S., Bare, B., Hinkle, J., & Cheever, K. (2008). *Brunner & Suddarth's Textbook of Medical-Surgical Nursing* (11th ed., p. 1773). Philadelphia: Lippincott Williams & Wilkins.

---

951. **EBP** A nurse is obtaining a health history on a client with a possible varicocele. What should be the nurse's priority assessment question?

1. "Did your father have any testicular problems?"
2. "Does the left side of your scrotum feel different from the right side?"
3. "Do you have any children?"
4. "Do you have any discomfort in your groin?"

ANSWER: 3

The most common cause of male infertility is a varicocele. Approximately 15% to 20% of the healthy, fertile male population is estimated to have varicoceles. However, 40% of infertile men may have them. Varicoceles are not inherited. A varicocele does occur most frequently on the left side due to retrograde blood flow from the renal vein; however, this is not the priority question. A varicocele rarely produces any symptoms and is usually diagnosed during physical examinations related to infertility. If symptoms do occur, pain or groin tenderness are the most common symptoms.

➧ ***Test-taking Tip:*** *"Priority" is the key term. Infertility is a major concern with a varicocele and thus the question about the client's ability to reproduce is the priority.*

Content Area: Adult Health; *Category of Health Alteration:* Reproductive Management; *Integrated Processes:* Nursing Process Assessment; *Client Need:* Safe and Effective Care Environment/Management of Care/Establishing Priorities; Physiological Integrity/Physiological Adaptation/Alterations in Body Systems; *Cognitive Level:* Application

References: Smeltzer, S., Bare, B., Hinkle, J., & Cheever, K. (2008). *Brunner & Suddarth's Textbook of Medical-Surgical Nursing* (11th ed., p. 1773). Philadelphia: Lippincott Williams & Wilkins; Lewis, S., Heitkemper, M., Dirksen, S., O'Brien, P., & Bucher, L. (2007). *Medical-Surgical Nursing: Assessment and Management of Clinical Problems* (7th ed., p. 1431). St. Louis, MO: Mosby/Elsevier.

EBP References: Institute for Clinical Systems Improvement. (2004). *Diagnosis and Management of Basic Infertility.* Available at: www.guideline.gov/summary/summary.aspx?doc_id=5567&nbr=003764&string=varicocele; Barclay, L., & Hghiem, H. (2008). Embolization of varicoceles may improve male infertility. *Medscape Medical News.* Available at: www.medscape.com/viewarticle/577841

952. EBP A client tells a nurse that he and his wife really want a child but that he has learned he has a sperm count of "only 40 million." He wonders if there is anything that would improve his ability to impregnate his wife. In planning care for the client, which factor should the nurse consider?

1. The client's lifestyle can be examined to determine if he is in contact with any gonadotoxins.
2. This sperm count is very low, and the chances of the client impregnating his wife are low.
3. The health-care practitioner may recommend testosterone supplementation.
4. The incidence of impregnation is decreased with a sperm count below 20 million.

ANSWER: 4

The normal sperm count is 60 to 100 million sperm/mL of semen, but the incidence of impregnation is lessened only when the sperm count decreases to less than 20 million/mL. Gonadotoxins are chemicals, drugs, or other substances that have a toxic or suppressive effect on sperm production, motility, or morphology. Their effect is usually reversible if exposure is discontinued, so no further action is needed for this client since his sperm count is adequate to achieve fertilization. There is no need to utilize testosterone supplements for this client.

➧ *Test-taking Tip: Note that options 1, 2, and 3 all assume that the client needs further treatment. Option 4 is different. Recall the sperm count needed for fertilization and select option 4.*

Content Area: Adult Health; *Category of Health Alteration:* Reproductive Management; *Integrated Processes:* Nursing Process Planning; *Client Need:* Physiological Integrity/Reduction of Risk Potential/Laboratory Values; *Cognitive Level:* Analysis

Reference: Smeltzer, S., Bare, B., Hinkle, J., & Cheever, K. (2008). *Brunner & Suddarth's Textbook of Medical-Surgical Nursing* (11th ed., p. 1650). Philadelphia: Lippincott Williams & Wilkins.

EBP Reference: Institute for Clinical Systems Improvement (2004). *Diagnosis and Management of Basic Infertility.* Available at: www.guideline.gov/summary/summary.aspx?doc_id=5567&nbr=003764&string=varicocele

---

953. EBP While volunteering at a prenatal education booth at a health and wellness fair, a young married couple tells a nurse they have been attempting to achieve a pregnancy and have been unsuccessful. They are wondering if they should begin treatment for infertility. In response, which *initial* question should the nurse ask?

1. "How long have you been having regular intercourse without contraception?"
2. "How old are you both?"
3. "Do either of you smoke cigarettes?"
4. "Have either of you ever had an infection in your reproductive tract?"

ANSWER: 1

The definition of *infertility* is the inability to achieve a pregnancy after 1 year of regular intercourse without contraception. If the couple has not been attempting to achieve a pregnancy for that length of time, then there is no need for infertility testing. The other questions address risk factors for infertility, but those questions would be inconsequential if the criterion in option 1 were not met.

➧ *Test-taking Tip: Read the question carefully; options 2, 3, and 4 are risk factors for infertility; however, the client's answer to option 1 would impact whether the other questions should be asked.*

Content Area: Adult Health; *Category of Health Alteration:* Reproductive Management; *Integrated Processes:* Nursing Process Assessment; *Client Need:* Health Promotion and Maintenance/Health and Wellness; *Cognitive Level:* Analysis

Reference: Lewis, S., Heitkemper, M., Dirksen, S., O'Brien, P., & Bucher, L. (2007). *Medical-Surgical Nursing: Assessment and Management of Clinical Problems* (7th ed., p. 1382). St. Louis, MO: Mosby/Elsevier.

EBP Reference: Quallich, S. (2006). Examining male infertility. *Urologic Nursing*, 26(4), 277–288.

---

954. A nurse is discharging a client after an elective abortion by suction curettage. Which statement should the nurse include in the client's discharge instructions?

1. Sexual intercourse can be resumed once vaginal discharge has stopped.
2. A vaginal douche with clean tap water should be performed bid for 48 hours.
3. If the vaginal discharge develops a foul odor, the health-care practitioner should be notified.
4. Plan to return to work in 1 week.

ANSWER: 3

Infection, hemorrhage, and retained tissue are among the more common complications of abortions that are performed via suction curettage. Foul-smelling vaginal discharge is a sign of vaginal infection and/or retained tissue and should be reported as soon as it is noted by the client. Nothing should be placed in the vagina until the client has been re-examined in 2 weeks by the health-care practitioner. Many women resume their usual activities the same day as the abortion. There is no evidence to support the need to wait a week before returning to work.

➧ *Test-taking Tip: Options 1 and 2 are similar in that they involve placing something into the vagina. If one were true the other also should be true, therefore eliminate both of these options.*

Content Area: Adult Health; *Category of Health Alteration:* Reproductive Management; *Integrated Processes:* Nursing Process Implementation; Teaching and Learning; *Client Need:* Physiological Integrity/Reduction of Risk Potential/Potential for Complications from Surgical Procedures and Health Alterations; *Cognitive Level:* Application

Reference: Lewis, S., Heitkemper, M., Dirksen, S., O'Brien, P., & Bucher, L. (2007). *Medical-Surgical Nursing: Assessment and Management of Clinical Problems* (7th ed., pp. 1340, 1385). St. Louis, MO: Mosby/Elsevier.

955. EBP A 15-year-old female client is placed on oral contraceptives (OCPs) to control dysmenorrhea. The girl's mother is concerned about this medical decision and asks a nurse why the physician would choose this mode of treatment. When formulating a response to the mother, which fact about oral contraceptives should the nurse consider?

1. Oral contraceptives inhibit uterine inflammation which indirectly causes dysmenorrhea.
2. Oral contraceptives increase blood flow to the uterus during menstruation and promote uterine relaxation.
3. Oral contraceptives inhibit progesterone production, which stimulates uterine contractions and causes pain.
4. Oral contraceptives suppress ovulation and therefore prostaglandin production.

ANSWER: 4

Dysmenorrhea is caused by excessive endometrial prostaglandin production, which increases myometrial contraction and constriction of small endometrial blood vessels resulting in ischemia and pain. OCPs block ovulation by preventing the release of follicle-stimulating hormone from the pituitary. The absence of ovulation decreases the sequential stimulation of the endometrium by estrogen and progesterone. This results in a decrease in the prostaglandin production by the endometrium and thus a decrease in pain. Treatment of dysmenorrhea is a well-accepted off-label use for OCPs. OCPs do not inhibit inflammation, and they do not increase uterine blood flow; in fact, the amount of menstrual discharge may decrease with OCP usage as a result of decreased endometrial stimulation. OCPs do inhibit progesterone production, but it is not progesterone that stimulates uterine contractions and pain; rather, it is prostaglandins.

Test-taking Tip: *The key to answering this question correctly is to recall the action of OCPs, which is to suppress ovulation. This knowledge makes option 4 the only choice.*

Content Area: Adult Health; *Category of Health Alteration:* Reproductive Management; *Integrated Processes:* Nursing Process Planning; *Client Need:* Physiological Integrity/Pharmacological and Parenteral Therapies/Expected Actions or Outcomes; *Cognitive Level:* Application

References: Smeltzer, S., Bare, B., Hinkle, J., & Cheever, K. (2008). *Brunner & Suddarth's Textbook of Medical-Surgical Nursing* (11th ed., p. 1641). Philadelphia: Lippincott Williams & Wilkins; Lewis, S., Heitkemper, M., Dirksen, S., O'Brien, P., & Bucher, L. (2007). *Medical-Surgical Nursing: Assessment and Management of Clinical Problems* (7th ed., p. 1386). St. Louis, MO: Mosby/Elsevier.

EBP Reference: Penney, G., Brechin, S., & Allerton, L. (2005). The use of contraception outside the terms of the product license. *Journal of Family Planning and Reproductive Health Care,* 31(3), 225–241. Available at: www.guideline.gov/summary/summary.aspx?doc_id=7488&nbr=004433&string=dysmenorrhea

956. Which laboratory result should a nurse carefully review when completing a health assessment of a female client with menorrhagia of unknown origin?

1. Calcium level
2. Blood urea nitrogen (BUN)
3. Hemoglobin level
4. White blood cell value

ANSWER: 3

Menorrhagia is excessive or prolonged bleeding at the time of the regular menstrual flow. Persistent heavy bleeding can result in anemia, which would be reflected in the client's hemoglobin. Calcium, BUN, and white blood cells should not be affected by menorrhagia.

Test-taking Tip: *The term "menorrhagia" is the key to this question. Apply knowledge of medical terminology and use the meaning of this term (excessive or prolonged bleeding) as a clue to the correct option.*

Content Area: Adult Health; *Category of Health Alteration:* Reproductive Management; *Integrated Processes:* Nursing Process Assessment; *Client Need:* Physiological Integrity/Reduction of Risk Potential/Laboratory Values; *Cognitive Level:* Application

Reference: Smeltzer, S., Bare, B., Hinkle, J., & Cheever, K. (2008). *Brunner & Suddarth's Textbook of Medical-Surgical Nursing* (11th ed., p. 1639). Philadelphia: Lippincott Williams & Wilkins.

957. A nurse is obtaining a health history from a 30-year-old female client who describes multiple concerns. Which concerns should alert the nurse to the possibility of endometriosis? SELECT ALL THAT APPLY.

1. Bleeding between periods
2. Vaginal dryness
3. Premenstrual tension headache
4. Pain during her menstrual period
5. Inability to conceive
6. Dyspareunia

ANSWER: 4, 5, 6

Endometriosis is the presence of normal endometrial tissue in sites outside the endometrial cavity. The tissue responds to hormonal influence, and therefore during menstruation the tissue bleeds. This bleeding causes inflammation and pain at the time of menstruation. Women with endometriosis are at increased risk for infertility. There are several theories about the cause of this infertility. One theory is that scarring and adhesion in and around the reproductive organs affect the fertilization and implantation process. Another theory is that women with endometriosis lack a substance in the uterus that is necessary for implantation of the fertilized ovum. A third theory is that the endometrial cysts produce substances that inhibit conception. Depending on the location of the endometrial tissue, clients may experience pain with intercourse. Vaginal dryness and bleeding between periods and premenstrual tension headaches are not symptoms of endometriosis.

Test-taking Tip: *Focus on symptoms that would arise when endometrial tissue appears in sites outside of the endometrial cavity.*

Content Area: Adult Health; *Category of Health Alteration:* Reproductive Management; *Integrated Processes:* Nursing Process Assessment; *Client Need:* Physiological Integrity/Physiological Adaptation/Alterations in Body Systems; *Cognitive Level:* Application

References: Smeltzer, S., Bare, B., Hinkle, J., & Cheever, K. (2008). *Brunner & Suddarth's Textbook of Medical-Surgical Nursing* (11th ed., pp. 1680, 1681). Philadelphia: Lippincott Williams & Wilkins; Lewis, S., Heitkemper, M., Dirksen, S., O'Brien, P., & Bucher, L. (2007). *Medical-Surgical Nursing: Assessment and Management of Clinical Problems* (7th ed., p. 1396). St. Louis, MO: Mosby/Elsevier.

958. A health-care practitioner has prescribed mifepristone (Mifeprex®) for a 35-year-old female as treatment for a leiomyoma. Before beginning the medication, which information is most important for the nurse to obtain?

1. A baseline blood pressure
2. Results of a blood test for liver enzymes
3. Results of a pregnancy test
4. A baseline weight

ANSWER: 3

Mifepristone is a synthetic steroid that blocks receptors for progesterone. Therefore it would decrease the hormonal supply to the leiomyoma and cause it to shrink. However, because it is also used in conjunction with other medications for termination of early intrauterine pregnancy, the pregnancy test results should be known. The drug does not cause changes in blood pressure, liver enzymes, or weight.

Test-taking Tip: *The focus of this question is the treatment of leiomyomas. Because leiomyomas are tumors associated with the uterus, it is most likely they would be treated with reproductive hormones. Select the option most closely associated with female reproductive hormones.*

Content Area: Adult Health; *Category of Health Alteration:* Reproductive Management; *Integrated Processes:* Nursing Process Planning; *Client Need:* Safe and Effective Care Environment/Safety and Infection Control/Injury Prevention; Physiological Integrity/Pharmacological and Parenteral Therapies/Expected Actions or Outcomes; *Cognitive Level:* Application

References: Lehne, R. (2007). *Pharmacology for Nursing Care* (6th ed., pp. 730, 732). St. Louis, MO: Elsevier/Saunders; Smeltzer, S., Bare, B., Hinkle, J., & Cheever, K. (2008). *Brunner & Suddarth's Textbook of Medical-Surgical Nursing* (11th ed., p. 1679). Philadelphia: Lippincott Williams & Wilkins.

959. A female client has an abdominal hysterectomy to remove a uterine fibroid. Which action should a nurse include when caring for the client postoperatively?

1. Monitor the perineal pad for bleeding
2. Administer hormone replacement therapy
3. Maintain bed rest for 48 hours
4. Start a regular diet 6 hours postsurgery

ANSWER: 1

Infection and hemorrhage are the major risks of hysterectomy. Monitoring the perineal pad will alert the nurse to any increase in vaginal bleeding. Hormone replacement therapy is only needed if the ovaries have been removed (oophorectomy). Development of deep vein thrombosis is a concern after abdominal hysterectomy, and the client should be encouraged to ambulate in the early postoperative period. Peristalsis is typically suppressed after abdominal hysterectomy, and the client will be on restricted oral intake until physical signs of the return of peristalsis are present.

➧ *Test-taking Tip: Read the question carefully: the client has had her uterus removed. There is no mention of removal of the ovaries; therefore there is no reason for hormone replacement. Therefore option 2 can be eliminated. Of the remaining options, focus on selecting an option specific to the woman's surgical procedure.*

Content Area: Adult Health; *Category of Health Alteration:* Reproductive Management; *Integrated Processes:* Nursing Process Implementation; *Client Need:* Physiological Integrity/Physiological Adaptation/Illness Management; *Cognitive Level:* Application

References: Monahan, F., Sands, J., Neighbors, M., Marek, J., & Green, C. (2007). *Phipps' Medical-Surgical Nursing: Health and Illness Perspectives* (8th ed., p. 1710). St. Louis, MO: Mosby/Elsevier; Smeltzer, S., Bare, B., Hinkle, J., & Cheever, K. (2008). *Brunner & Suddarth's Textbook of Medical-Surgical Nursing* (11th ed., pp. 1692–1693). Philadelphia: Lippincott Williams & Wilkins.

---

960. A 21-year-old college female, who has been diagnosed with polycystic ovary syndrome (PCOS), asks a nurse if there are any lifestyle changes that she could initiate to help to control her disease. Which statement is the nurse's best response?

1. "Decrease the amount of caffeine in your diet."
2. "Avoid using oral contraceptives for birth control."
3. "Avoid multiple sexual partners."
4. "Maintain your weight within the acceptable parameters for your height."

ANSWER: 4

Obesity exacerbates the problems of PCOS, especially related to insulin resistance. Oral contraceptives are useful in regulating the menstrual cycle for clients with PCOS and are utilized to treat this syndrome. Limiting caffeine in the diet and maintaining a monogamous sexual relationship will not impact PCOS.

➧ *Test-taking Tip: Recall the relationship of weight to PCOS. Use the process of elimination to rule out incorrect options.*

Content Area: Adult Health; *Category of Health Alteration:* Reproductive Management; *Integrated Processes:* Nursing Process Implementation; Communication and Documentation; *Client Need:* Health Promotion and Maintenance/Lifestyle Choices; *Cognitive Level:* Application

Reference: Lewis, S., Heitkemper, M., Dirksen, S., O'Brien, P., & Bucher, L. (2007). *Medical-Surgical Nursing: Assessment and Management of Clinical Problems* (7th ed., pp. 1399, 1400). St. Louis, MO: Mosby/Elsevier.

---

961. A student is preparing a seminar for college-age women about ways to decrease the risk of developing ovarian cancer. A registered nurse (RN) is reviewing the content the student nurse is planning to present. Which statement should the nurse delete from the student's prepared content?

1. Bear children if physically and psychologically able.
2. Decrease the fat in your diet.
3. Avoid using oral contraceptives for birth control.
4. Plan to breastfeed if you have children.

ANSWER: 3

The statement about avoiding oral contraceptives should be removed. Using oral contraceptives is associated with a lower ovarian cancer risk if they are used for more than 5 years. All other statements are correct. Nulliparity increases the risk of developing the disease, as does a high-fat diet. Breastfeeding does reduce the risk of developing the disease.

➧ *Test-taking Tip: The fact that the stem says the RN "deletes" indicates a false-response item. Look for the incorrect statement.*

Content Area: Adult Health; *Category of Health Alteration:* Reproductive Management; *Integrated Processes:* Nursing Process Implementation; Teaching and Learning; *Client Need:* Health Promotion and Maintenance/Lifestyle Choices; Health Promotion and Maintenance/Health and Wellness; *Cognitive Level:* Application

Reference: Lewis, S., Heitkemper, M., Dirksen, S., O'Brien, P., & Bucher, L. (2007). *Medical-Surgical Nursing: Assessment and Management of Clinical Problems* (7th ed., pp. 1399, 1402). St. Louis, MO: Mosby/Elsevier.

---

962. A primary care provider has written orders for a client who is 24 hours post–vulvectomy surgery. Which order should the nurse question?

1. Cleanse perineal wound with warm saline daily.
2. Remove Foley catheter; straight catheterize if unable to void.
3. Begin low-residue diet when tolerating oral intake.
4. Position in low Fowler's position.

ANSWER: 2

Because of perineal trauma and edema, a Foley catheter should be placed in surgery to provide urinary drainage. After the surgery, the Foley catheter may be needed for a prolonged period. To promote healing and prevent infection the perineal wound is cleansed with saline or the client is given sitz baths for cleansing. A low Fowler's position decreases postoperative discomfort. A low residue diet prevents straining at stool and wound contamination.

➧ *Test-taking Tip: Focus on the client's safety. Select the option that could potentially cause perineal trauma.*

Content Area: Adult Health; *Category of Health Alteration:* Reproductive Management; *Integrated Processes:* Nursing Process Implementation; *Client Need:* Safe and Effective Care Environment/ Safety and Infection Control/Injury Prevention; *Cognitive Level:* Application

References: Lewis, S., Heitkemper, M., Dirksen, S., O'Brien, P., & Bucher, L. (2007). *Medical-Surgical Nursing: Assessment and Management of Clinical Problems* (7th ed., pp. 1399, 1406). St. Louis, MO: Mosby/ Elsevier; Smeltzer, S., Bare, B., Hinkle, J., & Cheever, K. (2008). *Brunner & Suddarth's Textbook of Medical-Surgical Nursing* (11th ed., p. 1687). Philadelphia: Lippincott Williams & Wilkins.

963. A male client, who had been prescribed sildenafil (Viagra®) 2 weeks previously for erectile dysfunction, calls a urologic clinic to report that he takes his medication orally and waits for his erection to develop but nothing happens. When responding to the client's comment, which fact should form the basis for the nurse's response?

1. In clinical trials, the drug was only effective 20% of the time.
2. The drug is supposed to be inserted rectally and is not effective if taken orally.
3. In the absence of sexual stimuli, the drug will not cause an erection.
4. If taken with a high-fat meal, the drug is ineffective.

ANSWER: 3

The drug enhances the normal erectile response to sexual stimuli by promoting relaxation of arterial and trabecular smooth muscle. The resultant arterial dilation causes engorgement of sinusoidal spaces in the corpus cavernosum. In the absence of sexual stimuli however, nothing will happen. At least some improvement in erectile hardness and duration was reported by 70% of men taking the drug. The drug should be taken orally. A fatty meal delays absorption, and, as a result, plasma levels peak in 2 hours instead of an hour.

➧ ***Test-taking Tip:*** *Focus on the pharmacological action of sildenafil.*

Content Area: Adult Health; *Category of Health Alteration:* Reproductive Management; *Integrated Processes:* Nursing Process Planning; *Client Need:* Physiological Integrity/Pharmacological and Parenteral Therapies/Expected Actions or Outcomes; *Cognitive Level:* Application

Reference: Lehne, R. (2007). *Pharmacology for Nursing Care* (6th ed., p. 761). St. Louis, MO: Elsevier/Saunders.

964. **EBP** A client with erectile dysfunction is instructed on the use of alprostadil (Caverject®) via subcutaneous penile injection. A nurse determines that the client needs further instruction about alprostadil and its administration. Which statement was most likely made by the client to lead the nurse to this conclusion?

1. "I know I will have to keep the needle sterile before I inject my penis."
2. "I know I will not experience prolonged erections."
3. "I know the injection will produce an erection in 20 to 30 minutes.
4. "If feeling dizzy after an injection, I should report this."

ANSWER: 2

Clients using intracavernous injection therapy should be informed of the potential occurrence of prolonged erections and have a plan for the urgent treatment of prolonged erections. The client is correct in using sterile technique for the injection. The medication will begin to produce the desired effect within 30 minutes, and dizziness is a side effect of the medication and should be reported.

➧ ***Test-taking Tip:*** *The phrase "needs further instruction" is a false-response item. Look for the incorrect statement. Note that option 2 is different in that it contains the word "not."*

Content Area: Adult Health; *Category of Health Alteration:* Reproductive Management; *Integrated Processes:* Nursing Process Evaluation; *Client Need:* Physiological Integrity/Pharmacological and Parenteral Therapies/Expected Actions or Outcomes; *Cognitive Level:* Application

Reference: Lewis, S., Heitkemper, M., Dirksen, S., O'Brien, P., & Bucher, L. (2007). *Medical-Surgical Nursing: Assessment and Management of Clinical Problems* (7th ed., pp. 1435–1436). St. Louis, MO: Mosby/Elsevier.

EBP Reference: Montague, D., Jarow, J., Broderick, G., Dmochowski, R., Heaton, J., et al. (2006). *The Management of Erectile Dysfunction: An Update.* American Urologic Association Education and Research, Erectile Dysfunction Guideline Update Panel. Available at: www.guideline.gov/ summary/summary.aspx?doc_id=10018&nbr=005332&string=erectile+ AND+dysfunction

965. While presenting a seminar on reproductive health to a group of college-age women, a seminar participant asks a nurse if there is a way that a woman can recognize when she is ovulating. The nurse should respond that, at ovulation:

1. the mucus produced by the cervix becomes abundant and stretchy.
2. the body temperature drops and stays low for the rest of the menstrual cycle.
3. over-the-counter urine tests will be negative for luteinizing hormone.
4. the libido will decrease.

ANSWER: 1

At the time of ovulation, the mucus produced by the cervix becomes more abundant and stretchy. It looks and feels like egg whites. The ability of the mucus to be stretched indicates the period of maximum fertility. At the time of ovulation, the basal body temperature drops slightly and then, under the influence of progesterone, increases and stays elevated until 2 to 4 days before menstruation starts. Home measurement of luteinizing hormone (LH) is now possible with dip-stick urine tests. The correlation between urine LH levels and ovulation has been close to 100%. At the time of ovulation, most females note an increase in libido.

▶ ***Test-taking Tip:*** *Focus on physiological signs of ovulation*

Content Area: Adult Health; *Category of Health Alteration:* Reproductive Management; *Integrated Processes:* Nursing Process Implementation; Teaching and Learning; *Client Need:* Health Promotion and Maintenance/Health and Wellness; *Cognitive Level:* Application

Reference: Wong, L., Hockenberry, M., Perry, S., Lowdermilk, D., & Wilson, D. (2006). *Maternal Child Nursing Care* (3rd ed., pp. 92, 162–163). St. Louis, MO: Mosby.

966. A healthy 56-year-old female client who is menopausal tells a nurse that she has been experiencing vaginal itching, burning, and increased vaginal infections over the last 2 years. Which statement is the nurse's best response?

1. "Frequent vaginal infections could be a precursor to vulvar cancer."
2. "Vaginal itching could be related to a contact allergy."
3. "Your vagina becomes more acidic after menopause. This could be causing your symptoms."
4. "An increase in vaginal pH during menopause predisposes you to these symptoms."

ANSWER: 4

Decreased estrogen in menopausal women causes thinning of the vaginal mucosa and an increase in pH of vaginal secretions. As a result, the vagina is easily traumatized and more susceptible to infection. Vaginal infections do not predispose a female to vulvar cancer. Vaginal itching may be related to a contact allergy; however, this could be ultimately related to the increased fragility of the vaginal tissue after menopause.

▶ ***Test-taking Tip:*** *Focus on vaginal changes related to menopause.*

Content Area: Adult Health; *Category of Health Alteration:* Reproductive Management; *Integrated Processes:* Nursing Process Implementation; *Client Need:* Health Promotion and Maintenance/Aging Process; *Cognitive Level:* Application

References: Lewis, S., Heitkemper, M., Dirksen, S., O'Brien, P., & Bucher, L. (2007). *Medical-Surgical Nursing: Assessment and Management of Clinical Problems* (7th ed., p. 1391). St. Louis, MO: Mosby/Elsevier; Smeltzer, S., Bare, B., Hinkle, J., & Cheever, K. (2008). *Brunner & Suddarth's Textbook of Medical-Surgical Nursing* (11th ed., p. 1633). Philadelphia: Lippincott Williams & Wilkins.

967. EBP A female nurse is sitting at a table across from a Latino male she has been educating about the process of testicular self-examination. After a period of discussion, the client successfully verbalizes the process. The nurse excitedly praises the client, leans over the table, and makes the "OK" sign with her thumb and forefinger. The client immediately gets up and leaves the room. What caused the client's discomfort?

1. The client was uncomfortable discussing private body areas with a female nurse.
2. A nurse invaded the client's personal space inappropriately.
3. Many Latinos consider the "OK" gesture obscene.
4. Latinos consider the "OK" gesture to be demeaning.

ANSWER: 3

Gestures can be a source of misunderstanding among cultures. In much of Latin America, the North American "OK" sign (i.e., pinched thumb and forefinger) may be considered obscene. Latin Americans are not uncomfortable with close personal space; in fact, some Latinos perceive Anglos as distant because they prefer more personal space during a conversation. Since the client had participated in the discussion up to the point of leaving the room, he obviously was not uncomfortable with the discussion.

▶ ***Test-taking Tip:*** *Read the question carefully and focus on the nurse's actions at the end of the instruction session. Eliminate option 1 because the client had not been uncomfortable until the very end of the session.*

Content Area: Adult Health; *Category of Health Alteration:* Reproductive Management; *Integrated Processes:* Nursing Process Evaluation; Caring; *Client Need:* Psychosocial Integrity/Cultural Diversity; *Cognitive Level:* Application

Reference: Harkreader, H., Hogan, M., & Thobaben, M. (2007). *Fundamentals of Nursing* (3rd ed., pp. 52–53). St. Louis, MO: Saunders/Elsevier.

EBP Reference: Jucket, G. (2005). Cross-cultural medicine. *American Family Physician,* 72(11), 1–8.

Test 25: **Adult Health: Respiratory Management**

968. EBP A client with asthma has pronounced wheezing upon auscultation. Suspecting an impending asthma attack, a nurse should:

1. have the client cough and deep breathe.
2. prepare to intubate the client.
3. prepare to administer a nebulized beta-2 adrenergic agonist.
4. have the client lay on his or her right side.

ANSWER: 3

A client with asthma who is experiencing wheezing and an impending attack is best treated with inhaled beta-2 adrenergic agonist drugs such as albuterol (Ventolin®). Oxygen and corticosteroids may also be used. Neither coughing and deep breathing nor positioning will stop the attack. Intubation is not effective in treating the underlying cause of the attack, which is an inflammatory response and would not be a first-line intervention.

➧ ***Test-taking Tip:*** *Knowledge of mainstay therapies for asthma and emergency asthma management are essential. Note that the question does not indicate that the client is having a respiratory arrest, but rather the nurse suspects impending asthma attack. Do not read into the question or assume information.*

Content Area: Adult Health; *Category of Health Alteration:* Respiratory Management; *Integrated Processes:* Nursing Process Implementation; *Client Need:* Physiological Integrity/Physiological Adaptation/Medical Emergencies; *Cognitive Level:* Application

Reference: Lewis, S., Heitkemper, M., Dirksen, S., O'Brien, P., & Bucher, L. (2007). *Medical-Surgical Nursing: Assessment and Management of Clinical Problems* (7th ed., p. 626). St. Louis, MO: Mosby.

EBP Reference: Kaiser Permanente Care Management Institute. (2007). Adult asthma clinical practice guidelines. Available at: www.guideline.gov/summary/summary.aspx?doc_id=11247&nbr=005880&string=asthma

969. A nurse is teaching an elderly client about the importance of using the item that is attached to the inhaler. The nurse should explain that this item:

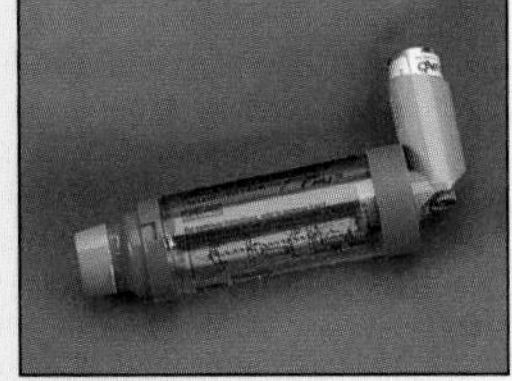

1. allows for a greater amount of medication to be delivered.
2. lets the client see the medication as it is delivered.
3. keeps the mouthpiece sterile.
4. allows for activating the medication canister by simply inhaling.

ANSWER: 1

The item pictured is a spacer or extender. These devices hold the medication in suspension for a few moments longer, allowing improved medication delivery. These devices are recommended for children or older adults who might not have the dexterity or knowledge to time an inhalation with medication delivery. Visual confirmation of delivery is not the main reason that the device is attached. The mouthpiece may be kept cleaner with a spacer but does not ensure sterility. Although some inhalers allow for inhalation "trigger" delivery, this is not the purpose of the spacer/extender.

➧ ***Test-taking Tip:*** *If unfamiliar with the item pictured, think logically about the situation and link it to the aspects of the question that you do know. In this case, some of the options do not seem to fit with the functions of what appears in the picture.*

Content Area: Adult Health; *Category of Health Alteration:* Respiratory Management; *Integrated Processes:* Nursing Process Implementation; Teaching and Learning; *Client Need:* Physiological Integrity/Pharmacological and Parenteral Therapies/Medication Administration; *Cognitive Level:* Analysis

Reference: Wilkinson, J., & Van Leuven, K. (2007). *Fundamentals of Nursing: Thinking & Doing* (Vol. 1, pp. 504–506). Philadelphia: F. A. Davis.

970. EBP A client, newly diagnosed with asthma is preparing for discharge. Which point should a nurse emphasize during the client's teaching?

1. Contact care provider only if nighttime wheezing becomes a concern
2. Limit exposure to sources that trigger an attack
3. Use peak flow meter only if symptoms are worsening
4. Use inhaled steroid medication as a rescue inhaler

ANSWER: 2

A client newly diagnosed with asthma has a large number of educational concerns that need to be addressed. Of primary importance is knowing ways to prevent an attack, such as avoiding known triggers. A peak flow meter is generally used on a daily basis to help document and identify worsening symptoms over time. Symptoms, such as worsening peak flow meter readings and nighttime wheezing, are one of many health changes that should signal the client to contact his or her care provider. Generally speaking, inhalers with steroid medications are not to be used as a rescue inhaler in the event of an attack.

➧ *Test-taking Tip: Knowledge of asthma self-care and pharmacology helps to reduce the number of possible answers. Consider also that options 1, 3, and 4 are responses to worsening symptoms, whereas option 2 is aimed at prevention, which is a primary goal of asthma education.*

Content Area: Adult Health; *Category of Health Alteration:* Respiratory Management; *Integrated Processes:* Teaching and Learning; *Client Need:* Health Promotion and Maintenance/Self-Care; *Cognitive Level:* Application

Reference: Lewis, S., Heitkemper, M., Dirksen, S., O'Brien, P., & Bucher, L. (2007). *Medical-Surgical Nursing: Assessment and Management of Clinical Problems* (7th ed., pp. 621–629). St. Louis, MO: Mosby.

EBP Reference: National Asthma Education and Prevention Program. (2007). Control of environmental factors and comorbid conditions that affect asthma. In *National Asthma Education and Prevention Program (NAEPP). Expert Panel Report 3: Guidelines for the Diagnosis and Management of Asthma* (pp. 165–212). Available at: www.guideline.gov/summary/summary.aspx?doc_id=11673&nbr=006022

971. EBP A nurse is working with a client to update the client's asthma action plan. The nurse knows that this action plan should include information on:

1. medication adjustments that should be made if peak flow is less than 50% normal.
2. timeline for allergy skin testing.
3. the most direct route when the client drives to the hospital.
4. the best methods for chest physiotherapy (CPT).

ANSWER: 1

The asthma action plan is intended to help clients determine how and when to adjust care if their asthma worsens; primarily through adjustment of medication regimen. The plan also identifies the best ways to access and alert emergency personnel if an acute attack occurs but the client should not be driving him- or herself to the hospital. Allergy skin testing would be done in the early phases of diagnosis. CPT is not usually a part of asthma therapy.

➧ *Test-taking Tip: Read what the question is specifically asking and consider which items would logically be a part of an asthma action plan.*

Content Area: Adult Health; *Category of Health Alteration:* Respiratory Management; *Integrated Processes:* Nursing Process Implementation; *Client Need:* Health Promotion and Maintenance/Self-Care; *Cognitive Level:* Application

Reference: Lewis, S., Heitkemper, M., Dirksen, S., O'Brien, P., & Bucher, L. (2007). *Medical-Surgical Nursing: Assessment and Management of Clinical Problems* (7th ed., pp. 621–629). St. Louis, MO: Mosby.

EBP Reference: Institute for Clinical Systems Improvement. (2008). *Diagnosis and Management of Asthma.* Available at: www.guideline.gov/summary/summary.aspx?doc_id=12293&nbr=006368&string=asthma

972. Which finding should a nurse expect when completing an assessment on a client with chronic bronchitis?

1. Minimal sputum with cough
2. Pink, frothy sputum
3. Barrel chest
4. Stridor on expiration

ANSWER: 3

Barrel chest is indicative of a client with chronic bronchitis because of lung hyperinflation. Pink, frothy sputum is indicative of pulmonary edema. Minimal sputum with cough is more indicative of emphysema than chronic bronchitis, which usually is characterized by copious secretions. Stridor indicates some type of upper respiratory edema that would not be an expected finding in this scenario.

➧ *Test-taking Tip: Knowledge of the typical assessment findings for a client with chronic bronchitis is required to answer this question.*

Content Area: Adult Health; *Category of Health Alteration:* Respiratory Management; *Integrated Processes:* Nursing Process Assessment; *Client Need:* Physiological Integrity/Physiological Adaptation/Alterations in Body Systems; *Cognitive Level:* Application

References: Smeltzer, S., Bare, B., Hinkle, J., & Cheever, K. (2008). *Brunner & Suddarth's Textbook of Medical-Surgical Nursing* (11th ed., pp. 689–690). Philadelphia: Lippincott Williams & Wilkins; Sommers, M., Johnson, S., & Beery, T. (2007). *Diseases and Disorders: A Nursing Therapeutics Manual* (3rd ed., pp. 158–161, 310–314). Philadelphia: F. A. Davis.

973. EBP A client learning about chronic obstructive pulmonary disease self-care at a community health class, asks a nurse why the participants are being taught about the "lip-breathing." The nurse should respond by explaining that pursed-lip breathing can help to:

1. reduce upper airway inflammation.
2. reduce anxiety through humor.
3. strengthen respiratory muscles.
4. increase effectiveness of inhaled medications.

ANSWER: 3

Pursed-lip breathing increases the strength of respiratory muscles and helps to keep alveoli open. It does not have an affect on upper airway inflammation, provide humor therapy, and is not a part of medication administration.

Test-taking Tip: *Note that two of the items deal directly with the respiratory nature of the disease. Consider knowledge of the disease process to select the correct option.*

Content Area: Adult Health; *Category of Health Alteration:* Respiratory Management; *Integrated Processes:* Nursing Process Implementation/Teaching and Learning; *Client Need:* Health Promotion and Maintenance/Principles of Teaching and Learning; Physiological Integrity/Physiological Adaptation/Illness Management; *Cognitive Level:* Analysis

Reference: Doenges, M., Moorhouse, M., & Murr, A. (2006). *Nursing Care Plans* (p. 126). Philadelphia: F. A. Davis.

EBP Reference: Ries, A., Bauldoff, G., Carlin, B., Casaburi, R., Emery, C., et al. (2007). Pulmonary rehabilitation: Joint ACCP/AACVPR evidence-based clinical practice guidelines. *Chest,* 131(5 Suppl), 4S–42S.

974. A home health nurse is visiting a client whose chronic bronchitis has recently worsened. Which instruction should the nurse reinforce with this client?

1. Increase amount of bedrest
2. Increase fluid intake
3. Decrease caloric intake
4. Reduce home oxygen use

ANSWER: 2

Adequate fluids may help liquefy secretions for easier expectoration. Imposing bedrest on a client with shortness of breath may worsen the situation. Physical activity interspersed with adequate rest can improve respiratory functioning. A diet high in calories can compensate for these client's hypermetabolic state, dyspnea, and poor appetite. Reducing home oxygen use, in this situation, would most likely exacerbate the client's symptoms.

Test-taking Tip: *Knowledge of the common nursing interventions for chronic obstructive pulmonary disease is essential for answering a question of this type. Consider the implications for the client when trying to select or narrow down the options.*

Content Area: Adult Health; *Category of Health Alteration:* Respiratory Management; *Integrated Processes:* Teaching and Learning; *Client Need:* Physiological Integrity/Physiological Adaptation/Illness Management; *Cognitive Level:* Application

References: Smeltzer, S., Bare, B., Hinkle, J., & Cheever, K. (2008). *Brunner & Suddarth's Textbook of Medical-Surgical Nursing* (11th ed., pp. 702–708). Philadelphia: Lippincott Williams & Wilkins; Doenges, M., Moorhouse, M., & Murr, A. (2006). *Nursing Care Plans* (7th ed., pp. 121–125). Philadelphia: F. A. Davis.

975. A client with chronic obstructive pulmonary disease (COPD) is in the third postoperative day following right-sided thoracotomy. During the day shift, the client has required 10 L oxygen by mask to keep his or her oxygen saturations greater than 88%. Based on this information, which action should be taken by the evening shift nurse?

1. Work to wean oxygen down to 3 L by mask
2. Call respiratory therapy for a nebulizer treatment
3. Check respiratory rate and notify the physician
4. Administer dose of ordered pain medications

ANSWER: 3

The night shift nurse should check the client's respiratory rate and report abnormal findings to the physician. Although uncommon, clients with COPD on high flow oxygen can lose their respiratory drive. Working to wean down oxygen by mask below 3 L will cause retention of CO_2; oxygen by mask generally should be set at 4 L or greater. Although a nebulizer and pain medications may assist the client, the immediate need is to determine if the high flow oxygen is affecting the client's respiratory drive and to further determine the cause of the low oxygen saturations.

Test-taking Tip: *An option that includes an assessment is often the correct answer because the nursing process is driven by the information collected in an assessment.*

Content Area: Adult Health; *Category of Health Alteration:* Respiratory Management; *Integrated Processes:* Nursing Process Implementation; *Client Need:* Physiological Integrity/Reduction of Risk Potential/Potential for Alterations in Body Systems; *Cognitive Level:* Application

Reference: Williams, L., & Hopper, P. (2007). *Understanding Medical-Surgical Nursing* (3rd ed., p. 561). Philadelphia: F. A. Davis.

976. A nurse enters a client's room after hearing the pulse oximeter alarm and sees the following tracing on the screen. Which action should be immediately taken by the nurse?

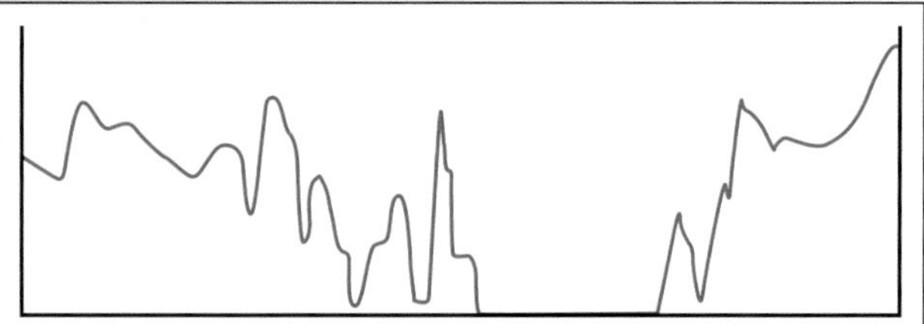

1. Call a code
2. Remove the machine and call maintenance
3. Administer oxygen through a nasal cannula or mask
4. Assess the client's level of consciousness and skin color

ANSWER: 4

The pleth wave tracing pictured is generally the result of artifact that is caused by the client moving the finger rather than signaling that the client is coding or that the machine is broken. By immediately evaluating the client's mental status and skin color, the nurse can quickly determine whether the tracing constitutes an emergency or if it is just artifact. A pulse oximeter, or any other technology should never replace the direct assessment of a client by the nurse. The nurse should always treat the client and not the monitor. Although applying oxygen would be a good choice if the nurse continued to be unable to determine the client's pulse oximetry reading within a few seconds, it may not be necessary or appropriate.

➧ *Test-taking Tip: Consider the steps of the nursing process in answering this question. An intervention is generally guided by the nurse's assessment findings.*

Content Area: Adult Health; *Category of Health Alteration:* Respiratory Management; *Integrated Processes:* Nursing Process Assessment; *Client Need:* Physiological Integrity/Reduction of Risk Potential/Vital Signs; Safe and Effective Care Environment/Safety and Infection Control/Safe Use of Equipment; *Cognitive Level:* Analysis

References: Wilkinson, J., & Van Leuven, K. (2007). *Fundamentals of Nursing: Theory, Concepts & Applications* (Vol. 2, pp. 809–811, 861). Philadelphia: F. A. Davis; Clark, A., Giuliano, K., & Chen, H. (2006). Legal and ethical pulse oximetry revisited: "But his O_2 sat was normal!" *Clinical Nurse Specialist: The Journal for Advanced Nursing Practice,* 20, 268–272; Lewis, S., Heitkemper, M., Dirksen, S., O'Brien, P., & Bucher, L. (2007). *Medical-Surgical Nursing: Assessment and Management of Clinical Problems* (7th ed., pp. 514–515). St. Louis, MO: Mosby; Smeltzer, S., Bare, B., Hinkle, J., & Cheever, K. (2008). *Brunner & Suddarth's Textbook of Medical-Surgical Nursing* (11th ed., p. 579). Philadelphia: Lippincott Williams & Wilkins.

977. A client with a suspected pulmonary embolus receives a ventilation and quantification nuclear medicine (VQ) scan to evaluate regional lung ventilation of airflow and regional lung blood flow. In consulting with a physician, a nurse learns that there is a VQ mismatch. Based on this information, which action should be taken by the nurse?

1. Tell the client that tuberculosis treatment will be needed
2. Reassure the client that he/she does not have a pulmonary embolus
3. Explain to the client that further testing will be needed
4. Inform the client that the test was normal

ANSWER: 3

An imbalanced or mismatched VQ scan indicates some type of problem with either ventilation or perfusion. Further testing is required, especially in the case of suspected pulmonary embolus. A chest x-ray, sputum culture, and Gram stain are used to diagnose tuberculosis; treatment should not be initiated. A VQ mismatch is highly suspicious, but not diagnostic of multiple lung diseases, including pulmonary embolus. A VQ mismatch is not a normal finding.

➧ *Test-taking Tip: Consider the pathophysiology and complexity of the condition discussed in the question to help narrow down the options. Look at key words so that even if the procedure is unfamiliar, the key descriptions will help to select the correct option.*

Content Area: Adult Health; *Category of Health Alteration:* Respiratory Management; *Integrated Processes:* Nursing Process Implementation; *Client Need:* Physiological Integrity/Physiological Adaptation/Alterations in Body Systems; *Cognitive Level:* Application

References: Lewis, S., Heitkemper, M., Dirksen, S., O'Brien, P., & Bucher, L. (2007). *Medical-Surgical Nursing: Assessment and Management of Clinical Problems* (7th ed., pp. 526–528). St. Louis, MO: Mosby; Kee, J. (2005). *Laboratory and Diagnostic Tests with Implications* (7th ed., pp. 632–633). Upper Saddle River, NJ: Prentice Hall.

978. A nurse is assessing lung sounds on a client with pneumonia who is having pain during inspiration and expiration. The nurse hears loud grating sounds over the lung fields. The nurse should document the client's pain level and should document that:

1. lung sounds were clear upon auscultation.
2. fine crackles were heard upon auscultation.
3. wheezing was heard upon auscultation.
4. pleural friction rub was heard upon auscultation.

ANSWER: 4

The client with pneumonia may have crackles, rhonchi, and wheezes as well as a pleural friction rub. A pleural friction rub has a distinctive sound that tends to be loud and grating and heard easily over the lung fields upon auscultation. Pleural friction rubs are also often associated with painful breathing. Fine or course crackles will have a moist, bubbling, or Velcro-tearing sound. Wheezing tends to have a high-pitched sound.

Test-taking Tip: *Consider the expected assessment findings for the condition described in the question.*

Content Area: Adult Health; *Category of Health Alteration:* Respiratory Management; *Integrated Processes:* Communication and Documentation; *Client Need:* Health Promotion and Maintenance/Techniques of Physical Assessment; *Cognitive Level:* Application

References: Lewis, S., Heitkemper, M., Dirksen, S., O'Brien, P., & Bucher, L. (2007). *Medical-Surgical Nursing: Assessment and Management of Clinical Problems* (7th ed., p. 625). St. Louis, MO: Mosby; Dillon, P. (2007). *Nursing Health Assessment* (2nd ed., pp. 425–429). Philadelphia: F. A. Davis.

---

979. EBP A nurse is helping a client with obstructive sleep apnea to apply a continuous positive airway pressure (CPAP) mask before going to sleep. The nurse knows that CPAP is intended to:

1. breathe for the client during sleep.
2. reduce intrathoracic pressure.
3. deliver high concentrations of oxygen.
4. prevent alveolar collapse.

ANSWER: 4

CPAP devices are intended for clients who can breathe on their own but need assistance in maintaining adequate oxygenation. The CPAP device keeps the alveoli open, allowing for maximal perfusion to occur. Although oxygen can be administered with a CPAP device, it is not always necessary. CPAP is not intended to reduce intrathoracic pressure.

Test-taking Tip: *Consider the client's health condition in the context of the question. In this case, a client with obstructive sleep apnea has periods of time where the airway is closed off. The client is able to breathe but needs assistance in keeping the airway open to allow for maximal perfusion.*

Content Area: Adult Health; *Category of Health Alteration:* Respiratory Management; *Integrated Processes:* Nursing Process Implementation/Caring; *Client Need:* Physiological Integrity/Reduction of Risk Potential/Therapeutic Procedures; *Cognitive Level:* Application

Reference: Lewis, S., Heitkemper, M., Dirksen, S., O'Brien, P., & Bucher, L. (2007). *Medical-Surgical Nursing: Assessment and Management of Clinical Problems* (7th ed., p. 543). St. Louis, MO: Mosby.

EBP Reference: Giles, T., Lasserson, T., Smith, B., White, J., Wright, J., & Cates, C. (2006). Continuous positive airways pressure for obstructive sleep apnea in adults. *Cochrane Database of Systematic Reviews*, Issue 3, Art. No. CD001106. DOI: 10.1002/14651858.CD001106.pub3. Available at: www.cochrane.org/reviews/en/ab001106.html

---

980. EBP A nurse begins to hear high-pressure alarms in the room of a client requiring respiratory assistance with a ventilator. Which is the best action by the nurse?

1. Wait and allow the client time to regulate breathing in coordination with the ventilator
2. Check ventilator tubing and connections
3. Silence the alarm and restart the ventilator
4. Lower the tidal volumes being delivered to the client

ANSWER: 2

High-pressure alarms should be immediately investigated by the nurse. Tubing and connections are often a source of both high- and low-pressure alarms. The causes may include the client biting on the endotracheal tube or fighting the ventilator-delivered breaths or migration of the endotracheal tube, which can cause coughing. Changing the ventilator settings would not change the cause of the problem if it is indeed external to the client. Waiting or silencing alarms is a threat to client safety.

Test-taking Tip: *Rule out any option that might threaten client safety, such as turning off an alarm or just waiting.*

Content Area: Adult Health; *Category of Health Alteration:* Respiratory Management; *Integrated Processes:* Nursing Process Implementation; *Client Need:* Safe and Effective Care Environment/ Safety and Infection Control/Safe Use of Equipment; *Cognitive Level:* Application

Reference: Smeltzer, S., Bare, B., Hinkle, J., & Cheever, K. (2008). *Brunner & Suddarth's Textbook of Medical-Surgical Nursing* (11th ed., p. 745). Philadelphia: Lippincott Williams & Wilkins.

EBP Reference: Couchman, B., Wetzig, S., Coyer, F., & Wheeler, M. (2007). Nursing care of the mechanically ventilated patient: What does the evidence say? Part one. *Intensive & Critical Care Nursing,* 23(1), 4–14.

---

981. A nurse is caring for a client requiring positive pressure mechanical ventilation. The client has been fighting the ventilator-assisted breaths, and the client's blood pressure has been steadily decreasing. Which would be the most appropriate intervention by the nurse?

1. Place the client in the prone position
2. Notify the respiratory therapist to increase the positive pressure settings
3. Call the physician to suggest sedatives and paralytics
4. Prepare to administer intravenous aminophylline

ANSWER: 3

Positive pressure ventilation can lead to decreased cardiac output and a drop in blood pressure. Administering appropriate levels of sedation and a paralytic will allow the client to be more relaxed physically and mentally. This state of psychological and physical relaxation allows for greater synchrony with the ventilator. Adjusting the ventilator settings may assist in reducing client response to ventilation, but in many cases sedatives and paralytics are necessary. Placing the client in the prone position or administering intravenous aminophylline will not be a primary part of correcting the underlying issue.

Test-taking Tip: *Do not read into the question. Put the needs of the client first. In this case, consider the psychosocial and physiological responses to mechanical ventilation.*

Content Area: Adult Health; *Category of Health Alteration:* Respiratory Management; *Integrated Processes:* Nursing Process Implementation; *Client Need:* Physiological Integrity/Physiological Adaptation/Unexpected Response to Therapies; *Cognitive Level:* Analysis

Reference: Smeltzer, S., Bare, B., Hinkle, J., & Cheever, K. (2008). *Brunner & Suddarth's Textbook of Medical-Surgical Nursing* (11th ed., p. 745). Philadelphia: Lippincott Williams & Wilkins.

---

982. On the third postoperative day following a total laryngectomy, a client's family asks a nurse when the client will be able to eat. Which response by the nurse is best?

1. "We are going to start with a feeding tube, but eventually he should be able to eat normally."
2. "We are going to start with a feeding tube, but eventually he will have to learn a different way of swallowing to prevent aspiration."
3. "Because of his surgery, it will be several more days before his gastrointestinal tract begins functioning again."
4. "He will probably always have to be fed through a gastrostomy tube in his stomach."

ANSWER: 1

A feeding tube is generally placed during the surgical procedure and used for stomach decompression and then eventually as a means of feeding the client. The client should be able to swallow normally once healing is near completion. The client is on the third postoperative day, at which point bowel functioning should be returning, especially since there was no manipulation of the bowel itself. Unless there were major complications, the client should be able to return to eating normally and should not need a permanent gastrostomy tube.

Test-taking Tip: *Watch for words such as "always" or "never," which can sometimes indicate an incorrect option. Knowledge of the client's physiological functioning after this procedure is essential.*

Content Area: Adult Health; *Category of Health Alteration:* Respiratory Management; *Integrated Processes:* Nursing Process Implementation; Teaching and Learning; *Client Need:* Physiological Integrity/Basic Care and Comfort/Nutrition and Oral Hydration; *Cognitive Level:* Analysis

References: Doenges, M., Moorhouse, M., & Murr, A. (2006). *Nursing Care Plans: Guidelines for Individualizing Client Care Across the Life Span* (7th ed., pp. 166–167). Philadelphia: F. A. Davis; Sommers, M., Johnson, S., & Beery, T. (2007). *Diseases and Disorders: A Nursing Therapeutics Manual* (3rd ed., pp. 553–556). Philadelphia: F. A. Davis.

983. A nurse is designing the plan of care for a client following total laryngectomy. Included in the plan of care is a referral to a nutritional support staff/dietician. The nurse understands that the referral is essential because the client:

1. is most likely depressed and uninterested in eating.
2. will have to relearn how to swallow.
3. may have lost his or her sense of smell and taste.
4. must learn strategies for preventing aspiration.

ANSWER: 3

After a total laryngectomy, the client loses the sense of smell and possibly the sense of taste, which may reduce the desire to eat and may change how certain foods taste. Putting together a balanced diet that addresses alterations in nutrition from the loss of smell and taste are important to maximize healing. Following total laryngectomy, the client may be depressed and uninterested in eating, but it is not the primary reason for such a consultation. Mental health concerns would not be handled by nutrition support staff. Re-learning how to swallow is more a concern with a partial laryngectomy than a total laryngectomy. Aspiration is no longer a concern because there is no continuity between the lungs and the esophagus.

➧ ***Test-taking Tip:*** *Consider the physiological impact of the procedure on the client's nutrition and functioning of the upper airway and respiratory system.*

Content Area: Adult Health; *Category of Health Alteration:* Respiratory Management; *Integrated Processes:* Nursing Process Planning; *Client Need:* Physiological Integrity/Basic Care and Comfort/Nutrition and Oral Hydration; Safe and Effective Care Environment/Management of Care/Referrals; *Cognitive Level:* Analysis

References: Doenges, M., Moorhouse, M., & Murr, A. (2006). *Nursing Care Plans: Guidelines for Individualizing Client Care Across the Life Span* (7th ed., pp. 165–167). Philadelphia: F. A. Davis; Smeltzer, S., Bare, B., Hinkle, J., & Cheever, K. (2008). *Brunner & Suddarth's Textbook of Medical-Surgical Nursing* (11th ed., pp. 616–620). Philadelphia: Lippincott Williams & Wilkins.

---

984. A nurse is evaluating discharge teaching that has been completed for a client following total laryngectomy. Which statement made by the client indicates that the client *does not* accept or understand the teaching?

1. "I will be sure to carry an extra supply of facial tissue with me."
2. "I probably will not be able to go swimming."
3. "I will schedule an appointment for closure of my tracheostomy."
4. "I will check the batteries on our smoke detectors."

ANSWER: 3

The client's tracheostomy is permanent because the larynx and part of the trachea are removed. Stating to schedule an appointment for closure of the tracheostomy indicates the client *does not* accept or understand the teaching. Following total laryngectomy, the client will frequently have a runny nose and potentially problems managing oral secretions. By carrying extra facial tissue he or she can reduce a sense of embarrassment and be prepared for these situations. Swimming puts the client at risk for aspirating water and should be avoided. The client's loss of smell can be a safety concern in the home.

➧ ***Test-taking Tip:*** *Knowledge of physiological alterations following total laryngectomy is essential for answering this question.*

Content Area: Adult Health; *Category of Health Alteration:* Respiratory Management; *Integrated Processes:* Nursing Process Evaluation; *Client Need:* Safe and Effective Care Environment/Safety and Infection Control/Home Safety; Physiological Integrity/Physiological Adaptation/Alterations in Body Systems; *Cognitive Level:* Analysis

References: Doenges, M., Moorhouse, M., & Murr, A. (2006). *Nursing Care Plans: Guidelines for Individualizing Client Care Across the Life Span* (7th ed., pp. 168–169). Philadelphia: F. A. Davis; Sommers, M., Johnson, S., & Beery, T. (2007). *Diseases and Disorders: A Nursing Therapeutics Manual* (3rd ed., pp. 553–556). Philadelphia: F. A. Davis.

---

985. A client with a large facial tumor is scheduled for a radical neck dissection. A nurse in the preoperative area is explaining the procedure. Which action will best help the client considering the potential for an alteration in body image from the procedure?

1. Show multiple photographs of clients who have had similar procedures.
2. Closely assess and monitor the client's verbal and nonverbal communication.
3. Direct the client's significant other to allow for the client's complete dependence on him or her.
4. Remind the client that it is what is on the inside that counts.

ANSWER: 2

Watching for signs of distress or concerns through the client's verbal and nonverbal communication will help determine if there are in fact any concerns and to what degree they may need to be addressed. The client may not be ready for photographs of other clients who have had the procedure, especially since not all of the incisions or drains used will be the same and could give the client a false sense of what to expect. The photographs may also be frightening and have the opposite of the intended effect. Directing the spouse to allow the client's total dependence on another encourages maladaptive behaviors. The nurse and significant others should be supportive but not encourage dependence. Some statements such as stating it is what's on the inside that counts could be misconstrued as condescending.

➧ ***Test-taking Tip:*** *Nursing care should begin with an assessment, which should help guide the selection of the correct option.*

Content Area: Adult Health; *Category of Health Alteration:* Respiratory Management; *Integrated Processes:* Nursing Process Implementation; *Client Need:* Psychosocial Integrity/Coping Mechanisms; *Cognitive Level:* Application

References: Lewis, S., Heitkemper, M., Dirksen, S., O'Brien, P., & Bucher, L. (2007). *Medical-Surgical Nursing: Assessment and Management of Clinical Problems* (7th ed., p. 555). St. Louis, MO: Mosby; Dochterman, J., & Bulecheck, G. (2004). *Nursing Interventions Classification* (pp. 209, 633). St. Louis, MO: Mosby.

986. EBP A 17-year-old client with cystic fibrosis (CF) is visiting with a nurse in preparation for leaving home for college. The nurse knows that the client needs further education if the client states:

1. "I will bring extra cough medicine so as to not wake up my roommate at night."
2. "I will contact the college's health center and pass on my medical records."
3. "I will check to make sure they have good workout facilities."
4. "I will be really careful about washing my hands and staying away from sick friends."

ANSWER: 1

A client with CF should not be using cough suppressants because of the high importance of expectorating secretions. Letting the health center know of special care needs and familiarizing them with the client can help begin the therapeutic relationship and reduce the anxieties of both the client and the care providers. It is important for clients with CF to exercise regularly and maintain physical strength in order to facilitate loosening and clearing secretions. Hand hygiene and avoiding sick friends will help to reduce the risk of respiratory illness.

Test-taking Tip: *Think through the impact of each option as it relates to the question being asked and the medical condition of the client. Select the option that would have negative consequences for a client whose health relies on frequent productive coughing.*

Content Area: Adult Health; *Category of Health Alteration:* Respiratory Management; *Integrated Processes:* Nursing Process Evaluation; *Client Need:* Physiological Integrity/Physiological Adaptation/Illness Management; Health Promotion and Maintenance/Self-Care; *Cognitive Level:* Analysis

Reference: Sommers, M., Johnson, S., & Beery, T. (2007). *Diseases and Disorders: A Nursing Therapeutics Manual* (3rd ed., pp. 260–264). Philadelphia: F. A. Davis.

EBP Reference: Bradley, J., & Moran, F. (2008). Physical training for cystic fibrosis. *Cochrane Database of Systematic Reviews*, Issue 1, Art. No. CD002768. DOI: 10.1002/14651858.CD002768.pub2. Available at: www.cochrane.org/reviews/en/ab002768.html

987. EBP A public health nurse is planning a flu shot clinic. The nurse is working on advertising. Which groups should be the highest priority to target when advertising the flu shot clinic? SELECT ALL THAT APPLY.

1. Pregnant women
2. Grade school children
3. Nursing assistants at a nursing home
4. A hypertension clinic population
5. Outpatient psychiatric population
6. Spinal cord–injured population at an assisted living facility

ANSWER: 1, 3, 6

The Centers for Disease Control and Prevention (CDC) provides guidelines for identifying those clients at high risk for influenza-related complications and severe disease. These groups include children aged 6 to 59 months, pregnant women, and clients older than 50 years of age. Those who have chronic respiratory conditions, their caregivers and household contacts, and those in the health-care field are also considered high priorities for vaccination. Clients with spinal cord injury are at high risk for respiratory complications and are prone to complications of flu related to immobilization and difficulty with clearing secretions. Grade school children, clients with hypertension, and persons receiving outpatient psychiatric care are not considered high risk by the CDC.

Test-taking Tip: *Select the groups who are at a higher risk for influenza-related complications.*

Content Area: Adult Health; *Category of Health Alteration:* Respiratory Management; *Integrated Processes:* Nursing Process Planning; *Client Need:* Health Promotion and Maintenance/Disease Prevention; *Cognitive Level:* Analysis

EBP References: Centers for Disease Control and Prevention. (2006). *Prevention and Control of Influenza: Recommendations of the Advisory Committee on Immunization Practices (ACIP).* Available at: www.cdc.gov/mmwr/preview/mmwrhtml/rr5510a1.htm; Rivetti, D., Jefferson, T., Thomas, R., Rudin, M., Rivetti, A., et al. (2006). Vaccines for preventing influenza in the elderly. *Cochrane Database of Systematic Reviews*, Issue 3, Art. No. CD004876. DOI: 10.1002/14651858.CD004876.pub2. Available at: www.cochrane.org/reviews/en/ab004876.html

988. A nurse is working at a telephone health service. Which advice should the nurse give to a client who has had 3 days of symptoms that strongly suggest influenza?

1. Return to work after another day of rest
2. Rest and increase fluid intake to 3 liters of fluid per day
3. Use over-the-counter antihistamines
4. Make an appointment to get the flu shot

ANSWER: 2

Rest and increased fluid intake are essential. Influenza is generally a self-limiting condition, but one that is also highly contagious, so returning to work should not occur until the client is symptom-free. Antihistamines are not the over-the-counter medications of choice. Generally antitussives and antipyretics are optimal for symptom control. Clients who have an active case of influenza should not get the shot.

▶ ***Test-taking Tip:*** *Knowledge of the best treatments and course of influenza will help to narrow the options.*

Content Area: Adult Health; *Category of Health Alteration:* Respiratory Management; *Integrated Processes:* Nursing Process Implementation; *Client Need:* Physiological Integrity/Physiological Adaptation/Illness Management; *Cognitive Level:* Analysis

References: Sommers, M., Johnson, S., & Beery, T. (2007). *Diseases and Disorders: A Nursing Therapeutics Manual* (3rd ed., pp. 518–520). Philadelphia: F. A. Davis; Lewis, S., Heitkemper, M., Dirksen, S., O'Brien, P., & Bucher, L. (2007). *Medical-Surgical Nursing: Assessment and Management of Clinical Problems* (7th ed., pp. 538–540). St. Louis, MO: Mosby.

---

989. A client, hospitalized for a severe case of pneumonia, is asking a nurse why a sputum sample is needed. The nurse should reply that the primary reason is to:

1. complete the first of three samples to be collected.
2. differentiate between pneumonia and atelectasis.
3. encourage expectoration of secretions.
4. help select the appropriate antibiotic.

ANSWER: 4

Culturing the causative organism and testing sensitivities for the most effective antibiotic is the main reason that a sample is collected. Three samples are taken for a client with suspected tuberculosis. A client with atelectasis may get pneumonia, but generally this is not a test used to diagnose atelectasis. Although secretions are expectorated to obtain a sputum sample, the collection itself does not encourage future expectoration of secretions.

▶ ***Test-taking Tip:*** *Consider the most basic reason why any sample for microorganisms is taken.*

Content Area: Adult Health; *Category of Health Alteration:* Respiratory Management; *Integrated Processes:* Nursing Process Implementation; *Client Need:* Physiological Integrity/Reduction of Risk Potential/Diagnostic Tests; *Cognitive Level:* Application

References: Smeltzer, S., Bare, B., Hinkle, J., & Cheever, K. (2008). *Brunner & Suddarth's Textbook of Medical-Surgical Nursing* (11th ed., p. 636). Philadelphia: Lippincott Williams & Wilkins; Kee, J. (2005). *Laboratory and Diagnostic Tests with Implications* (7th ed., p. 647). Upper Saddle River, NJ: Prentice Hall.

---

990. EBP A nurse is preparing to admit a client with a confirmed case of tuberculosis. Which action is essential to infection control for this client?

1. Providing a positive-pressure airflow room
2. Wearing gown and gloves when handling the client's stool or urine
3. Using a National Institute for Occupational Safety and Health (NIOSH)–approved N95 respirator mask for staff and visitors
4. Keeping the client quarantined in the room until antibiotic therapy has been initiated

ANSWER: 3

Clients with a confirmed or suspected case of tuberculosis are generally placed on some type of isolation precautions when hospitalized. These precautions include the use of high-efficiency particulate masks by those coming in contact with the client to prevent inhalation of potentially infectious respiratory secretions. The client should be placed in a negative-airflow room, which pulls the air out of the room and is vented externally. Gown and gloves may be appropriate if there is expected exposure to respiratory secretions. Although the client's movements around the hospital should be somewhat limited, the client can travel wearing a mask to reduce transmission risk and need not be quarantined.

▶ ***Test-taking Tip:*** *Carefully review each of the options. In this case, option 2 has elements that are correct, but the entire statement is not correct. Consider what is best psychologically for the client by using Maslow's Hierarchy of Needs, whereby quarantining the client would not be psychologically positive.*

Content Area: Adult Health; *Category of Health Alteration:* Respiratory Management; *Integrated Processes:* Nursing Process Planning; *Client Need:* Safe and Effective Care Environment/Safety and Infection Control/Standard/Transmission-based/Precautions/Surgical Asepsis; *Cognitive Level:* Application

Reference: Smeltzer, S., Bare, B., Hinkle, J., & Cheever, K. (2008). *Brunner & Suddarth's Textbook of Medical-Surgical Nursing* (11th ed., p. 645). Philadelphia: Lippincott Williams & Wilkins.

EBP Reference: Paul, A., Jensen, P., Lambert, L., Iademarco, M., & Ridzon, R. (2005). Guidelines for preventing the transmission of mycobacterium tuberculosis in health care settings. *Morbidity and Mortality Weekly Report,* 54(RR17), 1–141. Available at: www.cdc.gov/mmwr/preview/mmwrhtml/rr5417a1.htm?s_cid=rr5417a1_e

---

991. EBP A client requires intravenous vancomycin (Vancocin®) for antibiotic-resistant pneumonia. The order calls for 500 mg to be administered, and the medication is supplied in a 100 mL piggyback that contains 5 mg per 1 mL to run over 1 hour. In order to administer the correct dose, a nurse should set the infusion pump to run at a rate of _____ mL per hour.

ANSWER: 100

Use the formula for calculating intravenous flow rates.

Formula: **Infuse rate (in mL/hour) = Volume to be infused / Infusion time**

$$100 \text{ mL/hr} = \frac{100 \text{ mL}}{1 \text{ hr}}$$

➧ ***Test-taking Tip:*** *Identify the volume to be infused. The time over which it needs to be infused allows for quick and easy infusion rate calculations using the equation shown.*

Content Area: Adult Health; *Category of Health Alteration:* Respiratory Management; *Integrated Processes:* Nursing Process Implementation; *Client Need:* Physiological Integrity/Pharmacological and Parenteral Therapies/Dosage Calculation; *Cognitive Level:* Application

References: Deglin, J., & Vallerand, A. (2007). *Davis's Drug Guide for Nurses* (10th ed., pp. 1185–1187). Philadelphia: F. A. Davis; Wilkinson, J., & Van Leuven, K. (2007). *Fundamentals of Nursing: Thinking & Doing* (Vol. 2, p. 886). Philadelphia: F. A. Davis.

EBP Reference: Siegel, J., Rhinehart, E., Jackson, M., & Chiarellos, L. (2006). Management of multidrug-resistant organisms in healthcare settings, 2006. *CDC.* Available at: www.cdc.gov/ncidod/dhqp/pdf/ar/mdroGuideline2006.pdf

---

992. A nurse is planning care for a client with AIDS who has been hospitalized for a *Pneumocystis carinii* infection. Which nursing diagnosis should be the nurse's first priority for this client?

1. Fatigue related to hypermetabolism
2. Imbalanced nutrition, more than body requirements related to hypometabolism
3. Ineffective coping related to HIV diagnosis
4. Fluid volume excess related to oral and intravenous fluid intake

ANSWER: 1

Clients hospitalized for a *Pneumocystis carinii* infection are often acutely ill and fatigued. Hypermetabolism from AIDS and the illness state contribute to fatigue. The client would most likely be too fatigued to eat and would be at risk for nutritional deficit rather than body requirements. The client in this scenario, as stated in the question, has already been diagnosed with AIDS; thus ineffective coping related to HIV diagnosis is not correct. Clients with *P. carinii* infection are generally hypovolemic because of sweating, diarrhea, and vomiting, thus have a fluid volume deficit and not excess.

➧ ***Test-taking Tip:*** *Carefully review the stem. Although many of the options may be correct, cues from the stem can help eliminate choices.*

Content Area: Adult Health; *Category of Health Alteration:* Respiratory Management; *Integrated Processes:* Nursing Process Analysis; *Client Need:* Physiological Integrity/Physiological Adaptation/Illness Management; *Cognitive Level:* Application

References: Sommers, M., Johnson, S., & Beery, T. (2007). *Diseases and Disorders: A Nursing Therapeutics Manual* (3rd ed., pp. 736–739). Philadelphia: F. A. Davis; Doenges, M., Moorhouse, M., & Murr, A. (2006). *Nursing Care Plans: Guidelines for Individualizing Client Care Across the Life Span* (7th ed., pp. 728–743). Philadelphia: F. A. Davis.

993. A client presents to an emergency department following a motorcycle crash. A nurse assesses the client and notes uncoordinated or paradoxical chest rise and fall as well as multiple bruises across the client's chest and torso, crepitus, and tachypnea. Based on this assessment, the nurse should:

1. assist in the placement of a cervical collar.
2. anticipate the need to intubate the client.
3. provide chest compressions.
4. tape the chest wall.

ANSWER: 2

The assessment data implies a client with multiple broken ribs and potentially flail chest. In the case of flail chest, more invasive interventions are generally required, including management of the client's airway with intubation. The client would most likely already have a cervical collar on, and this is not the intervention that would address the assessment data. There is no evidence to suggest that chest compressions are warranted. Taping the chest wall is an intervention for broken ribs that has proven to not be as effective as once believed.

➧ ***Test-taking Tip:*** *In emergency situations or in a situation where the client is in distress, the ABCs (airway, breathing, circulation) should be a priority for assessment and intervention.*

Content Area: Adult Health; *Category of Health Alteration:* Respiratory Management; *Integrated Processes:* Nursing Process Planning; *Client Need:* Physiological Integrity/Physiological Adaptation/Medical Emergencies; *Cognitive Level:* Analysis

Reference: Smeltzer, S., Bare, B., Hinkle, J., & Cheever, K. (2008). *Brunner & Suddarth's Textbook of Medical-Surgical Nursing* (11th ed., pp. 676–677). Philadelphia: Lippincott Williams & Wilkins.

---

994. EBP A nurse is caring for a client in an emergency department who has five fractured ribs from blunt chest trauma. The client is rating pain at 9 out of 10 on a 0 to 10 numeric scale. For which pain management modality should the nurse advocate?

1. NSAIDs
2. Oral analgesics (narcotic + acetaminophen)
3. Regional/local analgesia (epidural or intercostal injection)
4. Intravenous (IV) bolus meperidine (Demerol®)

ANSWER: 3

Epidural analgesics and intercostal nerve blocks are the most optimal modality for blunt chest trauma because they directly target the injury site. Oral analgesics generally are not adequate to manage the pain associated with rib fractures. Meperidine is not the ideal narcotic for managing this type of pain because of its multiple adverse side effects.

➧ ***Test-taking Tip:*** *Consider the physiological implications of the injury in selecting the best option and the most directed type of intervention.*

Content Area: Adult Health; *Category of Health Alteration:* Respiratory Management; *Integrated Processes:* Nursing Process Planning; Caring; *Client Need:* Physiological Integrity/Pharmacological and Parenteral Therapies/Pharmacological Pain Management; *Cognitive Level:* Application

Reference: Smeltzer, S., Bare, B., Hinkle, J., & Cheever, K. (2008). *Brunner & Suddarth's Textbook of Medical-Surgical Nursing* (11th ed., p. 676). Philadelphia: Lippincott Williams & Wilkins.

EBP Reference: Eastern Association for the Surgery of Trauma. (2004). *Pain Management in Blunt Thoracic Trauma.* Available at: www.guideline.gov/summary/summary.aspx?doc_id=6229&nbr=004000&string=pain+AND+chest+AND+trauma

---

995. Following an unrestrained motor vehicle crash, a client presents to an emergency department with multiple injuries, including chest trauma. A physician notifies the care team that the client has progressed to acute respiratory distress syndrome (ARDS) and requests that the family be updated on the client's condition. The nurse should plan to discuss with the family that:

1. the condition generally stabilizes with positive prognosis.
2. the client can be discharged with home oxygen.
3. the condition is always fatal.
4. the condition is highly life-threatening and that end-of-life concerns should be addressed.

ANSWER: 4

ARDS has a reported mortality rate of 50% to 70% and family should be prepared for the possibility that their loved one may not survive the injury or diagnosis. The nurse must be able to discuss the care to be given, the progression of the syndrome, and make appropriate referrals as needed (such as pastoral care). The condition often does not have a positive prognosis and, if the client survives, home oxygen may or may not be needed. ARDS is not always fatal.

➧ ***Test-taking Tip:*** *Watch for absolute words such as "always" or "never" and eliminate these options.*

Content Area: Adult Health; *Category of Health Alteration:* Respiratory Management; *Integrated Processes:* Nursing Process Planning; Caring; *Client Need:* Physiological Integrity/Physiological Adaptation/Medical Emergencies; Psychosocial Integrity/Family Dynamics; *Cognitive Level:* Application

Reference: Smeltzer, S., Bare, B., Hinkle, J., & Cheever, K. (2008). *Brunner & Suddarth's Textbook of Medical-Surgical Nursing* (11th ed., pp. 646–659). Philadelphia: Lippincott Williams & Wilkins.

996. A nurse is caring for a client with a left-sided chest tube attached to a wet suction chest tube system. Which observation by the nurse would require immediate intervention?

1. Bubbling in the suction chamber
2. Dependent loop hanging off the edge of the bed
3. Banded connections between tubing sections
4. Occlusive dressing over chest tube insertion site

ANSWER: 2

A dependent loop creates pressure back up and prevents fluid from draining; this requires immediate intervention to prevent lung collapse. Bubbling in a wet suction chest tube system indicates that the suction is working and is an expected finding as are banded connections between sections of tubing. An occlusive dressing helps to prevent air from leaking into the subcutaneous space and maintains integrity of the closed drainage system.

▶ ***Test-taking Tip:*** *Visualize the different parts of a chest tube system and consider which of the options do not fit or seem negative.*

Content Area: Adult Health; *Category of Health Alteration:* Respiratory Management; *Integrated Processes:* Nursing Process Assessment; *Client Need:* Safe and Effective Care Environment/Safety and Infection Control/Safe Use of Equipment; Physiological Integrity Reduction of Risk Potential/Potential for Complications from Surgical Procedures and Health Alterations; *Cognitive Level:* Application

Reference: Smeltzer, S., Bare, B., Hinkle, J., & Cheever, K. (2008). *Brunner & Suddarth's Textbook of Medical-Surgical Nursing* (11th ed., pp. 759–761). Philadelphia: Lippincott Williams & Wilkins.

997. A nurse checks on a client following lower lobectomy for lung cancer. The nurse finds that the client is dyspneic with respirations in the 40s, is hypotensive, has a SaO_2 at 86% on 10 L close-fitting oxygen mask, has a trachea that is deviated slightly to the left, and notes that the right side of chest is not expanding. Which action should be taken by the nurse *first*?

1. Notify the physician
2. Give the client whatever medication was ordered to decrease anxiety
3. Check the chest tube to make sure it is not obstructed
4. Turn up the oxygen liter flow

ANSWER: 3

The scenario presented implies that the client is suffering from a tension pneumothorax as a result of a kinking of the tubing or other blockage in the chest tube system. Although notifying the physician would be warranted, unkinking tubing would give some immediate relief and would be the best initial action. Neither turning up the oxygen flow nor treating the client for anxiety would correct this problem.

▶ ***Test-taking Tip:*** *Use the steps of the nursing process; assessment should be considered as the best answer.*

Content Area: Adult Health; *Category of Health Alteration:* Respiratory Management; *Integrated Processes:* Nursing Process Implementation; *Client Need:* Physiological Integrity/Physiological Adaptation/Medical Emergencies; Physiological Integrity/Reduction of Risk Potential/Potential for Complications from Surgical Procedures and Health Alterations; *Cognitive Level:* Analysis

References: Wilkinson, J., & Van Leuven, K. (2007). *Fundamentals of Nursing: Thinking & Doing* (Vol. 2, p. 852). Philadelphia: F. A. Davis; Smeltzer, S., Bare, B., Hinkle, J., & Cheever, K. (2008). *Brunner & Suddarth's Textbook of Medical-Surgical Nursing* (11th ed., pp. 771–775). Philadelphia: Lippincott Williams & Wilkins; Goolsby, M., & Grubbs, L. (2006). *Advanced Assessment: Interpreting Findings and Formulating Differential Diagnoses* (p. 163). Philadelphia: F. A. Davis.

998. On the first postoperative day following right-sided thoracotomy, a nurse is assisting a client with arm and shoulder exercises. The client reports pain with the exercises and wants to know why they must be performed. The nurse should explain that the exercises:

1. promote respiratory function.
2. increase blood flow back to the heart and venous system.
3. improve muscle mass to compensate for muscle removed during the procedure.
4. prevent stiffening and loss of function.

ANSWER: 4

Because of the location of the incision, disuse can cause contractures and loss of muscle tone. The exercises help to preserve function of the arm and shoulder. Activity will promote respiratory function and improve venous return, but these are not the reasons for the exercises. Although the girdle muscles are cut, they are generally not removed.

▶ ***Test-taking Tip:*** *The key words "right-sided thoracotomy" points to the main reason for the exercises.*

Content Area: Adult Health; *Category of Health Alteration:* Respiratory Management; *Integrated Processes:* Teaching and Learning; *Client Need:* Physiological Integrity/Basic Care and Comfort/Mobility/Immobility; *Cognitive Level:* Application

Reference: Smeltzer, S., Bare, B., Hinkle, J., & Cheever, K. (2008). *Brunner & Suddarth's Textbook of Medical-Surgical Nursing* (11th ed., pp. 767–769). Philadelphia: Lippincott Williams & Wilkins.

999. Following a thoracotomy to remove a lung tumor, a nurse is preparing a client to be discharged to home. Which are appropriate teaching points for the client? SELECT ALL THAT APPLY.

1. Avoid lifting greater than 20 pounds
2. Build up exercise endurance
3. Continue to build endurance even when dyspneic
4. Expect return to normal activity level and strength within 1 month
5. Make time for frequent rest periods with activity

ANSWER: 1, 2, 5

With discharge after thoracotomy, the client should be instructed to avoid lifting more than 20 pounds until healing is complete. The client should work up to an appropriate exercise level and take rest periods during activity. The client should stop activity if he or she becomes short of breath, overly fatigued, or begins having chest pain. Clients can expect to be weaker than normal for up to 3 to 6 months.

▶ ***Test-taking Tip:*** *Visualize the surgical procedure and consider its physiological implications in anticipating the discharge instructions.*

Content Area: Adult Health; *Category of Health Alteration:* Respiratory Management; *Integrated Processes:* Teaching and Learning; *Client Need:* Physiological Integrity/Physiological Adaptation/Alterations in Body Systems; *Cognitive Level:* Application

Reference: Smeltzer, S., Bare, B., Hinkle, J., & Cheever, K. (2008). *Brunner & Suddarth's Textbook of Medical-Surgical Nursing* (11th ed., p. 770). Philadelphia: Lippincott Williams & Wilkins.

1000. A nurse is partnered with a patient care assistant (PCA) on a medical-surgical floor. The PCA provides information about the clients for whom the PCA has been caring. Based on the information from the PCA, which client should the nurse attend to first?

1. The client with a pulmonary embolus who has not had a bowel movement in 2 days
2. The client who underwent a video thoracoscopy with oxygen saturation readings from 88% to 90% on oxygen at 4 L/NC
3. The client who underwent a wedge resection of right lung and has a blood pressure of 100/65 mm Hg
4. The client who has rib fractures and has not voided for 6 hours after the urinary catheter was removed

ANSWER: 2

The most concerning report from the PCA is regarding the client who is not maintaining oxygen saturations despite receiving oxygen. None of the other clients have potentially life-threatening conditions or concerns that could not later be addressed. Although the blood pressure is low in option 3, it is only one data point and obtaining a repeat reading should be delegated to the PCA.

▶ ***Test-taking Tip:*** *Items requiring care prioritization should start with concerns that deal with the client's airway, breathing, and then circulation.*

Content Area: Adult Health; *Category of Health Alteration:* Respiratory Management; *Integrated Processes:* Nursing Process Planning; *Client Need:* Safe and Effective Care Environment/Management of Care/Establishing Priorities; *Cognitive Level:* Analysis

Reference: Lewis, S., Heitkemper, M., Dirksen, S., O'Brien, P., & Bucher, L. (2007). *Medical-Surgical Nursing: Assessment and Management of Clinical Problems* (7th ed., pp. 592–594). St. Louis, MO: Mosby.

1001. A nurse is caring for a client following an open thoracotomy for removal of a large tumor. Extensive blood loss during the procedure required fluid resuscitation of the client. The client is cyanotic and in respiratory distress with pink, frothy sputum coming from the mouth. The nurse should immediately:

1. put the client in high Fowler's position.
2. give a 200 mL fluid bolus.
3. activate the respiratory code system.
4. have the client cough and deep breathe.

ANSWER: 3

The scenario is suggestive of pulmonary edema most likely as a result of fluid overload. Calling a respiratory code in this emergency situation is essential so that intubation and appropriate pharmacological intervention such as vasopressors and diuretics can be administered. Sitting the client up does not address the immediate problem, and giving a fluid bolus would exacerbate the problem. Having the client cough and deep breathe would also not address the central issue.

▶ ***Test-taking Tip:*** *Determine the condition being hinted at in the stem in order to determine the best option.*

Content Area: Adult Health; *Category of Health Alteration:* Respiratory Management; *Integrated Processes:* Nursing Process Implementation; *Client Need:* Physiological Integrity/Physiological Adaptation/Medical Emergencies; *Cognitive Level:* Application

References: Smeltzer, S., Bare, B., Hinkle, J., & Cheever, K. (2008). *Brunner & Suddarth's Textbook of Medical-Surgical Nursing* (11th ed., p. 655). Philadelphia: Lippincott Williams & Wilkins; Lewis, S., Heitkemper, M., Dirksen, S., O'Brien, P., & Bucher, L. (2007). *Medical-Surgical Nursing: Assessment and Management of Clinical Problems* (7th ed., p. 379). St. Louis, MO: Mosby.

1002. A nurse observes for early manifestations of acute respiratory distress syndrome (ARDS) in a client being treated for smoke inhalation. Which signs indicates the possible onset of ARDS in this client?

1. Cough with blood-tinged sputum and respiratory alkalosis
2. Decrease in both white and red blood cell counts
3. Diaphoresis and low SaO_2 unresponsive to increased oxygen administration
4. Hypertension and elevated PaO_2

ANSWER: 3

ARDS is manifested and similar to an extreme state of respiratory distress that would include diaphoresis, tachypnea, and use of accessory muscles. Because of damage and alterations in lung tissue, the client would not be able to increase his or her oxygenation despite an increase in the flow or amount of oxygen. Blood pressure and acid-base imbalances vary depending on the stage of ARDS.

➧ ***Test-taking Tip:*** *Look at key words to help determine the best answer choices. First, eliminate the two options that do not suggest impaired oxygenation.*

Content Area: Adult Health; *Category of Health Alteration:* Respiratory Management; *Integrated Processes:* Nursing Process Analysis; *Client Need:* Physiological Integrity/Reduction of Risk Potential/Potential for Alterations in Body Systems; *Cognitive Level:* Application

References: Sommers, M., Johnson, S., & Beery, T. (2007). *Diseases and Disorders: A Nursing Therapeutics Manual* (3rd ed., pp. 41–44). Philadelphia: F. A. Davis; Kane, C., & Galanes, S. (2004). Adult respiratory distress syndrome. *Critical Care Nursing Quarterly,* 27(4), 325–335.

Test 26: **Adult Health: Vascular Management**

1003. Elevated homocysteine levels are associated with the development of arteriosclerosis and venous thrombosis. A clinic nurse should teach a client that the dietary therapy to decrease homocysteine levels includes eating foods rich in:

1. monosaturated fats.
2. B-complex vitamins.
3. vitamin C.
4. calcium.

ANSWER: 2

Homocysteine interferes with the elasticity of the endothelial layer in blood vessels. Foods rich in B-complex vitamins, especially folic acid, have been found to lower serum homocysteine levels. Monosaturated fats, vitamin C, and calcium are included in a healthy diet but have not been found to affect the homocysteine levels.

➧ ***Test-taking Tip:*** *Key words in the stem are "decrease homocysteine." The question is "What foods would lower high levels of homocysteine?"*

Content Area: Adult Health; *Category of Health Alteration:* Vascular Management; *Integrated Processes:* Nursing Process Analysis; *Client Need:* Health Promotion and Maintenance/Disease Prevention; Physiological Integrity/Basic Care and Comfort/Nutrition and Oral Hydration; *Cognitive Level:* Application

Reference: Ignatavicius, D., & Workman, M. (2006). *Medical-Surgical Nursing: Critical Thinking for Collaborative Care* (5th ed., pp. 780–781). St. Louis, MO: Elsevier/Saunders.

1004. An adult client has laboratory tests drawn during a routine physical examination. A nurse determines that the client has an increased risk for cardiovascular disease. Which laboratory value most likely led the nurse to this conclusion?

Laboratory Test	Client's Value	Normal Parameters
White blood cell count	4,900/µL	5000–10,000/µL
Red blood cell count	3.8 million/µL	4.2–5.4 million/µL
Hemoglobin	11.6 g/dL	12–16 g/dL
Hematocrit	36%	37–47%
Platelet count	149,000/µL	150,000–300,000/µL
Total cholesterol	210 mg/dL	122–200 mg/dL
Triglycerides	135 mg/dL	35–135 mg/dL

1. White blood cell count
2. Red blood cell count
3. Hemoglobin and hematocrit
4. Platelet count
5. Total cholesterol
6. Triglyceride level

ANSWER: 5

Only the total cholesterol level is within the risk range. Total cholesterol should be less than 200 mg/dL. Lipid profile studies are part of assessment for cardiovascular disease risk. Elevated triglyceride levels are considered an emerging lipid risk factor. The other abnormal laboratory results are not related to hematological functioning.

➧ ***Test-taking Tip:*** *The key words are "increased cardiovascular risk for cardiovascular disease." Evaluate each test and its relationship to cardiovascular risk (total cholesterol, triglycerides). Determine if the client's laboratory results from these tests is within the normal range.*

Content Area: Adult Health; *Category of Health Alteration:* Vascular Management; *Integrated Processes:* Nursing Process Analysis; *Client Need:* Physiological Integrity/Reduction of Risk Potential/Diagnostic Tests; *Cognitive Level:* Analysis

Reference: Ignatavicius, D., & Workman, M. (2006). *Medical-Surgical Nursing: Critical Thinking for Collaborative Care* (5th ed., pp. 695, 780, 882). St. Louis, MO: Elsevier/Saunders.

1005. EBP A client tests positive for factor V Leiden (FVL). A nurse recognizes that because the genetic trait is associated with venous thromboembolism (VTE) the client is:

1. also at a greater risk for myocardial infarction.
2. more likely to be of African American heritage.
3. at risk for premature death.
4. at risk for VTE if taking estrogen as an oral contraceptive or hormone replacement.

ANSWER: 4

FVL is a genetic trait that increases risk of VTE. There is no associated risk of arterial thrombosis associated with myocardial infarction. FVL is predominantly found in Caucasians and is common in older adult clients.

➧ ***Test-taking Tip:*** *Key words in the stem are "genetic trait" and "VTE." Use the process of elimination because it is well known that the risk of thromboembolism is associated with taking oral contraceptives.*

Content Area: Adult Health; *Category of Health Alteration:* Vascular Management; *Integrated Processes:* Nursing Process Analysis; *Client Need:* Health Promotion and Maintenance/Disease Prevention; Physiological Integrity/Reduction of Risk Potential/Diagnostic Tests; *Cognitive Level:* Application

Reference: Smeltzer, S., Bare, B., Hinkle, J., & Cheever, K. (2008). *Brunner & Suddarth's Textbook of Medical-Surgical Nursing* (11th ed., pp. 1095, 1099). Philadelphia: Lippincott Williams & Wilkins.

EBP Reference: Horne, M., & McCloskey, D. (2006). Factor V Leiden as a common genetic risk factor for venous thromboembolism. *Journal of Nursing Scholarship*, 38(1), 19–25.

1006. A client taking medication for treatment of essential hypertension has a serum potassium level of 3.2 mEq/L. A nurse is reviewing the list of medications being taken by the client. Which medication on the list should the nurse conclude to be the causative factor for this serum potassium level?

1. Spironolactone (Aldactone®)
2. Potassium chloride (K-Dur®)
3. Enalapril (Vasotec®)
4. Hydrochlorothiazide (Esidrix®, HydroDIURIL®)

ANSWER: 4

Hydrochlorothiazide is a thiazide diuretic that blocks sodium and water reabsorption in the distal tubule of the kidney and promotes potassium excretion, putting the client at risk for hypokalemia. Spironolactone acts by inhibiting sodium reabsorption in exchange for potassium (potassium-sparing diuretic). Potassium chloride is a potassium supplement. Enalapril is an angiotensin-converting enzyme (ACE) inhibitor that causes some clients to retain potassium.

▶ ***Test-taking Tip:*** *Hypokalemia is a below normal level of potassium in the blood. Consider each medication separately, its action, and relationship to potassium. Use the medication name as a clue to identify the thiazide diuretic. Thiazide diuretics promote potassium excretion.*

Content Area: Adult Health; *Category of Health Alteration:* Vascular Management; *Integrated Processes:* Nursing Process Analysis; *Client Need:* Physiological Integrity/Pharmacological and Parenteral Therapies/Adverse Effects/Contradictions; *Cognitive Level:* Application

Reference: Ignatavicius, D., & Workman, M. (2006). *Medical-Surgical Nursing: Critical Thinking for Collaborative Care* (5th ed., pp. 788–792). St. Louis, MO: Elsevier/Saunders.

1007. A nurse teaches individuals at a seminar that essential hypertension, if untreated, predisposes a client to: SELECT ALL THAT APPLY.

1. stroke.
2. cirrhosis.
3. renal failure.
4. myocardial infarction.
5. peripheral arterial disease.

ANSWER: 1, 3, 4, 5

Sustained blood pressure elevation damages blood vessels, causing hyperplasia of arterioles. The end result is damage to the involved body organs: stroke (brain), renal failure (kidney), myocardial infarction (heart), and the peripheral arterial system. Cirrhosis is extensive scarring of the liver caused by irreversible reaction to liver inflammation and necrosis. Common causes include alcoholic liver disease and hepatitis B and C.

▶ ***Test-taking Tip:*** *Focus on selecting the conditions that can occur from impaired blood supply.*

Content Area: Adult Health; *Category of Health Alteration:* Vascular Management; *Integrated Processes:* Teaching and Learning; *Client Need:* Health Promotion and Maintenance/Disease Prevention; *Cognitive Level:* Application

Reference: Ignatavicius, D., & Workman, M. (2006). *Medical-Surgical Nursing: Critical Thinking for Collaborative Care* (5th ed., pp. 784, 1368). St. Louis, MO: Elsevier/Saunders.

1008. A nurse is assessing a blood pressure of an adult client with a manual sphygmomanometer. The nurse places the bell diaphragm of the stethoscope over the brachial artery and pumps the cuff up to 180 mm Hg. The valve is released to allow a drop of 2 mm Hg per second. At 162 mm Hg the nurse hears the first tapping sound. The sound becomes muffled at 148 mm Hg. The sound changes to a soft thumping at the 138 mm Hg. The sound fades to a muffled blowing sound at 128 mm Hg and is last heard at 94 mm Hg. There is silence at 92 mm Hg. The nurse should document the blood pressure as:

1. 138/92 mm Hg.
2. 148/94 mm Hg.
3. 162/92 mm Hg.
4. 162/94 mm Hg.

ANSWER: 4

The systolic blood pressure is elicited at the pressure where the first clear tapping sound is heard. The diastolic blood pressure is elicited at the pressure where the last sound is heard.

➧ ***Test-taking Tip:*** *Consider the skill of auscultation of blood pressure. Phase 1 of Korotkoff sounds begins when the first faint clear tapping sound is heard (systolic blood pressure). The sounds change as the cuff is deflated through phases 2, 3, 4, and 5 and then silence. The diastolic blood pressure is the pressure at which the last sound is heard.*

Content Area: Adult Health; *Category of Health Alteration:* Vascular Management; *Integrated Processes:* Nursing Process Implementation; Communication and Documentation; *Client Need:* Physiological Integrity/Reduction of Risk Potential/Vital Signs; *Cognitive Level:* Application

Reference: Berman, A., Snyder, S., Kozier, B., & Erb, G. (2008). *Kozier & Erb's Fundamentals of Nursing: Concepts, Process, and Practice* (8th ed., pp. 553–558). Upper Saddle River, NJ: Pearson Education.

1009. A primary care provider prescribes lisinopril (Zestril®, Prinivil®) to treat a client with hypertension. The client returns to the clinic for a follow-up appointment. A nurse should evaluate the client for adverse effects by asking the client if he or she is experiencing:

1. muscle weakness.
2. bleeding gums.
3. persistent cough.
4. petechiae.

ANSWER: 3

Coughing is a common adverse effect of angiotensin-converting enzyme (ACE) inhibitors and warrants discontinuing the medication. The cough occurs from the action of ACE inhibitors in inhibition of kinase II and accumulation of bradykinin. Muscle weakness can be associated with statin therapy and warrants discontinuing the medication. Bleeding gums and petechiae are associated with bleeding. Petechiae are signs of low platelet counts.

➧ ***Test-taking Tip:*** *Use the suffix "-pril" as a cue that the medication is an ACE inhibitor. Evaluate each option for relevance to the ACE inhibitor and then use the process of elimination to rule out incorrect options. Eliminate options that pertain to bleeding.*

Content Area: Adult Health; *Category of Health Alteration:* Vascular Management; *Integrated Processes:* Nursing Process Evaluation; *Client Need:* Physiological Integrity/Pharmacological and Parenteral Therapies/Adverse Effects/Contradictions; *Cognitive Level:* Application

Reference: Lehne, R. (2007). *Pharmacology for Nursing Care* (6th ed., p. 466). St. Louis, MO: Elsevier Saunders.

1010. EBP A client's blood pressure is being taken at a screening clinic. Which client statement to a nurse demonstrates awareness of having a risk factor for hypertension?

1. "My doctor told me my body mass index is 23."
2. "I usually have a glass of wine or two to unwind when I come home from work."
3. "I should get my blood pressure checked more often because I am African American."
4. "I have colds during the winter, so I see my physician to get the flu vaccine every year."

ANSWER: 3

Research of clients with hypertension has shown that clients who are aware of their personal risk factors are more motivated to achieve adequate control of blood pressure. Being African American is a known risk factor for hypertension. A body mass index (BMI) of 25 or higher is considered a risk factor for hypertension. A BMI of 23 is normal. Excessive alcohol intake is a risk factor for hypertension; consuming two glasses of wine daily increases the risk for hypertension. Having frequent colds and taking the influenza vaccine does not increase the risk for hypertension. Medications for treating colds, if taken frequently, can increase the risk for hypertension.

➧ ***Test-taking Tip:*** *Key words in the stem are "risk factors." Evaluate each option to determine whether it describes an awareness of a risk factor for hypertension.*

Content Area: Adult Health; *Category of Health Alteration:* Vascular Management; *Integrated Processes:* Nursing Process Analysis; *Client Need:* Health Promotion and Maintenance/Disease Prevention; *Cognitive Level:* Application

Reference: Ignatavicius, D., & Workman, M. (2006). *Medical-Surgical Nursing: Critical Thinking for Collaborative Care* (5th ed., pp. 784–788). St. Louis, MO: Elsevier Saunders.

EBP Reference: Fongwa, M., Evangelista, L., & Doering, L. (2006). Adherence to treatment factors in hypertensive African American women. *Journal of Cardiovascular Nursing,* 21(3), 201–207.

1011. An 85-year-old female client seeks medical attention in an emergency department because of chest pain. She tells a nurse that the chest pain is stabbing through the chest into her back. Her blood pressure is 230/130 mm Hg. The nurse realizes that these findings are most suggestive of

1. pulmonary embolism.
2. subclavian steal syndrome.
3. acute arterial occlusion.
4. aortic dissection.

ANSWER: 4

With aortic dissection, the intimal layer of the aorta is torn and blood enters and further separates the layers of the aorta. This causes ripping, moving pain as the process occurs. The blood pressure is significantly elevated until complications occur. Pulmonary embolism produces sudden dyspnea with pleuritic chest pain (occurs with breathing movement). Acute arterial occlusion produces sudden pain in the area distal to the occlusion with loss of pulses. Subclavian steal syndrome is a slowly developing condition that produces weakness and ischemia in an upper extremity.

➧ ***Test-taking Tip:*** *The issue of the question is that the condition causes severe stabbing chest and back pain, and elevated blood pressure. The back pain, along with the other symptoms, should be a clue that this involves the aorta. Select the only option that pertains to the aorta.*

Content Area: Adult Health; *Category of Health Alteration:* Vascular Management; *Integrated Processes:* Nursing Process Analysis; *Client Need:* Physiological Integrity/Physiological Adaptation/Medical Emergencies; Physiological Integrity/Physiological Adaptation/Pathophysiology; *Cognitive Level:* Application

Reference: Ignatavicius, D., & Workman, M. (2006). *Medical-Surgical Nursing: Critical Thinking for Collaborative Care* (5th ed., p. 808). St. Louis, MO: Elsevier/Saunders.

1012. A client is discovered to have a popliteal aneurysm. Because of the aneurysm, a nurse should closely monitor the client for:

1. thoracic outlet syndrome.
2. ischemia in the lower limb.
3. pulmonary embolism.
4. Raynaud's phenomenon.

ANSWER: 2

A popliteal aneurysm (located in the space behind the knee) may cause ischemia in the leg distal to the aneurysm due to thrombus forming inside the aneurysm and potential emboli. Thoracic outlet syndrome is compression of the subclavian artery due to anatomic structures leading to pain and ischemia in the arm. Pulmonary embolism develops from deep venous thromboses in the leg or pelvic veins. Raynaud's phenomenon consists of vasospasms in small arteries of the extremities causing intermittent ischemia.

➧ ***Test-taking Tip:*** *Apply knowledge of medical terminology (popliteal) and note the relationship to option 2.*

Content Area: Adult Health; *Category of Health Alteration:* Vascular Management; *Integrated Processes:* Nursing Process Assessment; *Client Need:* Physiological Integrity/Reduction of Risk Potential/System Specific Assessments; Physiological Integrity/Physiological Adaptation/Pathophysiology; *Cognitive Level:* Application

Reference: Ignatavicius, D., & Workman, M. (2006). *Medical-Surgical Nursing: Critical Thinking for Collaborative Care* (5th ed., p. 809). St. Louis, MO: Elsevier/Saunders.

1013. EBP A nurse admits a client to a hospital and obtains a nursing history. The client tells the nurse that he had an endovascular repair of an abdominal aortic aneurysm found 1 year earlier during a routine screening. The nurse understands that this procedure consists of:

1. excision of the aneurysm and placement of a graft percutaneously.
2. an angioplasty with placement of a stent around the outside of the aorta.
3. placement of a filter within the aneurysm to block clots from becoming emboli.
4. placement of a stent graft inside the aorta that excludes the aneurysm from circulation.

ANSWER: 4

The endovascular repair consists of placement of the endovascular stent graft inside the aorta extending above and below the aneurysmal area to seal it off from the circulation. The aneurysm is left in place. Angioplasty (ballooning of plaque from the inside) is not involved and the stent is placed inside the aorta. Filters are not involved.

➧ ***Test-taking Tip:*** *Apply knowledge of medical terminology: the prefix "endo-" means internal. Use the process of elimination, eliminating all but options 3 and 4. Then eliminate option 3 after noting the word "repair" in the question.*

Content Area: Adult Health; *Category of Health Alteration:* Vascular Management; *Integrated Processes:* Nursing Process Analysis; *Client Need:* Physiological Integrity/Reduction of Risk Potential/Potential for Complications from Surgical Procedures and Health Alterations; *Cognitive Level:* Application

Reference: Smeltzer, S., Bare, B., Hinkle, J., & Cheever, K. (2008). *Brunner and Suddarth's Textbook of Medical-Surgical Nursing* (11th ed., pp. 998–1000). Philadelphia: Lippincott Williams & Wilkins.

EBP Reference: Cosford, P., & Leng, G. (2007). Screening for abdominal aortic aneurysm. *Cochrane Database of Systematic Reviews*, Issue 2, Art. No. CD002945. DOI: 10.1002/14651858.CD002945.pub2. Available at: www.cochrane.org/reviews/en/ab002945.html

1014. A client with an abdominal aortic aneurysm is having a high resolution computed tomography (CT) scan to determine the feasibility for an endovascular repair. Which collaborative interventions should a nurse anticipate to decrease the client's likelihood of developing nephrotoxicity? SELECT ALL THAT APPLY.

1. Administration of sodium bicarbonate 1 hour before injection of the intravenous (IV) contrast dye
2. Administration of 0.9% NaCl at 100 mL per hour before and after the CT scan
3. Administration of acetylcysteine (Mucomyst®) orally before and after the study
4. Monitoring aPTT level before and after the CT scan
5. Placing the client on a low potassium diet

ANSWER: 1, 2, 3

The contrast dye used in a high resolution presents a risk to the client's renal function. Intravenous fluids are administered to maintain hydration and enhance excretion of the dye. Sodium bicarbonate is administered 1 hour before and 6 hours after the IV contrast dye. Acetylcysteine is administered orally the day before and the day of the CT scan to prevent acute renal failure. Both sodium bicarbonate and acetylcysteine are free-radical scavengers that sequester the contract by-products that are destructive to renal cells. The aPTT (activated thromboplastin time) is a measure of blood coagulation and is not related to nephrotoxicity. A low potassium diet may be ordered for a client with renal failure but is not a preventive measure.

➧ ***Test-taking Tip:*** *Key words in the stem are "high resolution CT scan" and "decrease nephrotoxicity." Consider that high resolution CT involves the injection of a contrast media. Select options that will either enhance excretion or sequester the by-products of the contrast media. Eliminate options 4 and 5, which are irrelevant.*

Content Area: Adult Health; *Category of Health Alteration:* Vascular Management; *Integrated Processes:* Nursing Process Analysis; *Client Need:* Physiological Integrity/Physiological Adaptation/Unexpected Response to Therapies; *Cognitive Level:* Analysis

References: Smeltzer, S., Bare, B., Hinkle, J., & Cheever, K. (2008). *Brunner & Suddarth's Textbook of Medical-Surgical Nursing* (11th ed., p. 1133). Philadelphia: Lippincott Williams & Wilkins; Springhouse Publishing Company Staff. (2007). *Springhouse Nurse's Drug Guide 2007* (8th ed., pp. 103–104). Philadelphia: Lippincott Williams & Wilkins.

1015. A nurse is preparing a client for a thoracic aneurysm repair. Which assessment findings lead the nurse to suspect that a rupture has occurred? SELECT ALL THAT APPLY.

1. Severe chest pain radiating to the back
2. Abdominal distention
3. Hypotension
4. Dyspnea
5. Oliguria

ANSWER: 1, 3, 4, 5

A thoracic aneurysm that ruptures will cause pain in the thoracic area. Blood loss will lead to low blood pressure and scant urinary output. The pressure from the hemorrhage will interfere with the client's breathing. A thoracic aneurysm does not cause abdominal distention because the bleeding is in the thoracic area.

➧ ***Test-taking Tip:*** *The focus of the question is signs and symptoms of a ruptured thoracic aneurysm. Think about each option and its relationship to bleeding into the thoracic cavity and loss of blood volume.*

Content Area: Adult Health; *Category of Health Alteration:* Vascular Management; *Integrated Processes:* Nursing Process Analysis; *Client Need:* Physiological Integrity/Physiological Adaptation/Medical Emergencies; *Cognitive Level:* Application

Reference: Ignatavicius, D., & Workman, M. (2006). *Medical-Surgical Nursing: Critical Thinking for Collaborative Care* (5th ed., p. 808). St. Louis, MO: Elsevier/Saunders.

1016. EBP A client with symptoms of intermittent claudication receives treatment with a peripheral percutaneous transluminal angioplasty procedure with placement of an endovascular stent. During a follow-up home visit, a nurse determines that the client is making lifestyle changes to decrease the likelihood of re-stenosis and arterial occlusion. Which observations of the client's actions support this conclusion? SELECT ALL THAT APPLY.

1. States participating in an exercise program
2. Abstaining from nicotine
3. Wearing support hose
4. States receiving foot care from a podiatrist
5. Following a low saturated fat diet
6. Taking the medication rosuvastatin calcium (Crestor®)

ANSWER: 1, 2, 5, 6

Reducing client risk factors in order to slow the arteriosclerotic process may delay progression of the disease. Exercising promotes collateral circulation. Smoking cessation, following a low saturated fat diet, and taking medications to lower cholesterol also deter the arteriosclerotic process. There is evidence that more than 30% of clients having procedures to improve claudication seek further intervention within a year. Wearing support hose may impede circulation. Receiving professional foot care is a positive factor but does not prevent the progressive nature of peripheral arterial disease.

➧ ***Test-taking Tip:*** *The issue of the question is "factors to prevent re-occlusion after a peripheral percutaneous transluminal angioplasty with stent procedure." Use the process of elimination, eliminating options 3 and 4 because these do not reduce the client's risk for developing atherosclerosis.*

Content Area: Adult Health; *Category of Health Alteration:* Vascular Management; *Integrated Processes:* Nursing Process Evaluation; *Client Need:* Physiological Integrity/Physiological Adaptation/Illness Management; Health Promotion and Maintenance/Lifestyle Choices; *Cognitive Level:* Application

Reference: Smeltzer, S., Bare, B., Hinkle, J., & Cheever, K. (2008). *Brunner & Suddarth's Textbook of Medical-Surgical Nursing* (11th ed., pp. 994–995). Philadelphia: Lippincott Williams & Wilkins.

EBP References: Yellen, E. (2007). Synergy and peripheral percutaneous transluminal angioplasty. *Journal of Vascular Nursing*, XXV(1), 7–11; Watson, L., Ellis, B., & Leng, G. (2008). Exercise for intermittent claudication. *Cochrane Database of Systematic Reviews*, Issue 4, Art. No. CD000990. DOI: 10.1002/14651858.CD000990.pub2. Available at: www.cochrane.org/reviews/en/ab000990.html

---

1017. EBP A client seeks medical attention because of pain that develops while walking. An ankle-brachial index (ABI) test is ordered, and the results show that the client has ratios of 1.4 and 1.3 bilaterally. Based on these results, a nurse determines that the client:

1. has severe peripheral arterial disease.
2. would benefit from the medication ticlopidine hydrochloride (Ticlid®).
3. is experiencing pain that is psychological in origin.
4. needs further medical consultation to determine the cause of pain.

ANSWER: 4

The client requires further medical consultation because the ABI (comparison of blood pressure in ankle to the brachial blood pressure) is normal in each leg. A result of less than 0.9 is diagnostic of peripheral arterial disease. Based on the results of the ABI, the client has normal arterial circulation and would not benefit from ticlopidine hydrochloride. There is no information relating the pain to a psychological concern.

➧ ***Test-taking Tip:*** *Apply knowledge of normal ABI values (greater than 0.9) to select the correct option.*

Content Area: Adult Health; *Category of Health Alteration:* Vascular Management; *Integrated Processes:* Nursing Process Analysis; *Client Need:* Safe and Effective Care Environment/Management of Care/Consultation; *Cognitive Level:* Analysis

Reference: Ignatavicius, D., & Workman, M. (2006). *Medical-Surgical Nursing: Critical Thinking for Collaborative Care* (5th ed., pp. 795–796). St. Louis, MO: Elsevier/Saunders.

EBP Reference: Bonham P., & Flemister, B. (2008). *Guideline for Management of Wounds in Patients with Lower-Extremity Arterial Disease.* Available at: www.guideline.gov/summary/summary.aspx?doc_id=12613&nbr=006521&string=cellulitis

---

1018. A client has an appointment at a vascular clinic after being treated with pentoxifylline (Trental®) for 6 weeks. A nurse determines the pentoxifylline has been effective by noting that the client:

1. has a decrease in lower extremity edema.
2. is experiencing less symptoms of withdrawal after quitting smoking.
3. has a venous ulcer on the ankle that has decreased in size and depth.
4. is able to walk a greater distance without claudication.

ANSWER: 4

Pentoxifylline is thought to act by improving capillary blood flow and is prescribed to improve intermittent claudication. Effects are usually seen in 2 to 4 weeks. A diuretic medication is used to decrease edema. Nicotine substitutes are commonly prescribed to control withdrawal symptoms after the client quits smoking. Venous ulcers resulting from prolonged venous hypertension are not treated with pentoxifylline.

➧ ***Test-taking Tip:*** *Focus on the issue: evaluating the effectiveness of pentoxifylline. Consider the action of the pentoxifylline to improve circulation and use the process of elimination. Only option 4 indicates an improvement in circulation. If unsure, focus on the fact that the client is being seen in a vascular clinic.*

Content Area: Adult Health; *Category of Health Alteration:* Vascular Management; *Integrated Processes:* Nursing Process Evaluation; *Client Need:* Physiological Integrity/Pharmacological and Parenteral Therapies/Expected Actions or Outcomes; *Cognitive Level:* Analysis

Reference: Ignatavicius, D., & Workman, M. (2006). *Medical-Surgical Nursing: Critical Thinking for Collaborative Care* (5th ed., p. 796). St. Louis, MO: Elsevier/Saunders.

1019. A 31-year-old male client seeks care at a vascular clinic because of painful fingers and toes. He is diagnosed with Buerger's disease (thromboangiitis obliterans). A nurse is teaching the client ways to prevent progression of the disease. Which prevention measure should be the nurse's initial focus when teaching the client?

1. Avoiding exposure to cold
2. Maintaining meticulous hygiene practices
3. Abstaining from all tobacco products in all forms
4. Following a low-fat diet

ANSWER: 3

Buerger's disease is an uncommon vascular occlusive disease that affects the medial and small arteries and veins, initially in the distal limbs. It is strongly associated with tobacco smoking, which causes vasoconstriction. The most important action to communicate to the client is that he must abstain from tobacco in all forms to prevent progression of the disease. The other interventions are correct but not as important as abstaining from tobacco. Avoiding exposure to cold will reduce the pain. Meticulous hygiene and a low-fat diet are also positive actions to follow.

➧ ***Test-taking Tip:*** *The key words are "painful fingers and toes" and "prevent progression of the disease." The words "initial focus" identify the need to prioritize. Recall that the etiology of Buerger's disease is unknown so avoiding agents that cause vasoconstriction is priority.*

Content Area: Adult Health; *Category of Health Alteration:* Vascular Management; *Integrated Processes:* Teaching and Learning; *Client Need:* Physiological Integrity/Physiological Adaptation/Illness Management; *Cognitive Level:* Application

Reference: Ignatavicius, D., & Workman, M. (2006). *Medical-Surgical Nursing: Critical Thinking for Collaborative Care* (5th ed., p. 810). St. Louis, MO: Elsevier/Saunders.

1020. A client with Raynaud's disease is seen in a vascular clinic 6 weeks after nifedipine (Procardia®) has been prescribed. A nurse evaluates that the medication has been effective when which findings are noted?

1. The client's blood pressure is 110/68 mm Hg.
2. The client states experiencing less pain and numbness.
3. The client states that tolerance to heat is improved.
4. The client walks without claudication.

ANSWER: 2

Raynaud's disease is a disease in which cutaneous arteries in the extremities have recurrent episodes of vasospasm with blanching and then redness. The episodes are brought on by cold and result in pain and numbness. Nifedipine, a calcium channel blocker, causes vasodilation, which reduces pain and numbness. Nifedipine is used as an antihypertensive agent but that is not the purpose here. The client is at risk to develop hypotension as an adverse effect. Tolerance to cold, not heat, should improve. Claudication is not associated with Raynaud's disease but is associated with arteriosclerotic changes in the larger arteries.

➧ ***Test-taking Tip:*** *The issue of the question is "expected effects of Procardia® on Raynaud's disease." Consider the action of nifedipine and how it relates to the symptoms of Raynaud's disease.*

Content Area: Adult Health; *Category of Health Alteration:* Vascular Management; *Integrated Processes:* Nursing Process Evaluation; *Client Need:* Physiological Integrity/Pharmacological and Parenteral Therapies/Expected Actions or Outcomes; *Cognitive Level:* Analysis

Reference: Ignatavicius, D., & Workman, M. (2006). *Medical-Surgical Nursing: Critical Thinking for Collaborative Care* (5th ed., p. 811). St. Louis, MO: Elsevier/Saunders.

1021. A primary care provider orders that a client have an elastic bandage applied to the lower extremity to reduce edema. At which position on the client's leg should the nurse start wrapping the elastic bandage?

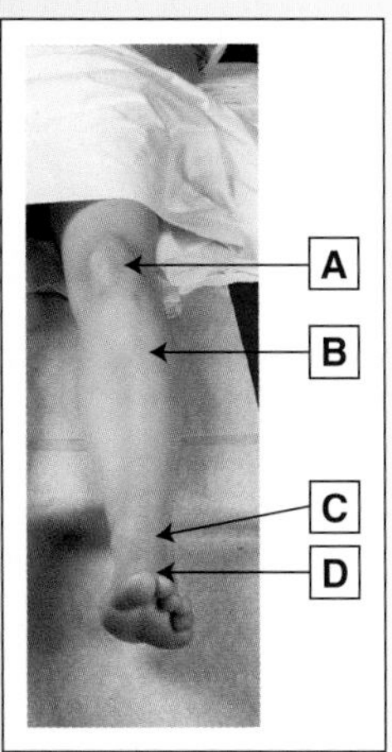

1. Location A
2. Location B
3. Location C
4. Location D

ANSWER: 4

The nurse should begin to apply the bandage at the distal point and proceed proximally. By starting at this point, trapping fluid atop the foot is avoided. The nurse should still be able to palpate the dorsalis pedis pulse underneath the bandage. The purpose of the bandage is to apply compression evenly to the lower leg. Applying the bandage at the knee, calf, or ankle will decrease venous return and increase edema in the lower extremity.

➧ ***Test-taking Tip:*** *Consider the purpose of the elastic bandage. Consider the venous flow in the leg: distal to proximal.*

Content Area: Adult Health; *Category of Health Alteration:* Vascular Management; *Integrated Processes:* Nursing Process Implementation; *Client Need:* Physiological Integrity/Basic Care and Comfort/Nonpharmacological Interventions; *Cognitive Level:* Application

Reference: Berman, A., Snyder, S., Kozier, B., & Erb, G. (2008). *Kozier & Erb's Fundamentals of Nursing: Concepts, Process, and Practice* (8th ed., pp. 928–930). Upper Saddle River, NJ: Pearson Education.

1022. A client is receiving continuous heparin therapy. The infusion is 25,000 units of heparin in 500 mL of 5% dextrose and is infusing at 12 mL per hour. The aPTT laboratory test result is 92 seconds. According to the heparin infusion protocol, the nurse should administer the heparin infusion at a rate of _____ mL/hr.

Heparin Infusion Protocol Adjustment Table

aPTT Results	Bolus Dose	Stop Infusion	Rate Change	Repeat aPTT
Less than 50	5,000 units	0 minutes	+3 mL/hr	6 hr
50–59	0	0 minutes	+2 mL/hr	6 hr
60–85	0	0 minutes	No change	Next a.m.
86–100	0	0 minutes	–1 mL/hr	Next a.m.
101–120	0	30 minutes	–2 mL/hr	6 hr
120–150	0	60 minutes	–3 mL/hr	6 hr
Greater than 150	0	60 minutes	–5 mL/hr	6 hr

ANSWER: 11

According to the protocol, with an aPTT value of 92 seconds, the rate should be decreased by 1 mL per hour. If the infusion was previously infusing at 12 mL per hour, the new rate is 11 mL/hr.

➧ ***Test-taking Tip:*** *Read the information carefully and follow the directions of the heparin infusion protocol to determine the new rate.*

Content Area: Adult Health; *Category of Health Alteration:* Vascular Management; *Integrated Processes:* Nursing Process Implementation; *Client Need:* Analysis; *Cognitive Level:* Physiological Integrity/Pharmacological and Parenteral Therapies/Dosage Calculation; Physiological Integrity/Reduction of Risk Potential/Laboratory Values

Reference: Springhouse Publishing Company Staff. (2007). *Springhouse Nurse's Drug Guide 2007* (8th ed., pp. 654–657). Philadelphia: Lippincott Williams & Wilkins.

1023. A nurse is discussing healthy lifestyle practices with a client who has chronic venous insufficiency. Which practices should be emphasized with this client? SELECT ALL THAT APPLY.

1. Avoid eating an excess of dark green vegetables.
2. Elevate the legs while sitting.
3. Wear elastic stockings (TEDS®) daily, applying them before getting out of bed.
4. Increase standing time and shift weight from one leg to the other when standing in one place.
5. Sleep with legs elevated above the level of the heart.

ANSWER: 2, 3, 5

Chronic venous insufficiency develops because of damaged valves in the veins, resulting in venous hypertension. Interventions focus on management of edema by elevating the legs and wearing elastic stockings. Eating excessive amounts of dark green vegetables could affect the anticoagulant effect of warfarin, but there is no indication the client is taking an anticoagulant. Clients who have chronic venous insufficiency should avoid prolonged standing.

➧ ***Test-taking Tip:*** *Recall that venous insufficiency impairs return of blood to the heart. Select options that will improve venous return.*

Content Area: Adult Health; *Category of Health Alteration:* Vascular Management; *Integrated Processes:* Teaching and Learning; *Client Need:* Physiological Integrity/Physiological Adaptation/Illness Management; *Cognitive Level:* Analysis

Reference: Ignatavicius, D., & Workman, M. (2006). *Medical-Surgical Nursing: Critical Thinking for Collaborative Care* (5th ed., pp. 816–818). St. Louis, MO: Elsevier/Saunders.

1024. After seeing a primary care provider for a routine appointment, a 48-year-old client tells a nurse that she experienced pain in the calf of her left leg earlier in the week, but she is pain-free now. The nurse assesses the client and finds the dorsalis pedis pulses palpable and no pain upon dorsiflexion bilaterally. A few varicose veins are visible in each leg. There is very slight swelling in the left foot and none in the right foot. Which is the best action by the nurse?

1. Ask the client if she has been walking more lately.
2. Notify the primary care provider.
3. Ask the client if she has thought about taking a baby aspirin once a day.
4. Explain to the client that there are no significant findings but to call the office if the pain returns.

ANSWER: 2

The nurse should notify the primary care provider about the client's additional concern. A possible deep venous thrombosis (DVT) is taken seriously because it can lead to pulmonary embolism (PE). Clients with DVT may be asymptomatic. Unilateral swelling of one leg, a classic symptom of DVT, is suggested with the slight swelling in the left foot. The primary care provider may order a noninvasive test, venous ultrasound, to determine whether the client has a DVT. With the unilateral swelling in the extremities, the nurse does not need additional assessment data (recent activity level). Advising aspirin is not within the scope of nursing and has possible negative consequences. Waiting until the pain returns would delay diagnosis, needed treatment, and expose the client to risk of PE if the client has a DVT.

➧ ***Test-taking Tip:*** *Key words in the stem are "pain in the calf" and "very slight swelling in the left foot, none in the right." The phrase "best action" identifies the need to prioritize. Consider the assessment in the stem carefully, noting that the negative Homan's sign is not significant. Research has shown that the Homan's sign is not an accurate indicator of the presence of a DVT. Consider the consequences of each action. Notifying the primary care provider offers the safest option. Therefore, select option 2.*

Content Area: Adult Health; *Category of Health Alteration:* Vascular Management; *Integrated Processes:* Nursing Process Implementation; *Client Need:* Safe and Effective Care Environment/Management of Care/Collaboration with Interdisciplinary Team; Physiological Integrity/Reduction of Risk Potential/System Specific Assessments; *Cognitive Level:* Analysis

Reference: Ignatavicius, D., & Workman, M. (2006). *Medical-Surgical Nursing: Critical Thinking for Collaborative Care* (5th ed., pp. 812–813). St. Louis, MO: Elsevier/Saunders.

1025. A nurse is caring for multiple clients on a medical unit. Which client, who has been diagnosed with a lower extremity deep venous thrombosis (DVT), should the nurse plan for possible placement of a filter in the inferior vena cava to protect against pulmonary embolism?

1. A 22-year-old female who has been taking oral contraceptives
2. A 65-year-old client admitted with a bleeding gastric ulcer
3. A 55-year-old client who had a total knee joint replacement
4. A 52-year-old female who had a vaginal hysterectomy 6 weeks earlier

ANSWER: 2

The client with the bleeding gastric ulcer is not a candidate for anticoagulant therapy and, therefore, needs the inferior vena cava filter to prevent an embolus from the DVT reaching the pulmonary circulation. The other clients have no contraindications listed for anticoagulant therapy.

➧ ***Test-taking Tip:*** *The issue of the question is "criteria for clients with DVT to be treated with a vena cava filter instead of anticoagulation." Consider each option separately regarding risk from anticoagulation.*

Content Area: Adult Health; *Category of Health Alteration:* Vascular Management; *Integrated Processes:* Nursing Process Planning; *Client Need:* Physiological Integrity/Reduction of Risk Potential/Therapeutic Procedures; *Cognitive Level:* Analysis

Reference: Ignatavicius, D., & Workman, M. (2006). *Medical-Surgical Nursing: Critical Thinking for Collaborative Care* (5th ed., p. 815). St. Louis, MO: Elsevier/Saunders.

1026. A client returns to a unit after undergoing placement of a vena cava filter. When caring for this client, a nurse should anticipate:

1. beginning anticoagulation therapy as soon as possible.
2. assessing the dressing over the abdominal incision.
3. checking the orders to determine the client's ordered activity.
4. forcing oral fluids to promote excretion of the dye used during the procedure.

ANSWER: 3

The procedure for placement of a vena cava filter is done percutaneously; usually through the subclavian or femoral vein approach. The client will have activity included in the postprocedural orders. Anticoagulation is not necessary if a vena cava filter is in place. There is no abdominal incision with the percutaneous approach. Dye is not used during the procedure.

➧ ***Test-taking Tip:*** *Think about how the procedure is performed and the potential complications before making a selection. Recall that a percutaneous approach is used.*

Content Area: Adult Health; *Category of Health Alteration:* Vascular Management; *Integrated Processes:* Nursing Process Planning; *Client Need:* Physiological Integrity/Reduction of Risk Potential/Therapeutic Procedures; *Cognitive Level:* Application

Reference: Ignatavicius, D., & Workman, M. (2006). *Medical-Surgical Nursing: Critical Thinking for Collaborative Care* (5th ed., p. 815). St. Louis, MO: Elsevier/Saunders.

1027. EBP An experienced nurse tells a new nurse that lymphedema is a complication that commonly occurs after women have received surgery for breast cancer. Which statement to the new nurse regarding lymphedema is correct?

1. Lymphedema is characterized by severe swelling in the arm and hand on the affected side.
2. Lymphedema usually resolves after the cancer treatment is completed when collateral lymph circulation develops.
3. Lymphedema is mainly controlled by encouraging women to keep their arm elevated.
4. Lymphedema frequently signifies that there is a recurrence of the malignancy.

ANSWER: 1

Lymphedema is a chronic condition characterized by extreme edema in the involved extremity. The lymph circulation is disrupted by the lymph node dissection (even 20% of persons with sentinel node biopsy develop lymphedema) that is part of the treatment of breast cancer. Collateral lymph circulation does not develop. Lymphedema is best controlled by wearing compression sleeves and/or gloves. Lymphedema occurs from the lymph node dissection and is not associated with recurrence of the malignancy.

➧ ***Test-taking Tip:*** *The question identifies lymphedema as a complication of breast cancer treatment. This implies that it is an undesirable effect of treatment. Select the only option that relates to an adverse effect.*

Content Area: Adult Health; *Category of Health Alteration:* Vascular Management; *Integrated Processes:* Nursing Process Analysis; *Client Need:* Physiological Integrity/Reduction of Risk Potential/Potential for Complications from Surgical Procedures and Health Alterations; *Cognitive Level:* Application

EBP References: Fu, M. (2005). Breast cancer survivors' intentions of managing lymphedema. *Cancer Nursing,* 28(6), 446–457; Revis, D. (2008). Lymphedema. *E-Medicine from WebMD.* Available at: www.emedicine.com/med/TOPIC 2722.HTM

1028. EBP A nurse is evaluating female clients who have been diagnosed with arm lymphedema. Which client demonstrates acceptance of her diagnosis and has included lymphedema management in her lifestyle?

1. A client who inspects her involved arm and hand only when pain occurs and the swelling worsens
2. The client who continues to knit because she enjoys making sweaters even though the repeated activity is painful
3. The client who never wears the compression sleeve and glove in public places
4. The client who asks her family members to perform tasks that include heavy lifting because the tasks have increased swelling in the past

ANSWER: 4

The client who asks for assistance with heavy lifting demonstrates acceptance of lymphedema as a chronic condition that can be managed with lifestyle changes. The woman with lymphedema should include daily inspection of the involved extremity as part of effective management. The woman who continues to knit despite worsening symptoms of lymphedema is not dealing effectively with the condition. The woman who avoids wearing the compression sleeve and glove in public will experience the recurrence of severe edema.

➧ ***Test-taking Tip:*** *Use the process of elimination, noting that option 1 contains the key word "only" and option 3 contains the key word "never." Eliminate these options because they contain absolute words. Then choose between options 2 and 4. Note that option 4 focuses on swelling and option 2 focuses on pain. Because lymphedema is associated with swelling, eliminate option 2.*

Content Area: Adult Health; *Category of Health Alteration:* Vascular Management; *Integrated Processes:* Nursing Process Evaluation; *Client Need:* Physiological Integrity/Physiological Adaptation/Illness Management; *Cognitive Level:* Analysis

Reference: Smeltzer, S., Bare, B., Hinkle, J., & Cheever, K. (2008). *Brunner & Suddarth's Textbook of Medical-Surgical Nursing* (11th ed., pp. 1016–1017). Philadelphia: Lippincott Williams & Wilkins.

EBP Reference: Fu, M. (2005). Breast cancer survivors' intentions of managing lymphedema. *Cancer Nursing,* 28(6), 446–457.

1029. EBP A client receives treatment for uncomplicated lower extremity cellulitis. A nurse notes improvement in the client's condition when which observation is noted on assessment?

1. Strong dorsalis pedis pulses palpated bilaterally
2. Increased erythema in the involved area
3. Temperature of 101.3°F (38.5°C) orally
4. Decreased swelling in the involved area

ANSWER: 4

Cellulitis is an infection with diffuse inflammation occurring in the tissue just under the skin. Observing a decrease in swelling is evidence of improvement. Circulation is not involved with cellulitis. Persons with diabetes or paralysis who have sensory and circulatory deficits may be less apt to experience the pain associated with cellulitis. Increased erythema (redness) and a fever are findings consistent with infection and inflammation.

➧ ***Test-taking Tip:*** *The suffix "-itis" indicates inflammation. Focus on the issue: improvement in the cellulitis. Eliminate options 2 and 3 because these indicate inflammation and infection are still present; option 1 is unrelated to uncomplicated cellulitis.*

Content Area: Adult Health; *Category of Health Alteration:* Vascular Management; *Integrated Processes:* Nursing Process Evaluation; *Client Need:* Physiological Integrity/Physiological Adaptation/Illness Management; *Cognitive Level:* Analysis

Reference: Smeltzer, S., Bare, B., Hinkle, J., & Cheever, K. (2008). *Brunner & Suddarth's Textbook of Medical-Surgical Nursing* (11th ed., p. 1017). Philadelphia: Lippincott Williams & Wilkins.

EBP Reference: Curtis, D. (2008). Cellulitis. *E-Medicine from WebMD*. Available at: www.emedicine.com/emerg/topic88.htm#section~Miscellaneous

---

1030. A nurse is completing a health history on a client admitted to a hospital with recurrent lower extremity cellulitis. The client tells the nurse that he has athlete's foot (tinea pedis). The nurse concludes that this is significant because:

1. the cellulitis is commonly caused by a fungus.
2. the cellulitis should resolve with topical fungicide therapy.
3. the client is at risk for developing a painful neuralgia after the infection has resolved.
4. the loss of skin integrity that occurs with tinea pedis allows bacteria to enter the tissue.

ANSWER: 4

Cellulitis is an infection with diffuse inflammation occurring in the tissue just under the skin. Chronic athlete's foot causes minute breaks in the skin, allowing bacteria on the skin to enter the tissue and cause the infectious process. Cellulitis is caused by a bacterial infection, most commonly *Streptococcus pyogenes*. Cellulitis is treated with antibiotics. Herpes zoster (shingles) infection is sometimes complicated by neuralgic pain after the acute infection.

➧ ***Test-taking Tip:*** *The suffix "-itis" indicates inflammation. Consider the usual symptoms associated with athlete's foot and the loss of skin integrity.*

Content Area: Adult Health; *Category of Health Alteration:* Vascular Management; *Integrated Processes:* Nursing Process Analysis; *Client Need:* Physiological Integrity/Physiological Adaptation/System Specific Assessments; *Cognitive Level:* Analysis

References: Smeltzer, S., Bare, B., Hinkle, J., & Cheever, K. (2008). *Brunner & Suddarth's Textbook of Medical-Surgical Nursing* (11th ed., p. 1017). Philadelphia: Lippincott Williams & Wilkins; Curtis, D. (2008). Cellulitis. *E-Medicine from WebMD*. Available at: www.emedicine.com/emerg/topic88.htm#section~Miscellaneous

---

1031. A nurse admits a client with a diagnosis of severe cellulitis in a lower extremity. The nurse anticipates the prescribed treatment will include:

1. obtaining baseline coagulation laboratory tests and initiating anticoagulation therapy.
2. applying sequential compression devices.
3. administering intravenous antibiotic therapy.
4. débriding the involved area.

ANSWER: 3

Cellulitis is an infection with diffuse inflammation occurring in the tissue just under the skin. Infections are treated with antibiotic therapy. Anticoagulants are not indicated for infection. Compression devices would be detrimental to the cellulitis. Débridement involves removal of nonviable tissue, which is not usually associated with cellulitis.

➧ ***Test-taking Tip:*** *The suffix "-itis" indicates inflammation. Consider each option separately and relate each to a decrease in inflammation. Use the process of elimination.*

Content Area: Adult Health; *Category of Health Alteration:* Vascular Management; *Integrated Processes:* Nursing Process Planning; *Client Need:* Physiological Integrity/Physiological Adaptation/Illness Management; *Cognitive Level:* Analysis

References: Smeltzer, S., Bare, B., Hinkle, J., & Cheever, K. (2008). *Brunner & Suddarth's Textbook of Medical-Surgical Nursing* (11th ed., p. 1017). Philadelphia: Lippincott Williams & Wilkins; Curtis, D. (2008). Cellulitis. *E-Medicine from WebMD*. Available at: www.emedicine.com/emerg/topic88.htm#section~Miscellaneous

1032. A nurse reviews the symptoms of acute graft occlusion with a client who has had a revascularization graft procedure of the lower extremity. Which symptom of acute arterial occlusion stated by the client indicates further teaching is needed?

1. Severe pain
2. Redness and warmth along the incisions
3. Paresthesia
4. Inability to move the foot

ANSWER: 2

Redness and warmth along the incision line is associated with inflammation or infection, not graft occlusion. Lack of blood supply to a body extremity may result in pain, pallor, pulselessness, paresthesia (numbness), paralysis (decreased ability to move), and poikilothermia (coolness).

➧ ***Test-taking Tip:*** *Key words in the stem are "acute arterial occlusion." Focus on the symptoms associated with decreased circulation and eliminate all but option 2.*

Content Area: Adult Health; *Category of Health Alteration:* Vascular Management; *Integrated Processes:* Teaching and Learning; *Client Need:* Physiological Integrity/Reduction of Risk Potential/Potential for Complications from Surgical Procedures and Health Alterations; *Cognitive Level:* Application

Reference: Ignatavicius, D., & Workman, M. (2006). *Medical-Surgical Nursing: Critical Thinking for Collaborative Care* (5th ed., p. 805). St. Louis, MO: Elsevier/Saunders.

1033. The report of a chest x-ray of a client who has had aortic femoral bypass graft surgery indicates that the client has atelectasis. Which priority intervention should a nurse plan to include in the client's care?

1. Assessing breath sounds
2. Monitoring oxygen saturation
3. Assisting the client to use the incentive spirometer every hour
4. Monitoring respiratory rate

ANSWER: 3

The chest x-ray indicates atelectasis—collapse of the alveoli that result from shallow breathing. Planning to assist the client to use the incentive spirometer every hour should reinflate the alveoli. The intervention to treat the atelectasis is the priority. Assessing breath sounds, oxygen saturation, and respiratory rate are correct assessments but are not interventions that will improve the atelectasis.

➧ ***Test-taking Tip:*** *The key word "priority" indicates the need to prioritize. Evaluate each option separately to determine whether it will improve the atelectasis. Eliminate options 1, 2, and 4 because these refer only to assessment and monitoring, which will not decrease the atelectasis.*

Content Area: Adult Health; *Category of Health Alteration:* Vascular Management; *Integrated Processes:* Nursing Process Planning; *Client Need:* Physiological Integrity/Reduction of Risk Potential/Potential for Complications from Surgical Procedures and Health Alterations; *Cognitive Level:* Analysis

Reference: Berman, A., Snyder, S., Kozier, B., & Erb, G. (2008). *Kozier & Erb's Fundamentals of Nursing: Concepts, Process, and Practice* (8th ed., pp. 962–963). Upper Saddle River, NJ: Pearson Education.

1034. A nurse is caring for a male client the night before the client is scheduled for an amputation. The client has a 7-year history of peripheral artery disease. Recent surgeries have failed to revascularize the client's leg. The client tells the nurse that he is a failure and all the efforts of his family and physician have been wasted. The most appropriate action by the nurse at this time is to:

1. explain that the hospital staff will help him through the surgery and recovery.
2. stay with the client, listen carefully, and encourage him to express his feelings.
3. offer to contact pastoral care.
4. offer to contact the primary care provider to obtain an antidepressant.

ANSWER: 2

The nurse should offer compassionate understanding to the client by being present and listening. This provides an opportunity for the client to express his feelings and begin to deal with the amputation and his loss. The other responses offer solutions without dealing with the emotional needs and loss the client is experiencing.

➧ ***Test-taking Tip:*** *The issue of the question is a client facing an amputation after enduring chronic peripheral arterial diseases. The question calls for a caring intervention by the nurse. Apply the therapeutic communication skills, including silence and presence, in answering this question.*

Content Area: Adult Health; *Category of Health Alteration:* Vascular Management; *Integrated Processes:* Caring; *Client Need:* Psychosocial Integrity/Grief and Loss; Psychosocial Integrity/Therapeutic Communications; *Cognitive Level:* Analysis

References: Berman, A., Snyder, S., Kozier, B., & Erb, G. (2008). *Kozier & Erb's Fundamentals of Nursing: Concepts, Process, and Practice* (8th ed., p. 447). Upper Saddle River, NJ: Pearson Education; Ignatavicius, D., & Workman, M. (2006). *Medical-Surgical Nursing: Critical Thinking for Collaborative Care* (5th ed., p. 1220). St. Louis, MO: Elsevier/Saunders.

1035. A nurse in the postanesthesia care unit (PACU) is monitoring a client who has had a repair of an aortic aneurysm with graft surgery. The nurse is unable to palpate the posterior tibial pulse of one leg that was palpable 15 minutes earlier. The most appropriate initial action for the nurse is to:

1. recheck the pulse in 15 minutes.
2. reposition the leg.
3. notify the surgeon.
4. remove the surgical dressing.

ANSWER: 3

The nurse should notify the surgeon immediately. The loss of the pulse could signify graft occlusion or embolization. The surgeon needs to reassess the client. The primary nursing intervention in the PACU is continual surveillance of clients. Rechecking the pulse in 15 minutes could allow ischemia to progress. The leg should already be in an appropriate position, so repositioning is not indicated. There is no need to remove the abdominal dressing because of an absent pulse.

➧ ***Test-taking Tip:*** *Use the ABCs (airway, breathing, circulation) to establish that circulation is a priority concern. Thus, notifying the surgeon would be the most immediate action so that the impaired circulation can be corrected.*

Content Area: Adult Health; *Category of Health Alteration:* Vascular Management; *Integrated Processes:* Nursing Process Implementation; *Client Need:* Physiological Integrity/Physiological Adaptation/Medical Emergencies; *Cognitive Level:* Analysis

Reference: Ignatavicius, D., & Workman, M. (2006). *Medical-Surgical Nursing: Critical Thinking for Collaborative Care* (5th ed., pp. 798, 807–808). St. Louis, MO: Elsevier/Saunders.

1036. Two days ago, a client had a femoral-popliteal artery bypass graft surgery. A priority nursing action at this time should be to:

1. monitor intake and output.
2. report any edema that develops in the operative leg.
3. maintain the client at a 60-degree sitting position when resting in bed.
4. monitor the dorsalis pedis and posterior tibial pulses bilaterally every 4 hours.

ANSWER: 4

The priority nursing action should be to monitor the pulses in the feet to detect graft occlusion. Intake and output is important but not the priority. Because of the surgery and improved circulation, edema in the operative leg is an expected outcome. Bending from the hip or knee should be limited to avoid graft occlusion.

➧ ***Test-taking Tip:*** *Use the ABCs (airway, breathing, circulation) to select the priority action of circulation and option 4.*

Content Area: Adult Health; *Category of Health Alteration:* Vascular Management; *Integrated Processes:* Nursing Process Implementation; *Client Need:* Physiological Integrity/Reduction of Risk Potential/System Specific Assessments; *Cognitive Level:* Application

Reference: Ignatavicius, D., & Workman, M. (2006). *Medical-Surgical Nursing: Critical Thinking for Collaborative Care* (5th ed., pp. 798–804). St. Louis, MO: Elsevier/Saunders.

1037. EBP Which intervention should a nurse plan to incorporate in the care of a surgical client to decrease the risk of deep venous thrombosis (DVT) and pulmonary embolism (PE)?

1. Use of intermittent compression devices on the lower extremities
2. Administration of heparin intravenously
3. Coughing and deep breathing exercises
4. Isometric leg exercises

ANSWER: 1

Recommendations to prevent DVT and PE address the need to improve circulation and counter any states of hypercoagulopathy. Intermittent compression devices improve circulation. While administration of heparin will achieve anticoagulation, a low dose of unfractionated or low-molecular-weight heparin is usually ordered subcutaneous, and not intravenous, administration. Coughing and deep breathing exercises and isometric leg exercises are positive actions but do not decrease the risk for DVT and PE.

➧ ***Test-taking Tip:*** *Focus on actions to decrease the risk for deep venous thrombosis and pulmonary embolism. Evaluate each option to determine its effect on improving circulation and reducing hypercoagulation.*

Content Area: Adult Health; *Category of Health Alteration:* Vascular Management; *Integrated Processes:* Nursing Process Planning; *Client Need:* Physiological Integrity/Basic Care and Comfort/Nonpharmacological Interventions; *Cognitive Level:* Application

Reference: Smeltzer, S., Bare, B., Hinkle, J., & Cheever, K. (2008). *Brunner & Suddarth's Textbook of Medical-Surgical Nursing* (11th ed., pp. 1008–1009). Philadelphia: Lippincott Williams & Wilkins.

EBP Reference: Daniels, S. (2007). Improving hospital care for surgical patients. *Nursing 2007*, 37(8), 36–42.

Test 27: **Adult Health: Pharmacological and Parenteral Therapies**

1038. A client is to receive a scheduled dose of digoxin (Lanoxin®). A nurse determines that the client's apical pulse is irregular at 92 beats per minute and that the client's serum potassium level is 3.9 mEq/L. Which documentation by the nurse reflects the most appropriate action based on this information?

1. Serum potassium level within normal limits. Digoxin administered for rapid apical pulse.
2. Digoxin withheld because the client's heart rate is irregular.
3. Digoxin withheld to prevent toxicity due to the low serum potassium level.
4. Physician notified to report the irregular heart rate and low serum potassium level.

ANSWER: 1

Digoxin, a cardiac glycoside, slows and strengthens the heart. It is used for rate control in clients with atrial fibrillation. Atrial fibrillation produces an irregular rhythm. A normal serum potassium level is 3.8 to 5.5 mEq/L. Dysrhythmias can occur if digoxin is administered when the serum potassium level is low; the serum potassium level is within a normal range. Withholding the digoxin and notifying the physician are unnecessary.

▶ ***Test-taking Tip:*** *Recall that the normal serum potassium level is 3.8 to 5.5 mEq/L. Review the nursing considerations/actions of digoxin if this question seems difficult.*

Content Area: Adult Health; *Category of Health Alteration:* Pharmacological and Parenteral Therapies; *Integrated Processes:* Communication and Documentation; *Client Need:* Physiological Integrity/Pharmacological and Parenteral Therapies/Expected Actions or Outcomes; *Cognitive Level:* Analysis

Reference: Lehne, R. (2007). *Pharmacology for Nursing Care* (6th ed., pp. 515–519). St. Louis, MO: Elsevier/Saunders.

1039. A hospitalized client has been receiving clonidine (Catapres®) 0.1 mg via transdermal patch once every 7 days. When bathing the client, a nursing assistant removes the patch thinking it is tape. Eight hours later, an on-coming nurse discovers that the transdermal patch is no longer on the client as prescribed. Based on this information, which assessment finding should be most concerning to the nurse?

1. Skin tear noted on the client's upper chest.
2. Excruciating headache reported.
3. Blood pressure is 182/100 mm Hg.
4. Electrocardiogram shows a heart rate of 120 beats per minute.

ANSWER: 3

Clonidine is an antihypertensive medication. Rebound hypertension occurs from abrupt withdrawal. Immediate intervention is required to lower the blood pressure. Though a skin tear is concerning and could have occurred during removal, it is not the most concerning. Headache can occur from the abrupt removal of clonidine, but is not the most concerning. Tachycardia is an adverse effect of clonidine.

▶ ***Test-taking Tip:*** *The key words are "most concerning." Use the ABCs (airway, breathing, circulation) to determine the most concerning finding. Select option 3 because it pertains to circulation.*

Content Area: Adult Health; *Category of Health Alteration:* Pharmacological and Parenteral Therapies; *Integrated Processes:* Nursing Process Assessment; *Client Need:* Physiological Integrity/ Pharmacological and Parenteral Therapies/Adverse Effects/Contradictions and Side Effects; *Cognitive Level:* Analysis

Reference: Lehne, R. (2007). *Pharmacology for Nursing Care* (6th ed., p. 177). St. Louis, MO: Elsevier/Saunders.

1040. A client, diagnosed with chronic, stable angina, telephones a clinic nurse. The client reports a headache lasting for several days after taking one dose of isosorbide mononitrate (Imdur®). The client also reports symptoms of orthostatic hypotension and palpitations. Which is the nurse's best action?

1. Recommend that the client make an appointment with the health-care provider
2. Have the client retime the dose to take it later in the day when the client is more active
3. Instruct the client to take two acetaminophen 325-mg tablets when taking the Imdur® dose
4. Teach the client that the headaches will subside over time with continued medication use

ANSWER: 1

Isosorbide mononitrate is a long-acting coronary vasodilator. Severe headaches, orthostatic hypotension, and palpitations may be a sign of isosorbide mononitrate toxicity, thus the client should be evaluated by a health-care provider. Other signs include syncope, dizziness, blurred vision, and light-headedness. Isosorbide mononitrate should be taken in the morning to improve blood flow to the heart and prevent angina attacks that can occur due to the increased oxygen demand from activity. A headache (but not a severe headache) can be treated with or prevented by analgesics taken either before or at the same time as the isosorbide mononitrate. Although the headaches will subside over time, the client is experiencing symptoms of isosorbide mononitrate toxicity.

▶ ***Test-taking Tip:*** *The key words are the client's symptoms of "severe headache, orthostatic hypotension, and palpitations" and "best action." Think about the toxic effects of isosorbide mononitrate. Select option 1 because this is the only option that evaluates the cause of the client's symptoms. Options 3 and 4 are similar. When two options are similar in a multiple choice question, either one or both of the options are incorrect.*

Content Area: Adult Health; *Category of Health Alteration:* Pharmacological and Parenteral Therapies; *Integrated Processes:* Nursing Process Implementation; *Client Need:* Physiological Integrity/Pharmacological and Parenteral Therapies/Adverse Effects/Contradictions and Side Effects; *Cognitive Level:* Application

Reference: Wilson, B., Shannon, M., Shields, K., & Stang, C. (2008). *Prentice Hall Nurse's Drug Guide 2008* (pp. 831–832). Upper Saddle River, NJ: Pearson Education.

1041. A client is taking metalazone (Zaroxolyn®) and diltiazem (Cardizem®) for treatment of hypertension. A home health nurse is reviewing the medications with the client. Which client statement indicates that the client needs teaching about these medications?

1. "I make sure that I eat foods high in potassium every day."
2. "Because metalazone makes me urinate more, I take my last dose at suppertime."
3. "I take my medications with a healthy breakfast of eggs, toast, grapefruit juice, and milk."
4. "Because ibuprofen (Motrin®) seems to affect my urine output, I prefer to take acetaminophen (Tylenol®) for pain."

ANSWER: 3

Grapefruit juice should be avoided because it inhibits the metabolism of diltiazem and can cause toxicity. Thiazide diuretics can result in hypokalemia. Consuming foods daily that are high in potassium is recommended. Diuretics should be avoided at bedtime to avoid nocturia and the loss of sleep. NSAIDs such as ibuprofen can decrease the diuretic and antihypertensive effects of thiazide diuretics.

▸ ***Test-taking Tip:*** *The key words are "needs teaching." Select the option that is a false statement.*

Content Area: Adult Health; *Category of Health Alteration:* Pharmacological and Parenteral Therapies; *Integrated Processes:* Nursing Process Evaluation; *Client Need:* Physiological Integrity/Pharmacological and Parenteral Therapies/Pharmacological Interactions; *Cognitive Level:* Application

References: Lehne, R. (2007). *Pharmacology for Nursing Care* (6th ed., p. 62). St. Louis, MO: Elsevier/Saunders; Lewis, S., Heitkemper, M., Dirksen, S., O'Brien, P., & Bucher, L. (2007). *Medical-Surgical Nursing: Assessment and Management of Clinical Problems* (7th ed., pp. 773–776). St. Louis, MO: Mosby.

1042. A health-care provider (HCP) adds a second medication for blood pressure control for a client whose blood pressure has not been well-controlled with one antihypertensive medication. If the HCP orders the following medication combinations, which combination should the nurse question?

1. Atenolol (Tenormin®) and metoprolol (Lopressor®)
2. Metolazone (Zaroxolyn®) and valsartan (Diovan®)
3. Captopril (Capoten®) and furosemide (Lasix®)
4. Bumetanide (Bumex®) and diltiazem (Cardizem®)

ANSWER: 1

When two medications are used to treat hypertension, each medication should be from different drug classifications. Atenolol and metroprolol are both beta-adrenergic blockers and would essentially have the same mechanism of action. Metolazone is a thiazide-like diuretic, and valsartan is an angiotensin II receptor blocker (ARB). Captopril is an angiotensin-converting enzyme (ACE) inhibitor, and furosemide is a loop diuretic. Bumetanide is a loop diuretic, and diltiazem is a calcium channel blocker.

▸ ***Test-taking Tip:*** *Recall that beta blockers end in "lol." Use this as a cue to identify the two medications that are within the same drug classification and would be inappropriately prescribed.*

Content Area: Adult Health; *Category of Health Alteration:* Pharmacological and Parenteral Therapies; *Integrated Processes:* Nursing Process Planning; *Client Need:* Physiological Integrity/Pharmacological and Parenteral Therapies/Pharmacological Interactions; *Cognitive Level:* Application

Reference: Lehne, R. (2007). *Pharmacology for Nursing Care* (6th ed., p. 501). St. Louis, MO: Elsevier/Saunders.

1043. A nurse is assessing a client who is taking atorvastatin (Lipitor®). For which manifestations should the nurse specifically assess?

1. Constipation and hemorrhoids
2. Muscle pain and weakness
3. Fatigue and dysrhythmias
4. Flushing and postural hypotension

ANSWER: 2

Atorvastatin is a 3-hydroxy-3-methylglutaryl coenzyme A (HMG-CoA) reductase inhibitor (statin) used to lower lipid levels. Statins can cause muscle tissue injury manifested by muscle ache or weakness. Muscle injury can progress to myositis (muscle inflammation) or rhabdomyolysis (muscle disintegration). Bile acid sequestrants may cause constipation and hemorrhoids because they are not absorbed from the small intestine. Diarrhea, not constipation, is a side effect of statin medications. Side effects of niacin, a lipid-lowering agent, include flushing, dysrhythmias, and postural hypotension.

▸ ***Test-taking Tip:*** *The key words are "specifically assess." The nurse should be monitoring for side effects. Select the option that includes the side effect for the HMG-CoA reductase inhibitors (statins).*

Content Area: Adult Health; *Category of Health Alteration:* Pharmacological and Parenteral Therapies; *Integrated Processes:* Nursing Process Assessment; *Client Need:* Physiological Integrity/Pharmacological and Parenteral Therapies/Adverse Effects/Contradictions and Side Effects; *Cognitive Level:* Application

References: Lehne, R. (2007). *Pharmacology for Nursing Care* (6th ed., pp. 557–565). St. Louis, MO: Elsevier/Saunders; Wilson, B., Shannon, M., Shields, K., & Stang, C. (2008). *Prentice Hall Nurse's Drug Guide 2008* (pp. 1067–1069). Upper Saddle River, NJ: Pearson Education.

1044. A nurse is reviewing the chart of a client with a diagnosis of stage II heart failure (see abbreviated chart). The data should suggest to the nurse that:

Admitting History & Physical	Serum Laboratory Data	Diagnostic Data Results	Medications
• Experiencing dyspnea on exertion • Lung sounds: crackles in bilateral bases • Reports seeing yellow halo when visualizing objects	• BNP: 886 ng/L* • aPTT: 55 sec** • K^+: 2.9 mEq/L	• 12-lead ECG results: Atrial fibrillation with frequent PVCs. • Chest x-ray: Pulmonary infiltrated bilateral bases. Cardiomegaly	• Buffered aspirin 325 mg oral daily • Digoxin (Lanoxin®) 0.25 mg oral daily • Furosemide (Lasix®) 40 mg oral daily • Atenolol (Tenormin®) 25 mg oral • Heparin intravenous infusion per protocol

*B-natriuretic peptide (BNP) normal value 100 ng/L
**Activated partial thromboplastin time (aPTT) normal range 24 to 33 seconds

1. medications should be administered as ordered.
2. the client may be experiencing digoxin toxicity.
3. hyperkalemia likely caused the client's cardiac dysrhythmias.
4. the client's visual disturbance likely resulted from the atrial fibrillation rhythm or effects of the anticoagulants.

ANSWER: 2

Signs of digoxin toxicity include yellow vision and dysrhythmias. The furosemide diuretic increases urinary excretion of potassium and can cause hypokalemia. A low serum potassium level can contribute to both cardiac dysrhythmias and digoxin toxicity. The digoxin should be held until a serum digoxin level is determined. A serum potassium level of 2.9 mEq/L indicates hypokalemia, not hyperkalemia. The yellow vision is a characteristic sign of digoxin toxicity and not a sign of cerebral damage from an infarct or bleeding.

Test-taking Tip: *Carefully read the information in the client's chart and then read each of the options. Use the key words in the options to analyze the information provided in the client's chart, which are, respectively, "medications...appropriate," "digoxin toxicity," "hyperkalemia," and "visual disturbances." Then use the process of elimination.*

Content Area: Adult Health; *Category of Health Alteration:* Pharmacological and Parenteral Therapies; *Integrated Processes:* Nursing Process Analysis; *Client Need:* Physiological Integrity/ Pharmacological and Parenteral Therapies/Adverse Effects/Contradictions and Side Effects; *Cognitive Level:* Application

References: Lehne, R. (2007). *Pharmacology for Nursing Care* (6th ed., pp. 515–519). St. Louis, MO: Elsevier/Saunders; Monahan, F., Sands, J., Neighbors, M., Marek, J., & Green, C. (2007). *Phipps' Medical-Surgical Nursing: Health and Illness Perspectives* (8th ed., pp. 816–821). St. Louis, MO: Mosby/Elsevier.

1045. EBP Which points should the nurse plan to include when teaching a client receiving a thiazide diuretic? SELECT ALL THAT APPLY.

1. Take the radial pulse before setting up the medication.
2. Include fruits such as melons and bananas in the diet.
3. Report side effects such as muscle cramps, nausea, or a skin rash.
4. Self-administer the last dose at bedtime when fluid tends to be at the highest levels.
5. Keep appointments for laboratory monitoring, including serum electrolytes, glucose, creatinine, blood urea nitrogen (BUN), and uric acid levels.
6. Minimize intake of high-fat foods because thiazide diuretics can increase serum cholesterol, low-density lipoprotein (LDL), and triglyceride levels.

ANSWER: 2, 3, 5, 6

Thiazide diuretics can cause hypokalemia. Encouraging potassium-rich foods can help maintain potassium levels. Muscle cramps are a sign of possible medication side effects of hypokalemia and hypocalcemia. Nausea and rash are also medication side effects. Laboratory results to be monitored during thiazide diuretic therapy include serum electrolytes, glucose, creatinine, BUN, and uric acid levels because thiazide diuretics are excreted mainly unchanged by the kidneys and can increase glucose levels. Reminders regarding keeping appointments promote medication adherence. Thiazide diuretics can increase serum cholesterol, LDL, and triglyceride levels, so teaching the client to minimize high-fat foods will help maintain cholesterol levels. It is unnecessary for a client to monitor the pulse before taking thiazide diuretics. A diuretic taken at bedtime can cause nocturia and loss of sleep. The usual timing of the last daily dose of a diuretic is at suppertime.

▸ ***Test-taking Tip:*** *Recall that thiazide diuretics lower blood pressure through diuresis, which can result in hypokalemia. Focus on the common thiazide diuretic, hydrochlorothiazide, and its effects and side effects when reading each of the options.*

Content Area: Adult Health; *Category of Health Alteration:* Pharmacological and Parenteral Therapies; *Integrated Processes:* Teaching and Learning; *Client Need:* Physiological Integrity/ Pharmacological and Parenteral Therapies/Medication Administration; *Cognitive Level:* Application

Reference: Lehne, R. (2007). *Pharmacology for Nursing Care* (6th ed., pp. 441–442). St. Louis, MO: Elsevier/Saunders.

EBP Reference: Haynes, R., Ackloo, E., Sahota, N., McDonald, H., & Yao X. (2007). Interventions for enhancing medication adherence. *Cochrane Database of Systematic Reviews 2007*, Issue 1, Art. No. CD000011. DOI: 10.1002/14651858.CD000011.pub3. Available at: www.cochrane.org/reviews/en/ab000011.html

1046. EBP A home health nurse visiting an older adult client for the first time is reviewing the client's medication list prepared by the client's daughter (see exhibit). Which finding in the client's medication list should be of most concern to the nurse and should be discussed first with the client?

Client's Medication List

Aspart insulin 1 unit per 1 carbohydrate choice (CHO) taken at meals	Captopril (Capoten®) 25 mg three times daily
Aspirin 1 tab. every AM	Glyberide (Diabeta®) 1 at breakfast
Atenolol (Tenormin®) 25 mg oral at breakfast	Hydrochlorothiazide 25 mg twice daily
Hydrochlorothiazide + captopril (Capozide®) 1 daily	Simvastatin (Zocor®) 10 mg daily in the evening

1. Some doses of medication are missing.
2. Some routes of medication are missing.
3. Some medications are duplicated.
4. Some medications have drug–drug interactions.

ANSWER: 3

Hydrochlorothiazide + captopril (Capozide®) is a combination product of hydrochlorothiazide and captopril. The nurse should first determine if the client is taking the combination product along with the individual products due to the potential for overdosing. Duplication of medications needs to be identified before missing dosages, missing routes, or drug–drug interactions are determined. The client may be clear regarding the dose and the route, but may not realize that two medications were replaced with one combination product.

▸ ***Test-taking Tip:*** *The key word is "first." The greatest safety risk for the client is medication overdosing.*

Content Area: Adult Health; *Category of Health Alteration:* Pharmacological and Parenteral Therapies; *Integrated Processes:* Nursing Process Evaluation; *Client Need:* Physiological Integrity/ Pharmacological and Parenteral Therapies/Pharmacological Interactions; *Cognitive Level:* Application

Reference: Lehne, R. (2007). *Pharmacology for Nursing Care* (6th ed., p. 496). St. Louis, MO: Elsevier/Saunders.

EBP Reference: Zwicker, D., & Fulmer, T. (2008). Reducing adverse drug events. In: E. Capezuti, D. Zwicker, M. Mezey, & T. Fulmer (eds.). *Evidence-Based Geriatric Nursing Protocols for Best Practice* (3rd ed., pp. 257–308). New York: Springer Publishing. Available at: www.guideline.gov/summary/summary.aspx?doc_id=12258&nbr=006342&string=Medication+AND+older+AND+adults.

1047. A client, following a total hip replacement, asks a nurse why she is receiving enoxaparin (Lovenox®) for prevention of deep vein thrombosis (DVT) when, with her last hip surgery, she received heparin subcutaneously. What is the nurse's best response?

1. "Enoxaparin is less expensive and easier to administer than the heparin."
2. "There is less risk of bleeding with enoxaparin, and it doesn't affect your laboratory results."
3. "Enoxaparin is a low-molecular-weight heparin that lasts twice as long as regular heparin."
4. "Enoxaparin can be administered orally whereas heparin is only administered by injection."

ANSWER: 3

Because enoxaparin is more specific in inhibiting active factor X, the response is more stable and the effect is two to four times longer than that of heparin. The cost of enoxaparin is more than twice the cost of the equivalent dose of heparin per injection. Both enoxaparin and heparin are administered by subcutaneous injection, and both are available in prefilled syringes for injection. Both enoxaparin and heparin increase activated partial thromboplastin time (aPTT). Enoxaparin is only administered subcutaneously.

▶ ***Test-taking Tip:*** *Focus on the issue: the difference between enoxaparin and heparin. Note that options 1, 2, and 4 are similar, addressing the supposed benefits of enoxaparin, whereas option 3 is different, describing the action of enoxaparin. The option that is different is usually the answer.*

Content Area: Adult Health; *Category of Health Alteration:* Pharmacological and Parenteral Therapies; *Integrated Processes:* Teaching and Learning; *Client Need:* Physiological Integrity/ Pharmacological and Parenteral Therapies/Expected Actions or Outcomes; *Cognitive Level:* Application

References: Adams, M., Holland, L., & Bostwick, P. (2008). *Pharmacology for Nurses: A Pathophysiologic Approach* (pp. 381–384). Upper Saddle River, NJ: Pearson Education; Deglin, J., & Vallerand, A. (2009). *Davis's Drug Guide for Nurses* (11th ed., pp. 616–623). Philadelphia: F. A. Davis.

1048. A client, diagnosed with chronic renal failure (CRF), is receiving epoetin alfa (Epogen®). Which finding should indicate to a nurse that the action of the medication has been effective?

1. Urine output increased to 30 mL per hour.
2. Hemoglobin is 12 g/dL, and hematocrit is 42%.
3. Blood pressure is 110/70, and heart rate is 68 bpm.
4. Client reports increased energy level and less fatigue.

ANSWER: 2

Epoetin alfa stimulates erythropoiesis or the production of red blood cells (RBCs). It is used in treating anemias associated with decreased RBC production, such as renal failure. Hemoglobin and hematocrit are used to evaluate the medication's effectiveness. The target hemoglobin for a client with CRF is 12 g/dL. Epoetin alfa does not have an effect on urine output or blood pressure. Clients may report increased energy and less fatigue because of the increased hemoglobin levels, but these findings are not used to evaluate the medication's action.

▶ ***Test-taking Tip:*** *Focus on the action of the medication in selecting an option. Recall that epoetin alfa affects the production of RBCs.*

Content Area: Adult Health; *Category of Health Alteration:* Pharmacological and Parenteral Therapies; *Integrated Processes:* Nursing Process Evaluation; *Client Need:* Physiological Integrity/ Pharmacological and Parenteral Therapies/Expected Actions or Outcomes; *Cognitive Level:* Application

References: Adams, M., Holland, L., & Bostwick, P. (2008). *Pharmacology for Nurses: A Pathophysiologic Approach* (p. 396). Upper Saddle River, NJ: Pearson Education; Lehne, R. (2007). *Pharmacology for Nursing Care* (6th ed., pp. 637–639). St. Louis, MO: Elsevier/Saunders.

1049. A client with a diagnosis of tonsillar cancer is receiving filgrastim (Neupogen®). Prior to administering the next dose of the medication the nurse notes that the client's absolute neutrophil count is 11,000/mm^3. What is the nurse's best action?

1. Administer the medication as ordered.
2. Place the client on neutropenic precautions.
3. Notify the health-care provider because treatment will likely be discontinued.
4. Apply gown, gloves, and a mask when entering the room to administer the medication.

ANSWER: 3

Filgrastim is a granulocyte colony-stimulating factor for treatment of neutropenia. Treatment is usually discontinued when the absolute neutrophil count reaches 10,000/mm^3. Unnecessary doses can cause leukocytosis (white blood cells above 100,000/mm^3), an adverse effect of the medication. A normal neutrophil count is greater than 2,000/mm^3. Neutropenic precautions and protective wear are unnecessary because the filgrastim (Neupogen®) has been effective in increasing the neutrophil count. A high-efficiency particulate air (HEPA) mask rather than a regular mask should be worn if the client is severely neutropenic (less than 100/mm^3).

▶ ***Test-taking Tip:*** *Apply knowledge of the action of filgrastim to answer this question. Treatment for neutropenia in the stem is a cue to the correct answer. Recall that a normal neutrophil count is greater than 2,000/mm^3.*

Content Area: Adult Health; *Category of Health Alteration:* Pharmacological and Parenteral Therapies; *Integrated Processes:* Nursing Process Implementation; *Client Need:* Physiological Integrity/Pharmacological and Parenteral Therapies/Medication Administration; *Cognitive Level:* Application

Reference: Lehne, R. (2007). *Pharmacology for Nursing Care* (6th ed., pp. 643–644). St. Louis, MO: Elsevier/Saunders.

1050. For which client should a nurse question a physician's order to administer 5% albumin?

1. A client of the Catholic faith who has refractory edema
2. An African American client experiencing hypovolemic shock
3. A client of the Jehovah's Witnesses faith who has cerebral edema
4. An Asian client experiencing adult respiratory distress syndrome (ARDS)

ANSWER: 3

Albumin is a blood derivative obtained by fractionating pooled venous and placental human plasma. Persons of the Jehovah's Witnesses faith usually do not accept blood or blood products. Albumin is used in the treatment of refractory edema, hypovolemic shock, cerebral edema, and ARDS. Persons of the Catholic faith or African American and Asian ethnic groups usually accept blood and blood products.

Test-taking Tip: *Recall that albumin is a blood derivative. Think about the religious group who does not accept blood or blood products.*

Content Area: Adult Health; *Category of Health Alteration:* Pharmacological and Parenteral Therapies; *Integrated Processes:* Nursing Process Analysis; *Client Need:* Physiological Integrity/Pharmacological and Parenteral Therapies/Blood and Blood Products; *Cognitive Level:* Analysis

References: Berman, A., Snyder, S., Kozier, B., & Erb, G. (2008). *Kozier & Erb's Fundamentals of Nursing: Concepts, Process, and Practice* (8th ed., p. 1052). Upper Saddle River, NJ: Pearson Education; Wilson, B., Shannon, M., Shields, K., & Stang, C. (2008). *Prentice Hall Nurse's Drug Guide 2008* (pp. 1097–1098). Upper Saddle River, NJ: Pearson Education.

1051. Which assessment finding should a nurse expect following administration of phenylephrine (Neosynephrine®) eye drops to perform an ophthalmoscopic eye examination?

1. Tremor
2. Hypotension
3. Pupil miosis
4. Pupil mydriasis

ANSWER: 4

Phenylephrine, an adrenergic agonist, produces pupil dilation (mydriasis) by activating alpha$_1$-adrenergic receptors on the dilator muscles of the iris. Tremors are a side effect if absorbed systemically. Because phenylephrine absorbed systemically is a vasoconstrictor, hypertension can occur. Miosis is pupil constriction, not an effect of phenylephrine.

Test-taking Tip: *If unsure of the action of phenylephrine, use the key words "ophthalmoscopic eye examination" to select the best option. A memory aid to remember the difference between miosis and mydriasis is using the "o" in mi**o**sis to refer to c**o**nstriction and the "d" in my**d**riasis to refer to **d**ilation.*

Content Area: Adult Health; *Category of Health Alteration:* Pharmacological and Parenteral Therapies; *Integrated Processes:* Nursing Process Assessment; *Client Need:* Physiological Integrity/Pharmacological and Parenteral Therapies/Expected Actions or Outcomes; *Cognitive Level:* Application

Reference: Lehne, R. (2007). *Pharmacology for Nursing Care* (6th ed., p. 103). St. Louis, MO: Elsevier/Saunders.

1052. A concerned client using latanoprost (Xalatan®) eye drops for treatment of glaucoma calls a clinic after noting a brown pigmentation of the iris. Which nursing action is most appropriate?

1. Inform the client that the brown pigmentation is a side effect of latanoprost and that he/she should be seen as soon as possible.
2. Schedule an appointment for the client to see an internist for liver function studies.
3. Tell the client that the brown pigmentation is from the latanoprost, but will eventually regress.
4. Recommend that the client wear sunglasses when outdoors to decrease iris pigmentation.

ANSWER: 1

A side effect of latanoprost, a prostaglandin, includes a heightened brown pigmentation of the iris, which stops progressing when latanoprost is discontinued. Jaundice sclera, and not brown iris pigmentation, would suggest the need to evaluate liver function. The brown iris pigmentation from the latanoprost does not usually regress. Wearing sunglasses will have no effect on the iris pigmentation.

Test-taking Tip: *Recall that brown pigmentation of the iris is a side effect of latanoprost.*

Content Area: Adult Health; *Category of Health Alteration:* Pharmacological and Parenteral Therapies; *Integrated Processes:* Nursing Process Implementation; *Client Need:* Physiological Integrity/Pharmacological and Parenteral Therapies/Adverse Effects/Contradictions and Side Effects; *Cognitive Level:* Application

Reference: Lehne, R. (2007). *Pharmacology for Nursing Care* (6th ed., p. 1194). St. Louis, MO: Elsevier/Saunders.

1053. Tazarotene (Tzorac®) topical medication is prescribed for a client with psoriasis vulgaris. Place an X on the illustration that shows the area about which a nurse should document applying a thin film of the medication.

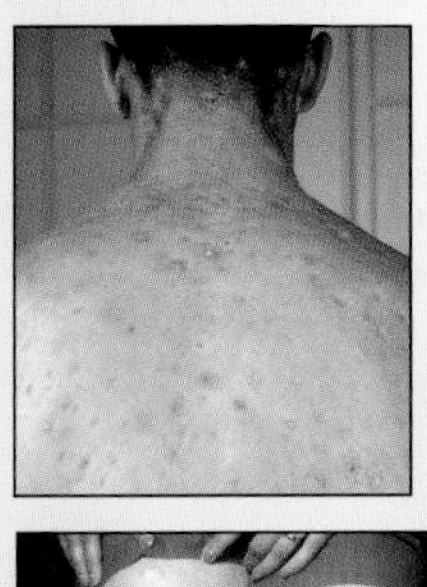
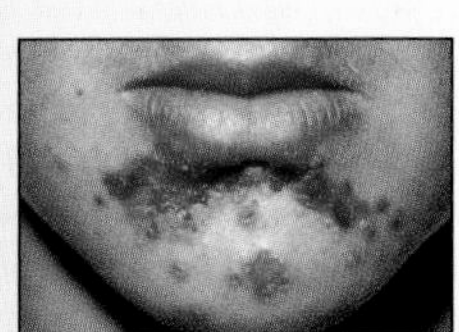
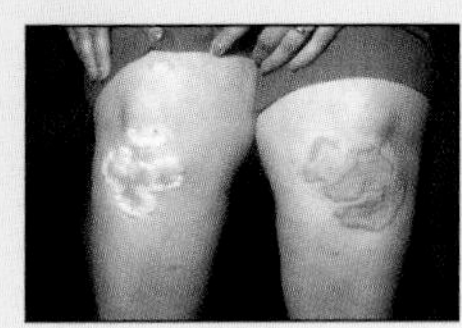
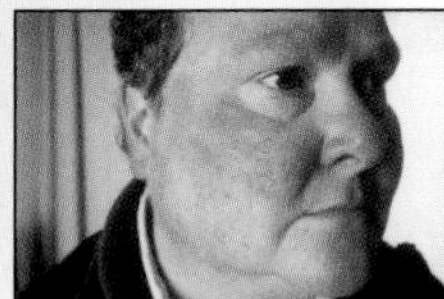

ANSWER:

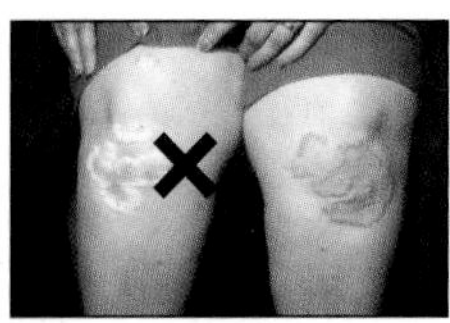

Psoriasis, a noninfectious inflammatory disorder, is characterized by red, raised patches of skin covered with flaky, thick, slivery scales. Psoriasis vulgaris usually occurs on extensor surfaces of the knees, elbows, and scalp.

Test-taking Tip: *Recall that psoriasis is characterized by flaky, thick, slivery scales.*

Content Area: Adult Health; *Category of Health Alteration:* Pharmacological and Parenteral Therapies; *Integrated Processes:* Communication and Documentation; *Client Need:* Physiological Integrity/Pharmacological and Parenteral Therapies/Medication Administration; *Cognitive Level:* Application

References: Adams, M., Holland, L., & Bostwick, P. (2008). *Pharmacology for Nurses: A Pathophysiological Approach* (pp. 766–767). Upper Saddle River, NJ: Pearson Education; Dillon, P. (2007). *Nursing Health Assessment: A Critical Thinking, Case Studies Approach* (2nd ed., pp. 257, 260–261). Philadelphia: F. A. Davis.

1054. A nurse receives a physician's order to start total parenteral nutrition (TPN) for a client who has a peripherally inserted central catheter (PICC). Into which type of catheter illustrated should the nurse plan to administer the TPN?

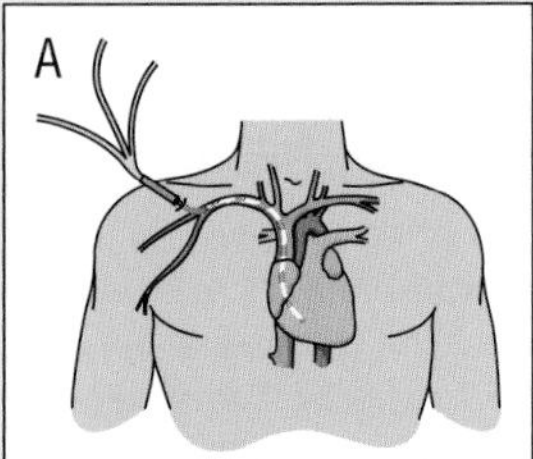

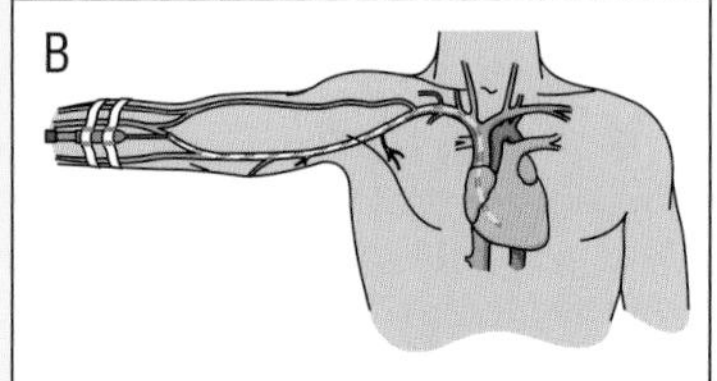

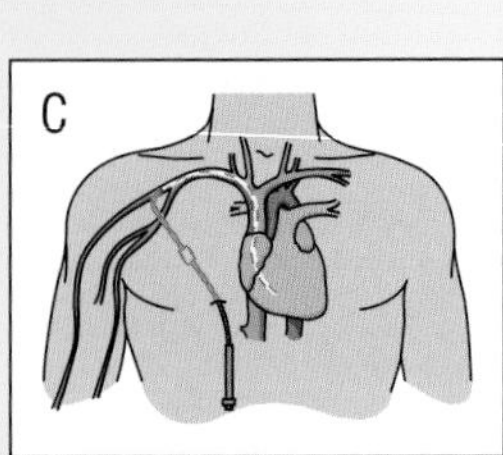

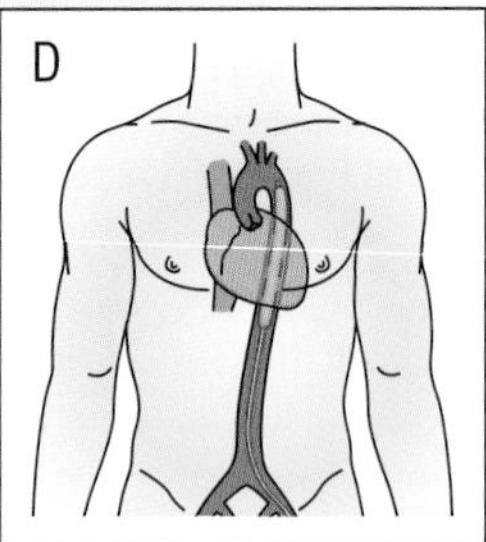

1. A
2. B
3. C
4. D

ANSWER: 2

Illustration B is a PICC, which is inserted into the arm and terminates in the central circulation. A PICC is used when medications or solutions are too caustic to be peripherally administered or when therapy lasts more then 2 weeks. Illustration A is a central line that is percutaneously inserted into the jugular or subclavian vein and terminates in the central circulation. These are intended for short-term venous access. Illustration C is a tunneled catheter inserted into the upper chest wall, threaded through the cephalic vein, and terminates in the central circulation. Illustration D is an intra-aortic balloon pump catheter that is inserted into the femoral artery and positioned in the descending aortic arch. The balloon on the end inflates during diastole. It is not used for medication or fluid administration.

Test-taking Tip: *Focus on the illustrations. Note that only options 2 and 4 are peripherally inserted catheters. Then note that only option 2 is inserted into a vein, whereas the catheter in option 4 is inserted into an artery.*

Content Area: Adult Health; *Category of Health Alteration:* Pharmacological and Parenteral Therapies; *Integrated Processes:* Nursing Process Planning; *Client Need:* Physiological Integrity/Pharmacological and Parenteral Therapies/Central Venous Access Devices; *Cognitive Level:* Application

Reference: Smeltzer, S., Bare, B., Hinkle, J., & Cheever, K. (2008). *Brunner & Suddarth's Textbook of Medical-Surgical Nursing* (11th ed., pp. 967, 1194–1199). Philadelphia: Lippincott Williams & Wilkins.

1055. A nurse has just completed teaching for a client who will be receiving total parenteral nutrition at home. Which client statement indicates that further teaching is needed?

1. "My refrigerator is large enough to accommodate several bags of the parenteral solution."
2. "I will keep my portable phone with me for emergency purposes."
3. "Because I will have an infusion pump, I plan on using the main floor bedroom."
4. "It will be easiest to remove my intravenous catheter cap and then attach the tubing if I am sitting at the table."

ANSWER: 4

The central catheter lumen is capped with a needleless port. The IV infusion tubing is connected to the insertion site cap and not removed during infusion therapy. Caps are changed every 3 to 7 days during dressing changes, with the client in a flat position. An air embolus can occur if the cap is removed while the client is in a sitting position. Several total nutrient solution bags are kept on hand and require refrigeration. A home telephone is necessary for contacting home health personnel, arranging for supply deliveries, and for emergency use. The TPN is delivered through an infusion pump, which can limit the client's mobility.

▶ *Test-taking Tip: The key words are "further teaching is needed." This is a false-response item. Select the client's statement that is incorrect.*

Content Area: Adult Health; *Category of Health Alteration:* Pharmacological and Parenteral Therapies; *Integrated Processes:* Nursing Process Evaluation; *Client Need:* Physiological Integrity/Pharmacological and Parenteral Therapies/Central Venous Access Devices; *Cognitive Level:* Application

Reference: Smeltzer, S., Bare, B., Hinkle, J., & Cheever, K. (2008). *Brunner & Suddarth's Textbook of Medical-Surgical Nursing* (11th ed., pp. 1194–1199). Philadelphia: Lippincott Williams & Wilkins.

1056. A physician orders 1,200 milliliters (mL) of total parenteral nutrition (TPN) solution to be administered over 24 hours for a homebound client. A home health nurse should instruct the client to set the infusion pump to deliver TPN at _______ mL per hour.

ANSWER: 50

Use the formula:

$$\frac{\text{Total mL ordered}}{\text{Total hours ordered}} = \text{mL/hr}$$

$$\frac{1{,}200}{24} = 50 \text{ mL/hr}$$

▶ *Test-taking Tip: Use the formula for calculating intravenous (IV) flow rates with electronic regulators. Verify the answer with a calculator.*

Content Area: Adult Health; *Category of Health Alteration:* Pharmacological and Parenteral Therapies; *Integrated Processes:* Nursing Process Implementation; *Client Need:* Physiological Integrity/Pharmacological and Parenteral Therapies/Parenteral/Intravenous Therapies; *Cognitive Level:* Application

Reference: Pickar, G. (2007). *Dosage Calculations: A Ratio-Proportion Approach* (2nd ed., p. 344). Clifton Park, NY: Thomson Delmar Learning.

1057. A nurse who is initiating an intravenous infusion of lactated Ringer's (LR) for a client in shock recognizes that the purpose of LR for the client is to:

1. increase fluid volume and urinary output.
2. draw water from the cells into the blood vessels.
3. provide dextrose and nutrients to prevent cellular death.
4. replace electrolytes of sodium, potassium, calcium, and magnesium for cardiac stabilization.

ANSWER: 1

LR is an isotonic crystalloid solution containing multiple electrolytes in approximately the same concentration as plasma. It enters the cells from the blood, replacing fluids and increasing urinary output. A hypertonic solution draws fluid from the cells into the vascular compartment. LR alone does not contain dextrose. Formulations with dextrose are available. Magnesium is not a component of LR.

▶ *Test-taking Tip: Apply knowledge of the components of LR and use the process of elimination. Eliminate options 3 and 4 because neither dextrose nor magnesium is a component of LR.*

Content Area: Adult Health; *Category of Health Alteration:* Pharmacological and Parenteral Therapies; *Integrated Processes:* Nursing Process Evaluation; *Client Need:* Physiological Integrity/Pharmacological and Parenteral Therapies/Parenteral/Intravenous Therapies; *Cognitive Level:* Application

References: Adams, M., Holland, L., & Bostwick, P. (2008). *Pharmacology for Nurses: A Pathophysiologic Approach* (pp. 411–413, 421, 832). Upper Saddle River, NJ: Pearson Education; Smeltzer, S., Bare, B., Hinkle, J., & Cheever, K. (2008). *Brunner & Suddarth's Textbook of Medical-Surgical Nursing* (11th ed., p. 311). Philadelphia: Lippincott Williams & Wilkins.

1058. EBP A client is receiving multiple medications for treatment of Parkinson's disease. Which signs and symptoms should a nurse recognize as adverse effects of carbidopa-levodopa (Sinemet®)?

1. Dystonia and akinesia
2. Bradykinesia and agitation
3. Muscle rigidity and cardiac dysrhythmias
4. Orthostatic hypotension and dry mouth

ANSWER: 4

Orthostatic hypotension and dry mouth are common adverse effects to carbidopa-levodopa and can be minimized by slow position changes and sucking on sugarless candy or chewing gum. While dystonia, agitation, and cardiac dysrhythmias are adverse effects, akinesia, bradykinesia, and muscle rigidity are signs and symptoms of Parkinson's disease.

Test-taking Tip: *Read each option carefully. Eliminate options that include a sign or symptom of Parkinson's disease.*

Content Area: Adult Health; *Category of Health Alteration:* Pharmacological and Parenteral Therapies; *Integrated Processes:* Nursing Process Evaluation; *Client Need:* Physiological Integrity/ Pharmacological and Parenteral Therapies/Adverse Effects/ Contraindications; *Cognitive Level:* Application

Reference: Aschenbrenner, D., & Venable, S. (2009). *Drug Therapy in Nursing* (3rd ed., pp. 247–248). Philadelphia: Lippincott Williams & Wilkins.

EBP Reference: Schoffer, K., Henderson, R., O'Maley, K., & O'Sullivan, J. (2007). Nonpharmacological treatment, fludrocortisone, and domperidone for orthostatic hypotension in Parkinson's disease. *Movement Disorders: Official Journal of the Movement Disorder Society,* 22(11), 1543–1549.

1059. A client calls a clinic 2 weeks after beginning to use oral carbidopa-levodopa (Parcopa®), stating that the medication has been ineffective in controlling the symptoms of Parkinson's disease. What nursing action is most appropriate?

1. Review the correct procedure for taking the medication.
2. Contact the physician to change the dose of the medication.
3. Remind the client that it may take 1 to 2 months to note any effects of the medication.
4. Ensure that the client is eating a diet high in protein and vitamin B_6 (pyridoxine).

ANSWER: 3

With oral administration of carbidopa-levodopa, it usually takes 1 to 2 months before noting an effect, although in some cases it may require up to 6 months. Reviewing the procedure, including foods to avoid, may be important, but option 3 is most important because effects usually are not seen within 2 weeks. A high-protein diet can slow or prevent absorption of carbidopa-levodopa. Vitamin B_6 (pyridoxine) increases the action of decarboxylases that destroys levodopa in the body's periphery, reducing the effects of carbidopa-levodopa. Foods high in pyridoxine should be avoided.

Test-taking Tip: *Apply knowledge of the delayed onset of the medication to select the correct option and eliminate other options.*

Content Area: Adult Health; *Category of Health Alteration:* Pharmacological and Parenteral Therapies; *Integrated Processes:* Nursing Process Implementation; *Client Need:* Physiological Integrity/ Pharmacological and Parenteral Therapies/Expected Effects/Outcomes; *Cognitive Level:* Analysis

Reference: Aschenbrenner, D., & Venable, S. (2009). *Drug Therapy in Nursing* (3rd ed., pp. 246–250). Philadelphia: Lippincott Williams & Wilkins.

1060. A nurse teaches a client with relapsing-remitting multiple sclerosis about glatiramer (Copaxone®). Which information addressed by the client indicates that the nurse's teaching has been effective? SELECT ALL THAT APPLY.

1. Keep the medication vial refrigerated until it is to be used.
2. Glatiramer is administered by injection into the subcutaneous tissue.
3. Injection sites should be rotated so that no one spot is used more than once a week.
4. The thigh and abdomen are the appropriate subcutaneous injection sites.
5. Used syringes can be washed, air dried, and reused until the needle becomes dull.
6. Adverse effects to report immediately include chest pain and unusual muscle weakness.

ANSWER: 1, 2, 3, 6

Glatiramer is used to delay the progression of multiple sclerosis. To maximize the therapeutic effects of glatiramer, the medication should be refrigerated and reconstituted correctly. Glatiramer is only administered subcutaneously; accidental intravenous administration must be avoided. Injection sites are rotated to prevent skin breakdown or lumps at the injection sites. The most serious adverse effects include chest pain or tightness, breathing difficulties, hives or severe rash, or unusual muscle weakness. Appropriate subcutaneous injection sites for glatiramer include the thigh, back of the hip, abdomen, and upper arm. Used syringes should be placed in a puncture-resistant container for proper disposal. Syringes and needles should not be reused.

Test-taking Tip: *Focus on the fact that glatiramer is only administered subcutaneously. Eliminate options that increase the risk for tissue trauma, infection, or injury.*

Content Area: Adult Health; *Category of Health Alteration:* Pharmacological and Parenteral Therapies; *Integrated Processes:* Teaching and Learning; *Client Need:* Health Promotion and Maintenance/ Principles of Teaching and Learning; *Cognitive Level:* Analysis

Reference: Aschenbrenner, D., & Venable, S. (2009). *Drug Therapy in Nursing* (3rd ed., pp. 258–259). Philadelphia: Lippincott Williams & Wilkins.

1061. A nurse on a medical unit receives multiple medication orders for adult clients with seizure disorders. Which order should the nurse clarify with a physician?

1. Administer fosphenytoin (Cerebyx®) 150 mg orally three times daily.
2. Obtain phenytoin level prior to administering additional doses of anticonvulsant medications.
3. Administer intravenous phenytoin (Dilantin®) 1 g in 100 mL 0.9% NaCl via intravenous piggyback (IVPB).
4. Document effectiveness of carbamazepine (Tegretol®) for the client's seizure control and restless leg syndrome.

ANSWER: 1

Because fosphenytoin is only administered intravenously, the order should be clarified with the physician. The phenytoin level should be checked periodically to determine therapeutic levels. Administering 1 g of phenytoin is within a therapeutic dosing range. Phenytoin is compatible with NaCl. It is incompatible with dextrose solutions. The primary use for carbamazepine is treating partial, tonic-clonic, or mixed seizures. Off-label uses include treatment for restless legs syndrome.

➧ ***Test-taking Tip:*** *The key word "clarify" indicates a false-response item. Select the order that is incorrect. Focus on how medications should be administered and the multiple uses of various anticonvulsant medications.*

Content Area: Adult Health; *Category of Health Alteration:* Pharmacological and Parenteral Therapies; *Integrated Processes:* Nursing Process Implementation; *Client Need:* Physiological Integrity/Pharmacological and Parenteral Therapies/Medication Administration; *Cognitive Level:* Analysis

References: Aschenbrenner, D., & Venable, S. (2009). *Drug Therapy in Nursing* (3rd ed., pp. 338–340). Philadelphia: Lippincott Williams & Wilkins; Deglin, J., & Vallerand, A. (2009). *Davis's Drug Guide for Nurses* (11th ed., pp. 976–980). Philadelphia: F. A. Davis.

1062. A client with multiple sclerosis is prescribed baclofen (Lioresol®). Which information is most important for a nurse to assess when caring for this client?

1. Serum baclofen levels
2. Muscle rigidity and pain
3. Intake and urine output
4. Client's weight

ANSWER: 2

Baclofen is used primarily to treat spasticity in multiple sclerosis and spinal cord injuries. The nurse should assess for muscle rigidity, movement, and pain to evaluate medication effectiveness. There is no serum baclofen level. Baclofen can cause urinary urgency. Measurements of urine output and weight are aspects of daily nursing care.

➧ ***Test-taking Tip:*** *Focus on the actions of baclofen, a medication commonly used in treating symptoms associated with multiple sclerosis.*

Content Area: Adult Health; *Category of Health Alteration:* Pharmacological and Parenteral Therapies; *Integrated Processes:* Nursing Process Assessment; *Client Need:* Physiological Integrity/Pharmacological and Parenteral Therapies/Expected Actions or Outcomes; *Cognitive Level:* Application

Reference: Adams, M., Holland, L., & Bostwick, P. (2008). *Pharmacology for Nurses: A Pathophysiologic Approach* (2nd ed., p. 276). Upper Saddle River, NJ: Prentice Hall.

1063. A client with cerebral palsy is taking dantrolene (Dantrium®). A nurse evaluates that the medication is effective when noting that the client has: SELECT ALL THAT APPLY.

1. increased muscle spasticity.
2. increased urinary frequency.
3. increased mobility.
4. increased ability to maintain balance.
5. increased alertness.

ANSWER: 3, 4

Dantrolene acts directly on skeletal muscles to inhibit muscle contraction, improving mobility and the ability to maintain balance. Increased muscle spasticity indicates the medication is not effective. Common adverse effects include urinary frequency, drowsiness, orthostatic hypotension, and diarrhea. Dantrolene does not increase alertness.

➧ ***Test-taking Tip:*** *Read each option carefully to determine the key words in the options. Eliminate options that are not associated with the use of dantrolene, a direct-acting skeletal muscle relaxant.*

Content Area: Adult Health; *Category of Health Alteration:* Pharmacological and Parenteral Therapies; *Integrated Processes:* Nursing Process Evaluation; *Client Need:* Physiological Integrity/Pharmacological and Parenteral Therapies/Expected Actions or Outcomes; *Cognitive Level:* Analysis

Reference: Karch, A. (2008). *Focus on Nursing Pharmacology* (4th ed., pp. 409–410). Philadelphia: Lippincott Williams & Wilkins.

1064. A nurse prepares to administer naloxone (Narcan®) 0.4 mg intravenously (IV) to a client experiencing respiratory depression from morphine sulfate administered by patient-controlled analgesia (PCA). Naloxone is supplied in a 1 mg/mL vial. In order to give the correct dose, the nurse should administer ____ mL to the client.

ANSWER: 0.4

Use a proportion formula to calculate the correct amount:
1 mg : 1 mL :: 0.4 mg : X mL
Multiply the extremes and then the means and solve for X.
X = 0.4 mL

➧ ***Test-taking Tip:*** *Use a medication formula to calculate the correct dosage. Double-check answers that seem unusually large.*

Content Area: Adult Health; *Category of Health Alteration:* Pharmacological and Parenteral Therapies; *Integrated Processes:* Nursing Process Implementation; *Client Need:* Physiological Integrity/ Pharmacological and Parenteral Therapies/Pharmacological Pain Management; *Cognitive Level:* Application

Reference: Lehne, R. (2007). *Pharmacology for Nursing Care* (6th ed., pp. 274–275). St. Louis, MO: Elsevier/Saunders.

1065. EBP A nurse is caring for a group of clients all in need of pain medication. The nurse has determined the most appropriate pain medication for each client based on the client's level of pain. Prioritize the order in which the nurse should plan to administer the pain medications beginning with the analgesic for the client with the most severe pain.

______ Ketorolac (Toradol®) 10 mg oral
______ Fentanyl (Sublimaze®) intravenously (IV) per patient-controlled analgesia (PCA) with a bolus dose
______ Hydromorphone (Dilaudid®) 5 mg oral
______ Morphine sulfate 4 mg IV
______ Propoxyphene (Darvon®) 65 mg oral

ANSWER: 4, 1, 3, 2, 5

The most potent of the medications is fentanyl (Sublimaze®), an opioid narcotic analgesic that binds to opiate receptors in the central nervous system (CNS), altering the response to and perception of pain. A dose of 0.1 to 0.2 mg is equivalent to 10 mg of morphine sulfate. Morphine sulfate is also an opioid analgesic. Hydromorphone, another opioid analgesic, would be third in priority. The oral dosing of this medication would indicate that the client's pain is less severe than the client receiving fentanyl or morphine sulfate. Hydromorphone 7.5 mg oral is an equianalgesic dose to 30 mg of oral morphine or 10 mg parenteral morphine. Ketorolac is a NSAID and nonopioid analgesic that inhibits prostaglandin synthesis, producing peripherally mediated analgesia. Propoxyphene is last in priority. It also binds to opiate receptors in the CNS but is used in treating mild to moderate pain. It has analgesic effects similar to acetaminophen.

➧ ***Test-taking Tip:*** *Focus on ordering the medications starting with the most potent opioid analgesics and ending with the nonopioid analgesic.*

Content Area: Adult Health; *Category of Health Alteration:* Pharmacological and Parenteral Therapies; *Integrated Processes:* Nursing Process Planning; *Client Need:* Physiological Integrity/ Pharmacological and Parenteral Therapies/Pharmacological Pain Management; *Cognitive Level:* Analysis

Reference: Aschenbrenner, D., & Venable, S. (2009). *Drug Therapy in Nursing* (3rd ed., pp. 379–389, 394). Philadelphia: Lippincott Williams & Wilkins.

EBP Reference: Institute for Clinical Systems Improvement. (2008). *Assessment and Management of Acute Pain.* Available at: www.guideline.gov/summary/summary.aspx?view_id=1&doc_id=12302

1066. EBP A nurse applies a fentanyl (Sublimaze®) transdermal patch to a client for the first time. Shortly after application, the client is experiencing pain. Which nursing action is most appropriate?

1. Remove the transdermal patch and apply a new one.
2. Administer a short-acting opioid analgesic.
3. Rub the transdermal patch to enhance absorption of the medication.
4. Call the physician to request a fentanyl transdermal patch with a higher dosage.

ANSWER: 2

When the first fentanyl transdermal patch is applied, effective analgesia may take 12 to 24 hours to develop because absorption is slow. Removing the patch is unnecessary. Transdermal patches should not be rubbed to enhance absorption because it can cause the delivery of the medication to fluctuate. It is premature to request a higher dose of fentanyl.

➧ ***Test-taking Tip:*** *Focus on that fact that absorption from a fentanyl transdermal patch is slow.*

Content Area: Adult Health; *Category of Health Alteration:* Pharmacological and Parenteral Therapies; *Integrated Processes:* Nursing Process Implementation; *Client Need:* Physiological Integrity/Pharmacological and Parenteral Therapies/Pharmacological Pain Management; *Cognitive Level:* Application

Reference: Lehne, R. (2007). *Pharmacology for Nursing Care* (6th ed., p. 290). St. Louis, MO: Elsevier/Saunders.

EBP Reference: Herr, K., Bjoro, K., Steffensmeier, J., & Rakel, B. (2006). *Acute Pain Management in Older Adults.* Available at: www.guideline.gov/summary/summary.aspx?doc_id=10198&nbr=005382&string=pain

1067. EBP A nurse evaluates that sumatriptan (Imitrex®) has been an effective treatment when a client reports:

1. an improvement in mood.
2. a decrease in muscle spasms.
3. an increased ability to fall asleep and stay asleep.
4. relief of migraine headache attacks.

ANSWER: 4

Sumatriptan is a serotonin receptor agonist and a first-line medication for terminating a migraine or cluster headache attack. Sumatriptan is not used in the treatment of mood alterations, muscle spasms, or insomnia.

➧ ***Test-taking Tip:*** *The key words are "effective treatment." Apply knowledge of the use of sumatriptan to answer this question*

Content Area: Adult Health; *Category of Health Alteration:* Pharmacological and Parenteral Therapies; *Integrated Processes:* Nursing Process Evaluation; *Client Need:* Physiological Integrity/ Pharmacological and Parenteral Therapies/Pharmacological Pain Management; *Cognitive Level:* Application

Reference: Lehne, R. (2007). *Pharmacology for Nursing Care* (6th ed., pp. 304–305). St. Louis, MO: Elsevier/Saunders.

EBP Reference: Institute for Clinical Systems Improvement (2007). *Diagnosis and Treatment of Headache*. Available at: www.guideline.gov/summary/summary.aspx?doc_id=11082&nbr=005845&string=migraine

1068. A nurse is caring for a client with osteoarthritis receiving piroxicam (Feldene®). Which instruction is most important for the nurse to include in the medication teaching plan?

1. "Take the medication with food to decrease gastric irritation."
2. "If your pain is severe, you can take an additional dose of the medication."
3. "Lie down until the medication begins to be effective for pain control."
4. "If you feel you are lacking energy, you can safely take ginkgo for an energy boost."

ANSWER: 1

Piroxicam should be taken with food and a full glass of water to prevent gastric irritation and possible bleeding. Piroxicam is administered in a once-daily dose, and additional doses should not be taken. Because of the gastric irritation and possible reflux, the client should sit upright after taking the medication. Ginkgo interacts with piroxicam, increasing the risk for bleeding.

➧ ***Test-taking Tip:*** *Focus on the gastric irritation that occurs with many anti-inflammatory medications. Note that options 1 and 3 address gastric irritation. Eliminate one of these options.*

Content Area: Adult Health; *Category of Health Alteration:* Pharmacological and Parenteral Therapies; *Integrated Processes:* Communication and Documentation; *Client Need:* Physiological Integrity/Pharmacological and Parenteral Therapies/Medication Administration; Health Promotion and Maintenance/Principles of Teaching and Learning; *Cognitive Level:* Application

Reference: Abrams, A., Lammon, C., & Pennington, S. (2007). *Clinical Drug Therapy: Rationales for Nursing Practice* (8th ed., pp. 120–121). Philadelphia: Lippincott Williams & Wilkins.

1069. A nurse identifies the nursing diagnosis of *Disturbed body image related to a client's long-term use of prednisone (Deltasone®)*. Which observations should support this diagnosis? SELECT ALL THAT APPLY.

1. Weight gain
2. Increased muscle mass
3. Fragile skin
4. Acne
5. Alopecia

ANSWER: 1, 3, 4

Weight gain, muscle atrophy, fragile skin, acne, and facial redness are possible body changes that may occur with long-term glucocorticoid therapy. Muscle wasting (not increased muscle mass) and hirsutism (not alopecia) are additional side effects of prednisone.

➧ ***Test-taking Tip:*** *Use the memory aid that glucocorticoids end in "-asone." Focus on the side effects of glucocorticoids to answer this question.*

Content Area: Adult Health; *Category of Health Alteration:* Pharmacological and Parenteral Therapies; *Integrated Processes:* Nursing Process Analysis; *Client Need:* Psychosocial Integrity/Unexpected Body Image Changes; Physiological Integrity/Pharmacological and Parenteral Therapies/Adverse Effects/Contraindications; *Cognitive Level:* Analysis

Reference: Karch, A. (2008). *Focus on Nursing Pharmacology* (4th ed., p. 568). Philadelphia: Lippincott Williams & Wilkins.

1070. EBP Which is the priority nursing diagnosis for a client taking doxorubicin (Doxil®) for recurrent ovarian cancer?

1. Risk for fluid volume deficit
2. Risk for imbalanced nutrition: Less than body requirements
3. Risk for alteration in cardiac output
4. Risk for self-care deficit

ANSWER: 3

Doxorubicin is a chemotherapeutic agent and can cause dysrhythmias and chest pain within minutes of administration. Cardiomyopathy can develop months to years after therapy. Chemotherapy-related side effects of nausea, vomiting, and fatigue are addressed by the nursing diagnoses Risk for fluid volume deficit, Risk for imbalanced nutrition, and Risk for self-care deficit. These are important, but not the priority.

➧ *Test-taking Tip: Focus on the key word "priority." Use the ABCs (airway, breathing, circulation) to select the priority nursing diagnosis.*

Content Area: Adult Health; *Category of Health Alteration:* Pharmacological and Parenteral Therapies; *Integrated Processes:* Nursing Process Planning; *Client Need:* Safe and Effective Care Environment/Safety and Infection Control/Injury Prevention; Physiological Integrity/Pharmacological and Parenteral Therapies/Adverse Effects/Contraindications; *Cognitive Level:* Analysis

Reference: Karch, A. (2008). *Focus on Nursing Pharmacology* (4th ed., pp. 220–221). Philadelphia: Lippincott Williams & Wilkins.

EBP Reference: Moore, K., Johnson, G., Fortner, B., & Houts, A. (2008). The AIM Higher Initiative: New procedures implemented for assessment, information, and management of chemotherapy toxicities in community oncology clinics. *Clinical Journal of Oncology Nursing,* 12(2), 229–238.

1071. A client with advanced prostate cancer is receiving abarelix (Plenaxis®). Due to the effects of the medication, what should be the priority nursing action?

1. Review with the client strategies to reduce constipation.
2. Monitor the client for breast pain and tenderness.
3. Observe the client for at least 30 minutes after abarelix administration.
4. Teach the client ways to improve sleep hygiene.

ANSWER: 3

Observe the client for at least 30 minutes after administration due to the risks of severe allergic reaction that increase with each dose and can occur within a short time after administration. Abarelix suppresses testicular testosterone production and is administered deeply intramuscularly (IM). Constipation, breast pain and tenderness, and sleep disturbances are common side effects of abarelix.

➧ *Test-taking Tip: Recall the adverse reactions of abarelix and use the process of elimination. Use the steps of the nursing process to eliminate options. Assessment should be priority.*

Content Area: Adult Health; *Category of Health Alteration:* Pharmacological and Parenteral Therapies; *Integrated Processes:* Nursing Process Assessment; *Client Need:* Physiological Integrity/Pharmacological and Parenteral Therapies/Adverse Effects/Contraindications; *Cognitive Level:* Application

Reference: Lehne, R. (2007). *Pharmacology for Nursing Care* (6th ed., p. 1175). St. Louis, MO: Elsevier/Saunders.

1072. Cyclosporine (Sandimmune®) and methotrexate (Rheumatrex®) are prescribed for a client with severe rheumatoid arthritis. Which points should a nurse address when teaching the client about these medications? SELECT ALL THAT APPLY.

1. Drinking grapefruit juice is best because the medications' effects are enhanced.
2. Keep well hydrated to maximize the therapeutic effects of methotrexate.
3. Avoid use of St. John's wort, echinacea, and melatonin, as these may interfere with immunosuppression.
4. These medications are administered weekly by subcutaneous injection.
5. Both methotrexate and cyclosporine suppress the immune system.

ANSWER: 2, 3, 5

Adequate hydration minimizes the risk of adverse effects. St. John's wort decreases cyclosporine levels. Echinacea and melatonin interact with cyclosporine to alter immunosuppression. Methotrexate and cyclosporine both have immunosuppressive effects. Grapefruit juice should be avoided because it can increase the concentration of cyclosporine. Methotrexate and cyclosporine can be taken orally instead of by injection. It is incorrect that both medications are taken weekly. Only methotrexate is taken weekly, whereas cyclosporine is usually taken twice daily.

➧ *Test-taking Tip: Read each option carefully and apply knowledge of the immunosuppressant medications to answer this question.*

Content Area: Adult Health; *Category of Health Alteration:* Pharmacological and Parenteral Therapies; *Integrated Processes:* Teaching and Learning; *Client Need:* Physiological Integrity/Pharmacological and Parenteral Therapies/Pharmacological Interactions; *Cognitive Level:* Analysis

References: Aschenbrenner, D., & Venable, S. (2009). *Drug Therapy in Nursing* (3rd ed., pp. 432–436). Philadelphia: Lippincott Williams & Wilkins; Wilson, B., Shannon, M., Shields, K., & Stang, C. (2008). *Prentice Hall Nurse's Drug Guide 2008* (pp. 397–400, 967–970). Upper Saddle River, NJ: Pearson Education.

1073. A nurse is assessing the laboratory test results for a male client receiving testosterone replacement therapy for treatment of hypogonadism. Which laboratory finding is most important for the nurse to review?

1. Fasting lipid profile
2. Partial thromboplastin time
3. Urinalysis
4. Serum potassium

ANSWER: 1

The most important test is the fasting lipid profile because testosterone can lower plasma levels of high-density lipoproteins (HDLs) and elevate plasma levels of low-density lipoproteins (LDLs), increasing the risk of atherosclerosis. Testosterone has little effect on partial thromboplastin time, urine, or serum potassium.

➧ ***Test-taking Tip:*** *Focus on testosterone's action of lowering HDL and raising LDL levels to select the correct option.*

Content Area: Adult Health; *Category of Health Alteration:* Pharmacological and Parenteral Therapies; *Integrated Processes:* Nursing Process Assessment; *Client Need:* Physiological Integrity/Pharmacological and Parenteral Therapies/Adverse Effects/Contraindications; *Cognitive Level:* Application

Reference: Lehne, R. (2007). *Pharmacology for Nursing Care* (6th ed., p. 757). St. Louis, MO: Elsevier/Saunders.

1074. **EBP** A client calls a clinic to renew the prescription for insulin being administered subcutaneously via an insulin pump. Which insulin type, if prescribed by a physician, should the nurse question?

1. Insulin lispro (Humolog®)
2. Insulin aspart (Novolog®)
3. Insulin glulisine (Apidra®)
4. Insulin glargine (Lantus®)

ANSWER: 4

Glargine is long-duration insulin not suited to delivery by an infusion pump; the order should be questioned. Four types of insulin may be delivered through an insulin pump: regular, lispro, aspart, and glulisine. These are short-duration and short or rapid-acting types of insulin that can be administered at a basal rate for continuous infusion at a slow but steady rate. The pump can also be triggered manually to provide a bolus dose to accommodate insulin needs to match the caloric contents of a meal.

➧ ***Test-taking Tip:*** *Recall that only short-duration and short- or rapid-acting types of insulin can be administered through an insulin pump. Thus, select the option with a long-duration insulin.*

Content Area: Adult Health; *Category of Health Alteration:* Pharmacological and Parenteral Therapies; *Integrated Processes:* Nursing Process Implementation; *Client Need:* Physiological Integrity/Pharmacological and Parenteral Therapies/Medication Administration; *Cognitive Level:* Analysis

Reference: Lehne, R. (2007). *Pharmacological and Parenteral Therapies for Nursing Care* (6th ed., pp. 654, 657). St. Louis, MO: Elsevier/Saunders.

EBP Reference: Farrar, D., Tuffnell, D., & West, J. (2007). Continuous subcutaneous insulin infusion versus multiple daily injections of insulin for pregnant women with diabetes. *Cochrane Database of Systematic Reviews*, Issue 3, Art. No. CD005542. DOI: 10.1002/14651858.CD005542.pub2. Available at: www.mrw.interscience.wiley.com/cochrane/clsysrev/articles/CD005542/frame.html

1075. **EBP** Exenatide (Byetta®) is prescribed for a client with type 2 diabetes mellitus in addition to a combination of metformin (Glucophage®) and glyburide (Micronase®). Which focus should be a nurse's priority when teaching the client about exenatide?

1. Teaching the client how to administer exenatide subcutaneously
2. Informing the client that exenatide helps to reduce body weight due to slower gastric emptying
3. Discussing exenatide's action in reducing hemoglobin $A1_C$ and fasting plasma glucose levels
4. Discussing the signs and symptoms of hypoglycemia

ANSWER: 1

Exenatide is an incretin mimetic used for type 2 diabetes mellitus only. The priority is to teach the client how to self-administer exenatide, since metformin and glyberide are oral medications. All instructions are correct, but teaching the client how to administer the medication is priority because it may take a few teaching sessions for the client to demonstrate self-administration correctly.

➧ ***Test-taking Tip:*** *To select the priority option, determine which teaching point would take the most time with the client.*

Content Area: Adult Health; *Category of Health Alteration:* Pharmacological and Parenteral Therapies; *Integrated Processes:* Teaching and Learning; *Client Need:* Physiological Integrity/Pharmacological and Parenteral Therapies/Medication Administration; *Cognitive Level:* Analysis

Reference: Aschenbrenner, D., & Venable, S. (2009). *Drug Therapy in Nursing* (3rd ed., p. 1078). Philadelphia: Lippincott Williams & Wilkins.

EBP Reference: American Diabetes Association (ADA). (2007). *Standards of Medical Care in Diabetes. VIII. Diabetes Care in Specific Settings.* Available at: www.guideline.gov/summary/summary.aspx?doc_id=10403&nbr=005449&string=diabetes+and+insulin

1076. An unresponsive client with diabetes mellitus is admitted to an emergency department with a serum glucose level of 35 mg/dL. Which medication should a nurse plan to administer?

1. Exenatide (Byetta®)
2. Pramlintide (Symlin®)
3. Miglitol (Glyset®)
4. Glucagon (GlucaGen®)

ANSWER: 4

Normal serum glucose is 70 to 110 mg/dL. Glucagon, administered intramuscularly, intravenously, or subcutaneously, is used in unconscious clients with diabetes to reverse severe hypoglycemia from insulin overdose. Exenatide, a synthetic incretin mimetic, is used as an adjunct in type 2 diabetes to decrease blood glucose levels. Pramlintide lowers postprandial glucose levels by slowing gastric emptying. Miglitol, an alpha-glucosidase inhibitor, lowers postprandial serum glucose levels.

▶ ***Test-taking Tip:*** *Eliminate options that will lower the blood glucose level further. If unsure of the hypoglycemic agents, note that two options end in "-tide." Use this clue to eliminate these.*

Content Area: Adult Health; *Category of Health Alteration:* Pharmacological and Parenteral Therapies; *Integrated Processes:* Nursing Process Planning; *Client Need:* Physiological Integrity/ Pharmacological and Parenteral Therapies/Expected Actions or Outcomes; *Cognitive Level:* Analysis

Reference: Aschenbrenner, D., & Venable, S. (2009). *Drug Therapy in Nursing* (3rd ed., pp. 1078–1079). Philadelphia: Lippincott Williams & Wilkins.

1077. A 40-year-old client is receiving levothyroxine (Synthroid®) for treatment of hypothyroidism. Which serum laboratory results should lead a nurse to conclude that the client's dose is adequate?

Serum Laboratory Value	Normal Value	Client Value
WBC	3.9–11.9 K/µL	11 K/µL
TSH	0.3–5.4 µU/mL	0.4 µU/mL
T_3	70–204 ng/dL	80 ng/dL
Free T_4	0.8–2.3 ng/dL	2.1 ng/dL
Cortisol	5–25 mcg/dL	10 mcg/dL
Glucose	70–110 mg/dL	80 mg/dL
K	3.8–5.3 mEq/L	4.5 mEq/L

1. Thyroid-stimulating hormone (TSH) and cortisol
2. TSH and free T_4
3. Triiodothyronine (T_3) and free thyroxine (T_4)
4. White blood cells (WBCs), glucose, and potassium (K)

ANSWER: 2

Restoration of normal laboratory values for TSH and free T_4 indicate that the dose of levothyroxine is therapeutic. T_3 is used to evaluate the effectiveness of liothyronine and propylthiouracil used in the treatment of thyroid disorders. Cortisol levels are used to evaluate adrenal function. The WBC count is used to determine if the client has an infection. Evaluation of serum glucose and potassium levels are unrelated to the use of levothyroxine.

▶ ***Test-taking Tip:*** *Recall that levothyroxine is a synthetic preparation of T_4, a naturally ocurring thyroid hormone. Thus eliminate options 1 and 4, and focus on options 2 and 3.*

Content Area: Adult Health; *Category of Health Alteration:* Pharmacological and Parenteral Therapies; *Integrated Processes:* Nursing Process Evaluation; *Client Need:* Physiological Integrity/ Reduction of Risk Potential/Laboratory Values; Physiological Integrity/ Pharmacological and Parenteral Therapies/Medication Administration; *Cognitive Level:* Analysis

Reference: Lehne, R. (2007). *Pharmacological and Parenteral Therapies for Nursing Care* (6th ed., pp. 678, 683–684). St. Louis, MO: Elsevier/ Saunders.

1078. A client is receiving fludrocortisone (Florinef®) for treatment of adrenocortical insufficiency. A nurse is evaluating the client's serum laboratory values for adverse effects of the medication. Place an X in the box for the laboratory values that the nurse should specifically assess related to the adverse effects of fludrocortisone.

Serum Laboratory Value	Normal Value	Client Value	Values Affected by Fludrocortisone
WBC	3.9–11.9 K/μL	11 K/μL	
Glucose	70–110 mg/dL	180 mg/dL	
K	3.8–5.3 mEq/L	3.5 mEq/L	
Ca	8.5–10.5 mg/dL	8.0 mg/dL	
Platelets (PLT)	179–450 K/μL	165 K/μL	
TSH	0.3–5.4 μU/mL	0.4 μU/mL	
T_3	70–204 ng/dL	80 ng/dL	
Free T_4	0.8–2.3 ng/dL	2.1 ng/dL	

ANSWER:

Serum Laboratory Value	Normal Value	Client Value	Values Affected by Fludrocortisone
WBC	3.9–11.9 K/μL	11 K/μL	
Glucose	70–110 mg/dL	180 mg/dL	X
K	3.8–5.3 mEq/L	3.5 mEq/L	X
Ca	8.5–10.5 mg/dL	8.0 mg/dL	X
Platelets (PLT)	179–450 K/μL	165 K/μL	X
TSH	0.3–5.4 μU/mL	9.4 μU/mL	
T_3	70–204 ng/dL	80 ng/dL	
Free T_4	0.8–2.3 ng/dL	0.1 ng/dL	

Adverse effects of fludrocortisones include hyperglycemia, hypocalcemia, hypokalemia, and thrombocytopenia. White blood cells (WBCs) and thyroid hormones, though abnormal, are unaffected by fludrocortisone administration. The abnormal thyroid hormones suggest hypothyroidism.

➧ ***Test-taking Tip:*** *Recall that the adverse effects of fludrocortisones include those related to the metabolic and hematological systems.*

Content Area: Adult Health; *Category of Health Alteration:* Pharmacological and Parenteral Therapies; *Integrated Processes:* Nursing Process Evaluation; *Client Need:* Physiological Integrity/Pharmacological and Parenteral Therapies/Adverse Effects/Contraindications; *Cognitive Level:* Analysis

Reference: Wilson, B., Shannon, M., Shields, K., & Stang, C. (2008). *Prentice Hall Nurse's Drug Guide 2008* (pp. 646–649). Upper Saddle River, NJ: Pearson Education.

1079. Oral terbutaline (Brethaire®) is prescribed for a client with bronchitis. Which comorbidity should prompt a nurse to monitor the client closely following administration of this medication?

1. Strabismus
2. Hypertension
3. Diabetes insipidus
4. Hypothyroidism

ANSWER: 2

Terbutaline is a bronchodilator with relative selectivity for beta$_2$-adrenergic (pulmonary) receptor sites, with less effect on beta$_1$-adrenergic (cardiac) receptors and should be used with caution in clients with hypertension. It should also be used with caution in clients with glaucoma (not strabismus), diabetes mellitus (not diabetes insipidus), hyperthyroidism (not hypothyroidism), impaired cardiac function, or a history of seizures. It is contraindicated in clients with hypersensitivity to sympathomimetics.

➧ ***Test-taking Tip:*** *Think about the action of terbutaline and the conditions that could be exacerbated by its use.*

Content Area: Adult Health; *Category of Health Alteration:* Pharmacological and Parenteral Therapies; *Integrated Processes:* Nursing Process Assessment; *Client Need:* Physiological Integrity/Pharmacological and Parenteral Therapies/Adverse Effects/Contraindications; *Cognitive Level:* Application

Reference: Deglin, J., & Vallerand, A. (2009). *Davis's Drug Guide for Nurses* (11th ed.). Philadelphia: F. A. Davis.

1080. A client is admitted to an emergency department with tachypnea, tachycardia, and hypotension. The client has been taking theophylline (Theo-Dur®) for treatment of asthma and erythromycin (Erythrocin®) for an upper respiratory tract infection. Which conclusion by the nurse and action taken is correct?

1. The client is experiencing an asthma attack and the nurse requests an order for albuterol.
2. The client is experiencing septicemia and the nurse requests an order for blood cultures.
3. The client is experiencing theophylline toxicity and the nurse requests an order for a serum theophylline level.
4. The client is experiencing an allergic reaction to erythromycin and the nurse requests an order for diphenhydramine (Benadryl®).

ANSWER: 3

Tachypnea, tachycardia, and hypotension are signs of theophylline toxicity. These occur because macrolide antibiotics such as erythromycin inhibit the metabolism of theophylline. Obtaining an order for a theophylline level will expedite the client's treatment. Symptoms of an asthma attack would include wheezing and other signs of air hunger. Additional signs would need to be present to suspect septicemia, such as an elevated temperature and skin flushing. Symptoms could suggest an allergic reaction, but epinephrine would be ordered; not diphenhydramine.

▶ ***Test-taking Tip:*** *Focus on information provided in the situation and avoid reading into the scenario.*

Content Area: Adult Health; *Category of Health Alteration:* Pharmacological and Parenteral Therapies; *Integrated Processes:* Nursing Process Analysis; *Client Need:* Physiological Integrity/Physiological Adaptation/Unexpected Response to Therapies; Physiological Integrity/Pharmacological and Parenteral Therapies/Adverse Effects/Contraindications; *Cognitive Level:* Analysis

Reference: Aschenbrenner, D., & Venable, S. (2009). *Drug Therapy in Nursing* (3rd ed., pp. 977–979). Philadelphia: Lippincott Williams & Wilkins.

1081. A client is admitted to an emergency department with a severe asthma attack. A nurse has a standing order to administer 0.5 mg epinephrine (Adrenalin®) subcutaneously. The medication is supplied in a vial for injection that contains 5 mg/mL. In order to administer the correct dose, the nurse should quickly inject ____ mL subcutaneously.

ANSWER: 0.1

Use a proportion to determine the amount in milliliters; then multiply the extremes and the means and solve for X.

5 mg : 1 ml :: 0.5 mg : X mL

5X = 0.5

X = 0.1 mL

▶ ***Test-taking Tip:*** *Use the calculator provided and double-check the calculations. Remember a subcutaneous injection is likely to be less than 1 mL.*

Content Area: Adult Health; *Category of Health Alteration:* Pharmacological and Parenteral Therapies; *Integrated Processes:* Nursing Process Implementation; *Client Need:* Physiological Integrity/Pharmacological and Parenteral Therapies/Dosage Calculation; *Cognitive Level:* Analysis

References: Lewis, S., Heitkemper, M., Dirksen, S., O'Brien, P., & Bucher, L. (2007). *Medical-Surgical Nursing: Assessment and Management of Clinical Problems* (7th ed., p. 619). St. Louis, MO: Mosby/Elsevier; Pickar, G. (2007). *Dosage Calculations: A Ratio-Proportion Approach* (2nd ed., p. 46). Clifton Park, NY: Thomson Delmar Learning.

1082. EBP A client is unable to control gastroesophageal reflux with lifestyle modifications. A nurse instructs the client that by using which over-the-counter medication the client's symptoms can be successfully decreased?

1. Aspirin once a day
2. Famotidine (Pepsid®)
3. Ibuprofen (Advil®)
4. Desloratadine (Claritin®, Tavist®, Alavert®)

ANSWER: 2

Famotidine blocks histamine 2 receptors on parietal cells, thus decreasing gastric acid production. Aspirin increases gastric acid secretion and NSAIDs do not reduce gastric acid. Desloratadine blocks only histamine 1 receptors and is not effective against histamine 2 receptors.

▶ ***Test-taking Tip:*** *Focus on the classification of medications used to control gastroesophageal reflux, a histamine receptor blocker, to select the correct option.*

Content Area: Adult Health; *Category of Health Alteration:* Pharmacological and Parenteral Therapies; *Integrated Processes:* Teaching and Learning; *Client Need:* Physiological Integrity/Pharmacological and Parenteral Therapies/Expected Actions or Outcomes; *Cognitive Level:* Application

Reference: Lehne, R. (2007). *Pharmacological and Parenteral Therapies for Nursing Care* (6th ed., pp. 804, 813, 815, 897). St. Louis, MO: Elsevier/Saunders.

EBP Reference: University of Michigan Health System. (2007). *Gastroesophageal Reflux Disease*. Available at: www.guideline.gov/summary/summary.aspx?doc_id=10631&nbr=5568

1083. A client has a new order for metoclopramide (Reglan®). On review of the client's chart, a nurse identifies that the client has a contraindication for the medication and that the order should be questioned. Which contraindication did the nurse most likely note?

1. Use of nasogastric suctioning
2. History of diabetes mellitus (DM)
3. History of seizure disorders
4. Chemotherapy treatment for cancer

ANSWER: 3

The nurse most likely noted a history of seizure disorder. Metoclopramide is a gastrointestinal stimulant and antiemetic. Because it blocks dopamine receptors in the chemoreceptor trigger zone of the central nervous system (CNS), it is contraindicated in seizure disorders and Parkinson's disease. It is also a gastrointestinal stimulant, thus contraindicated with gastrointestinal obstruction, hemorrhage, or perforation. It is used in the treatment of emesis after surgery, chemotherapy, and radiation. It should be used with caution with DM, but is not contraindicated.

➧ ***Test-taking Tip:*** *Think about the CNS affects of metoclopramide. Select the only option that is related to the CNS.*

Content Area: Adult Health; *Category of Health Alteration:* Pharmacological and Parenteral Therapies; *Integrated Processes:* Nursing Process Assessment; *Client Need:* Physiological Integrity/Pharmacological and Parenteral Therapies/Adverse Effects/Contraindications; *Cognitive Level:* Analysis

Reference: Wilson, B., Shannon, M., Shields, K., & Stang, C. (2008). *Prentice Hall Nurse's Drug Guide 2008* (pp. 983–985). Upper Saddle River, NJ: Pearson Education.

1084. A client with ulcerative colitis is started on the medication sulfasalazine (Azulfidine®). A nurse overhears the client talking with family members about this medication and recognizes the need for more teaching when the client says:

1. "This medication will help to control my diarrhea."
2. "Sulfasalazine will decrease the inflammation in my colon."
3. "After taking this medication for a year, I will be cured of the disease."
4. "The medication will help to prevent future exacerbations of my disease."

ANSWER: 3

Sulfasalazine is a medication commonly used to treat ulcerative colitis. It decreases inflammation in the colon; however, it will not cure the disease. Ulcerative colitis is a chronic illness; the only cure is a total protocolectomy.

➧ ***Test-taking Tip:*** *"Needs further teaching" is a false-response item. Select the incorrect statement. If unsure, focus on the option that includes the word "cured."*

Content Area: Adult Health; *Category of Health Alteration:* Pharmacological and Parenteral Therapies; *Integrated Processes:* Nursing Process Evaluation; *Client Need:* Physiological Integrity/Pharmacological and Parenteral Therapies/Expected Actions or Outcomes; *Cognitive Level:* Analysis

References: Lewis, S., Heitkemper, M., Dirksen, S., O'Brien, P., & Bucher, L. (2007). *Medical-Surgical Nursing: Assessment and Management of Clinical Problems* (7th ed., pp. 1051, 1054, 1055). St. Louis, MO: Mosby/Elsevier; Lehne, R. (2007). *Pharmacological and Parenteral Therapies for Nursing Care* (6th ed., p. 920). St. Louis, MO: Elsevier/Saunders.

1085. A nurse evaluates that pancrelipase (Pancrease®) is having the optimal intended benefit for a client with cystic fibrosis when assessing that the client has:

1. lost weight.
2. relief of heartburn.
3. increased steatorrhea.
4. improved nutritional status.

ANSWER: 4

Pancrelipase (Pancrease®) is a pancreatic enzyme used in clients with deficient exocrine pancreatic secretions, cystic fibrosis, chronic pancreatitis, or steatorrhea from malabsorption syndrome. Because it aids digestion, the nutritional status should be improved. Weight gain, not weight loss, is an intended effect. It is not used to treat abdominal heartburn. Pancrelipase reduces the amount of fatty stools (steatorrhea).

➧ ***Test-taking Tip:*** *The key words are "optimal intended benefit." Think about the role the pancreas plays in digestion when selecting the correct option.*

Content Area: Adult Health; *Category of Health Alteration:* Pharmacological and Parenteral Therapies; *Integrated Processes:* Nursing Process Evaluation; *Client Need:* Physiological Integrity/Pharmacological and Parenteral Therapies/Expected Actions or Outcomes; *Cognitive Level:* Application

Reference: Aschenbrenner, D., & Venable, S. (2009). *Drug Therapy in Nursing* (3rd ed., p. 1015). Philadelphia: Lippincott Williams & Wilkins.

1086. Medications are ordered for a client on admission to a hospital. A nurse notes that the client's serum creatinine level, which was normal upon admission, has now risen to 3.7 mg/dL. Which ordered medication should prompt the nurse to call a physician to request a change in dosage?

1. Ceftriaxone (Rocephin®)
2. Insulin glargine (Lantus®)
3. Diltiazem (Cardizem®)
4. Furosemide (Lasix®)

ANSWER: 1

Ceftriaxone, a third-generation cephalosporin antibiotic, is 33% to 67% excreted in the urine unchanged. Dosage reduction or increased dosing interval is recommended in renal insufficiency because it is nephrotoxic and can further damage the kidneys. Insulin glargine is partially metabolized at the site of injection to active insulin metabolites and by the liver, the spleen, the kidney, and muscle tissue; no dose reduction is necessary unless serum glucose levels fluctuate. Diltiazem is mostly metabolized by the liver. Furosemide is 30% to 40% metabolized by the liver, with some nonhepatic metabolism and renal excretion as unchanged medication.

➧ ***Test-taking Tip:*** *Think about how medications are excreted from the body. Remember that many antibiotics are nephrotoxic. If unsure select the antibiotic.*

Content Area: Adult Health; *Category of Health Alteration:* Pharmacological and Parenteral Therapies; *Integrated Processes:* Nursing Process Implementation; *Client Need:* Physiological Integrity/ Pharmacological and Parenteral Therapies/Adverse Effects/Contraindications; *Cognitive Level:* Analysis

Reference: Wilson, B., Shannon, M., Shields, K., & Stang, C. (2008). *Prentice Hall Nurse's Drug Guide 2008* (pp. 280–282, 478–480, 684–686, 782–791). Upper Saddle River, NJ: Pearson Education.

1087. EBP A nurse is to administer vancomycin (Vancocin®) to a client diagnosed with sepsis. The client is to have a peak and trough level completed on this dose of the medication. Which action should the nurse initiate *first*?

1. Determine if the trough level has been drawn on the client.
2. Determine medication compatibilities before infusing into an existing intravenous line.
3. Check the client's culture and sensitivity (C&S) report.
4. Check the amount of time over which the medication dose should infuse.

ANSWER: 1

A trough level must be drawn before medication administration. This is the first action because, if the trough level has not been drawn, it will delay administering the medication. Determining medication compatibilities and checking C&S reports and the infusion duration are important actions before administering vancomycin. However, these actions can be done while the laboratory is obtaining the trough level or after knowing that the level has been drawn.

➧ ***Test-taking Tip:*** *Note the key word "first" and focus on the situation "a peak and trough level." Eliminate options that do not pertain to obtaining a peak and trough level.*

Content Area: Adult Health; *Category of Health Alteration:* Pharmacological and Parenteral Therapies; *Integrated Processes:* Nursing Process Implementation; *Client Need:* Physiologic Integrity/ Pharmacological and Parenteral Therapies/Medication Administration; *Cognitive Level:* Application

Reference: Wilkinson, J., & Van Leuven, K. (2007). *Fundamentals of Nursing: Theory, Concepts & Applications* (Vol. 1, p. 486). Philadelphia: F. A. Davis.

EBP Reference: Murphy, J. (2006). Predictability of vancomycin trough concentrations using seven approaches for estimating pharmacokinetic parameters. *American Journal of Health-System Pharmacy*, 63(23), 2365–2370.

1088. A client is to receive a first dose of oral sulfamethoxazole (Gantanol®) 1 gram every 12 hours for treatment of recurrent urinary tract infections. Which information about the client should prompt the nurse to immediately notify the physician to question the medication order?

1. History of gastric ulcer
2. Type 1 diabetes mellitus
3. Urine culture positive for *Escherichia coli*
4. Near-term pregnancy

ANSWER: 4

Sulfamethoxazole, a sulfonamide antibiotic, is a Category D medication for near-term pregnancy. This means there is positive evidence of human fetal risk, but the benefits from use in pregnant women may be acceptable despite the risk (e.g., for a life-threatening illness or a serious disease for which safer medications cannot be used or are ineffective). History of gastric ulcer or type 1 diabetes does not prevent the use of sulfamethoxazole. A positive urine culture would be an indication for using sulfamethoxazole.

➧ ***Test-taking Tip:*** *First review option 3 because it is different from the other options. Eliminate this option knowing a positive urine culture would be an indication for antibiotic use. Of the three remaining options, think about the condition that would make the use of this medication most unsafe.*

Content Area: Adult Health; *Category of Health Alteration:* Pharmacological and Parenteral Therapies; *Integrated Processes:* Nursing Process Analysis; *Client Need:* Physiological Integrity/Pharmacological and Parenteral Therapies/Adverse Effects/Contraindications; *Cognitive Level:* Analysis

Reference: Wilson, B., Shannon, M., Shields, K., & Stang, C. (2008). *Prentice Hall Nurse's Drug Guide 2008* (pp. 1428–1429, 1639). Upper Saddle River, NJ: Pearson Education.

1089. A hospitalized client is being treated for tuberculosis (TB). When administering medications, which medication on the client's medication administration record (MAR) should a nurse conclude is used for the treatment of TB?

1. Isoniazid (Nydrazid®)
2. Fluconazole (Diflucan®)
3. Azithromycin (Zithromax®)
4. Acyclovir (Zovirax®)

ANSWER: 1

Isoniazid (INH) is an antimycobacterial medication affecting bacterial cell wall synthesis; it is used in the treatment of TB or other mycobacterial infections. Fluconazole is an antifungal agent that inhibits synthesis of fungal sterols, a necessary component of the cell membrane. Azithromycin is a macrolide antibiotic that is bacteriostatic against susceptible bacteria and is usually used for treating lower respiratory tract infections, skin infections, acute otitis media, tonsillitis, or *Mycobacterium avium*. Acyclovir is an antiviral agent limited to treatment of herpes viruses.

▶ ***Test-taking Tip:*** *Read each medication name carefully. Use key letters in each medication to determine the medications use ("-azone" is antifungal; "-vira" is antiviral) and eliminate options that do not pertain to a mycobacterium.*

Content Area: Adult Health; *Category of Health Alteration:* Pharmacological and Parenteral Therapies; *Integrated Processes:* Nursing Process Implementation; *Client Need:* Physiological Integrity/Pharmacological and Parenteral Therapies/Expected Actions or Outcomes; *Cognitive Level:* Application

Reference: Aschenbrenner, D., & Venable, S. (2009). *Drug Therapy in Nursing* (3rd ed., pp. 786–787, 830–831, 852–853, 866–867). Philadelphia: Lippincott Williams & Wilkins.

1090. EBP Ciprofloxacin (Cipro-XR®) is prescribed for a client to treat a urinary tract infection. Which point should a nurse stress when teaching the client about the medication?

1. Avoid taking ciprofloxacin with milk or yogurt.
2. Treat diarrhea, a side effect of ciprofloxacin, with bismuth subsalicylate (Pepto-Bismol®).
3. Avoid fennel because it will increase the absorption of the ciprofloxacin.
4. Take dietary calcium tablets 1 hour before or 2 hours after ciprofloxacin.

ANSWER: 1

Ciprofloxacin is a fluoroquinolone antibiotic. Milk or yogurt decreases its absorption and should be avoided. Bismuth subsalicylate also decreases the absorption of ciprofloxacin and should be avoided. Extended release ciprofloxacin significantly reduces the frequency of nausea and diarrhea. Fennel will decrease the absorption of the ciprofloxacin. Dietary calcium can be taken at any time; it is unaffected by ciprofloxacin.

▶ ***Test-taking Tip:*** *Eliminate actions that will cause a decrease in the absorption of ciprofloxacin.*

Content Area: Adult Health; *Category of Health Alteration:* Pharmacological and Parenteral Therapies; *Integrated Processes:* Teaching and Learning; *Client Need:* Physiological Integrity/Pharmacological and Parenteral Therapies/Medication Administration; *Cognitive Level:* Application

Reference: Aschenbrenner, D., & Venable, S. (2009). *Drug Therapy in Nursing* (3rd ed., pp. 807–812). Philadelphia: Lippincott Williams & Wilkins.

EBP Reference: American College of Obstetricians and Gynecologists. (2008). *Treatment of Urinary Tract Infections in Nonpregnant Women.* Available at: www.guideline.gov/summary/summary.aspx?doc_id=12628&nbr=006536&string=ciprofloxacin

---

1091. Which finding should indicate to a nurse that acyclovir (Zovirax®), administered orally for treatment of herpes zoster, is effective?

1. Drying and crusting of genital lesions
2. Crusting and healing of vesicular skin lesions
3. Urticaria decreased and pruritus relieved
4. Decrease in intensity of chickenpox lesions

ANSWER: 2

Herpes zoster produces painful vesicular skin eruptions along the course of a nerve. Crusting and healing of the vesicular skin lesions indicates that the medication is effective. Drying and crusting of genital lesions would indicate the medications effectiveness for treating genital herpes, not herpes zoster. Urticaria (swollen, raised areas) and pruritus (itching) are not symptoms of herpes zoster. The lesions of chickenpox are generalized, whereas herpes zoster lesions occur along the course of a nerve. Herpes zoster occurs when the chickenpox (varicella zoster) virus that has incorporated itself into nerve cells is reactivated years after the initial infection, but it is not chickenpox.

▶ *Test-taking Tip: Apply knowledge of herpes zoster (shingles) to answer this question. Recall that herpes zoster, herpes simplex, and genital herpes are all caused by a virus and develop vesicles, but these occur in different body locations.*

Content Area: Adult Health; *Category of Health Alteration:* Pharmacological and Parenteral Therapies; *Integrated Processes:* Nursing Process Evaluation; *Client Need:* Physiological Integrity/ Pharmacological and Parenteral Therapies/Expected Effects/Outcomes; *Cognitive Level:* Analysis

References: Aschenbrenner, D., & Venable, S. (2009). *Drug Therapy in Nursing* (3rd ed., pp. 866–869). Philadelphia: Lippincott Williams & Wilkins; Lewis, S., Heitkemper, M., Dirksen, S., O'Brien, P., & Bucher, L. (2007). *Medical-Surgical Nursing: Assessment and Management of Clinical Problems* (7th ed., p. 468). St. Louis, MO: Mosby/Elsevier.

1092. A nurse is caring for various clients being seen in a clinic. Ganciclovir (Cytovene®) is prescribed for one of the clients for lesions that have not healed and are recurring (see illustrations). For which client with the problem illustrated should the nurse document that teaching about ganciclovir was completed?

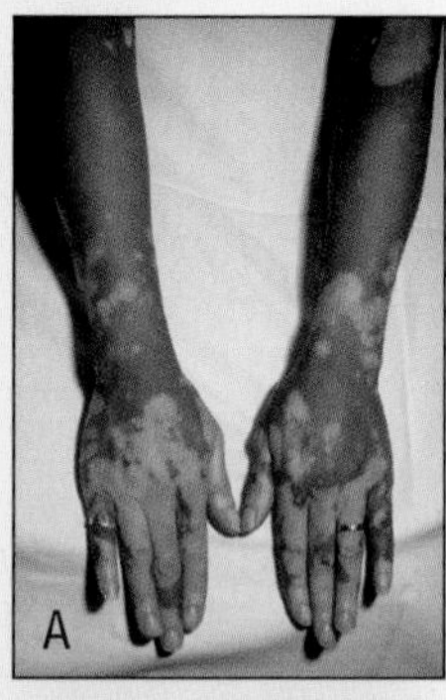

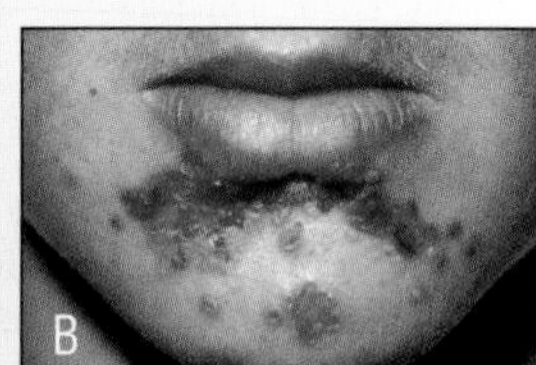

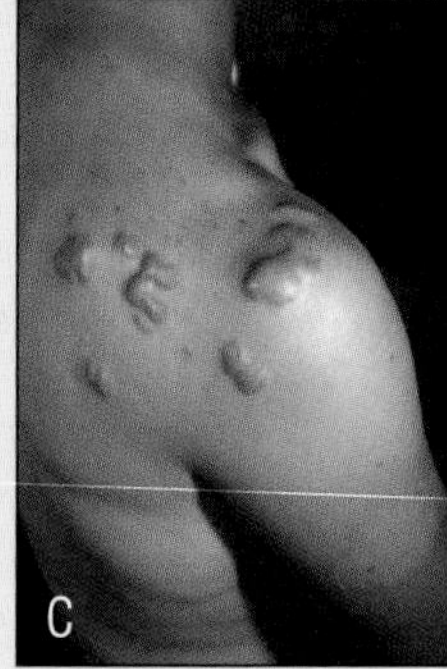

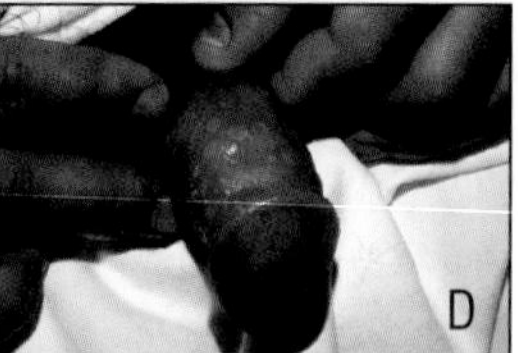

1. Client A
2. Client B
3. Client C
4. Client D

ANSWER: 4

Ganciclovir is an antiviral medication used in the treatment of recurrent genital herpes (client D). Client A has vitiligo, a skin disorder characterized by the patchy loss of skin pigment. Vitiligo is treated with topical steroids. Client B has dried herpes simplex, usually treated with the antiviral medication acyclovir (Zovirax®). Client C has keloids (hypertrophic scarring), which are usually not treated with medication.

▶ *Test-taking Tip: The key words are "not healing" and "recurring." Review each illustration and eliminate options 1 and 3 because these are not recurring lesions. Of options 2 and 4, determine which illustrates nonhealing lesions.*

Content Area: Adult Health; *Category of Health Alteration:* Pharmacological and Parenteral Therapies; *Integrated Processes:* Communication and Documentation; *Client Need:* Physiological Integrity/Pharmacological and Parenteral Therapies/Medication Administration; *Cognitive Level:* Analysis

References: Aschenbrenner, D., & Venable, S. (2009). *Drug Therapy in Nursing* (3rd ed., p. 867). Philadelphia: Lippincott Williams & Wilkins; Lewis, S., Heitkemper, M., Dirksen, S., O'Brien, P., & Bucher, L. (2007). *Medical-Surgical Nursing: Assessment and Management of Clinical Problems* (7th ed., pp. 457–458, 472). St. Louis, MO: Mosby/Elsevier.

Chapter Nine

Physiological Integrity: Care of Children and Families

Test 28: Child Health: Growth and Development

1093. Various children are being seen in the clinic for well-baby checks. By what age should a nurse expect a child to begin to use simple words to communicate needs?

1. Age 10–12 months
2. Age 1–2 years
3. Age 6–9 months
4. Age 2–3 years

ANSWER: 1
By age 10 to 12 months, a child is able to communicate simple words, using four to six words by 15 months of age. By age 1 to 2 years the child communicates in more than simple words, using about 50 words in two-word sentences. At 6 to 9 months, the child is learning to make sounds. At 2 to 3 years, the child's verbal language increases steadily, knowing full name, naming a color, and holding up fingers to show age.

➧ ***Test-taking Tip:*** *The word "begins" is a key word.*

Content Area: Child Health; *Category of Health Alteration:* Growth and Development; *Integrated Processes:* Nursing Process Assessment; *Client Need:* Health Promotion and Maintenance/Developmental Stages and Transitions; *Cognitive Level:* Application

Reference: Pillitteri, A. (2007). *Maternal & Child Health Nursing: Care of the Childbearing & Childrearing Family* (5th ed., p. 865). Philadelphia: Lippincott Williams & Wilkins.

1094. A nurse in a clinic is assessing the weight of an infant. Which infant's weight indicates to the nurse that the infant's weight is normal for the infant's age?

1. The baby's weight has tripled in the first 6 months of life
2. The baby's weight has doubled in the first year of life
3. The baby's weight has doubled in the first 6 months of life and tripled in the first year
4. The baby's weight has doubled in the first 6 months and doubled again in the next 6 months

ANSWER: 3
A baby's weight should double in the first 4 to 6 months of life and triple by the end of the first year. The weight needs to more than double the first year.

➧ ***Test-taking Tip:*** *As you read each option, take the normal weight of a newborn and apply the weight in the option before making a selection.*

Content Area: Child Health; *Category of Health Alteration:* Growth and Development; *Integrated Processes:* Nursing Process Evaluation; *Client Need:* Health Promotion and Maintenance/Developmental Stages and Transitions; *Cognitive Level:* Application

Reference: Pillitteri, A. (2007). *Maternal & Child Health Nursing: Care of the Childbearing & Childrearing Family* (5th ed., p. 827). Philadelphia: Lippincott Williams & Wilkins.

1095. A student explains to an instructor that the infant period is categorized as the "oral phase" according to Freud's theory. Which statements by the student suggest an understanding of this phase? SELECT ALL THAT APPLY.

1. An infant sucks for nourishment as well as pleasure
2. An infant does not find pleasure in sucking but does find enjoyment from the nourishment
3. An infant may have more pleasure in breastfeeding than bottle feeding because it expends more energy
4. An infant does not find pleasure in use of a pacifier
5. An infant explores the world through the mouth
6. An infant begins to explore the genital area to learn sexual identity

ANSWER: 1, 3, 5

An infant has the desire to suck, which may actually build the ego and self-esteem of an infant. There is more pleasure in breastfeeding because it expends more energy and also provides other comforting mechanisms, such as warmth. An infant explores the world through the mouth, especially the tongue. Freud believed the oral phase is important for both nutrition and pleasure in the first year of life. An infant finds pleasure in sucking on a pacifier, according to Freud. A preschooler learns sexual identity through awareness of the genital area.

➧ ***Test-taking Tip:*** *Look for key words in each option.*

Content Area: Child Health; *Category of Health Alteration:* Growth and Development; *Integrated Processes:* Teaching and Learning; *Client Need:* Growth and Development/Developmental Stages and Transitions; *Cognitive Level:* Analysis

Reference: Pillitteri, A. (2007). *Maternal & Child Health Nursing: Care of the Childbearing & Childrearing Family* (5th ed., pp. 814–815). Philadelphia: Lippincott Williams & Wilkins.

1096. An 8-month-old baby girl, who is developing appropriately, is admitted to a pediatric unit for respiratory syncytial virus (RSV). The baby is crying and being held by her mother. A nurse wants to provide appropriate care based on Erikson's developmental stages. In which stage is this baby, according to Erikson's theory?

1. Punishment versus obedience orientation
2. Oral stage
3. Initiative versus guilt
4. Trust versus mistrust

ANSWER: 4

Based on Erikson's stages of development, trust versus mistrust is appropriate for a child under a year old. The child learns to love and be loved. Experiences that add to security include soft sounds, touch, and visual stimulation for an active child. Punishment-versus-obedience orientation is not a developmental stage. Initiative versus guilt is a developmental task in the preschool stage. The oral phase is based on Freud not Erikson.

➧ ***Test-taking Tip:*** *Use the process of elimination. Recall that Erikson's developmental tasks include achievement of a task versus nonachievement of a task.*

Content Area: Child Health; *Category of Health Alteration:* Growth and Development; *Integrated Processes:* Nursing Process Assessment; *Client Need:* Health Promotion and Maintenance/Developmental Stages and Transitions; *Cognitive Level:* Application

Reference: Pillitteri, A. (2007). *Maternal & Child Health Nursing: Care of the Childbearing & Childrearing Family* (5th ed., p. 815). Philadelphia: Lippincott Williams & Wilkins.

1097. A nurse is caring for a 3-month-old infant. Based on the developmental age of the child, which motor skill should the nurse expect to see during an assessment?

1. Bangs objects held in hand
2. Begins to grab objects using a pincer grasp
3. Grabs objects using a palmar grasp
4. Looks and plays with own fingers

ANSWER: 4

Three-month-old babies can play with their own fingers. At 3 months, infants can reach for attractive objects in front of them, but because their grasp is unpracticed, they usually miss them. A 2-month-old infant will hold an object for a few minutes. A 10-month-old infant uses a pincer grasp. A 6-month-old infant uses a palmar grasp.

➧ ***Test-taking Tip:*** *Awareness of the developmental stages and age of a 3-month-old will assist with answering this question correctly.*

Content Area: Child Health; *Category of Health Alteration:* Growth and Development; *Integrated Processes:* Nursing Process Assessment; *Client Need:* Health Promotion and Maintenance/Growth and Development; *Cognitive Level:* Application

References: Ball, J., & Binder, R. (2006). *Clinical Handbook for Pediatric Nursing* (pp. 2–3). Upper Saddle River, NJ: Pearson Education; Pillitteri, A. (2007). *Maternal & Child Health Nursing: Care of the Childbearing & Childrearing Family* (5th ed., pp. 832–833). Philadelphia: Lippincott Williams & Wilkins.

1098. A 10-month-old child reaches the 9- to 12-month developmental stage. Which nursing action is most appropriate for providing tactile stimulation for this child?

1. Caress the child while diaper changing
2. Give the child a soft squeeze toy
3. Swaddle the child at nap time
4. Let the child squash and mash food while sitting in a high chair

ANSWER: 4

The most appropriate action is to let the child squash and mash food. At this age, an infant should be ready to touch and manipulate food and is capable of sitting up. Caressing a baby during diaper change, giving a baby a soft toy, and swaddling a baby at nap time are age-appropriate activities for providing tactile stimulation for younger babies.

➧ ***Test-taking Tip:*** *Note that the subject relates to age-appropriate tactile stimulation. Eliminate options that would be appropriate for a younger child.*

Content Area: Child Health; *Category of Health Alteration:* Growth and Development; *Integrated Processes:* Nursing Process Implementation; *Client Need:* Health Promotion and Maintenance/Developmental Stages and Transitions; *Cognitive Level:* Analysis

Reference: Pillitteri, A. (2007). *Maternal & Child Health Nursing: Care of the Childbearing & Childrearing Family* (5th ed., pp. 832–833). Philadelphia: Lippincott Williams & Wilkins.

1099. A clinic nurse is meeting with a mother and her 3-year-old son. The toddler is acting out, and the mother asks the nurse what a good form of discipline would be for her son. The nurse recommends a "time-out" for the child. Which statement regarding a time-out is most accurate?

1. The child should sit still for as many minutes as he misbehaved
2. The child should sit still at a time-out for as many minutes as his age in years
3. The child should be able to read a book during time-out
4. Children should not be expected to sit still until they are in school

ANSWER: 2

A 3-year-old should be expected to have a time-out of 3 minutes. Three minutes may not seem long to an adult, but to a toddler 3 minutes is an excellent form of discipline because it seems like a long time to be restricted from activity. The child should not have his time-out related to his minutes of misbehaving because the time-out may be too long an expectation. A child can act out for a long time. The time-out is a form of discipline, and reading a book should not be related to misbehaving. Reading a book should be a reward. Children can be expected to sit still for short periods of time at the toddler level.

➧ ***Test-taking Tip:*** *The key word is "discipline." Look for key words in each option related to discipline. Eliminate options that are different from the other options.*

Content Area: Child Health; *Category of Health Alteration:* Growth and Development; *Integrated Processes:* Teaching and Learning; *Client Need:* Psychosocial Integrity/Therapeutic Environment; *Cognitive Level:* Analysis

Reference: Pillitteri, A. (2007). *Maternal & Child Health Nursing: Care of the Childbearing & Childrearing Family* (5th ed., pp. 876–877). Philadelphia: Lippincott Williams & Wilkins.

1100. A clinic nurse is caring for a 2-year-old client. During the examination the child's parents ask the nurse when their toddler should be toilet trained. Which response by the nurse is most appropriate?

1. "Children should be placed on the potty chair often so they get used to the task and should be rewarded immediately for staying on the potty chair."
2. "Children need sphincter control, cognitive understanding of the task, and the ability to delay immediate gratification."
3. "Children should be ready to toilet train at about 2 years old."
4. "First put training pants on your child so the child gets used to not wearing a diaper."

ANSWER: 2

A child will be ready for toilet training based on his or her own readiness. Toilet training should not be pushed too soon or the child will become frustrated. A child's development is cephalocaudal, and therefore the child's body may not be able to control the rectal and urethral sphincters. A 2-year-old may not want to sit on a toilet when they do not feel it is necessary. There is no set age for potty training. A child may not be physiologically ready for controlling his or her bladder.

➧ ***Test-taking Tip:*** *Select an option that is individualized to the child.*

Content Area: Child Health; *Category of Health Alteration:* Growth and Development; *Integrated Processes:* Teaching and Learning; *Client Need:* Physiological Integrity/Basic Care and Comfort/Elimination; *Cognitive Level:* Application

Reference: Pillitteri, A. (2007). *Maternal & Child Health Nursing: Care of the Childbearing & Childrearing Family* (5th ed., p. 874). Philadelphia: Lippincott Williams & Wilkins.

1101. A nurse is preparing a 4-year-old boy for surgery. Which nursing action is appropriate for preoperative teaching based on Erikson's developmental stages?

1. Allowing the child to make a project related to the surgery
2. Having the child put a surgical mask on a doll
3. Asking the child how he feels about surgery
4. Allowing the child to listen to music without further instructions

ANSWER: 2

The child should practice putting a mask on the doll so he can feel the mask and know how it will fit on the doll. This will help to reduce the child's anxiety. The child is too young to do a project related to surgery. The child is not old enough to verbalize his feelings. Music may be helpful, but it cannot replace appropriate preoperative teaching based on the child's developmental stage.

➧ ***Test-taking Tip:*** *Focus on the age of the child. Recall that a 4-year-old likes doing things and relieves tension through play.*

Content: Child Health; *Category of Health Alteration:* Growth and Development; *Integrated Processes:* Nursing Process Implementation; *Client Need:* Health Promotion and Maintenance/Principles of Teaching and Learning; *Cognitive Level:* Application

Reference: Pillitteri, A. (2007). *Maternal & Child Health Nursing: Care of the Childbearing & Childrearing Family* (5th ed., p. 814). Philadelphia: Lippincott Williams & Wilkins.

1102. A nurse case manager is meeting with the parents of an 8-year-old client. The 8-year-old is scheduled for surgery to repair a cleft palate. The parents ask the case manager when they should discuss and explain the surgery to their child. Based on the child's developmental age, which is the best response by the nurse?

1. Explain the surgery immediately before it is carried out.
2. Explain the surgery 1 to 2 hours before it is carried out.
3. Explain the surgery up to 1 week before it is carried out.
4. Explain the surgery several days before it is carried out.

ANSWER: 4

An 8-year-old can receive teaching several days before surgery. School-age children have concrete operational thought and can remember events. A preschooler will remember explanations for only a couple of hours. A toddler has limited attention span and limited ability to remember things. An adolescent can handle information for the longest period of time.

➧ ***Test-taking Tip:*** *Focus on the length of time in each of the options and how long an 8-year-old should be able to remember events.*

Content Area: Child Health; *Category of Health Alteration:* Growth and Development; *Integrated Processes:* Communication and Documentation; *Client Need:* Health Promotion and Maintenance/ Developmental Stages and Transitions; *Cognitive Level:* Analysis

Reference: Ball, J., & Bindler, R. (2006). *Child Health Nursing: Partnering with Children and Families* (p. 179). Upper Saddle River, NJ: Pearson/ Prentice Hall.

1103. A 7-year-old child lived in foster homes when he was an infant. He was adopted at the age of 1 year to an intact family who provided him with love and security. Which developmental task was this child most likely unable to complete as an infant?

1. Trust versus mistrust
2. Industry versus inferiority
3. Autonomy versus shame and doubt
4. Initiative versus guilt

ANSWER: 1

Because the child lived in multiple foster homes, the child may have had delayed development in trust as an infant. The other options are not correct based on the developmental needs of an infant.

➧ ***Test-taking Tip:*** *Focus on the developmental stage for an infant, not that of a 7-year-old child.*

Content Area: Child Health; *Category of Health Alteration:* Growth and Development; *Integrated Processes:* Nursing Process Analysis; *Client Need:* Psychosocial Integrity/Therapeutic Environment; *Cognitive Level:* Analysis

Reference: Pillitteri, A. (2007). *Maternal & Child Health Nursing: Care of the Childbearing & Childrearing Family* (5th ed., p. 822). Philadelphia: Lippincott Williams & Wilkins.

1104. A clinic nurse is completing a school physical on an adolescent girl. The girl is concerned because she is 13 years old and has not yet started menstruating. Which statement by the nurse should be most helpful when addressing the girl's concerns?

1. "The average age for a girl to experience menarche is 12.5 years. That means some girls will be younger and some will be older than 12.5."
2. "Don't worry about it; your period will come."
3. "I can see why you are concerned, since some girls get their period when they are 10 years old."
4. "I can refer you to a specialist who can answer your questions."

ANSWER: 1

This response most directly answers the girl's question. An average age means some will be younger and some will be older. It is demeaning to make comments such as "don't worry about it." It is unnecessary to remind the client when some girls get their periods. There is no need for a specialist, because the girl is within the normal age range for the onset of menarche.

➧ ***Test-taking Tip:*** *Use principles of therapeutic communication. Eliminate options that are nontherapeutic.*

Content Area: Child Health; *Category of Health Alteration:* Growth and Development; *Integrated Processes:* Communication and Documentation; *Client Need:* Psychosocial Integrity/Therapeutic Communications; *Cognitive Level:* Application,

Reference: Pillitteri, A. (2007). *Maternal & Child Health Nursing: Care of the Childbearing & Childrearing Family* (5th ed., pp. 68–69). Philadelphia: Lippincott Williams & Wilkins.

1105. A nurse in a clinic is asked to teach a 13-year-old boy diagnosed with asthma. The nurse assesses that the child is developmentally on task. Which consideration should the nurse include when teaching this client?

1. The client is unable to differentiate cause and effect, so keep it simple.
2. The client is discovering new properties of objects and events, so expect many questions.
3. The client is not developmentally able to remember information, so handouts are necessary.
4. The client needs explanations of the physiology of asthma and demonstrations of appropriate interventions.

ANSWER: 4

The adolescent has formal operational thought and can understand the diagnosis and appropriate interventions both verbally and by demonstration. All other considerations are necessary for younger children.

➧ ***Test-taking Tip:*** *Recall that formal operational thought typically is a developmental state of the 13-year-old.*

Content Area: Child Health; *Category of Health Alteration:* Growth and Development; *Integrated Processes:* Nursing Process Analysis; *Client Need:* Health Promotion and Maintenance/Principles of Teaching and Learning; *Cognitive Level:* Analysis

Reference: Pillitteri, A. (2007). *Maternal & Child Health Nursing: Care of the Childbearing & Childrearing Family* (5th ed., p. 819). Philadelphia: Lippincott Williams & Wilkins.

1106. A clinic nurse assesses an infant diagnosed with thrush. Place an X on the photograph illustrating a thrush infection.

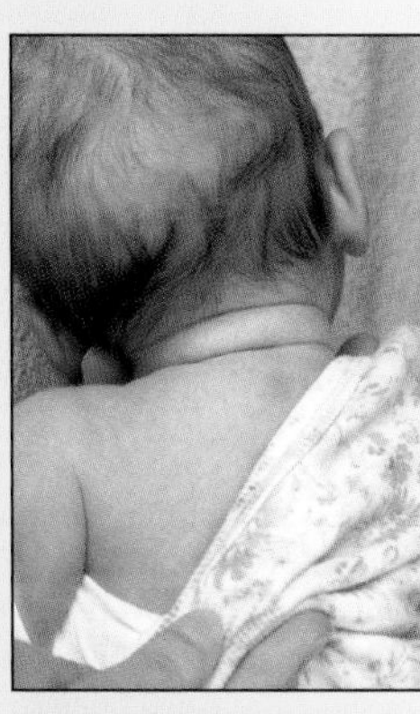

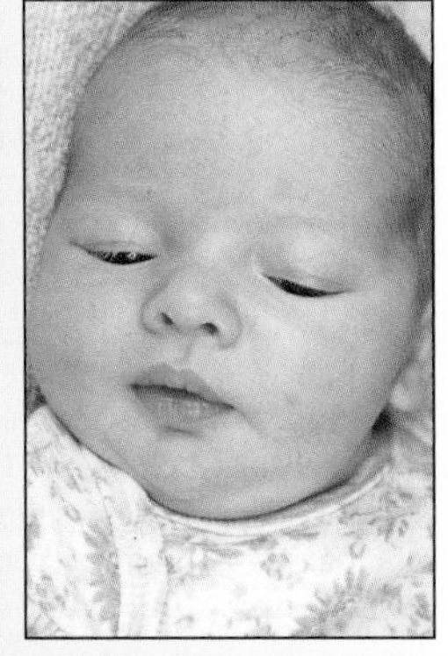

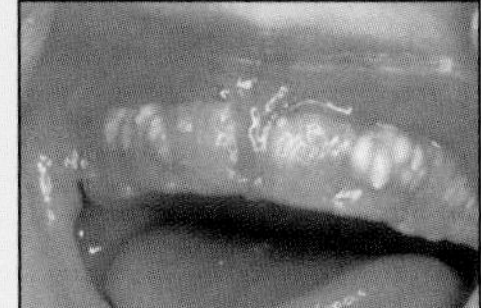

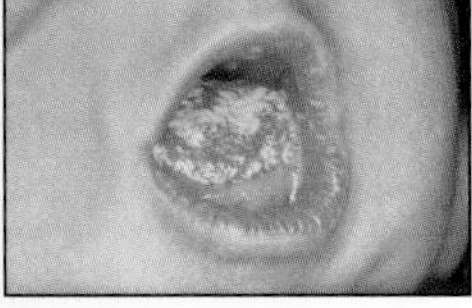

ANSWER:

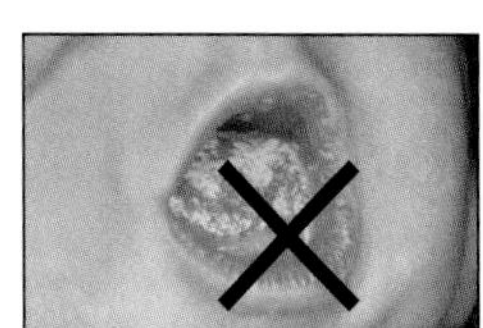

Candida albicans **(thrush) has characteristic white patches on the tongue. It can be contracted during vaginal delivery.** In the first illustrations, the infant has a flat hemangioma, or "stork bite," at the back of the neck. In the second illustration the infant has milia (white papules) on the face. In the third illustration the infant has Epstein's pearls: small, white, pearl-like epithelial cysts on the palate that usually disappear a few weeks after birth.

➧ ***Test-taking Tip:*** *Recall that thrush is a fungal infection. Focus on each illustration to determine if the infant has signs of an infection.*

Content Area: Child Health; *Category of Health Alteration:* Growth and Development; *Integrated Processes:* Nursing Process Evaluation; *Client Need:* Health Promotion and Maintenance/Health Screening; *Cognitive Level:* Application

Reference: Dillon, P. (2007). *Nursing Health Assessment: A Critical Thinking, Case Studies Approach* (2nd ed., pp. 859, 862). Philadelphia: F. A. Davis.

1107. A nurse is planning to use the Denver Articulation Screening Examination (DASE) for a 4-year-old child. To properly use the DASE, the nurse should plan to ask the child to:

1. read a favorite book at the child's developmental level.
2. read a phrase and tell the nurse the meaning of the phrase.
3. repeat familiar words that are read to the child.
4. ask the child to state the letters of the alphabet.

ANSWER: 3

The DASE is a 5-minute test to detect articulation disorders in children age 2½ to 6 years of age and involves having the child repeat words that are stated by the examiner. The other options are not components of the DASE.

➧ ***Test-taking Tip:*** *Use the key word "articulation" and eliminate options.*

Content Area: Child Health; *Category of Health Alteration:* Growth and Development; *Integrated Processes:* Nursing Process Planning; *Client Need:* Health Promotion and Maintenance/Health Screening; *Cognitive Level:* Application

Reference: Hockenberry, M., & Wilson, D. (2007). *Wong's Nursing Care of Infants and Children* (8th ed., p. 1849). St. Louis, MO: Mosby/Elsevier.

1108. Which result should a nurse expect if a 4-year-old child's visual acuity test is normal for the child's developmental age?

1. 10/10
2. 20/20
3. 20/40
4. 40/40

ANSWER: 3

Visual acuity is normally 20/40 during the toddler years. A visual acuity result of 10/10 or 20/20 is exceptional acuity for a toddler. Visual acuity would be 20/20 by age 6. A visual acuity result of 40/40 warrants further follow-up because the higher numbers indicate less visual acuity.

➧ ***Test-taking Tip:*** *Focus on the child's developmental age.*

Content Area: Child Health; *Category of Health Alteration:* Growth and Development; *Integrated Processes:* Nursing Process Evaluation; *Client Need:* Health Promotion and Maintenance/Health Screening; *Cognitive Level:* Application

Reference: Dillon, P. (2007). *Nursing Health Assessment: A Critical Thinking, Case Studies Approach* (2nd ed., pp. 894, 909). Philadelphia: F. A. Davis.

1109. A nurse has reviewed the upper arm blood pressure (BP) results for multiple children between the ages of 3 and 5 years. Which BP reading should the nurse evaluate as being an *abnormal* BP for this age group?

1. 96/42 mm Hg
2. 101/57 mm Hg
3. 112/66 mm Hg
4. 115/68 mm Hg

ANSWER: 1

Children between the ages of 1 month to 2 years have a mean BP of 95/58 mm Hg. A BP reading of 96/42 mm Hg has a mean arterial pressure (MAP) of 60, which indicates insufficient perfusion to tissues. MAP = (systolic blood pressure [SBP] + 2diastolic blood pressure [DBP])/3. The mean BP for a child 2 to 5 years is 101/57 (MAP = 74). The 90th percentile BP is 112/66 mm Hg (MAP = 82). The 95th percentile is 115/68 mm Hg (MAP = 85).

➧ ***Test-taking Tip:*** *If unsure of the BP values for this age group, calculate the MAP = (SBP + 2DBP)/3, and then select the option with a low MAP.*

Content Area: Child Health; *Category of Health Alteration:* Growth and Development; *Integrated Processes:* Nursing Process Analysis; *Client Need:* Health Promotion and Maintenance/Growth and Development; *Cognitive Level:* Analysis

Reference: Hockenberry, M., & Wilson, D. (2007). *Wong's Nursing Care of Infants and Children* (8th ed., p. 174). St. Louis, MO: Mosby/Elsevier.

1110. When taking an infant's blood pressure, which points are important for a nurse to remember? SELECT ALL THAT APPLY.

1. It is best to use an infant cuff on an infant.
2. The cuff used should be no more than two-thirds of the length of the upper arm.
3. The cuff used can be a Doppler ultrasound device.
4. The reading of the upper arm should be higher than the thigh.
5. A similar reading on the arm and the thigh could indicate coarctation of the aorta.

ANSWER: 1, 2, 3

An appropriately sized cuff should be used on an infant because a too-large cuff results in a lower blood pressure and a too-small cuff a higher blood pressure reading. The arm should be covered two-thirds or less with the cuff. A Doppler device can bounce off high frequency. The readings of the upper arm and thigh should be equal or close to equal in an infant. If they are not equal, it could be a sign of coarctation of the aorta. In coarctation of the aorta, the blood pressure in the upper extremities is higher (more than 15 mm Hg) than in the lower extremities.

➧ ***Test-taking Tip:*** *Visualize taking a blood pressure measurement on an infant prior to reading each of the options.*

Content Area: Child Health; *Category of Health Alteration:* Growth and Development; *Integrated Processes:* Nursing Process Assessment; *Client Need:* Physiological Integrity/Reduction of Risk Potential/Vital Signs; *Cognitive Level:* Application

References: Merenstein, G., & Gardner, S. (2006). *Handbook of Neonatal Intensive Care* (6th ed., p. 102). St. Louis, MO: Mosby/Elsevier; Pillitteri, A. (2007). *Maternal & Child Health Nursing: Care of the Childbearing & Childrearing Family* (5th ed., p. 1170). Philadelphia: Lippincott Williams & Wilkins.

1111. A 22-month-old toddler is walking into the examination room independently in front of the toddler's mother. Which method should the nurse plan to use to weigh the child?

1. A standing scale should be used because the toddler is able to stand independently.
2. Weigh using an infant scale because this is the method for all infants until the age of 2 years.
3. Ask the mother which would be best for the child.
4. Have the mother weigh herself and then weigh herself holding her child. Then subtract the mother's weight from the combined child and mother's weight.

ANSWER: 1

If the child is cooperative and able to stand, a standing scale should be used because it would be most accurate and allow for comparisons with later visits. A child's developmental ability and not age should be used to determine the most correct method to weigh the child. The mother depends on a nurse for the best suggestion. Weighing the baby and mother and then subtract the baby's weight is not as accurate.

Test-taking Tip: *Focus on the action of the toddler in making a decision.*

Content Area: Child Health; *Category of Health Alteration:* Growth and Development; *Integrated Processes:* Nursing Process Assessment; *Client Need:* Health Promotion and Maintenance/Techniques of Physical Assessment; *Cognitive Level:* Application

Reference: Pillitteri, A. (2007). *Maternal & Child Health Nursing: Care of the Childbearing & Childrearing Family* (5th ed., p. 992). Philadelphia: Lippincott Williams & Wilkins.

1112. EBP An experienced nurse is orienting a new nurse to the care of children in a clinic. Which immunizations should the experienced nurse inform the new nurse to plan to administer to normally healthy children between ages 1 and 5 years? SELECT ALL THAT APPLY.

1. Inactivated poliovirus
2. Diphtheria, tetanus, pertussis (DTaP)
3. Measles, mumps, rubella (MMR)
4. Hepatitis B (HepB)
5. Meningococcal

ANSWER: 1, 2, 3, 4

Inactivated poliovirus dose three is given between ages 12 and 18 months; dose four between ages 4 to 6 years. DTaP dose four is given between ages 12 and 18 months; dose five between ages 4 to 6 years. MMR dose one is given between ages 12 and 15 months; dose two between ages 2 to 6 years. Other immunizations include varicella zoster (chickenpox; VZV), given between ages 12 and 18 months or at any age after if the child has never had chickenpox, and *Haemophilus* influenza (Hib), whose dose four is given between ages 12 and 15 months. Meningococcal polysaccharide vaccine (MPSV4) is administered to children aged 2 to 10 years with terminal complement deficiencies or anatomic or functional asplenia and certain other high-risk groups.

Test-taking Tip: *If uncertain, recognize that there is a 5-year span of time in the question.*

Content Area: Child Health; *Category of Health Alteration:* Growth and Development; *Integrated Processes:* Teaching and Learning; *Client Need:* Health Promotion and Maintenance/Health and Wellness; *Cognitive Level:* Analysis

Reference: Dillon, P. (2007). *Nursing Health Assessment: A Critical Thinking, Case Studies Approach* (2nd ed., p. 898). Philadelphia: F. A. Davis.

EBP Reference: Department of Health and Human Services, Centers for Disease Control and Prevention. (2009). *Recommended Immunization Schedule for Persons Aged 0–6 Year.* Available at: www.cdc.gov/vaccines/recs/schedules/#child

1113. A nurse at a clinic is preparing the immunizations for a 6-month-old baby. The mother says, "My baby is afraid of strangers and afraid of separating from me. My mother-in-law is upset and thinks I am causing it." Which response by the nurse is most appropriate?

1. "Give your baby to strangers while you are present, so your baby gets used to strangers."
2. "Your mother-in-law is correct; you need to include her more in your baby's needs."
3. "Separation anxiety is an important component of a parent-child attachment."
4. "Just let your baby cry for a while; your baby will get used to being separated from you."

ANSWER: 3

It is a normal developmental stage when a baby exhibits separation anxiety. The mother can be reassured. Mothers are encouraged to have familiar people visit frequently; infants can then safely experience strangers. It is important to be patient through this stage of development. It is not appropriate to force the baby to be with strangers. The baby doesn't need to cry in order to get used to strangers. Eventually the baby will pass through this stage.

➧ ***Test-taking Tip:*** *Focus on the mother's comment and respond to her comment. The mother is not asking for advice.*

Content Area: Child Health; *Category of Health Alteration:* Growth and Development; *Integrated Processes:* Communication and Documentation; *Client Need:* Psychosocial Integrity/Coping Mechanisms; *Cognitive Level:* Application

Reference: Pillitteri, A. (2007). *Maternal & Child Health Nursing: Care of the Childbearing & Childrearing Family* (5th ed., p. 837). Philadelphia: Lippincott Williams & Wilkins.

1114. A nurse is assessing the nutritional needs of a 1-year-old client. According to recommendations for introducing milk products, which type of milk should a 1-year-old child be drinking?

1. 2% milk beginning at the age of 1
2. 1% milk
3. Whole milk until the age of 2 years
4. Skim milk

ANSWER: 3

A child should not have fat intake limited until the age of 2 years. Fats are necessary to ensure myelination of nerve fibers. Milk that is 2%, 1%, or skim has reduced amounts of fat.

➧ ***Test-taking Tip:*** *Select the option that has the highest amount of fat.*

Content Area: Child Health; *Category of Health Alteration:* Growth and Development; *Integrated Processes:* Nursing Process Assessment; *Client Need:* Physiological Integrity/Nutrition and Oral Hydration; *Cognitive Level:* Analysis

References: Ball, J., & Bindler, R. (2006). *Child Health Nursing: Partnering with Children and Families* (p. 327). Upper Saddle River, NJ: Pearson/Prentice Hall; Pillitteri, A. (2007). *Maternal & Child Health Nursing: Care of the Childbearing & Childrearing Family* (5th ed., p. 810). Philadelphia: Lippincott Williams & Wilkins.

1115. A nurse is teaching the parents of children between the ages of 2 and 3 years old about nutritional intake. The nurse should teach the parents that the percentage of the daily total intake of fat should be no more than which percentage?

1. 20% to 25%
2. 50%
3. 30%
4. 10% to 20%

ANSWER: 3

Toddlers can have a higher fat level in their diet than older children. Therefore 30% is acceptable for nutrition and digestive needs. A diet of 50% fat is too high for proper health. Any fat intake less than 30% is insufficient for the child's digestion and absorption of nutrients.

➧ ***Test-taking Tip:*** *Analyze each option, eliminating the very high and very low options.*

Content Area: Child Health; *Category of Health Alteration:* Growth and Development; *Integrated Processes:* Nursing Process Analysis; *Client Need:* Physiological Integrity/Nutrition and Oral Hydration; *Cognitive Level:* Analysis

Reference: Pillitteri, A. (2007). *Maternal & Child Health Nursing: Care of the Childbearing & Childrearing Family* (5th ed., pp. 810, 870). Philadelphia: Lippincott Williams & Wilkins.

1116. A mother brings her 5-month-old to the clinic for a well-child appointment. A nurse is doing an assessment when the mother asks when she can give her baby solid foods. What response is most appropriate?

1. Inquire if the baby can sit well with support and if the baby's tongue thrust has decreased.
2. Ask the mother is she feels the baby is ready for solids.
3. Ask the mother if the baby seems hungry after bottle feeding.
4. Tell the mother to ask the pediatrician.

ANSWER: 1

The baby needs to be physically and developmentally ready for solid foods. The baby should be able to sit up well and should have less tongue thrust so the food can stay in the mouth. The mother depends on information from the health-care providers (HCP) to help her with the decision. The criterion of a baby being hungry after bottle feeding may just mean the baby needs to take more formula or breast milk. The HCP can help with the decision, but the nurse has responsibility to conduct teaching within the registered nurse's scope of practice.

▸ ***Test-taking Tip:*** *Note that option 4 is different from the other options that ask a question. Eliminate this option and focus on actual physical information to support an answer to the mother's question.*

Content Area: Child Health; *Category of Health Alteration:* Growth and Development; *Integrated Processes:* Communication and Documentation; *Client Need:* Health Promotion and Maintenance/Growth and Development; *Cognitive Level:* Analysis

Reference: Ball, J., & Binder, R. (2006). *Clinical Handbook for Pediatric Nursing* (p. 324). Upper Saddle River, NJ: Pearson Education.

1117. EBP A school nurse is concerned about the lack of physical activity in the high school. The nurse has gathered data related to appropriate activity from the document *Healthy People 2010: Understanding and Improving Health*. Which recommendation for physical activity should the school nurse recommend for this age group?

1. Adolescents should get at least 60 minutes of physical activity daily.
2. High school students should be required to participate in physical education classes.
3. Teenagers should be exercising at least 30 minutes three to five times per week.
4. Adolescents should be exercising every day for at least 15 minutes.

ANSWER: 1

Getting at least 60 minutes of physical activity daily promotes healthy living related to consistent exercise. All students are not required to participate in high school activity. Adolescents need more exercise than twice per week. Daily exercise is recommended, but it should be for at least 60 minutes for children and 30 minutes for adults.

▸ ***Test-taking Tip:*** *Focus on recommendations from the Healthy People 2010 document.*

Content Area: Child Health; *Category of Health Alteration:* Growth and Development; *Integrated Processes:* Nursing Process Implementation; *Client Need:* Health Promotion and Maintenance/Health Promotion and Disease Prevention; *Cognitive Level:* Application

Reference: Ball, J., & Bindler, R. (2006). *Child Health Nursing: Partnering with Children and Families* (p. 485). Upper Saddle River, NJ: Pearson/Prentice Hall.

EBP Reference: U.S. Department of Health and Human Services. (2000). *Healthy People 2010: Understanding and Improving Health.* Available at: www.healthypeople.gov/Document/html/uih/uih_4.htm#physactiv

---

1118. A school nurse is teaching adolescents about oral care. Which point should the nurse address with the students?

1. The adolescent should floss daily, brush teeth twice a day, and see the dentist two times per year.
2. The adolescent should brush once a day and see the dentist twice per year.
3. The adolescent should see the dentist once a year and brush teeth twice a day.
4. The adolescent should floss daily, brush teeth twice a day, and see the dentist once a year.

ANSWER: 1

Adolescent and school-aged children should floss daily, brush teeth twice a day, and see the dentist two times per year.

▸ ***Test-taking Tip:*** *Apply the American Academy of Dentists and the American Academy of Pediatrics dental recommendations.*

Content Area: Child Health; *Category of Health Alteration:* Growth and Development; *Integrated Processes:* Nursing Assessment/Teaching and Learning; *Client Need:* Physiological Integrity/Basic Care and Comfort/Personal Hygiene; *Cognitive Level:* Application

Reference: Ball, J., & Bindler, R. (2006). *Child Health Nursing: Partnering with Children and Families* (p. 488). Upper Saddle River, NJ: Pearson/Prentice Hall.

1119. A nurse is caring for a 14-year-old client who was admitted for dehydration from nausea and vomiting. The client is ready for discharge and says to the nurse, "I will tell you something, but you can't tell anyone." Which nursing action is most appropriate?

1. Promise the client that the information will not be told to anyone due to Health Insurance Portability and Accountability Act (HIPAA) laws.
2. Tell the client that the information will be confidential unless it is life threatening or harmful.
3. Tell the client that only the physician will be told; otherwise the information will remain confidential.
4. Ask the client to tell a social worker who then can follow through with the information if it is concerning.

ANSWER: 2

The information can remain confidential unless there is adult abuse involved or if there are legal implications. The HIPAA law does not state that all information is to remain confidential. The nurse should not tell the physician unless the information is life threatening or could potentially result in harm to the client. The nurse should listen to the client. Though the client is willing to confide in the nurse, the client may not feel as comfortable with the social worker. Both the nurse and the social worker have the same obligation to report the information if it is life threatening or harmful.

▸ ***Test-taking Tip:*** *Think about the legal requirements for reporting information.*

Content Area: Child Health; *Category of Health Alteration:* Growth and Development; *Integrated Processes:* Communication and Documentation; Caring; *Client Need:* Psychosocial Integrity/Therapeutic Communications; *Cognitive Level:* Application

Reference: Ball, J., & Binder, R. (2006). *Clinical Handbook for Pediatric Nursing* (pp. 25–26). Upper Saddle River, NJ: Pearson Education.

1120. EBP A school nurse is teaching adolescents about sexual activity and how the human papilloma virus (HPV) is contracted and prevented. Which statements should the nurse include when teaching about HPV? SELECT ALL THAT APPLY.

1. HPV can be contracted by oral sex.
2. HPV can be contracted on the toilet seat.
3. HPV is so common that most people can get it soon after becoming sexually active.
4. HPV is contracted through vaginal sex.
5. HPV is contracted through anal sex.
6. Condom use can fully protect against contracting the HPV virus.

ANSWER: 4, 5

HPV is contracted by vaginal and anal sex and passed on by genital contact. It cannot be contracted by the other means, such as oral sex or the toilet seat. Condoms do not fully protect against contracting the HPV virus because HPV can infect areas that are not covered by a condom.

Test-taking Tip: *Apply knowledge of adolescent health and sexually transmitted diseases.*

Content Area: Child Health; *Category of Health Alteration:* Growth and Development; *Integrated Processes:* Teaching and Learning; *Client Need:* Health Promotion and Maintenance/Safe and Effective Care Environment/High Risk Behaviors; *Cognitive Level:* Application

Reference: Smeltzer, S., Bare, B., Hinkle, J., & Cheever, K. (2008). *Brunner & Suddarth's Textbook of Medical-Surgical Nursing* (11th ed., pp. 1666–1667). Philadelphia: Lippincott Williams & Wilkins.

EBP Reference: Department of Health and Human Services, Centers for Disease Control and Prevention. (2008). *Genital HPV Infection–CDC Fact Sheet*. Available at: www.cdc.gov/STD/HPV/STDFact-HPV.htm#howget

---

1121. EBP A school nurse is presenting the latest information related to driving under the influence (DUI) of alcohol to high school students. The nurse informs the students that all 50 states and the District of Columbia have laws defining it as a crime to drive with a blood alcohol concentration (BAC) at or above a prescribed level of:

1. 0.1%.
2. 1.0%.
3. 0.08%.
4. 0.8%.

ANSWER: 3

The level of 0.08% is considered an impaired blood alcohol level. A 0.1% blood level is too low, and 0.8% and 1.0% blood levels are too high.

Test-taking Tip: *Knowledge of certain laboratory values is expected on the licensure examination, including a BAC that suggests impairment.*

Content Area: Child Health; *Category of Health Alteration:* Growth and Development; *Integrated Processes:* Teaching and Learning; *Client Need:* Health Promotion and Maintenance/High Risk Behaviors; *Cognitive Level:* Application

Reference: Craven, R., & Hirnle, C. (2007). *Fundamentals of Nursing: Human Health, and Function* (5th ed., p. 679). Philadelphia: Lippincott Williams & Wilkins.

EBP Reference: Insurance Institute for Highway Safety. (2008). *DUI/DWI Laws.* Available at: www.iihs.org/laws/dui.aspx

---

1122. EBP The American Academy of Pediatrics lists safety tips for adolescents who drive a motor vehicle. When teaching a group of parents with teenagers, which statement should a nurse include in the teaching?

1. Nighttime driving is okay as long as the teenager is not fatigued.
2. A lack of experience will motivate the teenager to want to practice driving longer.
3. Transportation of other teenagers by a teenage driver should be avoided.
4. Although teenagers tend to use safety belts, reminders are always important.

ANSWER: 3

The teenager should be discouraged from transporting other teenagers because the driver's alertness is decreased from the distraction. Motor vehicle accidents are the most frequent cause of unintentional accidents for adolescents. Nighttime driving is not okay for teenagers because it is more difficult to judge and to see objects at night. Although teenagers need practice driving with a reliable, adult teacher, the lack of experience does not motivate them to practice longer. Teenagers continue to be inconsistent with wearing of safety belts.

Test-taking Tip: *Apply knowledge regarding evidence related to teenage motor vehicle drivers.*

Content Area: Child Health; *Category of Health Alteration:* Growth and Development; *Integrated Processes:* Nursing Process Implementation; *Client Need:* Health Promotion and Maintenance/High Risk Behaviors; *Cognitive Level:* Analysis

Reference: Pillitteri, A. (2007). *Maternal & Child Health Nursing: Care of the Childbearing & Childrearing Family* (5th ed., pp. 947, 950–951). Philadelphia: Lippincott Williams & Wilkins.

EBP Reference: Committee on Injury, Violence, and Poison Prevention, American Academy of Pediatrics, Committee on Adolescence, American Academy of Pediatrics, Weiss, J. (2006). The teen driver. *Pediatrics,* 118(6), 2570–2581. Available at: www.guideline.gov/summary/summary.aspx?doc_id=10390&nbr=005436&string=Teen+AND+Driver

1123. A 4-year-old child is hospitalized with a high fever. While the child is in bed, the child comforts himself by sucking the thumb. The mother of the child becomes concerned because her child has not sucked his thumb for 6 months. Which nursing response to the mother's concerns is most appropriate?

1. "I don't know why he is sucking his thumb; maybe your child just needs more attention."
2. "This is a form of developmental regression and can be a normal response for a child who is hospitalized. Continue to love and support your child."
3. "Is there anything else going on in your family right now that may be causing your child to feel anxious?"
4. "Where is the child's father? Maybe the child wants his father?"

ANSWER: 2

It is common for preschoolers to revert to a behavior they have outgrown in an effort to cope with difficult situations. Sucking a thumb is a comfort measure for the child. Thumb-sucking does not indicate that the child is not getting enough attention. Thumb-sucking does not mean there are other contributing factors. The hospitalization is enough stress in a child's life. Having a father present may or may not be helpful to the child.

▶ ***Test-taking Tip:*** *Consider the developmental stages of the 4-year-old.*

Content Area: Child Health; *Category of Health Alteration:* Growth and Development; *Integrated Processes:* Nursing Process Assessment; *Client Need:* Psychosocial Integrity/Coping Mechanisms; *Cognitive Level:* Application

Reference: Pillitteri, A. (2007). *Maternal & Child Health Nursing: Care of the Childbearing & Childrearing Family* (5th ed., p. 900). Philadelphia: Lippincott Williams & Wilkins.

1124. A pediatric nurse is to perform a head-to-toe assessment on a toddler who is admitted to a hospital for nausea and vomiting. Which is most important for the nurse to consider before beginning the examination?

1. Making sure the parents are present
2. Using a firm tone to settle the child down for the examination
3. Waiting until the child is ready to cooperate
4. Preparing for a physical examination based on the child's developmental age

ANSWER: 4

The nurse should relate to the child based on the developmental age of the child. Considering the developmental level of the child will help the nurse to know how to proceed with the examination. Each individual family can decide which family members should be present. It may be perceived as threatening to the child to be told to settle down. Many times an assessment may have to be completed before a child is ready to cooperate.

▶ ***Test-taking Tip:*** *The key phrase is "most important to consider." Look for a key word in the correct options indicating that the nurse should "consider."*

Content Area: Child Health; *Category of Health Alteration:* Growth and Development; *Integrated Processes:* Nursing Process Planning; *Client Need:* Health Promotion and Maintenance/Growth and Development; *Cognitive Level:* Application

Reference: Hockenberry, M. (2005). *Wong's Essentials of Pediatric Nursing* (7th ed., p. 132). St. Louis, MO: Mosby.

1125. A nurse is assessing an infant for attachment behavior with a parent. Which observations are important in assessing this relationship? SELECT ALL THAT APPLY.

1. The kind of body contact between the parent and infant
2. If the parent is holding and cuddling the infant
3. The kind of comfort techniques being used by the parent
4. The comfort level of the parent while interacting with the baby
5. Whether the infant is crying

ANSWER: 1, 2, 3, 4

Body contact, holding and cuddling, comforting techniques, comfort in the interaction, and the infant's temperament can affect attachment. The infant and parents will both show an ability to interact if their relationship is healthy. The fact that the infant may be crying is not a sole indication of the relationship between the infant and the parent; however, the way the parent interacts with the crying infant is an indication of this relationship.

▶ ***Test-taking Tip:*** *Focus on behaviors that promote attachment.*

Content Area: Child Health; *Category of Health Alteration:* Growth and Development; *Integrated Processes:* Nursing Process Assessment; *Client Need:* Health Promotion and Maintenance/Developmental Stages and Transitions; *Cognitive Level:* Analysis

Reference: Hockenberry, M. (2005). *Wong's Essentials of Pediatric Nursing* (7th ed., p. 193). St. Louis, MO: Mosby.

1126. A nurse is preparing to consult with an adolescent being seen in a clinic. Which principle is most important for the nurse to consider when interacting with the client?

1. Avoid a straightforward approach because adolescents cannot fully process their health needs.
2. Reassure the teenager that it is unnecessary to answer all questions; however, before the examination is complete the client will need to provide all information.
3. Avoid conveying surprise over comments made by the client.
4. Because adolescents want to be treated as adults, the same cognitive information should be provided as if they were an adult.

ANSWER: 3

The adolescent needs the trust of the registered nurse (RN). If the RN appears surprised over comments or information provided, the client may not feel safe or valued and may not be forthright in giving information. It is important to provide honest, straightforward information to the client. There may be questions the client does not want to answer, and that is acceptable. Adolescents are not adults, and they should not be addressed in the same manner as adults.

➧ ***Test-taking Tip:*** *Apply knowledge of adolescent development.*

Content Area: Child Health; *Category of Health Alteration:* Growth and Development; *Integrated Processes:* Communication and Documentation; *Client Need:* Psychosocial Integrity/Therapeutic Communication; *Cognitive Level:* Application

Reference: Ball, J., & Bindler, R. (2006). *Child Health Nursing: Partnering with Children and Families* (p. 178). Upper Saddle River, NJ: Pearson/Prentice Hall.

1127. A nurse in a clinic is caring for a 16-year-old mother and her baby. The mother seems anxious about her new role as a mother. She looks at the nurse and says, "I don't think I can do this." What are some conclusions that the nurse might make about this situation? SELECT ALL THAT APPLY.

1. There may be a concern for postpartum depression.
2. This mother may be at risk for abandoning her baby.
3. An intervention could be providing information for the nearest safe house for the baby.
4. The mother should have been taught how to deal with this situation in prenatal classes.
5. The mother should be encouraged to give up the infant for adoption.

ANSWER: 1, 2, 3

This mother is at risk for postpartum depression and should be followed by a specialist if needed. This mother also may be at risk for abandoning her baby. There are many safe houses, such as emergency departments at hospitals, where a mother can leave her baby and not be held liable. Though information may have been presented in prenatal classes, there is no indication that the mother attended these. The nurse's role includes providing support and information to the mother about how to cope with a new baby and options if she decides to not keep her baby.

➧ ***Test-taking Tip:*** *The key word is "conclusions." Read each option to determine if it fits with the situation. Avoid reading into the situation.*

Content Area: Child Health; *Category of Health Alteration:* Growth and Development; *Integrated Processes:* Nursing Process Analysis; *Client Need:* Psychosocial Integrity/Crisis Intervention; *Cognitive Level:* Analysis

Reference: Ball, J., & Binder, R. (2006). *Clinical Handbook for Pediatric Nursing* (p. 226). Upper Saddle River, NJ: Pearson Education.

Test 29: **Child Health: Cardiovascular Management**

1128. A nurse is performing a physical assessment of a pediatric client. While auscultating the heart, the nurse hears physiological splitting of S_2 when the child takes a deep breath. Which action should be taken by the nurse?

1. Notify the provider of suspected atrial-septal defect.
2. Notify the provider of suspected pulmonary stenosis.
3. Follow institutional policy for initiating an emergency response.
4. Document the findings as a normal finding.

ANSWER: 4

The physiological splitting of S_2 on deep inspiration is normal in pediatric clients. Normally, the aortic valve closes just before the pulmonary valve, but the valves are so close together that the S_2 sound is uniform and instantaneous. When a person takes in a deep breath, the decrease in intrathoracic pressure increases venous return. The right atrium and ventricle then fill slightly more than usual. With the extra blood, the pulmonary valve stays open slightly longer than usual, and the normally small difference between aortic and pulmonary valve closure becomes a noticeable split S_2. If this occurs during normal respiration, it is abnormal and may indicate an atrial-septal defect or pulmonary stenosis. Initiating an emergency response is unnecessary because the findings are normal.

▶ ***Test-taking Tip:*** *Apply knowledge of normal assessment findings in pediatric clients. Recall that a split S_2 is normal in children if it occurs only during deep inspiration.*

Content Area: Child Health; *Category of Health Alteration:* Cardiovascular Management; *Integrated Processes:* Nursing Process Assessment; *Client Need:* Health Promotion and Maintenance/Growth and Development; *Cognitive Level:* Analysis

References: Berman, A., Snyder, S., Kozier, B., & Erb, G. (2008). *Kozier & Erb's Fundamentals of Nursing: Concepts, Process, and Practice* (8th ed., p. 624). Upper Saddle River, NJ: Pearson/Prentice Hall; Dillon, P. (2007). *Nursing Health Assessment: Clinical Pocket Guide* (2nd ed., p. 385). Philadelphia: F. A. Davis.

1129. A nurse assesses the pain level of a Native American pediatric client recovering from cardiac surgery. Knowing that Native American pediatric clients may not express pain, the nurse reviews the child's pulse and blood pressure readings following analgesic administration. Which finding should indicate to the nurse that the client's pain is not well-controlled?

1. Decreased heart rate and decreased blood pressure
2. Increased heart rate and increased blood pressure
3. Increased heart rate and decreased blood pressure
4. Decreased heart rate and increased blood pressure

ANSWER: 2

Increased heart rate and blood pressure may be indicative of postoperative pain in a pediatric client. A decreased heart rate and blood pressure could indicate that analgesics are effective for pain control. An increased heart rate and decreased blood pressure could be signs of bleeding. A decreased heart rate and increased blood pressure could be a sign of a neurological complication associated with cardiac surgery.

▶ ***Test-taking Tip:*** *Note that options 1 and 2 are opposites and 3 and 4 are opposites. First examine the options that are opposites and eliminate one or both of these.*

Content Area: Child Health; *Category of Health Alteration:* Cardiovascular Management; *Integrated Processes:* Nursing Process Evaluation; *Client Need:* Physiological Integrity/Reduction of Risk Potential/Vital Signs; Psychosocial Integrity/Cultural Diversity; *Cognitive Level:* Analysis

Reference: Berman, A., Snyder, S., Kozier, B., & Erb, G. (2008). *Kozier & Erb's Fundamentals of Nursing: Concepts, Process, and Practice* (8th ed., pp. 952, 1193–1194). Upper Saddle River, NJ: Pearson/Prentice Hall.

1130. An emergency department nurse is assessing a pediatric client suspected of having acute pericarditis. Which assessment finding should the nurse conclude supports the diagnosis of acute pericarditis?

1. Bilateral lower extremity pain
2. Pain on expiration
3. Pleural friction rub
4. Pericardial friction rub

ANSWER: 4

Inflammation of the pericardial sac from acute pericarditis produces a pericardial friction rub. Decreased perfusion to the extremities can cause extremity pain, but this does not occur with pericarditis. Pain on inspiration, not expiration, is present with pericarditis. The friction rub is pericardial, not pleural.

▶ ***Test-taking Tip:*** *Focus on the word "pericarditis." "Peri-" is around, "cardio-" pertains to the heart, and "-itis" is inflammation. Eliminate options 1, 2, and 3 because option 4 pertains to the heart.*

Content Area: Child Health; *Category of Health Alteration:* Cardiovascular Management; *Integrated Processes:* Nursing Process Assessment; *Client Need:* Physiological Integrity/Reduction in Risk Potential/System Specific Assessments; *Cognitive Level:* Analysis

Reference: Monahan, F., Sands, J., Neighbors, M., Marek, J., & Green, C. (2007). *Phipps' Medical-Surgical Nursing: Health and Illness Perspectives* (8th ed., p. 805). St. Louis, MO: Mosby/Elsevier.

1131. A new nurse is managing the care of a pediatric client preparing for a cardiac catheterization under the supervision of an experienced nurse. Which factor identified by the new nurse demonstrates an understanding of the information that can be collected during cardiac catheterization? SELECT ALL THAT APPLY

1. Oxygen saturation of blood within the chambers and great vessels
2. Pressure of blood flow within the heart chambers
3. Cardiac output (CO)
4. Anatomic abnormalities
5. Ankle brachial index (ABI)
6. Ejection fraction

ANSWER: 1, 2, 3, 4, 6

In cardiac catheterization, a small radiopaque catheter is passed through the major vein in the arm, leg, or neck into the heart. Blood specimens can be obtained to determine oxygen saturation levels, and contrast dye can be injected for angiography and to assess for anatomic abnormalities such as septal defects or obstruction of flow. Pressure of blood flow in the heart chambers, CO, stroke volume, and ejection fraction can be evaluated during the procedure. ABI is a ratio of the ankle systolic pressure to the arm systolic pressure and an objective measurement of arterial disease that quantifies the degree of stenosis. It is not related to a cardiac catheterization procedure.

➧ ***Test-taking Tip:*** *Apply knowledge of a cardiac catheterization procedure to answer this question. Eliminate the one option that is unrelated to a cardiac catheterization.*

Content Area: Child Health; *Category of Health Alteration:* Cardiovascular Management; *Integrated Processes:* Nursing Process Evaluation; *Client Need:* Safe and Effective Care Environment/ Management of Care/Supervision; *Cognitive Level:* Analysis

References: Hockenberry, M., & Wilson, D. (2007). *Wong's Nursing Care of Infants and Children* (8th ed., p. 1443). St. Louis, MO: Mosby/Elsevier; Pillitteri, A. (2007). *Maternal & Child Health Nursing: Care of the Childbearing & Childrearing Family* (5th ed., pp. 1286–1288). Philadelphia: Lippincott Williams & Wilkins.

1132. A nurse is interpreting an ECG rhythm strip for a 2-year-old child with heart failure secondary to a congenital heart defect. In analyzing the rhythm, the nurse notes the measurements of PR interval is 0.26 seconds, the QRS is 0.08 seconds, and the QT is 0.28. The ventricular rate is 126 bpm. A nurse interprets the rhythm as:

1. sinus bradycardia.
2. sinus rhythm with a bundle branch block.
3. sinus rhythm with a first-degree AV block.
4. sinus tachycardia with a first-degree AV block.

ANSWER: 3

The normal heart rate for a 2-year-old is 80 to 130 bpm. A normal PR interval measures 0.12 to 0.20 seconds. The QRS is normal (0.6 to 0.10 seconds), and the QT is rate dependent. If the rate is fast, the QT will be shorter. It is within the normal range for the ventricular rate. The ventricular rate in sinus bradycardia for a 2-year-old should be less than 80. In a bundle branch block, the QRS interval should be greater than or equal to 0.12 seconds. In sinus tachycardia, the ventricular rate should be greater than 130 bpm for a 2-year-old.

➧ ***Test-taking Tip:*** *In order to answer this question, knowledge of the normal ECG waveforms and the measurements is necessary. If this is unknown, then begin to eliminate options. The heart rate is normal for a 2-year-old. Eliminate options 1 and 4. This increases the chance of getting a right answer to 50%.*

Content Area: Child Health; *Category of Health Alteration:* Cardiovascular Management; *Integrated Processes:* Nursing Process Implementation; *Client Need:* Physiological Integrity/Physiological Adaptation/Hemodynamics; *Cognitive Level:* Analysis

Reference: Pillitteri, A. (2007). *Maternal & Child Health Nursing: Care of the Childbearing & Childrearing Family* (5th ed., pp. 1282–1283, 1814). Philadelphia: Lippincott Williams & Wilkins.

1133. A nurse is caring for a pediatric client who has congestive heart failure (CHF). The client is receiving digoxin therapy. Which laboratory test result is most important to evaluate when preparing to administer digoxin?

1. Serum potassium levels
2. Serum magnesium levels
3. Serum sodium levels
4. Serum chloride levels

ANSWER: 1

The serum potassium level is the most important result when preparing to administer digoxin. Hypokalemia increases the risk of digoxin toxicity and life-threatening dysrhythmias. Though important, magnesium, sodium, and chloride levels are not as essential.

➧ ***Test-taking Tip:*** *Think of the electrolyte that would have the greatest effect on the heart. Applying knowledge of basic pharmacological principles will direct you to the correct response.*

Content Area: Child Health; *Category of Health Alteration:* Cardiovascular Management; *Integrated Processes:* Nursing Process Planning; *Client Need:* Physiological Integrity/Pharmacological and Parenteral Therapies/Medication Administration; Physiological Integrity/Reduction of Risk Potential/Laboratory Values; *Cognitive Level:* Application

References: Hockenberry, M., & Wilson, D. (2007). *Wong's Nursing Care of Infants and Children* (8th ed., p. 1451). St. Louis, MO: Mosby/Elsevier; Pillitteri, A. (2007). *Maternal & Child Health Nursing: Care of the Childbearing & Childrearing Family* (5th ed., p. 1309). Philadelphia: Lippincott Williams & Wilkins.

1134. EBP A nurse is caring for a pediatric client recently diagnosed with hypertension. Which diagnostic tests should the nurse anticipate being ordered for this client? SELECT ALL THAT APPLY.

1. Complete blood count (CBC)
2. Serum chemistry
3. Renal ultrasound
4. Drug screen
5. Glucose tolerance test (GTT)

ANSWER: 1, 2, 3, 4

The nurse should anticipate that a CBC, serum chemistry, renal ultrasound, and drug screen may be ordered for this client. A CBC would be important to rule out anemia and a serum chemistry to evaluate for altered blood urea nitrogen, creatinine, and electrolytes, which could be consistent with chronic renal disease secondary to hypertension. A renal ultrasound may help identify a renal scar, congenital anomaly, or disparate renal size. Drug screening is important to identify substances associated with hypertension. If a metabolic condition such as diabetes mellitus is suspected as a causative factor, a fasting serum glucose level should be drawn and, based on the test results, the need for a GTT should be determined.

➧ ***Test-taking Tip:*** *Use the process of elimination, ruling out the one test in which a screening test should be performed first.*

Content Area: Child Health; *Category of Health Alteration:* Cardiovascular Management; *Integrated Processes:* Nursing Process Planning; *Client Need:* Physiological Integrity/Reduction of Risk Potential/Diagnostic Tests; *Cognitive Level:* Analysis

Reference: Hockenberry, M., & Wilson, D. (2007). *Wong's Nursing Care of Infants and Children* (8th ed., p. 1487). St. Louis, MO: Mosby/Elsevier.

EBP Reference: Luma, G., & Spiotta, R. (2006). Hypertension in children and adolescents. *American Academy of Family Physicians,* 73(9), 1558–1568.

1135. A nurse is preparing to perform an electrocardiogram (ECG) on several pediatric clients. Which client would not benefit from an ECG?

1. A 4-year-old with tachycardia
2. A 3-year-old with bradycardia
3. A 10-year-old with an irregular pulse
4. An infant with a splitting of the S_2 heart sound only when the infant takes a deep breath

ANSWER: 4

An infant with a splitting of the S_2 heart sound when the child takes a deep breath would not benefit from an ECG because it is a normal finding in infants and young children. ECG is useful in diagnosing tachycardia, bradycardia, and irregular pulses. These rhythms can be recorded through an ECG.

➧ ***Test-taking Tip:*** *Note that three options are similar and one is different. Often the option that is different is the answer.*

Content Area: Child Health; *Category of Health Alteration:* Cardiovascular Management; *Integrated Processes:* Nursing Process Implementation; *Client Need:* Physiological Integrity/Reduction of Risk Potential/Diagnostic Tests; *Cognitive Level:* Analysis

References: Monahan, F., Sands, J., Neighbors, M., Marek, J., & Green, C. (2007). *Phipps' Medical-Surgical Nursing: Health and Illness Perspectives* (8th ed., p. 733). St. Louis, MO: Mosby/Elsevier; Pillitteri, A. (2007). *Maternal & Child Health Nursing: Care of the Childbearing & Childrearing Family* (5th ed., p. 1315). Philadelphia: Lippincott Williams & Wilkins.

1136. Which method should a nurse use to assess the arterial oxygen saturation of a pediatric client?

1. Finger pulse oximetry
2. Arterial blood gases
3. Hemoglobin levels
4. Peak flow

ANSWER: 1

Finger pulse oximetry should be used to assess the arterial oxygen saturation of a pediatric client. Finger pulse oximetry is a noninvasive measure of arterial oxygen saturation. The hemoglobin absorbs light waves from the sensor on the device. Because the hemoglobin absorbs light waves differently when it is bound to oxygen than when it is not, the oximeter can detect the degree of oxygen saturation in the hemoglobin. When the oxygen saturation is 95%, the Po_2 is in the normal range of 80 to 100 mm Hg. Arterial blood gases are invasive, involving an arterial puncture. The hemoglobin level measures the amount of oxygen-carrying protein in the blood. Peak flow determines the amount of airflow through the bronchi.

▶ ***Test-taking Tip:** If appropriate, noninvasive methods are the best choice when caring for pediatric clients. Focus on the noninvasive methods and eliminate the other options. Of the two remaining options, decide which is best for determining the arterial oxygen saturation.*

Content Area: Child Health; *Category of Health Alteration:* Cardiovascular Management; *Integrated Processes:* Nursing Process Assessment; *Client Need:* Physiological Integrity/Reduction of Risk Potential/Laboratory Values; *Cognitive Level:* Application

References: Monahan, F., Sands, J., Neighbors, M., Marek, J., & Green, C. (2007). *Phipps' Medical-Surgical Nursing: Health and Illness Perspectives* (8th ed., pp. 574–575). St. Louis, MO: Mosby/Elsevier; Pillitteri, A. (2007). *Maternal & Child Health Nursing: Care of the Childbearing & Childrearing Family* (5th ed., p. 1230). Philadelphia: Lippincott Williams & Wilkins.

1137. A nurse documented a nursing outcome of oxygen saturation (SaO_2) greater than 95% for a pediatric client diagnosed with heart failure. When the nurse obtains a SaO_2 value of 90%, the nurse determines that the outcome was not achieved and intervenes by administering oxygen. The nurse's intervention is based on the nurse's knowledge that the 90% SaO_2 value indicates a Pao_2 value of:

1. 40 mm Hg.
2. 60 mm Hg.
3. 80 mm Hg.
4. 90 mm Hg.

ANSWER: 2

When the Sao_2 value drops to 90%, the Pao_2 value is 60 mm Hg. A Pao_2 value of 40 mm Hg is too low. When the SaO_2 is 95%, the Pao_2 is in the normal range of 80 to 100 mm Hg.

▶ ***Test-taking Tip:** Remember the relationship of SaO_2 to Pao_2 is the 60 to 30 and 90 to 60 rule. When the SaO_2 is 60 mm, the Pao_2 is 30; when the SaO_2 is 90, the Pao_2 is 60.*

Content Area: Child Health; *Category of Health Alteration:* Cardiovascular Management; *Integrated Processes:* Nursing Process Evaluation; *Client Need:* Physiological Integrity/Physiological Adaptation/Illness Management; *Cognitive Level:* Application

References: Monahan, F., Sands, J., Neighbors, M., Marek, J., & Green, C. (2007). *Phipps' Medical-Surgical Nursing: Health and Illness Perspectives* (8th ed., pp. 574–575). St. Louis, MO: Mosby/Elsevier; Pillitteri, A. (2007). *Maternal & Child Health Nursing: Care of the Childbearing & Childrearing Family* (5th ed., p. 1230). Philadelphia: Lippincott Williams & Wilkins.

1138. **EBP** A school nurse is educating school-aged children on modifiable risk factors for coronary artery disease (CAD). Which modifiable risk factors should the nurse include in the presentation? SELECT ALL THAT APPLY.

1. Diabetes mellitus
2. Hypertension
3. Age
4. Family history
5. Sedentary lifestyle
6. Obesity

ANSWER: 1, 2, 5, 6

Diabetes mellitus, hypertension, sedentary lifestyle, and obesity are modifiable risk factors for CAD. While age and family are risk factors, they are nonmodifiable.

▶ ***Test-taking Tip:** The words "modifiable risk factors" and "CAD" are the key words in the stem.*

Content Area: Child Health; *Category of Health Alteration:* Cardiovascular Management; *Integrated Processes:* Teaching and Learning; *Client Need:* Health Promotion and Maintenance/Health Promotion and Disease Prevention; *Cognitive Level:* Application

Reference: Monahan, F., Sands, J., Neighbors, M., Marek, J., & Green, C. (2007). *Phipps' Medical-Surgical Nursing: Health and Illness Perspectives* (8th ed., pp. 746–747). St. Louis, MO: Mosby/Elsevier.

EBP Reference: Paridon, S., Alpert, B., Boas, S., Cabrera, M., Caldarera, L., et al. (2006). Clinical stress testing in the pediatric age group: A statement from the American Heart Association Council on Cardiovascular Disease in the Young, Committee on Atherosclerosis, Hypertension, and Obesity in Youth. *Circulation,* 113(15), 1905–1920.

1139. A nurse is taking a history on an adolescent client who has a new onset of hypertension. The nurse is aware that a history of substance abuse may contribute to this condition and questions the adolescent. Which abused substances acknowledged by the adolescent could contribute to hypertension? SELECT ALL THAT APPLY.

1. Amphetamines
2. Cocaine
3. Hallucinogens
4. Alcohol
5. Ecstasy
6. Marijuana

ANSWER: 1, 2, 3, 5, 6

Amphetamines, cocaine, hallucinogens, ecstasy, and marijuana may cause hypertension. Cocaine is a powerful vasoconstrictor that can lead to hypertension. Amphetamines and ecstasy (3, 4-methylenedioxymethamphetamine) are powerful sympathetic stimulants that may mimic the action of cocaine. Hallucinogens, such as LSD and PCP, will also often cause hypertension through autonomic stimulation. Alcohol is a depressant and is the least likely to contribute to new-onset hypertension.

➧ ***Test-taking Tip:*** *The words "hypertension" and "substance abuse" are the key words in the stem. Apply knowledge of the effects of each substance.*

Content Area: Child Health; *Category of Health Alteration:* Cardiovascular Management; *Integrated Processes:* Nursing Process Assessment; *Client Need:* Physiological Integrity/Reduction of Risk Potential/Vital Signs; *Cognitive Level:* Analysis

Reference: Hockenberry, M., & Wilson, D. (2007). *Wong's Nursing Care of Infants and Children* (8th ed., pp. 901–902). St. Louis, MO: Mosby/Elsevier.

1140. A nurse is educating the parents of a pediatric client with a cardiovascular disorder in preparation for home electrocardiogram (ECG) monitoring. The nurse uses a picture to explain the different components of a normal ECG tracing. Place an X on the illustration where the nurse should be pointing when explaining repolarization of the ventricles.

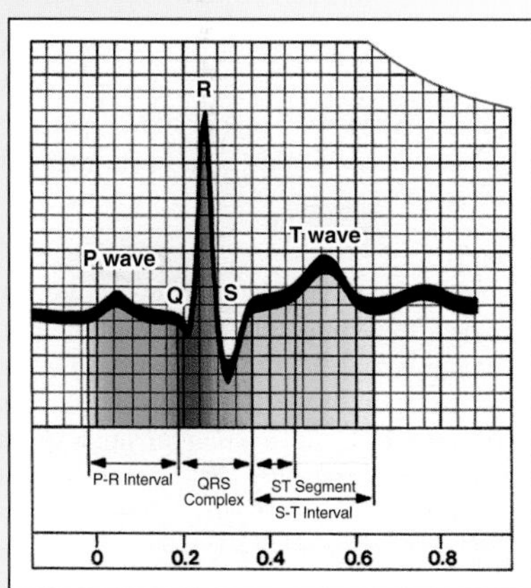

ANSWER:

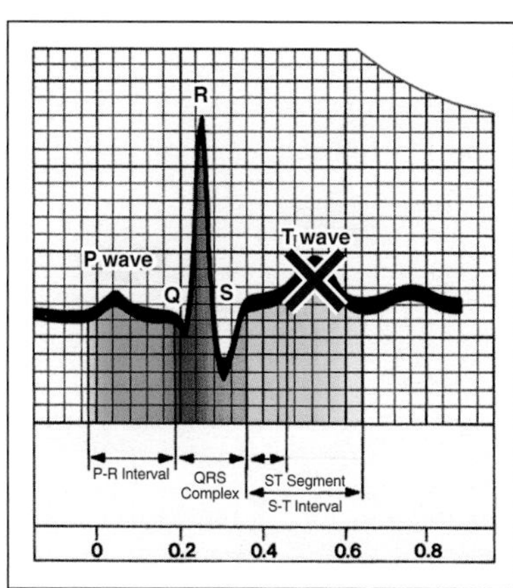

The T wave represents repolarization of the ventricles. Repolarization is the process whereby the cell is polarized again with positive charges on the outer surface and negative charges on the inner surface.

➧ ***Test-taking Tip:*** *Recall that the QRS represents ventricular depolarization. The next waveform would be repolarization.*

Content Area: Child Health; *Category of Health Alteration:* Cardiovascular Management; *Integrated Processes:* Teaching and Learning; *Client Need:* Physiological Integrity/Physiological Adaptation/Hemodynamics; *Cognitive Level:* Analysis

Reference: Smeltzer, S., Bare, B., Hinkle, J., & Cheever, K. (2010). *Brunner and Suddarth's Textbook of Medical-Surgical Nursing* (12th ed., p. 724). Philadelphia: Lippincott Williams & Wilkins.

1141. A nurse is caring for a pediatric client immediately following a permanent pacemaker placement. Which intervention should be the nurse's first priority for this client?

1. Initiate continuous electrocardiogram (ECG) monitoring.
2. Administer only non-narcotic analgesic medications to avoiding masking signs and symptoms of complications.
3. Transport the child to the radiology department for a chest x-ray.
4. Administer antibiotic therapy to prevent infection.

ANSWER: 1

The nurse's first priority should be to initiate continuous ECG monitoring. Continuous ECG monitoring during the recovery phase is important to assess pacemaker function immediately following placement. Analgesics, including narcotics, are administered as needed to control pain. A chest x-ray is performed within 24 hours for future comparison, but it is not the priority. While the nurse should carefully monitor the site for signs of infection; prophylactic antibiotic therapy is not the priority.

▶ ***Test-taking Tip:*** *Use the ABCs (airway, breathing, circulation) to establish priority. Recall that the pacemaker initiates an impulse to stimulate the electrical conduction of a person's heart.*

Content Area: Child Health; *Category of Health Alteration:* Cardiovascular Management; *Integrated Processes:* Nursing Process Implementation; *Client Need:* Safe and Effective Care Environment/ Management of Care/Establishing Priorities; *Cognitive Level:* Analysis

Reference: Hockenberry, M., & Wilson, D. (2007). *Wong's Nursing Care of Infants and Children* (8th ed., p. 1494). St. Louis, MO: Mosby/Elsevier.

1142. The parents of a pediatric client report that their child is experiencing palpitations, dizziness, diaphoresis, and chest pain. The client is diagnosed with supraventricular tachycardia (SVT). A nurse instructs the parents on techniques to reverse future episodes of SVT. Which technique stated by a parent indicates further teaching is needed?

1. Wrap the child's head with a cold, wet towel.
2. Massage the child's carotid arteries bilaterally.
3. Have the child perform the Valsalva's maneuver.
4. Administer medications after taking the child's pulse for 1 full minute.

ANSWER: 2

Further teaching is needed when a parent states to bilaterally massage the carotid arteries. This should not be employed to reverse SVT because it may restrict blood flow. Massaging the carotid arteries unilaterally, however, is a technique used to convert SVT and should be included in the teaching plan. Wrapping the child's head with a cold, wet towel, having the child perform the Valsalva's maneuver (bearing down), and taking the pulse prior to administering medications are techniques that the nurse should teach the parents to use when symptoms of SVT are present because these can potentially convert the SVT rhythm to a sinus rhythm.

▶ ***Test-taking Tip:*** *Read each option carefully. Think about how each option will affect the SVT rhythm as well as blood flow to the brain.*

Content Area: Child Health; *Category of Health Alteration:* Cardiovascular Management; *Integrated Processes:* Teaching and Learning; Nursing Process Evaluation; *Client Need:* Physiological Integrity/Physiological Adaptation/Hemodynamics; *Cognitive Level:* Application

Reference: Hockenberry, M., & Wilson, D. (2007). *Wong's Nursing Care of Infants and Children* (8th ed., p. 1494). St. Louis, MO: Mosby/Elsevier.

1143. EBP A nurse is taking the health and social history of an adolescent client experiencing episodes of palpitations. Which components of the social history could contribute to the palpitations? SELECT ALL THAT APPLY.

1. Alcohol intake
2. Sexual history
3. Nicotine use
4. Caffeine intake
5. A sports injury to the chest

ANSWER: 1, 3, 4, 5

Alcohol, nicotine, and caffeine could contribute to the palpitations. Nicotine and caffeine are stimulants that increase the heart rate. Although alcohol is a depressant, it has been shown to be linked with supraventricular tachycardia (SVT) and heart palpitations because it irritates the cardiac muscle. Chest trauma during a sports event can induce dysrhythmias. A sexual history is an important part of the social history, although it does not likely contribute to the client experiencing palpitations.

▶ ***Test-taking Tip:*** *Use knowledge of the physical effects of alcohol, nicotine, caffeine, and trauma. Use the process of elimination to select the correct options.*

Content Area: Child Health; *Category of Health Alteration:* Cardiovascular Management; *Integrated Processes:* Nursing Process Assessment; *Client Need:* Physiological Integrity/Reduction in Risk Potential/Potential for Alterations in Body Systems; *Cognitive Level:* Application

Reference: Pillitteri, A. (2007). *Maternal & Child Health Nursing: Care of the Childbearing & Childrearing Family* (5th ed., p. 1315). Philadelphia: Lippincott Williams & Wilkins.

EBP Reference: Drezner, J., Courson, R., Roberts, W., Mosesso, V., Link, M., et al. (2007). Inter-association task force recommendations on emergency preparedness and management of sudden cardiac arrest in high school and college athletic programs: A consensus statement. *Journal of Athletic Training,* 42(1), 143–158.

1144. A hospitalized preterm infant diagnosed with tetralogy of Fallot is experiencing a hypercyanotic spell. Which actions should be taken by the nurse? SELECT ALL THAT APPLY.

1. Place the infant in a knee-chest position.
2. Administer 2 L of oxygen via nasal cannula.
3. Administer intramuscular morphine sulphate.
4. Use a calm and comforting approach.
5. Administer oral propranolol (Inderal®).
6. Prepare for emergency surgery.

ANSWER: 1, 3, 4, 5

During a hypercyanotic episode, the infant becomes hypoxic and should be placed in a knee-chest position. This traps blood in the lower extremities and keeps the heart from being overwhelmed. Morphine sulfate decreases preload and afterload. A calm approach is also useful in settling the infant and decreasing the infant's oxygen demand. Propranolol may be given to aid pulmonary artery dilation. The infant should receive 100% oxygen via face mask in this condition. Emergency surgery is delayed for preterm infants. However, if the episodes increase, a temporary or palliative surgical repair can be done to create a shunt between the aorta and the pulmonary artery to enable blood to leave the aorta, enter the pulmonary artery, oxygenate the lungs, and return to the left side of the heart, the aorta, and the body.

➧ ***Test-taking Tip:*** *Applying basic knowledge of nursing care during a hypercyanotic spell in an infant will direct you to the correct responses.*

Content Area: Child Health; *Category of Health Alteration:* Cardiovascular Management; *Integrated Processes:* Nursing Process Implementation; *Client Need:* Physiological Integrity/Physiological Adaptation/Medical Emergencies; *Cognitive Level:* Application

References: Hockenberry, M., & Wilson, D. (2007). *Wong's Nursing Care of Infants and Children* (8th ed., p. 1458). St. Louis, MO: Mosby/Elsevier; Pillitteri, A. (2007). *Maternal & Child Health Nursing: Care of the Childbearing & Childrearing Family* (5th ed., pp. 1304–1305). Philadelphia: Lippincott Williams & Wilkins.

1145. A nurse is using a picture to educate the parents of a child with a congenital murmur about the etiology of the condition. The nurse demonstrates the location of the tricuspid valve. Place an X on the valve that the nurse is locating for the child's parents.

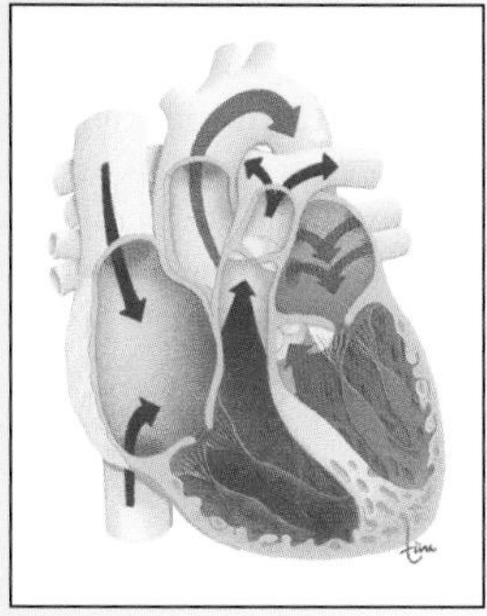

ANSWER:

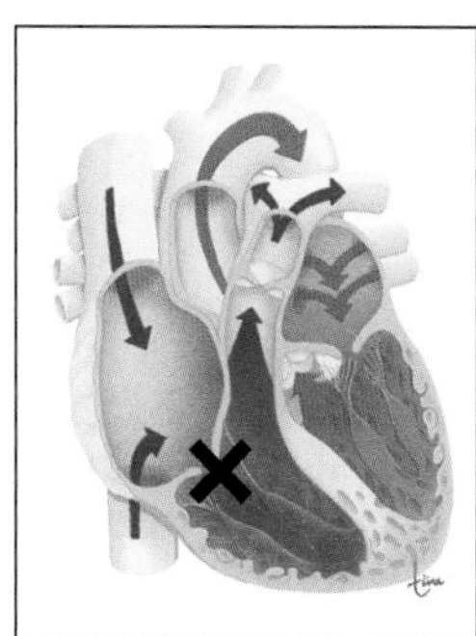

Blood is pumped from the right atrium to the right ventricle through the tricuspid valve. Backflow (regurgitation) or stenosis may result in a murmur.

➧ ***Test-taking Tip:*** *Apply basic knowledge of the anatomy and physiology of the heart to identify the tricuspid valve. A mnemonic for recalling the valves and the abnormal finding is APTM: **A**ll **P**oint **T**o a **M**urmur. The letters signify the heart valves: A is for aortic, P for pulmonic, T for tricuspid, and M for mitral.*

Content Area: Child Health; *Category of Health Alteration:* Cardiovascular Management; *Integrated Processes:* Teaching and Learning; *Client Need:* Physiological Integrity/Reduction in Risk Potential/Potential for Alterations in Body Systems; *Cognitive Level:* Application

Reference: Smeltzer, S., Bare, B., Hinkle, J., & Cheever, K. (2008). *Brunner and Suddarth's Textbook of Medical-Surgical Nursing* (11th ed., p. 782). Philadelphia: Lippincott Williams & Wilkins.

1146. EBP A nurse is managing the care of an infant with an unrepaired heart defect. Which health promotion strategy should the nurse recommend to the parent in planning for discharge?

1. Vaccinate against the respiratory syncytial virus (RSV) monthly during the RSV season.
2. Restrict the child's level of physical activity.
3. Encourage weight loss by restricting caloric intake.
4. Delay immunizations as the child's immune system may be too impaired.

ANSWER: 1

RSV vaccine is administered monthly during RSV season to infants with unrepaired heart defects. Children generally do not need to restrict activity and, in most cases, are anorexic and require high-nutrient foods. Infants should receive scheduled childhood immunizations according to current guidelines.

▶ ***Test-taking Tip:*** *Note the key words "health promotion." Eliminate options 2 and 3 because these are illness interventions and option 4 because without immunizations illness can occur.*

Content Area: Child Health; *Category of Health Alteration:* Cardiovascular Management; *Integrated Processes:* Teaching and Learning; *Client Need:* Physiological Integrity/Physiological Adaptation/Illness Management; *Cognitive Level:* Analysis

EBP Reference: Feltes, T. (2007). Palivizumab and the prevention of respiratory synctial viral illness. *Expert Opinion on Biological Therapy, 7*(9), 1471–1480.

1147. A pediatric nurse is providing discharge instructions to the parents of an infant with a history of hypoxemia. The nurse teaches the parents about the signs and symptoms associated with hypoxemia. Which signs or symptoms should prompt the parents to notify the practitioner immediately?

1. Weight loss or gain
2. Excessive crying
3. Dehydration and respiratory infection
4. Not achieving developmental milestones

ANSWER: 3

Hypoxemia is decreased oxygen concentration of arterial blood. Dehydration can increase the risk of stroke in hypoxemic children. Respiratory infection may compromise pulmonary function and increase an infant's hypoxemia. Weight changes, excessive crying, or concerns over developmental milestones should be reported to the practitioner but often are not immediate concerns.

▶ ***Test-taking Tip:*** *If unsure of the term hypoxemic, break the word down. "Oxy-" means oxygen, and "-emia" pertains to blood. "Hypo-" refers to low. Of the options, only 2 and 3 potentially affect oxygenation. Select option 3 because it is the most severe.*

Content Area: Child Health; *Category of Health Alteration:* Cardiovascular Management; *Integrated Processes:* Teaching and Learning; *Client Need:* Physiological Integrity/Physiological Adaptation/Illness Management; *Cognitive Level:* Application

Reference: Hockenberry, M., & Wilson, D. (2007). *Wong's Nursing Care of Infants and Children* (8th ed., p. 1459). St. Louis, MO: Mosby/Elsevier.

1148. A nurse is managing the care of a pediatric client in congestive heart failure (CHF). Which medically delegated interventions should be included in the care of the client? SELECT ALL THAT APPLY.

1. Oral positive inotropic agents
2. Diuretics
3. ACE inhibitors
4. Hypolipidemic agents
5. Oral positive chronotropic agents
6. Beta blockers

ANSWER: 1, 2, 3, 6

Therapeutic management of a client with congestive heart failure may include oral positive inotropic agents, diuretics, ACE inhibitors, and beta blockers. Positive inotropic agents increase the strength of muscular contraction. Diuretics increase urine excretion and reduce volume overload. ACE inhibitors (antihypertensive agents) relax arteries and promote renal excretion of salt and water by inhibiting the activity of an angiotensin-converting enzyme. Beta blockers decrease the workload of the heart by decreasing the amount of pressure against which it has to pump. Hypolipidemic agents are not standard management of CHF for pediatric clients. These agents are used to treat hyperlipidemia (elevated cholesterol and triglycerides), which contribute to coronary artery disease. Positive chronotropic agents will increase the heart rate.

▶ ***Test-taking Tip:*** *Recall that heart failure is inability of the heart to pump enough blood to meet the body's demand for energy. Select options that decrease the workload of the heart and improve cardiac output.*

Content Area: Child Health; *Category of Health Alteration:* Cardiovascular Management; *Integrated Processes:* Nursing Process Intervention; *Client Need:* Physiological Integrity/Physiological Adaptation/Illness Management; *Cognitive Level:* Application

Reference: Hockenberry, M., & Wilson, D. (2007). *Wong's Nursing Care of Infants and Children* (8th ed., pp. 1449–1450). St. Louis, MO: Mosby/Elsevier.

1149. A nurse is planning the care of a pediatric client with congenital heart disease. For which specific complications related to congenital heart disease should the nurse plan to monitor the client?

1. Congestive heart failure and pulmonary hypotension
2. Congestive heart failure and hypoxemia
3. Hypoxemia and pulmonary hypotension
4. Pulmonary hypotension and cyanosis

ANSWER: 2

Clients with congenital heart disease are at risk for developing congestive heart failure and hypoxemia. Congenital heart disease lessens the effectiveness of the heart's pumping action (heart failure), causing blood pooling in the heart or in the pulmonary circulation. Hypoxemia results when the blood is inadequately oxygenated. Pulmonary hypertension, not hypotension, is another possible complication.

➧ ***Test-taking Tip:*** *Use the process of elimination and eliminate options 1, 3, and 4 because pulmonary hypotension appears in each of these options.*

Content Area: Child Health; *Category of Health Alteration:* Cardiovascular Management; *Integrated Processes:* Nursing Process Planning; *Client Need:* Physiological Integrity/Reduction of Risk Potential/Potential for Alterations in Body Systems; *Cognitive Level:* Analysis

Reference: Hockenberry, M., & Wilson, D. (2007). *Wong's Nursing Care of Infants and Children* (8th ed., p. 1447). St. Louis, MO: Mosby/Elsevier.

1150. A pediatric client presents with tachycardia, edema, dyspnea, orthopnea, and crackles. A nurse performs a physical assessment of the client and notifies a physician immediately. Which condition does the nurse most likely suspect?

1. Right-sided heart failure
2. Rheumatic fever
3. Kawasaki disease
4. Left-sided heart failure

ANSWER: 4

The nurse suspects that the client has left-sided heart failure. A child in left-sided heart failure will present with pulmonary symptoms of dyspnea, orthopnea, and crackles because of the fluid accumulation in the lungs from the ineffective pumping action of the heart. In right-sided heart failure, the child would present with jugular venous distention, liver enlargement, splenomegaly, or ascites due to a reduced preload to the right side of the heart. In rheumatic fever, the child would present with an elevated temperature and a systolic murmur, mitral insufficiency, and a prolonged PR and QT interval. In Kawasaki disease, the child would present with fever, rash, and lymph node enlargement.

➧ ***Test-taking Tip:*** *Options 1 and 4 are opposites, so one of these is incorrect. Focus on the client's symptoms and cardiac anatomy and physiology to select the correct option.*

Content Area: Child Health; *Category of Health Alteration:* Cardiovascular Management; *Integrated Processes:* Nursing Process Assessment; *Client Need:* Physiological Integrity/Reduction of Risk Potential/System Specific Assessment; *Cognitive Level:* Analysis

Reference: Pillitteri, A. (2007). *Maternal & Child Health Nursing: Care of the Childbearing & Childrearing Family* (5th ed., pp. 1305–1313). Philadelphia: Lippincott Williams & Wilkins.

1151. A nurse is providing discharge teaching to the parents of a pediatric client following cardiac surgery. Which information should the nurse include in the discharge teaching? SELECT ALL THAT APPLY.

1. Action and side effects of medications
2. Care of the incision and circumstances in which to contact the health-care provider
3. Activity restrictions and follow-up appointments
4. Age-appropriate diet with vitamin C to promote wound healing
5. Prevention of pericarditis following dental procedures and prophylactic antibiotic use

ANSWER: 1, 2, 3, 4

Discharge teaching would include medications, wound care, activity, appointments, dietary guidance, and circumstances in which to contact the health-care provider. Discharge instructions should include the importance of prophylactic antibiotic therapy prior to dental procedures to prevent bacterial endocarditis (not pericarditis).

➧ *Test-taking Tip: Read the question carefully and consider each answer option. Look for key words in an option that makes it incorrect and eliminate that option.*

Content Area: Child Health; *Category of Health Alteration:* Cardiovascular Management; *Integrated Processes:* Teaching and Learning; *Client Need:* Physiological Integrity/Physiological Adaptation/ Illness Management; *Cognitive Level:* Application

Reference: Hockenberry, M., & Wilson, D. (2007). *Wong's Nursing Care of Infants and Children* (8th ed., p. 1477). St. Louis, MO: Mosby/Elsevier.

1152. A pediatric nurse evaluates that a nursing assistant knows emergency procedures when the nursing assistant activated the emergency response system for a 6-year-old child admitted with a diagnosis of heart failure. The sign observed by the nurse indicating that lifesaving measures were necessary likely was:

1. gagging.
2. coughing.
3. inability to speak.
4. heart rate of 125 bpm.

ANSWER: 3

A 6-year-old child should be able to speak. Inability suggests that the airway is compromised. Lifesaving measures are needed to clear the airway of an obstruction. Gagging indicates a patent airway, and coughing indicates that air is being exchanged. In both situations the child should be observed for possible vomiting or signs that the airway is compromised. The nurse should be notified, but the emergency response system does not need to be activated. The heart rate is a little high for a 6-year-old. The nurse should be notified, but the emergency response system does not need to be activated.

➧ *Test-taking Tip: Use the ABCs (airway, breathing, circulation) to establish priority. Absence of the ability to speak in a child likely indicates an airway problem.*

Content Area: Child Health; *Category of Health Alteration:* Cardiovascular Management; *Integrated Processes:* Nursing Process Evaluation; *Client Need:* Safe and Effective Care Environment/ Management of Care/Supervision; *Cognitive Level:* Analysis

Reference: Lewis, S., Heitkemper, M., Dirkson, S., O'Brien, P., & Bucher, L. (2007). *Medical-Surgical Nursing: Assessment and Management of Clinical Problems* (7th ed., p. 838). St. Louis, MO: Mosby/Elsevier.

1153. A nurse is suctioning a pediatric client who has just had cardiac surgery. The nurse observes tachypnea, the use of accessory muscles to breathe, and restlessness. Which action should be taken by the nurse?

1. Continue suctioning, as these are expected during the procedure.
2. Continue suctioning, but monitor closely as these could be signs of distress.
3. Discontinue suctioning, carefully monitor the client, and notify the physician immediately.
4. Discontinue suctioning and notify the physician to insert a chest tube.

ANSWER: 3

Because tachypnea, using accessory muscles to breathe, and restlessness are signs of hypoxia, suctioning should be discontinued, the client carefully monitored, and the physician notified immediately. Continuing with the suctioning further removes oxygen and can worsen the child's status. The child's status should be monitored, but there is no indication that a lung has collapsed; inserting a chest tube should not be indicated.

➧ *Test-taking Tip: Focus on the client's symptoms that indicate hypoxia and then select the option that is safest for the client.*

Content Area: Child Health; *Category of Health Alteration:* Cardiovascular Management; *Integrated Processes:* Nursing Process Implementation; *Client Need:* Safe and Effective Care Environment/ Safety and Infection Control/Safe Use of Equipment; *Cognitive Level:* Analysis

Reference: Hockenberry, M., & Wilson, D. (2007). *Wong's Nursing Care of Infants and Children* (8th ed., p. 1473). St. Louis, MO: Mosby/Elsevier.

1154. The parent of a child diagnosed with rheumatic heart disease questions the nurse following the doctor's statement that the child has a heart murmur. The nurse explains that a heart murmur is an abnormal or extra heart sound produced by which malfunctioning structure of the heart?

1. Heart valve
2. Heart vessel
3. Heart chamber
4. Heart conduction

ANSWER: 1

A heart murmur is an abnormal or extra heart sound caused by an incomplete closure of the heart valve. In rheumatic fever, the heart valves are damaged by an abnormal response by the immune system. Erosion of the valves makes them leaky and inefficient, and a murmur of backflowing blood will be heard. A malfunctioning vessel, chamber, or conduction would not produce a heart murmur but would likely affect blood flow, contractility, or cardiac rhythm.

Test-taking Tip: *Apply knowledge of anatomy and physiology to answer this question.*

Content Area: Child Health; *Category of Health Alteration:* Cardiovascular Management; *Integrated Processes:* Teaching and Learning; *Client Need:* Physiological Integrity/Reduction in Risk Potential/Potential for Alterations in Body Systems; *Cognitive Level:* Application

Reference: Pillitteri, A. (2007). *Maternal & Child Health Nursing: Care of the Childbearing & Childrearing Family* (5th ed., pp. 1311–1312). Philadelphia: Lippincott Williams & Wilkins.

1155. EBP A nurse is caring for a child who has liver enlargement secondary to infectious endocarditis. For which associated cardiac condition should the nurse assess the client?

1. Dysrhythmia
2. Right-sided heart failure
3. Myocardial infarction (MI)
4. Tetralogy of Fallot

ANSWER: 2

The nurse should assess for the presence of right-sided heart failure. Back pressure in the portal circulation occurs in right-sided heart failure. Dysrhythmias may occur due to impaired cardiac function. Chest pain, dyspnea, and dysrhythmias would be initial signs of a MI. Tetralogy of Fallot occurs as a result of the malformation of the right ventricular infundibulum, which can lead to heart failure.

Test-taking Tip: *The key word is liver enlargement. Visualize each of the conditions presented to determine which is likely to result in back pressure and fluid accumulation in the liver.*

Content Area: Child Health; *Category of Health Alteration:* Cardiovascular Management; *Integrated Processes:* Nursing Process Assessment; *Client Need:* Physiological Integrity/Physiological Adaptation/Pathophysiology; *Cognitive Level:* Analysis

Reference: Pillitteri, A. (2007). *Maternal & Child Health Nursing: Care of the Childbearing & Childrearing Family* (5th ed., pp. 1304–1306). Philadelphia: Lippincott Williams & Wilkins.

EBP Reference: Spektor, M., & Pflieger, K. (2006). Tetralogy of Fallot. *E-Medicine by WebMD*. Available at: www.emedicine.com/EMERG/topic575.htm

---

1156. A school nurse assesses a child who was stung by an insect and is beginning to exhibit signs of distress. The nurse is aware of the child's severe allergy to bee stings and immediately contacts emergency medical services (EMS). Which assessment finding reported to the EMS personnel should be questioned?

1. Signs of airway obstruction
2. Bronchospasm
3. Hypertension
4. Weak thready pulse

ANSWER: 3

Life-threatening reactions may begin within 5 to 10 minutes after a bee sting. The report of hypertension should be questioned because hypotension, and not hypertension, occurs with anaphylactic shock. Signs of airway obstruction secondary to laryngeal edema, bronchospasm, and cardiovascular collapse are signs of anaphylaxis due to immunological mechanisms and the toxin's effect in stimulating mast cells.

Test-taking Tip: *The key word is "questioned." Select the option that is not typically seen in an anaphylactic reaction.*

Content Area: Child Health; *Category of Health Alteration:* Cardiovascular Management; *Integrated Processes:* Nursing Process Intervention; *Client Need:* Physiological Integrity/Physiological Adaptation/Illness Management; *Cognitive Level:* Analysis

Reference: Hockenberry, M., & Wilson, D. (2007). *Wong's Nursing Care of Infants and Children* (8th ed., p. 787). St. Louis, MO: Mosby/Elsevier.

1157. EBP A nurse arrives at a local park to find a group of people surrounding a pediatric victim. Witnesses report the child collapsed just seconds ago. The child is not breathing and is without a pulse. While another person dials for emergency assistance, the nurse prepares to initiate single rescuer CPR. Which compression-to-ventilation ratio should be used by the nurse?

1. 30:2
2. 15:2
3. 30:1
4. 15:1

ANSWER: 1

Current guidelines for single rescuer CPR have the compression-to-ventilation ratio of 30:2 for both pediatric and adult victims. All other options are incorrect.

➧ ***Test-taking Tip:*** *Applying basic knowledge of CPR guidelines will direct you to the correct response.*

Content Area: Child Health; *Category of Health Alteration:* Cardiovascular Management; *Integrated Processes:* Nursing Process Implementation; *Client Need:* Physiological Integrity/Physiological Adaptation/Medical Emergencies; *Cognitive Level:* Application

EBP Reference: Sherman, M. (2007). The new American Heart Association cardiopulmonary resuscitation guidelines: Should children and adults have to share? *Current Opinions in Pediatrics,* 19(3), 253–257.

1158. An emergency department nurse receives a pediatric client who has just been in ventricular fibrillation (VF) and has been defibrillated. The nurse is informed that the child is currently in normal sinus rhythm (NSR) with a blood pressure of 95/51. Which action should be taken by the nurse?

1. Carefully assess the child's cardiac status.
2. Prepare for cardioversion.
3. Begin CPR.
4. Prepare the client for transfer to the pediatric unit.

ANSWER: 1

The nurse should carefully assess the child's cardiac status. VF is a medical emergency that was quickly corrected with defibrillation to prevent death. In VF the fibrillating ventricles are unable to pump blood and cardiac output decreases sharply. Though the rhythm has converted, the child is unstable and needs further assessment and monitoring. Cardioversion is used for atrial fibrillation, not VF. CPR is not indicated at this time. The child's heart rhythm should be monitored, so the child would likely be transferred to a pediatric unit with telemonitoring.

➧ ***Test-taking Tip:*** *Use the nursing process. When a nurse receives a new client, the nurse's first action should be an assessment.*

Content Area: Child Health; *Category of Health Alteration:* Cardiovascular Management; *Integrated Processes:* Nursing Process Implementation; *Client Need:* Physiological Integrity/Physiological Adaptation/Medical Emergencies; *Cognitive Level:* Application

Reference: Pillitteri, A. (2007). *Maternal & Child Health Nursing: Care of the Childbearing & Childrearing Family* (5th ed., pp. 1316–1319). Philadelphia: Lippincott Williams & Wilkins.

1159. A nurse receives an order to administer oral digoxin 10 micrograms/kilogram (mcg/kg) to a full-term infant. Knowing that the infant weighs 8 lbs, the nurse carefully calculates the dosage and administers _______mcg oral digoxin.

ANSWER: 36

The infant weighs 8 lbs or 3.6 kg (8 lbs divided by 2.2 lb per kg = 3.6 kg). Multiplying 3.6 and 10 mcg/kg will give you a correct response of 36 mcg.

➧ ***Test-taking Tip:*** *Recall that 2.2 lb equals 1 kg. Apply knowledge of the basic principles of medication calculation to lead you to the correct response.*

Content Area: Child Health; *Category of Health Alteration:* Cardiovascular Management; *Integrated Processes:* Nursing Process Analysis; *Client Need:* Physiological Integrity/Pharmacological and Parenteral Therapies/Dosage Calculation; *Cognitive Level:* Analysis

Reference: Hockenberry, M., & Wilson, D. (2007). *Wong's Nursing Care of Infants and Children* (8th ed., p. 1450). St. Louis, MO: Mosby/Elsevier.

1160. A nurse receives an order to administer digoxin to a 6-year-old child. Prior to administering the medication, the nurse reviews the child's laboratory report. Which laboratory value should concern the nurse and be reported to the physician?

Serum Laboratory Test	Client's Value	Normal Values
K	3.2 mEq/L	3.5–5.5 mEq/L
Hgb	10 g/dL	11.5–15.5 g/dL
Glucose	60 mg/dL	60–105 mg/dL
Na	140 mEq/L	135–145 mEq/L
Creatinine	0.3 mg/dL	0.3–0.7 mg/dL
Digoxin level	1.8 ng/mL	0.8–2.0 ng/mL

1. K 3.2 mEq/L
2. Hgb 10 g/dL
3. Digoxin level 1.8 ng/mL
4. Creatinine 0.3 mg/dL

ANSWER: 1

The low serum potassium level should concern the nurse and be reported to the physician. A low serum potassium level would increase the risk of digoxin toxicity. Although the hemoglobin level is a little low, this is not most concerning. The digoxin level is on the high side of normal, thus administering digoxin while the serum potassium level is low increases the risk further. The serum creatinine level is a measure of renal function. It is within normal limits and not concerning.

➧ ***Test-taking Tip:*** *Focus on the abnormal values and eliminate options 3 and 4 because these are normal values. Recall that potassium is involved in the conduction system of the heart.*

Content Area: Child Health; *Category of Health Alteration:* Cardiovascular Management; *Integrated Processes:* Nursing Process Analysis; *Client Need:* Physiological Integrity/Pharmacological and Parenteral Therapies/Adverse Effects/Contradictions/Interactions; *Cognitive Level:* Analysis

Reference: Hockenberry, M., & Wilson, D. (2007). *Wong's Nursing Care of Infants and Children* (8th ed., p. 1451). St. Louis, MO: Mosby/Elsevier.

1161. Before administering oral digoxin (Lanoxin®) to a pediatric client, a nurse notes that the child has bradycardia and mild vomiting. Which is the nurse's most appropriate action?

1. Explain to the parent that bradycardia is an expected effect of the digoxin.
2. Administer the medication, document the observations, and reevaluate after the next dose.
3. Withhold the medication and immediately notify the prescriber because these are signs of toxicity.
4. Administer an oral beta-blocker medication.

ANSWER: 3

The nurse should hold the medication and immediately notify the prescriber because these are signs of digoxin toxicity. Digoxin slows and strengthens the heart. Though digoxin slows the heart rate, bradycardia is a side effect. The medication should be held if the heart rate is slow. Continuing to administer the medication would be unsafe. A beta-blocking agent should not be administered because it may further slow the rate. If symptomatic, epinephrine would be prescribed to increase the heart rate.

➧ ***Test-taking Tip:*** *Look for key words in each option: "expected effects," "administer," "withhold," or "administer another medication." If unsure if these are signs of drug toxicity, recognize that the client is vomiting and would likely vomit the medication if administered.*

Content Area: Child Health; *Category of Health Alteration:* Cardiovascular Management; *Integrated Processes:* Nursing Process Implementation; *Client Need:* Physiological Integrity/Pharmacological and Parenteral Therapies/Adverse Effects/Contradictions/Interactions; *Cognitive Level:* Analysis

Reference: Hockenberry, M., & Wilson, D. (2007). *Wong's Nursing Care of Infants and Children* (8th ed., p. 1452). St. Louis, MO: Mosby.

1162. A sexually active female adolescent has been diagnosed with hyperlipidemia. After several months of lifestyle changes, the levels have not significantly decreased, and a statin medication is prescribed. A nurse is educating the client about this class of medications. Which instruction should be included in the nurse's teaching plan for this client?

1. Discontinue therapy and contact the prescriber if having new-onset muscle aches or dark urine.
2. Continue therapy even if she becomes pregnant.
3. Take the medication in the morning because it would be most effective.
4. Discontinue lifestyle modifications because these are ineffective in treating the condition.

ANSWER: 1

The nurse should instruct the client to discontinue therapy and contact the prescriber if having muscle aches or dark urine. Muscle aches and dark urine could be a sign of a dangerous side effect of statins, rhabdomyolysis, which is the rapid breakdown of skeletal muscle tissue due to the chemical effects of the medication. The drug should be discontinued immediately and the prescriber notified. The drug should be discontinued if the client becomes pregnant because the drug is teratogenic. Oral contraceptive therapy should be initiated in conjunction with a statin in clients who are at risk for becoming pregnant. Statins are most effective if taken in the evening. The client should proceed with lifestyle modifications as these are to be used in conjunction with statin therapy in order to receive the greatest benefit of therapy.

➧ ***Test-taking Tip:*** *Apply knowledge of the statin classification of antilipidemic medications to select the correct options.*

Content Area: Child Health; *Category of Health Alteration:* Cardiovascular Management; *Integrated Processes:* Teaching and Learning; *Client Need:* Physiological Integrity/Pharmacological and Parenteral Therapies/Medication Administration; *Cognitive Level:* Application

Reference: Hockenberry, M., & Wilson, D. (2007). *Wong's Nursing Care of Infants and Children* (8th ed., p. 1491). St. Louis, MO: Mosby/Elsevier.

1163. A nurse is administering medications to a pediatric client with hypertension. Which oral antihypertensive medication ordered for a child should the nurse question?

1. ACE inhibitor
2. Calcium channel blocker
3. Diuretic
4. Nitrate

ANSWER: 4

Nitrates are used to treat angina and not prescribed to treat hypertension in children. ACE inhibitors, beta blockers, calcium channel blockers, angiotensin-receptive blockers, and diuretics are all oral antihypertensive medications used in treating hypertension in children.

➧ ***Test-taking Tip:*** *Think about the action of each class of medications. Eliminate options that are known antihypertensive medications.*

Content Area: Child Health; *Category of Health Alteration:* Cardiovascular Management; *Integrated Processes:* Nursing Process Implementation; *Client Need:* Physiological Integrity/Pharmacological and Parenteral Therapies/Expected Actions or Outcomes; *Cognitive Level:* Application

Reference: Hockenberry, M., & Wilson, D. (2007). *Wong's Nursing Care of Infants and Children* (8th ed., p. 1488). St. Louis, MO: Mosby/Elsevier.

Test 30: **Child Health: Endocrine Management**

1164. A 12-year-old child's medication regimen for treating type 1 diabetes mellitus is changed from administering NPH and rapid-acting insulin to a basal-bolus insulin regimen. To achieve tight glucose control and for therapy to be effective, the nurse should instruct that the child and/or parent to: SELECT ALL THAT APPLY.

1. administer a once daily dose of a long-acting insulin such as glargine (Lantus®).
2. administer rapid-acting insulin such as aspart (NovoLog®) with each meal and snack based on the carbohydrate grams consumed.
3. administer extra rapid-acting insulin when the amount of the child's daily exercise increases.
4. consistently count the amount of carbohydrates the child consumes throughout the day.
5. monitor the child's blood glucose four to eight times a day.
6. monitor the child's blood glucose at midnight and 3 a.m. once a week.

ANSWER: 1, 2, 4, 5, 6

With basal-bolus insulin therapy, basal insulin is administered once a day using glargine, and then a bolus of rapid-acting insulin is administered with each meal and snack based on the number of carbohydrates eaten and the child's blood glucose level. Depending on the amounts of snacks eaten, blood glucose could be monitored up to eight times a day, and the child may get six to seven injections a day. Because of the potential for hypoglycemia at night, the child's blood glucose should be monitored at midnight and 3 a.m. once a week. Exercise increases the need for carbohydrates and not insulin.

▶ ***Test-taking Tip:*** *Read each option carefully. The duration of glargine insulin is 24 hours. The onset of aspart insulin is 5 to 10 minutes. Recall that aspart administration can be either subcutaneously or through an insulin infusion pump.*

Content Area: Child Health; *Category of Health Alteration:* Endocrine Management; *Integrated Processes:* Teaching and Learning; *Client Need:* Health Promotion and Maintenance/Self-Care; *Cognitive Level:* Analysis

Reference: Ball, J., & Bindler R. (2008). *Pediatric Nursing: Caring for Children* (4th ed., pp. 1226–1227). Upper Saddle River, NJ: Prentice Hall.

1165. **EBP** A nurse understands that to modify the risk for early cardiovascular disease in children diagnosed with type 1 diabetes mellitus a child should:

1. exercise at least 30 minutes every day.
2. eat a diet that is low in fat and high in protein.
3. maintain optimal management of blood sugar levels.
4. have a cardiac workup at each visit for the diabetes.

ANSWER: 3

Research indicates that hyperglycemia is the primary mediator for atherosclerosis in children with type 1 diabetes. Since the risk is only modified, the child needs to avoid hyperglycemia. Exercise and a healthy diet are a part of any growing child's needs. There is no need for a cardiac workup with each diabetes visit.

▶ ***Test-taking Tip:*** *Note that one option is more global than other options. Often a global option is the answer.*

Content Area: Child Health; *Category of Health Alteration:* Endocrine Management; *Client Need:* Physiological Integrity/Physiological Adaptation/Pathophysiology; *Cognitive Level:* Application

EBP Reference: Kavey, R., Allada, V., Daniels, S., Hayman, L., McCrindle, B., et al. (2007). Cardiovascular risk reduction in high-risk pediatric patients: A scientific statement from the American Heart Association expert panel on population and prevention science. *Journal of Cardiovascular Nursing,* 22(3), 218–253.

1166. A 9-year-old child with a history of type 1 diabetes mellitus for the past 6 years is admitted with a diagnosis of diabetic ketoacidosis (DKA). In preparing for the child's arrival to the nursing unit, the nurse should prepare to:

1. add sodium bicarbonate to the current IV fluids.
2. add potassium chloride to the current IV fluids.
3. use either 0.9% or 0.45% saline for the base IV fluid.
4. administer insulin by subcutaneous injection.

ANSWER: 3

Both water and sodium are depleted in DKA, thus the child will require intravenous saline. Research has shown no benefit to giving sodium bicarbonate to children with DKA to reverse metabolic acidosis. Potassium is added only after laboratory studies have confirmed that the plasma potassium is low. Usually there is not a drop in plasma potassium. Insulin is always given IV in DKA for rapid effect and close monitoring. Insulin onset by subcutaneous route is 15 to 30 minutes and can cause hypoglycemia from potential excessive dosing when attempting to reduce the hyperglycemia.

▶ ***Test-taking Tip:*** *Recall that high blood glucose levels causes osmotic diuresis and the loss of fluids. DKA is a life-threatening condition, and the nurse needs to be ready to act when the child is admitted.*

Content Area: Child Health; *Category of Health Alteration:* Endocrine Management; *Integrated Processes:* Nursing Process Implementation; *Client Need:* Physiological Integrity/Physiological Adaptation/Illness Management; *Cognitive Level:* Application

Reference: Lehne, R. (2007). *Pharmacology for Nursing Care* (6th ed., p. 668). St. Louis, MO: Saunders.

1167. A pediatric nurse is administering metformin (Glucophage®) to a child at risk for developing type 2 diabetes mellitus. The nurse understands that an important use of metformin in children is to:

1. delay the development of type 2 diabetes mellitus in high-risk children.
2. restore fertility in adolescent females.
3. reduce blood sugars in children who have type 1 diabetes mellitus.
4. restore renal function in children who have type 1 diabetes mellitus.

ANSWER: 1

When a family member has been diagnosed with type 2 diabetes mellitus, children in the family who are overweight will often be given metformin and placed on a weight-reduction diet.

➧ ***Test-taking Tip:*** *Knowledge of type 2 diabetes mellitus is needed to respond to this question.*

Content Area: Child Health; *Category of Health Alteration:* Endocrine Management; *Integrated Processes:* Nursing Process Implementation; *Client Need:* Physiological Integrity/Pharmacological and Parenteral Therapies/Expected Actions or Outcomes; *Cognitive Level:* Application

Reference: Lehne, R. (2007). *Pharmacology for Nursing Care* (6th ed., pp. 662–663). St. Louis, MO: Saunders.

1168. The parents of a 7-year-old child diagnosed with type 1 diabetes mellitus are planning to drive 1,200 miles for a vacation at the beach. They question the nurse about insulin storage for the trip. Which response by the nurse is most accurate?

1. "Because insulin must be refrigerated, you will need to obtain the medication from a pharmacy at your destination."
2. "Freeze the insulin before you leave home and take it in a cooler; it should be thawed by the time you get to the beach."
3. "Keep the insulin in a cooler with an ice pack and out of direct heat and sunlight for the trip. Store unopened insulin in the refrigerator at your destination."
4. "Because it is illegal to transport needles and syringes across most state lines, you will need to obtain a prescription from your doctor and purchase the insulin and the syringes at your destination."

ANSWER: 3

Because insulin should be kept out of direct sunlight and extreme heat, it should be transported in a cooler with an ice pack. Insulin is destroyed when frozen. Although it is not illegal to transport needles and syringes, the child should have a prescription to identify the medication and justify the syringes. The prescription also provides a means to obtain additional supplies if needed.

➧ ***Test-taking Tip:*** *Focus on what the question is asking: insulin storage. Eliminate options 1 and 4 because these responses do not address insulin storage. Decide the best option, 2 or 3. Note that option 3 is more complete, thus eliminate option 2.*

Content Area: Child Health; *Category of Health Alteration:* Endocrine Management; *Integrated Processes:* Teaching and Learning; *Client Need:* Health Promotion and Maintenance/Self-Care; *Cognitive Level:* Application

Reference: Lehne, R. (2007). *Pharmacology for Nursing Care* (6th ed., p. 670). St. Louis, MO: Saunders.

1169. A nurse explains to a parent who has a child with type 1 diabetes mellitus that the most important reason for counting the child's grams of carbohydrate intake is to:

1. lower blood glucose levels.
2. supply energy for growth and development.
3. provide consistent glucose to prevent hypoglycemia.
4. attain metabolic control of glucose and lipid levels.

ANSWER: 4

Children need energy for growth and development. A child who has type 1 diabetes mellitus needs a consistent intake of carbohydrate; but the overall goal of nutritional management is to achieve and maintain control of glucose and lipids metabolism. The other alternatives are only a partial answer to the question.

➧ ***Test-taking Tip:*** *Focus on what the question is asking, the reason for counting carbohydrates. Select option 4, which is the most complete. Apply knowledge of the goal of nutritional management to answer the question.*

Content Area: Child Health; *Category of Health Alteration:* Endocrine Management; *Integrated Processes:* Teaching and Learning; *Client Need:* Health Promotion and Maintenance/Self-Care; *Cognitive Level:* Application

Reference: Hockenberry, M., & Wilson, D. (2007). *Wong's Nursing Care of Infants and Children* (8th ed., p. 1113). St. Louis, MO: Elsevier/Mosby.

1170. An adolescent client is taught how to use a continuous subcutaneous insulin infusion pump for tight glucose control of type 1 diabetes mellitus. Which statement by the client indicates the need for additional teaching?

1. "I can put in the number of carbohydrates that I consume, and the insulin pump will calculate the bolus insulin dose that I will receive."
2. "I must still check my blood glucose levels with meals and snacks and calculate the amount of carbohydrates I consume to ensure I get the correct bolus dose of insulin."
3. "As my blood glucose control improves with the use of the insulin pump, I should see a drop in the weight that I have gained."
4. "Every 2 to 4 days, I will need to change the syringe, catheter, and site moving the site away at least 1 inch from the last site."

ANSWER: 3

Weight gain, and not weight loss, commonly occurs as blood glucose control improves. Newer pumps calculate bolus insulin dose to the carbohydrates consumed. Monitoring blood glucose levels and carbohydrates consumed is still necessary with an insulin pump. About every 2 to 4 days when a syringe is empty, a new syringe and tubing is attached to the pump along with a new skin setup. The site is also changed to prevent lipoatrophy.

▸ ***Test-taking Tip:*** *The key phrase "need for additional teaching" indicates that this is a false-response question. Select the option that is incorrect. Note that options 1, 2, and 4 relate to the pump operation, whereas option 3 is different. Often the option that is different is the answer.*

Content Area: Child Health; *Category of Health Alteration:* Endocrine Management; *Integrated Processes:* Nursing Process Evaluation; *Client Need:* Health Promotion and Maintenance/Principles of Teaching and Learning; *Cognitive Level:* Analysis

Reference: Ball, J., & Bindler R. (2008). *Pediatric Nursing: Caring for Children* (4th ed., pp. 1226–1227). Upper Saddle River, NJ: Prentice Hall.

1171. EBP A 10-year-old child with a 6-year history of type 1 diabetes mellitus has been seen in a clinic for enuresis over the past 2 weeks. Which conclusion by the nurse regarding the likely cause of the enuresis is correct?

1. Sustained blood sugar levels lower than normal
2. Acquired adrenocortical hyperfunction
3. Sustained blood sugar levels higher than normal
4. Acquired syndrome of inappropriate antidiuretic hormone (SIADH)

ANSWER: 3

Research indicates that children with type 1 diabetes mellitus who have higher hemoglobin A_{1c} levels, higher fasting blood sugar levels, and who experience polydipsia and polyuria are at risk for enuresis. Sustained hypoglycemia will not cause enuresis and neither should adrenal hyperfunction. SIADH will cause enuresis; however, a child with type 1 diabetes will most likely develop enuresis due to sustained, elevated blood glucose levels.

▸ ***Test-taking Tip:*** *Think about the pathophysiology of type 1 diabetes to respond to this question. Note that options 1 and 3 are opposites so either one or both of these are incorrect.*

Content Area: Child Health; *Category of Health Alteration:* Endocrine Management; *Integrated Processes:* Nursing Process Analysis; *Client Need:* Physiological Integrity/Physiological Adaptation/ Pathophysiology; *Cognitive Level:* Application

EBP Reference: Geffken, G., Williams, L., Silverstein, J., Monaco, L., Rayfield, A., et al. (2007). Metabolic control and nocturnal enuresis in children with type 1 diabetes. *Journal of Pediatric Nursing,* 22(1), 4–8.

1172. Which laboratory test results should a nurse monitor in evaluating the long-term success of a child's control of type 1 diabetes mellitus?

1. Hemoglobin A_{1c} levels
2. Blood insulin levels
3. Blood glucose levels
4. Urinary glucose levels

ANSWER: 1

Glycated hemoglobin (hemoglobin A_{1c}) is used to measure long-term success because glycated hemoglobin provides an index of average blood glucose levels over the past 2 to 3 months. The results of the other laboratory tests provided will evaluate only short-term success.

▸ ***Test-taking Tip:*** *The key word is "long-term." Select an option that, if drawn only once, provides information about blood glucose levels over the past 2 to 3 months.*

Content Area: Child Health; *Category of Health Alteration:* Endocrine Management; *Integrated Processes:* Nursing Process Evaluation; *Client Need:* Physiological Integrity/Reduction of Risk Potential/Laboratory Values; *Cognitive Level:* Application

References: Hockenberry, M., & Wilson, D. (2007). *Wong's Nursing Care of Infants and Children* (8th ed., p. 1117). St. Louis, MO: Elsevier/Mosby; Lehne, R. (2007). *Pharmacology for Nursing Care* (6th ed., p. 650). St. Louis, MO: Saunders.

1173. A child with a history of type 1 diabetes mellitus presents in the school nurse's office about an hour before the lunch period reporting disorientation. Which information is most important for the nurse to obtain?

1. Blood sugar
2. Temperature
3. Morning insulin dose
4. Urine ketones

ANSWER: 1

Children who become disoriented or sleepy within an hour of a meal are most likely experiencing hypoglycemia. Urine ketones are not indicated because ketones are not spilled at low plasma glucose levels. The temperature and insulin dose will not provide the information needed to intervene.

▸ ***Test-taking Tip:*** *Note the key words "most important." Look for the option that provides the information needed for the nurse to intervene immediately.*

Content Area: Child Health; *Category of Health Alteration:* Endocrine Management; *Integrated Processes:* Nursing Process Assessment; *Client Need:* Physiological Integrity/Reduction of Risk Potential/System Specific Assessments; *Cognitive Level:* Application

References: Hockenberry, M., & Wilson, D. (2007). *Wong's Nursing Care of Infants and Children* (8th ed., p. 1708). St. Louis, MO: Elsevier/Mosby; McCance, K., & Huether, S. (2006). *Pathophysiology: The Biologic Basis for Disease in Adults and Children* (5th ed., pp. 710–712). St. Louis, MO: Elsevier/Mosby.

1174. The mother of a 12-year-old child diagnosed with type 1 diabetes mellitus asks a nurse what changes in the daily routine should be made during attendance at summer camp. The child will be at camp for 4 weeks. Which is the best response by the nurse?

1. "The child will have an increased need for insulin due to the high carbohydrate content of camp food."
2. "The child's food intake should be decreased by 10% while the insulin should be increased by 10%."
3. "The child's food intake should be increased as activity increases; monitor blood glucose levels three to four times a day to evaluate results."
4. "The child's insulin injection should be given before every meal and snack to ensure that the food being consumed at camp can be utilized by the body."

ANSWER: 3

Increases in muscle activity promote a more efficient utilization of glucose. School-aged children are more physically active in the summer months than during the school year. An increase of insulin with an increase in physical activity and/or a decrease in food consumption will result in profound hypoglycemia. Giving regular insulin before every meal and snack is an option for older individuals who are usually engaged in regular, high-intensity physical activity; it would not be recommended for a 12-year-old child attending 4 weeks of camp.

▸ ***Test-taking Tip:*** *Knowledge of the physiological mechanism of insulin utilization by the body is needed, as well as the relationship of food to insulin needs and the metabolic needs of a 12-year-old child.*

Content Area: Child Health; *Category of Health Alteration:* Endocrine Management; *Integrated Processes:* Teaching and Learning; *Client Need:* Physiological Integrity/Physiological Adaptation/Illness Management; *Cognitive Level:* Application

References: Ball, J., & Bindler, R. (2006). *Child Health Nursing: Partnering with Children & Families* (pp. 1270–1278). Upper Saddle River, NJ: Prentice Hall; McCance, K., & Huether, S. (2006). *Pathophysiology: The Biologic Basis for Disease in Adults and Children* (5th ed., p. 670). St. Louis, MO: Elsevier/Mosby.

1175. A health-care provider prescribes for an 8-year-old child to receive 1 unit of aspart insulin for every 15 grams of carbohydrates consumed at mealtime. Additionally, the client is to receive insulin per the sliding scale insulin as noted below. The 8-year-old child's fingerstick blood glucose before breakfast is 82, and the child ate 30 grams of carbohydrates at breakfast. Based on this information and the sliding scale below, the nurse should administer ______ unit(s) to the child.

Mealtime Glucose Level mg/dL	Mealtime Units of Aspart Insulin for Glucose Level
70–79	−2 and call
80–89	−1
90–180	0
181–200	1
201–250	2
251–300	3
More than 300	Call

ANSWER: 1

One unit of insulin aspart should be administered. The client should receive 2 units for the 30 grams of carbohydrates (CHO) minus 1 unit for the blood glucose of 82 mg/dL, for a total of 1 unit.

▸ ***Test-taking Tip:*** *Carefully read what the question is asking. Be sure to note both the insulin "coverage dose" for the carbohydrate intake and the insulin "correction dose" for the blood sugar.*

Content Area: Child Health; *Category of Health Alteration:* Endocrine Management; *Integrated Processes:* Nursing Process Implementation; *Client Need:* Physiological Integrity/Pharmacological and Parenteral Therapies/Dosage Calculation; *Cognitive Level:* Analysis

Reference: Ball, J., & Bindler, R. (2008). *Pediatric Nursing: Caring for Children* (4th ed., pp. 1228–1229). Upper Saddle River, NJ: Prentice Hall.

1176. EBP A nursing assistant reports to a nurse that a 4-year-old child diagnosed with type 1 diabetes consumed ½ cup of oatmeal, 60 mL of orange juice, and 60 mL of milk for breakfast. The child's blood glucose was 150 mg/dL before breakfast, and the child did not receive insulin before breakfast. The nurse should conclude that: SELECT ALL THAT APPLY.

1. the total volume of fluid intake should be recorded as 120 mL.
2. insulin will need to be administered to cover for the carbohydrates eaten.
3. insulin will not be needed because the child's blood glucose was normal before breakfast.
4. a double-check of the amounts of carbohydrate eaten is needed before administering insulin.
5. the child should have received insulin before breakfast because the blood sugar is elevated.

ANSWER: 1, 2, 4

The nurse should record the fluid intake of 120 mL for the child. Because insulin is not being produced in type 1 diabetes, insulin is needed to transport the glucose into the cells. A double-check is done for all medications that have a high potential for error. For insulin, this includes calculating the amount of carbohydrates eaten as well as the insulin dose. While the blood glucose of 150 mg/dL is within the normal before-meal target range of 100 to 180 mg/dL for children under 6 years, insulin is still needed to transport the glucose into the cells. A serum glucose of 150 mg/dL is within the normal range.

***Test-taking Tip:** Recall that the normal before-meal target range for blood glucose is 100 to 180 mg/dL for children less than 6 years of age.*

Content Area: Child Health; *Category of Health Alteration:* Endocrine Management; *Integrated Processes:* Nursing Process Analysis; *Client Need:* Physiological Integrity/Pharmacological and Parenteral Therapies/Medication Administration; *Cognitive Level:* Analysis

Reference: Ball, J., & Bindler, R. (2008). *Pediatric Nursing: Caring for Children* (4th ed., pp. 1228–1229). Upper Saddle River, NJ: Prentice Hall.

EBP Reference: Institute for Safe Medication Practices. (2008). *ISMP's List of High-Alert Medications*. Available at: www.ismp.org/Tools/highalertmedications.pdf

---

1177. A health-care provider prescribes glucagon 0.5 mg subcutaneously for a client with type 1 diabetes mellitus. A nurse determines that glucagon is used to treat:

1. hypoglycemia resulting from too little food intake.
2. hyperglycemia resulting from too much food intake.
3. hypoglycemia resulting from too much insulin intake.
4. hyperglycemia resulting from too little insulin intake.

ANSWER: 3

Glucagon is a hormone produced by the pancreas that helps release stored glucose from the liver. Since glucagon acts by promoting glycogen breakdown, it will not treat hypoglycemia related to starvation because there is no glycogen. Glucagon does not treat hyperglycemia.

***Test-taking Tip:** Knowledge of pancreatic hormones and actions is needed to respond to this question.*

Content Area: Child Health; *Category of Health Alteration:* Endocrine Management; *Integrated Processes:* Nursing Process Implementation; *Client Need:* Physiological Integrity/Pharmacological and Parenteral Therapies/Expected Actions or Outcomes; *Cognitive Level:* Application

References: Lehne, R. (2007). *Pharmacology for Nursing Care* (6th ed., p. 668). St. Louis, MO: Saunders; Ball, J., & Bindler, R. (2008). *Pediatric Nursing: Caring for Children* (4th ed., p. 1240). Upper Saddle River, NJ: Prentice Hall.

1178. EBP A child's parents inform a nurse about how they care for their 12-year-old child with type 1 diabetes mellitus, including sick day management, treating hyperglycemia, and managing ketosis. In which situation could the parents safely manage the child's care at home?

1. Child's blood glucose level is 280 mg/dL; skin turgor very poor; lips and mouth parched.
2. Child's blood glucose level is 250 mg/dL; vomiting and dizziness; complains of double vision.
3. Child's blood glucose level is 240 mg/dL; large amounts of urine output decreasing to 100 mL total output for the last 8 hours.
4. Child's blood glucose level is 300 mg/dL; urine tested positive for ketones; skin is hot, flushed, and dry.

ANSWER: 4

According to the consensus statement from the American Diabetes Association, children who have established diabetes and who are in DKA without vomiting and severe dehydration can be managed at home if the parents are trained in sick day, hyperglycemia, and ketoacidosis management. In addition, the care must be supervised through the emergency department by an experienced diabetes team. The child should be managed in the hospital if showing signs of severe dehydration, vomiting, or cerebral involvement. Poor skin turgor and parched mucous membranes are signs of severe dehydration. Dizziness, double vision, and vomiting could be signs of cerebral involvement. Urine output less than 30 mL per hour is a sign of severe dehydration.

***Test-taking Tip:** Read each option carefully. Consider the complications that are occurring in each option and the parent's ability to care for their child.*

Content Area: Child Health; *Category of Health Alteration:* Endocrine Management; *Integrated Processes:* Nursing Process Evaluation; *Client Need:* Safe and Effective Care Environment/Management of Care/Continuity of Care; *Cognitive Level:* Analysis

References: Ball, J., & Bindler, R. (2006). *Child Health Nursing: Partnering with Children & Families* (pp. 1263–1285). Upper Saddle River, NJ; Prentice Hall: Hockenberry, M., & Wilson, D. (2007). *Wong's Nursing Care of Infants and Children* (8th ed., pp. 1705–1711). St. Louis, MO: Elsevier/Mosby.

EBP Reference: Wolfsdorf, J., Glaser, N., & Sperling, M. (2006). Diabetic ketoacidosis in infants, children, and adolescents: A consensus statement from the American Diabetes Association. *Diabetes Care,* 29(5), 1150.

1179. An infant diagnosed with hypothyroidism is prescribed levothyroxine sodium (Synthroid®). Which independent nursing intervention would assist the nurse in evaluating the effectiveness of this medication?

1. Monthly assessments of growth and development
2. Monthly serum calcium and thyroxin levels
3. Bimonthly catecholamine levels and electrocardiogram (ECG)
4. Absence of thyroid excess

ANSWER: 1

The nurse should independently monitor the medication's effectiveness by assessing for normal growth and development. If the medication is effective, the child will grow and develop at a normal rate for age. Serum calcium, thyroxin, catecholamines, and ECG require medical prescription. Assessing the absence of thyroid excess is too vague.

Test-taking Tip: *Note the key word "independent" and use the process of elimination to eliminate options 2 and 3. Eliminate any options that are vague.*

Content Area: Child Health; *Category of Health Alteration:* Endocrine Management; *Integrated Processes:* Nursing Process Implementation; *Client Need:* Physiological Integrity/Pharmacological and Parenteral Therapies/Expected Actions or Outcomes; *Cognitive Level:* Application

Reference: Lehne, R. (2007). *Pharmacology for Nursing Care* (6th ed., p. 683). St. Louis, MO: Saunders.

1180. A child is admitted in thyrotoxic crisis. Which manifestations should a nurse expect to observe during assessment? SELECT ALL THAT APPLY.

1. Delirium
2. Hypothermia
3. Bradycardia
4. Nausea
5. Vomiting

ANSWER: 1, 4, 5

Thyrotoxic crisis, or thyroid storm, is a medical emergency resulting from highly elevated circulating levels of thyroid hormone. Additional manifestations of thyrotoxic crisis are hyperpyrexia, tachycardia, hypertension, mental status changes, and multisystem organ failure.

Test-taking Tip: *Note the similarities in options 2 and 3; both are low (low temperature, low heart rate). Thyrotoxic crisis is extreme hyperthyroidism. Think about the effect of hyperthyroidism on the body and eliminate these options.*

Content Area: Child Health; *Category of Health Alteration:* Endocrine Management; *Integrated Processes:* Nursing Process Assessment; *Client Need:* Physiological Integrity/Physiological Adaptation/Alterations in Body Systems; *Cognitive Level:* Application

References: Ball, J., & Bindler, R. (2006). *Child Health Nursing: Partnering with Children & Families* (p. 1253). Upper Saddle River, NJ: Prentice Hall; Hockenberry, M., & Wilson, D. (2007). *Wong's Nursing Care of Infants and Children* (8th ed., p. 1693). St. Louis, MO: Elsevier/Mosby; McCance, K., & Huether, S. (2006). *Pathophysiology: The Biologic Basis for Disease in Adults and Children* (5th ed., p. 694). St. Louis, MO: Elsevier/Mosby.

1181. A nurse is educating the parents of a school-aged child newly diagnosed with hyperthyroidism. Until the disease is under control, which instruction should be included in the education provided by the nurse?

1. Discontinue physical education classes at school.
2. Increase stimulation in the school environment.
3. Restrict the number of calories from carbohydrate foods.
4. Dress your child in cold weather clothing even in warm weather.

ANSWER: 1

The child should avoid any vigorous activity and unnecessary external stimulation and should wear clothing that is comfortable. The child may experience heat intolerance and should be provided with warm weather clothing, even in winter. The child's appetite may increase, but the child will continue to lose weight until the problem is controlled.

Test-taking Tip: *Knowledge of hyperthyroidism is needed to respond to this question. Note that options 1 and 2 are somewhat opposite; option 1 decreases stimulation and option 2 increases stimulation. Either one or both are incorrect.*

Content Area: Child Health; *Category of Health Alteration:* Endocrine Management; *Integrated Processes:* Teaching and Learning; *Client Need:* Physiological Integrity/Physiological Adaptation/Illness Management; Health Promotion and Maintenance/Principles of Teaching and Learning; *Cognitive Level:* Application

References: Ball, J., & Bindler, R. (2006). *Child Health Nursing: Partnering with Children & Families* (pp. 1254–1255). Upper Saddle River, NJ: Prentice Hall; Hockenberry, M., & Wilson, D. (2007). *Wong's Nursing Care of Infants and Children* (8th ed., p. 1693). St. Louis, MO: Elsevier/Mosby; McCance, K., & Huether, S. (2006). *Pathophysiology: The Biologic Basis for Disease in Adults and Children* (5th ed., pp. 692–694). St. Louis, MO: Elsevier/Mosby.

1182. Which gland illustrated should a nurse palpate if Graves' disease is suspected?

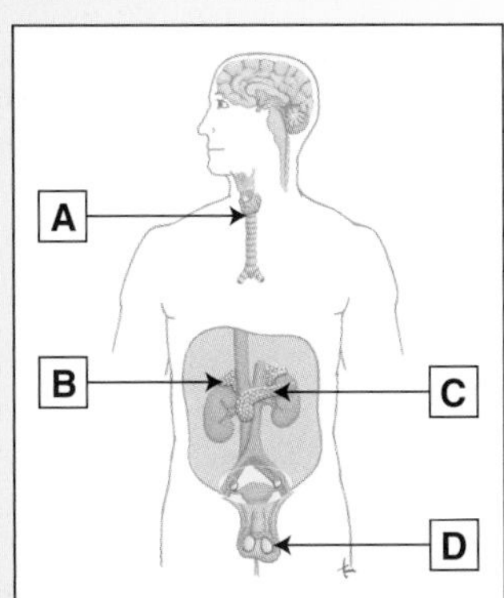

1. Gland A
2. Gland B
3. Gland C
4. Gland D

ANSWER: 1

The nurse should palpate the thyroid gland. The only other glands in the endocrine system that can be palpated are the ovaries and testes; neither have anything to do with Graves' disease.

➧ ***Test-taking Tip:*** *Note the word "gland" and use the process of elimination to rule out incorrect options.*

Content Area: Child Health; *Category of Health Alteration:* Endocrine Management; *Integrated Processes:* Nursing Process Assessment; *Client Need:* Health Promotion and Maintenance/Techniques of Physical Assessment; *Cognitive Level:* Application

Reference: McCance, K., & Huether, S. (2006). *Pathophysiology: The Biologic Basis for Disease in Adults and Children* (5th ed., p. 666). St. Louis, MO: Elsevier/Mosby.

1183. Which instruction should a nurse include when teaching parents who have a child diagnosed with hypoparathyroidism?

1. Monitor for muscle spasms, tingling around the mouth, and muscle cramps.
2. Monitor for side effects of excess medication therapy, including dry, scaly, coarse skin.
3. Decrease intake of foods high in calcium and phosphorus.
4. Increase environmental stimuli and encourage participation in high-energy activities.

ANSWER: 1

In hypoparathyroidism, insufficient amounts of parathyroid hormone is produced and this affects serum calcium regulation. Muscle spasms, tingling around the mouth, and muscle cramps are signs of hypocalcemia which could indicate that treatment with vitamin D and calcium is ineffective. Dry, scaly, and coarse skin are signs of hypoparathyroidism, not medication overdose. Calcium-rich foods, such as dark green vegetables, soybeans, and tofu, should be encouraged (not decreased in amounts). Foods high in oxalic acid (e.g., spinach and rhubarb) and phytic acid (e.g., bran and whole grains) should be avoided because these reduce calcium absorption. Phosphorus-rich foods (dairy products) are also high in calcium and are usually not restricted unless serum phosphorus levels are exceptionally high. During crisis episodes the environmental stimuli needs to be decreased (not increased) and the child kept quiet.

➧ ***Test-taking Tip:*** *Focus on looking for key words in the options that are opposite of the expected findings and treatment for hypoparathyroidism and eliminate the options.*

Content Area: Child Health; *Category of Health Alteration:* Endocrine Management; *Integrated Processes:* Teaching and Learning; *Client Need:* Physiological Integrity/Physiological Adaptation/Illness Management; Physiological Integrity/Reduction of Risk Potential/Potential for Complications from Surgical Procedures and Health Alterations; *Cognitive Level:* Analysis

Reference: Hockenberry, M., & Wilson, D. (2007). *Wong's Nursing Care of Infants and Children* (8th ed., p. 1695). St. Louis, MO: Elsevier/Mosby.

1184. Which nursing diagnosis has the highest priority for a child diagnosed with Addison's disease?

1. Potential excess fluid volume
2. Disturbed body image
3. Altered development
4. Altered sleep and rest

ANSWER: 2

There is a high incidence of body image disturbances related to changes in skin pigmentation associated with Addison's disease. There is a potential for fluid volume deficit, but there is not usually a problem with development or sleep and rest patterns.

➧ ***Test-taking Tip:*** *Apply knowledge of Addison's disease and use of the key word "priority." Remember that potential problems are of a lesser priority than actual problems.*

Content Area: Child Health; *Category of Health Alteration:* Endocrine Management; *Integrated Processes:* Nursing Process Analysis; *Client Need:* Physiological Integrity/Physiological Adaptation/Alterations in Body Systems; *Cognitive Level:* Analysis

References: Ball, J., & Bindler, R. (2006). *Child Health Nursing: Partnering with Children & Families* (p. 1262). Upper Saddle River, NJ: Prentice Hall; McCance, K., & Huether, S. (2006). *Pathophysiology: The Biologic Basis for Disease in Adults and Children* (5th ed., pp. 725–726). St. Louis, MO: Elsevier/Mosby.

1185. An adolescent is admitted with a diagnosis of suspected Addison's disease. Which assessment manifestations should the nurse expect to find if Addison's disease is the correct diagnosis?

1. Long history of fatigue, weight loss, and muscle tetany
2. Sudden onset of skin hypopigmentation, polydipsia, and hyperactivity
3. Gradual onset of salt craving, decreased pubic and axillary hair, and irritability
4. Sudden onset of increasing weight gain, hirsurtism, and skin hyperpigmentation

ANSWER: 3

Signs and symptoms of Addison's disease do not usually appear until about 90% of the adrenal tissue is nonfunctional, so the onset is very gradual. There is weight loss, fatigue, hyperpigmentation, muscle weakness, decreased pubic hair, and irritability, as well as a craving for salt. It usually occurs from lesions or neoplasms or the cause may be idiopathic. Previously healthy children exhibit the first signs during periods of stress. Options 2 and 4 are incorrect because they describe symptoms that are sudden in onset. Muscle tetany does not occur with Addison's disease.

Test-taking Tip: *Apply knowledge of adrenocortical insufficiency pathology and recall that Addison's disease, in the chronic state, is rare in children. Note that options 2 and 4 describe symptoms of sudden onset, whereas option 3 is gradual. Eliminate options 2 and 4.*

Content Area: Child Health; *Category of Health Alteration:* Endocrine Management; *Integrated Processes:* Nursing Process Assessment; *Client Need:* Physiological Integrity/Reduction of Risk Potential/System Specific Assessments; *Cognitive Level:* Application

References: Ball, J., & Bindler, R. (2006). *Child Health Nursing: Partnering with Children & Families* (pp. 1261–1262). Upper Saddle River, NJ: Prentice Hall; Hockenberry, M., & Wilson, D. (2007). *Wong's Nursing Care of Infants and Children* (8th ed., pp. 1698–1699). St. Louis, MO: Elsevier/Mosby.

1186. A nurse teaches the parents of a child diagnosed with Addison's disease signs of Addisonian crisis. Which sign identified by the parents indicates that further teaching is needed?

1. Severe hypertension
2. Abdominal pain
3. Seizures
4. Coma

ANSWER: 1

Addisonian crisis can lead to circulatory collapse with severe hypotension, not hypertension, Other signs include fever, generalized and pronounced weakness, dehydration, seizures, shock, and coma. Immediate intervention is needed.

Test-taking Tip: *The key words are "further teaching." Select the option that is not a sign of Addisonian crisis.*

Content Area: Child Health; *Category of Health Alteration:* Endocrine Management; *Integrated Processes:* Teaching and Learning; *Client Need:* Physiological Integrity/Physiological Adaptation/Alterations in Body Systems; *Cognitive Level:* Application

References: Ball, J., & Bindler, R. (2006). *Child Health Nursing: Partnering with Children & Families* (pp. 1261–1262). Upper Saddle River, NJ: Prentice Hall; Hockenberry, M., & Wilson, D. (2007). *Wong's Nursing Care of Infants and Children* (8th ed., pp. 1698–1699). St. Louis, MO: Elsevier/Mosby.

1187. A nurse instructs the parents of a child diagnosed with Addison's disease. Which instructions should be included by the nurse? SELECT ALL THAT APPLY.

1. Have the child wear a medical alert bracelet.
2. Encourage the child to ingest adequate fluids, particularly on hot summer days.
3. Include emergency cortisone treatment for Addisonian crisis on the school medical care plan.
4. If the child vomits the dose of cortisone within 1 hour, the dose is not repeated but the health-care provider notified.
5. Administer epinephrine subcutaneously immediately if Addisonian crisis should occur.

ANSWER: 1, 2, 3

The child should wear identification at all times so that personnel can identify potential problems in emergency situations. The school medical plan should include emergency treatment of the condition and the school nurse instructed on appropriate emergency measures. The child with Addison's disease is highly susceptible to dehydration. If the child vomits the medication within 1 hour, the dose is repeated. Epinephrine is used for allergic reactions, such as bee stings, and not for Addisonian crisis.

➧ ***Test-taking Tip:*** *Knowledge of the interventions for Addison disease is needed to respond to this question.*

Content Area: Child Health; *Category of Health Alteration:* Endocrine Management; *Integrated Processes:* Teaching and Learning; *Client Need:* Health Promotion and Maintenance/Principles of Teaching and Learning; *Cognitive Level:* Analysis

References: Ball, J., & Bindler, R. (2006). *Child Health Nursing: Partnering with Children & Families* (p. 1262). Upper Saddle River, NJ: Prentice Hall; McCance, K., & Huether, S. (2006). *Pathophysiology: The Biologic Basis for Disease in Adults and Children* (5th ed., pp. 725–726). St. Louis, MO: Elsevier/Mosby.

1188. Glucocorticoids are prescribed for a child diagnosed with congenital adrenal hyperplasia. Which manifestation should indicate to a nurse that therapy is successful?

1. Feminization in girls
2. Absence of symptoms of Cushing's syndrome
3. Precocious penile enlargement in boys
4. Increased growth rate in both boys and girls

ANSWER: 1

In congenital adrenal hyperplasia the body lacks the enzyme to produce cortisol and aldosterone. Without these hormones, the body produces more androgen, a type of male sex hormone. The goal of therapy is to reduce virilization (masculine characteristics) in girls. The presence of Cushing's syndrome is an adverse reaction and does not indicate if therapy is successful. Precocious penile enlargement in males and increased growth rate in both girls and boys indicates the medication is not successful.

➧ ***Test-taking Tip:*** *Associate "hyper" in hyperplasia with "more androgen." Recall that androgen is associated with the development of male characteristics. Select the option that emphasizes female characteristics.*

Content Area: Child Health; *Category of Health Alteration:* Endocrine Management; *Integrated Processes:* Nursing Process Evaluation; *Client Need:* Physiological Integrity/Pharmacological and Parenteral Therapies/Expected Effects/Outcomes; *Cognitive Level:* Analysis

Reference: Lehne, R. (2007). *Pharmacology for Nursing Care* (6th ed., pp. 699–700). St. Louis, MO: Saunders.

1189. Which nursing diagnosis has the highest priority for an infant diagnosed with congenital adrenal hypoplasia?

1. Disproportionate growth
2. Excess fluid volume
3. Impaired parent-infant attachment
4. Knowledge deficit of lifelong medication requirements

ANSWER: 3

There is a high risk for impaired parental-infant attachment due to underdetermined gender identity. Although there may be growth issues later as the child grows and the parents must be able to demonstrate understanding of the treatments to provide appropriate care, these are of lesser priority. Fluid volume excess is not a problem.

➧ ***Test-taking Tip:*** *Note the key words "highest priority." Look for an immediate concern and use the process of elimination. Physiological needs are priority, but because excess fluid volume is not a concern, eliminate option 2. Note growth in option 1 and lifelong in option 4; eliminate these because they would be later concerns.*

Content Area: Child Health; *Category of Health Alteration:* Endocrine Management; *Integrated Processes:* Nursing Process Analysis; *Client Need:* Physiological Integrity/Physiological Adaptation/Illness Management; *Cognitive Level:* Analysis

References: Ball, J., & Bindler, R. (2006). *Child Health Nursing: Partnering with Children & Families* (pp. 1260–1261). Upper Saddle River, NJ: Prentice Hall; McCance, K., & Huether, S. (2006). *Pathophysiology: The Biologic Basis for Disease in Adults and Children* (5th ed., p. 726). St. Louis, MO: Elsevier/Mosby.

1190. Which outcomes should a nurse plan for a child diagnosed with adrenal insufficiency? SELECT ALL THAT APPLY.

1. Child demonstrates a positive body image.
2. Child demonstrates no complications related to inactivity.
3. Child responds to oxygen regimes to avoid hospitalization.
4. Child and family verbalizes causes of the disease and treatment regimen.
5. Child responds to activity restrictions to conserve energy.

ANSWER: 1, 4

Adrenal insufficiency is associated with stress, fluid volume regulation, and hyperpigmentation of the skin which can affect body image. Verbalizing causes and treatments is a statement that can be measured. There are not usually problems related to oxygenation or activity.

➧ ***Test-taking Tip:*** *Knowledge of the outcomes of care for children with Addison's disease is needed to respond to this question.*

Content Area: Child Health; *Category of Health Alteration:* Endocrine Management; *Integrated Processes:* Nursing Process Planning; *Client Need:* Physiological Integrity/Physiological Adaptation/Illness Management; *Cognitive Level:* Analysis

References: Ball, J., & Bindler, R. (2006). *Child Health Nursing: Partnering with Children & Families* (p. 1262). Upper Saddle River, NJ: Prentice Hall; McCance, K., & Huether, S. (2006). *Pathophysiology: The Biologic Basis for Disease in Adults and Children* (5th ed., pp. 725–726). St. Louis, MO: Elsevier/Mosby.

1191. A 10-year-old child is admitted for testing to diagnose Cushing's syndrome. For which initial test should a nurse prepare the child and parents?

1. Glucose tolerance test (GTT)
2. Urine or saliva cortisol level
3. Dexamethasone suppression test
4. Serum 17-hydroxyprogesterone level

ANSWER: 2

A cortisol level, which is increased in Cushing's syndrome, is used in the initial screening for the syndrome. Hyperglycemia is associated with, but not diagnostic of, Cushing's syndrome; a GTT is used to diagnose diabetes mellitus. If the results for cortisol levels are borderline, a dexamethasone suppression test may be done. The serum 17-hydroxyprogesterone level is used to evaluate for adrenal hyperplasia.

➧ ***Test-taking Tip:*** *Recall that Cushing's syndrome is associated with increased levels of cortisone.*

Content Area: Child Health; *Category of Health Alteration:* Endocrine Management; *Integrated Processes:* Nursing Process Planning; *Client Need:* Physiological Integrity/Reduction of Risk Potential/Diagnostic Tests; *Cognitive Level:* Application

Reference: Ward, S., & Hisley, S. (2009). *Maternal-Child Nursing Care* (pp. 902–903). Philadelphia: F. A. Davis.

1192. Based on a child's growth chart from birth to age 12 months (illustrated below), which diagnostic test should a nurse expect a health-care provider to prescribe?

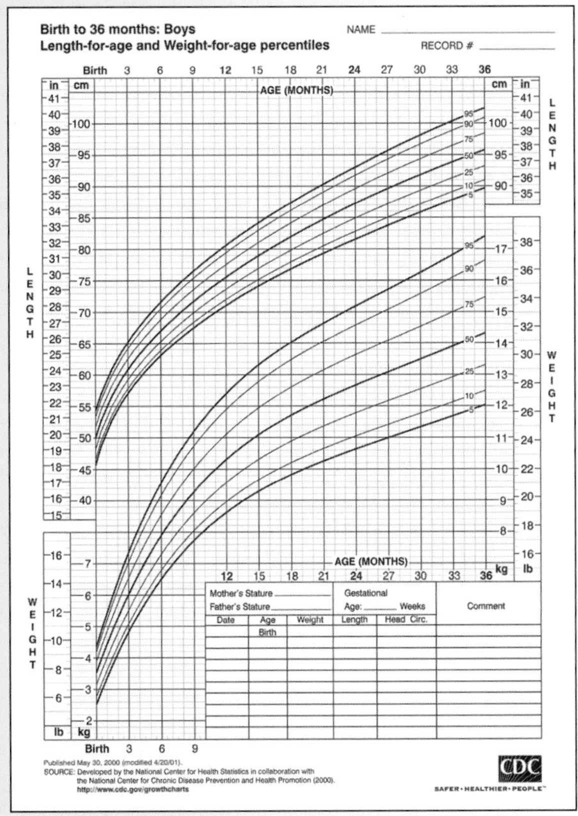

1. Radiographic views of the sella turcica
2. Bone age
3. Insulin-like growth factors (IGFs)
4. 17-alpha-hydroxyl progesterone

ANSWER: 3

IGF-1 and IGF binding protein-3 evaluate the levels of growth hormone deficiency. Any child who was a normal height and weight at birth but is below the third percentile by 12 months should be evaluated for growth hormone deficiency. If the IGF-1 levels are normal, then x-rays of the sella turcica (site of the pituitary gland) and bone age tests are requested. The 17-alpha-hydroxyl progesterone test evaluates adrenal hyperplasia.

➧ *Test-taking Tip: Knowledge of interpreting growth charts is needed, as well as an understanding of growth hormone deficiency.*

Content Area: Child Health; *Category of Health Alteration:* Endocrine Management; *Integrated Processes:* Nursing Process Analysis; *Client Need:* Physiological Integrity/Reduction of Risk Potential/Diagnostic Tests; *Cognitive Level:* Analysis

References: Ball, J., & Bindler, R. (2006). *Child Health Nursing: Partnering with Children & Families* (pp. 1242, 1260). Upper Saddle River, NJ: Prentice Hall; Hockenberry, M., & Wilson, D. (2007). *Wong's Nursing Care of Infants and Children* (8th ed., p. 1682). St. Louis, MO: Elsevier/Mosby.

1193. A 12-year-old child is being treated for growth hormone deficiency. The child is angry and refusing to go to school because all the other children are taller. In addition, this child is belligerent toward the mother, who gives the daily injection of growth hormone. Which initial intervention should be attempted by the nurse?

1. Teach the child self-administration of growth hormone.
2. Refer the family for counseling with particular emphasis on anger management.
3. Assist the parents to contact the school district so that home schooling can begin and last until the child has reached normal height.
4. Talk to the mother about requesting an Individual Educational Planning (IEP) team to assist in planning school interventions.

ANSWER: 1

Allowing the child to participate in the care fosters a sense of control over the problem. The family may ultimately be referred to counseling, but the anger this child is displaying is a normal reaction to seeing himself as different from other children the same age. This should decrease if participation in treatment is promoted. The child should not be removed from the school setting because that will just reinforce to the child that there is a difference. There is no need for an IEP team unless there are additional issues that could interfere with learning. At this point no additional issues have been established.

➧ *Test-taking Tip: Note the key word "first," the age of the child, and the fact that the mother is giving the injections. Only option 1 addresses the immediate concern; completing a referral or working with the school delays intervening immediately. Apply knowledge of the growth and developmental needs of 12-year-old children and treatment with long-term growth hormone therapy.*

Content Area: Child Health; *Category of Health Alteration:* Endocrine Management; *Integrated Processes:* Nursing Process Implementation; *Client Need:* Safe and Effective Care Environment/Management of Care/Establishing Priorities; *Cognitive Level:* Analysis

References: Hockenberry, M., & Wilson, D. (2007). *Wong's Nursing Care of Infants and Children* (8th ed., pp. 1684–1687). St. Louis, MO: Elsevier/Mosby; Lehne, R. (2007). *Pharmacology for Nursing Care* (6th ed., pp. 688, 689). St. Louis, MO: Saunders; Ormrod, J. (2006). *Educational Psychology: Developing Learners* (5th ed., pp. 68–79). Upper Saddle River, NJ: Prentice Hall.

1194. Which assessment findings should the nurse expect for a child diagnosed with diabetes insipidus? SELECT ALL THAT APPLY.

1. Polydipsia
2. Polyphagia
3. Polyuria
4. Glycosuria
5. Ketonuria

ANSWER: 1, 3

Children who are diagnosed with diabetes insipidus produce large amounts of very dilute urine and are constantly thirsty. There is an absence or insufficiency of antidiuretic hormone, so the body cannot concentrate urine. There is no associated increase in appetite, and the amount of glucose and ketones in the urine is not elevated. Children diagnosed with diabetes mellitus will exhibit polydipsia, polyphagia, polyuria, glycosuria, and ketonuria because the body is metabolizing fats and excreting glucose due to the lack of insulin.

▶ ***Test-taking Tip:*** *Be sure to differentiate between diabetes insipidus and diabetes mellitus. Eliminate options related to the body's ability to metabolize and use glucose.*

Content Area: Child Health; *Category of Health Alteration:* Endocrine Management; *Integrated Processes:* Nursing Process Analysis; *Client Need:* Physiological Integrity/Physiological Adaptation/Alterations in Body Systems; *Cognitive Level:* Analysis

References: Ball, J., & Bindler, R. (2006). *Child Health Nursing: Partnering with Children & Families* (p. 1068). Upper Saddle River, NJ: Prentice Hall; Hockenberry, M., & Wilson, D. (2007). *Wong's Nursing Care of Infants and Children* (8th ed., pp. 1688–1690). St. Louis, MO: Elsevier/Mosby.

1195. A nurse is assessing a 4-year-old child diagnosed with precocious puberty. Which physical assessment manifestation should the nurse expect to find?

1. Short stature
2. Hypothalmic tumor
3. Advanced bone age
4. Pubic and axillary hair

ANSWER: 4

Secondary sex characteristics are present in children under 8 years of age. They may also have a hypothalamic tumor and advanced bone age, but the nurse will not be able to assess those on physical exam. Children with precocious puberty do not have short stature, but are tall for their age.

▶ ***Test-taking Tip:*** *Knowledge of normal puberty is needed, as well as an understanding of the clinical manifestations of precocious puberty.*

Content Area: Child Health; *Category of Health Alteration:* Endocrine Management; *Integrated Processes:* Nursing Process Assessment; *Client Need:* Physiological Integrity/Physiological Adaptation/Alterations in Body Systems; *Cognitive Level:* Application

References: Ball, J., & Bindler, R. (2006). *Child Health Nursing: Partnering with Children & Families* (pp. 1248–1250). Upper Saddle River, NJ: Prentice Hall; McCance, K., & Huether, S. (2006). *Pathophysiology: The Biologic Basis for Disease in Adults and Children* (5th ed., p. 725). St. Louis, MO: Elsevier/Mosby.

1196. An older adolescent is diagnosed with acromegaly. Which medication should the nurse expect to be prescribed for this individual?

1. Somatropin (Genotropin®)
2. Desmopressin (Desmotabs®)
3. Somatostatin (Sandostatin®)
4. Clozapine (Clozaril®)

ANSWER: 3

Somatostatin suppresses growth hormone release. Somatropin is human growth hormone, desmopressin is used to treat diabetes insipidus, and clozapine is an antipsychotic medication used in the treatment of schizophrenia.

▶ ***Test-taking Tip:*** *Recall that acromegaly is a disorder caused by excess production of growth hormone. Select the medication that suppresses the release of growth hormone.*

Content Area: Child Health; *Category of Health Alteration:* Endocrine Management; *Integrated Processes:* Nursing Process Planning; *Client Need:* Physiological Integrity/Pharmacological and Parenteral Therapies/Expected Actions or Outcomes; *Cognitive Level:* Application

Reference: Lehne, R. (2007). *Pharmacology for Nursing Care* (6th ed., pp. 692–693). St. Louis, MO: Saunders.

1197. A 6-year-old child is diagnosed with pheochromocytoma. Which manifestations should lead a nurse to conclude that this child is in crisis?

1. Systolic blood pressure of 120 mm Hg
2. Rhabdomyolysis
3. Urine output of 30 mL/hr
4. Hyperexcitability

ANSWER: 2

During a pheochromocytoma crisis, there is skeletal muscle destruction (rhabdomyolysis). There is also profound hypertension, up to 250 mm Hg; acute renal failure with less than 30 mL/hr urine output; and decreased level of consciousness (not hyperexcitability).

➧ ***Test-taking Tip:*** *Eliminate options that are within normal or near normal parameters for a 6-year-old child.*

Content Area: Child Health; *Category of Health Alteration:* Endocrine Management; *Integrated Processes:* Nursing Process Assessment; *Client Need:* Physiological Integrity/Physiological Adaptation/Alterations in Body Systems; *Cognitive Level:* Analysis

Reference: Ball, J., & Bindler, R. (2006). *Child Health Nursing: Partnering with Children & Families* (pp. 1262–1263). Upper Saddle River, NJ: Prentice Hall.

Test 31: **Child Health: Gastrointestinal Management**

1198. A nurse is reviewing the laboratory report results for an infant who has diarrheal stools. Which analysis of the laboratory report results is correct?

Characteristic	Stool Sample
Color	Yellow
pH (less than 7 normal)	6.8
Odor	Sweet smelling
Occult blood	Positive

1. The color is more characteristic of normal stools than diarrheal stools.
2. The pH is abnormal and the stool is alkaline.
3. The odor is uncharacteristic for diarrheal stools.
4. The stools are discolored from the presence of visible blood.

ANSWER: 1

An infant's normal stool color is yellow. Diarrheal stools are green from lack of time for bile to be modified in the intestine, While the pH is abnormal, it is acidic rather than alkalotic because the pH is less than 7. Diarrheal stools can be either sweet or foul smelling. Only overt blood is visible in the stools, and a stool color change is dependent on the amount of blood and its source.

▶ **Test-taking Tip:** *Note that the client is an infant. Identify the normal finding for an infant's stool.*

Content Area: Child Health; *Category of Health Alteration:* Gastrointestinal Management; *Integrated Processes:* Nursing Process Analysis; *Client Need:* Physiological Integrity/Reduction of Risk Potential/Diagnostic Tests; *Cognitive Level:* Analysis

Reference: Pillitteri, A. (2007). *Maternal & Child Health Nursing: Care of the Childbearing & Childrearing Family* (5th ed., pp. 1420–1421). Philadelphia: Lippincott Williams & Wilkins.

1199. A child is to have a breath hydrogen test to evaluate for malabsorption syndrome. Which instruction is most important for a nurse to include when teaching the parents about the preparation needed for the test?

1. "Be sure to administer the prescribed antibiotics an hour before the test."
2. "The dinner the night before the test should consist of meat, rice, and water; avoid other starchy foods."
3. "Give the child an enema to cleanse the child's bowel the morning of the test."
4. "Encourage fluids just before the test to moisten the child's mouth for blowing into the mouthpiece."

ANSWER: 2

The breath hydrogen test is used to detect a rise in expired hydrogen after oral loading with a specific carbohydrate. A meal high in starch can interfere with test results. Antibiotics should not be given because they may reduce hydrogen levels. Bowel cleansing is not required because the colon is not being examined. The child should be NPO 12 hours before the test.

▶ **Test-taking Tip:** *If uncertain of a breath hydrogen test, focus on the words and eliminate any options not associated with the mouth. Of the three remaining options, note that two involve oral intake the morning of the test and the other is different. Often the option that is different is the answer.*

Content Area: Child Health; *Category of Health Alteration:* Gastrointestinal Management; *Integrated Processes:* Teaching and Learning; *Client Need:* Physiological Integrity/Reduction of Risk Potential/Diagnostic Tests; *Cognitive Level:* Analysis

Reference: Hockenberry, M., & Wilson, D. (2007). *Wong's Nursing Care of Infants and Children* (8th ed., pp. 1392–1393). St. Louis, MO: Mosby/Elsevier.

1200. A nurse is caring for a 2-month-old infant who has been admitted to a pediatric unit for hypovolemia secondary to gastroenteritis. The baby is irritable and will not calm when the parents hold the infant. The nurse's assessment findings include pulse, 180; respiratory rate, 48; blood pressure, 80/50 mm Hg; mucous membranes, dry; and decreased tears. The nurse interprets the information and determines that the child is moderately dehydrated. Which assessment finding further supports this conclusion?

1. Capillary refill greater than 2 seconds
2. Intense thirst
3. Normal to sunken anterior fontanel
4. Absence of tears

ANSWER: 3

The anterior fontanel closes between 16 and 18 months of age. In the infant with moderate dehydration, the fontanel will be normal or sunken. A moderately dehydrated infant will have slowed capillary refill time of between 2 and 4 seconds. Intense thirst and absence of tears are typical of severe, not moderate, dehydration.

▶ **Test-taking Tip:** *The key words are "moderately dehydrated." Be aware of the age-appropriate vital signs, and if they are altered, the likely causes. Analyze the similar options first and eliminate either one or both of these.*

Content Area: Child Health; *Category of Health Alteration:* Gastrointestinal Management; *Integrated Processes:* Nursing Process Analysis; *Client Need:* Physiologic Integrity/Physiological Adaptation/Alterations in Body Systems; *Cognitive Level:* Application

References: Ball, J., & Binder, R. (2006). *Clinical Handbook for Pediatric Nursing* (pp. 176–178; 389–390). Upper Saddle River, NJ: Pearson Education; Hockenberry, M., & Wilson, D. (2007). *Wong's Nursing Care of Infants and Children* (8th ed., p. 1147). St. Louis, MO: Mosby/Elsevier.

1201. EBP An infant is hospitalized with a diagnosis of infectious gastroenteritis and dehydration. A nurse determines that a nursing assistant caring for the infant understands the necessary precautions when the nursing assistant states: SELECT ALL THAT APPLY.

1. "I should put on a mask, gown, and gloves when I enter the room."
2. "I should put on gloves when I am holding the baby."
3. "I should wear gown and gloves to change the baby's diapers."
4. "I should keep the door to the baby's room closed most of the time."
5. "I should perform hand hygiene each time I change the baby's diaper."
6. "I should keep the baby in the room unless instructed otherwise."

ANSWER: 3, 5, 6

Because the organisms causing gastroenteritis are eliminated in the feces, contact precautions should be used. This includes the standard precautions plus wearing a gown and gloves when soiling may be possible or when in contact with infected surfaces or items. The infant's movement outside the room is limited to only what is absolutely necessary. A mask is worn for droplet precautions and is unnecessary; the microorganisms causing gastroenteritis are passed in the feces. If soiling is expected when holding the baby, then gloves and a gown should be worn. If soiling or contact with infected surfaces or items is unlikely, neither a gown nor gloves is needed. The door is closed for airborne precautions; gastroenteritis is not airborne.

➧ *Test-taking Tip: Because contact precautions are necessary with gastroenteritis, select options that pertain to this precaution.*

Content Area: Child Health; Category of Health Alteration: Gastrointestinal Management; Integrated Processes: Nursing Process Evaluation; Client Need: Safe and Effective Care Environment/ Management of Care/Supervision; Cognitive Level: Analysis

References: Berman, A., Snyder, S., Kozier, B., & Erb, G. (2008). *Kozier & Erb's Fundamentals of Nursing: Concepts, Process, and Practice* (8th ed., p. 689). Upper Saddle River, NJ: Pearson Education; Hockenberry, M., & Wilson, D. (2007). *Wong's Nursing Care of Infants and Children* (8th ed., pp. 1183, 1190). St. Louis, MO: Mosby/Elsevier.

EBP Reference: Siegel, J., Rhinehart, E., Jackson, M., & Chiarello, L. Healthcare Infection Control Practices Advisory Committee. (2007). *Guideline for Isolation Precautions: Preventing Transmission of Infectious Agents in Healthcare Settings.* Standard precautions. Available at: www.guideline.gov/summary/summary.aspx?doc_id=10986&nbr=005766&string=Clostridium+AND+difficile

1202. EBP A nurse is developing a teaching plan for the parents of a 5-month-old infant diagnosed with gastroenteritis caused by a rotavirus. Which instructions should the nurse include to reduce the risk for transmission? SELECT ALL THAT APPLY.

1. Vacuum carpets and upholstery daily to rid the house of the infectious organism.
2. Wash the child's clothing soiled with stool separately from other family clothing.
3. Tell family members to wash hands frequently, especially after changing the infant's diaper.
4. Once the child is well, take the child to the clinic to complete the rotavirus immunization series.
5. Use alcohol-based wipes to cleanse the infant after a stool to disinfect the skin.
6. Store toothbrushes, pacifiers, and other personal items away from the diaper-changing area.

ANSWER: 2, 3, 4, 6

Viral gastroenteritis is transmitted by the fecal oral route. Washing soiled clothing separately can prevent transmission, especially if using hot water and soap and cleaning the washer with a bleach solution after use. Proper hand-washing technique is essential to prevent transmission as is storing any items away from soiled areas that are easily contaminated and can cause reinfection or transmission to others. Infants documented to have had rotavirus gastroenteritis before receiving the full course of rotavirus immunizations at 2, 4, and 6 months of age should still initiate or complete the 3-dose schedule because the initial infection frequently provides only partial immunity. Vacuuming and spraying the house are measures taken for other infectious diseases. Alcohol-based wipes, though disinfecting, can irritate the child's skin.

➧ *Test-taking Tip: "Viral" is the key word in the stem. Eliminate measures that are used with other infectious diseases and not those caused by a virus.*

Content Area: Child Health; Category of Health Alteration: Gastrointestinal Management; Integrated Processes: Nursing Process Planning; Client Need: Physiological Integrity/Physiological Adaptation/ Alterations in Body Systems; Cognitive Level: Analysis

Reference: Hockenberry, M., & Wilson, D. (2007). *Wong's Nursing Care of Infants and Children* (8th ed., pp. 1183, 1187, 1189–1190). St. Louis, MO: Mosby/Elsevier.

EBP Reference: American Academy of Pediatrics Committee on Infectious Diseases. (2007). Prevention of rotavirus disease: Guidelines for use of rotavirus vaccine. *Pediatrics,* 119(1), 171–182.

1203. A nurse is recording intake for a child hospitalized with diarrhea who has now begun to eat. The nurse should document ____ mL for the 3 ounces of popsicle that the child consumed.

ANSWER: 90

One ounce is equal to 30 mL. Using the proportion formula:
1 oz : 30 mL :: 3 oz : X mL
Multiply the means and the extremes.
X = 90 mL.

➧ ***Test-taking Tip:*** *Recall that 1 ounce is equal to 30 mL. Visualize a medicine cup, which is 1 ounce or 30 mL.*

Content Area: Child Health; *Category of Health Alteration:* Gastrointestinal Management; *Integrated Processes:* Communication and Documentation; *Client Need:* Physiological Integrity/Basic Care and Comfort/Nutrition and Oral Hydration; *Cognitive Level:* Application

Reference: Ball, J., & Bindler, R. (2006). *Clinical Handbook for Child Health Nurses* (pp. 142–146). Upper Saddle River, NJ: Pearson/Prentice Hall; Pickar, G. (2007). *Dosage Calculations: A Ratio-Proportion Approach* (2nd ed., p. 46). Clifton Park, NY: Thomson Delmar Learning.

1204. A nurse is caring for a 12-month-old child who has been admitted to a pediatric unit for dehydration secondary to vomiting and diarrhea. The toddler weighs 22 pounds. The toddler is to receive D5½NS with 20 mEq KCL at 4 mL/kg/hr. The nurse should set the pump to deliver _____ mL per hour.

ANSWER: 40

Convert kg to lb and then calculate the mL/kg/hr.
1 kg = 2.2 lb.
22 lb = 10 kg
4 mL/kg/hr = 4 times 10 = 40

➧ ***Test-taking Tip:*** *Carefully read the question to ensure that the correct numbers are used in the calculation of the fluid to be administered. Use the calculator provided with the NCLEX-RN®.*

Content Area: Child Health; *Category of Health Alteration:* Gastrointestinal Management; *Integrated Processes:* Nursing Process Implementation; *Client Need:* Physiological Integrity/Pharmacological and Parenteral Therapies/Parenteral/Intravenous Therapies; *Cognitive Level:* Application

References: Ball, J., & Binder, R. (2006). *Clinical Handbook for Pediatric Nursing* (pp. 176–178, 389–390). Upper Saddle River, NJ: Pearson Education; Hockenberry, M., & Wilson, D. (2007). *Wong's Nursing Care of Infants and Children* (8th ed., pp. 1159, 1168). St. Louis, MO: Mosby/Elsevier.

1205. A clinic nurse is providing instructions to the parents of an 18-month-old child experiencing acute diarrhea. The child weighs 12 kilograms. When teaching the parents, which points should the nurse emphasize? SELECT ALL THAT APPLY.

1. "Have your child drink plenty of fluids, including apple juice and other fruit juices."
2. "Put your child on a diet of bananas, rice, applesauce, tea, and toast (BRATT) until the diarrhea resolves."
3. "Encourage your child to eat small amounts of foods included in the child's normal diet, except cow's milk or milk products."
4. "Avoid using commercial baby wipes that contain alcohol to cleanse your child's skin."
5. "Wash your hands often, especially after changing your toddler, and keep soiled articles away from clean areas."
6. "Give ½ glass (120 mL) of an oral replacement fluid, such as Pedialyte® for each diarrheal stool."

ANSWER: 3, 4, 5, 6

A normal diet and appropriate administration of fluids is advised. While a normal diet may increase stool output initially, the stool pattern is outweighed by the benefits of a better nutritional outcome with fewer complications and a shorter illness course. Cow's milk and milk products can be irritating to the gut. Hand washing prevents the spread of gastroenteritis. Oral replacement solutions are used during maintenance fluid therapy and replacing fluid losses from diarrheal stools. Rehydration is 50 mL/kg during the first 4 hours and 10 mL/kg for each diarrheal stool. Fruit juices should be avoided because these contain a high amount of carbohydrates, pull circulating fluids into the gut, and can prolong diarrhea. A BRATT diet is low in energy and protein and no longer recommended.

Content Area: Child Health; *Category of Health Alteration:* Gastrointestinal Management; *Integrated Processes:* Nursing Process Implementation; *Client Need:* Physiological Integrity/Basic Care and Comfort/Nutrition and Oral Hydration; *Cognitive Level:* Analysis

References: Ball, J., & Bindler, R. (2008). *Pediatric Nursing: Caring for Children* (4th ed., p. 944). Upper Saddle River, NJ: Prentice Hall; Hockenberry, M., & Wilson, D. (2007). *Wong's Nursing Care of Infants and Children* (8th ed., pp. 1182–1190). St. Louis, MO: Mosby/Elsevier.

1206. An experienced nurse is observing a new nurse providing care to an 11-month-old child who is 12 hours postoperative from a cleft palate repair. Which nursing action requires the experienced nurse to intervene?

1. Using a suction catheter to remove oral secretions
2. Feeding soft, blended foods
3. Removing an arm restraint to check the skin
4. Administering an analgesic

ANSWER: 1

The nurse should avoid allowing objects to be placed in the infant's mouth because it can disrupt the suture line and cause bleeding or injury. It is important the infant has blended food (no hard foods such as crackers or ice chips). The palate needs to heal and hard foods may disrupt the sutures in the mouth. The arm restraints can be removed periodically. When they are on for longer periods of time, the arms need to be evaluated for possibly skin breakdown. Pain management is important, and pain medication should be administered especially the first 24 hours.

▶ ***Test-taking Tip:*** *Note the key word "intervene." Select the option that is inappropriate and could cause injury.*

Content Area: Child Health; *Category of Health Alteration:* Gastrointestinal Management; *Integrated Processes:* Nursing Process Implementation; *Client Need:* Physiological Integrity/Physiological Adaptation/Alterations in Body Systems; *Cognitive Level:* Analysis

Reference: Kyle, T. (2008). *Essentials of Pediatric Nursing* (p. 675). Philadelphia: Lippincott Williams & Wilkins.

1207. EBP A 2-week-old infant born with cleft lip and palate is being discharged from a hospital. The infant's parents have each demonstrated the proper technique of feeding the infant with a special soft-sided bottle equipped with a cleft palate nipple. Which complication should a nurse inform the parents to monitor for with this type of feeding?

1. Overstimulation
2. Overfeeding
3. Aspiration
4. Hiccups

ANSWER: 3

Risk of aspiration is always present when feeding an infant, but in cases where positioning and special feeding equipment are used the risk is greater. In this case, the soft-sided bottle allows the fluid to be introduced into the infant's mouth while squeezing the bottle; this further increases the risk for aspiration. Coughing and sputtering are prime indicators that the fluid has been aspirated. Feeding is usually a time of increasing infant contentment and not a significant source of stimulation. The amount of the feeding has been determined as age appropriate. As hiccups may occur before, during, or after any feeding, and while the act of hiccupping may lead to aspiration, it is the aspiration itself that is the major complication associated with this type of feeding.

▶ ***Test-taking Tip:*** *The key word is "complication." Use the ABCs (airway, breathing, circulation) to determine a life-threatening risk.*

Content Area: Child Health; *Category of Health Alteration:* Gastrointestinal Management; *Integrated Processes:* Teaching and Learning; *Client Need:* Physiological Integrity/Basic Care and Comfort/Nutrition and Oral Hydration; *Cognitive Level:* Application

Reference: Ball, J., & Bindler, R. (2006). *Child Health Nursing: Partnering with Children and Families* (pp. 1091–1102). Upper Saddle River, NJ: Pearson/Prentice Hall.

EBP Reference: DiCenso, A., Guyatt, G., & Ciliska, D. (2005). *Evidence-Based Nursing: A Guide to Clinical Practice* (p. 32). St. Louis, MO: Mosby/Elsevier.

1208. A nurse is completing discharge teaching with the parents of a 12-month-old child who has undergone a cleft palate repair. Which topics should be discussed in the discharge teaching? SELECT ALL THAT APPLY.

1. Checking the temperature of foods
2. Administering prescribed pain medication routinely
3. Demonstrating how to use a regular baby bottle for feeding
4. Applying elbow restraints when the baby is not being monitored
5. Demonstrating how to suction the baby's mouth using a bulb syringe
6. Addressing financial concerns for long-term care

ANSWER: 1, 2, 4, 6

Monitoring the temperature of foods is important because the new palate has no nerve endings to sense when things are too hot, thus causing a burn. Administering prescribed pain medication routinely is very important; children cannot always tell a caregiver when they are in pain. Elbow restraints are used so that the child will not disrupt the suture line as it is healing. Elbow restraints need to be released at least every 2 hours to monitor skin integrity and provide the child with range of motion. Financial stressors often exist because of the hospitalization and the need for ongoing care and speech therapy. With cleft palate surgery soft nipples are recommended to maintain the approximation of the incision and intactness of the suture. Different types of specialty bottles are available and one should be used. A bulb syringe has a hard tip and can damage the surgical repair.

▶ ***Test-taking Tip:*** *Eliminate any options that could damage the surgical incision.*

Content Area: Child Health; *Category of Health Alteration:* Gastrointestinal Management; *Integrated Processes:* Teaching and Learning; *Client Need:* Physiological Integrity/Physiological Adaptation/Illness Management; *Cognitive Level:* Application

References: Muscari, M. (2005). *Pediatric Nursing* (4th ed., p. 186). Philadelphia: Lippincott Williams & Wilkins; Hockenberry, M., & Wilson, D. (2007). *Wong's Nursing Care of Infants and Children* (8th ed., p. 465). St. Louis, MO: Mosby/Elsevier.

1209. In an infant who has been tentatively diagnosed with esophageal atresia, what should be the priority nursing outcome?

1. Infant will maintain adequate fluid volume.
2. Infant will demonstrate effective breathing pattern.
3. Nutritional status will be maintained.
4. Parents will exhibit emotional health.

ANSWER: 2

In esophageal atresia, the infant has a high risk for aspiration if feedings are not withheld and if the infant is not evaluated before the next feeding. The infant also is at high risk for aspirating secretions if there is a fistula connecting the esophagus and the trachea. The other options are important but not the priority. Adequate fluid volume and nutrition are important because the infant is unable to take nourishment orally. The parents are concerned because surgical intervention will be required as there is no opening between the esophagus and the stomach and a fistula may exist between the esophagus and trachea.

➧ ***Test-taking Tip:*** *Use the ABCs (airway, breathing, circulation) to establish the priority. Airway is always priority.*

Content Area: Child Health; *Category of Health Alteration:* Gastrointestinal Management; *Integrated Processes:* Nursing Process Planning; *Client Need:* Physiological Integrity/Physiological Adaptation/Illness Management; *Cognitive Level:* Analysis

References: Pillitteri, A. (2007). *Maternal and Child Health Nursing* (5th ed., p. 1190). Philadelphia: Lippincott Williams & Wilkins; Kyle, T. (2008). *Essentials of Pediatric Nursing* (pp. 670–672). Philadelphia: Lippincott Williams & Wilkins.

1210. A novice nurse is assessing a newly born infant with respiratory distress and copious oral secretions. The nurse's initial thought is tracheoesophageal atresia (TEA). Which nursing action should confirm this?

1. Respiratory distress decreases with oral suctioning.
2. Nasogastric tube (NG) easily advances to obtain stomach contents.
3. Catheter tip noted to be in the stomach on x-ray.
4. Soft NG advances, but unable to obtain stomach contents.

ANSWER: 4

There is a pouch at the end of the esophagus that does not connect to the stomach, so the soft NG will not advance past the pouch. With TEA respiratory distress is caused by aspiration and will not improve with oral suctioning. In TEA a NG cannot be advanced to the stomach and would not be visible by x-ray.

➧ ***Test-taking Tip:*** *Carefully read the stem to know what is being asked. Note the similarities in options 2 and 3 and delete these options. Next look at options 1 and 4 and select the option with abnormal information.*

Content Area: Child Health; *Category of Health Alteration:* Gastrointestinal Management; *Integrated Processes:* Nursing Process Evaluation; *Client Need:* Physiological Integrity/Reduction of Risk Potential/Potential for Alterations in Body Systems; *Cognitive Level:* Analysis

Reference: Pillitteri, A. (2007). *Maternal and Child Health Nursing* (5th ed., p. 1190). Philadelphia: Lippincott Williams & Wilkins.

1211. A 39-week-old infant is postoperative day 1 after emergency surgery for tracheoesophageal atresia. Which nursing action would be unsafe for the infant?

1. Providing a pacifier during gastrostomy feedings
2. Performing both oral and tracheal suctioning
3. After a gastrostomy feeding, elevating the gastrostomy tube, covering it with sterile gauze, and leaving it unclamped
4. Turning the infant frequently

ANSWER: 2

Tracheal suctioning should be avoided because it can disrupt the suture line from the repair. To remove secretions, oral suctioning can be performed. A pacifier is provided during gastrostomy feedings for sucking pleasure. Gastrostomy feedings are administered below the level of the surgical repair, and the end of the tube is elevated, covered by sterile gauze, and kept unclamped to allow air introduced during the feeling to bubble from the tube and not enter the esophagus and pass the fresh suture line. Any vomitus will project into the gastrostomy tube and not contaminate the fresh sutures. Turning discourages fluid from accumulating in the lungs.

➧ ***Test-taking Tip:*** *The key word is "unsafe." This is a false-response item; select the action that should not be performed.*

Content Area: Child Health; *Category of Health Alteration:* Gastrointestinal Management; *Integrated Processes:* Nursing Process Implementation; *Client Need:* Physiological Integrity/Reduction of Risk Potential/Therapeutic Procedures; *Cognitive Level:* Analysis

Reference: Pillitteri, A. (2007). *Maternal & Child Health Nursing: Care of the Childbearing & Childrearing Family* (5th ed., pp. 1189–1191). Philadelphia: Lippincott Williams & Wilkins.

1212. EBP A nurse completes teaching the parents of a 3-month-old infant diagnosed with pyloric stenosis who underwent surgical correction. Which statement by the parents indicates teaching has been effective?

1. "We should use a special infant feeder, such as a Breck® feeder, so our baby does not get so much air."
2. "Increasing the amount of formula at each feeding will help to expand our baby's stomach."
3. "After feedings, our baby should be handled as little as possible."
4. "Once put back to bed after the feeding, our baby should be positioned on the right side."

ANSWER: 4

Positioning side lying will prevent aspiration of vomitus; the right side aids stomach emptying through the pyloric valve by gravity. A Breck® feeder is used in feeding children with cleft lip or palate and is unnecessary. Only the amount of prescribed fluid should be given to preserve the integrity of the surgical repair site. The infant should be bubbled well after a feeding so there is no pressure from air in the stomach.

Test-taking Tip: *The key word is "effective." Select the option that is a true statement.*

Content Area: Child Health; *Category of Health Alteration:* Gastrointestinal Management; *Integrated Processes:* Teaching and Learning; *Client Need:* Physiological Integrity/Basic Care and Comfort/Nutrition and Oral Hydration; *Cognitive Level:* Analysis

Reference: Pillitteri, A. (2007). *Maternal & Child Health Nursing: Care of the Childbearing & Childrearing Family* (5th ed., pp. 1424–1425). Philadelphia: Lippincott Williams & Wilkins.

EBP Reference: Cincinnati Children's Hospital Medical Center. (2007). *Evidence Based Clinical Practice Guideline for Hypertrophic Pyloric Stenosis.* Available at: www.guideline.gov/summary/summary.aspx?view_id=1&doc_id=12095

1213. An experienced nurse and a new nurse who is orienting to a pediatric unit are caring for an infant newly diagnosed with a pyloric stenosis. Using an illustration, the experienced nurse asks the new nurse to identify the area affected by a pyloric stenosis. Place an X on the area that the new nurse should identify as the affected area.

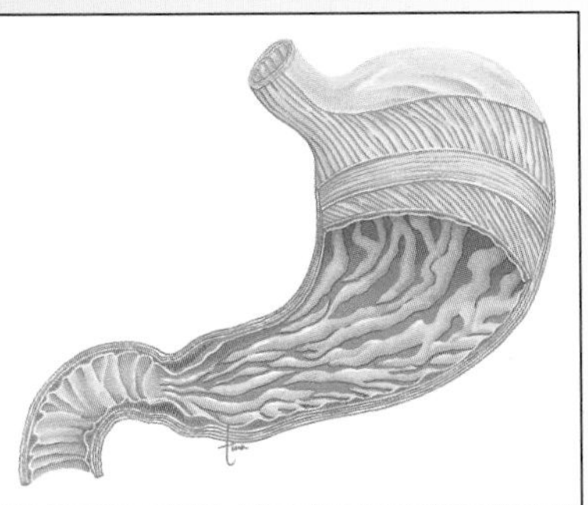

ANSWER:

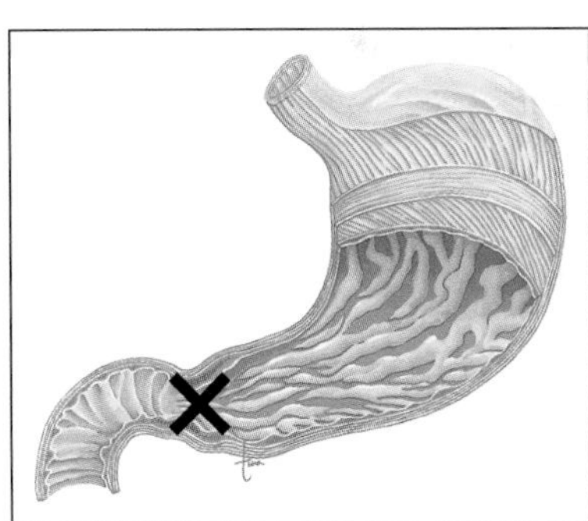

Fluid is unable to pass easily through the stenosed and hypertrophied pyloric valve (sphincter) at the lower portion of the stomach and the duodenum.

Test-taking Tip: *Carefully examine the illustration, noting the esophagus as the uppermost structure and the duodenum as the lowest structure on the illustration.*

Content Area: Child Health; *Category of Health Alteration:* Gastrointestinal Management; *Integrated Processes:* Teaching and Learning; *Client Need:* Safe and Effective Care Environment/Management of Care/Supervision; *Cognitive Level:* Application

Reference: Pillitteri, A. (2007). *Maternal & Child Health Nursing: Care of the Childbearing & Childrearing Family* (5th ed., pp. 1424–1425). Philadelphia: Lippincott Williams & Wilkins.

1214. An infant with prolonged vomiting secondary to pyloric stenosis has arterial blood gases (ABG) drawn. Which ABG results should a nurse expect when reviewing the laboratory report if the infant has an acid-base imbalance?

1. Increased pH and increased bicarbonate
2. Decreased pH and decreased bicarbonate
3. Increased pH and decreased bicarbonate
4. Decreased pH and increased bicarbonate

ANSWER: 1

An infant with pyloric stenosis often has been vomiting for 1 to 2 weeks, resulting in metabolic alkalosis as evidenced by an increase in both serum pH and bicarbonate. A decreased pH and bicarbonate are indicative of metabolic acidosis, which could result if overtreated for the acid-base imbalance or another complication. An increased pH and decreased bicarbonate could be from respiratory alkalosis with compensation. A decreased pH and increased bicarbonate could be from respiratory acidosis with compensation.

➧ ***Test-taking Tip:*** *First analyze the options with duplicate information and then eliminate either one or both of these. An acrostic memory cue is to label the mouth with the letter "a" for acid and the bottom or bowel movements with "b" for base to remember that acid is lost with vomiting and base is lost with diarrheal stool (bowel movements).*

Content Area: Child Health; *Category of Health Alteration:* Gastrointestinal Management; *Integrated Processes:* Nursing Process Assessment; *Client Need:* Physiological Integrity/Reduction of Risk Potential/Laboratory Values; *Cognitive Level:* Analysis

Reference: Hockenberry, M., & Wilson, D. (2007). *Wong's Nursing Care of Infants and Children* (8th ed., p. 1419). St. Louis, MO: Mosby/Elsevier.

1215. EBP Which interventions should a nurse include in the management of an infant newly diagnosed with pyloric stenosis? SELECT ALL THAT APPLY

1. Assess the amount, character, and frequency of vomitus
2. Keep the infant NPO
3. Administer parenteral solutions intravenously
4. Maintain patency of the nasogastric tube (NG)
5. Monitor for signs of hypokalemia
6. Maintain patency of the rectal tube

ANSWER: 1, 2, 3, 4, 5

Assessing the amount, character, and frequency of vomiting is very important in pyloric stenosis because infants dehydrate quickly. In pyloric stenosis, the frequent projectile vomiting from an overdistended stomach can be aspirated into the lungs. Thus the infant is kept NPO until surgical correction and may have a NG placed for gastric decompression. Frequent vomiting causes a lack in adequate hydration and a loss of potassium; fluids are replaced intravenously. Weakness, lethargy, and ECG changes can indicate hypokalemia from vomiting. A rectal tube would not be placed because stools will be minimal as a result of inadequate passage of food from the stomach to the duodenum due to constriction of the cardiac sphincter.

➧ ***Test-taking Tip:*** *If unsure, apply knowledge of medical terminology: pylorus is opening from the stomach into the intestine and stenosis is narrowing. Use this information to eliminate options not pertaining to the GI system from the end of the stomach and upward.*

Content Area: Child Health; *Category of Health Alteration:* Gastrointestinal Management; *Integrated Processes:* Nursing Process Implementation; *Client Need:* Physiological Integrity/Physiological Adaptation/Illness Management; *Cognitive Level:* Application

Reference: Hockenberry, M., & Wilson, D. (2007). *Wong's Nursing Care of Infants and Children* (8th ed., p. 1419). St. Louis, MO: Mosby/Elsevier.

EBP Reference: Cincinnati Children's Hospital Medical Center. (2007). *Evidence Based Clinical Practice Guideline for Hypertrophic Pyloric Stenosis.* Available at: www.guideline.gov/summary/summary.aspx?view_id=1&doc_id=12095

1216. A nurse is admitting a 5-week-old infant through an outpatient surgical unit for a laparoscopic correction of pyloric stenosis. Which manifestations should the nurse expect when asking the parents about the infant's symptoms? SELECT ALL THAT APPLY.

1. Projective vomiting
2. Bile-colored emesis
3. Sweet smelling vomitus
4. Weight loss
5. Absence of tears when crying
6. Hungry immediately after vomiting

ANSWER: 1, 4, 6

Because the sphincter is stenosed and the muscle hypertrophied, preventing emptying of the stomach into the duodenum, the infant would begin to vomit immediately after each feeding. Weight loss occurs due to lack of nourishment. With an empty stomach after vomiting, the infant feels hungry. The emesis should not be bile-colored because the feeding does not reach the duodenum to be mixed with bile. The vomitus is sour smelling and not sweet smelling because it has reached the stomach, where it is in contact with stomach enzymes. Absence of tears could indicate dehydration in an older infant, but infants younger than age 6 weeks do not tear.

➧ ***Test-taking Tip:*** *Focus on the age of the infant when selecting options. Eliminate any options that would suggest the passage of food into the duodenum.*

Content Area: Child Health; *Category of Health Alteration:* Gastrointestinal Management; *Integrated Processes:* Nursing Process Assessment; *Client Need:* Physiological Integrity/Reduction of Risk Potential/System Specific Assessments; *Cognitive Level:* Application

Reference: Pillitteri, A. (2007). *Maternal & Child Health Nursing: Care of the Childbearing & Childrearing Family* (5th ed., p. 1424). Philadelphia: Lippincott Williams & Wilkins.

1217. Based on assessment findings, a nurse thinks an infant may have developed necrotizing entercolitis (NEC) and plans interventions. In what order should a nurse plan to intervene for the infant? Place the items in order of priority.

______ Notify the health-care provider (HCP).
______ Immediately stop feedings.
______ Start prescribed antibiotics.
______ Prepare the infant for an abdominal x-ray.
______ Start prescribed intravenous fluids.

ANSWER: 2, 1, 4, 5, 3

It is critical to immediately stop feedings if NEC is suspected. The earlier the feedings are stopped, the better chance the infant has of preserving the bowel and not needing surgery. Next, notify the HCP, who will prescribe fluid replacement for the blood loss from bleeding from the bowel and prophylactic antibiotics. An x-ray will be prescribed; if perforation has occurred, there will be air in the abdominal cavity. If a portion of the bowel is necrosed and perforated, the infant needs immediate surgical intervention. The abdomen should also be handled gently to prevent bowel perforation.

➧ ***Test-taking Tip:*** *Use the ABCs (airway, breathing, circulation) to establish priority. The initial assessment requires an immediate intervention and then notifying the HCP. After notifying the HCP, focus on an intervention to preserve the circulation and then interventions that prevent harm.*

Content Area: Child Health; *Category of Health Alteration:* Gastrointestinal Management; *Integrated Processes:* Nursing Process Planning; *Client Need:* Physiological Integrity/Physiological Adaptation/Medical Emergencies; *Cognitive Level:* Analysis

References: Kyle, T. (2008). *Essentials of Pediatric Nursing* (pp. 688–689). Philadelphia: Lippincott Williams & Wilkins; Pillitteri, A. (2007). *Maternal & Child Health Nursing: Care of the Childbearing & Childrearing Family* (5th ed., p. 1435). Philadelphia: Lippincott Williams & Wilkins.

1218. A nurse is admitting an infant with a tentative diagnosis of intussusception. Which question to the mother would be most helpful in obtaining additional information to confirm the diagnosis?

1. "Does your baby vomit after each feeding?"
2. "What does the infant do when experiencing pain?"
3. "Is your infant passing ribbonlike stools?"
4. "Have you felt a mass in your infant's abdomen?"

ANSWER: 2

The diagnosis is suggested by the infant's history. In intussusception, infants suddenly draw up their legs and cry as if in severe pain due to a peristaltic wave that occurs from the invagination of one portion of the intestine into another. When the peristaltic wave passes, the infant is symptom free. Vomiting can occur with the pain from the peristaltic wave; this is unrelated to the time of feeding. Ribbonlike stools occur in Hirschsprung's disease because stool passes through areas of impacted feces and narrowed aganglionic distal segments of the bowel. The stools of intussusception are red, currant jelly–like in appearance from the mix of blood and mucous. A mass may be present and the baby's abdomen distended, but this is common to other gastrointestinal conditions and too general to confirm the diagnosis.

➧ ***Test-taking Tip:*** *Focus on the key words "additional information." Eliminate any options that elicit a "yes/no" response.*

Content Area: Child Health; *Category of Health Alteration:* Gastrointestinal Management; *Integrated Processes:* Communication and Documentation; *Client Need:* Physiological Integrity/Reduction of Risk Potential/System Specific Assessments; *Cognitive Level:* Analysis

Reference: Pillitteri, A. (2007). *Maternal & Child Health Nursing: Care of the Childbearing & Childrearing Family* (5th ed., pp. 1432–1433). Philadelphia: Lippincott Williams & Wilkins.

1219. A nurse is planning caring for an infant newly hospitalized with a diagnosis of intussusception. Which nursing diagnosis should the nurse establish as the immediate priority?

1. Pain related to abnormal abdominal peristalsis
2. Risk for deficient fluid volume related to bowel obstruction
3. Altered nutrition, less than body requirements related to vomiting
4. Risk for altered skin integrity related to bloody stools

ANSWER: 1

In intussusception, a portion of the intestine prolapses and then telescopes into another portion; this telescoping makes peristalsis difficult and intensely painful. The walls of the intestine also may rub together, causing inflammation, edema, and decreased blood flow, all of which can increase pain. Fluid can be lost through vomiting from the intense peristaltic waves or because of lack of absorption of fluids due to obstruction. Risk for deficient fluid volume is important, but not the priority, unless this were an actual problem. Vomiting can lead to altered nutrition, which is also important, but not the priority because the pain can cause the infant to be inconsolable and delay necessary interventions. Bloody stools, described as "currant jelly," occurs from inflammation and necrosis. Risk for altered skin integrity is important, but not the priority.

➧ ***Test-taking Tip:*** *Eliminate options that are risks and focus on the two actual problems. When determining priority, consider which problem could delay intervention for the other problem the most.*

Content Area: Child Health; *Category of Health Alteration:* Gastrointestinal Management; *Integrated Processes:* Nursing Process Planning; *Client Need:* Safe and Effective Care Environment/ Management of Care/Establishing Priorities; *Cognitive Level:* Analysis

Reference: Pillitteri, A. (2007). *Maternal & Child Health Nursing: Care of the Childbearing & Childrearing Family* (5th ed., pp. 1432–1434). Philadelphia: Lippincott Williams & Wilkins.

1220. A nurse is preparing a 4-month-old infant diagnosed with intussusception for surgery when the infant passes a normal brown stool. What is the nurse's most important action?

1. Notifying the health-care provider (HCP)
2. Palpating the infant's abdomen
3. Documenting the character of the stool
4. Checking the stool for the presence of blood

ANSWER: 1

The HCP should be notified because the passage of a normal brown stool may indicate reduction of the intussusception and the course of treatment may be altered and surgery cancelled. Palpating the infant's abdomen may indicate a change in the presence of a palpable mass and is important before notifying the HCP but not the most important action. The stools of intussusception are currant jelly–like in appearance from the mixture of mucous and blood due to inflammation and mechanical rubbing with the intussusception, and they now have changed to a normal appearance indicating the intussusception has been reduced. The documentation of the stool appearance and checking for blood in the stool are important but not the most important action.

➧ ***Test-taking Tip:*** *The key words are "most important." Select the option that is likely to alter the course of treatment.*

Content Area: Child Health; *Category of Health Alteration:* Gastrointestinal Management; *Integrated Processes:* Nursing Process Implementation; *Client Need:* Physiological Integrity/Physiological Adaptation/Alterations in Body Systems; *Cognitive Level:* Analysis

Reference: Ball, J., & Bindler, R. (2008). *Pediatric Nursing: Caring for Children* (4th ed., pp. 924–925). Upper Saddle River, NJ: Prentice Hall.

1221. A nurse is taking the history from a parent of an infant diagnosed with Hirschsprung's disease. Which statement is the parent most likely to make?

1. "My baby has ribbonlike stools that have a foul smell."
2. "My baby has projective vomiting and swollen arms and legs."
3. "My baby has gained weight faster than my other children."
4. "My baby cries for 4 hours every evening with leg and fist clenching."

ANSWER: 1

The common features of Hirschsprung's disease are ribbonlike, foul-smelling stools, chronic constipation, and abdominal distention. These occur from the absence of ganglion cells in affected bowel segments and resulting lack of peristalsis and loss of internal sphincter relaxation. Projective vomiting may occur from abdominal distention. Swollen arms and legs are not characteristics of Hirschsprung's disease. Weight loss and failure to thrive occurs due to malabsorption of nutrients. Recurrent evening crying with leg and fist clenching is more typical of colic, which is associated with increased peristalsis.

➧ ***Test-taking Tip:*** *Look for key words in the options that are inconsistent with Hirschsprung's disease, "swollen arms and legs," "gained weight," and "cries every evening."*

Content Area: Child Health; *Category of Health Alteration:* Gastrointestinal Management; *Integrated Processes:* Nursing Process Assessment; *Client Need:* Physiological Integrity/Physiological Adaptation/ Alterations in Body Systems; *Cognitive Level:* Application

Reference: Hockenberry, M., & Wilson, D. (2007). *Wong's Nursing Care of Infants and Children* (8th ed., pp. 1398–1399). St. Louis, MO: Mosby/ Elsevier.

1222. Which assessment findings might a nurse observe when assessing a neonate diagnosed with an anorectal malformation? SELECT ALL THAT APPLY.

1. Ribbonlike stools
2. Stenosed anal opening
3. Vomiting
4. Abdominal distention
5. Meconium in the urine
6. Poorly developed anal dimple

ANSWER: 1, 2, 3, 4, 5

Ribbonlike stools may occur with some malformations. The rectal opening can be narrowed or stenosed. Vomiting and abdominal distention can occur because stool has not passed. Meconium in the urine could indicate a fistula between the colon and urinary tract. A poorly developed anal dimple is suggestive of an anorectal malformation.

➧ ***Test-taking Tip:*** *Because anorectal malformations is a global term such that there may be many variations in findings related to the gastrointestinal system, eliminate this option.*

Content Area: Child Health; *Category of Health Alteration:* Gastrointestinal Management; *Integrated Processes:* Nursing Process Assessment; *Client Need:* Physiological Integrity/Reduction of Risk Potential/System Specific Assessments; *Cognitive Level:* Application

Reference: Ball, J., & Bindler, R. (2008). *Pediatric Nursing: Caring for Children* (4th ed., pp. 927–928). Upper Saddle River, NJ: Prentice Hall.

1223. A nurse is planning care for children diagnosed with inflammatory bowel diseases. After collecting and analyzing the information about the clients, which statement should best reflect the nurse's conclusion about the information?

1. All clients diagnosed with Crohn's disease are adolescent females.
2. None of the clients with a diagnosis of ulcerative colitis have a family history of the condition.
3. Most of the clients with either a diagnosis of Crohn's disease or ulcerative colitis are adolescent males.
4. Those clients diagnosed with Crohn's disease have more severe and bloody diarrhea than those diagnosed with ulcerative colitis.

ANSWER: 3

Both Crohn's disease and ulcerative colitis are more common in males, perhaps due to a familial or autoimmune tendency. Because Crohn's disease is more common in males, it is unlikely that all clients will be females. Both Crohn's disease and ulcerative colitis show familial tendencies. Because both diseases involve the development of ulcers of the mucosa or submucosal layers of the colon and rectum, both diseases manifest with diarrhea from irritation and unabsorbed fluids. The ileum is affected in Crohn's disease, whereas the colon and rectum are affected in ulcerative colitis. Because of the more severe ulcerations along the colon in ulcerative colitis, stools are more severe and bloody as compared with Crohn's disease.

➧ ***Test-taking Tip:*** *Eliminate the options with the absolute words "all" and "none," and then focus on the remaining two options.*

Content Area: Child Health; *Category of Health Alteration:* Gastrointestinal Management; *Integrated Processes:* Nursing Process Analysis; *Client Need:* Physiological Integrity/Physiological Adaptation/ Pathophysiology; *Cognitive Level:* Analysis

Reference: Pillitteri, A. (2007). *Maternal & Child Health Nursing: Care of the Childbearing & Childrearing Family* (5th ed., p. 1443). Philadelphia: Lippincott Williams & Wilkins.

1224. A parent is describing the stool number, consistency, appearance, and size for a child diagnosed with celiac disease to a nurse. Which changes in the child's stools should prompt the nurse to conclude that the child's ability to absorb nutrients is improving?

1. Disappearance of currant jelly–like stools
2. Reduction of ribbonlike stools
3. Absence of large, bulky, greasy stools
4. Absence of liquid green stools

ANSWER: 3

Large, bulky, greasy stools describe steatorrhea. When gluten is ingested in celiac disease, changes occur in the intestinal mucosa or villi that prevent the absorption of foods across the intestinal villi into the bloodstream and the inability to absorb fat. Currant jelly–like stools are characteristic of intussusception from the mixing of blood and mucous. Ribbonlike stools occur in Hirschsprung's disease because stool passes through areas of impacted feces and narrowed aganglionic distal segments of the bowel. Liquid green stools appear in diarrhea.

Test-taking Tip: *Carefully read what the question is asking. The key words are "absorb nutrients." Eliminate options that suggest bleeding or obstruction.*

Content Area: Child Health; *Category of Health Alteration:* Gastrointestinal Management; *Integrated Processes:* Nursing Process Evaluation; *Client Need:* Physiological Integrity/Reduction of Risk Potential/System Specific Assessments; *Cognitive Level:* Application

Reference: Pillitteri, A. (2007). *Maternal & Child Health Nursing: Care of the Childbearing & Childrearing Family* (5th ed., pp. 1420, 1433, 1439, 1442). Philadelphia: Lippincott Williams & Wilkins.

1225. A nurse is using a food list to address foods to be eliminated from a child's diet when counseling a parent of a child diagnosed with celiac disease. Which foods should appear on the elimination food list?

1. Cereal containing oat, wheat, or rye and certain frozen foods
2. Breads made with potato or corn and white whole or skim milk
3. Soups, sauces, and peanut butter
4. Cereals and breads containing rice, and cottage cheese

ANSWER: 1

Foods that contain gluten include wheat, rye, oats, and barley products should be eliminated. Packaged and frozen foods typically contain gluten as fillers. Potato bread or cornbread and whole, skim, or low-fat milk are acceptable. Chocolate milk and malt beverages contain gluten. Soups and sauces usually contain gluten used in the wheat flour for thickening. Peanut butter, cereals, and breads containing rice, and cottage cheese are acceptable foods.

Test-taking Tip: *Focus on what is being asked and select the foods that should be "eliminated" from the diet of a person with celiac disease.*

Content Area: Child Health; *Category of Health Alteration:* Gastrointestinal Management; *Integrated Processes:* Teaching and Learning; *Client Need:* Physiological Integrity/Basic Care and Comfort/Nutrition and Oral Hydration; *Cognitive Level:* Application

References: Lutz, C., & Przytulski, K. (2006). *Nutrition & Diet Therapy: Evidence-Based Applications* (4th ed., pp. 191–192). Philadelphia: F. A. Davis; Pillitteri, A. (2007). *Maternal & Child Health Nursing: Care of the Childbearing & Childrearing Family* (5th ed., pp. 1439–1440). Philadelphia: Lippincott Williams & Wilkins.

1226. A child is diagnosed with early hypovolemic shock following surgical intervention for a ruptured appendix. Which nursing assessment findings support this diagnosis?

1. Tachycardia, capillary refill greater than 2 seconds, cold extremities, and weak distal pulses
2. Bradycardia, hypotension, mottled color, and weak distal pulses
3. Irritability and anxiousness, capillary refill greater than 2 seconds, and absent distal pulses
4. Lethargy, cold extremities, decreased urine output, and absent distal pulses

ANSWER: 1

Signs and symptoms of early hypovolemic shock are tachycardia, increased respiratory rate, capillary refill time greater than 2 seconds, weak distal pulses, pallor or mottled color, cold extremities, blood pressure often normal for age, and decreased urine output (less than 1 to 2 mL/kg/hr in newborns and less than 0.5 to 1.0 mL/kg/hr in other age groups). Bradycardia and absent distal pulses are associated with a later stage of hypovolemic shock.

Test-taking Tip: *Analyze the options with the duplicate information first, weak distal pulses and absent distal pulses. Weak distal pulses are most likely in "early hypovolemic shock," thus eliminating options 3 and 4. Next examine the options with opposite information, tachycardia, and bradycardia to select the best option.*

Content Area: Child Health; *Category of Health Alteration:* Gastrointestinal Management; *Integrated Processes:* Nursing Process Assessment; *Client Need:* Physiological Integrity/Physiological Adaptation/Alterations in Body Systems; Physiological Integrity/Physiological Adaptation/Pathophysiology; *Cognitive Level:* Application

References: Ball, J., & Binder, R. (2006). *Clinical Handbook for Pediatric Nursing* (pp. 286–287). Upper Saddle River, NJ: Pearson Education; Hockenberry, M., & Wilson, D. (2007). *Wong's Nursing Care of Infants and Children* (8th ed., p. 1194). St. Louis, MO: Mosby/Elsevier.

1227. A nurse is caring for a 10-year-old child who has been diagnosed with peritonitis secondary to a ruptured appendix. Which prescription by the health-care provider (HCP) should the nurse question?

1. Irrigation of incision site bid with 0.9% NaCl solution
2. Empty and measure JP drain q8 hrs. or as needed
3. Continue IV fluids as previously requested and keep NPO
4. NG to high intermittent suction (HIS); empty and measure q8 hr.

ANSWER: 4

A nasogastric tube (NG) is needed until there is evidence of intestinal movement; however, the NG on a child this age would be kept on low intermittent suction (LIS) and not high intermittent suction (HIS) to ensure that there would be no injury to the gastric lining. Irrigating the incision site, emptying the Jackson-Pratt drain, and continuing IV fluids and keeping the client NPO are all appropriate interventions.

➧ ***Test-taking Tip:*** *The key words are "should question." This is a negative-response item. Select the prescription by the HCP that is not correct for this client.*

Content Area: Child Health; *Category of Health Alteration:* Gastrointestinal Management; *Integrated Processes:* Nursing Process Implementation; *Client Need:* Safe and Effective Care Environment/Safety and Infection Control/Accident and Injury Prevention; *Cognitive Level:* Analysis

Reference: Hockenberry, M., & Wilson, D. (2007). *Wong's Nursing Care of Infants and Children* (8th ed., p. 1405). St. Louis, MO: Mosby/Elsevier.

1228. A nurse is caring for a 5-year-old child who has been diagnosed with peritonitis secondary to a ruptured appendix. The child begins complaining of abdominal pain and nausea, even though a nasogastric tube (NG) is in place. When pulling back the covers, the nurse notes that the child's abdomen is distended. Which action should be taken by the nurse *first*?

1. Call the primary health-care provider (HCP).
2. Check the NG to determine if fluid is moving within the tubing to the drainage container.
3. Finish the abdominal assessment and check the child's vital signs.
4. Obtain and administer an antiemetic.

ANSWER: 2

The first action is to check the functionality of the NG, including suction and correct placement. Once it has been established that the NG is functioning, the nurse should complete the assessment and contact the primary HCP because nonmechanical paralytic ileus can develop in the immediate postoperative period. An antiemetic should be administered if prescribed, and reestablishment of a nonfunctioning NG does not relieve the nausea, but these are not the first action.

➧ ***Test-taking Tip:*** *The key words are "first." Focus on the client's symptoms.*

Content Area: Child Health; *Category of Health Alteration:* Gastrointestinal Management; *Integrated Processes:* Nursing Process Implementation; *Client Need:* Physiological Integrity/Reduction of Risk Potential/Therapeutic Procedures; *Cognitive Level:* Analysis

References: Hockenberry, M., & Wilson, D. (2007). *Wong's Nursing Care of Infants and Children* (8th ed., pp. 1128–1129). St. Louis, MO: Mosby/Elsevier; Lewis, S., Heitkemper, M., & Dirksen, S. (2007). *Medical-Surgical Nursing: Assessment and Management of Clinical Problems.* (7th ed., pp. 1060–1062). St. Louis, MO: Mosby.

1229. Before administering an enteral feeding to a 2-month-old infant, a nurse aspirates 5 mL of gastric contents. Which action should the nurse take *next*?

1. Return the aspirate and withhold the feeding.
2. Discard the aspirate and give the full feeding.
3. Return the aspirate before beginning the feeding.
4. Discard the aspirate and add an equal amount of normal saline to the feeding.

ANSWER: 3

If the amount aspirated is small (a few milliliters), the aspirate should be returned at the beginning of the feeding to prevent the loss of electrolytes and gastric enzymes. If the amount is large, as compared to the amount prescribed for the feeding, then the amount of the feeding should be reduced by the amount of the aspirate. Five milliliters is equivalent to a teaspoon, which is a small amount for a 2-month-old infant. With a small amount the feeding should not be withheld. Discarding the aspirate with each feeding can result in acid-base and electrolyte imbalances, and saline is not an electrolyte replacement for gastric contents.

➧ ***Test-taking Tip:*** *Examine options with duplicate words first. Determine whether the aspirate should be returned or discarded. After determining it should be returned, eliminate the discard options and then determine which of the two remaining options is best.*

Content Area: Child Health; *Category of Health Alteration:* Gastrointestinal Management; *Integrated Processes:* Nursing Process Implementation; *Client Need:* Physiological Integrity/Reduction of Risk Potential/Therapeutic Procedures; *Cognitive Level:* Application

Reference: Pillitteri, A. (2007). *Maternal & Child Health Nursing: Care of the Childbearing & Childrearing Family* (5th ed., p. 1129). Philadelphia: Lippincott Williams & Wilkins.

1230. An infant, who is unable to suck effectively, requires gavage feedings. Which statements best describes the proper protocol a nurse should follow when feeding an infant via gavage feedings? SELECT ALL THAT APPLY.

1. The gavage tube can be inserted in either the mouth or the nose.
2. The feedings should mimic the bottle feedings in amount.
3. Continuous feedings rather than intermittent feedings are preferred.
4. Aspirate stomach contents before the feeding and discard the aspirates.
5. Provide mouth care at least twice daily or more often to reduce bacterial growth.
6. Warm the gavage formula to room temperature before starting the feeding.

ANSWER: 1, 2, 5, 6

While orogastric insertion allows for easier breathing and less risk of vagal stimulation and is preferred, if the tube is to stay in place, it may be inserted nasally. The amount of gavage feeding should be similar in amount to what the child normally would ingest at a feeding to prevent overdistention or undernourishment. Oral care is necessary to prevent dryness and oral ulcers. Warming to room temperature will prevent chilling. Intermittent (not continuous) feedings are preferred to mimic the normal feeding pattern and allow the stomach to function more normally. Unless the amount is excessive, aspirates should be measured and reinserted (not discarded) so electrolytes are retained.

➧ ***Test-taking Tip:*** *Carefully read each option and look for key words in the options that are opposite of the actions in the protocol.*

Content Area: Child Health; *Category of Health Alteration:* Gastrointestinal Management; *Integrated Processes:* Nursing Process Implementation; *Client Need:* Integrity/Basic Care and Comfort/Nutrition and Oral Hydration; *Cognitive Level:* Application

Reference: Pillitteri, A. (2007). *Maternal & Child Health Nursing: Care of the Childbearing & Childrearing Family* (5th ed., p. 1127). Philadelphia: Lippincott Williams & Wilkins.

1231. A nurse is caring for a 1-year-old child who had surgery for a gastrostomy tube insertion. Which statement describes the nurse's best action in the care of the child?

1. Place thick dressings under the gastrostomy tube area to keep it clean and dry.
2. Apply the prescribed antibiotic ointment to the insertion site.
3. Apply tension on the gastrostomy device to ensure the balloon is against the stomach wall.
4. Begin tube feedings as soon as the child returns from surgery.

ANSWER: 2

Topical antibiotics and skin protective creams assist in preventing infections. While surgical sites carry a risk of infection and moist areas increase risk, a thick dressing puts tension on the tube, which could cause accidental removal or impaired tissue integrity from pressure. Tension should be avoided to prevent tissue trauma or accidental removal. Tube feedings are not begun until bowel function has returned.

➧ ***Test-taking Tip:*** *Identify the options that could cause harm and eliminate these.*

Content Area: Child Health; *Category of Health Alteration:* Gastrointestinal Management; *Integrated Processes:* Nursing Process Implementation; *Client Need:* Physiological Integrity/Basic Care and Comfort/Nutrition and Oral Hydration; *Cognitive Level:* Application

Reference: Hockenberry, M., & Wilson, D. (2007). *Wong's Nursing Care of Infants and Children* (8th ed., pp. 1132–1134). St. Louis, MO: Mosby/Elsevier.

1232. A public health nurse is caring for a 10-year-old child who is diagnosed with hepatitis A. The nurse is instructing the parents to avoid giving their child oral medications. Which is the nurse's rationale for giving this instruction?

1. The child does not need pain medications because there is no pain associated with hepatitis A.
2. The medication of choice is antibiotics, and the child will be on those only while hospitalized.
3. Normal medication doses may become dangerous due to the liver's inability to detoxify and excrete them.
4. The foods provided will contain all of the natural substances the child will need for recovery.

ANSWER: 3

The function of the liver is altered due to liver damage in hepatitis, and medications cannot be metabolized and detoxified by the liver and excreted from the body. The child is likely to experience epigastric or right upper-quadrant pain in hepatitis, so the child will need pain medication. The child probably will not need antibiotics because hepatitis is viral in origin. Foods are for nutritional needs and will not provide the necessary analgesia for pain control.

Test-taking Tip: *Note absolute words in two options (only and all) and delete these options. Rarely are options with absolute words the correct answer. Focusing on how medications are metabolized and excreted should lead you to select the correct option.*

Content Area: Child Health; *Category of Health Alteration:* Gastrointestinal Management; *Integrated Processes:* Nursing Process Analysis; *Client Need:* Physiological Integrity/Physiological Adaptation/Illness Management; Physiological Integrity/Pharmacological and Parenteral Therapies/Medication Administration; *Cognitive Level:* Analysis

Reference: Hockenberry, M., & Wilson, D. (2007). *Wong's Nursing Care of Infants and Children* (8th ed., pp. 1127–1129). St. Louis, MO: Mosby/Elsevier.

Test 32: **Child Health: Hematological and Oncological Management**

1233. A nurse is using an illustration to teach the parents of a child the location in which bone marrow will be aspirated for a bone marrow biopsy. Which anatomical site should the nurse identify to the parents as the site for a child's bone marrow aspiration? Place an X on the anatomical site.

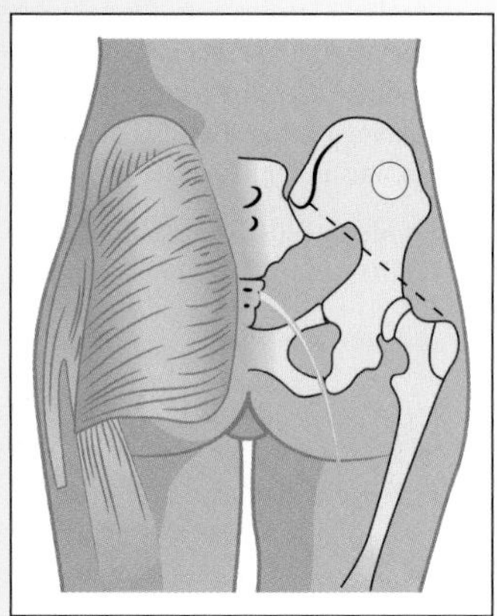

ANSWER:

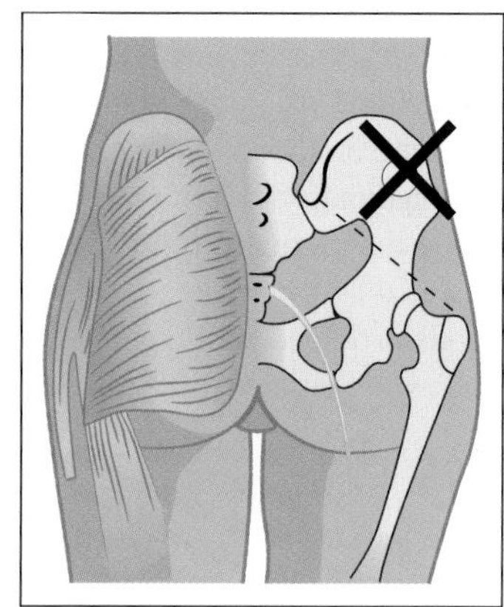

A common site used for bone marrow aspiration in children is the posterior superior iliac crest.

➧ ***Test-taking Tip:*** *Select an area in which the bone would be the largest and easily approached with a needle.*

Content Area: Child Health; *Category of Health Alteration:* Hematological and Oncological Management; *Integrated Processes:* Teaching and Learning; *Client Need:* Physiological Integrity/Reduction of Risk Potential/Diagnostic Tests; *Cognitive Level:* Application

Reference: Pillitteri, A. (2007). *Maternal & Child Health Nursing: Care of the Childbearing & Childrearing Family* (5th ed., pp. 1384–1385). Philadelphia: Lippincott Williams & Wilkins.

1234. Which nursing diagnosis should be the priority for a child hospitalized in sickle cell crisis?

1. Risk for deficient fluid volume related to inadequate fluid intake
2. Chronic pain related to chronic physical disability and clustering of sickled cells
3. Risk for infection related to ineffectively functioning spleen
4. Ineffective tissue perfusion related to pulmonary infiltrates of abnormal blood cells

ANSWER: 4

While all are appropriate nursing diagnoses, ineffective tissue perfusion is priority because it can be life threatening. Acute chest syndrome is a common cause of hospitalization for sickle cell disease. The other nursing diagnoses are not life threatening.

➧ ***Test-taking Tip:*** *Use the ABCs (airway, breathing, circulation) to establish priority. Problems with any of these can be life threatening.*

Content Area: Child Health; *Category of Health Alteration:* Hematological and Oncological Management; *Integrated Processes:* Nursing Process Analysis; *Client Need:* Safe and Effective Care Environment/Management of Care/Establishing Priorities; *Cognitive Level:* Analysis

Reference: Ball, J., & Bindler, R. (2008). *Pediatric Nursing: Caring for Children* (4th ed., pp. 814–815). Upper Saddle River, NJ: Pearson/Prentice Hall.

1235. The parents of an 8-year-old African American child diagnosed with sickle cell anemia are being taught pain control measures for their child. Which measure is most important to teach the parents to prevent the onset of vaso-occlusive pain?

1. Apply ice packs to all joints as soon as the child awakens.
2. Encourage drinking large amounts of fluids daily.
3. Administer acetaminophen (Tylenol®) 650 mg orally daily.
4. Increase outdoor exercise and exposure to the fresh air and sunshine.

ANSWER: 2

Hydration promotes hemodilution, reduces blood viscosity, and prevents vessel occlusion. Ice packs can cause vasoconstriction and decrease tissue perfusion, thereby increasing pain and sickling. Acetaminophen may be used for pain relief, but the dose is excessive for a child. Exercise increases oxygen demand, decreases oxygen tension, and increases sickling. Sunshine exposure can lead to dehydration, which increases blood viscosity.

Test-taking Tip: *The key phrase is "prevent the onset." Determine if each option would increase or decrease pooling of sickled cells and tissue hypoxia.*

Content Area: Child Health; *Category of Health Alteration:* Hematological and Oncological Management; *Integrated Processes:* Teaching and Learning; *Client Need:* Physiological Integrity/Basic Care and Comfort/Non-Pharmacological Comfort Interventions; *Cognitive Level:* Application

Reference: Pillitteri, A. (2007). *Maternal & Child Health Nursing: Care of the Childbearing & Childrearing Family* (5th ed., pp. 1396–1397). Philadelphia: Lippincott Williams & Wilkins.

1236. After 7 days of iron therapy, a child diagnosed with iron-deficiency anemia has serum laboratory tests completed. Which finding indicates that the medication is beginning to correct the anemia?

1. Increased reticulocyte count
2. Increased granulocytes
3. Increased indirect bilirubin
4. Increased erythropoietin levels

ANSWER: 1

Red blood cells (RBCs) are small and pale because of the stunted hemoglobin. Administering iron increases the production of RBCs. A reticulocyte count measures how fast the reticulocytes (slightly immature RBCs) are made by the bone marrow and released into the blood. Granulocytes (neutrophils, basophils, and eosinophils) are a type of white blood cell filled with microscopic granules and increase with infection or inflammation. Indirect bilirubin increases from the breakdown of the heme portion of RBCs. RBCs should not be breaking down. Erythropoietin is a hormone produced by the kidneys that is stimulated whenever a child has tissue hypoxia. If anemia is correcting, hypoxia should not occur and erythropoietin production not stimulated.

Test-taking Tip: *Eliminate options not directly related to the development of RBCs (options 2, 3, and 4).*

Content Area: Child Health; *Category of Health Alteration:* Hematological and Oncological Management; *Integrated Processes:* Nursing Process Evaluation; *Client Need:* Physiological Integrity/Reduction of Risk Potential/Laboratory Values; *Cognitive Level:* Analysis

Reference: Pillitteri, A. (2007). *Maternal & Child Health Nursing: Care of the Childbearing & Childrearing Family* (5th ed., pp. 1383, 1394). Philadelphia: Lippincott Williams & Wilkins.

1237. A child having recovered following ingestion of rat poison, develops aplastic anemia. Which assessment finding should a nurse conclude is specifically related to the aplastic anemia? SELECT ALL THAT APPLY.

1. Petechiae
2. Epistaxis
3. Easily fatigued
4. Pale skin color
5. Watery, itching eyes
6. Ulcerations around the mouth

ANSWER: 1, 2, 3, 4

Acquired aplastic anemia can result from chemicals, such as rat poisoning, that depress the hematopoietic activity in the bone marrow. Reduced platelet production results in easy bruising, petechiae, and bleeding, such as nose bleeds (epistaxis). The lower red blood cell count and resultant tissue hypoxia produce symptoms of fatigue and pallor. Watery, itching eyes are unrelated to aplastic anemia and could be from an allergic reaction. Mouth ulcerations could be burns from the rat poison ingestion.

Test-taking Tip: *Recall that aplastic anemia alters bone marrow function. Select the signs and symptoms that would be associated with a decreased bone marrow function.*

Content Area: Child Health; *Category of Health Alteration:* Hematological and Oncological Management; *Integrated Processes:* Nursing Process Assessment; *Client Need:* Physiological Integrity/Reduction of Risk Potential/System Specific Assessments; *Cognitive Level:* Application

Reference: Pillitteri, A. (2007). *Maternal & Child Health Nursing: Care of the Childbearing & Childrearing Family* (5th ed., p. 1390). Philadelphia: Lippincott Williams & Wilkins.

1238. A child diagnosed with aplastic anemia has had human leukocyte antigen (HLA) typing, evaluation of organ function, and laboratory studies completed as an outpatient. Which action should a nurse plan to implement *first* when the child is admitted to a transplant center for a hematopoietic stem cell transplant?

1. Checking the patency of the central line catheter
2. Placing the child in protective isolation
3. Ensuring that all food entering the child's room has been irradiated
4. Preparing the child to receive high doses of chemotherapy

ANSWER: 4

Preparing the child both physically and psychologically is priority. The child will be given high doses of chemotherapy and sometimes total body irradiation to destroy circulating blood cells and the diseased bone marrow before the transplantation of donor stem cells. Chemotherapy, and later donor stem cells, will be administered by intravenous infusion through a central line catheter. Although patency must be checked prior to administration, preparing the child is priority. During chemotherapy and pancytopenia, strict protective isolation is maintained. Strict isolation includes irradiating food and sterilizing utensils and other items used in the room.

➧ ***Test-taking Tip:** The key word is "first." All options are correct, but one option should occur first during the pretransplant phase.*

Content Area: Child Health; *Category of Health Alteration:* Hematological and Oncological Management; *Integrated Processes:* Nursing Process Planning; *Client Need:* Safe and Effective Care Environment/Management of Care/Establishing Priorities; *Cognitive Level:* Analysis

Reference: Ball, J., & Bindler, R. (2008). *Pediatric Nursing: Caring for Children* (4th ed., p. 833). Upper Saddle River, NJ: Pearson/Prentice Hall.

1239. EBP A child diagnosed with hemophilia is brought to a clinic due to pain and restricted movement of the left knee after tripping going upstairs. A nurse assesses that the knee is hot, swollen, and tender to touch. The nurse should initially conclude that the child is likely experiencing:

1. a Baker's cyst.
2. hemarthrosis.
3. a patella fracture.
4. disseminated intravascular coagulation (DIC).

ANSWER: 2

Hemarthrosis is bleeding into the joint. Signs include restricted movement, pain, tenderness, and a hot, swollen joint. A Baker's cyst is a bulge occurring in the popliteal bursa behind the knee from excess synovial fluid. A patella fracture is a broken kneecap. Signs include intense pain and swelling. Based on the child's history of hemophilia, patella fracture would be an unlikely initial conclusion for the nurse, although this could be the eventual diagnosis. DIC is widespread clotting throughout the body. Symptoms include diffuse bleeding from multiple sites.

➧ ***Test-taking Tip:** Focus on the child's history of hemophilia and note the similarities of "hem-" between the history and option 2.*

Content Area: Child Health; *Category of Health Alteration:* Hematological and Oncological Management; *Integrated Processes:* Nursing Process Assessment; *Client Need:* Physiological Integrity/Physiological Adaptation/Alterations in Body Systems; *Cognitive Level:* Analysis

Reference: Hockenberry, M., & Wilson, D. (2007). *Wong's Nursing Care of Infants and Children* (8th ed., pp. 1536–1540). St. Louis, MO: Mosby/Elsevier.

EBP Reference: Lamoureux, C., & Kilcoyne, R. (2007). Patella, fractures. *E-Medicine*. Available at: www.emedicine.com/radio/topic528.htm

---

1240. Which actions should a school nurse include in the emergency treatment of a child diagnosed with von Willebrand's disease who is experiencing epistaxis? SELECT ALL THAT APPLY.

1. Have the child lie down.
2. Elevate the child's feet.
3. Apply pressure to the child's nose with the thumb and forefinger.
4. Keep pressure applied for at least 10 minutes.
5. Apply ice or a cold cloth to the bridge of the child's nose.
6. Ask the child if he or she is carrying medication to treat the nosebleed.

ANSWER: 3, 4, 5

Most of the bleeding occurs in the anterior part of the nasal septum; therefore, compression helps stop the flow of blood. Because of delayed clotting due to insufficient clotting factors, pressure needs to be prolonged for at least 10 minutes. The application of cold constricts blood vessels and reduces bleeding. The child should sit and lean forward to protect the airway from being obstructed by the blood. Elevating the feet is unnecessary and if the child is lying down can increase the blood flow to the head. Usually a single dose of desmopressin acetate (DDAVP) is effective in stopping the nosebleed. The medication and supplies, if available at school, should be kept in a locked medication cupboard in the nurse's office and would not be carried by the student.

➧ ***Test-taking Tip:** Use principles from the ABCs (airway, breathing, circulation) to eliminate the options that compromise the child's airway, breathing, or circulation.*

Content Area: Child Health; *Category of Health Alteration:* Hematological and Oncological Management; *Integrated Processes:* Nursing Process Implementation; *Client Need:* Physiological Integrity/ Physiological Adaptation/Medical Emergencies; *Cognitive Level:* Application

Reference: Hockenberry, M., & Wilson, D. (2007). *Wong's Nursing Care of Infants and Children* (8th ed., pp. 1540–1541). St. Louis, MO: Mosby/ Elsevier.

1241. Which finding should a nurse expect when reviewing the laboratory results of an infant newly diagnosed with hemophilia A?

1. Prolonged prothrombin time (PT)
2. Decreased hemoglobin level
3. Decreased hematocrit level
4. Prolonged activated partial thromboplastin time (aPTT)

ANSWER: 4

Hemophilia A results from a deficiency of factor VIII. Because aPTT measures the activity of thromboplastin and factor VIII is deficient, the aPTT is prolonged. The PT measures the action of prothrombin and will be prolonged with deficiencies of prothrombin and factors V, VII, and X. The hemoglobin and hematocrit is not used to diagnose hemophilia A and should be normal unless the child is bleeding.

➧ ***Test-taking Tip:*** *Use a memory aid to remember the aPTT is prolonged in hemophilia A. Note the "A" in hemophilia A and the "a" in aPTT.*

Content Area: Child Health; *Category of Health Alteration:* Hematological and Oncological Management; *Integrated Processes:* Nursing Process Assessment; *Client Need:* Physiological Integrity/ Reduction of Risk Potential/Laboratory Values; *Cognitive Level:* Application

References: Ball, J., & Bindler, R. (2008). *Pediatric Nursing: Caring for Children* (4th ed., pp. 824-826). Upper Saddle River, NJ: Pearson/Prentice Hall; Pillitteri, A. (2007). *Maternal & Child Health Nursing: Care of the Childbearing & Childrearing Family* (5th ed., p. 1385). Philadelphia: Lippincott Williams & Wilkins.

1242. EBP A new nurse is telling an experienced nurse about treatments that a physician discussed with the parents of a child who has thalassemia major. Which statement by the new nurse should the experienced nurse question?

1. "Plasmapheresis will help remove the toxins that are destroying the red blood cells."
2. "Blood transfusions will need to be administered about every 2 to 4 weeks."
3. "A splenectomy may become necessary to reduce the child's abdominal discomfort."
4. "Bone marrow stem cell transplant can possibly cure this child's thalassemia major."

ANSWER: 1

Thalassemia major occurs from a deficiency in the synthesis of the beta-chain of the hemoglobin resulting in defective hemoglobin that damages the red blood cells. Plasmapheresis, selective removal of the plasma, would be ineffective in treating thalassemia because the cells are not being destroyed by toxins in the plasma. Blood transfusion, splenectomy, and bone marrow stem cell transplant are all treatments for thalassemia major. Bone marrow stem cell transplantation can offer a cure.

➧ ***Test-taking Tip:*** *This is a false-response item. Select the statement that would be incorrect. Note the commonalities between options 2, 3, and 4. Often the option that is different is the answer.*

Content Area: Child Health; *Category of Health Alteration:* Hematological and Oncological Management; *Integrated Processes:* Nursing Process Evaluation; *Client Need:* Physiological Integrity/ Physiological Adaptation/Illness Management; *Cognitive Level:* Analysis

References: Hockenberry, M., & Wilson, D. (2007). *Wong's Nursing Care of Infants and Children* (8th ed., pp. 1529, 1532–1534). St. Louis, MO: Mosby/Elsevier; Pillitteri, A. (2007). *Maternal & Child Health Nursing: Care of the Childbearing & Childrearing Family* (5th ed., pp. 1401–1402). Philadelphia: Lippincott Williams & Wilkins.

EBP Reference: Schrier, S., & Angelucci, E. (2005). New strategies in the treatment of the thalassemias. *Annual Review Medicine*, 56, 157–171.

1243. A child has iron overload from receiving multiple blood transfusions for treating thalassemia major. A nurse should anticipate the physician will likely:

1. order intravenous (IV) fluids to dilute the excess iron and increase urinary excretion.
2. change the type of blood product being transfused.
3. reduce the frequency of blood transfusions.
4. begin chelation therapy.

ANSWER: 4

In chelation therapy, an iron-chelating drug, such as deferoxamine, is administered to bind excess iron so it can be excreted by the kidneys. Hemodilution, changing blood products, and reducing the frequency of transfusions do not treat the iron overload. IV fluids will not increase the urinary excretion of iron.

➧ ***Test-taking Tip:*** *Focus on treating the problem, iron overload. Eliminate options 2 and 3, which do not treat the problem. Of options 1 and 4, determine which treatment will be effective.*

Content Area: Child Health; *Category of Health Alteration:* Hematological and Oncological Management; *Integrated Processes:* Nursing Process Planning; *Client Need:* Physiological Integrity/Physiological Adaptation/Unexpected Response to Therapies; *Cognitive Level:* Application

Reference: Ball, J., & Bindler, R. (2008). *Pediatric Nursing: Caring for Children* (4th ed., p. 821). Upper Saddle River, NJ: Pearson/Prentice Hall.

1244. EBP During a routine physical examination, a parent states to a nurse, "When I am taking pictures of my baby using the camera flash, I see a red coloration to my baby's left eye but the right eye has a white reflection. Is this normal?" Which response by the nurse is correct?

1. "Yes, the white reflection is normal; sometimes the light from the camera flash only catches one eye directly."
2. "Interesting. Your baby's eyes may be changing color. Many babies are born with what appears to be blue eyes but later they change to brown."
3. "It is good that you brought this to our attention because it is not the usual response. After further examining your baby's eyes, we can discuss what the white reflection may suggest."
4. "You seem concerned that your baby's eyes have different responses to the flash of the camera. Tell me more about your concern."

ANSWER: 3

The presence of a white reflection, rather than the normal red pupillary reflex, is a classic sign of retinoblastoma. Further examination is needed to specify a diagnosis. This response acknowledges the mother's concern, yet lets the mother know that this is not the usual response and that further follow-up is needed before her question can be answered. The nurse should not tell the mother that a white reflection is normal when it is not a normal finding. Stating the baby's eyes may be changing color is an incorrect interpretation by the nurse. Stating that the mother seems concerned is using a therapeutic communication technique but does not address the mother's question.

➧ ***Test-taking Tip:*** *First, eliminate any options that do not address the mother's question. Next, eliminate options that are known to be incorrect. For option 1, thinking about your own experience with taking pictures should direct you to eliminate this option.*

Content Area: Child Health; *Category of Health Alteration:* Hematological and Oncological Management; *Integrated Processes:* Communication and Documentation; *Client Need:* Physiological Integrity/Physiological Adaptation/Alterations in Body Systems; *Cognitive Level:* Analysis

Reference: Hockenberry, M., & Wilson, D. (2007). *Wong's Nursing Care of Infants and Children* (8th ed., p. 1572). St. Louis, MO: Mosby/Elsevier.

EBP References: American Academy of Ophthalmology Pediatric Ophthalmology/Strabismus Panel. (2007). *Pediatric Eye Evaluations: I. Screening; II. Comprehensive Ophthalmic Evaluation*. Available at: www.guideline.gov/summary/summary.aspx?doc_id=11753&nbr=006057&string=Retinoblastoma; Aventura, M. (2006). Retinoblastoma. *E-Medicine*. Available at: www.emedicine.com/oph/TOPIC346.HTM

1245. EBP A nurse is assessing a 6-year-old child newly diagnosed with acute lymphocytic leukemia (ALL). Which assessment findings should the nurse expect based on the child's diagnosis? SELECT ALL THAT APPLY.

1. Alopecia
2. Petechiae
3. Anorexia
4. Insomnia
5. Bleeding gums
6. Pallor

ANSWER: 2, 3, 5, 6

Petechiae, a sign of capillary bleeding, and bleeding gums result from decreased platelet production and the ability of the blood to clot. Anorexia occurs from enlarged lymph nodes and vague abdominal pain from inflammation within the intestinal tract. Pallor occurs from decreased production of erythrocytes. Alopecia (hair loss) may occur with chemotherapy but is not an expected sign with a new diagnosis. Because of the bone marrow depression, fatigue and increased time sleeping are signs associated with ALL.

➧ ***Test-taking Tip:*** *Recall that in leukemia the proliferation of immature white blood cells depress bone marrow production, decreasing erythrocytes, platelets, and the formation of mature white blood cells. Therefore, select options that relate to the functions of these blood cells.*

Content Area: Child Health; *Category of Health Alteration:* Hematological and Oncological Management; *Integrated Processes:* Nursing Process Assessment; *Client Need:* Physiological Integrity/Reduction of Risk Potential/System Specific Assessments; *Cognitive Level:* Application

Reference: Hockenberry, M., & Wilson, D. (2007). *Wong's Nursing Care of Infants and Children* (8th ed., p. 1584). St. Louis, MO: Mosby/Elsevier.

EBP Reference: Laningham, F., Kun, L., Reddick, W., Ogg, R., Morris E., et al. (2007). Childhood central nervous system leukemia: historical perspectives, current therapy, and acute neurological sequelae. *Neuroradiology,* 49(11), 873–888.

1246. A nurse is caring for a 5-year-old child diagnosed with acute lymphocytic leukemia (ALL). The nurse reviews the child's laboratory report after noting a large amount of blood on the bed linens and in tissues. Place an X on the specific laboratory value on the report illustrated that should be of greatest concern to the nurse.

Laboratory Report

Hematology	Client Value
Hgb (11.5–12.5 g/dL)	9.0 g/dL
Hct (35%–50%)	32%
WBC (5–15.5 K/μL)	22 K/μL
Platelets (PLT, 150–300 K/μL)	50 K/μL

ANSWER:

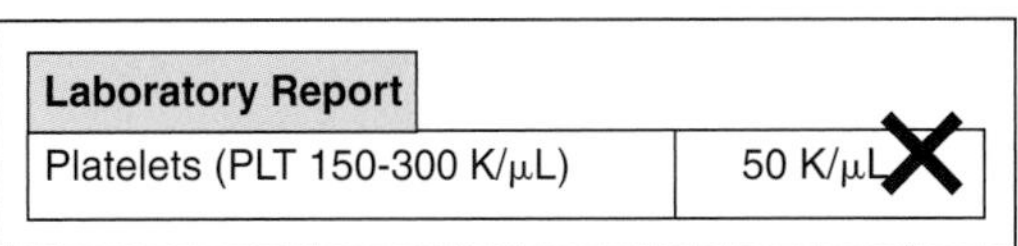

Laboratory Report	
Platelets (PLT 150-300 K/μL)	50 K/μL X

The low platelets are of primary concern because the child is bleeding and platelets are needed for coagulation. The low platelets are directly related to the leukemia, which causes a rapid proliferation of lymphocytes and a reduction in the production of platelets and red blood cells. The hemoglobin and hematocrit are decreased because of the bleeding. These are not of greatest concern because they do not provide information as to why the child is bleeding. The WBCs are elevated because of rapid proliferation of the lymphocytes that occurs in leukemia. However, the elevated WBCs are unrelated to the immediate concern of the bleeding.

▶ ***Test-taking Tip:*** *The key words are "greatest concern." Focus on the child's diagnosis of leukemia and the function of each of the blood components listed in the hematology report. Eliminate options not related to the bleeding.*

Content Area: Child Health; *Category of Health Alteration:* Hematological and Oncological Management; *Integrated Processes:* Nursing Process Evaluation; *Client Need:* Physiological Integrity/Reduction of Risk Potential/Laboratory Values; *Cognitive Level:* Application

Reference: Pillitteri, A. (2007). *Maternal & Child Health Nursing: Care of the Childbearing & Childrearing Family* (5th ed., p. 1811). Philadelphia: Lippincott Williams & Wilkins.

1247. A child diagnosed with leukemia is to receive a unit of platelets. The child's weight is 33 lbs. The ordered rate for the platelets is 10 mL/kg/hr. A nurse should plan to transfuse the platelets at a rate of _______ mL/hr.

ANSWER: 150

First convert pounds to kilograms using a proportion formula (2.2 lbs = 1 kg).
2.2 lbs : 1 kg :: 33 lbs : X kg
Multiply the extremes and then the means and solve for X.
2.2 X = 33
X = 15 kg. The child weighs 15 kilograms.
Next determine the rate: Milliliter per hour at 10 mL/kg/hr.
10 mL : 1 kg :: X mL : 15 kg
X = 150 mL/hr.
The commonly accepted rate for transfusions in a child is 10 mL/kg/hr.

▶ ***Test-taking Tip:*** *Read the question carefully to determine what is being asked. Recall that 2.2 pounds equals 1 kg.*

Content Area: Child Health; *Category of Health Alteration:* Hematological and Oncological Management; *Integrated Processes:* Nursing Process Planning; *Client Need:* Physiological Integrity/Pharmacological and Parenteral Therapies/Blood and Blood Products; *Cognitive Level:* Application

References: Pickar, G. (2007). *Dosage Calculations: A Ratio-Proportion Approach* (2nd ed., pp. 46, 344). Clifton Park, NY: Thomson Delmar Learning; Pillitteri, A. (2007). *Maternal & Child Health Nursing: Care of the Childbearing & Childrearing Family* (5th ed., pp. 1385–1386). Philadelphia: Lippincott Williams & Wilkins.

1248. A hospitalized child diagnosed with leukemia is being discharged after an initial treatment with chemotherapy. A nurse is teaching the parents about the allopurinol (Zyloprim®), which the child will continue to take at home. The nurse explains that the purpose of this medication is to:

1. help promote the child's sleep.
2. treat the joint pain and swelling caused by the child's gout.
3. prevent the child from developing gouty arthritis.
4. protect the child's kidneys by reducing the formation of uric acid.

ANSWER: 4

Rapid cell destruction from chemotherapy results in a high level of uric acid being excreted during treatment. This can plug the glomeruli and renal tubules, causing loss of kidney function. While allopurinol can cause drowsiness, this is not the purpose for this child. There is no indication that the child has gout or is likely to develop gout.

➧ ***Test-taking Tip:*** *Focus on the knowledge that chemotherapy will destroy multiple cells increasing uric acid levels. Use this cue to select the correct option.*

Content Area: Child Health; *Category of Health Alteration:* Hematological and Oncological Management; *Integrated Processes:* Teaching and Learning; *Client Need:* Physiological Integrity/ Pharmacological and Parenteral Therapies/Expected Actions or Outcomes; *Cognitive Level:* Application

Reference: Pillitteri, A. (2007). *Maternal & Child Health Nursing: Care of the Childbearing & Childrearing Family* (5th ed., p. 1692). Philadelphia: Lippincott Williams & Wilkins.

1249. **EBP** A child with Hodgkin's disease is treated with irradiation to the cervical area. The child's parent is concerned because the child lacks energy and is experiencing malaise. Based on this information, the nurse should further assess the child for: SELECT ALL THAT APPLY.

1. hypothyroidism.
2. anemia.
3. impaired nutrition.
4. difficulty swallowing.
5. difficulty voiding.

ANSWER: 1, 2, 3, 4

Irradiation to the cervical area could result in damage to the thyroid gland and cause hypothyroidism. Malaise and lack of energy can also be signs of anemia from decreased red blood cell production. Nutrition can be impaired with hypothyroidism, depression, or the effects of the radiation, which could influence the child's energy level. Though radiation results in few side effects, the inflammation from a mild skin reaction can cause difficulty swallowing. The cervical area is in the neck and is not associated with the renal system.

➧ ***Test-taking Tip:*** *Visualize the area that is being treated with radiation before reading each of the options.*

Content Area: Child Health; *Category of Health Alteration:* Hematological and Oncological Management; *Integrated Processes:* Nursing Process Assessment; *Client Need:* Physiological Integrity/ Reduction of Risk Potential/System Specific Assessments; *Cognitive Level:* Analysis

Reference: Hockenberry, M., & Wilson, D. (2007). *Wong's Nursing Care of Infants and Children* (8th ed., p. 1589). St. Louis, MO: Mosby/Elsevier.

EBP Reference: Monteleone, P., & Meadows, A. (2006). Late effects of childhood cancer and treatment. *E-Medicine*. Available at: www.emedicine.com/ped/TOPIC2591.HTM

1250. A child is neutropenic due to chemotherapy treatments. Which instructions should a nurse include when preparing the parents to take the child home? SELECT ALL THAT APPLY.

1. Prohibit visitors who have been recently vaccinated.
2. Keep the child's immediate surroundings free of plants and flowers.
3. Provide items such as goldfish, television, sanitized toys, or books for your child's playtime.
4. Arrange for the child to sleep alone, preferably in his or her own room.
5. Be sure the child bathes or showers daily.
6. Take your child's temperature, respiratory rate, and pulse four times daily.

ANSWER: 1, 2, 4, 5

If exposed to a recently vaccinated person, especially those vaccinated with a live virus, the child would be unable to mount an immune response and could develop an infection. Plants and flowers could harbor mold spores. Sleeping alone prevents exposure to those who may be developing an illness. Bathing or showering removes bacteria from the skin. Goldfish in the home should be placed in an area that is off limits to the child because they harbor mold spores. Temperature, respiratory rate, and pulse should be done daily; four times a day is unnecessary.

▸ ***Test-taking Tip:*** *Recall that neutropenia is a reduction of circulating neutrophils, the most common type of granular white blood cell (WBC). With a reduction in WBCs, there is an increased risk of infection. Select options that will reduce the child's risk of infection.*

Content Area: Child Health; *Category of Health Alteration:* Hematological and Oncological Management; *Integrated Processes:* Teaching and Learning; *Client Need:* Safe and Effective Care Environment/Safety and Infection Control/Home Safety; *Cognitive Level:* Analysis

Reference: Pillitteri, A. (2007). *Maternal & Child Health Nursing: Care of the Childbearing & Childrearing Family* (5th ed., p. 1696). Philadelphia: Lippincott Williams & Wilkins.

1251. EBP A 10-year-old pediatric client receiving treatment with aggressive combination chemotherapy has stomatitis. Which nursing actions should be taken to perform oral care for this child? SELECT ALL THAT APPLY.

1. Performing oral care with a soft sponge toothette
2. Mixing water with the alcohol-based mouthwash to be used to lessen irritation
3. Swabbing the child's mouth with viscous lidocaine before performing oral care
4. Massaging the area on the back of the child's hands between the thumb and index finger with an ice cube for 5 to 7 minutes
5. Providing oral care every 2 to 4 hours, especially after the child eats
6. Cleansing the child's gums using a piece of gauze soaked in saline or plain water

ANSWER: 1, 4, 5, 6

Soft toothbrushes or sponges are used to reduce trauma to the oral mucosa. Massaging the area on the backs of both hands between the thumb and index finger with an ice cube for 5 to 7 minutes until numb is a reflexology strategy to reduce oral pain. Frequent oral care rids mucosal surfaces of debris, which is an excellent medium for bacterial and fungal growth. A moistened gauze is appropriate for cleaning the gums. Alcohol-based mouthwash increases pain and tissue trauma because it has a drying effect. Viscous lidocaine is not recommended for young children because it may depress the gag reflex, increasing the risk of aspiration.

▸ ***Test-taking Tip:*** *Focus on selecting options that will cleanse the mouth of debris, reduce pain, and decrease the risk of infection.*

Content Area: Child Health; *Category of Health Alteration:* Hematological and Oncological Management; *Integrated Processes:* Nursing Process Implementation; *Client Need:* Physiological Integrity/Physiological Adaptation/Illness Management; *Cognitive Level:* Analysis

Reference: Hockenberry, M., & Wilson, D. (2007). *Wong's Nursing Care of Infants and Children* (8th ed., pp. 1578–1579). St. Louis, MO: Mosby/Elsevier.

EBP Reference: Keefe, D., Schubert, M., Elting, L., Sonis, S., Epstein, J., et al. (2007). Mucositis study section of the Multinational Association of Supportive Care in Cancer, International Society for Oral Oncology. Updated clinical practice guidelines for the prevention and treatment of mucositis. *Cancer*, 109(5), 820–831. Available at: www.guideline.gov/summary/summary.aspx?view_id=1&doc_id=12094

1252. Four parents call a clinic to have their children seen for unusual lumps or swelling. A nurse is trying to work the children into a physician's overbooked schedule. Which child should the nurse schedule to be seen *first*?

1. A child with Down's syndrome
2. A child who lives close to power lines
3. A child who has had chronic ear infections
4. A child whose sibling was treated for an osteosarcoma

ANSWER: 1

A correlation exists between some genetic disorders, such as Down's syndrome (trisomy 21), and childhood cancer. In a child with Down's syndrome, the probability of developing leukemia is about 20 times greater than that of other children. Studies have found marginally significant relationships between electromagnetic exposure and developing childhood cancer. Chronic infections do not automatically increase the risk for cancer. Studies suggest that in general there is not a strong constitutional genetic component for childhood cancers other than retinoblastoma.

➧ ***Test-taking Tip:*** *Consider an option that would show a genetic correlation between cancer and the child's data.*

Content Area: Child Health; *Category of Health Alteration:* Hematological and Oncological Management; *Integrated Processes:* Nursing Process Implementation; *Client Need:* Safe and Effective Care Environment/Management of Care/Establishing Priorities; *Cognitive Level:* Analysis

Reference: Hockenberry, M., & Wilson, D. (2007). *Wong's Nursing Care of Infants and Children* (8th ed., p. 1560). St. Louis, MO: Mosby/Elsevier.

1253. EBP Following diagnostic testing for an enlarged cervical lymph node, a health-care provider informs a 20-year-old female client of a diagnosis of Hodgkin's disease and explains the disease process and recommended treatment. Which statement, overhead by a nurse when the client telephoned her parents, indicates that the client understands the diagnosis and treatment?

1. "I am so relieved; I was worried that I had cancer and there wasn't anything that could be done to treat it."
2. "I have a good chance of being cured with radiation therapy, chemotherapy, or a combination of both."
3. "I will need to have a laparotomy to stage the disease before I can start irradiation and chemotherapy."
4. "I am so upset; I wanted to go to college, marry, and raise a family. Now, I won't be able to do any of this."

ANSWER: 2

Hodgkin's lymphoma, which peaks at 20 years of age, is potentially curable with radiation therapy alone or with a combination of several chemotherapeutic agents. The overall 10-year survival rate is as high as 90%. However, 30% of persons who survive pediatric Hodgkin's lymphoma develop a secondary malignancy 30 years after their Hodgkin's lymphoma is diagnosed. Hodgkin's disease is a B-cell malignant disorder (cancer) that affects the reticuloendothelial and lymphatic systems. A laparotomy and splenectomy are no longer performed to determine the staging. However, if lesions found on imaging performed for staging are suspicious and if the findings might alter the treatment regimen, then a biopsy may be performed. There is no indication that the client has an advanced stage of lymphoma.

➧ ***Test-taking Tip:*** *Select the statement that is a true statement. Eliminate options that include a client's emotional response to the diagnosis.*

Content Area: Child Health; *Category of Health Alteration:* Hematological and Oncological Management; *Integrated Processes:* Nursing Process Analysis; *Client Need:* Physiological Integrity/Physiological Adaptation/Illness Management; *Cognitive Level:* Analysis

Reference: Hockenberry, M., & Wilson, D. (2007). *Wong's Nursing Care of Infants and Children* (8th ed., pp. 1587–1589). St. Louis, MO: Mosby/Elsevier.

EBP Reference: de Alarcon, P., Albers, W., & Metzger, M. (2008). Hodgkin disease. *E-Medicine from WebMD.* Available at: emedicine.medscape.com/article/987101-overview

1254. EBP A nurse is completing a health history and an assessment for a male adolescent client tentatively diagnosed with Hodgkin's lymphoma. Which findings should the nurse conclude support this diagnosis? SELECT ALL THAT APPLY.

1. Firm, nontender lymph node enlargement in the axillary area
2. Drenching night sweats
3. Unexplained fever with temperatures above 100.4°F (38°C) for 3 consecutive days
4. Unexplained weight loss of 10% or more in the previous 6 months
5. A diet consisting mostly of seafood and saturated fats
6. A brother who was also diagnosed with Hodgkin's disease when an adolescent

ANSWER: 1, 2, 3, 4, 6

Hodgkin's disease is characterized by painless enlarged lymph nodes most commonly in the cervical area and less frequently in the axillary and inguinal areas. Drenching night sweats, unexplained fever with temperatures above 100.4°F (38°C) for 3 consecutive days, and unexplained weight loss of 10% or more in the previous 6 months are three symptoms that are recognized by the Ann Arbor Staging System as having prognostic significance in Hodgkin's disease. There is a genetic predisposition with an increased incidence among same-sex siblings. There is no conclusive association between dietary habits and the development of Hodgkin's disease.

➧ ***Test-taking Tip:*** *If uncertain, select options that suggest an illness. Apply knowledge that the malignancy begins in the lymphoid system.*

Content Area: Child Health; *Category of Health Alteration:* Hematological and Oncological Management; *Integrated Processes:* Nursing Process Assessment; *Client Need:* Physiological Integrity/ Physiological Adaptation/Alterations in Body Systems; *Cognitive Level:* Analysis

Reference: Hockenberry, M., & Wilson, D. (2007). *Wong's Nursing Care of Infants and Children* (8th ed., pp. 1587–1589). St. Louis, MO: Mosby/ Elsevier.

EBP Reference: de Alarcon, P., Albers, W., & Metzger, M. (2008). Hodgkin's disease. *E-Medicine from WebMD.* Available at: emedicine.medscape.com/article/987101-overview

---

1255. A nurse suspects that a 10-year-old client diagnosed with non-Hodgkin's lymphoma (NHL) has superior vena cava syndrome when assessing that the client has:

1. thrombocytopenia and leukocytosis.
2. hyperuricemia, hypocalcemia, and hyperphosphatemia.
3. tingling and paresthesias of the lower extremities and pain on light touch.
4. cyanosis of the upper chest, neck, face, upper extremity edema, and distended neck veins.

ANSWER: 4

Mediastinal tumors, especially from NHL, may cause compression of the great vessel (superior vena cava syndrome). Signs of compression include cyanosis of the upper chest, neck, face, upper extremity edema, and distended neck veins. Thrombocytopenia and leukocytosis increases the risk for vascular damage and life-threatening hemorrhage. Hyperuricemia, hypocalcemia, and hyperphosphatemia are signs of tumor lysis syndrome. A mass obstructing the spinal cord can be manifested by symptoms of tingling and paresthesias of the lower extremities and pain on light touch.

➧ ***Test-taking Tip:*** *Recognize that the options present signs and symptoms of life-threatening complications that may develop in children with cancer. Think about the possible complications and then use the process of elimination.*

Content Area: Child Health; *Category of Health Alteration:* Hematological and Oncological Management; *Integrated Processes:* Nursing Process Analysis; *Client Need:* Physiological Integrity/ Reduction of Risk Potential/Potential for Complications from Surgical Procedures and Health Alterations; *Cognitive Level:* Application

Reference: Hockenberry, M., & Wilson, D. (2007). *Wong's Nursing Care of Infants and Children* (8th ed., p. 1571). St. Louis, MO: Mosby/Elsevier.

1256. An experienced nurse and a new nurse are providing preoperative care for a 5-year-old child diagnosed with Wilms' tumor. The experienced nurse should intervene when observing the new nurse:

1. inform the child that water is not allowed because the procedure will be performed soon.
2. palpate the child's abdomen during assessment.
3. provide the child with a doll for play that has removable kidneys.
4. state to the child, "You'll get some medicine that you breathe or get through your arm to make you sleep."

ANSWER: 2

Wilms' tumor (nephroblastoma) is an intrarenal abdominal tumor. Palpating the abdomen can potentially spread the cancerous cells. A 5-year-old child would typically be NPO for 2 hours prior to the procedure, although this time period can vary. Play therapy is an appropriate means for teaching the child about the surgical procedure and assisting the child to cope. When explaining the surgery and anesthesia, words that the child understands should be used.

➧ ***Test-taking Tip:*** *Consider both the age of the child and the type of tumor when reading the options.*

Content Area: Child Health; *Category of Health Alteration:* Hematological and Oncological Management; *Integrated Processes:* Nursing Process Evaluation; *Client Need:* Safe and Effective Care Environment/Management of Care/Supervision; *Cognitive Level:* Application

Reference: Ball, J., & Bindler, R. (2008). *Pediatric Nursing: Caring for Children* (4th ed., pp. 419–428, 881–883). Upper Saddle River, NJ: Pearson/Prentice Hall.

1257. EBP While an experienced nurse is orienting a new nurse to a pediatric oncology unit, the new nurse asks why there seems to be so many adolescents with osteosarcoma and not other age groups. The experienced nurse explains that osteosarcoma has a peak incidence during adolescence because of the:

1. increase in hormonal production.
2. epiphyseal growth plates have closed.
3. rapid growth spurt experienced during adolescence.
4. increase in sports-related injuries that occurs during this time.

ANSWER: 3

Although younger children can develop osteosarcoma, the peak incidence is during the rapid growth years: at 13 years for girls and 14 years for boys. Adolescent growth spurts may be influenced by hormones, but the hormones are not directly related to the development of bone tumors. Osteosarcoma can occur before or after epiphyseal plate closure. Bone tissue of osteosarcoma never matures into compact bone. The diagnosis of osteosarcoma may be made when the client seeks medical attention for a sports-related injury.

➧ ***Test-taking Tip:*** *Use association to select the correct option. Associate the rapid cell production that occurs with cancer with the rapid growth of adolescence.*

Content Area: Child Health; *Category of Health Alteration:* Hematological and Oncological Management; *Integrated Processes:* Teaching and Learning; *Client Need:* Safe and Effective Care Environment/Management of Care/Continuity of Care; *Cognitive Level:* Application

Reference: Ball, J., & Bindler, R. (2008). *Pediatric Nursing: Caring for Children* (4th ed., pp. 883–884). Upper Saddle River, NJ: Pearson/Prentice Hall.

EBP Reference: Hartford, C., Wodowski, K., Rao, G., Khoury, J., Neel, M., et al. (2006). Osteosarcoma among children age 5 years and younger. *Journal of Pediatric Hematology and Oncology*, 28, 43–47.

1258. A 5-year-old child, hospitalized following surgical intervention for osteosarcoma, is uninterested in eating. Which nursing action would best support the child's nutrition?

1. Providing only foods that the child likes best
2. Asking the child's parents to visit at mealtime
3. Turning on the television so the child is distracted while eating
4. Offering juice, popsicles, or ice cream every 2 hours

ANSWER: 2

Meals at home are often a time for family socialization. Mealtime visiting with the parents may offer the emotional, social, and physical support to enhance the child's nutritional intake. While allowing the child to select only best-liked foods may increase the child's intake, a young child is unlikely to select the most nutritious foods. Distractions may inhibit the child's intake. Juices, popsicles, and ice cream lack protein, and offering these this frequently may decrease the child's intake of nutritious foods.

➧ ***Test-taking Tip:*** *The key phrase is "best support . . . nutrition." Eliminate any options that would increase intake but would not be nutritious.*

Content Area: Child Health; *Category of Health Alteration:* Hematological and Oncological Management; *Integrated Processes:* Nursing Process Implementation; *Client Need:* Physiological Integrity/Basic Care and Comfort/Nutrition and Oral Hydration; *Cognitive Level:* Application

Reference: Pillitteri, A. (2007). *Maternal & Child Health Nursing: Care of the Childbearing & Childrearing Family* (5th ed., p. 1079). Philadelphia: Lippincott Williams & Wilkins.

1259. A nurse is planning care for a child following removal of brain tumor. The child is confused, disoriented, and restless. Which nursing diagnosis should receive the highest priority?

1. Sensory perceptual alterations related to neurological surgery
2. Self-care deficit related to confusion and restlessness
3. Impaired verbal communication related to confusion
4. Risk for injury related to disorientation and restlessness

ANSWER: 4

Because the child is experiencing altered cognition, the priority is promoting client safety and preventing injury. The remaining nursing diagnoses are pertinent but not the priority.

➧ ***Test-taking Tip:*** *The key word is "priority." Use Maslow's Hierarchy of Needs theory to establish the priority nursing diagnosis. Safety and security is a priority.*

Content Area: Child Health; *Category of Health Alteration:* Hematological and Oncological Management; *Integrated Processes:* Nursing Process Analysis; *Client Need:* Safe and Effective Care Environment/Management of Care/Establishing Priorities; *Cognitive Level:* Application

Reference: Ball, J., & Bindler, R. (2008). *Pediatric Nursing: Caring for Children* (4th ed., pp. 878–880). Upper Saddle River, NJ: Pearson/Prentice Hall.

1260. A 6-year-old child is being seen in a clinic after discharge from a hospital for removal of a brain tumor. Which finding, reported by a parent, best suggests the child has likely developed a complication?

1. Reports occasional headaches
2. Voiding large amount of dilute urine
3. Able to walk with use of crutches
4. Ventricular–peritoneal shunt tubing palpable under the skin

ANSWER: 2

Voiding large amounts of dilute urine is a sign of diabetes insipidus caused by a deficiency in antidiuretic hormone (ADH) secreted by the posterior pituitary gland. When ADH is inadequate, the renal tubules do not reabsorb water, leading to polyuria. Headaches may be a symptom associated with a complication but also may occur due to the neurosurgical procedure. Physical mobility may be impaired because of the location of the tumor. Being able to walk with crutches is an expected outcome if mobility was affected. The ventricular–peritoneal shunt tubing is inserted into the ventricle, and a tract is made that travels behind the ear, along the neck and chest wall, and into the peritoneal cavity. The shunt may be felt under the skin behind the ear and along the neck.

➧ ***Test-taking Tip:*** *If unsure, select an option that is atypical for any person regardless of surgery.*

Content Area: Child Health; *Category of Health Alteration:* Hematological and Oncological Management; *Integrated Processes:* Nursing Process Evaluation; *Client Need:* Physiological Integrity/Reduction of Risk Potential/Potential for Complications from Surgical Procedures and Health Alterations; *Cognitive Level:* Analysis

Reference: Ball, J., & Bindler, R. (2008). *Pediatric Nursing: Caring for Children* (4th ed., pp. 877, 1063–1065, 1209). Upper Saddle River, NJ: Pearson/Prentice Hall.

1261. EBP Leukemic cells have invaded a 16-year-old male's testes and irradiation of the testes is planned. The client asks a nurse if this means he will be sterile. The nurse's best response to the client is based on knowing that: SELECT ALL THAT APPLY.

1. the irradiation to the testes will lead to sterilization.
2. the irradiation of the testes will decrease sperm production but not cause sterilization.
3. this is a question that only the oncologist and radiologist would be able to answer.
4. a lead shield will be used to protect the pelvic area and preserve reproductive organs.
5. if the male is past puberty and is forming sperm, sperm banking may be an option before treatment.

ANSWER: 1, 5

Because irradiation of the testes leads to sterilization, sperm banking might be suggested before chemotherapy and radiation to preserve sperm for reproduction later in life. No sperm will be produced after irradiation of the testes. A nurse would be expected to answer the client's question and not defer the question. Deferring could cause distrust between the client and nurse or lead the client to suspect that there is more that is not being told to him. The testes are reproductive organs of the male.

➧ ***Test-taking Tip:*** *Narrow the options by using the process of elimination, eliminating either option 1 or option 2. Visualize the area to be irradiated and think about the function of the male testes.*

Content Area: Child Health; *Category of Health Alteration:* Hematological and Oncological Management; *Integrated Processes:* Communication and Documentation; *Client Need:* Physiological Integrity/Physiological Adaptation/Alterations in Body Systems; *Cognitive Level:* Analysis

Reference: Pillitteri, A. (2007). *Maternal & Child Health Nursing: Care of the Childbearing & Childrearing Family* (5th ed., p. 1699). Philadelphia: Lippincott Williams & Wilkins.

EBP Reference: Hobbie, W., Ginsberg, J., Ogle, S., Carlson, C., & Meadows, A. (2005). Fertility in males treated for Hodgkin's disease with COPP/ABV hybrid. *Pediatric Blood Cancer*, 44(2), 193–196.

1262. Prior to administering L-asparaginase to a 12-year-old child with acute lymphocytic leukemia, a nurse reviews the child's laboratory report. Which lab value should prompt the nurse to notify a physician before administering the chemotherapeutic agent?

1. Hemoglobin (Hgb) 11.8 mg/dL
2. Blood glucose 252 mg/dL
3. Total bilirubin 1.2 mg/dL
4. Absolute neutrophil count (ANC) 1,078

ANSWER: 2

An adverse effect of L-asparaginase is hyperglycemia, which may need to be treated with insulin before administration of another dose. The normal Hgb for ages 6 to 12 years is 11.5 to 15.5 g/dL and total bilirubin is 0.3 to 1.2 mg/dL. An ANC of 1,078 is acceptable for L-asparaginase administration. An ANC of less that 1,000 increases the child's risk of infection.

➧ ***Test-taking Tip:*** *Eliminate options that are known to be within normal ranges. Of the remaining two options, 2 and 4, determine which would require intervention.*

Content Area: Child Health; *Category of Health Alteration:* Hematological and Oncological Management; *Integrated Processes:* Nursing Process Evaluation; *Client Need:* Physiological Integrity/Reduction of Risk Potential/Laboratory Values; *Cognitive Level:* Analysis

Reference: Ball, J., & Bindler, R. (2008). *Pediatric Nursing: Caring for Children* (4th ed., pp. 850, 888). Upper Saddle River, NJ: Pearson/Prentice Hall; Hockenberry, M., & Wilson, D. (2007). *Wong's Nursing Care of Infants and Children* (8th ed., pp. 1866–1869). St. Louis, MO: Mosby/Elsevier.

1263. Prednisone is ordered three times a day for a child receiving chemotherapy. Which is the best schedule for a nurse to suggest to a parent?

1. 6 a.m., 2 p.m., and 10 p.m.
2. 8 a.m., 1 p.m., and 6 p.m.
3. 10 a.m., 6 p.m., and 2 a.m.
4. 11 a.m., 4 p.m., and 9 p.m.

ANSWER: 2

Prednisone should be taken with meals or snacks to decrease or prevent gastrointestinal upset. This schedule is the closest of the options to meal time, yet it spaces the medication for effectiveness. While options 1 and 2 space the medication over a 24-hour time period, it is not given consistently in relation to meals. Option 4 would be administering prednisone before meals and at bedtime.

➧ ***Test-taking Tip:*** *Note that only one option gives the medication closest to meal time.*

Content Area: Child Health; *Category of Health Alteration:* Hematological and Oncological Management; *Integrated Processes:* Nursing Process Implementation; *Client Need:* Physiological Integrity/Pharmacological and Parenteral Therapies/Medication Administration; *Cognitive Level:* Analysis

Reference: Hockenberry, M., & Wilson, D. (2007). *Wong's Nursing Care of Infants and Children* (8th ed., p. 1567). St. Louis, MO: Mosby/Elsevier.

1264. EBP A 5-year-old girl with alopecia secondary to chemotherapy refuses to wear a wig. The child's mother consults a nurse because she thinks her daughter should wear a wig. She states feeling uncomfortable when people stare at her daughter. Which response is most appropriate?

1. "Have you tried having your child wear a colorful hat instead?"
2. "Does your child feel uncomfortable when others are looking at her?"
3. "You seem concerned about people looking at your daughter. Tell me more about what you are feeling."
4. "Your daughter only needs to wear a head covering when she is exposed to sunlight, wind, or the cold."

ANSWER: 3

Hair loss is often a greater problem for the parents than the child. The parent may be grieving the loss of a normal child. Option 3 acknowledges the parent's feelings and focuses the communication on the parent by using a therapeutic communication technique of a broad opening statement. Option 1 is giving advice. The mother already stated she would like her daughter to wear a wig. Option 2 focuses on the daughter's feelings rather than the mother's feelings. While option 4 is correct, this statement is ignoring the mother's concern of discomfort.

➧ ***Test-taking Tip:*** *The most appropriate response would be one that responds to the mother's feelings.*

Content Area: Child Health; *Category of Health Alteration:* Hematological and Oncological Management; *Integrated Processes:* Caring; *Client Need:* Psychosocial Integrity/Therapeutic Communications; *Cognitive Level:* Application

References: Berman, A., Snyder, S., Kozier, B., & Erb, G. (2008). *Kozier & Erb's Fundamentals of Nursing: Concepts, Process, and Practice* (8th ed., pp. 469–471). Upper Saddle River, NJ: Pearson Education; Hockenberry, M., & Wilson, D. (2007). *Wong's Nursing Care of Infants and Children* (8th ed., p. 1575). St. Louis, MO: Mosby/Elsevier; Pillitteri, A. (2007). *Maternal & Child Health Nursing: Care of the Childbearing & Childrearing Family* (5th ed., p. 1694). Philadelphia: Lippincott Williams & Wilkins.

EBP Reference: Ranmal, R., Prictor, M., & Scott, J. (2008). Interventions for improving communication with children and adolescents about their cancer. *Cochrane Database of Systematic Reviews*, Issue 4, Art. No. CD002969. DOI: 10.1002/14651858.CD002969.pub2. Available at: www.cochrane.org/reviews/en/ab002969.html

1265. A child is receiving radiation to the left thorax to treat metastases. A nurse adds a nursing diagnosis of *Risk for impaired skin integrity* to the child's plan of care. Which interventions should the nurse include for this nursing diagnosis? SELECT ALL THAT APPLY.

1. Avoid using soap on the irradiated area
2. Apply lotion to the target skin area after bathing
3. Use water to carefully wash the area, leaving markings on the skin
4. Wear a lead apron when in direct contact with the child
5. Apply a Tegaderm®-type dressing after irradiation to the target area

ANSWER: 1, 3

Radiation can cause burns to the skin. Soaps, lotions, and powders should not be applied to the irradiated area to prevent further skin irritation and possible skin breakdown. Talcum powder can potentially alter the radiation dosage. Only water should be used to gently cleanse the area. The markings outline the irradiation target area for precise positioning of the radiation and should remain until treatment is completed. Lotions and rubbing to apply the lotion can cause skin breakdown if applied to traumatized skin. A lead apron is unnecessary because radiation is not present in the client's body or in the room. The irradiated area should be left open to air. A Tegaderm®-type dressing is adherent and can cause skin tearing when removed.

▶ ***Test-taking Tip:*** *The focus of the question is interventions for Risk for impaired skin integrity. Eliminate option 4 because it is irrelevant to the nursing diagnosis. Of the remaining options, decide what is best to protect the skin.*

Content Area: Child Health; *Category of Health Alteration:* Hematological and Oncological Management; *Integrated Processes:* Nursing Process Analysis; *Client Need:* Physiological Integrity/ Physiological Adaptation/Alterations in Body Systems; *Cognitive Level:* Application

Reference: Ball, J., & Bindler, R. (2008). *Pediatric Nursing: Caring for Children* (4th ed., p. 867). Upper Saddle River, NJ: Pearson/Prentice Hall.

1266. A nurse is preparing a child for abdominal irradiation. Which medications should the nurse plan to administer to prevent nausea and vomiting?

1. Ondansetron (Zofran®) and dexamethasone (Decadron®)
2. Promethazine (Phenergan®) and cyclophosphamide (Cytoxan®)
3. Metoclopramide (Reglan®) and methotrexate (Amethopterin®)
4. Marijuana and L-asparaginase (Elspar®)

ANSWER: 1

Ondansetron is an antiemetic used to control nausea and vomiting. Dexamethasone is a corticosteroid anti-inflammatory agent used in the adjunctive management of nausea and vomiting from chemotherapy. Promethazine is a phenothiazine-type antiemetic, but cyclophosphamide is a chemotherapeutic agent. Metoclopramide is an antiemetic, but it causes extrapyramidal reactions in children. Methotrexate is a chemotherapeutic agent. Marijuana is not approved for use in the United States, but synthetic cannabinoids are now being used in children. L-asparaginase is a chemotherapeutic agent.

▶ ***Test-taking Tip:*** *Eliminate options that include chemotherapeutic agents.*

Content Area: Child Health; *Category of Health Alteration:* Hematological and Oncological Management; *Integrated Processes:* Nursing Process Planning; *Client Need:* Physiological Integrity/ Pharmacological and Parenteral Therapies/Expected Actions or Outcomes; *Cognitive Level:* Analysis

Reference: Hockenberry, M., & Wilson, D. (2007). *Wong's Nursing Care of Infants and Children* (8th ed., pp. 1564–1566, 1577–1578). St. Louis, MO: Mosby/Elsevier.

1267. A 15-year-old adolescent is scheduled to have total body irradiation in preparation for a bone marrow transplant. A nurse has completed teaching about care following irradiation. Which statements by the adolescent indicate correct understanding of the information? SELECT ALL THAT APPLY.

1. "I should report if I have any bleeding, such as after brushing my teeth, because my platelets will be low."
2. "I will work hard to improve my health by eating plenty of raw fruits and vegetables."
3. "To relieve the dry mouth, I can suck on lozenges or popsicles or drink cold liquids."
4. "I will need to take an antiemetic around the clock to help prevent nausea and vomiting."
5. "Once the irradiation is completed, I will no longer need to be in protective isolation."
6. "My friends know that I can't have live plants or flowers so they wanted to know if silk flowers are okay."

ANSWER: 1, 3, 4, 6

Irradiation results in bone marrow suppression and pancytopenia. Bleeding precautions are necessary. Xerostomia (dry mouth) is a side effect that can be combated by lozenges, liquids, or oral hygiene. Antiemetics are given around the clock to control nausea. Plants, flowers, and goldfish can harbor mold spores and are contraindicated. Visitors should check before bringing items from home. Raw fruits and vegetables should be avoided because these increase the risk of infection. Foods must be fully cooked. Protective isolation continues until after the bone marrow transplant.

➧ ***Test-taking Tip:*** *Correct understanding is a true response item. Select only the options that would be true statements.*

Content Area: Child Health; *Category of Health Alteration:* Hematological and Oncological Management; *Integrated Processes:* Nursing Process Evaluation; *Client Need:* Physiological Integrity/Physiological Adaptation/Alterations in Body Systems; *Cognitive Level:* Analysis

Reference: Hockenberry, M., & Wilson, D. (2007). *Wong's Nursing Care of Infants and Children* (8th ed., p. 1570). St. Louis, MO: Mosby/Elsevier.

Test 33: **Child Health: Integumentary Management and Other Health Alterations**

1268. A child is presenting with burn injuries. What should be the nurse's priority during the initial assessment?

1. Inspect location, extent, and shape of burn injuries.
2. Assess the child's and family's concerns regarding the child's appearance.
3. Assess for signs of smoke inhalation and burns to the face and neck.
4. Assess for signs and symptoms of infection.

ANSWER: 3

The initial emergency assessment should be the assessment of airway, breathing, and circulation (ABCs). It is imperative to ensure that the airway has not been compromised by smoke or edema related to neck and facial burns. Although inspecting burn injuries should be included in the initial assessment, it should not be the first priority. The child's and family's concerns should be addressed once the physiological status of the child is stabilized. Infection should be a concern after the first 24 hours.

➧ ***Test-taking Tip:*** *The words "priority" and "initial assessment" are important. Use the ABCs to determine priority. Remember that smoke inhalation can compromise the airway.*

Content Area: Child Health; *Category of Health Alteration:* Integumentary Management and Other Health Alterations; *Integrated Processes:* Nursing Process Assessment; *Client Need:* Physiological Integrity/Physiological Adaptation/Medical Emergencies; *Cognitive Level:* Application

Reference: Ball, J., & Bindler, R. (2006). *Clinical Handbook for Pediatric Nursing* (pp. 614–615). Upper Saddle River, NJ: Pearson Education.

1269. EBP A nurse is assessing a child who is presenting with burn injuries. Which injuries would *least* likely trigger the need for further assessment or evaluation for the potential of child abuse and mandatory reporting?

1. Rope burn with edema
2. Cigarette burns
3. Splash burns on the front torso, face, and neck
4. Scald burns of the feet and legs

ANSWER: 3

Splash burns on the front torso, face, and neck are consistent with a child pulling down a container of hot liquid. Burns that are a result of child abuse are injuries not consistent with burns seen in a child, such as rope, cigarette, and scalding burns. These types of burns should alert the nurse to further assess the situation. Physicians and nurses are mandated reporters, but the nurse need not conduct the investigation.

➧ ***Test-taking Tip:*** *Think about the injuries that would be inconsistent with a child's history and presentation prior to answering the question. If unfamiliar with signs and symptoms of child abuse (physical, sexual, and emotional), think logically about the situation and link it to the aspects of the question that you do know.*

Content Area: Child Health; *Category of Health Alteration:* Integumentary Management and Other Health Alterations; *Integrated Processes:* Nursing Process Analysis; *Client Need:* Safe and Effective Care Environment/Management of Care/Advocacy; Safe and Effective Care Environment/Management of Care/Legal Rights and Responsibilities; *Cognitive Level:* Application

Reference: Pillitteri, A. (2007). *Maternal and Child Health Nursing* (5th ed., pp. 1742, 1748). Philadelphia: Lippincott Williams & Wilkins.

EBP Reference: Kellogg, N. (2007). American Academy of Pediatrics Committee on Child Abuse and Neglect. Evaluation of suspected child physical abuse. *Pediatrics*, 119(6), 232–241. Available at: www.guideline.gov/summary/summary.aspx?doc_id=11057&nbr=005836&string=Burns.

1270. A 4-year-old girl has been hospitalized for moderate burns. A nurse plans care based on knowing that the most developmentally appropriate response to the injuries and resultant treatment for a child this age is likely to be:

1. anger and hostility while trying to not appear young.
2. pushing boundaries to further autonomy.
3. wanting clear instructions regarding details of treatment.
4. believing that she is responsible for the bad things that are happening to her.

ANSWER: 4

The preschool-aged child is increasingly verbal but has limitations. The preschool child may experience feelings of guilt, anxiety, and fear when thoughts or actions differ from perceived expected behavior. This may cause the child to believe that the injury was caused by that variation in expected behavior. Anger and hostility is an adolescent response. Pushing boundaries would be a response by a toddler. Wanting clear instructions would be characteristic of a school-aged child.

Test-taking Tip: *Think about the developmental stages outlined by Piaget, Erikson, and Freud and the responses expected by a toddler, a preschool-aged child, a school-aged child, and an adolescent when answering this question. Match options to the age groups and eliminate options not pertaining to a preschool-aged child.*

Content Area: Child Health; *Category of Health Alteration:* Integumentary Management and Other Health Alterations; *Integrated Processes:* Nursing Process Assessment; *Client Need:* Health Promotion and Maintenance/Developmental Stages and Transitions; *Cognitive Level:* Application

References: Ball, J., & Bindler, R. (2006). *Clinical Handbook for Pediatric Nursing* (pp. 2–4). Upper Saddle River, NJ: Pearson Education; Hockenberry, M., & Wilson, D. (2007). *Wong's Nursing Care of Infants and Children* (8th ed., pp. 645–646). St. Louis, MO: Mosby/Elsevier.

1271. EBP A nurse is caring for a 5-year-old child with secondary burns over 40% of the body. The child has just been diagnosed with disseminated intravascular coagulation (DIC). Which is the priority nursing diagnosis based on the most recent condition?

1. Ineffective tissue perfusion
2. Impaired urinary elimination
3. Risk for deficient fluid volume
4. Impaired physical mobility

ANSWER: 1

The most important consideration with this child is to ensure there is adequate tissue perfusion. Impaired urinary elimination, risk for deficient fluid volume, and impaired physical mobility are accurate nursing diagnoses, but not the priority in the acute phase of DIC.

Test-taking Tip: *Use the ABCs (airway, breathing, circulation) to determine priority. Note the vascular problem with DIC. This is a clue that there would be a perfusion problem, thus eliminate options 2 and 4. Eliminate option 3 because an actual problem (tissue perfusion) would be priority over a potential problem (risk).*

Content Area: Child Health; *Category of Health Alteration:* Integumentary Management and Other Health Alterations; *Integrated Processes:* Nursing Process Analysis; *Client Need:* Physiological Integrity/Physiological Adaptation/Illness Management; *Cognitive Level:* Analysis

Reference: Hockenberry, M., & Wilson, D. (2007). *Wong's Nursing Care of Infants and Children* (8th ed., pp. 1542–1543). St. Louis, MO: Mosby/Elsevier.

EBP Reference: Serour, F., Stein, M., Gorenstein, A., & Somekh, E. (2006). Early burn related gram positive systemic infection in children admitted to a pediatric surgical ward. *Burns*, 32(3), 352–356.

1272. A nurse is developing an educational program targeting parents of toddlers. The nurse should be able to present information aimed at preventing the majority of burn injuries in toddlers. Which is the most common cause of burns in toddlers?

1. Pulling pans of scalding liquid from the stove
2. Touching a curling iron
3. Burns from flames
4. Exposure to lighted candles

ANSWER: 1

The most common burn injury in the toddler population is scalding. Parents need to be educated regarding pots and pans on the stove, coffee pot cords hanging down that a toddler could pull, and hot liquid scalding the child. Burns from heat and flames are typically seen in an older child.

Test-taking Tip: *Think about the neuromuscular development of toddlers to identify the common type of burn injury. Note that options 3 and 4 are similar in that these are flame injuries, thus eliminate these options. Options 1 and 2 are heat-related injuries. Think about whether a toddler is more likely to touch or to pull down an object.*

Content Area: Child Health; *Category of Health Alteration:* Integumentary Management and Other Health Alterations; *Integrated Processes:* Nursing Process Planning; Teaching and Learning; *Client Need:* Safe and Effective Care Environment/Safety and Infection Control/ Accident and Injury Prevention; *Cognitive Level:* Application

References: Pillitteri, A. (2007). *Maternal and Child Health Nursing* (5th ed., p. 1668). Philadelphia: Lippincott Williams & Wilkins; Hockenberry, M., & Wilson, D. (2007). *Wong's Nursing Care of Infants and Children* (8th ed., pp. 636–637). St. Louis, MO: Mosby/Elsevier.

1273. EBP A nurse is reviewing orders received for a newly admitted child with second- and third-degree burns over 10% of the total body surface area (TBSA). The child weighs 20 kg. The nurse should seek further clarification from a physician when the physician's order is:

1. Ringer's lactate (RL) at 50 mL per hour for the next 8 hours.
2. insert a urinary catheter.
3. elevate the extremities above the level of the heart.
4. morphine sulfate IV prn for pain control.

ANSWER: 4

Because the order for morphine sulfate does not state a dose, the order should be clarified with the physician. If the physician intended the dose to be based on the weight of the child, then this should be included in the order. In the first 24 hours, fluid resuscitation is 4 mL/kg body weight per percentage of burn TBSA, with half over the first 8 hours and the remaining over the next 16 hours (4 mL $\times$ 20 kg = 80 mL; 80 mL $\times$ 10 = 800 mL for 24 hours; half of this is 400 mL over 8 hours; 400 $\div$ 8 = 50 mL). A Foley urinary catheter is inserted so that urine output can be closely monitored as a guide for volume status. During the resuscitation phase, edema formation can decrease perfusion. Elevating the limbs above the heart level promotes gravity-dependent drainage.

***Test-taking Tip:** Carefully read each option. Avoid reading into any option choice.*

Content Area: Child Health; *Category of Health Alteration:* Integumentary Management and Other Health Alterations; *Integrated Processes:* Nursing Process Analysis; *Client Need:* Safe and Effective Care Environment/Safety and Infection Control/Error Prevention; *Cognitive Level:* Analysis

Reference: Hockenberry, M., & Wilson, D. (2007). *Wong's Nursing Care of Infants and Children* (8th ed., pp. 1209–1212, 1217). St. Louis, MO: Mosby/Elsevier.

EBP Reference: Oliver, R., Spain, D., & Stadelmann, W. (2006). Burns, resuscitation, and early management. *E-Medicine from WebMD*. Available at: www.emedicine.com/plastic/TOPIC159.HTM

1274. A nurse is assessing a 16-year-old adolescent in an emergency department who has been admitted because of burns over 25% of the client's body. Upon initial examination, the nurse makes several observations. Which observation should be most concerning to the nurse?

1. Areas on upper extremities are mottled.
2. Areas on upper extremities are moist and red.
3. Areas on lower extremities are waxy white.
4. Red blistering on anterior lower extremities.

ANSWER: 3

Full-thickness or third-degree burns are most concerning, can present as waxy white or black, and are identified by a leathery appearance. These burns involve the entire epidermis and dermis and extend into the subcutaneous tissue. Hair follicles, nerve endings, and sweat glands are all destroyed. Full-thickness burns do not heal and will require some type of grafting. Mottled, moist-red, or blistering in appearance are consistent with partial-thickness burns, which will heal spontaneously within about 14 days, but scarring will occur.

***Test-taking Tip:** The most concerning burn should be a third-degree burn. The deeper the burn, the less viable the skin will be. Select the option in which the appearance is less like healthy skin.*

Content Area: Child Health; *Category of Health Alteration:* Integumentary Management and Other Health Alterations; *Integrated Processes:* Nursing Process Assessment; *Client Need:* Physiological Integrity/Physiological Adaptation/Medical Emergencies; *Cognitive Level:* Analysis

References: Hockenberry, M., & Wilson, D. (2007). *Wong's Nursing Care of Infants and Children* (8th ed., pp. 1203–1204). St. Louis, MO: Mosby/Elsevier; Pillitteri, A. (2007). *Maternal & Child Health Nursing: Care of the Childbearing & Childrearing Family* (5th ed., pp. 1668–1674). Philadelphia: Lippincott Williams & Wilkins.

1275. A nurse is caring for a 7-year-old client who has been hospitalized for several days with severe burn injuries in the lower extremities. On initial examination, the nurse makes the following assessments regarding the client's right leg: distal pulses are weak, capillary refill is greater than 3 seconds, and the child reports feelings of numbness and tingling in the leg. What should be the nurse's interpretation of this information?

1. This is to be expected during this phase of burn healing.
2. This is an emergency situation and a health-care provider should be notified.
3. Comparative assessment of the extremity in 1 hour is necessary.
4. Fluid has accumulated under the scab of the burn and is decreasing blood flow to the area.

ANSWER: 2

The information suggests inadequate circulation and impairment of nerve function. This is an emergency situation and an escharotomy needs to be performed. The tough, leathery scab (eschar) that forms over moderate to severe burns may create a tight band that constricts an area, such as the anterior and posterior portion of an extremity or the trunk. These are not expected findings during any phase of burn healing. Waiting an hour will delay treatment. This is not fluid, but an emergency situation because of constriction from the eschar.

➧ ***Test-taking Tip:*** *Recognize that the findings indicate impaired circulation and eliminate options that do not address this conclusion. Select the one option that interprets and acts on this information.*

Content Area: Child Health; *Category of Health Alteration:* Integumentary Management and Other Health Alterations; *Integrated Processes:* Nursing Process Analysis; *Client Need:* Physiological Integrity/Physiological Adaptation/Illness Management; *Cognitive Level:* Analysis

Reference: Pillitteri, A. (2007). *Maternal and Child Health Nursing* (5th ed., p. 1675). Philadelphia: Lippincott Williams & Wilkins.

1276. A nurse is in an emergency department when a parent calls sobbing hysterically and stating, "My baby has just put an electrical cord in her mouth! What do I do?" Which statement or question identifies the first priority of the nurse?

1. "Call 911 and have them bring your baby to the emergency department."
2. "Have you removed the cord from the baby's mouth?"
3. "Is there bleeding at or around the mouth?"
4. "What does your baby's mouth look like?"

ANSWER: 2

It is imperative to ensure that the cord has been removed from the baby's mouth to prevent further harm. Electrical current is conducted from the plug to the underlying tissue. The actual amount of tissue damage is much larger than where the cord actually touched. Telling the parent to call 911 or asking about the condition of the baby's mouth are correct actions, but not the first priority.

➧ ***Test-taking Tip:*** *The first priority should be to protect from further harm. Use this clue to select the correct option.*

Content Area: Child Health; *Category of Health Alteration:* Integumentary Management and Other Health Alterations; *Integrated Processes:* Nursing Process Implementation; *Client Need:* Physiological Integrity/Physiological Adaptation/Medical Emergencies; *Cognitive Level:* Analysis

References: Hockenberry, M., & Wilson, D. (2007). *Wong's Nursing Care of Infants and Children* (8th ed., pp. 558, 1202–1203). St. Louis, MO: Mosby/Elsevier; Pillitteri, A. (2007). *Maternal and Child Health Nursing* (5th ed., pp. 1670–1671). Philadelphia: Lippincott Williams & Wilkins.

1277. A nurse is caring for a 3-year-old burn victim who is the only child of a single parent. The parent has not visited the child for 2 days, and the child is crying and says, "I want my mommy! Where is she?" The nurse calls the parent, who says, "I cannot stand to see my baby in so much pain knowing that I am responsible for this." The best response of the nurse is:

1. "It sounds like you are feeling guilty. Can you come in to talk about how we can help you and your child?"
2. "I am sorry you are feeling responsible. I just wanted to know when you could be here."
3. "It is very important that your child see you. How can I help you to get here?"
4. "Why do you think that you are responsible for this?"

ANSWER: 1

Paraphrasing the mother's statements is a therapeutic response. Offering to help the mother demonstrates concern. A burn injury of a child is traumatic for the child and family. The parent acknowledges feeling responsible and may be grieving so deeply that she is unable to successfully support her child. The nurse should explore resources with the parent to assist in dealing with her own feelings so that she in turn can assist the child now and during the long course of treatments, surgeries, and rehabilitation. Option 2 acknowledges the mother's feelings, which is therapeutic, but changing the subject is a barrier to communication. Option 3 fails to acknowledge the mother's feelings. Asking a "why" question, as in option 4, is a barrier to therapeutic communication because it can initiate a defensive response.

➧ ***Test-taking Tip:*** *Identify the therapeutic communication with the parent that will support the parent during this time of ineffective coping.*

Content Area: Child Health; *Category of Health Alteration:* Integumentary Management and Other Health Alterations; *Integrated Processes:* Nursing Process Implementation; Caring; *Client Need:* Psychosocial Integrity/Coping Mechanisms; Psychosocial Integrity/Grief and Loss; Psychosocial Integrity/Therapeutic Communication; *Cognitive Level:* Analysis

Reference: Pillitteri, A. (2007). *Maternal and Child Health Nursing* (5th ed., pp. 1676–1677). Philadelphia: Lippincott Williams & Wilkins.

1278. A nurse is caring for a toddler with second- and third-degree burns over 20% of the body 8 hours postinjury. The most critical nursing diagnosis for this patient is:

1. impaired physical mobility.
2. imbalanced nutrition: less than body requirements.
3. risk for imbalanced body temperature.
4. deficient fluid volume.

ANSWER: 4

After burn injuries, hypovolemia occurs due to loss of plasma, which oozes from the vascular space and into the burn site. Physiologically this occurs during the first 6 hours, but it will continue for the first 24 hours. Impaired physical mobility, imbalanced nutrition: less than body requirements, and risk for imbalanced body temperature are also pertinent nursing diagnoses but not the most critical at this stage of treatment.

➧ ***Test-taking Tip:*** *Use the ABCs (airway, breathing, circulation) to establish priority. A nursing diagnosis related to circulation will be the priority in this situation.*

Content Area: Child Health; *Category of Health Alteration:* Integumentary Management and Other Health Alterations; *Integrated Processes:* Nursing Process Analysis; *Client Need:* Physiological Integrity/Physiological Adaptation/Fluid and Electrolyte Imbalances; *Cognitive Level:* Application

References: Ball, J., & Bindler, R. (2006). *Clinical Handbook for Pediatric Nursing* (pp. 2–4). Upper Saddle River, NJ: Pearson Education; Hockenberry, M., & Wilson, D. (2007). *Wong's Nursing Care of Infants and Children* (8th ed., pp. 1209–1210, 1218–1220). St. Louis, MO: Mosby/Elsevier.

1279. A nurse is planning the discharge of a pediatric burn victim to the child's home. The child is able to ambulate with assistance but is cognitively and developmentally unable to function at the age-appropriate milestones due to asphyxiation. Which component should the nurse include as most important in the discharge planning of this child?

1. Identifying support groups for the child's parents
2. Coordinating care and services for the child's rehabilitation
3. Assessing the child's home for safety concerns
4. Communicating with the school to ensure that the child will receive mandated services

ANSWER: 2

Identifying and making referrals to services for the rehabilitation of the child with neurological sequelae secondary to asphyxiation is imperative because the child will require assessments posthospitalization on a physical, emotional, cognitive, and social level. The parent will need support systems and support groups, but it is not the top priority because the initial focus should be on the child's needs. A home safety assessment is included in rehabilitation services. Communication with the school will need to occur but will likely happen postdischarge.

➧ ***Test-taking Tip:*** *This is a question in which all items are correct, but the focus is to identify the most important and the most global option. Understanding the need for care coordination for continued services posthospitalization will be necessary to answer this question.*

Content Area: Child Health; *Category of Health Alteration:* Integumentary Management and Other Health Alterations; *Integrated Processes:* Nursing Process Planning; *Client Need:* Safe and Effective Care Environment/Management of Care/Referrals; Safe and Effective Care Environment/Management of Care/Continuity of Care; *Cognitive Level:* Analysis

Reference: Hockenberry, M., & Wilson, D. (2007). *Wong's Nursing Care of Infants and Children* (8th ed., pp. 1621–1622). St. Louis, MO: Mosby/Elsevier.

1280. A nurse assesses the hand of a child who experienced a thermal burn from scalding (see exhibit). Which interventions should the nurse plan when caring for the child? SELECT ALL THAT APPLY.

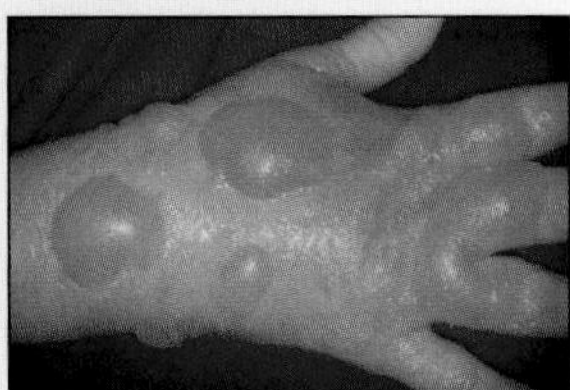

1. Administer analgesics prior to burn care.
2. Insert gauze between fingers.
3. Pierce blisters prior to dressing the hand.
4. Secure any dressings applied with netting.
5. Apply lotion to keep hand moist.

ANSWER: 1, 2, 4

Analgesics help relieve pain and decrease anxiety for subsequent dressing changes. Gauze should be inserted between fingers because burned surfaces should not touch. As healing takes place, webbing will form between burned surfaces that are touching. Netting rather than tape should be used to hold dressings in place because it expands easily, and tape can be painful to remove. Some burn centers keep blisters intact and others break them open. If blisters are broken, it is usually done by the health-care provider, and tissue is cut away to speed the healing process and prevent infection. Antibiotic creams may be prescribed, but lotion should not be applied because it can increase the risk of infection to the burn area.

➧ ***Test-taking Tip:*** *Focus on the illustration and then determine whether each option applies.*

Content Area: Child Health; *Category of Health Alteration:* Integumentary Management and Other Health Alterations; *Integrated Processes:* Nursing Process Planning; *Client Need:* Physiological Integrity/Reduction of Risk Potential/Therapeutic Procedures; *Cognitive Level:* Analysis

References: Ball, J., & Bindler, R. (2008). *Pediatric Nursing: Caring for Children* (4th ed., pp. 1289–1293). Upper Saddle River, NJ: Prentice Hall; Pillitteri, A. (2007). *Maternal & Child Health Nursing: Care of the Childbearing & Childrearing Family* (5th ed., pp. 1674–1675). Philadelphia: Lippincott Williams & Wilkins.

1281. A new nurse asks an experienced nurse during a child's dressing change, after the child had a skin graft, why the skin appears lattice-like and not smooth like the unburned areas of the child's body. Which is the experienced nurse's best response?

1. "The skin is an allograft from a cadaver donor, and the freezing of the skin causes this appearance."
2. "The skin is an autograft from a distal, unburned portion of the child's body, but the skin was meshed so it could be stretched to cover more area."
3. "After the grafting procedure, the area is covered by a bulky dressing. The lattice-like appearance is from the indentations of the dressing."
4. "The fluids that seep through the child's tissues cause the new skin to stretch and separate, but as it heals, the skin pulls back together."

ANSWER: 2

The lattice-like appearance is from a mesh graft. In a meshed autograft, a partial-thickness of skin is taken from another area of the body and is slit at intervals so that it can be stretched to cover a larger area. An allograft can be from a cadaver or a donor and is sterilized and frozen until needed. But unless it is meshed, it will not have a lattice-like appearance. Though bulky dressings applied too tightly can leave indentations, it will not be a uniform lattice-like appearance. Although fluid loss does occur with burn injuries, it does not cause the lattice-like appearance to a graft.

➧ ***Test-taking Tip:*** *Look for words that are a synonym to the lattice-like appearance when selecting the correct option.*

Content Area: Child Health; *Category of Health Alteration:* Integumentary Management and Other Health Alterations; *Integrated Processes:* Communication and Documentation; *Client Need:* Physiological Integrity/Reduction of Risk Potential/Therapeutic Procedures; *Cognitive Level:* Application

Reference: Pillitteri, A. (2007). *Maternal & Child Health Nursing: Care of the Childbearing & Childrearing Family* (5th ed., p. 1676). Philadelphia: Lippincott Williams & Wilkins.

1282. A 2-year-old child has a bulky dressing in place over 60% of the child's body following a skin-grafting procedure for a severe burn injury. A parent arrives to visit the child and is shocked to see the child's appearance. Which is the most caring action for a nurse?

1. Help the parent don the mask, gown, and gloves that are required to enter the child's room.
2. Bring the parent to a quiet place to allow the parent to talk about immediate concerns.
3. After the parent is appropriately attired, take the parent into the room and show the parent that it is okay to stroke the child's face and hold the child's hand.
4. Arrange for a member of the clergy to come visit with the parent for support.

ANSWER: 3

A parent may not ask spontaneously to touch the child or hold the child because the parent is likely in a state of grief, so he or she does not react in a normal manner. Both the parent and the child are supported by the nurse's gesture of caring. While assisting the parent to dress in appropriate attire, taking the parent to a quiet room, or arranging for the clergy may be supportive to the parent, the most caring response is offering support to both the parent and child.

➧ ***Test-taking Tip:*** *The key phrase is "most caring." Note that three options pertain to the parent and one option pertains to both the parent and the child. Select the option that pertains to both the parent and child.*

Content Area: Child Health; *Category of Health Alteration:* Integumentary Management and Other Health Alterations; *Integrated Processes:* Caring; *Client Need:* Psychosocial Integrity/Support Systems; *Cognitive Level:* Analysis

Reference: Pillitteri, A. (2007). *Maternal & Child Health Nursing: Care of the Childbearing & Childrearing Family* (5th ed., pp. 1676–1677). Philadelphia: Lippincott Williams & Wilkins.

1283. Parent education by a clinic nurse for home management of a toddler with eczema should include:

1. frequent bathing to remove flaking skin.
2. administering topical antibiotic medication.
3. identifying environmental triggers.
4. removal of the silvery scaling to promote healing.

ANSWER: 3

Eczema is characterized by superficial skin inflammation of erythema and local edema followed by vesicle formations that can ooze, crust, and scale. Dryness, change in environment or temperature, infection, stress, and substances in the environment can trigger the inflammation depending on the form of eczema. Frequent bathing can cause skin dryness and trigger eczema. Topical steroids are used to treat the inflammation and antibiotics are only used if excoriated skin becomes infected. Silvery scaling is a characteristic of psoriasis and not eczema.

➧ ***Test-taking Tip:*** *Visualize the appearance of eczema and then use the process of elimination.*

Content Area: Child Health; *Category of Health Alteration:* Integumentary Management and Other Health Alterations; *Integrated Processes:* Teaching and Learning; *Client Need:* Physiological Integrity/Physiological Adaptation/Illness Management; *Cognitive Level:* Application

References: Ball, J., & Bindler, R. (2006). *Child Health Nursing: Partnering within Children and Families* (pp. 1463–1465). Upper Saddle River, NJ: Pearson/Prentice Hall; Monahan, F., Sands, J., Neighbors, M., Marek, J., & Green, C. (2007). *Phipps' Medical-Surgical Nursing: Health and Illness Perspectives* (8th ed., pp. 1882–1888). St. Louis, MO: Mosby/Elsevier.

1284. A mother tells a clinic nurse that she has a history of eczema. Knowing this information, it is most important for the clinic nurse to assess the woman's infant for the presence of:

1. diaper rash, contact rash, seborrheic dermatitis, and eczema.
2. eczema, poison ivy rash, poison oak rash, and mite infestation.
3. scabies rash, eczema, diaper rash, and acne.
4. diaper rash, poison ivy rash, eczema, and mite infestation.

ANSWER: 1

"Dermatitis" and "eczema" are terms often used interchangeably. Because eczema can be hereditary, assessment should include other common types of dermatitis, including diaper rash, contact rash, seborrheic dermatitis, and eczema. Mite infestation and scabies are unrelated to the woman's history of eczema.

➧ ***Test-taking Tip:*** *Recall that eczema (dermatitis) can be hereditary. Eliminate options that have nonhereditary causes of dermatitis.*

Content Area: Child Health; *Category of Health Alteration:* Integumentary Management and Other Health Alterations; *Integrated Processes:* Nursing Process Assessment; *Client Need:* Physiological Integrity/Reduction of Risk Potential/System Specific Assessments; *Cognitive Level:* Analysis

References: Ball, J., & Bindler, R. (2006). *Child Health Nursing: Partnering with Children and Families* (p. 1460). Upper Saddle River, NJ: Pearson/Prentice Hall; Monahan, F., Sands, J., Neighbors, M., Marek, J., & Green, C. (2007). *Phipps' Medical-Surgical Nursing: Health and Illness Perspectives* (8th ed., pp. 1882–1888). St. Louis, MO: Mosby/Elsevier.

1285. EBP A child has a tentative diagnosis of Albright's disease (neurofibromatosis). A nurse assisting the child to disrobe prior to a physical exam should expect the presence of:

1. pediculosis.
2. café-au-lait spots.
3. tick bites.
4. congenital nevi.

ANSWER: 2

Neurofibromatosis is a neurocutaneous autosomal dominant disorder that causes tumors to grow along nerves. The presence of six café-au-lait spots or café-au-lait spots larger than 4 × 6 cm may indicate neurofibromatosis or Albright's disease. Pediculosis (lice infestations) and tick bites are not genetic disorders and have not been clinically shown to lead to neurofibromatosis. Congenital nevi (moles) are present at birth and result from a proliferation of benign melanocytes in the dermis, epidermis, or both and may lead to melanoma. Congenital nevi are different in appearance from café-au-lait spots of neurofibromatosis.

➧ ***Test-taking Tip:*** *Use the process of elimination and eliminate options 1 and 3, which are not indicative of an autosomal dominant disorder.*

Content Area: Child Health; *Category of Health Alteration:* Integumentary Management and Other Health Alterations; *Integrated Processes:* Nursing Process Planning; *Client Need:* Physiological Integrity/Physiological Adaptation/Pathophysiology; *Cognitive Level:* Application

References: Ball, J., & Bindler, R. (2006). *Child Health Nursing: Partnering with Children and Families* (p. 1484). Upper Saddle River, NJ: Pearson/Prentice Hall; Dillon, P. (2007). *Nursing Health Assessment: A Critical Thinking, Case Studies Approach* (2nd ed., p. 860). Philadelphia: F. A. Davis.

EBP Reference: Kam, J., & Helm, T. (2007). Neurofibromatosis. *E-Medicine from WebMD.* Available at: www.emedicine.com/derm/topic287.htm

1286. Which instructions should a nurse include when teaching a parent with a child diagnosed with contact dermatitis from poison ivy? SELECT ALL THAT APPLY.

1. Apply dressings moistened with either saline or water.
2. Apply a paste of baking soda and water.
3. Apply calamine or Caladryl® lotion.
4. Remove scabs to promote healing.
5. Inspect the yard for plants with three pointed leaflets that are different shapes.

ANSWER: 1, 3, 5

Applying moistened dressings and calamine or Caladryl® lotion should relieve itching. The allergen should be identified and eliminated. The yard should be inspected and poison ivy destroyed. Poison ivy has three pointed leaflets that are different shapes and shiny. The color varies by season. A baking soda bath can relieve itching, but applying a paste of baking soda can be harmful. Scabs should fall off naturally, not removed, so that healing tissues are protected.

➧ ***Test-taking Tip:*** *Read each option carefully, looking for key words that would make the option incorrect.*

Content Area: Child Health; *Category of Health Alteration:* Integumentary Management and Other Health Alterations; *Integrated Processes:* Teaching and Learning; *Client Need:* Physiological Integrity/Reduction of Risk Potential/Therapeutic Procedures; *Cognitive Level:* Application

Reference: Pillitteri, A. (2007). *Maternal & Child Health Nursing: Care of the Childbearing & Childrearing Family* (5th ed., pp. 1345–1346). Philadelphia: Lippincott Williams & Wilkins.

1287. A nurse is cleansing the skin of a hospitalized child with impetigo. Which action is most important for the nurse to take?

1. Apply clean gloves to prevent the spread of the infection to others.
2. Use sterile technique to prevent any further infection of the lesions.
3. Ensure the water is cold to help reduce pain during cleansing.
4. Keep the child in contact precautions until the child is discharged.

ANSWER: 1

Impetigo is transmitted by direct contact. Clean gloves are used to prevent the spread of infection to the nurse or others. Sterile technique is not needed because the infection is already present and the goal is to prevent spread of the infection to others. The water temperature should be tepid or one that is comforting to the child. Contact precautions can be discontinued 24 hours after initiation of therapy and do not need to continue during the entire hospitalization time period.

➧ ***Test-taking Tip:*** *The key phrase is "most important." Impetigo is transmissible from contact with the lesions.*

Content Area: Child Health; *Category of Health Alteration:* Integumentary Management and Other Health Alterations; *Integrated Processes:* Nursing Process Implementation; *Client Need:* Safe and Effective Care Environment/Safety and Infection Control/Standard or Transmission-based/Precautions/Surgical Asepsis; *Cognitive Level:* Application

Reference: Pillitteri, A. (2007). *Maternal & Child Health Nursing: Care of the Childbearing & Childrearing Family* (5th ed., p. 1367). Philadelphia: Lippincott Williams & Wilkins.

1288. EBP A 4-year-old child is being seen in a clinic. A parent explains that the child has been bumping into objects not directly in front of the child and complaining of seeing halos around objects and sometimes seeing two objects when there is only one. A referral is made for a tonometry test. A nurse explains to the parent that tonometry of the child's eyes will be testing for:

1. cataracts.
2. strabismus.
3. glaucoma.
4. lazy eye.

ANSWER: 3

The child's symptoms suggest glaucoma. Tonometry is a method for measuring intraocular pressure (IOP) and detecting glaucoma. Other symptoms of glaucoma include excessive tearing, light sensitivity (photophobia), closure of one or both eyes in the light, one eye may be larger than the other, vision loss, irritability, fussiness, poor appetite, blurred vision, and a cloudy, enlarged cornea. Although some symptoms exhibited are similar to those of cataracts, strabismus, and lazy eye, tonometry is not used to detect these. A characteristic of cataracts is lens opacity, which is not present. While symptoms of bumping into objects and diplopia can occur with strabismus (cross-eyes), it is not evaluated by tonometry. Lazy eye results when one eye does not receive sufficient stimulation and poor vision results in the affected eye; a child may bump into objects because of the poor vision or exhibited diplopia.

➧ ***Test-taking Tip:*** *If unfamiliar with tonometry, focus on the child's symptom of seeing halo's and eliminate options.*

Content Area: Child Health; *Category of Health Alteration:* Integumentary Management and Other Health Alterations; *Integrated Processes:* Teaching and Learning; *Client Need:* Physiological Integrity/Reduction of Risk Potential/Diagnostic Tests; *Cognitive Level:* Analysis

Reference: Hockenberry, M., & Wilson, D. (2007). *Wong's Nursing Care of Infants and Children* (8th ed., pp. 1012–1013). St. Louis, MO: Mosby/Elsevier.

EBP Reference: American Academy of Ophthalmology Pediatric Ophthalmology/Strabismus Panel. (2007). *Pediatric Eye Evaluations: I. Screening; II. Comprehensive Ophthalmic Evaluation*. Available at: www.guideline.gov/summary/summary.aspx?view_id=1&doc_id=11753

1289. A 4-year-old child is brought to an emergency department after being hit in the side of the head. Ear trauma is suspected, but the child is turning away from a nurse and burrowing against the parent, crying, and not allowing anyone near. Which action is best for the nurse to take to enable assessing the child's ear?

1. Administer an analgesic first and then proceed after it has taken effect.
2. Ask the parent to hold and restrain the child while the child's ear is inspected.
3. Ask the child to place the nurse's hand by the area that was hurt.
4. Lay the child on a bed and mummy wrap the child; have the parent hold the child's head for examination.

ANSWER: 3

Asking the child to place the nurse's hand will assist in gaining the child's cooperation. Crying can be from fear rather than pain. A pain assessment should be completed before administering an analgesic. Restraining the child (whether in the parent's arms or in a mummy wrap) increases fear, anxiety, and agitation and can cause injury.

Test-taking Tip: *The key word is "best," which indicates more than one option could be used to assess the child. Select the option that could decrease the child's anxiety and promote cooperation.*

Content Area: Child Health; *Category of Health Alteration:* Integumentary Management and Other Health Alterations; *Integrated Processes:* Nursing Process Implementation; *Client Need:* Psychosocial Integrity/Stress Management; *Cognitive Level:* Application

Reference: Hockenberry, M., & Wilson, D. (2007). *Wong's Nursing Care of Infants and Children* (8th ed., pp. 1052, 1087). St. Louis, MO: Mosby/Elsevier.

1290. A child with a tentative diagnosis of otitis externa is being evaluated in the clinic. A nurse should expect to prepare the child for: SELECT ALL THAT APPLY.

1. an otoscopic examination.
2. a complete blood count (CBC) with differential.
3. a culture of the external auditory canal.
4. x-rays of the face and skull.
5. ear curettage for removal of debris present in the ear canal.

ANSWER: 1, 3, 5

External otitis is inflammation of the external ear canal. An otoscopic examination allows visualization of the tympanic membrane to ensure that there is no extension of the external otitis into the middle ear. If there is any drainage in the ear, cultures are taken to identify the organism. Ear curettage for removal of debris present in the ear canal may be necessary to visualize the tympanic membrane. A CBC is usually not done because diagnosis is based on the symptoms and physical examination. X-rays are not beneficial.

Test-taking Tip: *Eliminate options that are not directly related to the ear.*

Content Area: Child Health; *Category of Health Alteration:* Integumentary Management and Other Health Alterations; *Integrated Processes:* Nursing Process Planning; *Client Need:* Physiological Integrity/Reduction of Risk Potential/Diagnostic Tests; *Cognitive Level:* Application

References: Hockenberry, M., & Wilson, D. (2007). *Wong's Nursing Care of Infants and Children* (8th ed., pp. 186, 1327). St. Louis, MO: Mosby/Elsevier; Pillitteri, A. (2007). *Maternal & Child Health Nursing: Care of the Childbearing & Childrearing Family* (5th ed., p. 1600). Philadelphia: Lippincott Williams & Wilkins.

1291. A nurse is assessing a child and notes that the child's eyes appear crossed. In reviewing the child's medical record, which medical diagnosis should the nurse expect to find noted for this child?

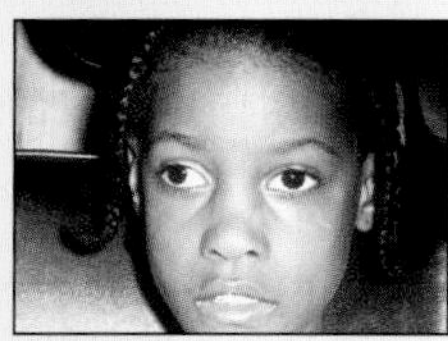

1. Strabismus
2. Diplopia
3. Hemianopsia
4. Pterygium

ANSWER: 1

Strabismus in children is noted when the two eyes fail to focus on the same image, and the brain may learn to ignore the input from one eye. After a period of disuse, visual acuity, already weak in the eye, deteriorates, resulting in a loss of vision in that eye. Children with hemangioma are noted to have a higher incidence of strabismus. Diplopia is double vision and can occur because each eye transmits the images received, but this is not the medical diagnosis for the condition. Hemianopia is seeing a portion of an object out of each eye. Pterygium is a triangular growth of the bulbar conjunctiva from the nasal side of the eye toward the pupil and can obstruct the vision if the growth occludes the pupil.

▶ ***Test-taking Tip:*** *Eliminate options that list symptoms.*

Content Area: Child Health; *Category of Health Alteration:* Integumentary Management and Other Health Alterations; *Integrated Processes:* Nursing Process Analysis; *Client Need:* Physiological Integrity/Reduction of Risk Potential/Potential for Alterations in Body Systems; *Cognitive Level:* Analysis

References: Dillon, P. (2007). *Nursing Health Assessment: A Critical Thinking, Case Studies Approach* (2nd ed., p. 362). Philadelphia: F. A. Davis; Pillitteri, A. (2007). *Maternal & Child Health Nursing: Care of the Childbearing & Childrearing Family* (5th ed., pp. 1589–1590). Philadelphia: Lippincott Williams & Wilkins.

1292. A child is diagnosed with strabismus and a school health nurse is meeting with the child's teacher. Which suggestions should the school nurse make to the teacher? SELECT ALL THAT APPLY.

1. Ensure that the child has preferential seating.
2. Seat the impaired child with other impaired children.
3. Allow extra time for assignments and test taking.
4. Order additional materials and books in large print.
5. Speak louder than usual when the child is present in the classroom.

ANSWER: 1, 3, 4

Strabismus is unequally aligned eyes (cross-eyes) due to unbalanced muscle control. By law, this is a disability that allows for school accommodations. Preferential seating will enable the child to see assignments, class presentations, and the teacher. Allowing for extra time to complete assignments ensures that the child has time to adjust and focus his or her vision to read the necessary documents. Federal and state laws provide educational plans to ensure that individuals with disabilities have the materials and equipment needed to attain an education like any other student in the system. Seating or grouping impaired children violates federal Individual with Disabilities Education Act (IDEA) guidelines. Speaking louder is unnecessary because this is a visual, not a hearing, problem.

▶ ***Test-taking Tip:*** *Think about the limitations a person with strabismus would have and then read the options carefully.*

Content Area: Child Health; *Category of Health Alteration:* Integumentary Management and Other Health Alterations; *Integrated Processes:* Nursing Process Implementation; *Client Need:* Safe and Effective Care Environment/Management of Care/Legal Rights and Responsibilities; *Cognitive Level:* Analysis

Reference: Ball, J., & Bindler, R. (2006). *Clinical Handbook for Pediatric Nursing* (p. 205). Upper Saddle River, NJ: Prentice Hall.

1293. An 8-year-old child is hospitalized with a femur fracture. A parent tells a nurse that the child's glasses for treating nearsightedness were damaged during the accident that resulted in the hospitalization. Which observations should the nurse expect due to the child's nearsightedness? SELECT ALL THAT APPLY.

1. Reads with a book held at arms length away from the eyes
2. Bends with head close to the table when coloring
3. Squints in an attempt to see objects clearly
4. One eye turns inward
5. Lens of the eye appears opaque

ANSWER: 2, 3

Nearsightedness is an ability to see objects clearly when at close range but not at a distance, so objects are brought closer to the eyes. Because objects farther away are not as visible, squinting may occur in an attempt to see objects more clearly. Holding a book farther away is observed in farsightedness because objects are better seen when farther away. In esotropia strabismus, an eye turns inward. An opaque lens is seen with cataracts.

▶ ***Test-taking Tip:*** *Use the memory aid that in nearsightedness objects need to be near to be seen. In farsightedness, objects are best seen if farther away.*

Content Area: Child Health; *Category of Health Alteration:* Integumentary Management and Other Health Alterations; *Integrated Processes:* Nursing Process Assessment; *Client Need:* Psychosocial Integrity/Sensory/Perceptual Alterations; *Cognitive Level:* Analysis

Reference: Hockenberry, M., & Wilson, D. (2007). *Wong's Nursing Care of Infants and Children* (8th ed., pp. 1012–1013). St. Louis, MO: Mosby/Elsevier.

1294. A school nurse has completed a second visual screen for preschool-aged and school-aged children. Which child should the nurse plan to complete a referral for follow-up evaluation of the child's vision?

1. A 4-year-old child who has 20/40 vision in both eyes
2. A 6-year-old child who has 20/30 vision in both eyes
3. A 7-year-old child who has 20/40 vision in both eyes
4. A 9-year-old child who has 20/15 vision in both eyes

ANSWER: 3

After a second screening, a child 6 years of age or older who has 20/40 vision or worse in one or both eyes should be referred to a physician for corrective eye care. A preschooler with 20/40 vision and a school-aged child with 20/30 vision should not be referred because these are normal findings for this age group. A result of 20/15 on visual acuity tests indicates vision that is better than normal.

➧ ***Test-taking Tip:*** *First, eliminate any options that are within normal or better than normal parameters.*

Content Area: Child Health; *Category of Health Alteration:* Integumentary Management and Other Health Alterations; *Integrated Processes:* Nursing Process Planning; *Client Need:* Safe and Effective Care Environment/Management of Care/Referrals; *Cognitive Level:* Application

Reference: Pillitteri, A. (2007). *Maternal & Child Health Nursing: Care of the Childbearing & Childrearing Family* (5th ed., p. 1014). Philadelphia: Lippincott Williams & Wilkins.

1295. A public health nurse is presenting an educational session to parents of preschool children about conjunctivitis. Which statement from a parent following the presentation indicates the parent understood the most important point about conjunctivitis?

1. "Viral conjunctivitis is self-limiting."
2. "The most common cause of conjunctivitis is presence of a foreign body."
3. "Prevention of infection in other family members is an important consideration with bacterial conjunctivitis."
4. "Conjunctivitis can occur during the birth process."

ANSWER: 3

The most common cause of conjunctivitis is a bacterial infection. With this infection, transmission to other family members and to people in direct contact with the child can easily occur. Therefore the washcloth and towel the child uses should be kept separate from the others, tissues used should be disposed of immediately, and good hand-washing techniques should be followed by everyone. Viral conjunctivitis is self-limiting, but the fact that bacterial conjunctivitis is extremely contagious is the most important information. Conjunctivitis can occur after birth because of exposure to bacteria during the birthing process, but the audience being addressed is parents of preschoolers.

➧ ***Test-taking Tip:*** *Recall that bacterial conjunctivitis is extremely contagious. Use this knowledge to select the correct option.*

Content Area: Child Health; *Category of Health Alteration:* Integumentary Management and Other Health Alterations; *Integrated Processes:* Nursing Process Evaluation; *Client Need:* Safe and Effective Care Environment/Safety and Infection Control/Standard or Transmission-based/Precautions/Surgical Asepsis; *Cognitive Level:* Application

References: Hockenberry, M., & Wilson, D. (2007). *Wong's Nursing Care of Infants and Children* (8th ed., pp. 283, 677). St. Louis, MO: Mosby/Elsevier; Pillitteri, A. (2007). *Maternal and Child Health Nursing* (5th ed., p. 998). Philadelphia: Lippincott Williams & Wilkins.

1296. A mother tells a nurse that her 1-month-old infant does not react to light. Which response to the parent is best?

1. "You should have your infant's vision tested; I can help you with arranging an appointment."
2. "It is normal for your infant not to react to light because visual acuity improves as the infant develops."
3. "All babies react to light differently. Try seeing what your baby's response is to different lighting."
4. "It is nothing to worry about, but I will let the doctor know in case further testing is needed."

ANSWER: 1

Parent concerns should be taken seriously. If the infant does not respond to light, it could indicate blindness. Visual acuity does improve with development, but a neonate is able to follow light or ceases body movement when a room is lighted. Infants respond differently based on level of alertness and age, but giving advice to try different lighting is inappropriate. The infant needs an eye examination and evaluation. Telling the mother that there is nothing to worry about is providing false reassurance.

➧ ***Test-taking Tip:*** *Focus on therapeutic communication skills. Eliminate options that use barriers to effective communication or do not address the parent's concern.*

Content Area: Child Health; *Category of Health Alteration:* Integumentary Management and Other Health Alterations; *Integrated Processes:* Communication and Documentation; *Client Need:* Physiological Integrity/Reduction of Risk Potential/Diagnostic Tests; *Cognitive Level:* Application

Reference: Hockenberry, M., & Wilson, D. (2007). *Wong's Nursing Care of Infants and Children* (8th ed., p. 1012). St. Louis, MO: Mosby/Elsevier.

1297. A nurse is counseling the parents of an infant who was born blind. Which statement indicates that a parent needs additional teaching?

1. "We or others will need to play with our infant so the infant will learn how to play."
2. "As our child grows we should attach Braille tags to clothing to help the child to learn to dress independently."
3. "We should seek the services of a speech therapist early because blind children also have difficulty with learning verbal skills."
4. "We have already discussed obtaining a seeing eye dog for our child so the child can get used to the animal at a young age."

ANSWER: 3

Verbalizing the need for a speech therapist indicates that further teaching is needed. Blind children have little difficulty in learning verbal skills and are able to communicate with age-mates and participate in suitable activities. Because blind children cannot imitate others or actively explore the environment, they rely much more on others to stimulate them and teach them to play. Braille tags to clothing and other articles will help the child to distinguish items, colors, and prints. The use of a dog guide helps the child become independent in navigation.

➧ ***Test-taking Tip:*** *The key phrase "needs additional teaching" indicates that this is a false-response item, so select the statement that is incorrect.*

Content Area: Child Health; *Category of Health Alteration:* Integumentary Management and Other Health Alterations; *Integrated Processes:* Teaching and Learning; Nursing Process Evaluation; *Client Need:* Psychosocial Integrity/Sensory/Perceptual Alterations; *Cognitive Level:* Analysis

Reference: Hockenberry, M., & Wilson, D. (2007). *Wong's Nursing Care of Infants and Children* (8th ed., p. 1014). St. Louis, MO: Mosby/Elsevier.

1298. A 12-year-old child is seen in a clinic after being hit in the eye by a baseball. A nurse assesses gross hyphema (hemorrhage into the anterior chamber) and a visible fluid meniscus across the iris. Which physician order should the nurse anticipate?

1. Immediate referral to an ophthalmologist
2. Immediate transfer to an emergency department
3. Home treatment with application of ice for 24 hours
4. Instillation of cortisone drops and application of an eye patch

ANSWER: 1

An ophthalmologist referral is necessary to evaluate for further injury. Transfer to an emergency department will delay evaluation and treatment. If hyphema was not present, then ice would be applied for 24 hours to reduce swelling. If eye contamination is suspected, antibiotic eye drops (not cortisone drops) may be ordered. The child should close and rest the affected eye. An eye patch is usually not necessary.

➧ ***Test-taking Tip:*** *Use Maslow's Hierarchy of Needs theory to establish the priority action. Focus on preservation of eye function.*

Content Area: Child Health; *Category of Health Alteration:* Integumentary Management and Other Health Alterations; *Integrated Processes:* Nursing Process Planning; *Client Need:* Physiological Integrity/Physiological Adaptation/Medical Emergencies; *Cognitive Level:* Application

Reference: Hockenberry, M., & Wilson, D. (2007). *Wong's Nursing Care of Infants and Children* (8th ed., p. 1011). St. Louis, MO: Mosby/Elsevier.

1299. A nurse is planning care for a 4-year-old child who is to have eye surgery. Which intervention should the nurse most definitely include in the plan to prepare the child for surgery?

1. Discuss the impending surgery with parents who should then discuss it with their child.
2. Provide a doll with an eye patch in place and allow time for the child to play with it.
3. Introduce the child to other children on the unit who have had surgery.
4. Show the child a 30-minute movie featuring a child being prepared for surgery.

ANSWER: 2

Allowing the child to play with a doll with an eye patch provides the opportunity to play out fears and concerns and allows clarification of misconceptions. Neutral words should be used to describe the procedure and explanations should be provided by both the nurse and parents. The child should also have the opportunity for rehearsing and handling items that will be used in providing care. A preschooler is egocentric and needs information on how surgery will affect him or her and not how it affects other children. A 30-minute movie is too long. A child has a limited concept of time, and a teaching session should be no more than 10 to 15 minutes.

➧ ***Test-taking Tip:*** *The key phrase is "most definitely," indicating that more than one answer may be right but that one is better than the others.*

Content Area: Child Health; *Category of Health Alteration:* Integumentary Management and Other Health Alterations; *Integrated Processes:* Nursing Process Planning; *Client Need:* Psychosocial Integrity/Stress Management; *Cognitive Level:* Application

Reference: Hockenberry, M., & Wilson, D. (2007). *Wong's Nursing Care of Infants and Children* (8th ed., pp. 1086–1087). St. Louis, MO: Mosby/Elsevier.

1300. EBP Which signs and symptoms should a nurse expect when assessing a toddler diagnosed with acute otitis media (AOM)? SELECT ALL THAT APPLY.

1. Fussy, restless
2. Irritable, crying
3. Pulling at the affected ear
4. Rhinitis, cough, and diarrhea
5. Rolls head from side to side

ANSWER: 1, 2, 3, 5

Fussiness, restlessness, irritability, crying, pulling on the affected ear, and rolling the head from side to side are classic signs and symptoms of acute otitis media from the pain and pressure in the ear. Rhinitis, cough, and diarrhea are symptoms that occur with otitis media effusion and are not usually associated with AOM.

➧ ***Test-taking Tip:*** *Read the question and think about the pathophysiology related to ear aches; consider the age of the child and the limitations in speech.*

Content Area: Child Health; *Category of Health Alteration:* Integumentary Management and Other Health Alterations; *Integrated Processes:* Nursing Process Assessment; *Client Need:* Physiological Integrity/Physiological Adaptation/Alterations in Body Systems; *Cognitive Level:* Application

Reference: Kyle, T. (2008). *Essentials of Pediatric Nursing* (pp. 538–542). Philadelphia: Wolters Kluwer/Lippincott Williams & Wilkins.

EBP Reference: Institute for Clinical Systems Improvement. (2008). *Diagnosis and Treatment of Otitis Media in Children.* Available at: www.guideline.gov/summary/summary.aspx?doc_id=12292&nbr=006367&string=Blindness

1301. A nurse is caring for a 4-year-old child who has drainage from the ears following insertion of tympanostomy tubes. Which interventions should the nurse include when caring for the child? SELECT ALL THAT APPLY.

1. Administer acetaminophen (Tylenol®) for mild pain.
2. Apply an ice compress over the ear.
3. Cleanse the exterior canal with sterile cotton swabs.
4. Insert ear plugs.
5. Apply moisture barriers to the ear lobes.

ANSWER: 1, 2, 3, 5

Analgesics, such as acetaminophen and ibuprofen, are used for minor pain, and codeine can be used for more severe episodes. Ice compresses are used to decrease inflammation. Keeping the exterior clean and dry prevents excoriation. Moisture barriers such as Aqua Vista® and Vaseline® can be applied to prevent excoriation from the exudate. Ear wicks, and not ear plugs, should be inserted to facilitate drainage and should be kept clean and dry and changed frequently as needed to help prevent infection from spreading to the mastoid process.

➧ ***Test-taking Tip:*** *Read each option carefully and eliminate the option that impairs the drainage from the ears.*

Content Area: Child Health; *Category of Health Alteration:* Respiratory Management; *Integrated Processes:* Nursing Process Implementation; *Client Need:* Physiological Integrity/Reduction of Risk Potential/Potential for Complications of Diagnostic Tests/Treatments/Procedures; *Cognitive Level:* Application

Reference: Kyle, T. (2008). *Essentials of Pediatric Nursing* (pp. 538–542). Philadelphia: Wolters Kluwer/Lippincott Williams & Wilkins.

1302. A nurse is planning care for a toddler with otitis media who is returning from surgery following a tympanostomy. Which nursing diagnoses should be addressed by the nurse first? Prioritize the nursing diagnoses by placing each in the correct order.

______ Interrupted family process related to illness and/or hospitalization of child, temporary hearing loss

______ Acute pain related to pressure caused by inflammatory process

______ Infection related to presence of infective organisms

______ Risk for delayed growth and development related to potential hearing loss

ANSWER: 3, 1, 2, 4

Pain should be the primary nursing diagnosis immediately after surgery. The presence of pain influences vital signs and participation in measures needed for recovery. The next nursing diagnosis that should be addressed is infection related to the presence of infective organisms. This is second because measures should be taken to eliminate the infection. Next is interrupted family process related to illness and hospitalization. The final nursing diagnosis is risk for delayed growth and development.

➧ ***Test-taking Tip:*** *Use Maslow's Hierarchy of Needs to order the nursing diagnoses.*

Content Area: Child Health; *Category of Health Alteration:* Integumentary Management and Other Health Alterations; *Integrated Processes:* Nursing Process Planning; *Client Need:* Physiological Integrity/Reduction of Risk Potential/Potential for Complications from Surgical Procedures and Health Alterations; *Cognitive Level:* Analysis

References: Kyle, T. (2008). *Essentials of Pediatric Nursing* (pp. 538–542). Philadelphia: Wolters Kluwer/Lippincott Williams & Wilkins; Ball, J., & Bindler, R. (2008). *Pediatric Nursing: Caring for Children* (4th ed., pp. 654–655). Upper Saddle River, NJ: Prentice Hall; Berman, A., Snyder, S., Kozier, B., & Erb, G. (2008). *Kozier & Erb's Fundamentals of Nursing: Concepts, Process, and Practice* (8th ed., pp. 217–218). Upper Saddle River, NJ: Pearson Education.

1303. EBP A public health nurse is presenting an educational session to parents with one of the topics being hearing loss/deafness. Which is the most accurate statement that the nurse can make regarding this topic?

1. Routine screening for adequate hearing levels begins at age 1.
2. A child with an ear infection should be tested during the infection period to identify hearing loss.
3. Some children with a minimal hearing loss may be thought to have behavioral problems in school.
4. Cerumen in the ear canal has been documented to substantially decrease hearing.

ANSWER: 3

The child with a minimal hearing loss may be thought to have behavioral issues because he or she does not follow the instructions of the teacher, participate in discussions in the classroom, or interact with other students. A newborn hearing test is done soon after birth, with routine screenings for adequate hearing levels beginning usually at age 3, not age 1. Children with an ear infection should be tested after the ears are clear, not while infected, to identify a temporary hearing loss. There is no support that cerumen in the ear canal substantially decreases hearing.

➧ ***Test-taking Tip:*** *Consider the development of the child and what may impact hearing in that child. Consider where a hearing loss might first be identified.*

Content Area: Child Health; *Category of Health Alteration:* Integumentary Management and Other Health Alterations; *Integrated Processes:* Teaching and Learning; *Client Need:* Physiological Integrity/Physiological Adaptation/Pathophysiology; *Cognitive Level:* Analysis

References: Pillitteri, A. (2007). *Maternal and Child Health Nursing* (5th ed., pp. 1016–1018). Philadelphia: Lippincott Williams & Wilkins; Ball, J., & Bindler, R. (2006). *Clinical Handbook for Pediatric Nursing* (pp. 217–220). Upper Saddle River, NJ: Pearson Education.

EBP Reference: US Preventive Services Task Force. (2008). Universal screening for hearing loss in newborns: US Preventive Services Task Force recommendation statement. *Pediatrics*, 122(1), 143–148. Available at: www.guideline.gov/summary/summary.aspx?view_id=1&doc_id=12640.

1304. A nurse is working in a pediatric clinic where a physician has just removed a peanut from the ear of a preschool child. When teaching the child and parent postprocedure, what is the most important action for the nurse?

1. Discussing methods with the parent for preventing the child from placing a foreign body in the ear again
2. Talking to the child about potential complications of placing a foreign body in the ear again
3. Addressing postprocedural care with the child and the parent
4. Talking to the parents about foreign body objects that can cause obstructions in the ears and other orifices

ANSWER: 3

The immediate need for the parents is understanding postprocedure care for their child. Developmentally, the child should be involved in the teaching to provide some control over the situation. Discussing prevention measures, potential complications, and other objects that can cause obstruction are correct actions, but are more appropriately done in a follow-up visit with the primary care provider.

➧ ***Test-taking Tip:*** *The key phrase is "most important." All options are correct, but one is more important than the other options. Select the learning need that is the priority.*

Content Area: Child Health; *Category of Health Alteration:* Integumentary Management and Other Health Alterations; *Integrated Processes:* Nursing Process Implementation; *Client Need:* Safe and Effective Care Environment/Safety and Infection Control/Accident Prevention; *Cognitive Level:* Application

Reference: Pillitteri, A. (2007). *Maternal and Child Health Nursing* (5th ed., p. 1665). Philadelphia: Lippincott Williams & Wilkins.

1305. EBP A preschool-aged child who has purulent, foul-smelling drainage from the nares is brought to an urgent-care clinic. The first action a registered nurse should take is to:

1. ask the child to tell the story of what happened.
2. obtain a set of vital signs.
3. provide comfort for the child.
4. complete a focused physical examination.

ANSWER: 4

Judging by the quick interpretation of the presenting symptoms, the child most likely has a foreign body in one or two nare(s). The focused assessment would provide information to determine what instruments would be appropriate for removal of the object. The child could provide the story of what happened, but the needed information is the time frame in which the odor was noted by the parent. Preschoolers do not have the concept of time and could not provide that information. Obtaining a set of vital signs is not an appropriate first intervention. If there is concern for infection, obtaining a temperature could be significant. Providing comfort to the child is extremely important and should be done along with the physical examination.

➧ ***Test-taking Tip:*** *The foul odor and the age of the child are significant.*

Content Area: Child Health; *Category of Health Alteration:* Integumentary Management and Other Health Alterations; *Integrated Processes:* Nursing Process Assessment; *Client Need:* Physiological Integrity/Physiological Adaptation/Alterations in Body Systems; *Cognitive Level:* Analysis

Reference: Pillitteri, A. (2007). *Maternal and Child Health Nursing* (5th ed., p. 1665). Philadelphia: Lippincott Williams & Wilkins.

EBP Reference: Institute for Clinical Systems Improvement. (2008). Diagnosis and treatment of respiratory illness in children and adults. Available at: www.guideline.gov/summary/summary.aspx?doc_id=12294&nbr=006369&string=foreign+AND+body.

1306. A nurse is working in a clinic and answers a telephone call from a parent who states that a 6-year-old child has a nose bleed that is not stopping. Which direction should the nurse provide to the parent?

1. Tilt the child's head back.
2. Squeeze the child's nares below the nasal bone for 10 to 15 minutes.
3. Take the child to urgent care as soon as possible.
4. Immediately insert a cotton ball or swab in each nare.

ANSWER: 2

The nares should be squeezed for 10 to 15 minutes just below the nasal bone and the child should be instructed to breathe through the mouth. An ice pack may be placed on the back of the neck or on the nose. The child's head should be tilted forward to prevent blood from going down the throat, which can lead to vomiting. If the bleeding cannot be stopped, there may be a need to access health care through an urgent-care setting. If the bleeding cannot be controlled, one of the treatments is the insertion of a cotton ball or swab soaked with phenylephrine, which causes vasoconstriction.

➧ ***Test-taking Tip:*** *Identify the interventions that would be least invasive to most invasive. Think from a physiological standpoint the best position for the head to be in to decrease the risk of complications of epistaxis.*

Content Area: Child Health; *Category of Health Alteration:* Integumentary Management and Other Health Alterations; *Integrated Processes:* Nursing Process Implementation; *Client Need:* Physiological Integrity/Reduction of Risk Potential/Potential for Complications from Surgical Procedures and Health Alterations; *Cognitive Level:* Application.

Reference: Ball, J., & Bindler, R. (2006). *Clinical Handbook for Pediatric Nursing* (pp. 220–224). Upper Saddle River, NJ: Pearson Education.

1307. A malnourished child has cheilosis of the lips, burning and itching eyes, and seborrheic dermatitis. The child is diagnosed with a vitamin B_2 (riboflavin) deficiency. Which additional findings on the assessment should a nurse deem consistent with the diagnosis?

1. Parasthesia
2. Irregular heart rate
3. Acanthosis nigricans
4. Irritation and cracks at the nasal angles of the nose

ANSWER: 4

Vitamin B_2 functions in maintaining healthy skin, especially around the mouth, nose, and eyes. Irritation and cracks at the nasal angles of the nose is consistent with the diagnosis of a vitamin B_2 deficiency. Paresthesia, an abnormal sensation, is seen with vitamin B_2 excess. Cardiac arrhythmias that could present with an irregular heart rate are seen in niacin excess. Acanthosis nigricans—a brown to black, poorly defined, velvety hyperpigmentation in skin folds of the neck or under the arms—are seen with niacin excess.

➧ ***Test-taking Tip:*** *Eliminate the two options that do not pertain to skin changes. Of the two remaining options, determine which is most consistent with the skin changes in the situation.*

Content Area: Child Health; *Category of Health Alteration:* Integumentary Management and Other Health Alterations; *Integrated Processes:* Nursing Process Assessment; *Client Need:* Physiological Integrity/Physiological Adaptation/Alterations in Body Systems; *Cognitive Level:* Analysis

Reference: Hockenberry, M., & Wilson, D. (2007). *Wong's Nursing Care of Infants and Children* (8th ed., pp. 570–571). St. Louis, MO: Mosby/Elsevier.

Test 34: **Child Health: Neurological and Musculoskeletal Management**

1308. A child is being evaluated for possible increased intracranial pressure following head trauma. Which assessment finding associated with increased intracranial pressure (ICP) should a nurse report to a health-care provider?

1. Increasing alertness
2. Widened pulse pressure
3. Tachycardia
4. Decreased systolic blood pressure (SBP)

ANSWER: 2

A widened pulse pressure (increased SBP and a decreased diastolic blood pressure) is one of the signs of Cushing's triad and is indicative of ICP. Decreasing level of consciousness (not increasing alertness), bradycardia (not tachycardia) and an increased SBP (not decreased SBP) are other signs and symptoms of Cushing's triad.

➧ ***Test-taking Tip:*** *While it's helpful to know Cushing's triad, it's not necessary to answer the question. The widening pulse pressure so commonly associated with increased ICP is associated with a lowered pulse. Eliminate any options that show improvement.*

Content Area: Child Health; *Category of Health Alteration:* Neurological and Musculoskeletal Management; *Integrated Processes:* Nursing Process Assessment; *Client Need:* Physiological Integrity/ Physiological Adaptation/Unexpected Response to Therapies; *Cognitive Level:* Application

Reference: Potts, N., & Mandleco, B. (2007). *Pediatric Nursing: Caring for Children and their Families* (2nd ed., p. 1056). Clifton Park, NY: Thompson Delmar Learning.

1309. A nurse is caring for an adolescent diagnosed with new-onset generalized tonic-clonic seizures of unknown etiology. Which nursing actions should be initiated by the nurse? SELECT ALL THAT APPLY.

1. Teaching the parents care and safety measures should a seizure occur at home
2. Obtaining an oropharyngeal airway and placing it near the adolescent's bed
3. Padding the side rails on the bed
4. Placing the adolescent in droplet precaution isolation
5. Securing a tongue blade to the head of the bed
6. Setting up suction equipment in the adolescent's room

ANSWER: 1, 2, 3, 6

Generalized tonic-clonic seizures cause muscle rigidity and intense muscle jerking. Thus, teaching will help ensure that injury does not occur as a result of a seizure. Airway obstruction can occur during or after the seizure. An oropharyngeal airway should be available, but should not be inserted during the seizure. If the seizure has commenced, nothing should be forced into the adolescent's mouth. Padding protects the adolescent's limbs from injury against the hard side rails. Suctioning equipment may be needed to clear secretions after the seizure. The etiology is unknown. Only if an airborne or droplet infectious disease were the suspected cause would droplet precautions be considered. A tongue blade inserted into the adolescent's mouth during a seizure can cause injury.

➧ ***Test-taking Tip:*** *Select the options that will ensure the adolescent's safety should a seizure occur.*

Content Area: Child Health; *Category of Health Alteration:* Neurological and Musculoskeletal Management; *Integrated Processes:* Nursing Process Implementation; *Client Need:* Physiological Integrity/ Reduction of Risk Potential/Potential for Complications from Surgical Procedures and Health Alterations; *Cognitive Level:* Analysis

Reference: Pillitteri, A. (2007). *Maternal & Child Health Nursing: Care of the Childbearing & Childrearing Family* (5th ed., pp. 1565–1568). Philadelphia: Lippincott Williams & Wilkins.

1310. A nurse is administering multiple anticonvulsant medications to children. For which medication should a nurse teach the parents about ensuring that their child has good oral care to prevent gingival hyperplasia?

1. Carbamazepine (Tegretol®)
2. Valproic acid (Depakene®)
3. Phenobarbital
4. Phenytoin (Dilantin®)

ANSWER: 4

About 20% of people taking phenytoin have gingival hyperplasia. This can be minimized with thorough oral care. Gingival hyperplasia is unique to phenytoin among antiepileptic medications and is not a side effect of carbamazepine, valproic acid, or phenobarbital.

➧ ***Test-taking Tip:*** *Apply knowledge of medication side effects to answer this question.*

Content Area: Child Health; *Category of Health Alteration:* Neurological and Musculoskeletal Management; *Integrated Processes:* Teaching and Learning; *Client Need:* Physiological Integrity/ Pharmacological and Parenteral Therapies/Adverse Effects/Contradictions/ Interactions; *Cognitive Level:* Application

Reference: Lehne, R. (2007). *Pharmacology for Nursing Care* (6th ed., p. 222). St. Louis, MO: Elsevier/Saunders.

1311. A woman has just undergone a prenatal screening that indicates that her child might have a neural tube defect. In response to a question about neural tube defects, a nurse describes one possible defect. Which neural tube defect is the nurse describing when stating that the vertebral arch fails to close and the spinal cord and meninges stay within the vertebral canal?

1. Spina bifida occulta
2. Spina bifida cystica
3. Meningocele
4. Myelomeningocele

ANSWER: 1

In spina bifida occulta there is failure of the vertebrae to close without hernial protrusion. Because the central nervous system structures remain in the spinal canal, there are often no adverse physical sequelae, and the condition might remain undiagnosed, or hidden (occult). Spina bifida cystica is also known as myelomeningocele, and includes the protrusion of the spinal cord through incompletely arched vertebrae because of lack of union between the laminae of the vertebrae. In a meningocele, the meninges protrude, but the spinal cord is not involved.

➧ ***Test-taking Tip:*** *Use the word "occulta" as a clue that the spinal cord and meninges stay hidden.*

Content Area: Child Health; *Category of Health Alteration:* Neurological and Musculoskeletal Management; *Integrated Processes:* Teaching and Learning; *Client Need:* Physiological Integrity/Physiological Adaptation/Pathophysiology; *Cognitive Level:* Application

Reference: Ball, J., & Bindler, R. (2008). *Pediatric Nursing: Caring for Children* (4th ed., p. 1066). Upper Saddle River, NJ: Prentice Hall.

1312. A child with myelodysplasia has a TEV (talipes equinovarus) repair that requires a cast application. In the postoperative period, a nurse notes serosanguineous drainage on the cast. What should the nurse do when making this observation?

1. Cut a window where the drainage is seeping through the cast
2. Petal the cast to minimize skin irritation and decrease leakage
3. Measure the area of drainage and document this finding
4. Notify the surgeon

ANSWER: 3

The circumference of the drainage should be measured and the information documented for further comparisons. It is not the nurse's responsibility to place a window in the cast. Windowing may be used to relieve pressure. Petaling the cast, or bending the edges of the cast away from the skin, might make the cast more comfortable for the child, but it won't help with the drainage. Serosanguineous drainage on the cast is not an emergency situation unless it becomes bloody and copious.

➧ ***Test-taking Tip:*** *Focus on the color of the drainage on the cast to select the correct option. Recognize that this is not a medical emergency and that the nurse should not alter the cast.*

Content Area: Child Health; *Category of Health Alteration:* Neurological and Musculoskeletal Management; *Integrated Processes:* Communication and Documentation; *Client Need:* Physiological Integrity/Basic Care and Comfort/Mobility/Immobility; *Cognitive Level:* Application

Reference: Ball, J., & Bindler, R. (2006). *Clinical Handbook for Pediatric Nursing* (1st ed., p. 571). Upper Saddle River, NJ: Prentice Hall.

1313. A nurse is reinforcing teaching to the parents of a child with myelomeningocele, which was diagnosed at birth and surgically corrected, about safety considerations. The nurse's instructions should include:

1. making sure that braces lie smoothly against the child's skin.
2. teaching the child to shift position at least every 3 hours.
3. placing a blanket between the child and the wheelchair.
4. checking all of the child's skin daily for redness or irritation.

ANSWER: 4

Because with a myelomeningocele the spinal cord ended at the point where the spinal cord and the meninges protruded through the vertebrae, the child's motor and sensory function are absent beyond this point. A daily thorough skin check is the best way to evaluate circulatory and skin alterations due to the child's immobility, altered sensation, or therapeutic treatments, such as braces. Braces should never be directly against the skin; there should always be a cloth between the braces and the skin. The child should be taught to shift every hour (not every 3 hours). The child should sit on a gel cushion because blanket folds can interrupt circulation.

➧ ***Test-taking Tip:*** *The considerations for the child with myelomeningocele are similar to the child (and adult) with a spinal cord injury. Considering the effects of the disease will help in determining the answer.*

Content Area: Child Health; *Category of Health Alteration:* Neurological and Musculoskeletal Management; *Integrated Processes:* Teaching and Learning; *Client Need:* Safe and Effective Care Environment/Safety and Infection Control/Accident or Injury Prevention; *Cognitive Level:* Application

Reference: Ball, J., & Bindler, R. (2008). *Pediatric Nursing: Caring for Children* (4th ed., p. 1070). Upper Saddle River, NJ: Prentice Hall.

1314. A child is being screened for hydrocephalus. In teaching the parents about the condition, the nurse illustrates the location of the lateral ventricle. Place an X where the nurse should locate the lateral ventricle.

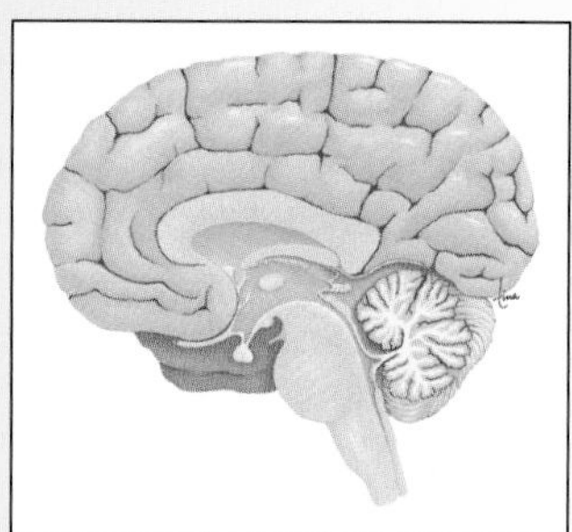

ANSWER:

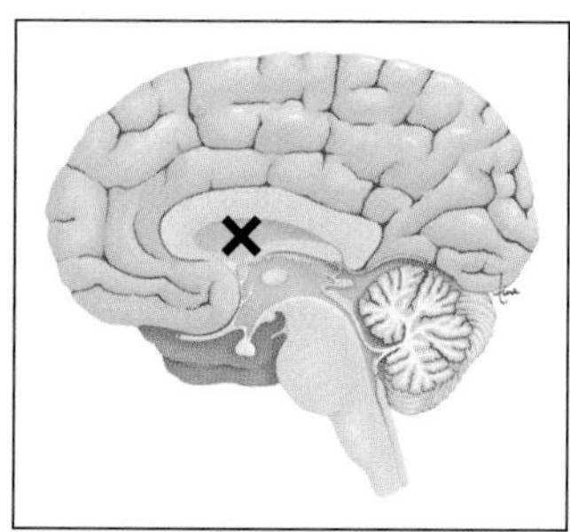

The two lateral ventricles, the largest of the four ventricles, are irregular in shape. Each consists of a central part, with anterior, posterior, and inferior horns. Cerebral spinal fluid forms in the choroid plexus of the pia mater, flows through the two lateral ventricles, through the foramen of Monro into the third ventricle, and through the aqueduct of Sylvius to the fourth ventricle. The lateral ventricle is large and often where a ventriculoperitoneal or ventriculoatrial shunt is inserted at the cephalic end.

➧ ***Test-taking Tip:*** *Don't confuse the lateral ventricles with the corpus collosum, the band of nerve fibers that connect the left and right cerebral hemispheres, which is adjacent to the lateral ventricles.*

Content Area: Child Health; *Category of Health Alteration:* Neurological and Musculoskeletal Management; *Integrated Processes:* Teaching and Learning; *Client Need:* Physiological Integrity/Physiological Adaptation/Pathophysiology; *Cognitive Level:* Application

Reference: Pillitteri, A. (2007). *Maternal & Child Health Nursing: Care of the Childbearing & Childrearing Family* (5th ed., pp. 1541–1542). Philadelphia: Lippincott Williams & Wilkins.

1315. A nurse is caring for multiple hospitalized children. In which conditions might the nurse assess for the presence of papilledema? SELECT ALL THAT APPLY.

1. Eczema
2. Craniosynostosis
3. Shaken baby syndrome
4. Hydrocephalus
5. Chest trauma

ANSWER: 2, 3, 4

Papilledema is edema and inflammation of the optic nerve caused by increased intracranial pressure (ICP). It can be assessed with the use of an ophthalmoscope. Any condition that increases ICP can cause papilledema. Eczema and chest trauma do not cause increased intracranial pressure.

➧ ***Test-taking Tip:*** *Determine the commonality in some of the conditions (increased ICP) and then eliminate options that are not associated with ICP.*

Content Area: Child Health; *Category of Health Alteration:* Neurological and Musculoskeletal Management; *Integrated Processes:* Nursing Process Assessment; *Client Need:* Physiological Integrity/Physiological Adaptation/Alterations in Body Systems; *Cognitive Level:* Application

Reference: Potts, N., & Mandleco, B. (2007). *Pediatric Nursing: Caring for Children and their Families* (2nd ed., pp. 923, 1215). Clifton Park, NY: Thompson Delmar Learning.

1316. A nurse is caring for a child immediately following insertion of a ventriculoperitoneal (VP) shunt for treatment of hydrocephalus. The nurse's postoperative care should include:

1. maintaining the head of the bed in an elevated position.
2. ensuring that the child minimizes movement of the extremities.
3. providing a pressure dressing over the cephalic insertion site.
4. changing the child's position every 2 hours.

ANSWER: 4

Because the child should be placed in a flat position following insertion of the shunt, it is necessary to protect the child's skin by turning the child every 2 hours. An elevation of the head of the bed is contraindicated because it will increase the flow from the shunt. Range of motion of the extremities should be done as the child recovers. A clear dressing (not a compression dressing) is placed over the incision sites to allow observation.

➧ ***Test-taking Tip:*** *Think about the immediate postoperative position of the child before making a selection.*

Content Area: Child Health; *Category of Health Alteration:* Neurological and Musculoskeletal Management; *Integrated Processes:* Nursing Process Implementation; *Client Need:* Physiological Integrity/ Physiological Adaptation/Illness Management; *Cognitive Level:* Application

Reference: Ball, J., & Bindler, R. (2006). *Clinical Handbook for Pediatric Nursing* (pp. 515–516). Upper Saddle River, NJ: Prentice Hall.

1317. A 7-year-old child may have hydrocephalus secondary to a malignancy. Which assessment findings should a nurse anticipate? SELECT ALL THAT APPLY.

1. Increased head circumference
2. Headache
3. Personality change
4. Vomiting
5. Angioedema

ANSWER: 2, 3, 4

Headache, personality change, and vomiting can each result from a space-occupying lesion that is applying pressure on brain structures. Because a 7-year-old child's sutures should be closed, there should be no increase in head circumference occurring with hydrocephalus. Angioedema is swelling and fluid accumulation under the skin.

▶ ***Test-taking Tip:*** *Focus on the age of the child and eliminate any option that is inconsistent with the child's age.*

Content Area: Child Health; *Category of Health Alteration:* Neurological and Musculoskeletal Management; *Integrated Processes:* Nursing Process Planning; *Client Need:* Physiological Integrity/ Physiological Adaptation/Alterations in Body Systems; *Cognitive Level:* Application

Reference: Ball, J., & Bindler, R. (2008). *Pediatric Nursing: Caring for Children* (4th ed., p. 1163). Upper Saddle River, NJ: Prentice Hall.

1318. A health-care provider's progress notes states that an infant with meningitis is in an opisthotonus position. The nurse should expect to observe:

1. resistance with specific leg movement.
2. knee or hip flexion with head flexion.
3. a high-pitched cry with neck flexion.
4. hyperextension of the head and neck.

ANSWER: 4

In an opisthotonus position the child's neck and head are hyperextended to relieve discomfort. Resistance with particular leg movement is Kernig's sign; Brudzinski's sign is knee or hip flexion with head flexion. The specific quality of cry with neck flexion is not characteristic of opisthotonus.

▶ ***Test-taking Tip:*** *Apply knowledge of medical terminology: "-tonus" is related to muscle tone. Select the option that would be caused from an extreme spasm of the muscles.*

Content Area: Child Health; *Category of Health Alteration:* Neurological and Musculoskeletal Management; *Integrated Processes:* Nursing Process Assessment; *Client Need:* Physiological Integrity/ Physiological Adaptation/Alterations in Body Systems; *Cognitive Level:* Application

Reference: Ball, J., & Bindler, R. (2008). *Pediatric Nursing: Caring for Children* (4th ed., pp. 1049–1050). Upper Saddle River, NJ: Prentice Hall.

1319. A child with autism has been admitted to a four-bed ward on a pediatric unit. The nurse admitting the child should:

1. request that the child be transferred to a private room.
2. request that the child be transferred to a double room.
3. admit the child to the assigned room.
4. request that the child be assigned to an isolation room.

ANSWER: 1

Because autistic children are unable to relate to other children or to respond to emotional or social cues appropriately, the child should be in a private room. Autistic children can have bizarre responses to the environment, repetitive hand movement, rocking, and rhythmic body movements that can frighten other children. A double room or a four-bed ward is an inappropriate room assignment. Isolation is unnecessary since autism is not a communicable disease.

▶ ***Test-taking Tip:*** *Recall that autism is a developmental disorder characterized by impairment of social and communication skills.*

Content Area: Child Health; *Category of Health Alteration:* Neurological and Musculoskeletal Management; *Integrated Processes:* Nursing Process Implementation; *Client Need:* Safe and Effective Care Environment/Safety and Infection Control/Accident or Injury Prevention; Psychosocial Integrity/Therapeutic Environment; *Cognitive Level:* Analysis

Reference: Pillitteri, A. (2007). *Maternal & Child Health Nursing: Care of the Childbearing & Childrearing Family* (5th ed., p. 1561). Philadelphia: Lippincott Williams & Wilkins.

1320. What is the most important factor for a nurse to consider when teaching a child with cerebral palsy (CP)?

1. Age
2. Type of cerebral palsy
3. The child's prior experiences with illness
4. Developmental level

ANSWER: 4

Many children with CP have some degree of cognitive impairment. This makes considerations of age and experience much less salient variables. Cognitive impairment also occurs across types of CP.

➧ ***Test-taking Tip:*** *Developmental level is almost always a better indicator than age in planning interactions with children.*

Content Area: Child Health; *Category of Health Alteration:* Neurological and Musculoskeletal Management; *Integrated Processes:* Nursing Process Planning; *Client Need:* Health Promotion and Maintenance/Growth and Development; *Cognitive Level:* Analysis

Reference: Potts, N., & Mandleco, B. (2007). *Pediatric Nursing: Caring for Children and their Families* (2nd ed., p. 1103). Clifton Park, NY: Thompson Delmar Learning.

1321. EBP A nurse is developing teaching materials for new mothers. The nurse should include information about which common practice that can increase the risk for developmental dysplasia of the hip (DDH)?

1. Carrying a child in a backpack
2. Carrying a child in a frontpack
3. Swaddling
4. Extended time in a car seat

ANSWER: 3

Although swaddling has many benefits (e.g., neurological and musculoskeletal development, less physiological distress, better motor organization, and more self-regulatory ability), it can cause DDH because the legs are in extension and adduction. Abduction, as in front, or backpacks, or in car seats does not increase this risk.

➧ ***Test-taking Tip:*** *Select the option that positions the legs in extension and adduction.*

Content Area: Child Health; *Category of Health Alteration:* Neurological and Musculoskeletal Management; *Integrated Processes:* Nursing Process Planning; *Client Need:* Physiological Integrity/ Reduction of Risk Potential/Potential for Alterations in Body Systems; *Cognitive Level:* Analysis

Reference: Ball, J., & Bindler, R. (2008). *Pediatric Nursing: Caring for Children* (4th ed., p. 1416). Upper Saddle River, NJ: Prentice Hall.

EBP Reference: Van Sleuwen, B., Engelberts, A., Boere-Boonekamp, M., Kuis, W., Schulpen, T., et al. (2007). Swaddling: A systematic review. *Pediatrics,* 120, 1097–1106.

1322. EBP Which screening test is a neonatal nurse likely to use to detect developmental dysplasia of the hip (DDH)?

1. Barlow's maneuver
2. Pavlik's maneuver
3. Gower's maneuver
4. Allis's maneuver

ANSWER: 1

The Barlow maneuver is performed by adducting the hip while pushing the thigh posterior. If the hip goes out of the socket, it is called "dislocatable" and is positive for DDH. A Pavlik harness is used to treat DDH. Gower's maneuver is used by children with muscular dystrophy to stand. An Allis's maneuver is used with children who can respond to positional instruction.

➧ ***Test-taking Tip:*** *If all the terms sound familiar, consider selecting the option that is your first instinct.*

Content Area: Child Health; *Category of Health Alteration:* Neurological and Musculoskeletal Management; *Integrated Processes:* Nursing Process Assessment; *Client Need:* Physiological Integrity/ Reduction of Risk Potential/System Specific Assessments; *Cognitive Level:* Application

Reference: Ball, J., & Bindler, R. (2008). *Pediatric Nursing: Caring for Children* (4th ed., p. 1416). Upper Saddle River, NJ: Prentice Hall.

EBP Reference: Schwend, R., Schoenecker, P., Richards, B., Flynn, J., & Vitale, M. (2007). Screening the newborn for developmental dysplasia of the hip: Now what do we do? *Journal of Pediatric Orthopedics,* 27, 607–610.

1323. A nurse is educating a family whose child is newly diagnosed with scoliosis. The nurse explains that the goal of therapy is to:

1. limit or stop progression of the curvature.
2. prepare the child for surgery.
3. minimize the psychosocial complications of prolonged immobilization.
4. develop a pain management protocol that will minimize complications of medications.

ANSWER: 1

The goal of screening is to limit progression of the curve, obviating the need for more aggressive interventions. Not all children with scoliosis need surgery, nor do most require prolonged immobilization. Most do not require aggressive pain management.

Test-taking Tip: *Focus on the diagnosis of scoliosis to select the option that relates to the skeletal system.*

Content Area: Child Health; *Category of Health Alteration:* Neurological and Musculoskeletal Management; *Integrated Processes:* Teaching and Learning; *Client Need:* Physiological Integrity/Reduction of Risk Potential/Therapeutic Procedures; *Cognitive Level:* Application

Reference: Ball, J., & Bindler, R. (2008). *Pediatric Nursing: Caring for Children* (4th ed., pp. 1168–1169). Upper Saddle River, NJ: Prentice Hall.

1324. EBP A nurse is asked to provide education for a 15-year-old who requires surgical treatment for scoliosis. Which should be an appropriate explanation for the adolescent? "The goal of surgery is to:

1. allow you to be taller."
2. prevent pain."
3. prevent problems with breathing."
4. allow clothes to fit you better."

ANSWER: 3

Surgery for scoliosis is to prevent future problems with breathing and to improve any current problems with breathing. While some height may be gained and pain decreased, these are not guaranteed, nor are they primary indications for the surgery. The same is true for wardrobe.

Test-taking Tip: *Use the ABCs (airway, breathing, circulation) to determine which goal has the highest priority.*

Content Area: Child Health; *Category of Health Alteration:* Neurological and Musculoskeletal Management; *Integrated Processes:* Teaching and Learning; *Client Need:* Physiological Integrity/Reduction of Risk Potential/Therapeutic Procedures; *Cognitive Level:* Application

Reference: Hockenberry, M., & Wilson, D. (2007). *Wong's Nursing Care of Infants and Children* (8th ed., pp. 1783–1784). St. Louis, MO: Mosby/Elsevier.

EBP Reference: Newton P., Perry, A., Bastrom, T., Lenke, L., Betz, R., et al. (2007). Predictors of change in postoperative pulmonary function in adolescent idiopathic scoliosis: A prospective study of 254 patients. *Spine,* 32, 1875–1882.

1325. A nurse is completing a thorough assessment of the spine. The nurse is concerned about a curve in a young child and records the exaggerated lumbar curve as:

1. scoliosis.
2. lordosis.
3. kyphosis.
4. kyphoscoliosis.

ANSWER: 2

Lordosis involves an exaggerated lumbar curve. Scoliosis is a lateral curve; kyphosis is an exaggerated thoracic curve. Kyphoscoliosis involves both curves in the same person.

Test-taking Tip: *The two (lordosis and lumbar) start with the same letter, making it easier to remember this type of curvature.*

Content Area: Child Health; *Category of Health Alteration:* Neurological and Musculoskeletal Management; *Integrated Processes:* Communication and Documentation; *Client Need:* Physiological Integrity/Reduction of Risk Potential/System Specific Assessments; *Cognitive Level:* Application

Reference: Potts, N., & Mandleco, B. (2007). *Pediatric Nursing: Caring for Children and their Families* (2nd ed., p. 407). Clifton Park, NY: Thompson Delmar Learning.

1326. A school-aged child has an Ilizarov external fixator applied to a lower extremity for bone lengthening. Which action should a nurse include when caring for the child?

1. Loosening the bolts and lengthen the rods on the fixator every other day
2. Cleansing the pin sites with sterile saline twice daily
3. Discouraging the child from bearing any weight on the involved extremity
4. Removing sections of the fixator apparatus when the child is positioned in bed

ANSWER: 2

An Ilizarov external fixator is an external fixation device that uses wires, rings, and telescoping rods to permit limb lengthening to occur by manual manipulation of the rods. Pins secure the device into the bone. Pin site care is necessary to prevent infection and allow inspection for loosening of the pins. Only the health-care provider should manipulate the rods to lengthen them. Partial weight bearing is allowed. The fixation device must remain intact and should be supported on pillows when the child is in bed.

Test-taking Tip: *If uncertain, select the simplest of the options.*

Content Area: Child Health; *Category of Health Alteration:* Neurological and Musculoskeletal Management; *Integrated Processes:* Nursing Process Implementation; *Client Need:* Physiological Integrity/Basic Care and Comfort/Mobility/Immobility; *Cognitive Level:* Application

Reference: Hockenberry, M., & Wilson, D. (2006). *Wong's Nursing Care of Infants and Children* (7th ed., p. 1763). St. Louis, MO: Mosby.

1327. EBP A nurse at the high school works with the trainers to develop early identification of injuries. The nurse teaches the trainers that adolescent soccer players are at increased risk for:

1. varus knee deformities.
2. valgus knee deformities.
3. varus ankle deformities.
4. valgus ankle deformities.

ANSWER: 1

Soccer players are at risk for varus knee deformities because of the planting and leaning involved in the game. A varus deformity means that the structures are further apart than expected; valgus means they are closer.

▶ ***Test-taking Tip:*** *The letter "l" in a valgus deformity can be a reminder that the knees or ankles are together.*

Content Area: Child Health; *Category of Health Alteration:* Neurological and Musculoskeletal Management; *Integrated Processes:* Teaching and Learning; *Client Need:* Physiological Integrity/Physiological Adaptation/Alterations in Body Systems; *Cognitive Level:* Application

Reference: Ball, J., & Bindler, R. (2008). *Pediatric Nursing: Caring for Children* (4th ed., p. 1449). Upper Saddle River, NJ: Prentice Hall.

EBP Reference: Yaniv, M., Becker, T., Goldwirt, M., Khamis, S., Steinberg, D., et al. (2006). Prevalence of bowlegs among child and adolescent soccer players. *Clinical Journal of Sport Medicine,* 16, 392–396.

1328. A 7-year-old has had hip pain for several months. Because it was mild pain, the parent did not pay a great deal of attention. The child was ultimately given a diagnosis of Legg-Calvé-Perthes disease. In preparing the child and family for treatment, the nurse should instruct the parents that:

1. most of the child's treatment will be done while the child is hospitalized.
2. activities that promote hip adduction are encouraged.
3. treatment is likely to continue for about 6 months.
4. the desired outcome is a pain-free joint with full range of motion.

ANSWER: 4

Legg-Calvé-Perthes disease is avascular necrosis of the proximal femoral epiphysis occurring in association with incomplete clotting factors. The treatment goal is full function. Treatment is community based rather than hospitalization. Abduction, not adduction, allows proper placement of the joint. Treatment of the disease is likely to occur for as long as 2 years.

▶ ***Test-taking Tip:*** *The long time to diagnosis should be a clue that the course of the disease is also likely to be longer.*

Content Area: Child Health; *Category of Health Alteration:* Neurological and Musculoskeletal Management; *Integrated Processes:* Nursing Process Planning; *Client Need:* Physiological Integrity/Reduction of Risk Potential/Therapeutic Procedures; *Cognitive Level:* Application

References: Potts, N., & Mandleco, B. (2007). *Pediatric Nursing: Caring for Children and Their Families* (2nd ed., pp. 1164–1165). Clifton Park, NY: Thompson Delmar Learning; Pillitteri, A. (2007). *Maternal & Child Health Nursing: Care of the Childbearing & Childrearing Family* (5th ed., p. 1621). Philadelphia: Lippincott Williams & Wilkins.

1329. The parents of a child with Duchenne muscular dystrophy have just learned that children with the disease have a limited life expectancy. They ask what this means for how they will raise their son. Which explanation by the nurse is best?

1. "Because he will be cognitively impaired, there is no reason to deal with the prognosis."
2. "Throughout his disease, we will focus on maximizing his abilities and keeping him comfortable."
3. "There is not enough known about this disease to know what will happen to your son."
4. "Nothing is likely to happen for a long time; we'll deal with it when the time comes."

ANSWER: 2

The answer acknowledges the prognosis, describes a plan, and gives the message that the family would not be abandoned. Much is known about the disease, so it is possible to maximize opportunities. Information can allow the family to begin planning, including genetic planning.

▶ ***Test-taking Tip:*** *Select the option that provides for continuous support.*

Content Area: Child Health; *Category of Health Alteration:* Neurological and Musculoskeletal Management; *Integrated Processes:* Communication and Documentation; *Client Need:* Physiological Integrity/Physiological Adaptation/Illness Management; *Cognitive Level:* Application

Reference: Potts, N., & Mandleco, B. (2007). *Pediatric Nursing: Caring for Children and Their Families* (2nd ed., p. 1162). Clifton Park, NY: Thompson Delmar Learning.

1330. A child who is crying and in pain is assessed by a school nurse. The child describes an injury in which another student twisted the child's right arm. The nurse should: SELECT ALL THAT APPLY.

1. elevate and apply ice at the site of the child's injury.
2. wrap the child's arm with an elastic bandage.
3. notify the child's parent.
4. call the child's health-care provider (HCP).
5. send the child for an x-ray of the arm.
6. have the student who caused the injury come to the nurse's office for questioning.

ANSWER: 1, 2, 3

A muscle strain is caused by excessive stretching of a muscle-tendon unit from an antagonist muscle group, an external object/person, or active muscle contraction. Rest, ice, compression, and elevation (RICE) are the initial treatments immediately after an injury. Ice reduces edema at the site, and an elastic wrap provides firm support. The parent should be notified to take the child to a HCP. The parent should contact the child's HCP, not the school nurse. The school nurse's scope of practice does not include prescribing; a HCP needs to request an x-ray. Appropriate channels should be used for reporting the incident rather than calling the offending student to the nurse's office.

▶ ***Test-taking Tip:*** *Consider that the child is describing a strain. Select options to treat a muscle strain.*

Content Area: Child Health; *Category of Health Alteration:* Neurological and Musculoskeletal Management; *Integrated Processes:* Nursing Process Implementation; *Client Need:* Physiological Integrity/Physiological Adaptation/Illness Management; *Cognitive Level:* Analysis

Reference: Ball, J., & Bindler, R. (2008). *Pediatric Nursing: Caring for Children* (4th ed., p. 1142). Upper Saddle River, NJ: Prentice Hall.

1331. A child is admitted to an emergency department with a dislocated kneecap that occurred while skiing. Which most immediate treatment by a health-care provider (HCP) should a nurse anticipate?

1. Realignment of the kneecap by sliding it back into position in the front of the knee
2. Open surgical intervention to repair the kneecap
3. Arthroscopy to surgically repair the torn cartilage
4. Application of a cast to the affected leg until the kneecap heals

ANSWER: 1

Dislocation of the kneecap causes it to move to the posterior surface of the knee. The kneecap is realigned by the HCP sliding it back into position. Open surgical intervention is unnecessary since the kneecap is movable. A kneecap dislocation in itself does not cause a torn cartilage. After realignment, a leg immobilizer is applied and used for about a week.

▶ ***Test-taking Tip:*** *The key words are "most immediate." Select an option that can be accomplished quickly. Remember that the kneecap is movable.*

Content Area: Child Health; *Category of Health Alteration:* Neurological and Musculoskeletal Management; *Integrated Processes:* Nursing Process Planning; *Client Need:* Physiological Integrity/Reduction of Risk Potential/Therapeutic Procedures; *Cognitive Level:* Analysis

Reference: Potts, N., & Mandleco, B. (2007). *Pediatric Nursing: Caring for Children and Their Families* (2nd ed., p. 1142). Clifton Park, NY: Thompson Delmar Learning.

1332. A 13-year-old is brought to the emergency department following a motor vehicle crash in which the child's head hit the dashboard. The child is diagnosed with a mild head injury. When assessing the child, which score on the Glasgow coma scale should the nurse expect?

1. 5
2. 10
3. 15
4. 20

ANSWER: 3

Glasgow coma scale scores range from 0 (dead) to 15 (intact). A score of 15 indicates that brain function is intact. A child with a mild head injury should have intact neurological function. The other options are either too low or beyond the score ranges.

▶ ***Test-taking Tip:*** *Knowing that a higher score is better will help to select the correct option. Remember that the highest attainable score is 15.*

Content Area: Child Health; *Category of Health Alteration:* Neurological and Musculoskeletal Management; *Integrated Processes:* Nursing Process Analysis; *Client Need:* Physiological Integrity/Reduction of Risk Potential/System Specific Assessments; *Cognitive Level:* Application

Reference: Potts, N., & Mandleco, B. (2007). *Pediatric Nursing: Caring for Children and Their Families* (2nd ed., p. 1092). Clifton Park, NY: Thompson Delmar Learning.

1333. A nurse has been asked to continue teaching with a group of parents of children with neurological and musculoskeletal conditions. For which condition should a nurse tell the parents that there is no genetic basis to the condition?

1. Osteomyelitis
2. Muscular dystrophy
3. Spina bifida
4. Tourette's Syndrome

ANSWER: 1

Osteomyelitis is an infection that might have long term sequelae; however, the cause is not genetic. The remaining conditions are genetic with varying inheritance patterns.

➧ ***Test-taking Tip:*** *Most words that end it "itis" indicate inflammation. The key words are "no genetic basis." Thus, select the option that refers to an infection.*

Content Area: Child Health; *Category of Health Alteration:* Neurological and Musculoskeletal Management; *Integrated Processes:* Teaching and Learning; *Client Need:* Health Promotion and Maintenance/ Health and Wellness; *Cognitive Level:* Application

Reference: Potts, N., & Mandleco, B. (2007). *Pediatric Nursing: Caring for Children and their Families* (2nd ed., p. 1156). Clifton Park, NY: Thompson Delmar Learning.

1334. A nurse explains to a child's parents that the role of methotrexate (Rheumatrex®) in treating children with juvenile arthritis is to:

1. decrease the inflammatory response.
2. improve functional ability.
3. control the febrile response.
4. minimize the effects of uveitis.

ANSWER: 1

Methotrexate is an immunosuppressant that decreases the inflammatory response. It is categorized as a disease-modifying drug. While decreasing inflammation may improve functional ability, this is not the action of the medication. Fever may be a sign of medication toxicity. Uveitis is a nonspecific term for any intraocular inflammatory disorder and is thought to be an autoimmune phenomenon; corticosteroids are prescribed for treating uveitis.

➧ ***Test-taking Tip:*** *Use your knowledge that arthritis has an inflammatory component to select the correct option.*

Content Area: Child Health; *Category of Health Alteration:* Neurological and Musculoskeletal Management; *Integrated Processes:* Nursing Process Implementation; *Client Need:* Physiological Integrity/ Pharmacological and Parenteral Therapies/Expected Actions or Outcomes; *Cognitive Level:* Analysis

Reference: Lehne, R. (2007). *Pharmacology for Nursing Care* (6th ed., p. 840). St. Louis, MO: Saunders/Elsevier.

1335. A 10-year-old is scheduled to receive methotrexate (Rheumatrex®) to treat juvenile arthritis. Which laboratory findings should lead the nurse to decide to withhold the dose and contact the health-care provider?

1. Urine pH 7.4
2. Hemoglobin 13 g/dL
3. Serum creatinine 2.2 mg/dL
4. Alanine aminotransferase (ALT) less than 40 international units/L (U/L)

ANSWER: 3

The serum creatinine is elevated, indicating a concern for excreting methotrexate. Urine pH should be kept above 7.0 to prevent renal damage. The hemoglobin and ALT values are normal. For a 10-year-old, normal hemoglobin is 10 to 15.5 g/dL and ALT is 4 to 36 U/L.

➧ ***Test-taking Tip:*** *Knowing how drugs are metabolized and excreted can give a clue as to which options should be considered.*

Content Area: Child Health; *Category of Health Alteration:* Neurological and Musculoskeletal Management; *Integrated Processes:* Nursing Process Planning; *Client Need:* Physiological Integrity/Reduction of Risk Potential/Laboratory Values; Physiological Integrity/Pharmacological and Parenteral Therapies/Medication Administration; *Cognitive Level:* Analysis

Reference: Wilson, B., Shannon, M., Shields, K., & Stang, C. (2008). *Prentice Hall Nurse's Drug Guide 2008* (pp. 967–970). Upper Saddle River, NJ: Pearson Education.

1336. An infant has been diagnosed with osteogenesis imperfecta (OI). The nurse is teaching the parents about how to care for their infant. Which information is most important for the nurse to include in the instructions to the parents?

1. Check the color of your infant's nailbeds and mucous membranes for signs of circulatory impairment.
2. If you note signs of infection, bring your infant to the clinic because the infant has a significant immune dysfunction.
3. Protect your infant from injury and handle your baby carefully because your infant's bones can break very easily.
4. Notify the health-care provider if your infant does not respond to sound because the infant's central nervous system (CNS) fails to develop completely.

ANSWER: 3

OI is also known as brittle bone disease, and the infant should be handled carefully and protected from injury. OI is not a disease of circulation, the immune system, or the CNS.

Test-taking Tip: *Use knowledge of medical terminology. "Osteo-" refers to bone. Select the option that refers to bone.*

Content Area: Child Health; *Category of Health Alteration:* Neurological and Musculoskeletal Management; *Integrated Processes:* Nursing Process Analysis; *Client Need:* Physiological Integrity/ Physiological Adaptation/Alterations in Body Systems; *Cognitive Level:* Application

Reference: Potts, N., & Mandleco, B. (2007). *Pediatric Nursing: Caring for Children and Their Families* (2nd ed., p. 1174). Clifton Park, NY: Thompson Delmar Learning.

1337. During a physical examination of a 1-month-old infant, a nurse notes that the infant has blue sclerae. The nurse suspects that the infant may have:

1. juvenile arthritis.
2. Tay-Sachs disease.
3. muscular dystrophy (MD).
4. osteogenesis imperfecta.

ANSWER: 4

Newborns not uncommonly have sclerae that appear blue; however, in children older than newborns, blue sclerae are an indicator for osteogenesis imperfecta, a genetic disorder that causes fragile bones as well as other health problems. For a child who has not yet fractured a bone, blue sclerae may be the first sign that promotes a further workup. Blue sclerae are not present in Tay-Sachs disease, MD, or juvenile arthritis. Juvenile arthritis is a chronic inflammation of the joints that can lead to damaged joint cartilage and bone, causing deformity and impaired use of the joint. It is believed to be caused by a combination of genetic and environmental factors. Tay-Sachs disease is a fatal genetic lipid storage disorder in which infants appear to develop normally for the first few months of life. Then, deterioration of mental and physical abilities occurs as nerve cells become distended with fatty material. MD is a genetic disease causing progressive weakness and skeletal muscle degeneration of muscles used during voluntary movement.

Test-taking Tip: *If uncertain, select the condition that results in fragile bones. Remember that "osteo-" pertains to bones.*

Content Area: Child Health; *Category of Health Alteration:* Neurological and Musculoskeletal Management; *Integrated Processes:* Nursing Process Assessment; *Client Need:* Physiological Integrity/ Physiological Adaptation/Alterations in Body Systems; *Cognitive Level:* Application

Reference: Potts, N., & Mandleco, B. (2007). *Pediatric Nursing: Caring for Children and Their Families* (2nd ed., p. 1174). Clifton Park, NY: Thompson Delmar Learning.

1338. A teen is brought to an emergency department with a likely spinal cord injury. To minimize the damage from the spinal cord injury, which classification of medications should a nurse expect a health-care provider to prescribe?

1. An antibiotic
2. An analgesic
3. A steroid medication
4. An antihypertensive medication

ANSWER: 3

Steroids, administered shortly after injury, help to decrease inflammation and prevent further injury. An antibiotic may be unnecessary; there is no indication of impaired skin integrity or an associated risk for infection that could further damage the spinal cord. Pain control is important, but not the most important medication for preventing swelling and compression of the spinal cord. While autonomic dysreflexia is a complication of a spinal cord injury, and the hypertensive crisis is treated with an antihypertensive medication, this will not protect the spinal cord from further injury.

Test-taking Tip: *The focus of the question is a medication that will minimize damage to the spinal cord. Eliminate options that do not have a direct effect on tissues surrounding the spinal cord.*

Content Area: Child Health; *Category of Health Alteration:* Neurological and Musculoskeletal Management; *Integrated Processes:* Nursing Process Planning; *Client Need:* Physiological Integrity/Physiological Adaptation/Illness Management; *Cognitive Level:* Application

Reference: Ball, J., & Bindler, R. (2008). *Pediatric Nursing: Caring for Children* (4th ed., p. 1358). Upper Saddle River, NJ: Prentice Hall.

1339. An adolescent client diagnosed with a T12 spinal cord injury (SCI) is admitted to a rehabilitation unit. A nurse is teaching the client about the need to be diligent in skin protection. The nurse explains that the primary reason for the client's increased risk for alterations in skin integrity is:

1. the inability to perceive extremes in temperature leading to burns.
2. the circulatory changes that cause vasoconstriction and decreased blood supply.
3. the inability to feel skin irritation such as wrinkled clothing.
4. the increased likelihood of bowel and bladder dysfunction and skin irritation.

ANSWER: 3

The most common cause of altered skin integrity is due to lack of perceived stimuli and sensations to promote movement. The person must be taught to plan movement, even in the lack of a physical prompt (e.g., discomfort) to move. While there are circulatory and sensation changes with a spinal cord injury, these are not the most common cause for altered skin integrity. There is usually a bowel and bladder dysfunction with an SCI; however, good hygiene and a bowel and catheterization regimen minimize the likelihood of this as a cause of skin breakdown.

Test-taking Tip: *Focus on the key word "primary." While several of the options have elements that are right, altered temperature, bowel and bladder dysfunction, or circulatory changes alone do not cause breakdown.*

Content Area: Child Health; *Category of Health Alteration:* Neurological and Musculoskeletal Management; *Integrated Processes:* Nursing Process Analysis; *Client Need:* Physiological Integrity/Basic Care and Comfort/Mobility/Immobility; *Cognitive Level:* Application

Reference: Taylor, C., Lillis, C., LeMone, P., & Lynn, P. (2008). *Fundamentals of Nursing: The Art and Science of Nursing Care* (6th ed., p. 1187). Philadelphia: Lippincott Williams & Wilkins.

1340. EBP An 11-year-old child is hospitalized for elective surgery. The child has a neurogenic bladder from a spinal cord injury with a lower motor neuron lesion occurring 2 years previously. In planning care, the nurse considers that the optimal treatment for neurogenic bladder in the hospitalized child is:

1. intermittent catheterization.
2. insertion of a retention catheter.
3. insertion of a suprapubic catheter.
4. administration of an anticholinergic medication.

ANSWER: 1

A neurogenic bladder from a lower motor neuron lesion produces a flaccid bladder. The bladder is unable to respond to changes in passive pressure, causing overdistention. Periodic emptying of the bladder with intermittent catheterization is necessary. Some facilities may have a procedure in place for using a clean versus sterile technique because research has shown there is no difference in infection rates, and the child uses a clean technique while at home. A retention catheter is unnecessary and can increase the risk of infection. There is no indication that a suprapubic catheter is needed. An anticholinergic medication, such as dicyclomine (Bentyl®), relaxes the bladder musculature and promotes increased bladder capacity and more adequate emptying, but it is used in persons with a spastic and not a flaccid bladder.

Test-taking Tip: *Recognize that a lower motor neuron lesion of the spinal cord produces a flaccid bladder. Eliminate any options that pertain to just a spastic bladder. Of the remaining options, determine which is optimal.*

Content Area: Child Health; *Category of Health Alteration:* Neurological and Musculoskeletal Management; *Integrated Processes:* Nursing Process Planning; *Client Need:* Physiological Integrity/Basic Care and Comfort/Elimination; *Cognitive Level:* Analysis

Reference: Hockenberry, M., & Wilson, D. (2007). *Wong's Nursing Care of Infants and Children* (8th ed., p. 1833). St. Louis, MO: Mosby/Elsevier.

EBP Reference: Lemke, J., Kasprowicz, K., & Worral, P. (2005). Neurogenic bladder: Sterile versus clean. Using evidence-based practice at the staff nurse level. *Journal of Nursing Care Quarterly,* 20, 302–306.

1341. A pediatric client with a spinal cord injury undergoes range of motion exercises several times each day. In teaching the parent how to do range of motion at home, the nurse observes the client increasing the angle between the extremity and the midline. The nurse concludes that the client is safely performing:

1. abduction.
2. adduction.
3. flexion.
4. extension.

ANSWER: 1

Abduction refers to increasing the angle between the extremity and the body's midline. Flexion and extension are not relative to midline. Adduction is decreasing the angle between the extremity and the body.

▶ ***Test-taking Tip:*** *"Ad"-duction means decreasing the angle between the extremity and midline, or "adding."*

Content Area: Child Health; *Category of Health Alteration:* Neurological and Musculoskeletal Management; *Integrated Processes:* Nursing Process Evaluation; *Client Need:* Physiological Integrity/Basic Care and Comfort/Mobility/Immobility; *Cognitive Level:* Comprehension

Reference: Taylor, C., Lillis, C., LeMone, P., & Lynn, P. (2008). *Fundamentals of Nursing: The Art and Science of Nursing Care* (6th ed., p. 1320). Philadelphia: Lippincott Williams & Wilkins.

1342. When preparing to complete a health history for a 9-year-old child diagnosed with mental retardation with an IQ level of 45, which level of participation should a nurse expect?

1. Able to communicate verbally only with two-letter words
2. Able to read and comprehend simple written instruction with large letters
3. Able to walk independently to perform a simple skill
4. Able to perform tasks that requires careful manual dexterity

ANSWER: 3

An IQ of 45 is considered to be moderate mental retardation. The range of IQ for moderate mental retardation is 36 to 49. At the level of IQ, a 9-year-old child can perform simple manual skills and should be able to walk independently. The child can use simple communication with more than the use of two-letter words. At an IQ level of 45, the child does not progress in functional reading or arithmetic, so would be unable to read and comprehend written instructions even with large lettering. While simple manual skills are able to be performed, skills requiring manual dexterity are not.

▶ ***Test-taking Tip:*** *An IQ level of 45 is considered moderate mental retardation. Select an option that is able to be performed by a younger child.*

Content Area: Child Health; *Category of Health Alteration:* Neurological and Musculoskeletal Management; *Integrated Processes:* Nursing Process Analysis; *Client Need:* Physiological Integrity/Physiological Adaptation/Alterations in Body Systems; *Cognitive Level:* Application

Reference: Hockenberry, M., Wilson, D., Winkelstein, M., & Kline, N. (2006). *Wong's Nursing Care of Infants and Children* (8th ed., p. 990). St. Louis, MO: Mosby.

Test 35: **Child Health: Renal and Urinary Management**

1343. EBP A nurse is analyzing a pediatric client's serum laboratory report. Based on the findings, which health-care provider's order should a nurse anticipate receiving *next*?

Serum Laboratory Test	Client's Value	Normal Values
BUN	26	5–25 mg/dL
Creatinine	2.0	0.5–1.5 mg/dL
Na	140	135–145 mEq/L
K	5.0	3.5–5.3 mEq/L
Cl	100	95–105 mEq/L
CO_2	28	22–30 mEq/L
Phosphate	2.0	1.7–2.6 mEq/L
Calcium	10	9–11 mg/dL
Hgb	15	13.5–17 g/dL
Hct	50	40%–54%
PTH	30	11–54 pg/mL

1. Obtain a urine culture.
2. Obtain a complete blood count (CBC).
3. Obtain a urinalysis.
4. Obtain liver function tests.

ANSWER: 3

The elevated blood urea nitrogen (BUN) and creatinine indicate abnormal kidney function; a urinalysis should be an additional study to further explore kidney function. A urine culture, CBC, or liver function tests would not be indicated at this time because these are not specific to kidney function.

▶ ***Test-taking Tip:*** *Note that only the BUN and creatinine are abnormal. Thus, another test of kidney function is needed next. Eliminate options 2 and 4 because these do not specifically evaluate kidney function.*

Content Area: Child Health; *Category of Health Alteration:* Renal and Urinary Management; *Integrated Processes:* Nursing Process Implementation; *Client Need:* Physiological Integrity/Reduction of Risk Potential/Laboratory Values; *Cognitive Level:* Application

Reference: Ball, J., & Bindler, R. (2008). *Pediatric Nursing: Caring for Children* (4th ed., pp. 977–978). Upper Saddle River, NJ: Prentice Hall.

EBP Reference: Miller, D., & MacDonald, D. (2006). Management of pediatric patients with chronic kidney disease. *Nephrology Nursing Journal,* 33(4), 415–422, 429.

1344. A nurse is educating the parent of a 6-month-old infant on bringing a urine sample to the health-care facility for examination. Which instruction indicates that the nurse is misinformed about the correct procedure?

1. Properly applying the collection device and storing the specimen is necessary.
2. Bring the specimen to the designated place as soon as possible.
3. Store the sample in a warm, dark place until brought to the facility.
4. Notify the examiner of the time lapsed between collecting and delivering the sample.

ANSWER: 3

When a urine sample is brought into a health-care facility for examination, it is stored in the refrigerator if there is any lapse in time between collection and delivery. It is important to instruct the parent on properly applying the collection device and delivering the specimen as soon as possible because delays may alter the results of the urine testing.

▶ ***Test-taking Tip:*** *The key word is "misinformed." This is a negative-response item. Select the option that is not correct.*

Content Area: Child Health; *Category of Health Alteration:* Renal and Urinary Management; *Integrated Processes:* Teaching and Learning; *Client Need:* Physiological Integrity/Reduction of Risk Potential/Diagnostic Tests; *Cognitive Level:* Application

Reference: Hockenberry, M., & Wilson, D. (2007). *Wong's Nursing Care of Infants and Children* (8th ed., p. 1115). St. Louis, MO: Mosby/Elsevier.

1345. A 3-year-old client presents with vomiting and diarrhea for 24 hours. On routine urinalysis, which finding should indicate to a nurse that the child is dehydrated?

1. Specific gravity 1.000.
2. Specific gravity 1.010.
3. Specific gravity 1.020.
4. Specific gravity 1.030.

ANSWER: 4

A specific gravity (SG) greater than 1.025 may indicate dehydration. The normal SG range is between 1.010 and 1.025. Options 1, 2, and 3 are less than 1.025. A low specific gravity can indicate dilute urine because as urine becomes more concentrated, its specific gravity increases.

▶ ***Test-taking Tip:*** *Comprehension of the normal ranges of key laboratory values would be expected on the NCLEX-RN®. Review the ranges for key laboratory values to answer this question.*

Content Area: Child Health; *Category of Health Alteration:* Renal and Urinary Management; *Integrated Processes:* Nursing Process Analysis; *Client Need:* Physiological Integrity/Reduction of Risk Potential/Laboratory Values; *Cognitive Level:* Application

Reference: Berman, A., Snyder, S., Kozier, B., & Erb, G. (2008). *Kozier & Erb's Fundamentals of Nursing: Concepts, Process, and Practice* (8th ed., p. 815). Upper Saddle River, NJ: Pearson Education.

1346. A nurse is preparing an adolescent client to conduct a 24-hour urine collection. The nurse instructs the client that the collection period always starts and ends with an empty bladder so that at the time the collection begins, the client should void and the specimen should be discarded. All urine voided in the subsequent 24 hours should be saved. Twenty-four hours after the precollection specimen was discarded, the client should void. What instruction should the nurse give to the client regarding the final specimen?

1. Add it to the container.
2. Discard it.
3. Measure it and discard it.
4. Store it separately in the refrigerator.

ANSWER: 1

At the completion of the 24-hour period, the client is asked to void and the specimen is added to the container. It would be inappropriate to discard the specimen or store it separately. If the specimen was discarded, the test would need to be restarted.

➧ ***Test-taking Tip:*** *Carefully read the situation. Visualize the instructions given to the client to select the correct option.*

Content Area: Child Health; *Category of Health Alteration:* Renal and Urinary Management; *Integrated Processes:* Teaching and Learning; *Client Need:* Physiological Integrity/Reduction of Risk Potential/Diagnostic Tests; *Cognitive Level:* Application

Reference: Hockenberry, M., & Wilson, D. (2007). *Wong's Nursing Care of Infants and Children* (8th ed., p. 1115). St. Louis, MO: Mosby/Elsevier.

1347. A nurse is preparing a 12-year-old female client for a renal/bladder ultrasound. In doing so, the nurse explains to the client:

1. that she cannot void before the procedure because a full bladder will facilitate the best visualization of important structures.
2. that she should void immediately before the procedure because a full bladder impairs the visualization of important structures.
3. that she will have to void during the procedure in order to obtain the best results.
4. that the fullness of the bladder is not relevant to the study findings.

ANSWER: 1

A full bladder is important during a renal ultrasound to permit the best visualization of structures. Voiding before or during the procedure is not recommended. The fullness of the bladder is quite relevant in properly obtaining desired results.

➧ ***Test-taking Tip:*** *Options 1 and 2 are opposite, and therefore one of these is most likely the correct response.*

Content Area: Child Health; *Category of Health Alteration:* Renal and Urinary Management; *Integrated Processes:* Teaching and Learning; *Client Need:* Physiological Integrity/Reduction of Risk Potential/Diagnostic Tests; Psychosocial Integrity/Therapeutic Environment; *Cognitive Level:* Application

Reference: Hockenberry, M., & Wilson, D. (2007). *Wong's Nursing Care of Infants and Children* (8th ed., pp. 1235–1236). St. Louis, MO: Mosby/Elsevier.

1348. A nurse is taking a history of a 9-month-old infant with altered urinary elimination. Which abnormal finding should the nurse report *first*?

1. Odorless urine
2. Dark amber urine
3. Not producing a wet diaper in a 24-hour period
4. Urinary output between 250 and 500 mL per day

ANSWER: 3

Anuria, or a lack of urine production, may be a sign of altered renal function. Infants often have odorless urine, and output is usually between 250 and 500 mL daily. Dark amber urine may require more inquiry, although it is not the priority item to report.

➧ ***Test-taking Tip:*** *Use the process of elimination, and eliminate options 1 and 4 because odorless urine and urinary output of 250 to 500 mL per day can be normal for an infant. Option 2, amber urine, may require further evaluation in an infant.*

Content Area: Child Health; *Category of Health Alteration:* Renal and Urinary Management; *Integrated Processes:* Nursing Process Implementation; *Client Need:* Physiological Integrity/Basic Care and Comfort/Elimination; *Cognitive Level:* Application

Reference: Berman, A., Snyder, S., Kozier, B., & Erb, G. (2008). *Kozier & Erb's Fundamentals of Nursing: Concepts, Process, and Practice* (8th ed., p. 1290). Upper Saddle River, NJ: Pearson Education.

1349. An adolescent male with a history of spinal cord injury reports a leaking of urine at fairly regular intervals. A nurse should document in the client's plan of care a nursing diagnosis of:

1. functional urinary incontinence.
2. reflex urinary incontinence.
3. stress urinary incontinence.
4. urge urinary incontinence.

ANSWER: 2

Reflex urinary incontinence is an involuntary loss of urine at fairly regular intervals. It occurs from an autonomic response when the bladder reaches a certain urine volume. Functional, stress, and urge incontinence do not occur at fairly regular intervals. Functional incontinence occurs when a usually continent person is unable to reach the toilet in time to avoid unintentional loss of urine. Stress incontinence occurs when activities that increase abdominal pressure cause a sudden leakage of urine. Urge incontinence occurs when there is involuntary passage of urine soon after feeling a strong sense of needing to void.

➧ ***Test-taking Tip:*** *Apply knowledge of medical terminology to eliminate options 1, 3, and 4.*

Content Area: Child Health; *Category of Health Alteration:* Renal and Urinary Management; *Integrated Processes:* Communication and Documentation; *Client Need:* Physiological Integrity/Basic Care and Comfort/Elimination; *Cognitive Level:* Application

Reference: Berman, A., Snyder, S., Kozier, B., & Erb, G. (2008). *Kozier & Erb's Fundamentals of Nursing: Concepts, Process, and Practice* (8th ed., p. 1295). Upper Saddle River, NJ: Pearson Education.

1350. A nurse is caring for multiple clients preparing for placement of an external diversional urinary system. Which client has the greatest need for interventions to promote a positive body image?

1. An infant with spina bifida
2. A toddler who has recently been toilet trained
3. A school-aged child in foster care
4. An adolescent who has recently become sexually active

ANSWER: 4

Because of the developmental stage, an external device would put an adolescent at the highest risk for body image disturbance, and therefore that age group has the greatest need for interventions. According to Havighurst's age periods, an adolescent's developmental task is accepting one's physique and using the body effectively. The developmental stage according to Erikson's Developmental Task Theory is to achieve a coherent sense of self. An infant's developmental stage is trust versus mistrust. The infant is unaware of body alterations. A toddler's developmental level is autonomy versus shame and doubt and he or she could be at risk for altered body image, depending on the response of parents and others. A school-aged child's developmental level is industry versus inferiority. The child would be at risk for body image disturbance if unable to develop competence with the device or not achieving a sense of wholeness (one of Havighurst's developmental tasks).

➧ ***Test-taking Tip:*** *Think about the developmental stage of each individual before making a selection. The key phrase is "greatest need."*

Content Area: Child Health; *Category of Health Alteration:* Renal and Urinary Management; *Integrated Processes:* Caring; Nursing Process Planning; *Client Need:* Health Promotion and Maintenance/Growth and Development; *Cognitive Level:* Analysis

References: Berman, A., Snyder, S., Kozier, B., & Erb, G. (2008). *Kozier & Erb's Fundamentals of Nursing: Concepts, Process, and Practice* (8th ed., pp. 353–354). Upper Saddle River, NJ: Pearson Education; Hockenberry, M., & Wilson, D. (2007). *Wong's Nursing Care of Infants and Children* (8th ed., p. 491). St. Louis, MO: Mosby/Elsevier.

1351. Which client would be most appropriate for a nurse to instruct on the use of intermittent self-urinary catheterization?

1. A 15-year-old female preparing to have a cesarian section
2. A 18-year-old female newly diagnosed with multiple sclerosis (MS)
3. A 13-year-old male with spinal cord injury and no awareness of urge to void
4. A 16-year-old female who is 8 months pregnant and reports dribbling

ANSWER: 3

A 13-year-old male with spinal cord injury and no awareness of urge to void would require a means to empty his bladder. The 15-year-old would need only temporary indwelling catheterization. A person newly diagnosed with MS would likely not have bladder involvement requiring intermittent catheterization. This may occur later in the disease process. Dribbling is common in the third trimester of pregnancy. Catheterization would be avoided.

➧ ***Test-taking Tip:*** *The key word is "intermittent." Eliminate options 1 and 4 because neither situation would be intermittent. Eliminate option 2 because option 3 is more appropriate.*

Content Area: Child Health; *Category of Health Alteration:* Renal and Urinary Management; *Integrated Processes:* Nursing Process Implementation; *Client Need:* Physiological Integrity/Basic Care and Comfort/Elimination; *Cognitive Level:* Analysis

Reference: Berman, A., Snyder, S., Kozier, B., & Erb, G. (2008). *Kozier & Erb's Fundamentals of Nursing: Concepts, Process, and Practice* (8th ed., pp. 1296–1297). Upper Saddle River, NJ: Pearson Education.

1352. EBP A nurse is educating the parent of a child newly diagnosed with vesicoureteral reflux. An important concept to include in the teaching is the therapeutic use of:

1. steroidal therapy for at least 3 to 6 months.
2. prophylactic antibiotic therapy until such an age as the condition resolves.
3. acetaminophen (Tylenol®) as needed.
4. growth hormone injections to prevent renal failure.

ANSWER: 2

Vesicoureteral reflux is retrograde flow of urine from the bladder into the ureters from an incompetent valve that prevents backflow. Because urine is retained in the ureters after voiding, stasis of this urine leads to infection. Infection is managed with prophylactic antibiotic therapy until such an age as the condition resolves. Steroids are anti-inflammatory agents and unnecessary. High doses of acetaminophen can lead to renal impairment. Growth hormone injections are used to treat a deficiency of growth hormone, which is unrelated.

▶ ***Test-taking Tip:*** *Think about what occurs in vesicoureteral reflux. If unsure, use knowledge of medical terminology. "Reflux" means backflow and "ureteral" refers to ureters.*

Content Area: Child Health; *Category of Health Alteration:* Renal and Urinary Management; *Integrated Processes:* Teaching and Learning; *Client Need:* Health Promotion and Maintenance/Disease Prevention; *Cognitive Level:* Application

Reference: Pillitteri, A. (2007). *Maternal & Child Health Nursing: Care of the Childbearing & Childrearing Family* (5th ed., pp. 1464–1465). Philadelphia: Lippincott Williams & Wilkins.

EBP Reference: Bray, L., & Saunders, C. (2006). Nursing management of pediatric urethral catheterization. *Nursing Standard,* 20(24), 51–60.

1353. A nurse is conducting preoperative counseling for the parents of a child diagnosed with hypospadias. Which principle objectives regarding surgical correction of hypospadias should be addressed? SELECT ALL THAT APPLY.

1. To circumcise immediately after the condition is identified
2. To enhance the child's ability to void in the standing position with a straight stream
3. To improve the physical appearance of the genitalia for psychological reasons
4. To preserve a sexually active organ
5. To promote bowel elimination
6. To descend an undescended testicle

ANSWER: 2, 3, 4

In hypospadias, the urethra does not properly exit the penis at the tip. It can be a mild defect, with the urethral opening slightly out of place, or a severe defect, with the urethral opening closer to the scrotum. Therefore, the principle objectives of hypospadias repair include voiding enhancement, improving the physical appearance of the genitalia for psychological reasons, and preserving a sexually active organ. Circumcision may be delayed to save the foreskin to use in the repair of this condition, if needed. An undescended testicle is unrelated to hypospadias repair.

▶ ***Test-taking Tip:*** *Apply knowledge of medical terminology. The words "objectives" and "hypospadias repair" are the key words in the stem.*

Content Area: Child Health; *Category of Health Alteration:* Renal and Urinary Management; *Integrated Processes:* Teaching and Learning; *Client Need:* Physiological Integrity/Reduction of Risk Potential/Potential for Complications from Surgical Procedures and Health Alterations; *Cognitive Level:* Application

Reference: Hockenberry, M., & Wilson, D. (2007). *Wong's Nursing Care of Infants and Children* (8th ed., pp. 486–487). St. Louis, MO: Mosby/Elsevier.

1354. A nurse is educating the parent of an infant male client with phimosis. Which important concept should the nurse include in teaching?

1. Occasionally, the narrowing obstructs the flow of urine, resulting in a dribbling stream.
2. Once the infant is older and begins toileting, urinating a straight stream will be impossible.
3. Retract the foreskin away from the glans penis daily to prevent urinary retention.
4. Watch for enlargement of the testicles because fluid is likely to accumulate.

ANSWER: 1

Phimosis is a narrowing of the preputial opening of the foreskin that prevents retraction of the foreskin over the glans penis. Occasionally, the narrowing obstructs the flow of urine, resulting in a dribbling stream or even ballooning of the foreskin with accumulated urine during voiding. Hypospadias is a condition in which the urethral opening is located below the glans penis or anywhere along the ventral surface. If not corrected, a straight stream may not be possible. Hypospadias is unrelated to phimosis. In phimosis, the foreskin is already retracted and is causing the urinary problems. A hydrocele is the presence of fluid in the processus vaginalis. Fluid does not accumulate in the testicles but can cause urinary retention.

▶ ***Test-taking Tip:*** *The word "phimosis" is the key in the stem. Apply knowledge of medical terminology to answer this question.*

Content Area: Child Health; *Category of Health Alteration:* Renal and Urinary Management; *Integrated Processes:* Teaching and Learning; *Client Need:* Physiological Integrity/Physiological Adaptation/Alterations in Body Systems; *Cognitive Level:* Application

Reference: Hockenberry, M., & Wilson, D. (2007). *Wong's Nursing Care of Infants and Children* (8th ed., pp. 483–486). St. Louis, MO: Mosby/Elsevier.

1355. Which of the following should a nurse expect in the plan of care for a client newly diagnosed with ambiguous genitalia? SELECT ALL THAT APPLY.

1. A physical examination by a pediatric urologist
2. Immediate surgical intervention
3. Chromosome analysis
4. Biochemical tests
5. Ultrasonography
6. Radiographic contrast studies

ANSWER: 1, 3, 4, 5, 6

Uncertain gender is a potential lifetime social tragedy for the child and family so the identification of appropriate gender must be done with precision and accuracy. Therefore, careful history and physical examination, chromosome analysis, biochemical tests, and ultrasonography and radiographic contrast studies are important components of the assessment to determine gender assignment. The assignment of a gender followed by immediate surgical intervention was the traditional approach to treatment for ambiguous genitalia. A multidisciplinary team approach is now used to assign gender, and surgical reconstruction may be delayed to avoid irreversible surgical interventions.

➧ ***Test-taking Tip:*** *Consider ramifications of all options and delete the one option that can have irreversible ramifications.*

Content Area: Child Health; *Category of Health Alteration:* Renal and Urinary Management; *Integrated Processes:* Nursing Process Planning; *Client Need:* Physiological Integrity/Physiological Adaptation/Illness Management; *Cognitive Level:* Application

Reference: Hockenberry, M., & Wilson, D. (2007). *Wong's Nursing Care of Infants and Children* (8th ed., p. 493). St. Louis, MO: Mosby/Elsevier.

1356. A nurse is caring for a pediatric client who will be going home with an indwelling catheter. Which important component should the nurse include in the instructions to the client and his or her parents?

1. Keeping the urine drainage bag below the level of the bladder
2. Pulling and taping the catheter securely down the length of the child's leg
3. Decreasing fluid intake to limit the need for frequent bag emptying
4. Taking tub baths in place of showers to minimize standing

ANSWER: 1

Keeping the drainage bag below the level of the bladder prevents reflux of urine back into the bladder, which increases the risk of a bladder infection. Placing tension on the catheter increases the risk of injury to the urinary meatus. Fluid intake should be increased to reduce bacterial growth. Showering minimizes the potential for contaminating the urinary drainage bag.

➧ ***Test-taking Tip:*** *Eliminate options that increase the child's risk for infection and injury.*

Content Area: Child Health; *Category of Health Alteration:* Renal and Urinary Management; *Integrated Processes:* Teaching and Learning; *Client Need:* Health Promotion and Maintenance/Self-Care; *Cognitive Level:* Application

Reference: Berman, A., Snyder, S., Kozier, B., & Erb, G. (2008). *Kozier & Erb's Fundamentals of Nursing: Concepts, Process, and Practice* (8th ed., p. 1308). Upper Saddle River, NJ: Pearson Education.

1357. EBP A pediatric client requires clean intermittent catheterization while at home. Which early signs of infection should the nurse teach the parents to report immediately?

1. Fever, pulse in the upper range of normal, foul-smelling urine
2. Increased appetite, anuria, sweet-smelling urine
3. Tachypnea, tachycardia, hypertension
4. Mental confusion, diarrhea, dehydration

ANSWER: 1

Fever, increased pulse rate, and foul-smelling urine are early signs of infection that the parent should report to the health-care provider. Changes in appetite and in the odor of urine could be signs of other conditions and need to be properly evaluated. Anuria, or the absence of producing urine, requires immediate evaluation and intervention. Elevated respiratory rate, pulse, and blood pressure could be related to infection but would not likely be the early signs parents would be instructed to monitor. Symptoms such as mental confusion, diarrhea, and dehydration would not be early signs of infection.

➧ ***Test-taking Tip:*** *The words "early signs of infection" are the key words in the stem.*

Content Area: Child Health; *Category of Health Alteration:* Renal and Urinary Management; *Integrated Processes:* Teaching and Learning; *Client Need:* Health Promotion and Maintenance/Self-Care; *Cognitive Level:* Application

EBP Reference: Miller, D., & MacDonald, D. (2006). Management of pediatric patients with chronic kidney disease. *Nephrology Nursing Journal,* 33(4), 415–422, 429.

1358. EBP A nurse is preparing to administer an analgesic for short-term, mild pain in a pediatric client with a history of acute renal insufficiency. Which pharmacological agent should the nurse select from the list of standing orders from the health-care provider?

1. Ibuprofen (Motrin®)
2. Acetaminophen (Tylenol®)
3. Morphine sulfate
4. Meperidine (Demerol®)

ANSWER: 2

Acetaminophen is an appropriate analgesic for short-term, mild to moderate pain in this client as it will not contribute to renal insufficiency. Ibuprofen could contribute to renal impairment. Morphine sulfate and meperidine are narcotic analgesics and are best used for moderate to severe pain.

➧ ***Test-taking Tip:*** *The key phrases are "short-term, mild pain" and "renal insufficiency." Apply knowledge of pharmacology to eliminate all but option 2.*

Content Area: Child Health; *Category of Health Alteration:* Renal and Urinary Management; *Integrated Processes:* Physiological Integrity/Pharmacological and Parenteral Therapies/Pharmacological Pain Management; *Client Need:* Nursing Process Implementation; *Cognitive Level:* Application

EBP Reference: Knapp Dlugosz, C., Chater, R., & Engle, J. (2006). Appropriate use of nonprescription analgesics in pediatric patients. *Journal of Pediatric Health Care, 20*(5), 316–325.

1359. A parent of a 4-year-old with acute poststreptococcal glomerulonephritis is concerned about care of the child after discharge. A nurse should educate the parent on which important concepts? SELECT ALL THAT APPLY.

1. That the recovery time is quick
2. Returning to pre-illness activities as soon as possible
3. Weighing the child daily to determine fluid retention or loss
4. Avoiding infection by avoiding contact with ill persons
5. Administering antibiotics that are likely to be prescribed
6. Administering antihypertensive medication because the diastolic blood pressure is 98 mm Hg

ANSWER: 3, 4, 6

Because diet is controversial, the best indicator of fluid loss or retention is daily weight. Salt restriction may be needed to control edema, but most children do well on a normal diet with normal salt and protein content. Because the child's system is already compromised, there is increased risk of contracting an infection. Antihypertensive therapy with calcium channel blockers is used to treat a diastolic pressure greater than 90 mm Hg. The recovery period may be as long as 2 years in acute glomerulonephritis. Fatigue may restrict the return to the previous activity level. After 1 to 2 weeks, the child can attend school and engage in normal activities, except competitive activities because these stress the kidneys. Antibiotics are usually ineffective because the disease is caused not by an active infection, but by an antigen–antibody inflammatory response to a past infection.

➧ ***Test-taking Tip:*** *"Education" and "acute poststreptococcal glomerulonephritis" are the key words in the stem. Read each option carefully to determine if it is associated with acute poststreptococcal glomerulonephritis.*

Content Area: Child Health; *Category of Health Alteration:* Renal and Urinary Management; *Integrated Processes:* Physiological Integrity/Physiological Adaptation/Illness Management; *Client Need:* Teaching and Learning; *Cognitive Level:* Application

References: Monahan, F., Sands, J., Neighbors, M., Marek, J., & Green, C. (2007). *Phipps' Medical-Surgical Nursing: Health and Illness Perspectives* (8th ed., p. 968). St. Louis, MO: Mosby/Elsevier; Pillitteri, A. (2007). *Maternal & Child Health Nursing: Care of the Childbearing & Childrearing Family* (5th ed., p. 1469). Philadelphia: Lippincott Williams & Wilkins.

1360. A nurse caring for a hospitalized 10-year-old child writes a nursing diagnosis *Altered urinary elimination*. Which outcome should the nurse include?

1. Urinates six to eight times per day
2. Enuresis diminishes to every other day
3. Related to diminished excretory function of the kidney
4. Ambulates to the bathroom independently

ANSWER: 1

The elimination system reaches maturity during school age, so the child should urinate six to eight times per day. Enuresis is no longer expected in this age group. A diminished excretory function may be the cause of the altered urinary elimination. If so, it should be included as part of the nursing diagnosis. It is not an outcome. Ambulating to the bathroom independently is an outcome for a nursing diagnosis pertaining to mobility and not urinary elimination.

➧ ***Test-taking Tip:*** *Use the nursing process. An expected outcome is a normal finding. Applying knowledge of this to the age of the child should direct you to option 1.*

Content Area: Child Health; *Category of Health Alteration:* Renal and Urinary Management; *Integrated Processes:* Nursing Process Planning; *Client Need:* Physiological Integrity/Basic Care and Comfort/Elimination; Safe and Effective Care Environment/Management of Care/Continuity of Care; *Cognitive Level:* Application

Reference: Berman, A., Snyder, S., Kozier, B., & Erb, G. (2008). *Kozier & Erb's Fundamentals of Nursing: Concepts, Process, and Practice* (8th ed., p. 1288). Upper Saddle River, NJ: Pearson Education.

1361. A child presents to an emergency department with periorbital edema, anorexia, and the passage of dark-colored urine. The most significant history reported by the parent related to the possible etiology is:

1. a "cold" approximately 10 days before onset of these symptoms.
2. a fall off a skateboard the night before.
3. eating fast food for lunch.
4. international travel to Europe 1 month ago.

ANSWER: 1

Periorbital edema, anorexia, and dark-colored urine (often tea colored, reddish-brown, or smoky from hematuria) are the initial signs of nephrotic reaction in a child with acute glomerulonephritis (AGN). Often, the child has been in good health with no history of infection except for symptoms described as a mild cold approximately 10 days before onset. A fall, fast food, and international travel are not likely significant in diagnosing this condition.

Test-taking Tip: *Use the process of elimination, and eliminate options 2, 3, and 4 because these are not significant components of a history in a child with AGN.*

Content Area: Child Health; *Category of Health Alteration:* Renal and Urinary Management; *Integrated Processes:* Nursing Process Analysis; *Client Need:* Physiological Integrity/Reduction of Risk Potential/Potential for Alterations in Body Systems; *Cognitive Level:* Analysis

Reference: Hockenberry, M., & Wilson, D. (2007). *Wong's Nursing Care of Infants and Children* (8th ed., p. 1244). St. Louis, MO: Mosby/Elsevier.

1362. A nurse is reviewing the laboratory report of a pediatric client suspected of having chronic glomerulonephritis. Along with proteinuria, which laboratory findings should the nurse expect?

1. Elevated blood urea nitrogen (BUN), creatinine, and uric acid levels
2. Decreased BUN, creatinine, and uric acid levels
3. Elevated BUN and creatinine and decreased uric acid levels
4. Decreased BUN and elevated creatinine and uric acid levels

ANSWER: 1

Expected laboratory findings in a client with chronic glomerulonephritis include proteinuria with casts and red and white blood cells. Failing renal function is evidenced by increased BUN, creatinine, and uric acid levels due to the accumulation of the by-products of metabolism. Electrolyte alterations include metabolic acidosis, increased potassium levels, increased phosphate levels, and decreased calcium levels.

Test-taking Tip: *Note that options 1 and 2 are opposites and that options 3 and 4 have a mixture of elevated and decreased levels. All options except 2 have an elevated serum creatinine. Recall that serum creatinine elevates with renal disorders, thus eliminate option 2. When serum creatinine elevates with renal conditions, BUN also elevates; thus eliminate option 4.*

Content Area: Child Health; *Category of Health Alteration:* Renal and Urinary Management; *Integrated Processes:* Nursing Process Assessment; *Client Need:* Physiological Integrity/Reduction of Risk Potential/Diagnostic Tests; *Cognitive Level:* Application

Reference: Hockenberry, M., & Wilson, D. (2007). *Wong's Nursing Care of Infants and Children* (8th ed., pp. 1246–1247). St. Louis, MO: Mosby/Elsevier.

1363. A nurse is caring for a 17-year-old client with renal insufficiency from impaired blood flow to the kidneys sustained during a motor vehicle accident. Which assessment finding related to renal insufficiency should be reported immediately to the health-care provider?

1. Oliguria
2. Dysuria
3. Frequency
4. Urgency

ANSWER: 1

Oliguria, or low urine output, could indicate impaired kidney function. Dysuria, frequency, and urgency often suggest infection. Dysuria means voiding that is either painful or difficult. Urinary frequency is voiding at frequent intervals. Urgency is the sudden strong desire to void.

Test-taking Tip: *The key phrase is "related to renal insufficiency." Use the process of elimination, and eliminate options 2, 3, and 4 because dysuria, frequency, and urgency are unrelated to renal insufficiency from impaired blood flow. These indicate another problem.*

Content Area: Child Health; *Category of Health Alteration:* Renal and Urinary Management; *Integrated Processes:* Nursing Process Implementation; *Client Need:* Safe and Effective Care Environment/Management of Care/Collaboration with Interdisciplinary Team; Physiological Integrity/Physiological Adaptation/Illness Management; *Cognitive Level:* Application

Reference: Berman, A., Snyder, S., Kozier, B., & Erb, G. (2008). *Kozier & Erb's Fundamentals of Nursing: Concepts, Process, and Practice* (8th ed., pp. 1290–1291). Upper Saddle River, NJ: Pearson Education.

1364. EBP For which associated complications should a nurse plan to monitor the pediatric client with chronic kidney disease? SELECT ALL THAT APPLY.

1. Dehydration
2. Hypocalcemia
3. Metabolic alkalosis
4. Bone disease
5. Anemia
6. Obesity

ANSWER: 1, 2, 4, 5

The few functioning nephrons cannot reabsorb enough sodium to maintain a functioning level of body fluid, so dehydration occurs. Hypocalcemia and hyperphosphatemia occur due to the kidney's inability to excrete phosphate. Osteodystrophy (bone disease) occurs as calcium is withdrawn from bones to compensate. Erythropoeitin, which is formed by the kidneys, stimulates red cell production. Anemia develops with decreased red blood cell production. Metabolic acidosis, not alkalosis, occurs from the kidney's inability to excrete the hydrogen ion. Growth failure, not obesity, occurs because of the alteration in calcium metabolism and the kidney's inability to synthesize vitamin D so that it can be used.

Test-taking Tip: *Focus on the issue: complications of chronic kidney disease. Recall the kidney's function in relation to fluid and electrolyte balance, vitamin D synthesis, and hydrogen ion excretion.*

Content Area: Child Health; *Category of Health Alteration:* Renal and Urinary Management; *Integrated Processes:* Nursing Process Planning; *Client Need:* Physiological Integrity/Physiological Adaptation/Illness Management; *Cognitive Level:* Application

Reference: Pillitteri, A. (2007). *Maternal & Child Health Nursing: Care of the Childbearing & Childrearing Family* (5th ed., pp. 1477–1478). Philadelphia: Lippincott Williams & Wilkins.

EBP Reference: Miller, D., & MacDonald, D. (2006). Management of pediatric patients with chronic kidney disease. *Nephrology Nursing Journal,* 33(4), 415–422, 429.

1365. EBP Nursing management of a pediatric client with chronic kidney disease includes knowledge that these clients will often demonstrate normochromic, normocytic anemia primarily caused by:

1. decreased erythropoietin production.
2. increased erythropoietin production.
3. decreased hemoglobin production.
4. increased hemoglobin production.

ANSWER: 1

Erythropoeitin, formed by the kidneys, stimulates red blood cell production. A decrease causes normochromic, normocytic anemia, where the size and hemoglobin content of red blood cells (RBCs) remain normal, but there are fewer RBCs. Increased erythropoietin would stimulate RBC production and not produce anemia. The hemoglobin production is not a cause of normochromic, normocytic anemia.

Test-taking Tip: *Note that options 1 and 2 are opposites, so one or both of these are incorrect; the same is true for options 3 and 4.*

Content Area: Child Health; *Category of Health Alteration:* Renal and Urinary Management; *Integrated Processes:* Nursing Process Analysis; *Client Need:* Physiological Integrity/Reduction of Risk Potential/Laboratory Values; *Cognitive Level:* Application

Reference: Pillitteri, A. (2007). *Maternal & Child Health Nursing: Care of the Childbearing & Childrearing Family* (5th ed., p. 1477). Philadelphia: Lippincott Williams & Wilkins.

EBP Reference: Miller, D., & MacDonald, D. (2006). Management of pediatric patients with chronic kidney disease. *Nephrology Nursing Journal,* 33(4), 415–422, 429.

1366. EBP A nurse is caring for a 3-year-old child with chronic renal failure. The nurse has established a nursing diagnosis of *Risk for interrupted family processes related to chronically ill family member.* The nurse evaluates that an outcome has been met for this nursing diagnosis when which observation is made?

1. Parents stay with the child continuously while hospitalized.
2. Parents participate in the care of their ill child.
3. Parents inform the nurses when they are unable to visit.
4. Parents find child care for children at home so they can visit.

ANSWER: 2

Because the parents should be assisting with the child's care if healthy, then participating in the child's care when ill should promote family processes. Continuously staying with the child doesn't demonstrate normal family processes where parents should be taking time for themselves. Informing the nurses when they are unable to visit is unrelated to the nursing diagnosis of risk for interrupted family processes. Although visiting an ill child is expected, it does interrupt normal family processes for children at home. However, the focus of this nursing diagnosis is the interruption of family processes between the child and the parent. In normal family processes, the parent should be involved with the child and not just visiting.

Test-taking Tip: *Focus on the nursing diagnosis: risk for interrupted family processes. Think about which actions should be normal for a parent in a family without an ill child.*

Content Area: Child Health; *Category of Health Alteration:* Renal and Urinary Management; *Integrated Processes:* Nursing Process Evaluation; *Client Need:* Physiological Integrity/Physiological Adaptation/Illness Management; *Cognitive Level:* Analysis

Reference: Pillitteri, A. (2007). *Maternal & Child Health Nursing: Care of the Childbearing & Childrearing Family* (5th ed., pp. 1477–1478). Philadelphia: Lippincott Williams & Wilkins.

EBP Reference: Miller, D., & MacDonald, D. (2006). Management of pediatric patients with chronic kidney disease. *Nephrology Nursing Journal,* 33(4), 415–422, 429.

1367. A nurse has assessed a 6-month-old boy illustrated below. Which nursing documentation is most accurate?

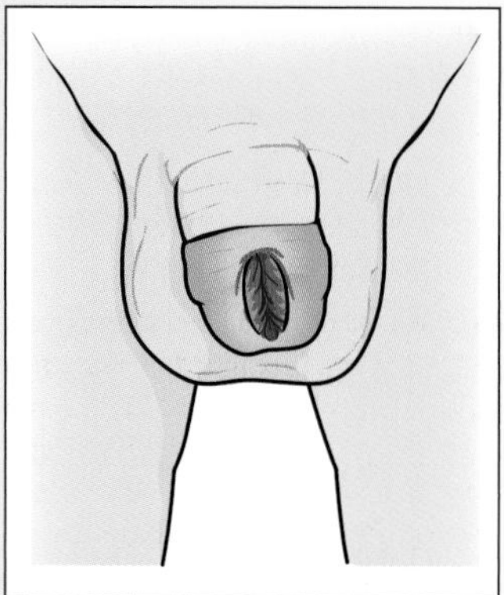

1. Altered urinary stream due to hypospadias
2. Urethral opening noted at the dorsum of the penis
3. Penis normal in color, size, and appearance for a 6-month-old male
4. Ulcerations noted at tip of penis extending to the suprapubic area

ANSWER: 2

The child is presenting with an epispadias. In epispadias the urethra ends in an opening on the upper aspect (the dorsum) of the penis. The urethral opening in hypospadias is on the lower aspect of the penis. Both epispadias and hypospadias alter the direction of the urinary stream. The penis is malformed because of the presence of an epispadias. The reddened area is the urethral opening and not ulcerations.

➧ ***Test-taking Tip:*** *Recall that "dorsum" means upper. Carefully analyze the illustration to select the correct option.*

Content Area: Child Health; *Category of Health Alteration:* Renal and Urinary Management; *Integrated Processes:* Communication and Documentation; *Client Need:* Safe and Effective Care Environment/Management of Care/Continuity of Care; *Cognitive Level:* Analysis

Reference: Hockenberry, M., & Wilson, D. (2007). *Wong's Nursing Care of Infants and Children* (8th ed., pp. 486–487). St. Louis, MO: Mosby/Elsevier.

1368. EBP A pediatric client with chronic kidney disease has elevations in serum blood urea nitrogen (BUN) and creatinine. A nurse interprets this to mean that the child has a reduction in:

1. serum erythropoietin.
2. growth hormone.
3. glomerular filtration rate.
4. blood flow to the kidneys.

ANSWER: 3

A reduction in glomerular filtration rate results in an accumulation of nitrogenous wastes. This is reflected in the serum BUN and creatinine. Serum erythropoietin, growth hormone, or the residual urine do not reflect elevations in BUN and creatinine. Serum erythropoietin is a measurement of the degree of hormonal stimulation to the bone marrow to stimulate the release of red blood cells (RBCs). Growth hormone is an anabolic hormone that promotes protein application and mobilizes glucose and free fatty acids. Reduced blood flow to the kidneys is but one cause of renal failure.

➧ ***Test-taking Tip:*** *Think about the function of the kidneys in filtering urine. Then use the process of elimination to eliminate all options except option 3 because the other options do not relate to filtering urine.*

Content Area: Child Health; *Category of Health Alteration:* Renal and Urinary Management; *Integrated Processes:* Nursing Process Analysis; *Client Need:* Physiological Integrity/Reduction of Risk Potential/Laboratory Values; *Cognitive Level:* Application

Reference: Pillitteri, A. (2007). *Maternal & Child Health Nursing: Care of the Childbearing & Childrearing Family* (5th ed., pp. 1453–1454). Philadelphia: Lippincott Williams & Wilkins.

EBP Reference: Miller, D., & MacDonald, D. (2006). Management of pediatric patients with chronic kidney disease. *Nephrology Nursing Journal,* 33(4), 415–422, 429.

1369. An emergency department nurse is triaging a group of pediatric clients. Which child should a nurse address *first*?

1. A child with periorbital edema that is worse in the morning
2. A previously well child who begins to gain weight insidiously over a period of days
3. A child with a recent renal transplant who has developed fever, local tenderness, decreased urinary output, and elevated blood pressure
4. A child with fever, foul-smelling urine, dysuria, and frequency and urgency on urination

ANSWER: 3

The child with recent renal transplantation with these symptoms needs to be evaluated immediately for possible rejection. All of the children presented in the other options require prompt evaluation, but are not the first client to be seen.

Test-taking Tip: *Use the process of elimination and eliminate option 1, as this child likely has acute glomerulonephritis. Almost all clients with this condition who are properly diagnosed and treated will recover completely. Eliminate option 2, as this client may have nephrotic syndrome for which the prognosis for ultimate recovery in most cases is good. Eliminate option 4, as this client likely has a urinary tract infection. Adequate treatment at the time of diagnosis will usually result in an excellent prognosis.*

Content Area: Child Health; *Category of Health Alteration:* Renal and Urinary Management; *Integrated Processes:* Nursing Process Assessment; *Client Need:* Safe and Effective Care Environment/ Management of Care/Establishing Priorities; *Cognitive Level:* Analysis

Reference: Hockenberry, M., & Wilson, D. (2007). *Wong's Nursing Care of Infants and Children* (8th ed., p. 1269). St. Louis, MO: Mosby/Elsevier.

1370. To allow a 10-year-old child receiving peritoneal dialysis a sense of control, a nurse should best allow the child to:

1. cleanse the abdomen before inserting the needle for administering the local anesthetic.
2. select liquids to drink during the dialysis procedure and for meals from a list of options.
3. engage in therapeutic play with a cloth doll that has a dialysis catheter.
4. play with a toy that is only allowed during the peritoneal dialysis procedure.

ANSWER: 2

Because the bulk of peritoneal fluid causes pressure on the stomach and causes a feeling of fullness, a child is provided with a liquid diet or small frequent feedings. Allowing the child to choose the preferred, allowable liquid ensures a sense of control. Other suggestions include allowing the child to record the amount of solution infused and drained and then compare this to the nurse's recordings. The nurse needs to ensure sterility of supplies and prevent infection. Allowing a 10-year-old to cleanse the abdomen is not the best option. Therapeutic play is used to enhance self-esteem and reduce anxiety. Playing with a toy allowed only during dialysis helps to reduce boredom.

Test-taking Tip: *The key words are "sense of control" and "best." Eliminate options 3 and 4 because these activities do not promote a sense of control.*

Content Area: Child Health; *Category of Health Alteration:* Renal and Urinary Management; *Integrated Processes:* Nursing Process Implementation; Caring; *Client Need:* Physiological Integrity/Physiological Adaptation/Illness Management; *Cognitive Level:* Application

Reference: Pillitteri, A. (2007). *Maternal & Child Health Nursing: Care of the Childbearing & Childrearing Family* (5th ed., pp. 1457–1458). Philadelphia: Lippincott Williams & Wilkins.

1371. A 9-year-old male client is about to undergo a kidney transplant. A nurse explains to the client and his family that kidney transplants: SELECT ALL THAT APPLY.

1. are restricted to blood relatives as donors.
2. eliminate dependence on dialysis.
3. may result in rejection, hypertension, or infection.
4. may involve living, non–heart beating, and deceased donors.
5. eliminate the need for dietary restrictions.
6. are more cost-effective than dialysis after the first year.

ANSWER: 2, 3, 4, 5, 6

Transplant does eliminate dependence on dialysis and the need to restrict diet. However, dialysis may be used postoperatively, depending on the type of kidney donor. Transplant may result in rejection, hypertension, or infection and is more cost-effective than dialysis after the first year. Kidney transplant donors are not restricted to blood relatives. Donors may be living, non–heart beating, or deceased. Blood and tissue typing is done to determine a match to prevent rejection.

Test-taking Tip: *Focus on the issue: a kidney transplant procedure. Carefully read each option to determine if it is related to kidney transplant.*

Content Area: Child Health; *Category of Health Alteration:* Renal and Urinary Management; *Integrated Processes:* Teaching and Learning; *Client Need:* Physiological Integrity/Reduction of Risk Potential/Potential for Complications from Surgical Procedures and Health Alterations; *Cognitive Level:* Application

Reference: Monahan, F., Sands, J., Neighbors, M., Marek, J., & Green, C. (2007). *Phipps' Medical-Surgical Nursing: Health and Illness Perspectives* (8th ed., pp. 1025–1033). St. Louis, MO: Mosby/Elsevier.

1372. An adolescent with a history of a renal transplant has not been adhering to the pharmacological regime. The result has been damage to the kidney and loss of the graft. The multidisciplinary team is considering whether the client should receive a second transplant. Which course of action is most appropriate for the nurse to consider *next*?

1. Allow the client to decide.
2. Allow the managing health-care provider (HCP) to decide.
3. Follow through with the procedure only if the client can cover the costs.
4. Refer the case to the institution's ethics committee.

ANSWER: 4

Because of a scarcity of donors, expense of the procedure, and costly medications, this case should be referred to the institutional ethics committee. Actions may include discussing the decision with the client and HCP, but allowing either to decide is not the next action. Performing another transplant only if the client can pay is unethical.

Test-taking Tip: *Comprehension of the ethic dilemmas posed by retransplantation should direct you to the correct option. Focus on the next and most appropriate action.*

Content Area: Child Health; *Category of Health Alteration:* Renal and Urinary Management; *Integrated Processes:* Nursing Process Analysis; Caring; *Client Need:* Safe and Effective Care Environment/Management of Care/Referrals; *Cognitive Level:* Analysis

Reference: Hockenberry, M., & Wilson, D. (2007). *Wong's Nursing Care of Infants and Children* (8th ed., p. 1269). St. Louis, MO: Mosby/Elsevier.

1373. A nurse is managing care of a pediatric client following renal trauma. The nurse should monitor the client *first* for:

1. electrolyte imbalance.
2. profuse bleeding.
3. hypertension.
4. hypotension.

ANSWER: 2

Following renal trauma, the client is at risk for profuse bleeding because the blood supply to the kidney constitutes approximately one-fifth of the total cardiac output. Changes in blood pressure or electrolyte imbalances are important considerations but these are not the first considerations for monitoring.

Test-taking Tip: *Note that options 3 and 4 are opposites; thus one or both must be incorrect. Use the ABCs (airway, breathing, circulation) to determine priority; thus, eliminate option 1.*

Content Area: Child Health; *Category of Health Alteration:* Renal and Urinary Management; *Integrated Processes:* Nursing Process Implementation; *Client Need:* Safe and Effective Care Environment/Management of Care/Establishing Priorities; *Cognitive Level:* Application

Reference: Hockenberry, M., & Wilson, D. (2007). *Wong's Nursing Care of Infants and Children* (8th ed., pp. 1254–1255). St. Louis, MO: Mosby/Elsevier.

1374. An emergency department nurse is triaging a group of pediatric clients. Which client should the nurse assess *first*?

1. A child with an oral temperature of 102.1°F (38.9°C)
2. A child with dyspnea and a palpable abdominal mass
3. A child with a 3-cm facial laceration
4. A child with vomiting and diarrhea for 24 hours

ANSWER: 2

Priority should be given to the child with respiratory compromise and a palpable mass. The most common presenting sign of Wilms' tumor is a swelling or mass in the abdomen. Priority nursing care of a client with this condition involves ensuring swift diagnosis and surgical intervention. Fever, facial lacerations, vomiting, and diarrhea may be symptoms requiring immediate care. However, the priority client has the abdominal mass.

Test-taking Tip: *Use the ABCs (airway, breathing, circulation) to determine priority. Option 2 is the only option that presents with oxygenation issues.*

Content Area: Child Health; *Category of Health Alteration:* Renal and Urinary Management; *Integrated Processes:* Nursing Process Analysis; *Client Need:* Safe and Effective Care Environment/Management of Care/Establishing Priorities; Physiological Integrity/Reduction of Risk Potential/Potential for Alterations in Body Systems; *Cognitive Level:* Application

Reference: Hockenberry, M., & Wilson, D. (2007). *Wong's Nursing Care of Infants and Children* (8th ed., pp. 1599–1601). St. Louis, MO: Mosby/Elsevier.

1375. EBP A nurse caring for a pediatric client with nephrotic syndrome should anticipate administering:

1. prednisone (Liquid Pred®).
2. ibuprofen (Children's Motrin®).
3. penicillin (Pen-Vee K®).
4. hydrochlorothiazide (Esidrix®).

ANSWER: 1

An immunological mechanism is involved in nephrotic syndrome. Corticosteroids reduce inflammation and proteinuria. It is given until diuresis without protein loss is accomplished. Ibuprofen is a NSAID used to treat mild inflammation. Penicillin is an antibiotic used to treat infection. Infection is not the cause. Hydrochlorothiazide is a diuretic used to treat hypertension or edema, although it is not commonly used because it tends to decrease blood volume, which is already decreased.

Test-taking Tip: *The words "nephrotic syndrome" and "standard" are the key words in the stem.*

Content Area: Child Health; *Category of Health Alteration:* Renal and Urinary Management; *Integrated Processes:* Nursing Process Planning; *Client Need:* Physiological Integrity/Pharmacological and Parenteral Therapies/Medication Administration; *Cognitive Level:* Application

Reference: Pillitteri, A. (2007). *Maternal & Child Health Nursing: Care of the Childbearing & Childrearing Family* (5th ed., pp. 1470–1471). Philadelphia: Lippincott Williams & Wilkins.

EBP Reference: Mills, M., White, S., Kershaw, D., Flynn, J., Brophy, P., et al. (2005). Developing clinical protocols for nursing practice: Improving nephrology care for children and their families. *Nephrology Nursing Journal*, 32(6), 599–607.

1376. A nurse is caring for a pediatric client with acute renal failure. A health-care practitioner prescribes a sodium biphosphate and sodium phosphate (Fleet®) enema. The next most appropriate nurse action is to:

1. administer the enema as ordered.
2. administer the enema as ordered after discussing the risks with the parent.
3. administer the enema as ordered after discussing the risks with the practitioner.
4. refuse administration of the enema without careful investigation because of the lethal risks.

ANSWER: 4

The use of sodium biphosphate and sodium phosphate enemas in children with renal failure is potentially lethal because of hyperphosphatemia and should not be implemented without careful investigation. The other actions are incorrect because these include administering the enema.

Test-taking Tip: *Note that option 4 is different from the other options (refusing administration). When three options are similar and one is different, the different option is likely the answer.*

Content Area: Child Health; *Category of Health Alteration:* Renal and Urinary Management; *Integrated Processes:* Nursing Process Implementation; *Client Need:* Safe and Effective Care Environment/ Management of Care/Legal Rights and Responsibilities; *Cognitive Level:* Application

Reference: Hockenberry, M., & Wilson, D. (2007). *Wong's Nursing Care of Infants and Children* (8th ed., p. 1233). St. Louis, MO: Mosby/Elsevier.

1377. A 6-year-old child is to receive 20 mcg intranasal desmopressin acetate (DDAVP) at bedtime for enuresis. The medication is supplied in a nasal spray pump of 10 mcg/spray in a 5-mL bottle (0.1 mg/mL), which contains 50 doses of DDAVP. A nurse should instruct the parent to deliver _____ nasal sprays at bedtime.

ANSWER: 2

10 mcg : 1 spray :: 20 mcg : X spray
10 X = 20
X = 2 sprays

Test-taking Tip: *Carefully read the question and the data provided to determine what is being asked. Sometimes more information is provided than is necessary for a drug calculation because the medication may contain all this information on the label.*

Content Area: Child Health; *Category of Health Alteration:* Renal and Urinary Management; *Integrated Processes:* Nursing Process Implementation; Teaching and Learning; *Client Need:* Physiological Integrity/Pharmacological and Parenteral Therapies/Dosage Calculation; *Cognitive Level:* Analysis

References: Pillitteri, A. (2007). *Maternal & Child Health Nursing: Care of the Childbearing & Childrearing Family* (5th ed., p. 1467). Philadelphia: Lippincott Williams & Wilkins; Olsen, J., Shrimpton, D., Giangrasso, A., & Dillon, P. (2007). *Medical Dosage Calculations* (9th ed., p. 264). Upper Saddle River, NJ: Prentice Hall.

Test 36: **Child Health: Respiratory Management**

1378. EBP A 2-year-old child, admitted to an acute care pediatric unit with a sore throat, is tentatively diagnosed with epiglottitis. Which diagnostic test should a nurse plan to review to confirm the diagnosis?

1. Blood culture
2. Complete blood count (CBC)
3. Throat culture
4. Lateral neck x-ray

ANSWER: 4

A lateral neck x-ray will show the enlarged epiglottis. A blood culture will identify the organism and suggest antibiotic selection, but results will be delayed until the microorganism grows in the culture media. The CBC will identify elevated white blood cells and the presence of an infection but will not confirm the diagnosis. A throat culture is usually not performed because gagging can cause complete airway obstruction.

▶ ***Test-taking Tip:*** *The key words are "confirm the diagnosis." Think about which results are available for each of the laboratory tests.*

Content Area: Child Health; *Category of Health Alteration:* Respiratory Management; *Integrated Processes:* Nursing Process Analysis; *Client Need:* Physiological Integrity/Reduction of Risk Potential/Diagnostic Tests; *Cognitive Level:* Analysis

References: Ball, J., & Bindler, R. (2006). *Clinical Handbook for Pediatric Nursing* (pp. 176–200). Upper Saddle River, NJ: Pearson Prentice Hall; Pillitteri, A. (2007). *Maternal & Child Health Nursing: Care of the Childbearing & Childrearing Family* (5th ed., p. 1252). Philadelphia: Lippincott Williams & Wilkins.

EBP Reference: Centers for Disease Control and Prevention. Division of Bacterial and Mycotic Diseases. (2008). Haemophilus influenzae *Serotype b (Hib) Disease. Division of Bacterial and Mycotic Diseases.* Available at: www.cdc.gov/ncidod/dbmd/diseaseinfo/haeminfluserob_t.htm

---

1379. A physician orders arterial blood gases (ABGs) on a 5-year-old client admitted with severe asthma. Which signs and symptoms noted during a nurse's assessment of the child are consistent with the blood gas findings of pH = 7.30, $Paco_2$ = 49 mm Hg, and HCO_3 = 24 mEq/L?

1. Diaphoresis, headache, tachycardia, confusion, restlessness, apprehension, and flushed face
2. Rapid and deep respirations, paresthesia, light-headedness, twitching, anxiety, and fear
3. Rapid and deep breathing, fruity breath, fatigue, headache, lethargy, drowsiness, nausea, vomiting, and abdominal pain
4. Slow and shallow breathing, hypertonic muscles, restlessness, twitching, confusion, irritability, apathy, tetany, and seizures

ANSWER: 1

Diaphoresis, headache, tachycardia, confusion, restlessness, apprehension, and flushed face are all signs and symptoms of respiratory acidosis without compensation. These occur because of the lack of oxygen and trapping of carbon dioxide in the lower airway from the narrowed airway passages. Rapid and deep respirations, paresthesia, light-headedness, twitching, anxiety, and fear are signs and symptoms of respiratory alkalosis. Respiratory alkalosis may occur in asthma if excess artificial ventilation is used in treatment. Rapid and deep breathing, fruity breath, fatigue, headache, lethargy, drowsiness, nausea, vomiting, and abdominal pain are signs and symptoms of metabolic acidosis. Slow and shallow breathing, hypertonic muscles, restlessness, twitching, confusion, irritability, apathy, tetany, and seizures are signs and symptoms of metabolic alkalosis. Metabolic acidosis and alkalosis are not associated with asthma but may occur from other complications.

▶ ***Test-taking Tip:*** *Analyze the ABG findings to determine if respiratory acidosis, respiratory alkalosis, metabolic acidosis, or metabolic alkalosis is present. Then think about how the bronchial constriction and bronchial spasms of asthma can cause these abnormal results. The assessment findings should be those noted in respiratory acidosis.*

Content Area: Child Health; *Category of Health Alteration:* Respiratory Management; *Integrated Processes:* Nursing Process Assessment; *Client Need:* Physiological Integrity/Reduction of Risk Potential/Laboratory Values; *Cognitive Level:* Analysis

Reference: Ball, J., & Bindler, R. (2006). *Clinical Handbook for Pediatric Nursing* (pp. 176–200). Upper Saddle River, NJ: Pearson Prentice Hall.

1380. EBP A triage nurse determines that a child brought to an emergency department is experiencing severe respiratory distress when observing:

1. diaphoresis, restlessness, tachypnea, and anorexia.
2. pallor, coughing, wheezing, and confusion.
3. retractions, grunting, cyanosis, and bradycardia.
4. agitation, decreased level of consciousness, diarrhea, and tachypnea.

ANSWER: 3

Emergency intervention is needed if a child exhibits retraction, indicating use of accessory muscles to breathe. Grunting is an involuntary response to end-stage respiratory effort. Cyanosis indicates that a state of hypoxia exists due to lack of circulating oxygen and progression to bradycardia is an ominous sign that the body is so overtaxed that it is wearing out. The diaphoresis, restlessness, and tachypnea indicate the possibility of an electrolyte imbalance and may indicate *mild* respiratory distress. Anorexia and other effects of impaired nutritional status exist in conditions of respiratory distress, but the dietary issue does not cause immediate concern. Options 2 and 4 may indicate *moderate* respiratory distress.

Test-taking Tip: Focus on signs of severe respiratory distress in selecting the correct option.

Content Area: Child Health; *Category of Health Alteration:* Respiratory Management; *Integrated Processes:* Nursing Process Assessment; *Client Need:* Physiological Integrity/Physiological Adaptation/Medical Emergencies; *Cognitive Level:* Application

Reference: Pillitteri, A. (2007). *Maternal & Child Health Nursing: Care of the Childbearing & Childrearing Family* (5th ed., p. 1252). Philadelphia: Lippincott Williams & Wilkins.

EBP Reference: Agency for Healthcare Research and Quality (AHRQ). (2007). *Highlights of AHRQ Children's Health Care Quality Findings.* AHRQ Publication No. 07-M013-1. Available at: www.ahrq.gov/child/qfindings.htm

---

1381. A clinic nurse receives a call from a mother of a 2-year-old child. The mother states that the child has a temperature of 104°F (40°C), a sore throat, and has been drooling for a few days. The child is now sleepy. Which is the best advice by the nurse?

1. "Take your child to an emergency department immediately."
2. "Bring your child into the clinic to be seen as soon as possible."
3. "Administer acetaminophen (Tylenol®) for the temperature and allow your child to sleep."
4. "Use a spoon to look inside your child's mouth and throat and tell me what you see."

ANSWER: 1

An elevated temperature and sore throat and drooling could suggest epiglottitis. The sleepiness could be from the effects of the elevated temperature or from respiratory depression. The child should be seen in an emergency department immediately because the infant could develop respiratory failure. Bringing the child to the clinic could delay emergency treatment if needed. Acetaminophen may reduce the child's temperature, but allowing the child to sleep without being assessed could be detrimental. If the epiglottis is swollen and inflamed, stimulating the gag reflex can cause complete obstruction of the glottis and respiratory failure, and it should never be checked for a person with suspected epiglottitis.

Test-taking Tip: A decreased level of consciousness can occur from impaired oxygenation. Use the ABCs (airway, breathing, circulation) to determine the best advice.

Content Area: Child Health; *Category of Health Alteration:* Respiratory Management; *Integrated Processes:* Nursing Process Implementation; *Client Need:* Physiological Integrity/Physiological Adaptation/Alterations in Body Systems; *Cognitive Level:* Application

Reference: Pillitteri, A. (2007). *Maternal & Child Health Nursing: Care of the Childbearing & Childrearing Family* (5th ed., p. 1252). Philadelphia: Lippincott Williams & Wilkins.

1382. A 4-year-old is hospitalized after experiencing a sore throat and difficulty swallowing for a week. Laboratory tests reveal elevated white blood cells (WBCs), bands, and neutrophils. A throat culture completed a week ago showed *Haemophilus influenzae* type B. Based on the information, which tentative medical diagnosis should a nurse expect to be documented in the client's chart?

1. Tonsillitis
2. Bronchiolitis
3. Epiglottitis
4. Tuberculosis

ANSWER: 3

Epiglottitis is an acute inflammation of the epiglottis and commonly results from *Haemophilus influenzae* type B. Diagnosis of tonsillitis is made on the basis of visual inspection and clinical manifestations. Inflammation of the tonsils often occurs with pharyngitis and may be viral or a Group A streptococcus bacterial infection. Viral infections require only symptomatic treatment. Diagnosis of bronchiolitis includes enzyme-linked immunosorbent assay or direct fluorescent assay that is performed on nasal wash specimens. Tuberculosis is diagnosed by intradermal purified protein derivative (PPD) and chest x-ray.

Test-taking Tip: Note the results of the child's throat culture and review diagnostic tests for respiratory problems.

Content Area: Child Health; *Category of Health Alteration:* Respiratory Management; *Integrated Processes:* Communication and Documentation; *Client Need:* Physiological Integrity/Reduction of Risk Potential/Laboratory Values; *Cognitive Level:* Analysis

Reference: Kyle, T. (2007). *Essentials of Pediatric Nursing* (pp. 572, 576, 581). Philadelphia: Wolters Kluwer/Lippincott Williams & Wilkins.

1383. A 3-year-old child, admitted with sudden onset of fever, lethargy, dyspnea, sore throat, and difficulty swallowing, has a suspected diagnosis of acute epiglottitis. A nurse's initial assessment should focus on: SELECT ALL THAT APPLY.

1. reviewing the vital sign results.
2. reviewing the past medical history (PMH).
3. auscultating the lungs.
4. obtaining a throat culture.
5. observing swallowing.
6. allaying anxiety and fear.

ANSWER: 1, 2, 3, 5, 6

Vital signs and a focused assessment of body systems are needed to establish a baseline for further assessment, and the PMH is required for prior health information. While assessing, the nurse should minimize the child's anxiety and fear. A throat culture is contraindicated in a diagnosis or suspected diagnosis of epiglottitis because performing a throat culture may cause a complete airway obstruction.

➧ ***Test-taking Tip:*** *Use the nursing process of assessment and only include the options that pertain to assessment. Eliminate options that would be contraindicated in epiglottitis.*

Content Area: Child Health; *Category of Health Alteration:* Respiratory Management; *Integrated Processes:* Nursing Process Assessment; *Client Need:* Physiological Integrity/Physiological Adaptation/Medical Emergencies; *Cognitive Level:* Analysis

References: Ball, J., & Bindler, R. (2008). *Clinical Handbook for Pediatric Nursing.* Upper Saddle River, NJ: Pearson Prentice Hall; Pillitteri, A. (2007). *Maternal & Child Health Nursing: Care of the Childbearing & Childrearing Family* (5th ed., p. 1252). Philadelphia: Lippincott Williams & Wilkins.

1384. A nurse notes substernal retractions when assessing a child. At which area on the illustration did the nurse make this observation?

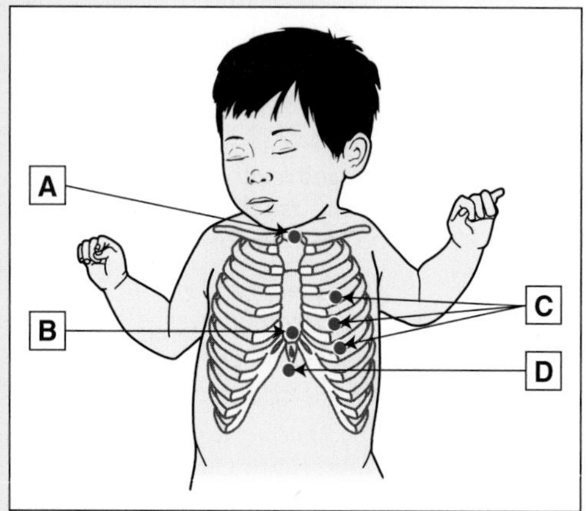

1. A
2. B
3. C
4. D

ANSWER: 4

Line D is pointing to the substernal locations, line A points to the suprasternal location, line B points to the xiphoid process, and line C points to intercostal spaces.

➧ ***Test-taking Tip:*** *Remember anatomical locations and consider the prefix "sub-" used for the word describing the location in the question; then, visualize the area to be assessed.*

Content Area: Child Health; *Category of Health Alteration:* Respiratory Management; *Integrated Processes:* Nursing Process Assessment; *Client Need:* Physiological Integrity/Reduction of Risk Potential/System Specific Assessments; *Cognitive Level:* Analysis

Reference: Kyle, T. (2007). *Essentials of Pediatric Nursing* (pp. 550–609). Philadelphia: Wolters Kluwer/Lippincott Williams & Wilkins.

1385. A 3-month-old child is hospitalized with acute laryngotracheobronchitis (LTB). In formulating a nursing care plan, which nursing diagnosis should be a nurse's priority?

1. Anxiety
2. Risk for deficient fluid volume
3. Ineffective breathing pattern
4. Deficient knowledge

ANSWER: 3

Ineffective breathing pattern is the most important prioritization based on physiological needs. Fear and anxiety, deficient fluid volume, and deficient knowledge are all applicable but not the priority.

➧ ***Test-taking Tip:*** *Use Maslow's Hierarchy of Needs theory to determine the physiological needs of the client to establish the priority need.*

Content Area: Child Health; *Category of Health Alteration:* Respiratory Management; *Integrated Processes:* Nursing Process Planning; *Client Need:* Physiological Integrity/Reduction of Risk Potential/Potential for Alterations in Body Systems; *Cognitive Level:* Analysis

Reference: Kyle, T. (2007). *Essentials of Pediatric Nursing* (pp. 550–609). Philadelphia: Wolters Kluwer/Lippincott Williams & Wilkins.

1386. An albuterol nebulizer treatment is ordered for a 6-month-old infant hospitalized with laryngotracheobronchitis (LTB). A nurse should understand that albuterol (Ventolin®), when used as a nebulizer treatment:

1. relaxes smooth muscles in the airways.
2. reduces inflammation and mucosal edema in airways.
3. removes excess fluid from the lungs.
4. loosens and thins pulmonary secretions.

ANSWER: 1

Albuterol binds to beta2-adrenergic receptors in the airway's smooth muscles, leading to activation of adenyl cyclase and increased levels of cyclic-3',5'-adenosine monophosphate (cAMP). Increases in cAMP activate kinases, which inhibits the phosphorylation of myosin and decreases intracellular calcium. Decreased intracellular calcium relaxes smooth muscles in the airways. Expectorants reduce inflammation by liquefying mucus and stimulating the natural lubricant fluids from the bronchial glands. Diuretics remove excess fluid by acting to increase renal function, which affects circulation, which facilitates removal of excess fluid from the lungs. Mucolytics reduce the thickness of pulmonary secretions by acting directly on the mucus plugs and dissolving them.

➧ ***Test-taking Tip:*** *Use basic pharmacology drug classifications and body system interactions for medications specific to the treatment of respiratory disorders.*

Content Area: Child Health; *Category of Health Alteration:* Respiratory Management; *Integrated Processes:* Nursing Process Analysis; *Client Need:* Physiological Integrity/Pharmacological and Parenteral Therapies/Expected Actions or Outcomes; *Cognitive Level:* Application

Reference: Wilson, B., Shannon, M., Shields, K., & Stang, C. (2008). *Prentice Hall Nurse's Drug Guide 2008* (pp. 30–31). Upper Saddle River, NJ: Pearson Education.

1387. An 18-month-old child is hospitalized with laryngotracheobronchitis (LTB). The child weighs 26.75 pounds, is 33 inches tall, and the body surface area (BSA) is 0.53. A physician orders prednisolone (Orapred®) 0.05 mg/kg oral daily, to be given with food or milk every 6 hours. A nurse should give _________ mg per dose to this client.

ANSWER: 0.15

Calculate the child's weight in kilograms (pounds ÷ 2.2) = 26.75 ÷ 2.2 = 12.159. Weight in kilograms × daily mg/kg: 12.159 × 0.05 = 0.607. Divide daily dose by 4 (ordered every 6 hours [24 ÷ 6 = 4]) = 0.607 ÷ 4 = 0.151 = 0.15 mg.

➧ ***Test-taking Tip:*** *Be sure to read the question carefully to determine what is being asked. First determine the child's weight in kilograms (2.2 pounds equals 1 kilogram). Then calculate the total daily dose. Next, calculate the individual dose. On the NCLEX-RN® exam, use the on-screen calculator to calculate your answer.*

Content Area: Child Health; *Category of Health Alteration:* Respiratory Management; *Integrated Processes:* Nursing Process Analysis; *Client Need:* Physiological Integrity/Pharmacological and Parenteral Therapies/Dosage Calculation; *Cognitive Level:* Analysis

References: Pickar, G. (2007). *Dosage Calculations: A Ratio-Proportion Approach* (2nd ed., pp. 46, 344). Clifton Park, NY: Thomson Delmar Learning; Wilson, B., Shannon, M., Shields, K., & Stang, C. (2008). *Prentice Hall Nurse's Drug Guide 2008* (pp. 1258–1261). Upper Saddle River, NJ: Pearson Education.

1388. EBP A nurse is formulating a plan of care for a 22-month-old child with a diagnosis of laryngotracheobronchitis (LTB). Which symptoms should indicate to the nurse that the child is experiencing impending respiratory failure?

1. Restlessness and irritability
2. Retractions of the accessory chest muscles
3. Decreased inspiratory breath sounds
4. Hoarseness

ANSWER: 3

Decreased inspiratory breath sounds are a sign of physical exhaustion and may indicate impending respiratory failure. Restlessness and irritability are signs and symptoms of LTB, and children may often prefer sitting upright or in a parent's lap. Retractions may also be noted in most children with LTB as they attempt to compensate for the varying degrees of airway obstruction. Hoarseness is usually associated with other respiratory disorders such as asthma or tonsillitis.

➧ ***Test-taking Tip:*** *Use the nursing process of assessment and pathophysiology to identify the physical symptoms related to inflammation of the respiratory tract.*

Content Area: Child Health; *Category of Health Alteration:* Respiratory Management; *Integrated Processes:* Nursing Process Assessment; *Client Need:* Physiological Integrity/Reduction of Risk Potential/Potential for Alterations in Body Systems; *Cognitive Level:* Analysis

References: Ball, J., & Bindler, R. (2008). *Pediatric Nursing Caring for Children* (4th ed. pp. 694–698). Upper Saddle River, NJ: Pearson Prentice Hall; Hockenberry, M., & Wilson, D. (2007). *Wong's Nursing Care of Infants and Children* (8th ed., pp. 1301–1303). St. Louis, MO: Mosby/Elsevier.

EBP Reference: King, L. (2007). Pediatrics, croup or laryngotracheobronchitis. *E-Medicine from WebMD.* Available at: www.emedicine.com/EMERG/topic370.htm

1389. A 6-month-old is hospitalized with a diagnosis of bronchiolitis. The infant's past medical history is as follows: recent admission (2 weeks ago) for streptococcus pneumonia and discharged to home on antibiotics. The mother states the baby has been sneezing, wheezing, and has had a runny nose for 2 days and has not eaten for over 8 hours. Vital signs are temperature 100.2°F (38°C), pulse 102, and respiratory rate 32. Place the nurse's actions in priority order.

_____ Promote desired fluid intake
_____ Assess respiratory distress
_____ Administer prescribed medications
_____ Promote adequate oxygenation
_____ Institute droplet isolation
_____ Provide family teaching

ANSWER: 5, 1, 4, 2, 3, 6

Assessing respiratory distress and promoting adequate oxygenation will promote basic physiological needs. Instituting droplet isolation will provide primary physiological integrity and promote disease prevention and transmission to others, and administering prescribed medications will maintain and facilitate the physiological needs of the client. It will also promote a safe and comfortable environment. Promoting health should be the next focus of the nurse, with promoting desired fluid intake to maintain physiological needs and help to maintain fluid and electrolyte balance. Finally, providing teaching to the child and family will ensure proper communication and patient and family education.

➧ ***Test-taking Tip:*** *Read the options carefully and place the statements that are immediate interventions first, and then consider the items that will promote a better physical environment for the client. Prioritization is placing items in the correct order.*

Content Area: Child Health; *Category of Health Alteration:* Respiratory Management; *Integrated Processes:* Nursing Process Application; *Client Need:* Physiological Integrity/Physiological Adaptation/Illness Management; *Cognitive Level:* Application

References: Berman, A., Snyder, S., Kozier, B., & Erb, G. (2008). *Kozier & Erb's Fundamentals of Nursing: Concepts, Process, and Practice* (8th ed., pp. 217–218). Upper Saddle River, NJ: Pearson Education; Hockenberry, M., & Wilson, D. (2007). *Wong's Nursing Care of Infants and Children* (8th ed., pp. 1334–1337). St. Louis, MO: Mosby/Elsevier.

1390. An 11-month-old infant is brought to the hospital after experiencing a respiratory infection and severe diarrhea for 5 days. The child has poor skin turgor, respirations 30, temperature 101.3°F (39°C), low serum potassium levels, and watery green stools. A physician orders an antipyretic and to begin intravenous (IV) fluid replacement of D5NS with a potassium additive. It is most important for a nurse to:

1. ensure the infant had urine output before beginning the ordered IV fluids.
2. apply oxygen because the child is experiencing rapid respirations.
3. change the infant's diaper to prevent skin breakdown.
4. administer the antipyretic first.

ANSWER: 1

It is imperative to know if the infant's kidneys are functioning before administering fluid replacement with a potassium additive because excess potassium is excreted by the kidneys. High levels of excess potassium can cause life-threatening events, such as cardiac dysrhythmias. A respiration rate of 20 to 40 breaths per minute is within the expected range for an infant. Preventing skin breakdown and administering an antipyretic are also important, but they may not result in a life-threatening event.

➧ *Test-taking Tip: Knowledge regarding how the body excretes and responds to excess potassium is necessary in order to answer this question.*

Content Area: Child Health; *Category of Health Alteration:* Respiratory Management; *Integrated Processes:* Nursing Process Implementation; *Client Need:* Physiological Integrity/Pharmacological and Parenteral Therapies/Parenteral/Intravenous Therapies; *Cognitive Level:* Analysis

Reference: Pillitteri, A. (2007). *Maternal & Child Health Nursing: Care of the Childbearing & Childrearing Family* (5th ed., pp. 1419–1422). Philadelphia: Lippincott Williams & Wilkins.

1391. Which goal should a nurse deem as essential when caring for a 14-month-old infant with bronchiolitis?

1. Promoting and maintaining adequate hydration
2. Setting up and facilitating the use of a mist tent
3. Ensuring that antibiotics are ordered
4. Providing a cough suppressant as necessary

ANSWER: 1

Hydration is very important in children with bronchiolitis (RSV) to loosen secretions, prevent shock, and maintain basic physiological needs. Independent studies have shown that mist tents offer no additional benefits such as keeping secretions moist to facilitate laboratory testing. Antibiotics do not treat illnesses with viral etiologies; they may be used to treat secondary causes but are not primary for viral diseases. Cough suppressants decrease a child's ability to effectively clear the airway.

➧ *Test-taking Tip: Note that three options are similar and one is different. The key word is "goal." Eliminate options that are interventions.*

Content Area: Child Health; *Category of Health Alteration:* Respiratory Management; *Integrated Processes:* Nursing Process Evaluation; *Client Need:* Physiological Integrity/Reduction of Risk Potential/Potential for Alterations in Body Systems; *Cognitive Level:* Analysis

References: Kyle, T. (2007). *Essentials of Pediatric Nursing* (pp. 575–580). Philadelphia: Lippincott Williams & Wilkins; Hockenberry, M., & Wilson, D. (2007). *Wong's Nursing Care of Infants and Children* (8th ed., p. 1849). St. Louis, MO: Mosby/Elsevier.

1392. A 5-month-old infant hospitalized with a diagnosis of *Pneumocystis carinii* pneumonia is being treated with trimethoprim-sulfamethoxazole (TMP-SMZ) with no adverse effects. A nurse assesses that the infant has thick tenacious secretions and poor cough effort, diarrhea, anorexia, and is diaphoretic. Which nursing diagnosis should the nurse establish as the priority?

1. Ineffective airway clearance related to increased secretions and inability to clear the respiratory tract
2. Altered nutrition: less than body requirements related to recurrent illness, diarrheal losses, loss of appetite, and oral candidiasis
3. Risk for infection related to impaired body defenses and presence of infective organisms
4. Risk for fluid volume deficit related to difficulty taking fluids, insensible fluid losses from hyperventilation, and diaphoresis

ANSWER: 1

Ineffective airway clearance related to increased secretions and inability to clear the respiratory tract is a basic physiological need and should be addressed first. Altered nutrition: less than body requirements related to recurrent illness, diarrheal losses, loss of appetite, oral candidiasis is essential to maintaining physiological needs of an immunocompromised child. Risk for infection related to impaired body defenses, presence of infective organisms, preventing infection in an infant/child with an immunological dysfunction is key to maintaining a healthy lifestyle. Immunocompromised children are susceptible to infection and every effort should be made to keep them risk free. There is risk for fluid volume deficit related to difficulty taking fluids, insensible fluid losses from hyperventilation, and diaphoresis. Preventing risk for volume deficit is secondary to physical needs and can be prevented by maintaining fluid volume and encouraging intake.

➧ *Test-taking Tip: Consider Maslow's Hierarchy of Needs theory and the ABCs (airway, breathing, circulation). Address physiological needs first and safety and security needs second.*

Content Area: Child Health; *Category of Health Alteration:* Respiratory Management; *Integrated Processes:* Nursing Process Planning; *Client Need:* Safe and Effective Care Environment/Management of Care/Establishing Priorities; *Cognitive Level:* Analysis

Reference: Kyle, T. (2007). *Essentials of Pediatric Nursing* (pp. 578–580). Philadelphia: Wolters Kluwer/Lippincott Williams & Wilkins.

1393. A 3-year-old child is brought to an emergency department with acute pulmonary edema. The child was seen in an emergency department 48 hours earlier for a near-drowning incident. Treatment was provided at that time, and the child was monitored and discharged home. Current chest radiography indicates diffuse bilateral infiltrates. There is no history of cardiopulmonary disease. Which pulmonary dysfunctions should a nurse think about when assessing the child?

1. Foreign body aspiration
2. Aspiration pneumonia
3. Bronchopneumonia
4. Acute respiratory distress syndrome

ANSWER: 4

Acute respiratory distress syndrome is recognized in children as well as adults and has been associated with clinical conditions and injuries such as sepsis, viral pneumonia, smoke inhalation, and near drowning. It is characterized by respiratory distress and hypoxemia occurring within 72 hours of the injury. Foreign body aspiration occurs when any solid or liquid substance is inhaled into the respiratory tract. It is common in infants and young children and can present in life-threatening acute situations. Aspiration pneumonia is caused by aspiration of meconium or amniotic fluids during the birth process. Bronchopneumonia is often basilar, affects the lower lobes of the lungs, and is often nosocomial or community acquired.

➧ ***Test-taking Tip:*** *Bilateral diffuse infiltrates on the chest radiograph are key to answering this question.*

Content Area: Child Health; *Category of Health Alteration:* Respiratory Management; *Integrated Processes:* Nursing Process Analysis; *Client Need:* Physiological Integrity/Reduction of Risk Potential/Potential for Alterations in Body Systems; *Cognitive Level:* Analysis

Reference: Kyle, T. (2007). *Essentials of Pediatric Nursing* (pp. 583–584). Philadelphia: Wolters Kluwer/Lippincott Williams & Wilkins.

1394. A child with asthma is being discharged to home and has an order for a bronchodilator (albuterol) to be administered via a metered dose inhaler (MDI). Which point should a nurse address for appropriate administration of this medication?

1. When administering medication via a MDI, avoid shaking the canister before discharging the medication.
2. Medication is ordered in two "puffs"; press on the canister twice in succession to discharge the medication.
3. There should be a tight seal around the mouthpiece of the inhaler before discharging the medication.
4. There should be a 2- to 3-inch space (or spacer device) between the inhaler and the open mouth of the child.

ANSWER: 4

Children often have difficulty learning to depress and inhale their medications at the same time, and holding the MDI 2 to 3 inches away from the mouth or utilizing a "spacer" (an attachable device that provides space and contains the medication in a confined area) improves the effects of the medication. Shaking the MDI canister well before use supplies a better delivery of the aerosolized medication. When using two "puffs" of medication, waiting 1 minute between puffs allows for better absorption of the inhaled medication. When using inhaled medications via an MDI, the client should be instructed that wrapping the lips tightly around the mouthpiece consolidates the medication in the buccal cavity and decreases the effectiveness of inhaled medications.

➧ ***Test-taking Tip:*** *Read each option carefully and attempt to visualize what is presented.*

Content Area: Child Health; *Category of Health Alteration:* Respiratory Management; *Integrated Processes:* Teaching and Learning; *Client Need:* Physiological Integrity/Reduction of Risk Potential/Therapeutic Procedures; *Cognitive Level:* Application

Reference: Kyle, T. (2007). *Essentials of Pediatric Nursing* (p. 593). Philadelphia: Wolters Kluwer/Lippincott Williams & Wilkins.

1395. A nurse is caring for a newly admitted 4-year-old client diagnosed with asthma who is pale, and has dry mucous membranes, cracked lips, and nasal flaring with inspiration. Which actions should the nurse perform? SELECT ALL THAT APPLY

1. Obtain a pulse oximetry
2. Obtain vital signs
3. Assess lung sounds
4. Administer a nebulizer treatment
5. Offer oral fluids
6. Elevate the head of the bed

ANSWER: 1, 2, 3, 6

Obtaining a pulse oximetry and assessing vital signs and lung sounds provide important information to assess the respiratory status and can safely be performed within the scope of nursing practice. Elevating the head of the bed promotes oxygenation. Before administering any medication or treatment, such as a nebulizer treatment, a nurse should determine if the treatment or medication has been ordered by a physician or other care provider. Before offering oral fluids, a nurse should check to see if oral fluids can be given.

➧ ***Test-taking Tip:*** *Use the nursing process to decide the appropriate actions. Recall scope of practice to determine safe and effective care measures.*

Content Area: Child Health; *Category of Health Alteration:* Respiratory Management; *Integrated Processes:* Nursing Process Implementation; *Client Need:* Physiological Integrity/Physiological Adaptation/Illness Management; *Cognitive Level:* Analysis

Reference: Hockenberry, M., & Wilson, D. (2007). *Wong's Nursing Care of Infants and Children* (8th ed., pp. 1360–1373). St. Louis, MO: Mosby/Elsevier.

1396. EBP A nurse determines that a mother understands the benefits of using a peak flow meter when the mother states:

1. "I will have my child lie flat and obtain the meter reading each morning before getting out of bed, with the meter set on the average peak flow."
2. "I will have my child obtain the meter reading after completing a morning exercise routine to encourage better airflow before testing the peak flow."
3. "I will encourage my child to test the peak flow meter every day and set the meter at zero before testing the peak flow and record the reading once a month."
4. "I will have my child stand and 'huff and cough' two or three times to clear the airway and set the meter gauge on zero before beginning to test the peak flow."

ANSWER: 4

Standing for the peak flow test provides for full expansion of the lungs; huff and cough clears the airways to allow for a complete full breath before testing a peak flow. Lying flat would not allow for full lung expansion and would not provide an accurate peak flow rate. Performing peak flow rates before exercise will help parents and children to determine if it would be safe to exercise. A peak flow rate tested after exercise is ineffective. Encouraging a child to test the peak flow meter every day and to set the meter at zero before testing is an accurate statement; however, recording peak flow rating on a daily basis is essential.

➧ ***Test-taking Tip:*** *Visualize the actions in each option and eliminate any options in which full lung expansion could not be best achieved.*

Content Area: Child Health; *Category of Health Alteration:* Respiratory Management; *Integrated Processes:* Teaching and Learning; Nursing Process Evaluation; *Client Need:* Health Promotion and Maintenance/ Principles of Teaching and Learning; *Cognitive Level:* Analysis

Reference: Bowden, V., & Greengerg, C. (2008). *Pediatric Nursing Procedures* (2nd ed., pp. 537–542). Philadelphia: Wolters Kluwer/ Lippincott Williams & Wilkins.

EBP Reference: Centers for Disease Control and Prevention. (2007). *Expert Panel Report 3 (EPR3): Guidelines for the Diagnosis and Management of Asthma.* Available at: www.nhlbi.nih.gov/guidelines/ asthma/asthgdln.htm

---

1397. A 4-year-old child is hospitalized and diagnosed with mild intermittent asthma. Oxygen is ordered via simple facemask. A nurse should plan to instruct the parents that which items can be harmful while oxygen is being administered?

1. Plastic blocks and handheld toys
2. Electronic educational toys and books
3. Cotton-filled toys and clothing
4. Synthetic toys and clothing

ANSWER: 4

Synthetic toys and clothing are restricted during oxygen use because these items can build up static electricity, create a spark, and start a fire. Plastic blocks, handheld toys, electronic toys, books, cotton-filled toys, and clothing are safe and entertaining toys to provide children while they are receiving oxygen therapy.

➧ ***Test-taking Tip:*** *Review the items listed and select an option with items that can cause static electricity.*

Content Area: Child Health; *Category of Health Alteration:* Respiratory Management; *Integrated Processes:* Nursing Process Planning; *Client Need:* Safe and Effective Care Environment/Safety and Infection Control/Safe Use of Equipment; *Cognitive Level:* Analysis

Reference: Bowden, V., & Greengerg, C. (2008). *Pediatric Nursing Procedures* (2nd ed., pp. 522–528). Philadelphia: Wolters Kluwer/Lippincott Williams & Wilkins.

1398. A nurse is caring for a 5-year-old child diagnosed with bronchial asthma. Which statement is most important for the nurse to make when teaching the parents?

1. "Bronchial asthma is also called hyperactive airway disease."
2. "Frequent occurrences of bronchiolitis before 5 years of age could be a sign of asthma."
3. "Severe respiratory alkalosis can result from respiratory failure in asthma."
4. "Severe bronchoconstriction can occur when exposed to cold air and irritating odors."

ANSWER: 4

Children with asthma can have sensitization to inhalant antigens such as pollens, molds, house dust, food, and exposure to cold air or irritating odors, such as turpentine, smog, or cigarette smoke. Although bronchial asthma is also called hyperactive airway disease, this is not the most important statement. Asthma tends to occur initially before 5 years of age, but in the early years it may be diagnosed as bronchiolitis rather than asthma. Severe respiratory acidosis, not alkalosis, can result from respiratory failure in asthma.

▶ ***Test-taking Tip:*** *The key words are "most important," indicating that more than one option is correct. Prioritize according to the ABCs (airway, breathing, circulation) to determine which statement is most important.*

Content Area: Child Health; *Category of Health Alteration:* Respiratory Management; *Integrated Processes:* Teaching and Learning; *Client Need:* Physiological Integrity/Physiological Adaptation/ Pathophysiology; *Cognitive Level:* Application

Reference: Pillitteri, A. (2007). *Maternal & Child Health Nursing: Care of the Childbearing & Childrearing Family* (5th ed., p. 1259). Philadelphia: Lippincott Williams & Wilkins.

1399. Which nursing assessment findings and therapy should a nurse expect for a child diagnosed with cystic fibrosis (CF)?

1. Pica appetite; increasing nutritional choices
2. Abnormal accumulation of mucus in respiratory and other mucous duct tracts; managing infection
3. Steatorrhea; increasing oral fluids
4. Decreased sodium and chloride secretion; vitamin and mineral supplements

ANSWER: 2

CF is an autosomal recessive disorder of the exocrine gland. The thick, stagnant, mucous secretions become a hospitable environment for bacteria, leading to infection. Pica appetite is an appetite for nonnutritive substances such as soil, chalk, coal, or paper. No research has linked a pica appetite directly with CF. Even though children with CF do manifest appetites for either sweet or salty foods on occasion, that appetite has not been termed "pica." Although steatorrhea may be present, the therapy does not include increasing oral fluids. With CF there is increased (not decreased) sodium chloride secretion. Vitamin and mineral supplements are important, but pancreatic enzyme supplementation is a much greater concern.

▶ ***Test-taking Tip:*** *Think about the function of exocrine glands. Because exocrine glands do not regulate appetite or fecal elimination, options 1 and 3 can be eliminated.*

Content Area: Child Health; *Category of Health Alteration:* Respiratory Management; *Integrated Processes:* Nursing Process Planning; *Client Need:* Physiological Integrity/Physiological Adaptation/Illness Management; *Cognitive Level:* Application

Reference: Lutz, C., & Przytulski, K. (2006). *Nutrition and Diet Therapy: Evidence-Based Applications* (pp. 496–497). Philadelphia: F. A. Davis.

1400. Which fact about cystic fibrosis (CF) should a nurse consider when formulating a plan of care for a child with the diagnosis?

1. Pulmonary secretions are abnormally thick.
2. CF is an autosomal dominant hereditary disorder.
3. Early in the disease, children with CF will also have diabetes mellitus.
4. Chronic constipation usually occurs in CF.

ANSWER: 1

Pulmonary secretions are abnormally thick, and the lungs are filled with mucus that the cilia cannot clear. CF is an autosomal recessive (not dominant) disorder. In CF the acinar cells of the pancreas producing lipase, trypsin, and amylase are plugged, causing atrophy of the acinar cells and an inability to produce the enzymes. The islets of Langerhans and insulin production are not involved until late in the disease because the islets have ductless activity. Children with CF characteristically have large, bulky, frothy, and foul-smelling stools from the inability to digest fats and protein.

▶ ***Test-taking Tip:*** *Read the question carefully. If uncertain, consider the priority physiological need based on Maslow's Hierarchy of Needs.*

Content Area: Child Health; *Category of Health Alteration:* Respiratory Management; *Integrated Processes:* Nursing Process Planning; *Client Need:* Physiological Integrity/Physiological Adaptation/Illness Management; *Cognitive Level:* Application

Reference: Ball, J., & Bindler, R. (2008). *Pediatric Nursing Caring for Children* (4th ed., pp. 726–728). Upper Saddle River, NJ: Pearson Prentice Hall.

1401. A nurse is preparing to perform chest physiotherapy on a 7-year-old client diagnosed with cystic fibrosis. When should the nurse plan to perform the treatment?

1. Before performing postural drainage
2. Before a nebulized aerosol treatment
3. After suctioning the upper respiratory tract
4. One hour before meals

ANSWER: 4

Chest physiotherapy is done between meals to prevent esophageal reflux. Postural drainage is most effective after treatments and chest physiotherapy because secretions have been loosened. Nebulizer treatments help to loosen secretions and are beneficial prior to chest physiotherapy. Suction is utilized after treatments and therapy to help clear the airways.

▶ ***Test-taking Tip:*** *Select the option that will prevent aspiration.*

Content Area: Child Health; *Category of Health Alteration:* Respiratory Management; *Integrated Processes:* Nursing Process Planning; *Client Need:* Physiological Integrity/Reduction of Risk Potential/Therapeutic Procedures; *Cognitive Level:* Application

Reference: Kyle, T. (2007). *Essentials of Pediatric Nursing* (pp. 597–604). Philadelphia: Wolters Kluwer/Lippincott Williams & Wilkins.

1402. EBP A nurse is preparing a 4-year-old child with cystic fibrosis (CF) for discharge to home. The nurse determines that a parent needs further education when the parent states:

1. "Playing on the backyard swings and hanging upside down are exercises our child will enjoy."
2. "If children at the day care center have a cough, fever or flu symptoms, we should keep our child home."
3. "No pancreatic enzyme supplements will be necessary if our child has a good appetite and regular bowel movements."
4. "Three to four times every day we will perform chest therapy and postural drainage, even if our child doesn't seem congested."

ANSWER: 3

Because children with CF suffer from absorption and nutrition problems due to lack of enzyme production from clogged and atrophied cells producing the enzymes, pancreatic enzymes must be taken before all meals and snacks. Backyard play, physical exercise, and "hanging upside down" should facilitate gravity drainage and can be considered with proper safety measures enforced. Children with CF should be kept away from areas of known communicable disease outbreaks because acquiring a respiratory disease can cause inflammation, tissue damage, and respiratory failure for a child with CF. Performing chest therapy and postural drainage three to four times a day will help to keep hospitalization for the child with CF at a minimum by loosening and clearing secretions.

▶ ***Test-taking Tip:*** *The key phrase is "further education." This is a false response option; select the option that is not correct.*

Content Area: Child Health; *Category of Health Alteration:* Respiratory Management; *Integrated Processes:* Teaching and Learning; *Client Need:* Physiological Integrity/Physiological Adaptation/Illness Management; *Cognitive Level:* Analysis

Reference: Kyle, T. (2007). *Essentials of Pediatric Nursing* (pp. 597–604). Philadelphia: Wolters Kluwer/Lippincott Williams & Wilkins.

EBP Reference: Cystic Fibrosis Foundation. (2007). *Building Strength: Therapies for CF.* Available at:www.cff.org/treatments/Therapies/

1403. A nurse is reviewing the laboratory report for a 6-year-old child hospitalized with hemoptysis. Based on the results of the laboratory report, the nurse should implement measures to treat the child for:

Laboratory Report

Serum Laboratory Test	Client Value	Normal Range
Potassium	4.0 mEq/L	3.5–5.0 mEq/L
Sodium	128 mEq/L	135–145 mEq/L
Chloride	88 mEq/L	94–106 mEq/L
Glucose	110 mg/dL	60–100 mg/dL
SCr	0.4 mg/dL	0.3–0.7 mg/dL
BUN	25 mg/dL	5–20 mg/dL
Hgb	10.8 g/dL	11.5–13.5 g/dL
Hct	34%	35%–50%
WBCs	11,500 cell/mm^3	4,500–10,500 cell/mm^3

Other Laboratory Test	Client Value	Normal Range
Sweat chloride levels	66 mEq/L	23–47.5 mEq/L

1. renal failure.
2. cardiac dysrhythmias.
3. type 1 diabetes mellitus.
4. cystic fibrosis (CF).

ANSWER: 4

The decreased sodium and chloride levels and elevated blood glucose levels are consistent with a diagnosis of CF. Because sodium and chloride are lost in the sweat, the serum levels are decreased, and the sweat test shows increased chloride levels. Chloride levels of more than 60 mEq/L in sweat are diagnostic of CF. Dehydration from loss of NaCl causes an increase in the blood urea nitrogen (BUN) level. The hemoglobin is a little low due to hemoptysis, and the white blood cells (WBCs) are elevated due to inflammation or infection. Hypernatremia (not low serum sodium) and elevated serum creatinine (not normal) are present in renal failure. An elevated serum potassium level could result in dysrhythmias. Random glucose levels of 200 mg/dL or fasting glucose levels of 126 mg/dL are diagnostic for diabetes mellitus.

➧ ***Test-taking Tip:*** *Focus on the two laboratory values that relate to chloride first and think about possible causative factors.*

Content Area: Child Health; *Category of Health Alteration:* Respiratory Management; *Integrated Processes:* Nursing Process Analysis; *Client Need:* Physiological Integrity/Reduction of Risk Potential/Diagnostic Tests; *Cognitive Level:* Analysis

Reference: Ball, J., & Bindler, R. (2006). *Clinical Handbook for Pediatric Nursing* (pp. 242–246). Upper Saddle River, NJ: Pearson Prentice Hall.

1404. Which specific expected outcomes should a nurse establish for a child diagnosed with cystic fibrosis (CF)?

1. Adequate urine output, absence of injury, and normal growth and development
2. Absence of pulmonary infection, adequate nutrition, and skin remains intact
3. Adequate hydration, absence of diarrhea, and eats at least 75% of meals
4. Absence of dehydration, maintains cleanliness, and adheres to medication regimen

ANSWER: 2

A child with CF has a generalized dysfunction of the exocrine glands such that mucus secretions, particularly in the pancreas and the lungs, are so tenacious that they have difficulty flowing through gland ducts. Thickened secretions in the bronchioles are a media for microorganism growth. Interventions are necessary to achieve the outcome of absence of pulmonary infection. Enzymes for digesting fat, protein, and some sugars are unavailable because the ducts in the pancreas for secreting the enzymes are plugged by the enzyme secretions. Interventions are necessary to achieve the outcome of adequate nutrition. Because of the high fat content, stools are bulky, foul-smelling, and irritating and can cause skin breakdown. Interventions are necessary to achieve the outcome of absence of skin breakdown. Although options 1 and 3 include outcomes, adequate urine output and absence of diarrhea are not specific to the child with CF. Absence of dehydration, maintains cleanliness, and adheres to medication regimen (option 4) are pertinent but are not the most specific outcomes to be achieved.

➧ ***Test-taking Tip:*** *The key word is "specific," indicating that more than one option is correct, but one option is better than all other options. Focus on the child's diagnosis when answering this question.*

Content Area: Child Health; *Category of Health Alteration:* Respiratory Management; *Integrated Processes:* Nursing Process Analysis; *Client Need:* Physiological Integrity/Physiological Adaptation/Illness Management; *Cognitive Level:* Analysis

Reference: Pillitteri, A. (2007). *Maternal & Child Health Nursing: Care of the Childbearing & Childrearing Family* (5th ed., pp. 1269–1273). Philadelphia: Lippincott Williams & Wilkins.

1405. A community health nurse is planning a follow-up visit to a family after their firstborn child died from sudden infant death syndrome (SIDS). Which action is most important for the nurse to include in the *initial* visit?

1. Help the family in making a plan for future children.
2. Allow time for the parents to express their anger and grief.
3. Make a referral for genetic counseling and education.
4. Educate the family on the causes of sudden infant death syndrome.

ANSWER: 2

Many families are unable to express their grief and loss openly. Helping the parents understand SIDS and that they are not to blame for the death of their child is the most important action at the current time. Helping families make plans for future children is essential once the grieving process resolves. There is no definitive etiology for SIDS, and making a referral for genetic counseling and education is not necessary. Educating the family on what are associated incidences of children who have died from SIDS can help the parents plan for and use safety precautions for their future children.

➧ ***Test-taking Tip:*** *Consider the stage of grief for the parents when selecting an option.*

Content Area: Child Health; *Category of Health Alteration:* Respiratory Management; *Integrated Processes:* Nursing Process Planning; *Client Need:* Psychosocial Integrity/Grief and Loss; *Cognitive Level:* Analysis

Reference: Videbeck, S. (2008). *Psychiatric Mental Health Nursing* (4th ed., pp. 215–225). Philadelphia: Lippincott Williams & Wilkins.

1406. EBP A nurse is evaluating the laboratory findings for a 7-year-old client being treated with isoniazid (INH) for tuberculosis. Which adverse effect of the medication should the nurse consider after reviewing the laboratory results report?

Serum Laboratory Test	Client's Value	Normal Ranges
BUN	18	5–25 mg/dL
Creatinine	0.9	0.4–1.2 mg/dL
Na	139	135–145 mEq/L
K	4.2	3.5–5.5 mEq/L
Cl	99	98–105 mEq/L
CO_2	28	20–28 mEq/L
Phosphate	4.9	4.5–5.5 mg/dL
Calcium	10	4.5–5.8 mEq/L
Hgb	14	11–16 g/dL
Hct	43	31%–43%
ALT/SGPT	38	10–35 unit/L

1. Renal insufficiency
2. Hepatotoxicity
3. Aplastic anemia
4. Heart failure

ANSWER: 2

Elevated ALT (alanine transaminase) or SGPT (serum glutamic pyruvic transaminase) suggests hepatotoxicity. Isoniazid (INH) is metabolized by the liver. The laboratory values do not support the other conditions. The serum creatinine level should be elevated (not normal) with renal insufficiency. Aplastic anemia is an adverse effect of isoniazid, but the hemoglobin and hematocrit are normal. A B-type natriuretic peptide (BNP) laboratory value would be needed to determine if heart failure was an adverse effect, but it is not reported.

➧ ***Test-taking Tip:*** *Eliminate all normal laboratory findings and focus on the abnormal values. Relate the abnormal laboratory value to the conditions listed in the options.*

Content Area: Child Health; *Category of Health Alteration:* Respiratory Management; *Integrated Processes:* Nursing Process Analysis; *Client Need:* Physiological Integrity/Pharmacological and Parenteral Therapies/Adverse Effects/Contraindications/Interactions; *Cognitive Level:* Analysis

Reference: Wilson, B., Shannon, M., Shields, K., & Stang, C. (2008). *Prentice Hall Nurse's Drug Guide 2008* (pp. 825–827). Upper Saddle River, NJ: Pearson Education.

EBP Reference: Centers for Disease Control and Prevention. (2008). Trends in tuberculosis–United States. *MMWR,* 57(11), 281–285. Available at: www.cdc.gov/mmwr/preview/mmwrhtml/mm5711a2.htm

1407. A child of African descent has a positive acid-fast bacillus sputum culture after returning to the United States from a trip to Africa to visit relatives. During a nursing assessment, a nurse observes that the parent refers to the child's diagnosis by using the impersonal pronoun "it." Which statement made by the nurse is best?

1. "Tell me how you feel about your child's diagnosis."
2. "If your child takes the prescribed medications, 'it' can be cured."
3. "Why do you call your child's tuberculosis 'it', rather than referring to the diagnosis of tuberculosis?"
4. "I need to find out more information about 'it'. How long has your child been having night sweats and a productive cough?"

ANSWER: 1

Asking the parent about feelings allows the parent time to express feelings and concerns, and a rationale may be provided for referring to the tuberculosis as "it." Some cultures avoid calling the disease by name for fear that it may cause further harm. Telling the parent that if the child takes the prescribed medication, the child will be cured is irrelevant during an assessment. Asking a "why" question is a barrier to therapeutic communication and can result in defensiveness. Although assessing the length of time the child may have had symptoms is important, this question ignores the parent's feelings.

➧ ***Test-taking Tip:*** *The key word is "best," indicating that more than one option is correct, but one option is better than all other options. Eliminate any options that do not pertain to the nursing process step of assessment.*

Content Area: Child Health; *Category of Health Alteration:* Respiratory Management; *Integrated Processes:* Communication and Documentation; *Client Need:* Psychosocial Integrity/Coping Mechanisms; Psychosocial Integrity/Cultural Diversity; *Cognitive Level:* Application

Reference: Berman, A., Snyder, S., Kozier, B., & Erb, G. (2008). *Kozier & Erb's Fundamentals of Nursing: Concepts, Process, and Practice* (8th ed., pp. 469–471). Upper Saddle River, NJ: Pearson Education.

1408. A nurse is caring for a newborn diagnosed with the most common type of esophageal atresia, esophageal atresia with lower tracheoesophageal fistula. Place an "X" on the illustration for the type of atresia that the nurse should visualize when thinking about esophageal atresia with lower tracheoesophageal fistula.

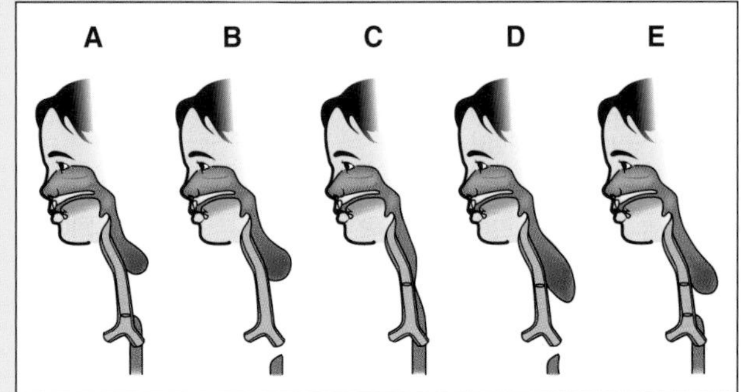

ANSWER:

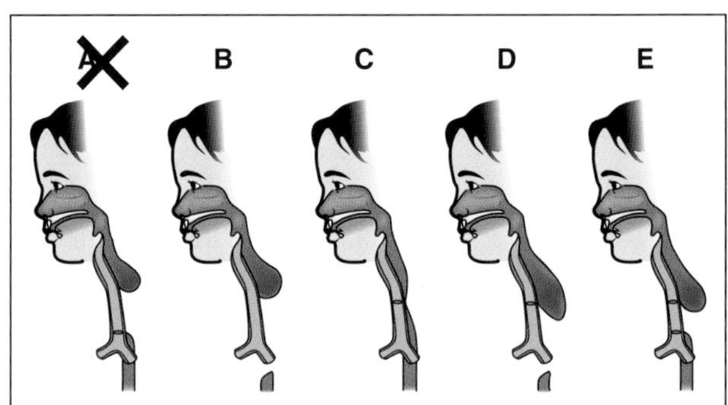

There are five classifications of esophageal atresia. In esophageal atresia with lower tracheoesophageal fistula, the proximal segment of the esophagus ends in a blind pouch and the distal segment connects with the trachea by way of a fistula. It is the most common type of esophageal atresia occurring in 80% to 90% of infants with this defect. In illustration B, both the upper and the lower segments end in blind pouches; there is no fistula. In illustration C, both the upper and the lower segments communicate with the trachea through a fistula. In illustration D, the upper segment ends in a blind pouch and communicates by a fistula to the trachea. In illustration E, separate fistulas connect the upper and lower segments of the esophagus to the trachea.

➧ ***Test-taking Tip:*** *Read the question carefully and analyze the pictures to determine which best illustrates atresia with a lower tracheoesophageal fistula.*

Content Area: Child Health; *Category of Health Alteration:* Respiratory Management; *Integrated Processes:* Nursing Process Analysis; *Client Need:* Physiological Integrity/Physiological Adaptation/Alterations in Body Sysems; *Cognitive Level:* Analysis

Reference: Ball, J., & Bindler, R. (2008). *Pediatric Nursing Caring for Children* (4th ed., pp. 915–917). Upper Saddle River, NJ: Pearson Prentice Hall.

1409. Which nursing diagnosis should have the highest priority for an infant newly diagnosed with trans-esophageal fistula?

1. Risk for impaired infant attachment
2. Risk for infection
3. Risk for imbalanced nutrition
4. Risk for aspiration

ANSWER: 4

Risk for aspiration reflects a basic physiological need according to Maslow's Hierarchy of Needs and is the priority nursing diagnosis. Though infection and impaired nutrition are also physiological problems, aspiration and subsequent respiratory malfunction would be a higher priority. Although impaired infant attachment may occur in this situation, it would be a second or third level of need.

▶ ***Test-taking Tip:*** *Note the key words "highest priority." Use Maslow's Hierarchy of Needs theory and ABCs (airway, breathing, circulation) to select the physiological need for air.*

Content Area: Child Health; *Category of Health Alteration:* Respiratory Management; *Integrated Processes:* Nursing Process Analysis; *Client Need:* Physiological Integrity/Reduction of Risk Potential/Potential for Complications from Surgical Procedures and Health Alterations; *Cognitive Level:* Analysis

Reference: Pillitteri, A. (2007). *Maternal & Child Health Nursing: Care of the Childbearing & Childrearing Family* (5th ed., pp. 1189–1191). Philadelphia: Lippincott Williams & Wilkins.

1410. In which position should a nurse place a child post-operative tonsil and adenoidectomy (T&A)?

1. Semi-Fowler with the head turned to the side
2. High Fowler, head slightly forward and to the side
3. Side-lying
4. Supine

ANSWER: 3

A side-lying position is best to facilitate drainage from the oropharynx. A semi-Fowler's position with the head turned to either side would hinder drainage and increase the risk for aspiration. A supine position would allow secretions to pool at the back of the throat or in the buccal cavity.

▶ ***Test-taking Tip:*** *Use the ABCs (airway, breathing, circulation) to determine the best position to facilitate drainage from the oropharynx.*

Content Area: Child Health; *Category of Health Alteration:* Respiratory Management; *Integrated Processes:* Nursing Process Implementation; *Client Need:* Physiological Integrity/Reduction of Risk Potential/Potential for Complications of Diagnostic Tests/Treatments/Procedures; *Cognitive Level:* Application

Reference: Kyle, T. (2007). *Essentials of Pediatric Nursing* (p. 572). Philadelphia: Wolters Kluwer/Lippincott Williams & Wilkins.

1411. A nurse is formulating a preoperative plan of care for a 5-year-old child who is scheduled for a tonsil and adenoidectomy (T&A). Which nursing diagnosis is priority?

1. Imbalanced nutrition: less than body requirements related to surgery
2. Pain related to surgery
3. Ineffective airway clearance related to hesitation or reluctance to cough secondary to pain
4. Anxiety related to surgery

ANSWER: 4

Anxiety related to surgery is a preoperative diagnosis. Anxiety is a key element for children admitted to the hospital. Options 1, 2, and 3 are all considered postoperative diagnoses and are applicable following the procedure.

▶ ***Test-taking Tip:*** *Read the situation carefully. Focus on the preoperative phase and eliminate nursing diagnoses for the postoperative phase.*

Content Area: Child Health; *Category of Health Alteration:* Respiratory Management; *Integrated Processes:* Nursing Process Planning; *Client Need:* Psychosocial Integrity/Stress Management; *Cognitive Level:* Analysis

Reference: Kyle, T. (2007). *Essentials of Pediatric Nursing* (p. 572). Philadelphia: Wolters Kluwer/Lippincott Williams & Wilkins.

1412. A nurse is caring for a 3-year-old client who is postoperative tonsil and adenoidectomy (T&A) surgery. The nurse should suspect complications when assessing:

1. complaints of sore throat and difficulty swallowing.
2. secretions and dried blood at the corners of the mouth.
3. frequent swallowing and clearing of the throat.
4. the presence of "dark coffee ground" emesis.

ANSWER: 3

Frequent swallowing and clearing of the throat are signs and symptoms of hemorrhage. Sore throat, difficulty swallowing, dried blood around the mouth, or "coffee ground" emesis are expected findings following a T&A.

➧ ***Test-taking Tip:*** *Eliminate the options that would be expected following a T&A.*

Content Area: Child Health; *Category of Health Alteration:* Respiratory Management; *Integrated Processes:* Nursing Process Assessment; *Client Need:* Physiological Integrity/Reduction of Risk Potential/Potential for Complications from Surgical Procedures and Health Alterations; *Cognitive Level:* Analysis

Reference: Kyle, T. (2007). *Essentials of Pediatric Nursing* (p. 572). Philadelphia: Wolters Kluwer/Lippincott Williams & Wilkins.

Test 37: **Child Health: Pharmacological and Parenteral Therapies**

1413. EBP A nurse is preparing an educational program on immunizations for parents of children 11 to 12 years of age. To ensure the information presented is accurate for this age group, which immunizations should the nurse plan to address?

1. Mumps, measles, and rubella (MMR); diphtheria-tetanus-pertussis (Dtap); and hepatitis B
2. Haemophilus influenza, varicella, and human papillomavirus (HPV)
3. Diphtheria-tetanus-pertussis (Dtap), meningococcal, and Haemophilus influenza
4. Mumps, measles, and rubella (MMR); pneumococcal (PPSV); and hepatitis A

ANSWER: 3

The recommended immunization schedule for children 11 to 12 years old include a Dtap booster and meningococcal and *Haemophilus influenzae* vaccines. Others include HPV, PPSV, and hepatitis A series. Both MMR and varicella vaccines are administered at 12 to 15 months, with the second dose at 4 to 6 years. A hepatitis B vaccine is administered to all newborns prior to hospital discharge, with the second dose at 1 to 2 months and the third dose at 6 to 18 months. The first dose of hepatitis A vaccine is administered before 1 year of age, with the second dose 6 months after the first dose.

➧ ***Test-taking Tip:*** *Identify those diseases that younger children are more likely to have exposure to and that require early immunizations, a series for the immunization, or a later booster.*

Content Area: Child Health; *Category of Health Alteration:* Pharmacological and Parenteral Therapies; *Integrated Processes:* Nursing Process Planning; *Client Need:* Health Promotion and Maintenance/Immunizations; Physiological Integrity/Pharmacological and Parenteral Therapies/Expected Actions or Outcomes; *Cognitive Level:* Analysis

Reference: Hockenberry, M., & Wilson, D. (2007). *Wong's Nursing Care of Infants and Children* (8th ed., pp. 841–842). St. Louis, MO: Mosby/Elsevier.

EBP References: Centers for Disease Control and Prevention (CDC). (2009). *Recommended Immunization Schedule for Persons Aged 0–6 Years—United States*. Available at: www.cdc.gov/vaccines/recs/schedules/downloads/child/2009/09_0-6yrs_schedule_pr.pdf; (CDC). (2009). *Recommended Immunization Schedule for Persons Aged 7–18 Years—United States.* Available at: www.cdc.gov/vaccines/recs/schedules/downloads/child/2009/09_7-18yrs_schedule_pr.pdf

1414. EBP In order to properly store vaccine for future use, a nurse should: SELECT ALL THAT APPLY.

1. refrigerate all vaccines.
2. place aluminum foil around the vial to protect light-sensitive vaccines from light.
3. place vaccines requiring refrigeration in the middle of the refrigerator.
4. establish periodic checks for expiration dates on the vaccines.
5. store bulk supplies of vaccines in a freezer.

ANSWER: 2, 3, 5

Aluminum foil can be used to protect light-sensitive vaccines. When refrigeration is required, a main shelf inside the refrigerator is best because a shelf in the door will have frequent temperature changes that will alter the potency of the vaccine. A schedule for checking expiration dates is necessary to ensure that out-dated vaccines are not administered. Some vaccines will be inactivated by refrigeration and freezing.

➧ ***Test-taking Tip:*** *Eliminate options that contain absolute words, such as "all."*

Content Area: Child Health; *Category of Health Alteration:* Pharmacological and Parenteral Therapies; *Integrated Processes:* Nursing Process Implementation; *Client Need:* Physiological Integrity/Pharmacological and Parenteral Therapies/Medication Administration; *Cognitive Level:* Analysis

EBP Reference: Centers for Disease Control and Prevention (2007). Vaccine Management. Recommendations for Storage and Handling of Selected Biologicals. Available at: www.cdc.gov/vaccines/pubs/downloads/bk-vac-mgt.pdf

1415. A new nurse asks an experienced nurse why the first dose of the measles, mumps, and rubella (MMR) vaccine is given only between 12 to 15 months of age and not any earlier. Which explanation by the experienced nurse is correct?

1. "The second dose of the vaccine is given before a child reaches puberty, and giving the first dose of the vaccine at 12 to 15 months of age allows the correct interval between vaccinations."
2. "Because a live virus is administered, the chance of developing measles, mumps, or rubella is much higher if given at an earlier age."
3. "A first dose at this age provides passive immunity and decreases the incidence of a child developing any of the diseases."
4. "If administered earlier, the vaccine will neutralize the passive immunity to measles from the child's mother and no immunity will result."

ANSWER: 4

Because the MMR vaccine is a live virus, a person develops a mild form of the diseases after administration, stimulating the body to develop immunity. The passively acquired antibodies to measles can interfere with the child's immune response to the vaccine, and no immunity will result. The second dose of the MMR vaccine can be given earlier, provided that at least 4 weeks has elapsed since the first dose. However, a second dose is usually not given earlier because sufficient immunity is usually present. The chance of developing measles is greater only if the vaccine is given at a younger age because the vaccine may neutralize the passive antibodies. The MMR provides active (not passive) immunity.

▸ *Test-taking Tip: Read each option carefully. Because the MMR vaccine is a live virus, think about how it acts within the body to produce immunity.*

Content Area: Child Health; *Category of Health Alteration:* Pharmacological and Parenteral Therapies; *Integrated Processes:* Teaching and Learning; *Client Need:* Safe and Effective Care Environment/ Management of Care/Staff Education; *Cognitive Level:* Analysis

Reference: Pillitteri, A. (2007). *Maternal & Child Health Nursing: Care of the Childbearing & Childrearing Family* (5th ed., p. 1025). Philadelphia: Lippincott Williams & Wilkins.

1416. EBP A nurse working on a pediatric unit has medications to give at 1000 hours. Which assessments should lead the nurse to conclude that the prescribed medication should be withheld and the health-care provider (HCP) contacted?

1. Oral hydrocodone with acetaminophen (Vicodin®) to a 10-year-old child with burn injuries who is complaining of being dizzy and light headed.
2. Oral acetaminophen (Tylenol®) to a 6-month-old infant with a fever of 102°F (38.9°C) due to an infection secondary to a motor vehicle accident who has developed a rash.
3. Intravenous (IV) clindamycin (Cleocin®) to a 16-year-old male with aspiration pneumonia secondary to a near-drowning experience whose blood pressure (BP) is 92/56 mm Hg.
4. IV phenobarbital to a 5-year-old child with intermittent seizures secondary to a closed head injury who is complaining of being tired and whom the parent reports is acting drowsy.

ANSWER: 3

An adverse effect of clindamycin is hypotension. A BP of 92/56 mm Hg is low for a 16-year-old. Normal BP for a 16-year-old male is 111/63 mm Hg to 136/90 mm Hg, depending on height percentile. The nurse should compare the previous BP readings with the current one to determine the degree of BP variation before notifying the HCP. In options 1, 2, and 4, the signs and symptoms are consistent with medication side effects. However, none of these would be potentially life threatening at this time. Monitoring all the children for increasing and/or changing side effects from the medications is necessary.

▸ *Test-taking Tip: Use the ABCs (airway, breathing, circulation) to establish priority. Avoid reading into the options. Eliminate options 1, 2, and 4 after noting that only option 3 deals with a potentially life-threatening circulatory alteration.*

Content Area: Child Health; *Category of Health Alteration:* Pharmacological and Parenteral Therapies; *Integrated Processes:* Nursing Process Evaluation; *Client Need:* Physiological Integrity/Pharmacological and Parenteral Therapies/Medication Administration; *Cognitive Level:* Analysis

Reference: Wilson, B., Shannon, M., Shields, K., & Stang, C. (2008). *Prentice Hall Nurse's Drug Guide 2008* (pp. 344–346). Upper Saddle River, NJ: Pearson Education.

EBP Reference: Hayman, L., Meininger, J., Daniels, S., McCrindle, B., Helden, L., et al. (2007). Primary prevention of cardiovascular disease in nursing practice: Focus on children and youth: A scientific statement [trunc]. *Circulation,* 116(3), 344–357.

1417. A hospitalized pediatric client has a blood lead level (BLL) of 50 mcg/dL and is diagnosed with acute lead poisoning. Succimer (Chemet®) 10 mg/kg oral q8h for 5 days is initially prescribed. The child weighs 20 kg. An experienced nurse should intervene when observing a new nurse:

1. administering one 100-mg succimer capsule with food.
2. opening a succimer capsule and sprinkling the beads on a small amount of food.
3. offering fluids frequently during the shift to increase the child's urine output.
4. explaining to a parent that chelation therapy removes the lead from the blood and some lead from tissues and organs.

ANSWER: 1

A 20 kg child should receive two capsules (not one). Use a proportion formula and then multiply the means (inside values) and extremes (outside values) and solve for X:
10 mg : 1 kg :: X mg : 20 kg
X = 200 mg.
Succimer capsules can be opened and sprinkled on a small amount of food or liquid to be swallowed. Fluids should be increased to prevent renal damage because succimer is excreted by the kidneys. Succimer forms a water-soluble compound with lead, allowing urinary elimination of excessive amounts of lead. Lead is removed from the blood and theoretically some lead is removed from tissues and organs.

➧ ***Test-taking Tip:*** *Calculate the amount of medication the child should receive, then read each option carefully.*

Content Area: Child Health; *Category of Health Alteration:* Pharmacological and Parenteral Therapies; *Integrated Processes:* Nursing Process Evaluation; *Client Need:* Physiological Integrity/ Pharmacological and Parenteral Therapies/Medication Administration; *Cognitive Level:* Analysis

Reference: Hockenberry, M., & Wilson, D. (2007). *Wong's Nursing Care of Infants and Children* (8th ed., pp. 694–695). St. Louis, MO: Mosby/ Elsevier.

1418. A child, admitted to an emergency department, is experiencing nausea and vomiting, salivation, respiratory muscle weakness, and depressed reflexes an hour after exposure to pesticides. Which medications should a nurse anticipate administering to the child?

1. Atropine and flumazenil (Romazicon®)
2. Atropine and pralidoxime (Protopam chloride®)
3. Epinephrine and naloxone (Narcan®)
4. Epinephrine and digoxin immune Fab (Digibind®)

ANSWER: 2

An organophosphate base in pesticides causes acetylcholine to accumulate at neuromuscular junctions. Atropine, an anticholinergic medication, and pralidoxime chloride, a cholinesterase reactivator, are effective antidotes to reverse the symptoms. Flumazenil antagonizes the effects of benzodiazepines on the central nervous system (CNS), such as sedation, impaired recall, and psychomotor impairment. Epinephrine is an alpha- and beta-adrenergic agonist and cardiac stimulant that strengthens myocardial contractions, increases systolic blood pressure and cardiac rate and output, and constricts bronchial arterioles, inhibiting histamine release. Naloxone is a narcotic antagonist that reverses the effects of opiates. Digibind is the antidote for digoxin and digitoxin, which acts by complexing with circulating digoxin or digitoxin, preventing the drug from binding at receptor sites.

➧ ***Test-taking Tip:*** *The focus of the question is an antidote for organophosphates in pesticides. Examine options with duplicate information first. Use the trade names as cues for identifying the antidote and eliminate the antidotes for benzodiazepines, opiates, and digoxin.*

Content Area: Child Health; *Category of Health Alteration:* Pharmacological and Parenteral Therapies; *Integrated Processes:* Nursing Process Planning; *Client Need:* Physiological Integrity/ Pharmacological and Parenteral Therapies/Expected Actions or Outcomes; *Cognitive Level:* Analysis

References: Pillitteri, A. (2007). *Maternal & Child Health Nursing: Care of the Childbearing & Childrearing Family* (5th ed., p. 1664). Philadelphia: Lippincott Williams & Wilkins; Wilson, B., Shannon, M., Shields, K., & Stang, C. (2008). *Prentice Hall Nurse's Drug Guide 2008* (pp. 132–135, 473–475, 553–554, 649, 1247). Upper Saddle River, NJ: Pearson Education.

1419. A 5-year-old client is receiving dextrose 5% in water and half-normal saline (D5 0.45 NaCl) solution at 100 mL/hr. Which findings during a nursing assessment suggest excessive parenteral fluid intake? SELECT ALL THAT APPLY.

1. Dyspnea
2. Gastric distention
3. Crackles
4. Lethargy
5. Temperature of 102°F (38.9°C)
6. Dry mucous membranes

ANSWER: 1, 3, 4

Dyspnea, crackles, and other signs of respiratory distress indicate fluid volume overload and occurs from fluid rapidly shifting between the intracellular and extracellular compartments. Lethargy and change in level of consciousness can occur from fluid shifting in brain cells. Gastric distention can occur from excessive oral fluid intake or infection. An elevated temperature and dry mucous membranes are signs of fluid volume deficit, not excess.

➧ ***Test-taking Tip:*** *Eliminate options that pertain to oral fluid intake or fluid volume deficit.*

Content Area: Child Health; *Category of Health Alteration:* Pharmacological and Parenteral Therapies; *Integrated Processes:* Nursing Process Assessment; *Client Need:* Physiological Integrity/Pharmacological and Parenteral Therapies/Parenteral/Intravenous Therapies; *Cognitive Level:* Analysis

Reference: Hockenberry, M., & Wilson, D. (2007). *Wong's Nursing Care of Infants and Children* (8th ed., p. 1144). St. Louis, MO: Mosby/Elsevier.

1420. A new nurse, under the supervision of an experienced nurse, is preparing to cannulate a 2-month-old infant's scalp vein for an intravenous infusion. In which order should the steps be performed to complete the procedure correctly. Prioritize the steps in the order that they should be performed by the new nurse.

______ Return in 60 minutes and reswaddle the infant in a mummy restraint.
______ Restrain the infant with a mummy restraint for preparing the site.
______ Cleanse the site over the temporal bone and shave the hair at the insertion site.
______ With an assistant holding the child's head, insert a scalp vein needle and observe for blood return.
______ Apply lidocaine/prilocaine cream (EMLA® cream) to the chosen site and unswaddle the infant after the EMLA application.
______ Ask the supervising nurse to turn the infant's head to the side and hold it firmly in position, with one hand on the occiput and the other on the front of the head.
______ Cleanse the shaved area with an antiseptic solution.
______ Remove the mummy restraint after initiating the infusion and comfort the infant.
______ Initiate the infusion and cover the infusion needle with a gauze dressing.

ANSWER: 5, 1, 3, 7, 4, 2, 6, 9, 8

The first step should be to restrain the infant with a mummy restraint for preparing the site. The next step for the new nurse is to ask the supervising nurse to turn the infant's head to the side and hold it firmly in position, with one hand on the occiput and the other on the front of the head. Next, the new nurse should cleanse the site over the temporal bone and shave the hair at the insertion site, apply EMLA cream to the chosen site, and unswaddle the infant. The new nurse should return in 60 minutes, reswaddle the infant in a mummy restraint, and cleanse the shaved area with an antiseptic solution. With an assistant holding the child's head, the scalp vein needle should be inserted and observed for blood return. The new nurse should then initiate the infusion and cover the infusion needle with a gauze dressing. Finally, the mummy restraints should be removed after initiating the infusion and the infant comforted.

➧ ***Test-taking Tip:*** *Visualize the procedure prior to placing the steps in the correct order. Look for key words in the options to determine if the step is an early or a later step.*

Content Area: Child Health; *Category of Health Alteration:* Pharmacological and Parenteral Therapies; *Integrated Processes:* Nursing Process Evaluation; *Client Need:* Physiological Integrity/Pharmacological and Parenteral Therapies/Parenteral/Intravenous Therapies; *Cognitive Level:* Application

Reference: Pillitteri, A. (2007). *Maternal & Child Health Nursing: Care of the Childbearing & Childrearing Family* (5th ed., pp. 1151–1152). Philadelphia: Lippincott Williams & Wilkins.

1421. An 8-year-old child with gastroenteritis is prescribed to receive 500 mL of lactated Ringer's (LR) solution over the next 10 hours. The rate in milliliters per hour that a nurse should infuse the solution is _______ mL.

ANSWER: 50

The 50 mL per hour is obtained by dividing 10 hours into 500 mL of LR.

➧ ***Test-taking Tip:*** *Use a known formula and check your answer, especially if it seems unusually large.*

Content Area: Child Health; *Category of Health Alteration:* Pharmacological and Parenteral Therapies; *Integrated Processes:* Nursing Process Implementation; *Client Need:* Physiological Integrity/Pharmacological and Parenteral Therapies/Dosage Calculation; *Cognitive Level:* Application

Reference: Ball, J., & Bindler, R. (2006). *Clinical Handbook for Child Health Nurses* (pp. 142–146). Upper Saddle River, NJ: Pearson/Prentice Hall.

1422. A new nurse is initiating total parenteral nutrition (TPN) for four hospitalized pediatric clients. An experienced nurse should intervene when the new nurse attaches the TPN infusion and tubing to:

1. a catheter inserted in the right external jugular vein of a 2-year-old child.
2. a catheter inserted in the right subclavian vein of a 4-year-old child.
3. a peripherally inserted intravenous catheter in a hand vein of a 12-year-old child.
4. a peripherally inserted central catheter in the right upper arm of a 6-year-old child.

ANSWER: 3

TPN is a concentrated hypertonic solution containing glucose, vitamins, electrolytes, trace minerals, and protein. Because it is hypertonic, it should be administered through a central intravenous access site or a peripherally inserted central venous catheter (PICC). A major vein is used to avoid inflammatory reactions and venous thrombosis from the high-caloric and high-osmotic fluid. The external jugular vein, subclavian vein, and a PICC are central intravenous access sites.

▶ ***Test-taking Tip:*** *The focus of the question is access sites appropriate for administration of TPN. Identify the central intravenous access sites and eliminate these because this is a false-response item.*

Content Area: Child Health; *Category of Health Alteration:* Pharmacological and Parenteral Therapies; *Integrated Processes:* Nursing Process Implementation; *Client Need:* Physiological Integrity/ Pharmacological and Parenteral Therapies/Total Parenteral Nutrition; *Cognitive Level:* Analysis

Reference: Pillitteri, A. (2007). *Maternal & Child Health Nursing: Care of the Childbearing & Childrearing Family* (5th ed., pp. 1131–1132). Philadelphia: Lippincott Williams & Wilkins.

1423. EBP A 4-year-old child with cystic fibrosis (CF) is prescribed vitamin A supplements. Which finding by a clinic nurse indicates that the vitamin has been effective?

1. Viscosity of secretions is decreased.
2. Pancreatic enzyme absorption is increased.
3. Skin is supple and healthy.
4. Number of bleeding episodes is reduced.

ANSWER: 3

A water-miscible form of vitamin A is given in children diagnosed with CF because the uptake of the fat-soluble vitamins is decreased. One of the functions of vitamin A is to keep epithelial tissue healthy by aiding the differentiation of specialty cells. Other treatments for CF, such as bronchodilators and recombinant human doxyribonuclease (Pulmozyme®), decrease the viscosity of secretions. Vitamin A has no effect on pancreatic enzyme absorption. Vitamin K, another fat-soluble vitamin administered in CF, increases coagulation.

▶ ***Test-taking Tip:*** *Eliminate options that pertain to outcomes for the treatments for CF. Of the two remaining options, determine which pertains to vitamin A and which to vitamin K.*

Content Area: Child Health; *Category of Health Alteration:* Pharmacological and Parenteral Therapies; *Integrated Processes:* Nursing Process Evaluation; *Client Need:* Physiological Integrity/Pharmacological and Parenteral Therapies/Expected Actions or Outcomes; *Cognitive Level:* Analysis

References: Hockenberry, M., & Wilson, D. (2007). *Wong's Nursing Care of Infants and Children* (8th ed., pp. 1378–1379). St. Louis, MO: Mosby/ Elsevier; Lutz, C., & Przytulski, K. (2006). *Nutrition & Diet Therapy: Evidence-Based Applications* (4th ed., pp. 98–99). Philadelphia: F. A. Davis.

EBP Reference: O'Neil, C., Shevill, E., & Chang, A. (2008). Vitamin A supplementation for cystic fibrosis. *Cochrane Database of Systematic Reviews*, Issue 2, Art. No. CD006751. DOI: 10.1002/14651858.CD006751.pub2. Available at: www.cochrane.org/reviews/en/ab006751.html

---

1424. A nurse is taking a history for a 4-year-old child diagnosed with Reye's syndrome. A parent states prior to hospitalization that multiple over-the-counter medications were administered to treat the child's influenza. Which medication stated by the parent is most important for the nurse to report to a health-care provider?

1. Acetaminophen (Tylenol®)
2. Bismuth subsalicylate (Pepto-Bismol®)
3. Pseudoephedrine (Dimetapp®)
4. Diphenhydramine (Benadryl®)

ANSWER: 2

Although the etiology of Reye's syndrome is unknown, the condition typically occurs after a viral illness, such as influenza, and is associated with aspirin (acetylsalicylic acid) use during the illness. Bismuth subsalicylate contains aspirin. Acetaminophen is an aspirin-free analgesic and antipyretic. Pseudoephedrine is an allergy and/or cold remedy used for nasal drying and decongestion, and diphenhydramine is an antihistamine. These do not contain aspirin.

▶ ***Test-taking Tip:*** *Use the generic name as a cue to select the correct option. Reye's syndrome is thought to be associated with aspirin use during a viral illness.*

Content Area: Child Health; *Category of Health Alteration:* Pharmacological and Parenteral Therapies; *Integrated Processes:* Communication and Documentation; *Client Need:* Physiological Integrity/Pharmacological and Parenteral Therapies/Adverse Effects/Contraindications/Interactions; *Cognitive Level:* Analysis

Reference: Hockenberry, M., & Wilson, D. (2007). *Wong's Nursing Care of Infants and Children* (8th ed., p. 1651). St. Louis, MO: Mosby/Elsevier.

1425. A nurse is caring for a 5-year-old child from Italy. The child is crying and the interpreter is stating that the child has extreme pain. The nurse's first priority should be to:

1. have the child's mother who knows limited English ask the child what hurts.
2. assess the level of the child's pain using an appropriate FACES pain rating scale.
3. administer morphine sulfate 1 mg IV as prescribed.
4. call the health-care provider to request a change in pain medication dosage as it is not adequately controlling the child's pain.

ANSWER: 2
The FACES pain-rating scale has been translated to a variety of languages. The nurse's judgment regarding the choice of pain medication and dose should be based on the reported level of pain. If possible, the nurse should do an independent assessment because sometimes information can be misinterpreted if there is limited knowledge of the language. Assessment should be completed prior to a pain intervention. There is no information indicating the need for the pain medication to be changed.

➧ ***Test-taking Tip:*** *Note the key word "priority." Use the nursing process. Assessment is the first step.*

Content Area: Child Health; *Category of Health Alteration:* Pharmacological and Parenteral Therapies; *Integrated Processes:* Nursing Process Assessment; Caring; *Client Need:* Physiological Integrity/Pharmacological and Parenteral Therapies/Pharmacological Pain Management; *Cognitive Level:* Application

References: Hockenberry, M., & Wilson, D. (2007). *Wong's Nursing Care of Infants and Children* (8th ed., pp. 209–217, 1876). St. Louis, MO: Mosby/Elsevier; Ball, J., & Bindler, R. (2006). *Child Health Nursing: Partnering with Children and Families* (pp. 568–575). Upper Saddle River, NJ: Prentice Hall.

1426. A health-care provider prescribed a dose of acetaminophen (Tylenol®) according to weight recommendations for a child. The package insert reads the recommended dose is 15 mg per kilogram. What dose should a nurse give if the child weighs 48 lbs?

1. 327 mg
2. 327 mL
3. 500 mg
4. 500 mL

ANSWER: 1
First, change 48 lbs into kilograms by dividing 48 by 2.2 to = 21.8 kg. Next multiply 21.8 kg by 15 = 327 mg. Option 2 gives an answer in milliliters not milligrams. The math is not correct in option 3. In option 4 the math is not correct, and the answer is given in milliliters not the required milligrams.

➧ ***Test-taking Tip:*** *Recall that 1 kg = 2.2 lbs.*

Content Area: Child Health; *Category of Health Alteration:* Pharmacological and Parenteral Therapies; *Integrated Processes:* Nursing Process Implementation; *Client Need:* Physiological Integrity/Pharmacological and Parenteral Therapies/Dosage Calculation; *Cognitive Level:* Analysis

Reference: Ball, J., & Bindler, R. (2006). *Clinical Handbook for Child Health Nurses* (pp. 142–146). Upper Saddle River, NJ: Pearson Prentice Hall.

1427. An adolescent, who is receiving morphine sulfate via a patient-controlled analgesia (PCA), complains of itching. Which medication should a nurse plan on administering to relieve the itching?

1. Naloxone hydrochloride (Narcan®)
2. Diazepam (Valium®)
3. Butenafine hydrochloride (Mentax®)
4. Diphenhydramine (Benadryl®)

ANSWER: 4
Diphenhydramine is an antihistamine that blocks histamine release by competing for the histamine receptors. Naloxone is a narcotic antagonist that reverses the effects of opiates. Diazepam acts on the central nervous system to produce sedation, hypnosis, skeletal muscle relaxation, and anticonvulsant activity. Butenafine is an antifungal antibiotic used to treat tinea pedis, tinea corporis, and tinea cruris.

➧ ***Test-taking Tip:*** *Knowledge of medications is needed to answer this question.*

Content Area: Child Health; *Category of Health Alteration:* Pharmacological and Parenteral Therapies; *Integrated Processes:* Nursing Process Planning; *Client Need:* Physiological Integrity/Pharmacological and Parenteral Therapies/Expected Actions or Outcomes; *Cognitive Level:* Application

Reference: Wilson, B., Shannon, M., Shields, K., & Stang, C. (2008). *Prentice Hall Nurse's Drug Guide 2008* (pp. 206, 455, 486, 1044). Upper Saddle River, NJ: Pearson Education.

1428. A nurse is preparing to administer morphine sulfate intravenously for a 6-year-old child in severe pain. The child has an intravenous (IV) infusion of D5W at 50 mL/hr through a peripherally inserted central catheter (PICC). Which action is best for the nurse to take to administer the medication?

1. Dilute the morphine sulfate with 5 mL of sterile water and administer over 5 minutes into the existing IV tubing's medication port closest to the client.
2. Administer the morphine sulfate undiluted into the existing IV tubing's medication port closest to the client.
3. Question the prescribed medication because morphine sulfate cannot be administered through a central line.
4. Disconnect the infusion, inject 3 mL of normal saline, and administer the morphine sulfate undiluted.

ANSWER: 1

The nurse should dilute the morphine sulfate before administration to prevent too-rapid administration and adverse effects. A single dose should be given over 4 to 5 minutes. To avoid too-rapid administration, a syringe pump should be used. Administering undiluted morphine sulfate to a child increases the risk of adverse effects. Morphine sulfate can be administered into a PICC access device. Unnecessary IV disconnections increase the risk for infection. Morphine sulfate is compatible with D5W.

➧ ***Test-taking Tip:*** *Select an option that is the most complete and the safest for the child.*

Content Area: Child Health; *Category of Health Alteration:* Pharmacological and Parenteral Therapies; *Integrated Processes:* Nursing Process Implementation; *Client Need:* Physiological Integrity/Pharmacological and Parenteral Therapies/Medication Administration; *Cognitive Level:* Application

Reference: Wilson, B., Shannon, M., Shields, K., & Stang, C. (2008). *Prentice Hall Nurse's Drug Guide 2008* (pp. 1022–1025). Upper Saddle River, NJ: Pearson Education.

1429. A health-care provider's (HCPs) progress notes state a plan to initiate an oral NSAID for a child's pain. Based on this information, a nurse should consult with the HCP when noting that which medication was prescribed?

1. Acetaminophen (Tylenol®)
2. Tolmetin (Tolectin®)
3. Hydromorphone (Dilaudid®)
4. Naproxen (Naprosyn®)

ANSWER: 3

Hydromorphone is an opioid analgesic, not an NSAID. Acetaminophen, tolmetin, and naproxen are all NSAIDs.

➧ ***Test-taking Tip:*** *This is a false-response item; select the medication that is not an NSAID.*

If uncertain, use the generic name of the medication as a cue to determine the answer.

Content Area: Child Health; *Category of Health Alteration:* Pharmacological and Parenteral Therapies; *Integrated Processes:* Communication and Documentation; *Client Need:* Physiological Integrity/Pharmacological and Parenteral Therapies/Pharmacological Pain Management; *Cognitive Level:* Application

Reference: Hockenberry, M., & Wilson, D. (2007). *Wong's Nursing Care of Infants and Children* (8th ed., pp. 226–227). St. Louis, MO: Mosby/Elsevier.

1430. A nurse is caring for a pediatric client experiencing wheezing from an asthma episode. A dose of albuterol (Proventil®) 5 mg by nebulization is prescribed. The medication vial contains 2.5 mg per 3 mL. The nurse should prepare ______ mL of medication for nebulization.

ANSWER: 6

Use a proportion formula:

2.5 mg : 3 mL :: 5 mg : X mL

Multiple the outside values and then the inside values and solve for X

2.5 X = 15

X = 6 mL

➧ ***Test-taking Tip:*** *Focus on the information in the question and use the on-screen calculator.*

Content Area: Child Health; *Category of Health Alteration:* Pharmacological and Parenteral Therapies; *Integrated Processes:* Nursing Process Implementation; *Client Need:* Physiological Integrity/Pharmacological and Parenteral Therapies/Dosage Calculation; *Cognitive Level:* Application

Reference: Pickar, G. (2007). *Dosage Calculations: A Ratio-Proportion Approach* (2nd ed., p. 46). Clifton Park, NY: Thomson Delmar Learning.

1431. A home care nurse is observing a 7-year-old client self-administer a dose of albuterol (Ventolin®) via a metered-dose inhaler with a spacer. Within a short time, the client begins to wheeze loudly. The nurse should:

1. consult with the health-care provider (HCP) to have the child's medication dosage increased.
2. report the findings to the HCP because it indicates paradoxical bronchospasms.
3. reassure the parent that this usually only occurs when the medication is initially begun.
4. reassess the child's technique; contact of the inhalation drug with the eyes can cause this reaction.

ANSWER: 2

The client's wheezing suggests paradoxical bronchospasms, which can occur with excessive use of adrenergic bronchodilators. The medication should be withheld and the HCP notified. A paradoxical bronchospasm can occur from excessive use, so the dosage should not be increased. Reassuring the parent is an inappropriate action. There is no indication that this is an initial dose. Contact with the eyes can cause eye irritation.

Test-taking Tip: *Examine options with duplicate words first (options 1 and 2) and eliminate one of these options. Then review the remaining options. Use the ABCs (airway, breathing, circulation) to determine that wheezing requires an immediate intervention.*

Content Area: Child Health; *Category of Health Alteration:* Pharmacological and Parenteral Therapies; *Integrated Processes:* Nursing Process Implementation; *Client Need:* Physiological Integrity/Pharmacological and Parenteral Therapies/Adverse Effects/Contraindications/Interactions; *Cognitive Level:* Analysis

Reference: Wilson, B., Shannon, M., Shields, K., & Stang, C. (2008). *Prentice Hall Nurse's Drug Guide 2008* (pp. 30–31). Upper Saddle River, NJ: Pearson Education.

1432. EBP An initial treatment regimen of isoniazid (Laniazid®), rifampin (Rifadin®), and ethambutol (Myambutol®) are prescribed for a 16-year-old client who has a positive tuberculin skin test. The client confides that she thinks she may have become pregnant since she was diagnosed and asks if she should be taking the medication while pregnant. On which rationale should a nurse base a response to the client's question?

1. These drugs cross the placental barrier and treatment should be withheld until the postpartum period.
2. The medications should be taken but the diagnosis is an indication for termination of the pregnancy.
3. The medications should be postponed because the risk for hepatitis is greatly increased in the intrapartum period.
4. The medications should be taken because untreated tuberculosis represents a far greater hazard to a pregnant woman and her fetus than does the treatment of the disease.

ANSWER: 4

Infants born to women with untreated tuberculosis may be of lower birth weight than those born to women without tuberculosis, and, rarely, the infant may acquire congenital tuberculosis. Isoniazid, rifampin, and ethambutol are all considered safe for use in pregnancy as reported by the Centers for Disease Control and Prevention (CDC). The medications do not cross the placental barrier, so treatment should not be withheld. Administering antituberculosis medications would not be an indication for termination of pregnancy because the medications are safe during pregnancy. The risk of hepatitis is slightly increased with the use of antituberculosis medications in pregnant women; however, the benefits of treatment strongly outweigh postponement of treatment.

Test-taking Tip: *Evaluate similar options first (not giving the medication) and eliminate one or both of these. Then examine the two remaining options. Think about the risk to others if the client is not treated.*

Content Area: Child Health; *Category of Health Alteration:* Pharmacological and Parenteral Therapies; *Integrated Processes:* Nursing Process Analysis; *Client Need:* Physiological Integrity/Pharmacological and Parenteral Therapies/Expected Actions or Outcomes; *Cognitive Level:* Analysis

Reference: Wilson, B., Shannon, M., Shields, K., & Stang, C. (2008). *Prentice Hall Nurse's Drug Guide* (pp. 604–606, 825–827, 1343–1346). Upper Saddle River, NJ: Pearson Education.

EBP Reference: National Collaborating Centre for Chronic Conditions. (2006). *Tuberculosis: Clinical Diagnosis and Management of Tuberculosis, and Measures for Its Prevention and Control.* London (UK): Royal College of Physicians. Available at: www.guideline.gov/summary/summary.aspx?doc_id=8993&nbr=004877&string=tuberculosis.

1433. A nurse practitioner prescribes amoxicillin (Amoxil®) for an 8-month-old client diagnosed with acute otitis media. A nurse correctly explains the primary purpose of the medication to a parent when stating it is prescribed to:

1. shrink swollen tissue in the eustachian tube.
2. reduce the severe pain.
3. treat the probable organism, *Haemophilus influenzae.*
4. reduce the fever.

ANSWER: 3

Acute otitis media is frequently caused by the *Haemophilus influenzae* and *Streptococcus pneumoniae* bacteria. The primary purpose of amoxicillin is to treat the infection caused by these two organisms. Reducing inflammation of the eustachian tube will occur, but this is not the primary purpose for treatment with amoxicillin. Treating the ear infection will reduce the pain but is not the primary purpose for treatment with amoxicillin. As the infection is treated, the fever will be reduced, but this is not the primary reason for treatment with amoxicillin.

Test-taking Tip: *The key words are "primary purpose." Focus on the main action of the medication.*

Content Area: Child Health; *Category of Health Alteration:* Pharmacological and Parenteral Therapies; *Integrated Processes:* Nursing Process Implementation; *Client Need:* Physiological Integrity/ Pharmacological and Parenteral Therapies/Expected Actions or Outcomes; *Cognitive Level:* Application

Reference: Hockenberry, M., & Wilson, D. (2007). *Wong's Nursing Care of Infants and Children* (8th ed., p. 1327). St. Louis, MO: Mosby/Elsevier.

1434. EBP A 6-year-old child weighing 20 kg is to receive ceftriaxone (Rocephin®) 2 g IV q12h and dexamethasone (Decadron®) 3 mg IVP q6h for 4 days to treat *Haemophilus influenzae* type b meningitis. A new nurse consults a drug reference and notes the usual dose of ceftriaxone is 100 mg/kg/ dose with a maximum daily dose of 4 g. The recommended dose of dexamethasone for treating *H. influenzae* type b meningitis is 0.15 mg/kg q6h for 2 to 4 days. Based on the medications prescribed and these findings, which conclusion by the nurse is correct?

1. The dose of ceftriaxone is too high.
2. The dose of dexamethasone is too low.
3. Both medications are safe to administer as prescribed.
4. The ceftriaxone should be administered before the dexamethasone.

ANSWER: 3

The doses of ceftriaxone and dexamethasone are at the recommended doses. To determine the dose, use a proportion formula and then calculate the dose for each medication by multiplying the means (inside values) and extremes (outside values) and solve for X.

Ceftriaxone Dose
100 mg : 1 kg :: X mg : 20 kg X = 2,000 mg 1,000 mg : 1 g :: 2,000 mg : X g 1,000 X = 2,000 X = 2 g

Dexamethasone Dose
0.15 mg : 1 kg :: X mg : 20 kg X = 3 mg

Guidelines recommend that the use of adjunctive dexamethasone in cases of *H. influenzae* type b meningitis to be initiated 10 to 20 minutes prior to or at least concomitant with the first antimicrobial dose.

► ***Test-taking Tip:*** *Use a medication calculation formula and calculate the doses to answer the question. An intravenous-push (IV-push) medication takes less time to administer than an intravenous piggyback (IVPB) medication.*

Content Area: Child Health; *Category of Health Alteration:* Pharmacological and Parenteral Therapies; *Integrated Processes:* Nursing Process Analysis; *Client Need:* Physiological Integrity/ Pharmacological and Parenteral Therapies/Dosage Calculation; *Cognitive Level:* Analysis

Reference: Wilson, B., Shannon, M., Shields, K., & Stang, C. (2008). *Prentice Hall Nurse's Drug Guide 2008* (pp. 279–280, 441–443). Upper Saddle River, NJ: Pearson Education.

EBP References: Miller, M., Gaur, A., & Kumar, A. (2008). Meningitis, bacterial. *E-Medicine from WebMD.* Available at: www.emedicine.com/ped/ TOPIC198.HTM; van de Beek, D., de Gans, J., McIntyre, P., & Prasad, K. (2006). Corticosteroids for acute bacterial meningitis. *Cochrane Database of Systematic Reviews*, Issue 4, Art. No: CD004405. DOI: 10.1002/14651858. CD004405.pub2. Available at: www.cochrane.org/reviews/en/ab004405.html.

1435. EBP A 17-year-old female is undergoing a drug screening test for employment. The client tells a nurse collecting the urine specimen of a recent complicated urinary tract infection that was treated with antibiotic therapy. Which antibiotic, if identified by the client, could produce a false positive urine screening test for opioids?

1. Amoxicillin (Amoxil®)
2. Cephalexin (Keflex®)
3. Ciprofloxacin (Cipro®)
4. Ceftazidime (Fortaz®)

ANSWER: 3

Fluoroquinolones, such as ciprofloxacin, can cause false-positive urine opiate screens. Amoxicillin (an aminopenicillin) and cephalexin and ceftazidime (cephalosporin) do not interfere with urine testing for opioids.

► ***Test-taking Tip:*** *Eliminate options from the same drug classification and then determine which of the two remaining medications is likely to cause false-positive opioid results.*

Content Area: Child Health; *Category of Health Alteration:* Pharmacological and Parenteral Therapies/Antimicrobials; *Integrated Processes:* Nursing Process Analysis; *Client Need:* Physiological Integrity/Pharmacological and Parenteral Therapies/Adverse Effects/ Contraindications/Interactions; *Cognitive Level:* Application

Reference: Wilson, B., Shannon, M., Shields, K., & Stang, C. (2008). *Prentice Hall Nurse's Drug Guide 2008* (pp. 82–84, 274–276, 284–285, 331–333). Upper Saddle River, NJ: Pearson Education.

EBP Reference: Reisfield, G., Salazar, E., & Bertholf, R. (2007). Rational use and interpretation of urine drug testing in chronic opioid therapy. *Annals of Clinical Laboratory Science,* 37(4), 301–314.

1436. EBP A 12-year-old child weighing 50 kg is hospitalized with bacterial pneumonia and an upper respiratory tract infection. The child is allergic to penicillin, azithromycin, and cefazolin sodium. A nurse is reviewing a serum laboratory report for the child before administering newly prescribed medications.

Serum Laboratory Test	Client's Value	Normal Values
BUN	36 mg/dL	7–18 mg/dL
Creatinine	1.2 mg/dL	0.3–0.7 mg/dL
Na	136 mEq/L	138–145 mEq/L
K	3.4 mEq/L	3.5–5.0 mEq/L
Cl	96 mEq/L	98–106 mEq/L
Hgb	11.5 g/dL	11.5–15.5 g/dL
Hct	35%	35%–45%
WBC	16.2 K/μL	4.5–13.5 K/μL
Osmolality	298 mOsm/kg	275–295 mOsm/kg H_2O

Based on the findings of the serum laboratory report, which health-care provider prescription is most important for the nurse to question?

1. Dextrose 5% in 0.25 NaCl with 20 mEq/L KCL at 65 mL/hr
2. Amikacin sulfate (Amikin®) 375 mg IVPB q12h
3. Guaifenesin (Robitussin®) 50–100 mg q4h prn for cough
4. Acetaminophen (Tylenol®) 325–650 mg q4–6h prn, not to exceed five doses/24 hr

ANSWER: 2

Amikacin is an aminoglycoside, which is nephrotoxic and should be questioned. The serum creatinine and blood urea nitrogen (BUN) levels are elevated, suggesting decreased renal function. The serum osmolality is high, suggesting dehydration and the potassium level is below normal. Daily fluid requirements may be met when dehydration occurs with dextrose 5% in 0.25 isotonic sodium chloride solution with 20 mEq/L added potassium. If the client weighs more than 20 kg, IV fluid replacement is 1,500 mL/day, plus 20 mL/kg/day for each kilogram over 20 kg, so the rate of 65 mL per hour is appropriate for maintenance. Guaifenesin is used for cough. The dose is within the range for a child of 12 years. The dose of acetaminophen is within the normal range (10–15 mg/kg/dose q4–6h as needed, not to exceed five doses/24 hr), but is also concerning because of the decreased renal function. Because this is a prn medication and amikacin is a timed medication, the amikacin is most important for the nurse to question.

***Test-taking Tip:** Carefully examine each laboratory value for abnormalities. Consider medications that are nephrotoxic.*

Content Area: Child Health; *Category of Health Alteration:* Pharmacological and Parenteral Therapies/Antimicrobials; *Integrated Processes:* Nursing Process Implementation; *Client Need:* Physiological Integrity/Pharmacological and Parenteral Therapies/Adverse Effects/Contraindications/Interactions; *Cognitive Level:* Analysis

References: Hockenberry, M., & Wilson, D. (2007). *Wong's Nursing Care of Infants and Children* (8th ed., pp. 1862, 1866–1873). St. Louis, MO: Mosby/Elsevier; Egland, A., & Egland, T. (2006). Pediatrics, dehydration. *E-Medicine from WebMD.* Available at: www.emedicine.com/emerg/TOPIC372.HTM.

EBP Reference: Schetz, M., Dasta, J., Goldstein, S., & Golper, T. (2005). Drug-induced acute kidney injury. *Current Opinion in Critical Care,* 11(6), 555–565.

1437. A nurse is caring for a 4-year-old child, diagnosed with sickle cell disease, who has undergone a splenectomy. The child is allergic to penicillin. Which medication should the nurse anticipate that the child will be required to take after discharge?

1. Morphine sulfate
2. Epoetin (Procrit®)
3. Amoxicillin (Amoxil®)
4. Erythromycin ethylsuccinate (EryPed®)

ANSWER: 4

There is a decreased capability to fight infection following a splenectomy. Daily prophylactic antibiotics are administered. Erythromycin is of the macrolide class of antibiotics. Opioids are administered in sickle cell crises or for severe pain; its use depends on the severity of pain and may not be required. Epoetin stimulates the bone marrow to produce red blood cells (erythropoiesis). In sickle cell disease, the red blood cells "sickle," increasing the levels of hemoglobin S (HbS). Increasing the production of sickled red blood cells can worsen the condition. Amoxicillin is an aminopenicillin and is contraindicated when allergies to penicillin are present.

***Test-taking Tip:** Note the penicillin allergy and eliminate any options that are contraindicated. Consider both the disease and the surgery when reviewing the remaining options.*

Content Area: Child Health; *Category of Health Alteration:* Pharmacological and Parenteral Therapies; *Integrated Processes:* Nursing Process Planning; *Client Need:* Physiological Integrity/Pharmacological and Parenteral Therapies/Expected Actions or Outcomes; *Cognitive Level:* Analysis

Reference: Ball, J., & Bindler, R. (2008). *Pediatric Nursing: Caring for Children* (4th ed., p. 811). Upper Saddle River, NJ: Prentice Hall.

1438. A nurse is caring for a 16-year-old client following a barbiturate overdose. The client's blood pressure is 94/48 mm Hg, heart rate 112, and urine output 200 mL for the past 8 hours. The client's cardiac rhythm is sinus tachycardia with premature atrial contractions (PACs). Dopamine 1 mcg/kg/min is prescribed. Which finding should prompt the nurse to conclude that the medication has been effective?

1. Increase in urine output
2. Increase in the diastolic blood pressure (DBP)
3. Decrease in pulse pressure
4. Decrease in PACs

ANSWER: 1

Low dose dopamine, 0.5–2.0 mcg/kg/min, acts on dopaminergic receptor sites along afferent arterioles in the glomerulus, dilates the renal vasculature, and improves urine output. Positive inotropic effects of dopamine include an increase in systolic blood pressure with little or no effect on DBP and an increase (not decrease) in pulse pressure. Dopamine will have no effect on decreasing the incidence of PACs.

Test-taking Tip: *The usual dose of dopamine for treating shock is 2–5 mcg/kg/min, increased gradually to 20–50 mcg/kg/min. Think about the effect of this low-dose dopamine. Note that three options involve the cardiovascular system, and one is different. Often the option that is different is the correct option.*

Content Area: Child Health; *Category of Health Alteration:* Pharmacological and Parenteral Therapies; *Integrated Processes:* Nursing Process Evaluation; *Client Need:* Physiological Integrity/Pharmacological and Parenteral Therapies/Expected Actions or Outcomes; *Cognitive Level:* Analysis

Reference: Wilson, B., Shannon, M., Shields, K., & Stang, C. (2008). *Prentice Hall Nurse's Drug Guide 2008* (pp. 505–507). Upper Saddle River, NJ: Pearson Education.

1439. A 12-year-old hospitalized child, diagnosed with type 1 diabetes mellitus, is learning to use insulin pens for basal-bolus insulin therapy with both a very long-acting insulin and rapid-acting insulin. The short-acting insulin is administered with each meal and snack based on the carbohydrate grams consumed, and the long-acting insulin is administered at bedtime. Which action by the child should indicate to a nurse that additional teaching is needed?

1. The child counts the number of carbohydrates eaten at breakfast and selects the insulin lispro (Humalog®) pen for covering the carbohydrates eaten.
2. The child determines that the blood glucose level at bedtime is within the normal range, eats a piece of turkey, and tells the nurse that rapid-acting insulin coverage is not needed.
3. The child holds the insulin glargine (Lantus®) pen against the skin for 10 seconds after administering the correct amount of insulin.
4. The child counts the number of carbohydrates eaten at lunch and selects the insulin glargine (Lantus®) pen for covering the carbohydrates eaten.

ANSWER: 4

Insulin glargine (Lantus®) is very long-acting insulin administered once daily. Insulin lispro (Humalog®) is rapid-acting insulin with an onset of 5 to 10 minutes. Either rapid-acting or short-acting (regular) insulin is administered with each meal and snack based on the carbohydrate grams consumed and the before-meal blood glucose level. Turkey does not contain carbohydrates; bolus insulin is only administered to cover the carbohydrates eaten. To ensure that the medication is administered with the insulin pens, the pen is held in place for 10 seconds after delivery of the medication.

Test-taking Tip: *Carefully read the situation. Examine the options that have duplicate information first and then eliminate either one or both of these.*

Content Area: Child Health; *Category of Health Alteration:* Pharmacological and Parenteral Therapies/Endocrine; *Integrated Processes:* Nursing Process Evaluation; *Client Need:* Physiological Integrity/Pharmacological and Parenteral Therapies/Medication Administration; *Cognitive Level:* Analysis

Reference: Ball, J., & Bindler, R. (2008). *Pediatric Nursing: Caring for Children* (4th ed., pp. 1226–1227). Upper Saddle River, NJ: Prentice Hall.

1440. A nurse completes teaching insulin administration to the parent of a toddler newly diagnosed with type 1 diabetes mellitus. The nurse concludes that the teaching was successful when the parent states:

1. "NPH insulin (Humulin N®) is only given at night immediately before the bedtime snack."
2. "It is okay to use only the buttocks for the insulin injections until the child is older."
3. "Insulin lispro (Humalog®) acts within 15 minutes and peaks 30 to 90 minutes after injection."
4. "Insulin detemir (Levenir®) can be added to the insulin lispro (Humalog®) pen to reduce the number of injections."

ANSWER: 3

Lispro is rapid-acting insulin that peaks in 30 to 90 minutes and may last as long as 5 hours in the blood. NPH insulin can be given in the morning, but there is better glucose control if given at night. NPH peaks in 4 to 14 hours, so there is no need to make sure food is available immediately after administration. Insulin injections should always be rotated to prevent subcutaneous tissue damage from giving the injections in the same location. Detemir is long-acting and lispro is rapid-acting insulin. An insulin pen uses pre-filled, multiple-use insulin cartridges; adding other types of insulins should not be attempted.

Test-taking Tip: *Eliminate options with absolute words such as "only." Focus on the type of insulin a newly diagnosed child with type 1 diabetes is most likely to receive.*

Content Area: Child Health; *Category of Health Alteration:* Pharmacological and Parenteral Therapies; *Integrated Processes:* Teaching and Learning; *Client Need:* Physiological Integrity/Pharmacological and Parenteral Therapies/Medication Administration; *Cognitive Level:* Application

References: Hockenberry, M., & Wilson, D. (2007). *Wong's Nursing Care of Infants and Children* (8th ed., p. 1720). St. Louis: Mosby/Elsevier; Lehne, R. (2007). *Pharmacology for Nursing Care* (6th ed., pp. 657–659). St. Louis, MO: Saunders.

1441. A 4-year-old child is brought to an emergency department by a parent. The parent states to a nurse, "My child's behavior isn't right. I think some of my medication is gone." The parent hands the nurse the medication bottle illustrated. Which action should the nurse take first?

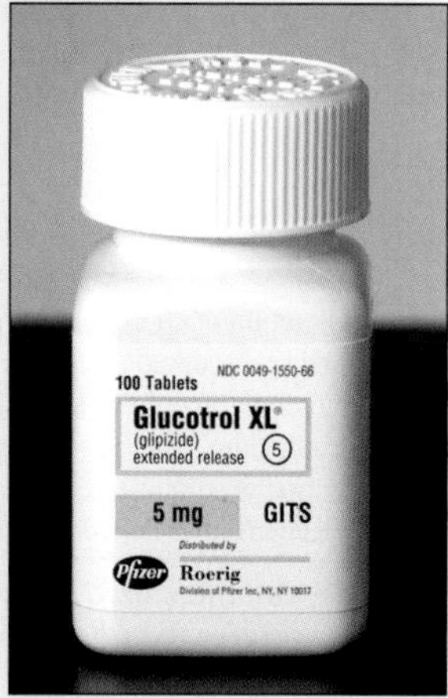

1. Ask the mother how many tablets the child may have taken.
2. Check the child's blood glucose level.
3. Administer glucagon (GlucaGen®) 1 mg subcutaneously.
4. Start an infusion of D5W at 40 mL/hr.

ANSWER: 2

Glipizide (Glucotrol XL®) is a sustained released second-generation sulfonylurea hypoglycemic agent with an onset of 15 to 30 minutes, a peak of 1 to 2 hours, and a duration of up to 24 hours. The child's behavior and the presence of the bottle suggest the child may have ingested some of the medication. The child's blood glucose level should be checked first because the mother "thinks" that the child may have ingested the medication. Questioning the mother about the number of tablets taken may delay the child's treatment. An oral form of glucose should be administered if the child is responsive and glucagon administered only if the child is unresponsive or too uncooperative or upset to take oral glucose. Glucagon stimulates the release of liver glycogen and releases glucose into the circulation. Initiating an intravenous access for glucose administration is more time-consuming than administering glucose by the oral route or glucagon subcutaneously to a child who is still responsive.

***Test-taking Tip:** Use the steps of the nursing process. Assessment should be completed to determine an appropriate intervention.*

Content Area: Child Health; *Category of Health Alteration:* Pharmacological and Parenteral Therapies; *Integrated Processes:* Nursing Process Assessment; *Client Need:* Safe and Effective Care Environment/Management of Care/Establishing Priorities; Physiological Integrity/Pharmacological and Parenteral Therapies/Medication Administration; *Cognitive Level:* Analysis

References: Berman, A., Snyder, S., Kozier, B., & Erb, G. (2008). *Kozier & Erb's Fundamentals of Nursing: Concepts, Process, and Practice* (8th ed., pp. 217–218). Upper Saddle River, NJ: Pearson Education; Pillitteri, A. (2007). *Maternal & Child Health Nursing: Care of the Childbearing & Childrearing Family* (5th ed., p. 1531). Philadelphia: Lippincott Williams & Wilkins; Wilson, B., Shannon, M., Shields, K., & Stang, C. (2008). *Prentice Hall Nurse's Drug Guide 2008* (pp. 707–710). Upper Saddle River, NJ: Pearson Education.

1442. Trimethoprim-sulfamethoxazole (TMP-SMZ or Bactrim®) is prescribed for a 6-year-old child who develops a urinary tract infection (UTI). Which points should a nurse address when teaching the parents about administering the medication? SELECT ALL THAT APPLY.

1. Weigh the child daily.
2. Encourage the child to drink plenty of fluids.
3. Take the child's temperature daily.
4. Administer the medication at the prescribed times.
5. Continue the medication until the full prescription is gone.
6. If a rash should occur report this immediately to the health-care provider.

ANSWER: 2, 4, 5, 6

Fluids should be increased to dilute bacterial toxins and increase urinary output. The medication should be given in the exact amount at the times directed to maintain a therapeutic blood level. If the therapeutic blood level falls, organisms can build a resistance to the medication. If the full prescription is not taken, the infection may return. Trimethoprim-sulfamethoxazole is a sulfonamide antibiotic. A rash can indicate an allergy to sulfonamides. Weighing is unnecessary; it is important with medications that affect fluid balance. Monitoring temperature would be important to evaluate the effectiveness of antipyretic medications.

***Test-taking Tip:** Use the child's diagnosis as a key, and eliminate options that do not pertain to a UTI or the medication.*

Content Area: Child Health; *Category of Health Alteration:* Pharmacological and Parenteral Therapies; *Integrated Processes:* Teaching and Learning; *Client Need:* Physiological Integrity/Pharmacological and Parenteral Therapies/Medication Administration; *Cognitive Level:* Analysis

References: Pillitteri, A. (2007). *Maternal & Child Health Nursing: Care of the Childbearing & Childrearing Family* (5th ed., p. 1464). Philadelphia: Lippincott Williams & Wilkins; Wilson, B., Shannon, M., Shields, K., & Stang, C. (2008). *Prentice Hall Nurse's Drug Guide 2008* (pp. 1554–1556). Upper Saddle River, NJ: Pearson Education.

1443. EBP A 6-year-old child is to start on medication therapy for enuresis that has not resolved with behavioral interventions. Which medication should a nurse anticipate being prescribed for the child?

1. Nitrofurantoin (Furadantin®)
2. Spironolactone (Aldactone®)
3. Lorazepam (Ativan®)
4. Desmopressin (DDAVP, Stimate®)

ANSWER: 4

Enuresis is involuntary passage of urine past the age when bladder control should be expected. Desmopressin is an analog of arginine vasopressin, which acts as an antidiuretic. It promotes resorption of water in the renal tubule or decreases bladder filling. Nitrofurantoin is a urinary tract antiseptic used to treat urinary tract infections. Spironolactone is a potassium-sparing diuretic that would promote, not inhibit, diuresis. Lorazepam is a benzodiazepine used to treat anxiety. A side effect is drowsiness, which could impair a child's ability to waken for voiding.

▶ *Test-taking Tip: Enuresis is involuntary passage of urine. Eliminate options that are a urinary antiseptic, diuretic, and antianxiety classification of medication.*

Content Area: Child Health; *Category of Health Alteration:* Pharmacological and Parenteral Therapies; *Integrated Processes:* Nursing Process Planning; *Client Need:* Physiological Integrity/ Pharmacological and Parenteral Therapies/Expected Actions or Outcomes; *Cognitive Level:* Application

References: Aschenbrenner, D., & Venable, S. (2009). *Drug Therapy in Nursing* (3rd ed., pp. 473, 821). Philadelphia: Lippincott Williams & Wilkins; Pillitteri, A. (2007). *Maternal & Child Health Nursing: Care of the Childbearing & Childrearing Family* (5th ed., pp. 1466–1467). Philadelphia: Lippincott Williams & Wilkins.

EBP Reference: Glazener, C., & Evans, J. (2006). Desmopressin for nocturnal enuresis in children. *Cochrane Database of Systematic Reviews*, Issue 2, Art. No. CD002112. DOI: 10.1002/14651858.CD002112. Available at: www.cochrane.org/reviews/en/ab002112.html

1444. A nurse records an infant's weight as 16 pounds 8 ounces at a clinic visit. Ranitidine (Zantac®) is prescribed for the infant. The prescription reads, "Give ranitidine 2 mg/kg twice daily." The medication is supplied as 15 mg/mL. The nurse should instruct the parent to withdraw ____ mL in the syringe to administer one dose.

ANSWER: 1

Use a proportion formula to calculate the dose. First, determine the dose for the child's weight.
16 pounds 8 ounces = 16.5 pounds divided by 2.2 pound/kg = 7.5 kg
Next, multiply the weight times the prescribed dose. 7.5 kg × 2 mg = 15 mg. The medication is supplied in 15 mg per 1 mL. The dose to administer is 1 mL.

▶ *Test-taking Tip: Convert pounds and ounces to kilograms: 1 pound equals 16 ounces and 1 kilogram equals 2.2 pounds.*

Content Area: Child Health; *Category of Health Alteration:* Pharmacological and Parenteral Therapies; *Integrated Processes:* Nursing Process Implementation; *Client Need:* Physiological Integrity/ Pharmacological and Parenteral Therapies/Dosage Calculation; *Cognitive Level:* Application

Reference: Wilkinson, J., & Van Leuven, K. (2007). *Fundamentals of Nursing: Thinking and Doing* (p. 521). Philadelphia: F. A. Davis.

1445. A nurse is caring for a 14-month-old child, hospitalized with a diagnosis of gastroenteritis and severe dehydration. Which prescriptions should a nurse determine are most appropriate for treating the child's diagnosed condition? SELECT ALL THAT APPLY.

1. An antidiarrheal medication to control the toddler's diarrhea
2. Intravenous (IV) fluid therapy for rehydration
3. IV antibiotic therapy to treat infection
4. Antipyretic therapy for fever
5. Oral fluid therapy for fluid rehydration
6. Analgesics for pain and discomfort

ANSWER: 2, 3, 4

The child who presents with severe dehydration at this age needs IV therapy to stabilize the balance of fluids and electrolytes. Frequently, a symptom of gastroenteritis is fever. Ensuring that the fever is controlled will provide some comfort to the child. There are many causes of gastroenteritis that do require a course of antibiotics to ensure complete recovery. An antidiarrheal medication is contraindicated in a toddler this age. Oral fluid rehydration is appropriate, but not when the toddler presents with severe dehydration. The pain and discomfort the toddler will have is due to fever and cramping from the gastrointestinal illness, thus analgesics will not usually be prescribed.

➧ *Test-taking Tip: Consider the fact that this is a 14-month-old who would quickly be at risk for dehydration. Also consider the pathophysiology of gastroenteritis and what the focus of treatment should be.*

Content Area: Child Health; *Category of Health Alteration:* Pharmacological and Parenteral Therapies; *Integrated Processes:* Nursing Process Evaluation; *Client Need:* Physiological Integrity/ Pharmacological and Parenteral Therapies/Medication Administration; Physiological Integrity/Pharmacological and Parenteral Therapies/ Parenteral/Intravenous Therapies; *Cognitive Level:* Analysis

References: Pillitteri, A. (2007). *Maternal & Child Health Nursing: Care of the Childbearing & Childrearing Family* (5th ed., pp. 1442–1443). Philadelphia: Lippincott Williams & Wilkins; Wilson, B., Shannon, M., Shields, K. & Stang, C. (2008). *Nurse's Drug Guide* (pp. 896–898). Upper Saddle River, NJ: Pearson Education.

1446. A nurse is preparing to administer intravenous (IV) fluids to a 13-kg child who has been diagnosed with dehydration secondary to gastroenteritis. The daily fluid requirement to administer IV fluid is 1,000 mL + 50 mL/kg weight more than 10 kg. The correct hourly rate to administer the IV therapy is:

1. 48 mL.
2. 54 mL.
3. 62.5 mL.
4. 69 mL.

ANSWER: 1

To calculate the correct hourly rate, it first must be determined what the daily fluid requirement is for this child. Because this child is 13 kilograms, the daily requirement is 1,000 mL plus 150 mL (50 mL × 3 = 150 mL) for a total of 1,150 mL in 24 hours. 1,150 mL is divided by 24 hours, thus 48 mL is the correct hourly rate. All other rates are incorrect.

➧ *Test-taking Tip: Refer to medication calculations and take into account all information provided. The daily fluid requirement is a cue that the total amount should be divided by 24 hours. Avoid multiplying the additional milliliter per kilogram by either 10 or 13 kg.*

Content Area: Child Health; *Category of Health Alteration:* Pharmacological and Parenteral Therapies; *Integrated Processes:* Nursing Process Implementation; *Client Need:* Physiological Integrity/ Pharmacological and Parenteral Therapies/Dosage Calculation; *Cognitive Level:* Application

Reference: Pillitteri, A. (2007). *Maternal & Child Health Nursing: Care of the Childbearing & Childrearing Family* (5th ed., pp. 1146–1151). Philadelphia: Lippincott Williams & Wilkins.

1447. A clinic nurse is educating a parent in administration of eye drops to a 3-year-old who has purulent drainage out of both eyes, swollen eye lids, and inflamed conjunctiva and has been diagnosed with bacterial conjunctivitis. The most important fact that the nurse needs to teach the parent is to:

1. have the child sitting when administering the medication.
2. have the child be in Trendelenburg's position when administering the medication.
3. restrain the child prior to administering the medication.
4. tell the child in detail exactly what will take place so that the child will be cooperative.

ANSWER: 3

It is necessary to secure the child prior to administering the medication to ensure that the child receives the entire prescribed dose. A 3-year-old child is able to understand what is occurring in relation to the limited amount of experiences the child has had. The child is likely to resist instillation of the eye drops because a child is told not to put anything in the eyes and is likely to remember painful experiences such as dust or a foreign object that has gotten into the eye. The child should be supine when ophthalmic medication administration occurs. Telling the child what is happening is extremely important, but at the age of 3 a detailed explanation will not make the child more cooperative.

➧ *Test-taking Tip: Logically process what would need to be done to be successful at administering ophthalmic medication to a child who is 3 years of age.*

Content Area: Child Health; *Category of Health Alteration:* Pharmacological and Parenteral Therapies; *Integrated Processes:* Teaching and Learning; *Client Need:* Physiological Integrity/ Pharmacological and Parenteral Therapies/Medication Administration; *Cognitive Level:* Application

Reference: Pillitteri, A. (2007). *Maternal & Child Health Nursing: Care of the Childbearing & Childrearing Family* (5th ed., pp. 998, 1147). Philadelphia: Lippincott Williams & Wilkins.

1448. A clinic nurse is reviewing prescriptions for a 5-year-old client who has a new diagnosis of generalized contact dermatitis. Which medication prescription should the nurse question?

1. Diphenhydramine (Benadryl®)
2. Prednisone (Deltasone®)
3. Calamine lotion
4. Hydrocortisone cream (Cortaid®)

ANSWER: 2

Children who have new diagnoses of contact dermatitis require medication that will relieve the symptoms and discomfort while the identified allergen is being removed from their environment. Prednisone would not be a first-line treatment for contact dermatitis. This medication potentially could be added at a later date if there has not been significant and expected resolution of the contact dermatitis. Diphenhydramine, calamine lotion, and hydrocortisone cream should all be expected medications for the treatment of contact dermatitis.

▶ ***Test-taking Tip:** The usual regime for treatment of contact dermatitis would start with those medications that would be least disruptive to the system. Take into account that this is the beginning course of treatment for this illness.*

Content Area: Child Health; *Category of Health Alteration:* Pharmacological and Parenteral Therapies; *Integrated Processes:* Nursing Process Intervention; *Client Need:* Physiological Integrity/ Pharmacological and Parenteral Therapies/Expected Actions or Outcomes; *Cognitive Level:* Analysis

Reference: Pillitteri, A. (2007). *Maternal & Child Health Nursing: Care of the Childbearing & Childrearing Family* (5th ed., pp. 1345–1346). Philadelphia: Lippincott Williams & Wilkins.

1449. Methylphenidate hydrochloride (Ritalin®) is prescribed for a 6-year-old child with attention deficit hyperactivity disorder (ADHD). A nurse should teach the parents to administer the medication:

1. whenever the child exhibits inattention behaviors.
2. whenever the child exhibits hyperactive behaviors.
3. with a snack before bed to calm the child for sleep.
4. during or after meals if the medication decreases appetite.

ANSWER: 4

A side effect of methylphenidate hydrochloride is anorexia. It should be given during or immediately after breakfast and lunch to prevent decreased intake of foods and fluids. Methylphenidate is usually administered twice daily at or before breakfast and at noon and not whenever inattention or hyperactive behaviors occur. Abrupt withdrawal of the medication may result in severe depression and psychotic behavior. The last dose of the medication should be given before 6 p.m. to prevent insomnia.

▶ ***Test-taking Tip:** Examine options with duplicate words first and eliminate one or both of these. Think about the effect of psychostimulants on sleep.*

Content Area: Child Health; *Category of Health Alteration:* Pharmacological and Parenteral Therapies; *Integrated Processes:* Teaching and Learning; *Client Need:* Physiological Integrity/ Pharmacological and Parenteral Therapies/Medication Administration; *Cognitive Level:* Application

Reference: Hockenberry, M., & Wilson, D. (2007). *Wong's Nursing Care of Infants and Children* (8th ed., pp. 799–800). St. Louis, MO: Mosby/ Elsevier.

1450. A nurse is administering phenobarbital (Luminal®) 300 mg intravenously (IV) to a child weighing 18 kg who is in status epilepticus. Which actions should the nurse take to safely administer the medication? SELECT ALL THAT APPLY.

1. Administer the phenobarbital over 20 minutes.
2. Monitor the IV site for signs of extravasation.
3. Dilute the phenobarbital in 10 mL D5W.
4. Prepare the phenobarbital for administration via an IV piggyback.
5. Identify incompatible medication or solutions being infused.
6. Administer the phenobarbital over 10 minutes in the port closest to the client.

ANSWER: 2, 5, 6

Whenever IV medications are being administered by any route, the site should be evaluated for irritation and extravasation. Intravenously administered phenobarbital that extravasates may cause necrotic tissue changes that necessitate skin grafting. Phenobarbital should be administered no faster than 1 mg/kg/min, with a maximum of 30 mg over 1 minute in infants and children. When administering IV medications, identification of medications or solutions that would be incompatible with that medication must occur so that the tubing can be flushed to ensure that crystallization does not occur in the IV tubing. This dose of phenobarbital should be administered as an IV-push medication over 10 minutes; administering it over 20 minutes will delay the medication's effects that treat status epilepticus. Phenobarbital, if diluted, should be mixed with sterile water for injection and not D5W. Phenobarbital should be prepared for direct IV administration and not as an IV piggybacked solution because this would delay the child's receiving the medication to terminate the seizure.

▶ ***Test-taking Tip:** Examine options with duplicate words first "administer the phenobarbital . . ." Eliminate one of these options. Then, consider if the medication should be administered via IV piggyback. Apply knowledge regarding administration of an IV medication as well as the pathophysiology of status epilepticus to identify the correct options.*

Content Area: Child Health; *Category of Health Alteration:* Pharmacological and Parenteral Therapies; *Integrated Processes:* Nursing Process Implementation; *Client Need:* Physiological Integrity/ Pharmacological and Parenteral Therapies/Medication Administration; *Cognitive Level:* Analysis

References: Wilson, B., Shannon, M., Shields, K., & Stang, C. (2008). *Nurse's Drug Guide* (pp. 1200–1203). Upper Saddle River, NJ: Pearson Education; Pillitteri, A. (2007). *Maternal & Child Health Nursing: Care of the Childbearing & Childrearing Family* (5th ed., pp. 1565–1566). Philadelphia: Lippincott Williams & Wilkins.

1451. An adolescent brought to an emergency department by the police is suspected of recent drug ingestion with possible overdose. Based on the table illustrated, for which drugs, if ingested, should a nurse expect drug residue to be present in a urine specimen taken within 6 hours of drug ingestion?

Suspected Drug Duration for Witnessed Urine Sample

Drug	Detection Duration
Amphetamines	4 hours
Barbiturates	24 hours to 7 days
Benzodiazepines	3 days
Cannabinoids	21 hours to 3 days
Cocaine	2 to 3 days
Codeine	4 hours
Methadone	3 days
Methaqualone	7 days
Morphine	4 hours
Phencyclidine	7 days

1. Phencyclidine, methaqualone, and morphine
2. Barbiturates, cocaine, and codeine
3. Benzodiazepines, cocaine, and methaqualone
4. Amphetamines, codeine, and morphine

ANSWER: 3

According to the table, benzodiazepines can be detected for up to 3 days; cocaine for up to 2 to 3 days; and methaqualone for up to 7 days. If drugs were ingested 6 hours ago, these still could be detected in the urine. Morphine, codeine, and amphetamines can only be detected in the urine for up to 4 hours.

➧ ***Test-taking Tip:*** *Focus on what the question is asking: presence of drug residue if the adolescent ingested drugs within the past 6 hours.*

Content Area: Child Health; *Category of Health Alteration:* Pharmacological and Parenteral Therapies; *Integrated Processes:* Nursing Process Analysis; *Client Need:* Physiological Integrity/ Reduction of Risk Potential/Diagnostic Tests; *Cognitive Level:* Application

Reference: Dillon, P. (2007). *Nursing Health Assessment: A Critical Thinking Case Studies Approach* (pp. 913–915). Philadelphia: F. A. Davis.

1452. A nurse is providing information to parents whose 3-year-old child has been treated with vincristine sulfate for the diagnosis of Wilms' tumor. In teaching the parents, the nurse should inform the parents to immediately notify the health-care provider if:

1. the child's hair begins to fall out.
2. the child develops diarrhea.
3. the child has signs or symptoms of depression.
4. the child develops dysphagia and paresthesias.

ANSWER: 4

Dysphagia and paresthesias are central nervous system adverse effects from vincristine that can result in injury to the child. Hair loss is a common adverse reaction to the medication and is reversible. Both diarrhea and severe constipation are adverse effects of vincristine, and prophylactic treatment is implemented at the beginning of therapy to decrease the potential of these occurring. Three-year-olds may not show signs or symptoms of depression. If present, the signs and symptoms should be distinguished as being associated with the neoplastic disease itself or side effects of the medication.

➧ ***Test-taking Tip:*** *The key words are "most important." Use Maslow's Hierarchy of Needs to identify a problem that has the potential for causing injury.*

Content Area: Child Health; *Category of Health Alteration:* Pharmacological and Parenteral Therapies; *Integrated Processes:* Teaching and Learning; *Client Need:* Physiological Integrity/ Pharmacological and Parenteral Therapies/Adverse Effects/Contraindications/ Interactions; *Cognitive Level:* Application

References: Pillitteri, A. (2007). *Maternal & Child Health Nursing: Care of the Childbearing & Childrearing Family* (5th ed., pp. 1711–1712). Philadelphia: Lippincott Williams & Wilkins; Wilson, B., Shannon, M., Shields, K., & Stang, C. (2008). *Nurse's Drug Guide* (pp. 1591–1593). Upper Saddle River, NJ: Pearson Education.

Chapter Ten

Psychosocial Integrity: Care of Adults and Children with Mental Health Disorders

Test 38: Mental Health: Anxiety and Mood Disorders

1453. A client reports becoming involved with legislation that promotes gun safety after the death of a child by accidental shooting. Which defense mechanism is the client exhibiting?

1. Sublimation
2. Identification
3. Denial
4. Intellectualization

ANSWER: 1

Sublimation involves redirecting unacceptable feelings or drives into an acceptable channel. Identification involves taking on attributes and characteristics of someone admired. Denial is the refusal to accept a painful reality by pretending that it did not happen. Intellectualization involves excessive focus on reasoning to avoid feelings associated with a situation.

Test-taking Tip: *Use the process of elimination with an understanding of defense mechanism terminology.*

Content Area: Mental Health; *Category of Health Alteration:* Anxiety and Mood Disorders; *Integrated Processes:* Nursing Process Analysis; *Client Need:* Psychosocial Integrity/Coping Mechanisms; *Cognitive Level:* Application

Reference: Pedersen, D. (2008). *Psych Notes* (2nd ed., p. 6). Philadelphia: F. A. Davis.

1454. A client reports becoming physically ill with frequent crying spells, intense feelings of worthlessness, and loss of appetite on the anniversary of the death of the client's spouse. The client reports this has occurred for the last 5 years. Based on the reported symptoms, what should a nurse conclude that the client is experiencing?

1. Uncomplicated grief
2. Delayed grief reaction
3. Distorted grief reaction
4. Depression

ANSWER: 3

The nurse should determine that the client is experiencing a distorted grief reaction. The symptoms reported by the client are exaggerated and prolonged. In uncomplicated grief, the client's self-esteem remains intact with symptom resolution. Delayed grief reaction is the absence of the expression of grief during situations when a grief reaction is expected. A depression disorder is a form of an exaggerated or distorted grief response.

Test-taking Tip: *Focus on the most important information in the scenario to answer the question: the client's symptoms occur only on the anniversary of the spouse's death and for the last 5 years. Removing less relevant information makes a question easier to answer.*

Content Area: Mental Health; *Category of Health Alteration:* Anxiety and Mood Disorders; *Integrated Processes:* Nursing Process Analysis; *Client Need:* Psychosocial Integrity/Grief and Loss; *Cognitive Level:* Analysis

Reference: Townsend, M. (2008). *Nursing Diagnoses in Psychiatric Nursing* (p. 368). Philadelphia: F. A. Davis.

1455. A client is being discharged after hospitalization for a suicide attempt. Which question asked by the nurse assesses the learned prevention and future coping strategies of the client?

1. "How did you try to kill yourself?"
2. "Do you have the phone number of the suicide prevention center?"
3. "What skills can you utilize if you experience problems again?"
4. "Why did you think life wasn't worth living?"

ANSWER: 3

Asking the client directly regarding what skills he or she could utilize if similar problems occurred in the future provides the client with an opportunity to reflect on learned behaviors and to determine a plan for future prevention. How suicide was initially attempted would have been addressed during the initial assessment and does not determine future coping. Although asking the client if the suicide prevention center number is known would be helpful, the question does not determine learned coping strategies. Asking the client a "why" question is not helpful and conveys a judgmental attitude.

➧ ***Test-taking Tip:*** *Focus on using therapeutic communication techniques, and eliminate any options that include barriers of probing and challenging statements. The key words in the stem are "discharged after hospitalization," "suicide attempt," and "learned prevention and future coping strategies."*

Content Area: Mental Health; *Category of Health Alteration:* Anxiety and Mood Disorders; *Integrated Processes:* Nursing Process Assessment; *Client Need:* Psychosocial Integrity/Coping Mechanisms; *Cognitive Level:* Application

References: Fortinash, K., & Holoday Worret, P. (2007). *Psychiatric Nursing Care Plans* (5th ed., p. 99). St. Louis, MO: Mosby; Berman, A., Snyder, S., Kozier, B., & Erb, G. (2008). *Kozier & Erb's Fundamentals of Nursing: Concepts, Process, and Practice* (8th ed., pp. 469–471). Upper Saddle River, NJ: Pearson Education.

1456. EBP Which nursing diagnosis should a nurse give highest priority when caring for a client with major depressive disorder?

1. Powerlessness
2. Potential for spiritual distress
3. Potential for injury
4. Disturbed sleep patterns

ANSWER: 3

The potential for suicidal behavior is the highest priority for clients diagnosed with major depressive disorder. The presence of powerlessness, spiritual distress, and disturbed sleep patterns are concerning but do not take priority over the potential for suicide.

➧ ***Test-taking Tip:*** *Use Maslow's Hierarchy of Needs theory to identify the priority. Safety is priority since it could result in life-threatening injury.*

Content Area: Mental Health; *Category of Health Alteration:* Anxiety and Mood Disorders; *Integrated Processes:* Nursing Process Analysis; *Client Need:* Safe and Effective Care Environment/Safety and Infection Control/Accident and Injury Prevention; *Cognitive Level:* Analysis

Reference: Varcarolis, E., Benner Carson, V., & Shoemaker, N. (2006). *Foundations of Psychiatric Mental Health Nursing* (5th ed., p. 331). St. Louis, MO: Saunders/Elsevier.

EBP Reference: Rudd, M., Berman, A., & Joiner, T. (2006). Warning signs for suicide. *Suicide and Life Threatening Behavior,* 36(3), 255–262. Available at: www.suicidology.org

1457. A nurse is interviewing a client at a mental health clinic. Which care setting should the nurse determine is most appropriate for the client who recently attempted suicide and continues to report suicidal ideation?

1. An outpatient clinic
2. A community mental health center
3. An inpatient mental health unit
4. A nursing home

ANSWER: 3

A client with a history of suicidal behavior with current suicidal ideation is at-risk and in need of hospitalization. The most appropriate setting is an inpatient mental health unit that is equipped to handle the safety issues of risky behaviors. The remaining choices do not provide the level of safety that is required for the client.

➧ ***Test-taking Tip:*** *The key words are "suicidal ideation." Focus on the safest environment for the client and eliminate other less-safe options. Focus on using Maslow's Hierarchy of Needs theory and the safest location for the client.*

Content Area: Mental Health; *Category of Health Alteration:* Anxiety and Mood Disorders; *Integrated Processes:* Nursing Process Planning; *Client Need:* Psychosocial Integrity/Therapeutic Environment; Safe and Effective Care Environment/Management of Care/Continuity of Care; *Cognitive Level:* Application

Reference: Fortinash, K., & Holoday Worret, P. (2007). *Psychiatric Nursing Care Plans* (5th ed., p. 89). St. Louis, MO: Mosby.

1458. EBP A nurse is meeting with a client who is being discharged after hospitalization for suicidal ideation. Based on knowledge of expert consensus of warning signs for suicide, the nurse should plan to advise the client to seek help by contacting a mental health professional or calling the national suicide prevention hotline if experiencing: SELECT ALL THAT APPLY

1. sadness.
2. hopelessness.
3. severe anxiety and agitation.
4. feeling of being trapped.
5. increasing alcohol or drug use.

ANSWER: 2, 3, 4, 5

Consensus warning signs are hopelessness, rage/anger or seeking revenge, acting reckless, feeling trapped (like there is no way out), increasing alcohol or drug use, withdrawing from family or friends, severe anxiety or agitation, dramatic changes in mood, and feeling no reason for living. Sadness can be a normal mood variation.

▶ ***Test-taking Tip:*** *Use the process of elimination to eliminate any option pertaining to normal mood variation.*

Content Area: Mental Health; *Category of Health Alteration:* Anxiety and Mood Disorders; *Integrated Processes:* Nursing Process Planning; *Client Need:* Safe and Effective Care Environment/Management of Care/Continuity of Care; *Cognitive Level:* Application

Reference: Varcarolis, E., Benner Carson, V., & Shoemaker, N. (2006). *Foundations of Psychiatric Mental Health Nursing* (5th ed., p. 480). St. Louis, MO: Saunders/Elsevier.

EBP Reference: Rudd, M., Bermann, A., & Joiner, T. (2006). Warning signs for suicide: Theory, research, and clinical applications. *Suicide and Life-Threatening Behavior*, 36(3), 255–262.

1459. A nurse is planning care for a client diagnosed with acute mania. What situation must occur prior to initiating treatment with lithium carbonate?

1. Room seclusion has proven ineffective in controlling the client's behavior.
2. The client has been fasting for 12 hours.
3. The client's history and physical results, including laboratory results, are reviewed.
4. Administration of benzodiazepine has been terminated.

ANSWER: 3

The use of lithium carbonate requires initial and ongoing health assessment and laboratory monitoring. Because lithium is excreted by the kidneys, a baseline evaluation has to be completed before treatment begins. Room seclusion is used as a last resort and is unrelated to medication administration. Having the client fast is unnecessary. Benzodiazepines are often used in treatment during the initiation phase to aid in controlling mania, as it can take up to a week for lithium to become effective.

▶ ***Test-taking Tip:*** *Use the process of elimination. Apply guidelines and side effects for the use of lithium carbonate.*

Content Area: Mental Health; *Category of Health Alteration:* Anxiety and Mood Disorders; *Integrated Processes:* Nursing Process Planning; *Client Need:* Physiological Integrity/Pharmacological and Parenteral Therapies/Medication Administration; *Cognitive Level:* Application

Reference: Fortinash, K., & Holoday Worret, P. (2007). *Psychiatric Nursing Care Plans* (5th ed., p. 497). St. Louis: MO: Mosby.

1460. A nurse is interpreting the serum laboratory report for a client in an emergency department. The history and reports reveal that the client has been diagnosed with bipolar disorder and receives lithium carbonate. Based on the findings of the serum laboratory report, which result would explain the client's condition of impaired consciousness, nystagmus, and seizures?

Serum Laboratory Test	Client's Value
Creatinine	0.8 mg/dL
BUN	10 mg/dL
Na	140 mEq/L
Lithium	3.8 mEq/L

1. Creatinine
2. BUN
3. Na
4. Lithium

ANSWER: 4

Symptoms of lithium toxicity appear at levels greater than 1.5 mEq/L. At a level greater than 3.5 mEq/L, the symptoms of toxicity include coma, nystagmus, seizures, and cardiovascular collapse. The results of kidney function tests (blood urea nitrogen [BUN] and creatinine) are within normal limits (normal BUN values are 5–25 mg/dL; normal creatinine is 0.5–1.5 mg/dL). Normal sodium (Na) is 135–145 mEq/L.

▶ ***Test-taking Tip:*** *Use the process of elimination with an understanding of the normal serum levels for lithium carbonate.*

Content Area: Mental Health; *Category of Health Alteration:* Anxiety and Mood Disorders; *Integrated Processes:* Nursing Process Evaluation; *Client Need:* Physiological Integrity/Pharmacological and Parenteral Therapies/Adverse Effects/Contradictions/Interactions; *Cognitive Level:* Analysis

Reference: Townsend, M. (2008). *Essentials of Psychiatric Mental Health Nursing* (4th ed., pp. 197, 199). Philadelphia: F. A. Davis.

1461. EBP A client is newly prescribed tramadol hydrochloride (Ultram®) for chronic pain. The client is also taking fluoxetine (Prozac®) 40 mg daily for depression. Which statement by the nurse accurately explains the interactions between the two drugs?

1. "There is no major concern with this drug combination."
2. "Tramadol hydrochloride (Ultram®) may decrease the effectiveness of fluoxetine (Prozac®)."
3. "This drug combination can increase the risk of serotonin syndrome."
4. "Selective serotonin reuptake inhibitors (SSRIs) should not be taken within 14 days of the last dose of tramadol hydrochloride (Ultram®)."

ANSWER: 3

Tramadol hydrochloride is a centrally acting analgesic that binds to mu-opioid receptors. It inhibits the reuptake of serotonin and norepinephrine in the central nervous system (CNS). Fluoxetine is an SSRI that selectively inhibits the reuptake of serotonin in the CNS. The combination of tramadol hydrochloride and fluoxetine can overactivate central serotonin receptors resulting in serotonin syndrome, a life-threatening but rare event. There is a significant potential for drug interaction with this drug combination. Tramadol hydrochloride intensifies the action of fluoxetine. SSRIs should not be taken within 14 days of an MAOI (monoamine oxidase inhibitor).

➧ ***Test-taking Tip:*** *Focus on the issue: the actions of tramadol and fluoxetine individually and then when combined. Recall that both medications inhibit the reuptake of serotonin in the CNS.*

Content Area: Mental Health; *Category of Health Alteration:* Anxiety and Mood Disorders; *Integrated Processes:* Nursing Process Evaluation; *Client Need:* Physiological Integrity/Pharmacological and Parenteral Therapies/Adverse Effects/Contradictions/Interactions; *Cognitive Level:* Analysis

Reference: Lippincott Williams & Wilkins. (2008). *Nursing 2008 Drug Handbook* (28th ed., pp. 416–417). Philadelphia: Author.

EBP Reference: Boyer, E., & Shannon, M. (2005). The serotonin syndrome. *The New England Journal of Medicine*, 352(11), 1112–1120. Available at: www.content.nejm.org

---

1462. A nurse is educating a client about prescription antidepressant medications and the appropriate expectations when taking these. Which statement by the nurse is accurate?

1. "It is important to continue taking antidepressant medication even after you feel better."
2. "Your symptoms will subside about 72 hours after starting the antidepressant medication."
3. "The most potent antidepressant is fluoxetine (Prozac®)."
4. "Some common side effects of SSRIs are dry mouth, blurred vision, and urinary retention."

ANSWER: 1

Evidence-based practice guidelines recommend continuing antidepressant medication a minimum of 6 months after recovery following the first episode of depression to decrease the chance of relapse. Symptom improvement begins approximately 2 weeks after medication is initiated and often takes 6 to 8 weeks at a therapeutic dose to achieve significant remission of symptoms. Antidepressants are equally efficacious. The individual's personal and family history and specific cluster of symptoms guide medication selection. Dry mouth, blurred vision, and urinary retention are anticholinergic side effects associated with tricyclic antidepressants (TCA), not a serotonin selective reuptake inhibitor (SSRI).

➧ ***Test-taking Tip:*** *Use the process of elimination with an understanding of depression and medication management.*

Content Area: Mental Health; *Category of Health Alteration:* Anxiety and Mood Disorders; *Integrated Processes:* Teaching and Learning; *Client Need:* Health Promotion and Maintenance/Self-Care; *Cognitive Level:* Analysis

Reference: Fortinash, K., & Holoday Worret, P. (2007). *Psychiatric Nursing Care Plans* (5th ed., pp. 91–92). St. Louis, MO: Mosby.

1463. A nurse is reviewing diet restrictions with a client taking a monoamine oxidase inhibitor (MAOI). Which symptom could occur with nonadherence to diet restrictions while taking a MAOI?

1. Agranulocytosis
2. Explosive occipital headache
3. Severe hypotension
4. Akathisia

ANSWER: 2

Explosive occipital headache is a symptom of hypertensive crisis, which is a major concern with the combination of a monoamine oxidase inhibitor (MAOI) and certain foods (e.g., aged cheeses, overripe fruit, and sausage). Agranulocytosis, hypotension, and akathisia (unpleasant sensations of "inner" restlessness that results in an inability to sit still) are not symptoms associated with MAOIs and food restrictions.

➧ ***Test-taking Tip:*** *Use the process of elimination and review diet restrictions with clients taking MAOIs.*

Content Area: Mental Health; *Category of Health Alteration:* Anxiety and Mood Disorders; *Integrated Processes:* Nursing Process Planning; *Client Need:* Physiological Integrity/Pharmacological and Parenteral Therapies/Adverse Effects/Contraindications/Interactions; *Cognitive Level:* Analysis

Reference: Fortinash, K., & Holoday Worret, P. (2007). *Psychiatric Nursing Care Plans* (5th ed., pp. 494–495). St. Louis, MO: Mosby.

1464. A client who is receiving amitriptyline (Elavil®) 150 mg daily is scheduled for surgery. Which statement reflects accurate understanding of safety concerns in this situation?

1. Client could be switched to doxepin (Sinequan®) instead of amitriptyline.
2. Amitriptyline should be continued as the stress of surgery will worsen depression.
3. Amitriptyline can cause hypertensive episodes during surgery.
4. Amitriptyline can be safely reduced to 100 mg daily rather than discontinuing it.

ANSWER: 3

Hypertensive episodes have occurred during surgery with tricyclic antidepressants (TCAs). Amitriptyline is in this drug category. For client safety, the dosage should be gradually decreased and discontinued several days prior to surgery. Doxepin is in the same drug category as amitriptyline. The remaining responses do not support the client safety requirements.

***Test-taking Tip:** Use the process of elimination and review side effects of tricyclic antidepressants.*

Content Area: Mental Health; *Category of Health Alteration:* Anxiety and Mood Disorders; *Integrated Processes:* Nursing Process Planning; *Client Need:* Safe and Effective Care Environment/Safety and Infection Control/Accident and Injury Prevention; Physiological Integrity/Reduction of Risk Potential/Potential for Complications from Surgical Procedures and Health Alterations; *Cognitive Level:* Analysis

Reference: Deglin, J., & Vallerand, A. (2007). *Davis's Drug Guide for Nurses* (10th ed., p. 127). Philadelphia: F. A. Davis.

1465. An experienced nurse is teaching a new nurse about establishing therapeutic relationships with clients on a mental health unit. Which intervention should the nurse suggest when attempting to establish a therapeutic relationship with a client diagnosed with major depressive disorder?

1. Sit with the client in silence.
2. Ask the client to join others to watch a 2-hour movie.
3. Invite the client to attend an exercise class.
4. Ask the client how his or her day should be scheduled.

ANSWER: 1

An effective therapeutic intervention is to sit with the client in silence. Nonverbal communication conveys respect, understanding, and interest. Clients diagnosed with depression have decreased attention spans and concentration. Lack of energy is a common symptom of depression. Clients with depression are often indecisive and dependent.

***Test-taking Tip:** Focus on therapeutic techniques to use with major depressive disorder. Eliminate options that would be ineffective due to the client's decreased attention span and concentration, lack of energy, and indecisiveness and dependency.*

Content Area: Mental Health; *Category of Health Alteration:* Anxiety and Mood Disorders; *Integrated Processes:* Teaching and Learning; *Client Need:* Psychosocial Integrity/Behavioral Interventions; Psychosocial Integrity/Therapeutic Communications; *Cognitive Level:* Application

References: Potter, P., & Perry, A. (2009). *Fundamentals of Nursing* (7th ed., pp. 352–355). St. Louis, MO: Mosby/Elsevier; Pedersen, D. (2008). *Psych Notes* (2nd ed., pp. 98–99). Philadelphia: F. A. Davis.

1466. A nurse is establishing a plan of care for a client scheduled for electroconvulsive therapy (ECT). Which planned action by the nurse is unsafe when caring for this client?

1. Administering a short-acting barbiturate prior to the procedure
2. Monitoring vital signs before, during, and after the procedure
3. Administering succinylcholine after the procedure to decrease recovery time
4. Educating the client that experiencing confusion, tiredness, headache, muscle pain, or back pain after the procedure is normal

ANSWER: 3

Succinylcholine is administered *before* the procedure to paralyze muscles and prevent fractures. If continued after the procedure it can result in respiratory arrest. Short-acting barbiturate is administered to induce sleep during the ECT. ECT can decrease blood pressure, increase heart rate, and/or cause heart rhythm disturbances. Vital signs need to be taken prior to the procedure and be continually monitored for safety. Mild disorientation, fatigue, headache, and muscle and back pain are expected and common symptoms after ECT.

***Test-taking Tip:** The key word is "unsafe." Eliminate safe nursing actions.*

Content Area: Mental Health; *Category of Health Alteration:* Anxiety and Mood Disorders; *Integrated Processes:* Nursing Process Implementation; *Client Need:* Physiological Integrity/Basic Care and Comfort/Non-Pharmacological Comfort Interventions; *Cognitive Level:* Analysis

Reference: Varcarolis, E., Benner Carson, V., & Shoemaker, N. (2006). *Foundations of Psychiatric Mental Health Nursing* (5th ed., pp. 351–352). St. Louis, MO: Saunders/Elsevier.

1467. A client recently diagnosed with depression tells a nurse that she is 2 months pregnant and is reluctant to take an antidepressant medication. The client asks what other treatment options are available. Which type of therapy should a nurse recommend as an alternate treatment for depression?

1. Client-centered therapy
2. Gestalt therapy
3. Therapeutic touch therapy
4. Cognitive behavioral therapy

ANSWER: 4

Cognitive behavioral therapy is a research-supported treatment that focuses on patterns of thinking that are maladaptive and the beliefs that underlie such thinking. The aim of therapy is to influence and change disturbed thinking patterns and the messages that the client gleans. Client-centered and gestalt therapies are psychoanalytic modalities and not evidenced-based practices for the treatment and management of depression. Client-centered therapy is a humanistic approach that emphasizes expression of feelings through reflection and clarification. Gestalt therapy emphasizes self-expression, self-exploration, and self-awareness in the present. Therapeutic touch is used to reduce pain and anxiety and to promote relaxation.

➧ ***Test-taking Tip:*** *Select the therapy that will influence and change disturbed thinking patterns.*

Content Area: Mental Health; *Category of Health Alteration:* Anxiety and Mood Disorders; *Integrated Processes:* Teaching and Learning; *Client Need:* Psychosocial Integrity/Mental Health Concepts; *Cognitive Level:* Application

Reference: Townsend, M. (2008). *Essentials of Psychiatric Mental Health Nursing* (4th ed., p. 342). Philadelphia: F. A. Davis.

1468. A client diagnosed with major depressive disorder has the nursing diagnosis of *Disturbed sleep pattern*. When developing a plan of care for this client, which nursing actions are most appropriate? SELECT ALL THAT APPLY.

1. Determine sleep patterns prior to hospitalization.
2. Discourage sleeping during the day.
3. Record and limit caffeinated drinks.
4. Reinforce reality thinking.
5. Encourage measures that aid in relaxation.

ANSWER: 1, 2, 3, 5

Determining past sleep patterns is important in determining what is normal for the client. Limiting daytime sleeping promotes nighttime sleep routines. Caffeine is a stimulant that interferes with sleep patterns. Measures such as soft music and relaxation exercises may be helpful in promoting sleep. Encouraging reality thinking would be an appropriate intervention for a thought disorder.

➧ ***Test-taking Tip:*** *Focus on the issue: interventions to promote sleep.*

Content Area: Mental Health; *Category of Health Alteration:* Anxiety and Mood Disorders; *Integrated Processes:* Nursing Process Planning; *Client Need:* Safe and Effective Care Environment/Management of Care/Case Management; Psychosocial Integrity/Behavioral Interventions; *Cognitive Level:* Application

Reference: Townsend, M. (2008). *Nursing Diagnoses in Psychiatric Nursing* (pp. 174–175). Philadelphia: F. A. Davis.

1469. A nurse is assessing a client with dysthymia who reports symptoms of depressed mood. Which assessment finding supports the essential feature of dysthymia?

1. Recurrent thoughts of death
2. Chronically depressed mood for most of the day for at least 2 years
3. Significant weight loss
4. Diminished ability to think or concentrate

ANSWER: 2

Individuals diagnosed with dysthymia describe their mood as sad or "down in the dumps" more days than not for at least 2 years. The depressive symptoms are chronic but less severe and may not be easily distinguished from the person's usual functioning. Recurrent thoughts of death, significant weight loss, and decreased concentration are neurovegetative symptoms most commonly associated with a major depressive disorder.

➧ ***Test-taking Tip:*** *Use the process of elimination and review diagnostic criteria for dysthymia.*

Content Area: Mental Health; *Category of Health Alteration:* Anxiety and Mood Disorders; *Integrated Processes:* Nursing Process Assessment; *Client Need:* Psychosocial Integrity/Mental Health Concepts; *Cognitive Level:* Knowledge

Reference: Townsend, M. (2008). *Essentials of Psychiatric Mental Health Nursing* (4th ed., p. 335). Philadelphia: F. A. Davis.

1470. A depressed client tells a nurse, "Nothing gives me joy. Things seem hopeless." Which actions should be taken by the nurse when caring for this client? Prioritize the nurse's actions by placing each step in the correct order.

______ Demonstrate genuine empathy and caring in discussing client's feelings about suicide.
______ Evaluate the client's risk for suicide by direct questioning (asking about suicide intent and plan).
______ Initiate suicide precautions as needed, according to policy and standards of care.
______ Continue to support and monitor prescribed medical and psychosocial treatment plans.
______ Assist client in maintaining nutritional needs, hygiene, and grooming.
______ Contact the client's support system in collaboration with case manager and/or social services.

ANSWER: 3, 1, 2, 5, 4, 6

First evaluate the client's risk for suicide by direct questioning (asking about suicide intent and plan). Then initiate suicide precautions as needed, according to policy and standards of care. Demonstrate genuine empathy and caring in discussing client's feelings about suicide. Next, assist client in maintaining nutritional needs, hygiene, and grooming. Continue to support and monitor prescribed medical and psychosocial treatment plans. Finally, contact the client's support system in collaboration with case manager and/or social services.

➧ ***Test-taking Tip:*** *Anhedonia and feelings of hopelessness are significant risk factors for suicide. Focus on the goal of suicide prevention; prioritizing is putting items in sequence (most important first) to achieve critical outcomes. Consider steps in the nursing process and phases of treatment.*

Content Area: Mental Health; *Category of Health Alteration:* Anxiety and Mood Disorders; *Integrated Processes:* Nursing Process Analysis; *Client Need:* Safe and Effective Care Environment/Management of Care/Establishing Priorities; *Cognitive Level:* Analysis

Reference: Fortinash, K., & Holoday Worret, P. (2007). *Psychiatric Nursing Care Plans* (5th ed., pp. 109–111). St. Louis, MO: Mosby.

1471. A nurse is educating a client diagnosed with depression who is experiencing insomnia. Which intervention should the nurse recommend to reduce episodes of insomnia?

1. Maintain regular bedtime hours.
2. Sleep late on weekends to catch up on missed sleep.
3. Fight insomnia when it occurs.
4. Establish a regular exercise program a few hours before bedtime.

ANSWER: 1

Maintaining a regular bedtime is a recommended sleep hygiene practice. Sleep experts recommend avoiding sleeping late on weekends and avoiding stimulating activities, including exercise, close to bedtime. Instead of fighting insomnia, the client should get out of bed and do something nonstimulating until feeling tired again.

➧ ***Test-taking Tip:*** *Use the process of elimination and review techniques to reduce/eliminate insomnia.*

Content Area: Mental Health; *Category of Health Alteration:* Anxiety and Mood Disorders; *Integrated Processes:* Teaching and Learning; *Client Need:* Physiological Integrity/Basic Care and Comfort/Rest and Sleep; *Cognitive Level:* Application

Reference: Fortinash, K., & Holoday Worret, P. (2007). *Psychiatric Nursing Care Plans* (5th ed., pp. 109–111). St. Louis, MO: Mosby

---

1472. A nurse is assessing a client with suspected major depression. Which findings would support a diagnosis of major depression? SELECT ALL THAT APPLY.

1. Loss of interest or pleasure nearly daily for at least 2 weeks
2. Presence of psychomotor agitation nearly daily for at least 2 weeks
3. Feelings of worthlessness nearly daily for at least 2 weeks
4. Having a depressed mood nearly daily for at least 2 weeks
5. Talking rapidly with pressured speech nearly daily for at least 2 weeks
6. Impaired concentration nearly daily for at least 2 weeks

ANSWER: 1, 2, 3, 4, 6

Loss of interest or pleasure, psychomotor agitation, feelings of worthlessness, depressed mood, and impaired concentration are symptoms that meet diagnostic criteria for a major depressive disorder. Rapid, pressured speech is a diagnostic criterion for bipolar disorder and not major depressive disorder.

➧ ***Test-taking Tip:*** *Use the process of elimination to eliminate the one option pertaining to bipolar disorder.*

Content Area: Mental Health; *Category of Health Alteration:* Anxiety and Mood Disorders; *Integrated Processes:* Nursing Process Assessment; *Client Need:* Psychosocial Integrity/Mental Health Concepts; *Cognitive Level:* Application

Reference: Townsend, M. (2008). *Essentials of Psychiatric Mental Health Nursing* (4th ed., p. 336). Philadelphia: F. A. Davis.

1473. EBP During a client education class, a nurse is asked: "What is an effective treatment for seasonal affective disorder?" Which intervention should the nurse recommend as an evidence-based practice for the first-line treatment of seasonal effective disorder?

1. A 2-week trial of lithium carbonate
2. Individual therapy with a psychologist
3. Prescribing quetiapine (Seroquel®)
4. Light therapy

ANSWER: 4

Light therapy is an evidence-based practice to use as a first-line treatment for seasonal affective disorder. This intervention has proven effectiveness compared to psychopharmacological treatments in various placebo controls. Lithium carbonate is used to treat bipolar disorder and not seasonal affective disorder. Although there may be situations in which a person with seasonal affective disorder could seek therapy with a psychologist, it is not a first-line treatment intervention. Quetiapine (Seroquel®) is an atypical antipsychotic used for treatment of schizophrenia.

▶ ***Test-taking Tip:*** *Use the process of elimination and review treatments for seasonal affective disorder.*

Content Area: Mental Health; *Category of Health Alteration:* Anxiety and Mood Disorders; *Integrated Processes:* Nursing Process Implementation; *Client Need:* Physiological Integrity/Basic Care and Comfort/Nonpharmacological Comfort Interventions; *Cognitive Level:* Comprehension

Reference: Varcarolis, E., Benner Carson, V., & Shoemaker, N. (2006). *Foundations of Psychiatric Mental Health Nursing* (5th ed., p. 352). St. Louis, MO: Saunders/Elsevier.

EBP Reference: Blumberger, D., & Levitt, M. (2005). The lighter side of treating seasonal affective disorder. *Psychiatric Times,* 22(11), 49. Available at: www.psychiatrictimes.com/print

1474. A client of Latino/Hispanic ethnicity reports of poor appetite, lack of energy, and feeling hopeless nearly every day for the past 3 weeks. An admitting nurse notices that the client does not make eye contact upon questioning. What is the most likely explanation for the client's behavior?

1. The client is suicidal.
2. The client is demonstrating respect.
3. The client is psychotic.
4. The client does not like the nurse.

ANSWER: 2

The most likely explanation for the client's lack of eye contact is that the client is demonstrating respect for the nurse. Persons of Latino/Hispanic ethnicity have traditionally been taught to avoid eye contact with figures of authority as a sign of respect.

▶ ***Test-taking Tip:*** *The key words in the stem are "Latino/Hispanic" and "eye contact." Use the process of elimination and review common practices within the Latino/Hispanic culture.*

Content Area: Mental Health; *Category of Health Alteration:* Anxiety and Mood Disorders; *Integrated Processes:* Nursing Process Analysis; *Client Need:* Psychosocial Integrity/Cultural Diversity; *Cognitive Level:* Analysis

References: Varcarolis, E., Benner Carson, V., & Shoemaker, N. (2006). *Foundations of Psychiatric Mental Health Nursing* (5th ed., p. 184). St. Louis, MO: Saunders/Elsevier; Edelman, C., & Mandle, C. (2006). *Health Promotion Throughout the Life Span* (6th ed., p. 84). St. Louis, MO: Mosby.

1475. A nurse is assessing a client, attempting to differentiate the client's symptoms between delirium and depression. Which symptoms of the client are unique to depression? SELECT ALL THAT APPLY.

1. Sadness
2. Disturbance in sleep patterns
3. Fluctuating levels of consciousness
4. Labile affect
5. Lack of motivation
6. Presence of hallucinations

ANSWER: 1, 5

Clients with depression experience sadness, depression, apathy/lack of motivation, and decreased energy to complete activities. Both clients with depression and clients with delirium experience sleep disturbances, fluctuating levels of consciousness, and labile affect. Presence of hallucinations is associated with delirium, not depression.

▶ ***Test-taking Tip:*** *Use the process of elimination and review signs and symptoms of depression.*

Content Area: Mental Health; *Category of Health Alteration:* Anxiety and Mood Disorders; *Integrated Processes:* Nursing Process Analysis; *Client Need:* Psychosocial Integrity/Psychopathology; *Cognitive Level:* Analysis

Reference: Fortinash, K., & Holoday Worret, P. (2007). *Psychiatric Nursing Care Plans.* (5th ed., pp. 84, 336). St. Louis, MO: Mosby.

1476. EBP A nurse is developing a care plan for an older adult female client diagnosed with depression. The inclusion of the nursing diagnosis *Risk for injury due to osteopenia* demonstrates that the nurse understands which evidence-based concept related to the client's medical diagnosis?

1. Geriatric female clients are more prone to injury.
2. Geriatric female clients diagnosed with depression tend to engage in self-destructive behavior.
3. Geriatric female clients with hip bone loss are at increased risk for depression.
4. Geriatric female clients have a higher incidence of confusion.

ANSWER: 3

Researchers have found a significant relationship between older female clients diagnosed with depression and increased loss of bone density. Options 1, 2, and 4 have no basis for evidence-based conclusions.

➧ ***Test-taking Tip:*** *Select an option that includes both depression and bone loss.*

Content Area: Mental Health; *Category of Health Alteration:* Anxiety and Mood Disorders; *Integrated Processes:* Nursing Process Planning; *Client Need:* Health Promotion and Maintenance/Aging Process; Safe and Effective Care Environment/Safety and Infection Control/Accident and Injury Prevention; *Cognitive Level:* Analysis

EBP Reference: Diem, S., Blackwell, T., & Stone, K. (2007). Depressive symptoms and rates of bone loss at the hip in older women. *Journal American Geriatric Society,* 55(6), 824–831. Available at: www.surgeongeneral.gov/library/bonehealth/Appendix_B.html

1477. A nurse is assessing a client for suspected depression. The client is recently divorced and has a court appearance for a driving while intoxicated (DWI) charge the following week. Which response by the nurse is most therapeutic?

1. "Were you surprised that your spouse left after you got a DWI?"
2. "You aren't thinking about hurting yourself, are you?"
3. "I think you should have a substance abuse evaluation before we treat your depression."
4. "I'm concerned about your drinking. I'd like you to talk with our chemical dependency staff."

ANSWER: 4

Stating concern and referring the client to someone specializing in chemical dependency is the most therapeutic response. The client needs to be assessed for substance abuse/dependence. Response 1 projects a judgmental attitude and is not a helpful comment. Any client with suspected depression should be screened for suicide risk. However, response 2 uses poor therapeutic technique. Response 3 fails to acknowledge that both chemical dependency and depression are considered primary and need simultaneous treatment.

➧ ***Test-taking Tip:*** *The key words are "most therapeutic." Eliminate options that elicit a "yes" or "no" response. Of the two remaining options, select the option that conveys concern and is most direct.*

Content Area: Mental Health; *Category of Health Alteration:* Anxiety and Mood Disorders; *Integrated Processes:* Communication and Documentation; *Client Need:* Psychosocial Integrity/Chemical and other Dependencies; Physiological Integrity/Physiological Adaptation/Illness Management; *Cognitive Level:* Analysis

Reference: Varcarolis, E., Benner Carson, V., & Shoemaker, N. (2006). *Foundations of Psychiatric Mental Health Nursing* (5th ed., p. 564). St. Louis, MO: Saunders/Elsevier.

1478. A nurse is teaching a class to assistive personnel on depression. Which statement(s) by the nurse provide accurate information about depression? SELECT ALL THAT APPLY.

1. Depression is a condition in which behaviors can fluctuate between low mood and euphoria.
2. Women are approximately twice as likely as men to develop depression.
3. The rate of depression among adolescents increases with age.
4. Children in all age groups can become depressed.
5. Symptoms of perfectionism and rigid thought patterns are indicative of depression.

ANSWER: 2, 3, 4

The reasons for gender susceptibility are unclear, with suspected reasons being stress, lifestyle, and hormonal factors. The rate of depression rises after puberty to the late teenage years. Fluctuating mood is characteristic of bipolar disorder and not depression. Perfectionism and rigid thought patterns are characteristic of obsessive-compulsive disorder, not depression.

➧ ***Test-taking Tip:*** *Carefully review the options that discuss behaviors associated with depression and note that these options are different from the other options. Eliminate options 1 and 5 because these behaviors are not characteristic of depression.*

Content Area: Mental Health; *Category of Health Alteration:* Anxiety and Mood Disorders; *Integrated Processes:* Teaching and Learning; *Client Need:* Psychosocial Integrity/Mental Health Concepts; *Cognitive Level:* Application

Reference: Edelman, C., & Mandle, C. (2006). *Health Promotion Throughout the Life Span* (6th ed., p. 515). St. Louis, MO: Mosby.

1479. EBP A nurse is assessing a client's alcohol intake as part of a routine screening examination. The client reports drinking 3 to 4 beers; five times per week. The client is being treated for depression with sertraline (Zoloft®) 100 mg daily. Which statement by the nurse about the client's alcohol consumption is accurate?

1. A moderate amount of alcohol helps the client forget problems and can decrease depression.
2. As long as the client does not exceed five drinks in any 24-hour period, alcohol intake is within normal limits.
3. Alcohol worsens depression and makes treatment of depression more difficult.
4. Alcohol is a stimulant that will help the client be more social.

ANSWER: 3

The nurse is correct when stating that alcohol worsens depression and makes treatment of depression more difficult. Alcohol is a central nervous system depressant. Combining alcohol and prescription medications can increase the risk of adverse effects. Additionally, alcohol blocks neurotransmitter receptor sites, decreasing effectiveness of antidepressant medication. Clients with depression use alcohol as an escape; however, avoiding problems undermines self-esteem and increases stressors which exacerbate depression. NIH guidelines define at-risk drinking as more than 14 drinks per week. Client's alcohol intake of 15–20 beers weekly exceeds that amount. Alcohol is a depressant, not a stimulant; it impairs judgment and increases impulsivity.

▶ *Test-taking Tip: Focus on the key word "accurate." Identify key words in the options ("forget problems," "five drinks in 24 hours," and "a stimulant") that make the option incorrect.*

Content Area: Mental Health; *Category of Health Alteration:* Anxiety and Mood Disorders; *Integrated Processes:* Nursing Process Assessment; *Client Need:* Health Promotion and Maintenance/High Risk Behaviors; *Cognitive Level:* Analysis

Reference: Townsend, M. (2008). *Essentials of Psychiatric Mental Health Nursing* (4th ed., pp. 267–271, 338). Philadelphia: F. A. Davis.

EBP Reference: National Institute on Alcohol Abuse and Alcoholism of the National Institute of Health. (2006). *National Epidemiologic Survey on Alcohol and Related Conditions*. Available at: http://pubs.niaaa.nih.gov/publications/arh29-2/toc29-2.htm

---

1480. EBP A nurse is developing a care plan for a client diagnosed with bipolar disorder. The inclusion of the nursing diagnosis *Risk for imbalanced nutrition* demonstrates that the nurse understands that clients diagnosed with bipolar disorder:

1. are compulsive eaters.
2. often suffer from poor nutrition.
3. have a greater risk for obesity.
4. take medications that can cause weight loss.

ANSWER: 3

Clients diagnosed with bipolar disorder have a greater risk for obesity. There is emerging data concerning weight gain in clients diagnosed with bipolar disorder. The reasons are multifactorial, and a client who understands the concept will be better prepared for self-monitoring and making healthy diet choices. Weight gain is a significant factor in medication noncompliance and relapse. Poor nutrition and compulsive eating are not evidence-based concepts related to bipolar disorder. Mood stabilizers cause weight gain, not weight loss.

▶ *Test-taking Tip: Note that options 3 and 4 are opposites; eliminate one of these options.*

Content Area: Mental Health; *Category of Health Alteration:* Anxiety and Mood Disorders; *Integrated Processes:* Nursing Process Planning; *Client Need:* Physiological Integrity/Basic Care and Comfort/Nutrition and Oral Hydration; Physiological Integrity/Physiological Adaptation/Illness Management; *Cognitive Level:* Analysis

EBP Reference: Simmons-Alling, S., & Talley, S. (2008). Bipolar disorder and weight gain: A multifactorial assessment. *Journal of the American Psychiatric Nurses Association,* 13(6), 345–352. Available at: www.sagepublications.com

---

1481. A client diagnosed with mania tells a nurse, "I think you're very pretty. Maybe we could go to my room." Which response by the nurse is most therapeutic?

1. "It's time for occupational therapy."
2. "That's not appropriate and I'm offended."
3. "I don't have that kind of relationship with clients."
4. "Let's walk down to the seclusion room."

ANSWER: 1

The most therapeutic response by the nurse is to redirect the client. Hypersexual behavior and impulsivity are symptoms of mania. Rather than confront the client or acknowledge the provocative comment, it is more effective to redirect the client as clients with mania are easily distracted. Secluding the client is unnecessary.

▶ *Test-taking Tip: Use the process of elimination with an understanding of the therapeutic responses necessary when working with a client exhibiting symptoms of bipolar disorder/manic state.*

Content Area: Mental Health; *Category of Health Alteration:* Anxiety and Mood Disorders; *Integrated Processes:* Communication and Documentation; *Client Need:* Psychosocial Integrity/Therapeutic Communications; *Cognitive Level:* Analysis

Reference: Fortinash, K., & Holoday Worret, P. (2007). *Psychiatric Nursing Care Plans* (5th ed., pp. 123–124). St. Louis, MO: Mosby.

1482. EBP A nursing assistant (NA) comments to the nurse about a recently admitted client. "I think the new admit is just faking being sick. Yesterday we couldn't get a word out of the client and today the client is talking nonstop." Which response by the nurse is most appropriate in reflecting empathy for the client?

1. "Thanks for letting me know. I think the client is just looking for attention."
2. "Please refer to the client by name and not as the new admission."
3. "The client has a condition called rapid-cycle bipolar disorder; quickly changing moods is part of the illness."
4. "The client has the right to be difficult to assess."

ANSWER: 3

About one in six clients seeking care for bipolar disorder present with a rapid-cycling pattern, with a significantly higher incidence among females. Stating that the client is seeking attention and/or is difficult does not convey client empathy. Although the information is correct in response 2, it is not the best response. Response 4 is likely to illicit defensiveness and a missed teaching opportunity with the NA.

➧ ***Test-taking Tip:*** *Use the process of elimination to select an option that teaches the NA about bipolar disorder.*

Content Area: Mental Health; *Category of Health Alteration:* Anxiety and Mood Disorders; *Integrated Processes:* Caring; Communication and Documentation; *Client Need:* Psychosocial Integrity/Therapeutic Communications; Psychosocial Integrity/Psychopathology; *Cognitive Level:* Analysis

EBP Reference: Antai-Otong, D. (2006). Treatment considerations for patients experiencing rapid-cycling bipolar disorder. *Perspectives in Psychiatric Care,* 42(1), 55–58. Available at: www.healthinternetwork.org

---

1483. A nurse is assessing a recently admitted client who is exhibiting agitation that appears to be related to acute mania. Which action should a nurse plan to utilize when caring for a client experiencing agitation related to acute mania?

1. Apply restraints to prevent the client from harming self or others
2. Involve the client in group activities to provide structure
3. Leave the client alone
4. Maintain a low level of stimuli in the client's environment

ANSWER: 4

Maintaining a low level of stimulation minimizes anxiety, agitation, and suspiciousness. The client should be offered the least restrictive treatment alternative. Restraints should be used as a last resort if other interventions are unsuccessful and the client presents imminent risk of harm to self or others. Group activities could increase level of stimuli and worsen agitation. The client's behavior must be closely observed to ensure safety. Correct nursing action is to stay with the client.

➧ ***Test-taking Tip:*** *Use the process of elimination and review treatment protocols for clients diagnosed with acute mania.*

Content Area: Mental Health; *Category of Health Alteration:* Anxiety and Mood Disorders; *Integrated Processes:* Nursing Process Planning; *Client Need:* Physiological Integrity/Reduction of Risk Potential/Therapeutic Procedures; *Cognitive Level:* Analysis

Reference: Townsend, M. (2008). *Essentials of Psychiatric Mental Health Nursing* (4th ed., p. 357). Philadelphia: F. A. Davis.

1484. A nurse assesses a client who reports feeling full of energy in spite of being awake for the past 48 hours. Which diagnosis is the nurse likely to find documented in the client's medical record?

1. Obsessive-compulsive disorder
2. Bipolar disorder/manic type
3. Bipolar disorder/mixed type
4. Korsakoff's psychosis

ANSWER: 2

The symptoms of increased psychomotor activity with diminished need for sleep are suggestive of bipolar disorder of the manic type. The client is not reporting recurrent and persistent thoughts or impulses. There is no mention of mood fluctuations of both depression and mania. The symptoms of confusion, loss of recent memory, and confabulation would be present in Korsakoff's psychosis.

➧ ***Test-taking Tip:*** *Use the process of elimination and review symptoms of bipolar disorder, manic type.*

Content Area: Mental Health; *Category of Health Alteration:* Anxiety and Mood Disorders; *Integrated Processes:* Nursing Process Analysis; *Client Need:* Psychosocial Integrity/Psychopathology; *Cognitive Level:* Application

Reference: Townsend, M. (2008). *Essentials of Psychiatric Mental Health Nursing* (4th ed., p. 356). Philadelphia: F. A. Davis.

1485. EBP A nurse observes that a client diagnosed with major depressive disorder who recently started on an antidepressant is acting differently. Two days ago, the client appeared sad and remained in bed. Now the client is awake at 4 a.m. and planning a unit party. What is the most likely explanation for the change in behavior?

1. The client is responding positively to the antidepressant.
2. The client was misdiagnosed and what was thought to be a depression is bipolar disorder.
3. The client is more familiar with the unit milieu and is able to be self-expressive.
4. The client is happy because the client expects to be discharged soon.

ANSWER: 2

The clinical presentation of unipolar and bipolar depression can be similar and both conditions should be considered when making treatment choices. Clients receiving an antidepressant without a concurrent mood stabilizer can have a manic episode precipitated. Option 1 could be correct if the client had been receiving an antidepressant for 3 to 4 weeks. The phrase of "recently started" would rule out this choice. The information given does not support the conclusions in options 3 or 4.

▸ ***Test-taking Tip:*** *Use the process of elimination and review signs/symptoms of depression and bipolar disorder. Review effects of antidepressant medication.*

Content Area: Mental Health; *Category of Health Alteration:* Anxiety and Mood Disorders; *Integrated Processes:* Nursing Process Analysis; *Client Need:* Psychosocial Integrity/Psychopathology; Physiological Integrity/Physiological Adaptation/Unexpected Response to Therapies; *Cognitive Level:* Analysis.

Reference: Varcarolis, E., Benner Carson, V., & Shoemaker, N. (2006). *Foundations of Psychiatric Mental Health Nursing* (5th ed., p. 347). St. Louis, MO: Saunders/Elsevier.

EBP Reference: Hirschfield, R., & Cass, A. (2005). Screening for bipolar disorder in patients treated for depression in a family medicine clinic. *Journal of American Board of Family Practice,* 18(4), 233–239. Available at: www.jabfp.org

1486. A nurse is assessing a client recently admitted to a psychiatric unit who is experiencing acute mania. Which nursing action should the nurse plan when caring for a client with acute mania?

1. Sustain conversations to improve the client's concentration.
2. Provide finger foods that the client can carry while moving around the unit.
3. Teach the client and family about available community resources.
4. Help the family understand that anger directed at them is likely to escalate unless they confront the client's behavior.

ANSWER: 2

Provide finger foods as nutritional status may be compromised because of hyperactive behaviors. This strategy provides a convenient method for eating and maintaining nutritional integrity for clients who may be too distracted to sit down for a meal. Conversations should be brief while the client is hypomanic or manic to minimize confusion and frustration. Client and family teaching about community resources is an appropriate nursing action but is not appropriate at this time (acute mania). Client's anger is likely to be transitory and will improve as mania subsides. Family should avoid sensitive or volatile topics while the client is in a manic phase.

▸ ***Test-taking Tip:*** *Use the process of elimination to eliminate options that will worsen the client's mania.*

Content Area: Mental Health; *Category of Health Alteration:* Anxiety and Mood Disorders; *Integrated Processes:* Nursing Process Planning; *Client Need:* Physiological Integrity/Basic Care and Comfort/Reduction of Risk Potential; *Cognitive Level:* Analysis

Reference: Fortinash, K., & Holoday Worret, P. (2007). *Psychiatric Nursing Care Plans* (5th ed., p. 93). St. Louis, MO: Mosby.

1487. A nurse is caring for a client diagnosed with acute mania. The nurse observes coarse hand tremors and learns that the client's serum lithium level is 1.8 mEq/L. Which action should be taken by the nurse?

1. Continue to administer lithium as ordered.
2. Advise the client to limit fluids.
3. Withhold the medication and notify the physician.
4. Acknowledge that the side effects are unpleasant.

ANSWER: 3

The nurse should withhold the medication and notify the physician. Lithium is at a toxic level. This is a medical emergency requiring rapid treatment. Limiting fluids would worsen lithium toxicity. Coarse hand tremor is a symptom of lithium toxicity. not an unpleasant side effect.

▸ ***Test-taking Tip:*** *Focus on the symptoms of lithium toxicity to select the correct option.*

Content Area: Mental Health; *Category of Health Alteration:* Anxiety and Mood Disorders; *Integrated Processes:* Nursing Process Implementation; *Client Need:* Physiological Integrity/Pharmacological and Parenteral Therapies/Adverse Effects/Contradictions/Interactions; *Cognitive Level:* Analysis

Reference: Varcarolis, E., Benner Carson, V., & Shoemaker, N. (2006). *Foundations of Psychiatric Mental Health Nursing* (5th ed., p. 506). St. Louis, MO: Saunders/Elsevier.

1488. A nurse is teaching an education class to clients with mild to moderate anxiety. Which teaching strategies should the nurse practice when educating the clients? SELECT ALL THAT APPLY.

1. Maintain a calm, nonthreatening manner.
2. Create an atmosphere of low stimuli.
3. Encourage the client to verbalize thoughts and feelings that could contribute to symptoms of anxiety.
4. Reinforce reality by focusing on the "here and now."
5. Limit the length of class time and the amount of provided information.
6. Create an environment free from hazardous objects that the client could use to cause harm.

ANSWER: 1, 2, 3, 5

A client with anxiety develops a sense of security when in the presence of a calm staff person. A client's anxiety level may increase in a stimulating environment. A client's verbalization of thoughts and feelings can assist in understanding and managing anxiety symptoms. A client with anxiety has a decreased attention span and diminished level of concentration. Reinforcing reality is a teaching strategy used with a thought disorder for a psychotic condition. Self-harming behavior in a client with mild to moderate anxiety would not be commonly present.

Test-taking Tip: *Use the process of elimination and review therapeutic approaches to working with clients diagnosed with anxiety.*

Content Area: Mental Health; *Category of Health Alteration:* Anxiety and Mood Disorders; *Integrated Processes:* Teaching and Learning; *Client Need:* Health Promotion and Maintenance/Principles of Teaching and Learning; *Cognitive Level:* Application

Reference: Townsend, M. (2008). *Nursing Diagnoses in Psychiatric Nursing* (pp. 149–150). Philadelphia: F. A. Davis.

1489. A nurse is admitting a client diagnosed with generalized anxiety disorder. During the client's assessment, the nurse determines that which findings would be consistent with generalized anxiety disorder? SELECT ALL THAT APPLY

1. Expansive mood with pressured speech
2. Restlessness or feeling keyed up or on edge
3. Difficulty controlling the anxiety
4. Irritability
5. Muscle tension

ANSWER: 2, 3, 4, 5

Restlessness or feeling keyed up, difficulty controlling anxiety, irritability, and muscle tension are DSM-IV criteria for generalized anxiety. Expansive mood and pressured speech are symptoms of bipolar disorder, not generalized anxiety.

Test-taking Tip: *Eliminate an option that relates to bipolar disorder.*

Content Area: Mental Health; *Category of Health Alteration:* Anxiety and Mood Disorders; *Integrated Processes:* Nursing Process Assessment; *Client Need:* Psychosocial Integrity/Psychopathology *Cognitive Level:* Application

Reference: Townsend, M. (2008). *Essentials of Psychiatric Mental Health Nursing* (4th ed., p. 382). Philadelphia: F. A. Davis.

1490. A recently discharged veteran reports symptoms of recurring intrusive thoughts, insomnia, and hypervigilance. Which mental health diagnosis would a nurse suspect for this client?

1. Narcolepsy
2. Posttraumatic stress disorder
3. Trichotillomania disorder
4. Obsessive compulsive disorder

ANSWER: 2

The reported symptoms are consistent with the diagnosis of posttraumatic stress disorder and are often present with veterans who have been exposed to combat trauma. Narcolepsy is a disorder that produces excessive sleepiness. Trichotillomania disorder is defined as the recurrent pulling out of one's own hair. Obsessive-compulsive disorder is characterized by involuntary recurring thoughts, but is not characterized by hypervigilance.

Test-taking Tip: *Focus on the fact that the client is a recently discharged veteran and the common disorder associated with trauma.*

Content Area: Mental Health; *Category of Health Alteration:* Anxiety and Mood Disorders; *Integrated Processes:* Nursing Process Assessment; *Client Need:* Psychosocial Integrity/Psychopathology; *Cognitive Level:* Application

Reference: Townsend, M. (2008). *Nursing Diagnoses in Psychiatric Nursing* (p. 146). Philadelphia: F. A. Davis.

1491. A client tells a nurse about an intense fear of dogs that causes the client to avoid visiting others unless it is confirmed that there are no dogs on the premises. The client further explains that these fears seem unreasonable, but the fear continues in spite of this acknowledgment. Based on the client's report, which conclusion by the nurse is accurate?

1. The client has a recognized fear, but there is no evidence of psychopathology.
2. A fear that is recognized as excessive and unreasonable is a DSM-IV criterion for phobias.
3. True phobias are rare in the general population.
4. Phobias begin in childhood and are diagnosed more often in men.

ANSWER: 2

Marked fear cued by the presence or anticipation of a specific object (e.g., dogs), recognition that the fear is excessive, and avoidance of the object/situation are diagnostic criteria for a specific phobia. The client's symptoms meet diagnostic criteria for a psychopathological disorder. Specific phobias frequently occur concurrently with other anxiety disorders and are common among the general population. Phobias can occur at any age. The disorder is diagnosed more often in women than in men. While phobias are common, people seldom seek treatment unless the phobia interferes with their ability to function.

➧ ***Test-taking Tip:*** *Look for similar words in the question and the options. Use the process of elimination and review DSM-IV criteria for phobias.*

Content Area: Mental Health; *Category of Health Alteration:* Anxiety and Mood Disorders; *Integrated Processes:* Nursing Process Analysis; *Client Need:* Psychosocial Integrity/Psychopathology; *Cognitive Level:* Analysis

Reference: Townsend, M. (2008). *Essentials of Psychiatric Mental Health Nursing* (4th ed., p. 388). Philadelphia: F. A. Davis.

1492. A client diagnosed with an anxiety disorder tells a nurse that being in crowds creates thoughts of losing control and the need to hurriedly leave. What should the nurse recommend as an effective, nonpharmacological therapy for managing the client's symptoms of anxiety?

1. Cognitive behavioral therapy (CBT)
2. Electroconvulsive therapy (ECT)
3. Family systems therapy
4. Psychoanalytical therapy

ANSWER: 1

Cognitive behavioral therapy is a treatment that focuses on patterns of thinking that are maladaptive and would be an effective choice for the described symptoms. Electroconvulsive therapy is primarily used as an intervention for major depression. Family systems therapy is an intervention warranted when a client's symptoms signal the presence of dysfunction within the whole family. Psychoanalytic therapy focuses on repressed conflicts that are both conscious and unconscious.

➧ ***Test-taking Tip:*** *The key words are "anxiety" and "crowds." Eliminate any option that includes multiple individuals.*

Content Area: Mental Health; *Category of Health Alteration:* Anxiety and Mood Disorders; *Integrated Processes:* Nursing Process Implementation; *Client Need:* Safe and Effective Care Environment/ Management of Care/Consultation; *Cognitive Level:* Application

Reference: Fortinash, K., & Holoday Worret, P. (2007). *Psychiatric Nursing Care Plans* (5th ed., pp. 37, 90, 471). St. Louis, MO: Mosby.

Test 39: **Mental Health: Cognitive, Schizophrenic, and Psychotic Disorders**

1493. A nurse engages an older adult client by describing the weather as "raining cats and dogs." The client looks bewildered and shows concern for the "animals." The nurse determines that the client is exhibiting concrete thinking. Which response by the nurse is most therapeutic?

1. Assure the client that the animals are not being hurt in any way.
2. Explain to the client that it is a way of saying it is raining heavily.
3. Alert the staff to the client's inability to understand abstract concepts.
4. Document the client's response to the conversation as concrete thinking.

ANSWER: 2

The most therapeutic response is to explain to the client that "raining cats and dogs" is a way of saying that it is raining heavily. A client who continually gives literal translations to verbal communication is exhibiting concrete thinking. Due to the client's inability to think in the abstract, care must be taken to avoid conversations that include abstract concepts. The nurse should attempt to clarify any confusion for the client. Even though option 1 addresses the client's concern for the well-being of the animals, it does not clarify the statement of "raining cats and dogs." While the staff needs to be aware of the client's limitation in understanding the abstract, alerting the staff does not address the issue of presenting information for the client in an acceptable manner. Documentation of the client's limitations is appropriate but does not address the issue of clarification of ideas and information.

➧ ***Test-taking Tip:*** *The key phrase is "most therapeutic." Eliminate options 3 and 4 because these are not therapeutic responses. Option 1 would falsely reinforce the idea that the cats and dogs are real; therefore, option 2 is the logical response.*

Content Area: Mental Health; *Category of Health Alteration:* Cognitive, Schizophrenic, and Psychotic Disorders; *Integrated Process:* Communication and Documentation; *Client Needs:* Psychosocial Integrity/Mental Health Concepts; *Cognitive Ability:* Application

Reference: Videbeck, S. (2006). *Psychiatric Mental Health Nursing* (3rd ed., p. 156). Philadelphia: Lippincott Williams & Wilkins.

1494. A nurse is assessing a 78-year-old postoperative client who is exhibiting signs of delirium. The nurse observes that the client is convinced that it is 1954 and is complaining about "the bugs in this hotel." The nurse's priority intervention should be to:

1. obtain a prn order for haloperidol (Haldol®).
2. transfer the client to a room near the nursing station.
3. call the client's family to come and stay with the client.
4. arrange for an unlicensed sitter to stay with the client.

ANSWER: 4

The nurse's priority intervention should be to arrange for someone to stay with the client. The client's immediate safety is the primary concern, and constant observation is the best means of providing a safe environment for this client. While medication may become appropriate, it should not be the first response to manage a client's behavior. It does not address the issue of observing the client for safety. Transferring the client closer to the nursing station does not provide the constant observation that is most appropriate for the client at this time. Asking the client's family to stay may not be a realistic expectation.

➧ ***Test-taking Tip:*** *Use Maslow's Hierarchy of Needs theory to determine the priority action. Client safety is always a high priority. Determine which option provides for the most thorough, reasonable, and speedy means of addressing the client's safety needs.*

Content Area: Mental Health; *Category of Health Alteration:* Cognitive, Schizophrenic, and Psychotic Disorders; *Integrated Process:* Nursing Process Implementation; *Client Needs:* Psychosocial Integrity/Behavioral Interventions; *Cognitive Ability:* Analysis

Reference: Mohr, W. (2006). *Psychiatric-Mental Health Nursing* (6th ed., pp. 726–734). Philadelphia: Lippincott Williams & Wilkins.

1495. A nurse is visiting the home of a client diagnosed with Alzheimer's disease. The nurse assesses the stress level of the client's spouse, the primary caregiver. Which question is most appropriate for assessing the spouse's stress level?

1. "So, what is a typical day like for you?"
2. "What do you do to relieve stress for yourself?"
3. "May I arrange for some part-time help for you?"
4. "Being a full-time caregiver must be very stressful, isn't it?"

ANSWER: 1

The nurse should ask the client's wife to describe a typical day. Using an open-ended questioning technique provides the client's wife with an opportunity to share any information she feels appropriate. Based on the information provided, the nurse can then ask questions that are more specific to the areas of concern. Option 2 presumes that the client's wife is experiencing stress and may cause her to become defensive. Option 3 is a close-ended question that limits the discussion. Option 4 again presumes that the wife is experiencing stress and limits discussion since it requires only a yes or no answer.

Test-taking Tip: *Focus on the issue of the question; the spouse's stress level. Select an option that uses therapeutic communication techniques to assess the stress level.*

Content Area: Mental Health; *Category of Health Alteration:* Cognitive, Schizophrenic, and Psychotic Disorders; *Integrated Process:* Nursing Process Assessment; *Client Needs:* Psychosocial Integrity/Coping Mechanisms; *Cognitive Ability:* Application

Reference: Mohr, W. (2006). *Psychiatric-Mental Health Nursing* (6th ed., pp. 65–76, 763–764). Philadelphia: Lippincott Williams & Wilkins.

1496. Which goals should be included in the plan of care for a client with dementia? SELECT ALL THAT APPLY.

1. The client will remain physically safe.
2. The client will receive emotional support.
3. The client will receive physical health care.
4. The client will show cognitive improvement.
5. The client will function at highest level of independence.
6. The client will perform activities of daily living independently.

ANSWER: 1, 2, 3, 5

The care of a client with dementia should include provisions for physical and emotional well-being and safety. The nurse should encourage and support the client's independence within the limit of his or her abilities. Alzheimer-type dementia is characterized by a progressive loss of both physical and cognitive function. Therefore, improvement and/or independent living are not realistic goals.

Test-taking Tip: *Use the process of elimination to eliminate options that are inconsistent with the diagnosis.*

Content Area: Mental Health; *Category of Health Alteration:* Cognitive, Schizophrenic, and Psychotic Disorders; *Integrated Process:* Nursing Process Planning; *Client Needs:* Psychosocial Integrity/Sensory/Perceptual Alterations; *Cognitive Ability:* Analysis

Reference: Mohr, W. (2006). *Psychiatric-Mental Health Nursing* (6th ed., p. 742). Philadelphia: Lippincott Williams & Wilkins.

1497. A client diagnosed with delirium is restrained in order to prevent the removal of a Foley catheter and an intravenous fluid line. Which response should the nurse expect after the client is restrained?

1. The client rests better at night.
2. The client becomes visibly agitated.
3. The client requires less pain medication.
4. The client experiences a decrease in blood pressure.

ANSWER: 2

The nurse should expect to observe the client becoming visibly agitated. Being physically restrained can be a humiliating and demoralizing experience. Typical responses to physical restraint include anger, anxiety, fear, depression, and stress-related responses. The client is more likely to be restless and experience insomnia with the potential for increased agitation, fear, and anxiety resulting in a heightened sense of pain. With the potential for increased agitation, fear, and anxiety, the client is more likely to have an increase in blood pressure.

Test-taking Tip: *The key words are "delirium" and "restrained." Focus on the responses most likely to occur when a client with delirium is restrained. Use the process of elimination and knowledge related to the effects of restraints and the care of the cognitively impaired.*

Content Area: Mental Health; *Category of Health Alteration:* Cognitive, Schizophrenic, and Psychotic Disorders; *Integrated Process:* Nursing Process Planning; *Client Needs:* Psychosocial Integrity/Behavioral Interventions; Safe and Effective Care Environment/Safety and Infection Control/Use of Restraints/Safety Devices; *Cognitive Ability:* Analysis

Reference: Varcarolis, E., Carson, V., & Shoemaker, N. (2006). *Foundations of Psychiatric Mental Health Nursing: A Clinical Approach* (5th ed., p. 701). St. Louis, MO: Saunders.

1498. A nurse is assessing a client recently admitted into a psychiatric unit for observation. Which client behavior is indicative of impaired cognition?

1. Mumbling
2. Asking repeatedly, "How did I get here?"
3. Spending hours staring out the window
4. Discussing "the voices" with another client

ANSWER: 2

The client's disorientation is indicative of impaired cognition. Cognitive impairment can affect an individual's orientation to person, place, time, or memory of recent events. Mumbling is observed in clients with impaired cognition, but it can be a response to any number of situations, including anger, bewilderment, or experiencing hallucinations. Staring is seen in clients with impaired cognition, but it can be a response to any number of situations including fatigue and/or attempts at social isolation. Clients experiencing impaired cognition do not typically experience auditory hallucinations.

➧ ***Test-taking Tip:*** *Focus on selecting the option that indicates that the client's orientation is impaired. Use the process of elimination and knowledge related to impaired cognition.*

Content Area: Mental Health; *Category of Health Alteration:* Cognitive, Schizophrenic, and Psychotic Disorders; *Integrated Process:* Nursing Process Assessment; *Client Needs:* Psychosocial Integrity/ Sensory/Perceptual Alterations; *Cognitive Ability:* Analysis

Reference: Varcarolis, E., Carson, V., & Shoemaker, N. (2006). *Foundations of Psychiatric Mental Health Nursing: A Clinical Approach* (5th ed., pp. 422–430). St. Louis, MO: Saunders.

1499. A nurse is caring for a client who states, "Lately I'm getting forgetful about things. I'm so afraid I'm getting Alzheimer's disease." Which response by the nurse is most therapeutic?

1. "Now, I don't think we really need to discuss this. I'm sure it is just normal aging."
2. "I'm forgetful, too. I have to make lists to remember everything."
3. "Although it's not unusual to experience some lapses of memory, let's discuss your concerns."
4. "Oh, what you are describing isn't Alzheimer's disease. It's much more complicated than that."

ANSWER: 3

The nurse is most therapeutic when attempting to discuss the client's concerns. With regard to memory functioning, the normal older adult will find that the time required for memory scanning is longer for both recent and remote memory recall. Dementia associated with Alzheimer's disease has a slow and insidious onset and is generally progressive and deteriorating in its course. The remaining responses provide false reassurance, which devalues the client's feelings, belittles valid concerns, and discourages the expression of feelings due to the anticipation of ridicule.

➧ ***Test-taking Tip:*** *The key phrase is "most therapeutic." Select the option that uses therapeutic communication techniques.*

Content Area: Mental Health; *Category of Health Alteration:* Cognitive, Schizophrenic, and Psychotic Disorders; *Integrated Process:* Communication and Documentation; *Client Needs:* Psychosocial Integrity/Therapeutic Communications; *Cognitive Ability:* Application

Reference: Varcarolis, E., Carson, V., & Shoemaker, N. (2006). *Foundations of Psychiatric Mental Health Nursing: A Clinical Approach* (5th ed., pp. 430–436). St. Louis, MO: Saunders.

1500. A nurse is caring for a client with a self-care deficit who exhibits behaviors associated with dementia. Which goals should be included in the plan of care for this client? SELECT ALL THAT APPLY.

1. The client will be provided with unlimited time to care for personal needs.
2. The client will consistently function at the highest possible level of personal independence.
3. The client will consistently complete all daily hygiene needs independently.
4. The client will receive assistance with daily hygiene needs by nursing staff.
5. The client's unmet hygiene needs will be addressed by members of the institution's multidisciplinary health-care team.
6. The client's family will receive instructions on supporting the client's independence and promoting self-care in regard to daily hygiene.

ANSWER: 2, 5, 6

The client's goals should be to function on the highest level of personal independence. The client's needs should be addressed by a team of health-care professionals with expertise in the areas related to the client. Supporting the family to encourage the client's independence contributes to the client's sense of control and well-being. While support in the form of sufficient time is appropriate, this response fails to address the fact that the client may never reach total independence. Assuming that the client will reach total independence may not be realistic. Not allowing for client autonomy by assisting with daily needs is not directed toward the client's best interest.

➧ ***Test-taking Tip:*** *Use the process of elimination and focus on knowledge regarding the care of the cognitively impaired.*

Content Area: Mental Health; *Category of Health Alteration:* Cognitive, Schizophrenic, and Psychotic Disorders; *Integrated Process:* Nursing Process Planning; *Client Needs:* Psychosocial Integrity/ Psychopathology; Physiological Integrity/Basic Care and Comfort/Personal Hygiene; *Cognitive Ability:* Analysis

Reference: Varcarolis, E., Carson, V., & Shoemaker, N. (2006). *Foundations of Psychiatric Mental Health Nursing: A Clinical Approach* (5th ed., p. 441). St. Louis, MO: Saunders.

1501. A cognitively impaired nursing home resident is beginning to show physical signs of agitation. Which activity would be most therapeutic to de-escalate the client's agitation?

1. Playing bingo with other residents
2. Spending time alone in the client's room
3. Taking a walk outside with the nurse
4. Watching television in the presence of staff

ANSWER: 3

The most therapeutic activity would be to take a walk with the nurse. Structured activities will provide the client with a release for physical tension as well as an opportunity to build a trusting relationship with the nurse. Bingo is competitive, which may accelerate the client's agitation and thus place the client and the other residents in a potentially unsafe environment. The other responses fail to provide a structured outlet to promote de-escalation.

► ***Test-taking Tip:*** *The key phrase is "most therapeutic." Use the process of elimination and focus on knowledge of impaired cognition, anger management, and therapeutic interventions to minimize the physical effects of agitation.*

Content Area: Mental Health; *Category of Health Alteration:* Cognitive, Schizophrenic, and Psychotic Disorders; *Integrated Process:* Nursing Process Implementation; *Client Needs:* Psychosocial Integrity/Behavioral Interventions; Safe and Effective Care Environment/Safety and Infection Control/Accident and Injury Prevention; *Cognitive Ability:* Analysis

Reference: Varcarolis, E., Carson, V., & Shoemaker, N. (2006). *Foundations of Psychiatric Mental Health Nursing: A Clinical Approach* (5th ed., pp. 439–446). St. Louis, MO: Saunders.

1502. A client is displaying behaviors consistent with stage 2 Alzheimer's disease. The client can no longer recognize family members and requires assistance with personal hygiene and dressing. The client is frequently incontinent of both urine and feces and displays violent outbursts during these times. Which nursing diagnoses should the nurse give highest priority to when developing the client's care plan?

1. Violence: directed at self or others
2. Incontinence: both bowel and bladder
3. Self-care deficient: hygiene, dressing, toileting
4. Altered thought processes with impaired memory

ANSWER: 1

The nurse should give the highest priority to diagnoses of violence. Safety is the first priority for any client. The client's memory loss and violent outbursts pose safety issues for both the client and others. While the other diagnoses are appropriate for this client, they do not have priority over the client's safety and the safety of others.

► ***Test-taking Tip:*** *The key phrase is "highest priority." Use the process of elimination and Maslow's Hierarchy of Needs theory to prioritize. Focus on nursing interventions directed toward ensuring client safety, especially of the cognitively impaired client.*

Content Area: Mental Health; *Category of Health Alteration:* Cognitive, Schizophrenic, and Psychotic Disorders; *Integrated Process:* Nursing Process Analysis; *Client Needs:* Psychosocial Integrity/Mental Health Concepts; Safe and Effective Care Environment/Safety and Infection Control/Accident and Injury Prevention; *Cognitive Ability:* Analysis

Reference: Varcarolis, E., Carson, V., & Shoemaker, N. (2006). *Foundations of Psychiatric Mental Health Nursing: A Clinical Approach* (5th ed., pp. 439–446, 449). St. Louis, MO: Saunders.

1503. A home health nurse caring for a client diagnosed with Alzheimer's disease is attempting to determine whether the client's daughter understands the client's prognosis. Which of the daughter's questions to the nurse will most accurately assess the daughter's understanding of Alzheimer's disease and its prognosis?

1. "What types of support services are available?"
2. "What can we do to improve our father's memory?"
3. "How long does it take for his medication to help?"
4. "Which local hospital has the best treatment program?"

ANSWER: 1

The daughter's question about support services indicates an understanding that her father will experience increased cognitive impairment that will require the support of outside personnel and/or agencies. While current drug therapy delays the progressive deterioration of cognitive function, there may not be any apparent improvement for this chronic, irreversible, progressive disease. Therefore, questions related to improving memory and medications do not elicit the needed response. Being able to identify the best treatment program does not mean that the daughter understands the disease.

► ***Test-taking Tip:*** *The key phrase is "most accurately." Use the process of elimination and focus on knowledge of Alzheimer's disease to identify the family member's question that most accurately represents understanding of the chronic, progressive nature of the disease.*

Content Area: Mental Health; *Category of Health Alteration:* Cognitive, Schizophrenic, and Psychotic Disorders; *Integrated Process:* Nursing Process Evaluation; *Client Needs:* Psychosocial Integrity/Psychopathology; *Cognitive Ability:* Analysis

Reference: Varcarolis, E., Carson, V., & Shoemaker, N. (2006). *Foundations of Psychiatric Mental Health Nursing: A Clinical Approach* (5th ed., pp. 439–446). St. Louis, MO: Saunders.

1504. EBP A nurse is discussing discharge plans with a homeless client diagnosed with paranoid schizophrenia. What is the primary factor that will affect the formulation of the discharge plan for this client?

1. The formulation of a support system for the homeless client
2. The nurse's ability to work effectively with the homeless client
3. The homeless client's ability to comply with the discharge plan
4. The existence of community resources such as homeless shelters

ANSWER: 2

Research has identified that a nurse–client relationship that is accepting, trusting, and mutually respectful is the most important factor in the therapeutic treatment of the homeless client. Compliance of a client with paranoid delusions is especially dependent on the ability to trust the health-care provider and the information and services he or she provides. While a strong, effective support system is important to any client with similar needs, the formulation of a therapeutic discharge plan is not solely dependent on it. While the availability of needed services and community acceptance is vital to discharge planning, it is not the primary factor in the formulation of an appropriate, effective discharge plan.

Test-taking Tip: *The key term is "primary factor." Use the process of elimination to select the option that best implies knowledge of the needs of a homeless client diagnosed with paranoid schizophrenia.*

Content Area: Mental Health; *Category of Health Alteration:* Cognitive, Schizophrenic, and Psychotic Disorders; *Integrated Process:* Nursing Process Planning; *Client Needs:* Psychosocial Integrity/Mental Health Concepts; *Cognitive Ability:* Analysis

References: Varcarolis, E., Carson, V., & Shoemaker, N. (2006). *Foundations of Psychiatric Mental Health Nursing: A Clinical Approach* (5th ed., pp. 163–169, 578). St. Louis, MO: Saunders; Boyd, M. A. (2005). *Psychiatric Nursing: Contemporary Practice* (3rd ed., pp. 712–725). Philadelphia: Lippincott Williams & Wilkins.

EBP Reference: Bonin, E., Brehove, T., Kline, S., Misgen, M., Post, P., et al. (2004). *Adapting Your Practice: General Recommendations for the Care of Homeless Patients.* Nashville, TN: Health Care for the Homeless Clinicians' Network, National Health Care for the Homeless Council. Available at: www.guideline.gov/summary/summary.aspx?doc_id=5272&nbr=003599&string=homeless+AND+mental+AND+illness#s23

1505. A client recently prescribed haloperidol (Haldol®) complains of severe muscle pain. Assessment findings include a heart rate of 104 beats per minute, blood pressure of 172/92 mm Hg, and an oral temperature of 101.2°F (38.4°C). Based on the assessment findings, what is the most appropriate nursing action?

1. Question the client concerning known cardiovascular health status.
2. Assure the client that the symptoms are unrelated to the new medication.
3. Immediately notify the client's health-care provider of the assessment findings and complaints.
4. Gather information concerning the client's possible exposure to a bacterial infection.

ANSWER: 3

Immediate notification of the health-care provider regarding the signs and symptoms is the most appropriate intervention for the client at this time. The assessment data combined with the use of haloperidol (Haldol®), an antipsychotic medication, suggest the possibility of a life-threatening condition called neuroleptic malignant syndrome (NMS). NMS is manifested by severe muscle spasms, muscle rigidity, hypertension, fever, and tachycardia. While the symptoms would indicate a possible cardiac problem, questioning the client does not address the immediate seriousness of the potential problem. Assuring the client is inappropriate because NMS is possible with the use of antipsychotic medication. The nurse should never ignore symptoms of tachycardia, hypertension, or hyperthermia. Although a bacterial infection may result in some of the symptoms, it would not account for the hypertension and severe muscle pain.

Test-taking Tip: *The key phrase is "most appropriate." Use the process of elimination and select the option that best relates to the nursing action that recognizes the potential side effects of antipsychotic medications as well as the seriousness of NMS.*

Content Area: Mental Health; *Category of Health Alteration:* Cognitive, Schizophrenic, and Psychotic Disorders; *Integrated Process:* Nursing Process Assessment; *Client Needs:* Psychosocial Integrity/Mental Health Concepts; Physiological Integrity/Pharmacological and Parenteral Therapies/Adverse Effects/Contraindications/Interactions; *Cognitive Ability:* Analysis

Reference: Mohr, W. (2006). *Psychiatric-Mental Health Nursing* (6th ed., p. 641). Philadelphia: Lippincott Williams & Wilkins.

1506. A nurse is assessing the mood and cognitive state of mind of a client diagnosed with schizophrenia. Which signs and symptoms is the nurse most likely to observe? SELECT ALL THAT APPLY.

1. Poor appetite
2. Disrupted sleep
3. Poor concentration
4. Incongruous affect
5. Compulsive behavior
6. Involuntary muscle movement

ANSWER: 1, 2, 3, 4

A client with schizophrenia can exhibit various signs and symptoms related to altered mood, affect, behavior, and cognitive status. A poor appetite, disturbed sleep patterns, and difficulty concentrating can all be indicators of depression, which is a common manifestation in such a client. The client may also exhibit inappropriateness in the expression of an emotion, such as giggling when describing a sad experience. While obsessive-compulsive behavior indicates a personality disorder, it does not relate to either mood or cognitive state of mind. The presence of involuntary, abnormal muscular movements known as tardive dyskinesia is not an indicator of mood or cognitive state of mind but rather a side effect of antipsychotic medication therapy.

➧ ***Test-taking Tip:*** *The key phrase is "most likely." Use the process of elimination to select the options that are generally identified as assessment findings indicative of schizophrenia.*

Content Area: Mental Health; *Category of Health Alteration:* Cognitive, Schizophrenic, and Psychotic Disorders; *Integrated Process:* Nursing Process Assessment; *Client Needs:* Psychosocial Integrity/ Mental Health Concepts; Safe and Effective Care Environment/Safety and Infection Control/Accident and Injury Prevention; *Cognitive Ability:* Analysis

Reference: Mohr, W. (2006). *Psychiatric-Mental Health Nursing* (6th ed., pp. 631, 640, 645). Philadelphia: Lippincott Williams & Wilkins.

1507. A nurse is educating a client diagnosed with schizophrenia on appropriate measures to help prevent the relapse of schizophrenic symptoms. Which interventions should the nurse encourage the client to use to help prevent symptom relapse? SELECT ALL THAT APPLY.

1. Ignore auditory hallucinations.
2. Engage in regular physical exercise.
3. Report changes in sleeping patterns.
4. Enroll in stress-management classes.
5. Avoid drinking alcoholic beverages.
6. Avoid employment that is demanding.

ANSWER: 2, 3, 4, 5

The nurse should educate the client on the recognition and management of the symptoms of a relapse. Maintaining good physical health through stress management, exercise, diet, and adequate sleep are important in the prevention of a relapse, as are the avoidance of alcohol and nonprescribed drugs. The client will need to intervene when hallucinations occur. While a client will need to recognize and manage stress, there is no known therapeutic value in avoiding certain types of employment.

➧ ***Test-taking Tip:*** *The key phrase is "appropriate measures." Look for the key words in the options "ignore," "engage," "report," "avoid," "enroll," and "avoid," respectively. Select the options that are positive in nature. Of the negative options, determine if these are appropriate measures in this specific scenario.*

Content Area: Mental Health; *Category of Health Alteration:* Cognitive, Schizophrenic, and Psychotic Disorders; *Integrated Process:* Nursing Process Planning; *Client Needs:* Psychosocial Integrity/Mental Health Concepts; *Cognitive Ability:* Analysis

Reference: Mohr, W. (2006). *Psychiatric-Mental Health Nursing* (6th ed., pp. 628, 643, 650, 652). Philadelphia: Lippincott Williams & Wilkins.

1508. A nurse is reviewing with the client's father the discharge plan of a client recently diagnosed with paranoid schizophrenia. Which of the father's statements indicates to the nurse that he understands the diagnoses and prognosis of paranoid schizophrenia?

1. "We will need to watch for signs of depression."
2. "He won't get worse if he continues to take his medication."
3. "There is a good chance that this will be his only hospitalization."
4. "We will need to keep him at home so we can monitor his illness closely."

ANSWER: 1

The nurse should determine that the father understands the risks of depression in relation to the client's diagnosis. Clients diagnosed with schizophrenia are at high risk for suicide when suffering from depression. While medication compliance is an important factor in managing paranoid schizophrenia, it does not guarantee an eradication of symptoms. Although there have been incidences of a sole schizophrenic episode, the course of this condition typically includes periods of exacerbation and remission of symptoms. The client diagnosed with schizophrenia will function best with a treatment plan that encourages independence within the capabilities of the client. A lifestyle that is too restrictive is likely to result in rebellion and noncompliance.

➧ ***Test-taking Tip:*** *Use the process of elimination to select the option that best reflects an understanding of schizophrenia and its relationship to depression.*

Content Area: Mental Health; *Category of Health Alteration:* Cognitive, Schizophrenic, and Psychotic Disorders; *Integrated Process:* Nursing Process Evaluation; *Client Needs:* Psychosocial Integrity/ Psychopathology; *Cognitive Ability:* Analysis

Reference: Mohr, W. (2006). *Psychiatric-Mental Health Nursing* (6th ed., pp. 634–635). Philadelphia: Lippincott Williams & Wilkins.

1509. The mother of a client diagnosed with paranoid schizophrenia visiting her son 2 days after his admission to the psychiatric unit approaches a nurse and states, "He is still talking about how the government is controlling his thoughts." What is the most accurate nursing appraisal of the mother's statement?

1. The mother's expectations of her son are realistic.
2. The mother's concern is reasonable.
3. The mother should request a medication adjustment.
4. The mother requires further education regarding the client's diagnosis.

ANSWER: 4

The nurse should assess that the mother needs further education regarding the client's diagnosis. Two days is not enough time for the client to experience the therapeutic benefits of treatment for paranoid schizophrenia. Improvement of symptoms usually occurs between 5 and 9 days. Expecting improvement in 2 days is not a realistic or reasonable expectation. A request for medication adjustment reflects a need to provide the mother with appropriate information related to her son's condition.

▶ ***Test-taking Tip:*** *The key phrase is "most accurate." Use the process of elimination and apply understanding of schizophrenia and its treatment outcomes.*

Content Area: Mental Health; *Category of Health Alteration:* Cognitive, Schizophrenic, and Psychotic Disorders; *Integrated Process:* Nursing Process Evaluation; *Client Needs:* Psychosocial Integrity/ Psychopathology; *Cognitive Ability:* Analysis

Reference: Mohr, W. (2006). *Psychiatric-Mental Health Nursing* (6th ed., pp. 619–656). Philadelphia: Lippincott Williams & Wilkins.

1510. A nurse is developing a plan of care for a client prescribed the traditional antipsychotic drug haloperidol (Haldol®) for the treatment of schizophrenia. Which medication should the nurse expect to administer if extrapyramidal side effects develop?

1. Olanzapine (Zyprexa®)
2. Benztropine (Cogentin®)
3. Chlorpromazine (Thorazine®)
4. Escitalopram oxalate (Lexapro®)

ANSWER: 2

Benztropine is an anticholinergic drug that is the drug of choice to control the extrapyramidal side effects caused by traditional antipsychotic medications. Olanzapine is an atypical antipsychotic drug that can cause extrapyramidal side effects. Chlorpromazine is in the same drug classification as haloperidol. Escitalopram oxalate is a selective serotonin reuptake inhibitor used to treat depression.

▶ ***Test-taking Tip:*** *Use the process of elimination and focus on the antidote for extrapyramidal side effects caused by traditional antipsychotic drugs used as pharmacological interventions for the treatment of schizophrenia.*

Content Area: Mental Health; *Category of Health Alteration:* Cognitive, Schizophrenic, and Psychotic Disorders; *Integrated Process:* Nursing Process Planning; *Client Needs:* Psychosocial Integrity/ Psychopathology; Physiological Integrity/Pharmacological and Parenteral Therapies/Expected Actions or Outcomes; *Cognitive Ability:* Analysis

Reference: Mohr, W. (2006). *Psychiatric-Mental Health Nursing* (6th ed., pp. 639–642). Philadelphia: Lippincott Williams & Wilkins.

1511. A client admitted to a behavioral medicine unit with a diagnosis of catatonic schizophrenia is constantly rearranging furniture and appears to be responding to internal stimuli. In addition to being free of physical injury during phases of hyperactivity, which short-term goal is appropriate for this client?

1. The client will sleep at least 6 hours per night.
2. The client will consume adequate food and fluid per day.
3. The client will engage in at least one client-to-client interaction daily.
4. The client will show decreased activity within 24 hours of onset of hyperactivity.

ANSWER: 2

The excited phase of catatonic schizophrenia is marked by periods of extreme activity and potential violent behavior. The primary nursing focus for the client during this phase is to prevent both physical exhaustion and injury. Nursing interventions should be directed toward providing adequate food and fluids and maintaining a safe, low-stimulus environment. The client needs constant monitoring and regular assessments to assure his nutritional, fluid, and safety needs are met. The remaining responses may not be realistic for the client at this time.

▶ ***Test-taking Tip:*** *Use the process of elimination and Maslow's Hierarchy of Needs theory to identify the correct responses. Prevention of exhaustion is a key issue.*

Content Area: Mental Health; *Category of Health Alteration:* Cognitive, Schizophrenic, and Psychotic Disorders; *Integrated Process:* Nursing Process Analysis; *Client Needs:* Psychosocial Integrity/ Psychopathology; *Cognitive Ability:* Analysis

Reference: Varcarolis, E., Carson, V., & Shoemaker, N. (2006). *Foundations of Psychiatric Mental Health Nursing: A Clinical Approach* (5th ed., pp. 414–416). St. Louis, MO: Saunders.

1512. A nurse includes the nursing diagnosis of *Disturbed thought processes secondary to paranoia* in the care plan for a newly admitted client diagnosed with schizophrenia. Which approach is most appropriate for this client?

1. Avoid laughing or whispering in front of the client.
2. Begin to identify social supports in the community.
3. Encourage the client to interact with others on the unit.
4. Have the client sign a written release of information form.

ANSWER: 1

The client is experiencing paranoia and is distrustful and suspicious of others. Laughing or whispering in front of the client would only serve to increase the client's suspicions. The client is not ready to identify information concerning community support. Asking the client to trust and to share personal information with strangers is unachievable at this time. Having the client sign a release may not be appropriate due to the client's current level of awareness.

Test-taking Tip: *The key phrase is "most appropriate." Use the process of elimination and focus on nursing interventions appropriate for the stated nursing diagnosis and psychiatric disorder.*

Content Area: Mental Health; *Category of Health Alteration:* Cognitive, Schizophrenic, and Psychotic Disorders; *Integrated Process:* Nursing Process Planning; *Client Needs:* Psychosocial Integrity/Psychopathology; *Cognitive Ability:* Application

Reference: Varcarolis, E., Carson, V., & Shoemaker, N. (2006). *Foundations of Psychiatric Mental Health Nursing: A Clinical Approach* (5th ed., p. 400). St. Louis, MO: Saunders.

1513. A nurse is discussing the importance of taking medication as prescribed with a client diagnosed with paranoid schizophrenia. Which response demonstrates that the nurse understands the importance of relapse prevention?

1. "Take your medications as ordered and you will not relapse."
2. "Your overall mental health will suffer with each relapse that occurs."
3. "Your medication may cause some side effects, but they will be mild."
4. "Contact your mental-health-care provider if the side effects become severe."

ANSWER: 2

The nurse should understand that with each relapse of psychosis, there is an increase in residual mental dysfunction and general mental deterioration. None of the remaining responses deal with the impact of relapse prevention.

Test-taking Tip: *The key word is "demonstrates." Use the process of elimination; only one option deals with the impact of a relapse.*

Content Area: Mental Health; *Category of Health Alteration:* Cognitive, Schizophrenic, and Psychotic Disorders; *Integrated Process:* Nursing Process Evaluation; *Client Needs:* Psychosocial Integrity/Psychopathology; *Cognitive Ability:* Application

Reference: Varcarolis, E., Carson, V., & Shoemaker, N. (2006). *Foundations of Psychiatric Mental Health Nursing: A Clinical Approach* (5th ed., p. 388). St. Louis, MO: Saunders.

1514. A nurse is evaluating a client diagnosed with paranoid schizophrenia who reports hearing a voice that says, "Do not remove your hat because they will be able to read your mind." Which response by the nurse is the most therapeutic?

1. "Who are 'they'?"
2. "Why would someone want to read your mind?"
3. "I do not believe that anyone can read another's mind."
4. "It must be very frightening to believe that someone can read your mind."

ANSWER: 4

It is most therapeutic for the nurse to empathize with the client's experience while engaging in therapeutic communication to discuss the true root of the client's concern. The main characteristic of paranoid schizophrenia is the presence of persecutory or grandiose delusions and hallucinations. Discussion concerning the hallucination itself has no therapeutic value. Disagreeing with the client may prompt the client to become defensive and thus hinder therapeutic communication between the nurse and client.

Test-taking Tip: *The key phrase is "most therapeutic." Use the process of elimination and focus on therapeutic communication with the paranoid client.*

Content Area: Mental Health; *Category of Health Alteration:* Cognitive, Schizophrenic, and Psychotic Disorders; *Integrated Process:* Nursing Process Implementation; *Client Needs:* Psychosocial Integrity/Therapeutic Communications; Safe and Effective Care Environment/Safety and Infection Control/Accident and Injury Prevention; *Cognitive Ability:* Application

Reference: Varcarolis, E., Carson, V., & Shoemaker, N. (2006). *Foundations of Psychiatric Mental Health Nursing: A Clinical Approach* (5th ed., pp. 400–402, 412–414). St. Louis, MO: Saunders.

1515. A client, who is experiencing both positive and negative symptoms of schizophrenia, is prescribed an atypical antipsychotic, risperidone (Risperdal®). The client asks the nurse to explain the common side effects of this medication. Which side effects should the nurse state to the client? SELECT ALL THAT APPLY.

1. Dizziness
2. Dystonia
3. Drowsiness
4. Weight gain
5. Constipation
6. Hypotension

ANSWER: 1, 3, 4, 5, 6

Risperidone is an atypical antipsychotic that blocks dopamine and serotonin blockers in the brain. It also has anticholinergic, antihistaminic, and alpha-adrenergic-blocking abilities. Common side effects include dizziness, drowsiness, weight gain, constipation, and hypotension. Dystonia (severe muscle spasm) is not a common side effect of atypical antipsychotic medications.

Test-taking Tip: *Use the process of elimination and focus on the side effects most commonly experienced when taking the atypical antipsychotic classification of drugs.*

Content Area: Mental Health; *Category of Health Alteration:* Cognitive, Schizophrenic, and Psychotic Disorders; *Integrated Process:* Teaching and Learning; *Client Need:* Physiological Integrity/Pharmacological and Parenteral Therapies/Adverse Effects/Contraindications/Interactions; *Cognitive Ability:* Application

Reference: Mohr, W. (2006). *Psychiatric-Mental Health Nursing* (6th ed., pp. 267, 641). Philadelphia: Lippincott Williams & Wilkins.

1516. A nurse is assessing a client diagnosed with a history of paranoid schizophrenia and chronic alcohol abuse. The client has been taking olanzapine (Zyprexa®) for 2 weeks and has not consumed alcohol in the last 5 days. The client reports shaky hands and trouble sleeping because of frequent nightmares. The client is concerned that the olanzapine is causing the problems. Which is the most therapeutic response given by the nurse?

1. "These are not typical side effects for that drug."
2. "Just ignore the symptoms. They will go away in just a few days."
3. "These symptoms are more likely a result of not drinking alcohol for 5 days."
4. "It is possible, since this medication is contraindicated in those who abuse alcohol."

ANSWER: 3

Nightmares and tremors are common in alcohol withdrawal, not as side effects of olanzapine. Olanzapine is more likely to cause sleeplessness, nausea, dizziness, constipation, weight gain, and headache. Dismissing the symptoms is not a therapeutic approach to the client's concerns. If the client were currently drinking alcohol, there might be an additive effect, but this is not true because the client is abstaining.

Test-taking Tip: *The key phrase is "most therapeutic." Use the process of elimination and focus on the therapeutic medication management of clients with a history of both schizophrenia and alcohol abuse. Understanding of the common side effects of both alcohol withdrawal and olanzapine are vital to the selection of the correct option.*

Content Area: Mental Health; *Category of Health Alteration:* Cognitive, Schizophrenic, and Psychotic Disorders; *Integrated Process:* Nursing Process Implementation; *Client Needs:* Psychosocial Integrity/Psychopathology; Physiological Integrity/Pharmacological Therapy/Adverse Effects/Contraindications/Interactions; *Cognitive Ability:* Analysis

Reference: Mohr, W. (2006). *Psychiatric-Mental Health Nursing* (6th ed., pp. 641–642, 698). Philadelphia: Lippincott Williams & Wilkins.

1517. A nurse is evaluating a client experiencing paranoid delusions. The client states, "Two men wearing gray shirts keep coming into the dayroom and watching me." Which of the nurse's responses is most therapeutic when communicating to a client with paranoid delusions?

1. "What makes you think they are interested in you?"
2. "I don't believe you have anything to worry about."
3. "Ignore them, and let's select a movie to watch after dinner."
4. "Those are maintenance personnel discussing the room remodeling."

ANSWER: 4

The primary intervention is directed toward therapeutic communication between the nurse and client that will help the client identify and express the reason(s) for anxiety while reinforcing reality. The remaining responses appear to support or ignore the client's delusion, fail to provide reinforcement of reality, and do not provide an opportunity to discuss the root of the client's true fears.

Test-taking Tip: *The key phrase is "most therapeutic." Use the process of elimination and focus on the therapeutic management of clients experiencing hallucinations and/or delusions.*

Content Area: Mental Health; *Category of Health Alteration:* Cognitive, Schizophrenic, and Psychotic Disorders; *Integrated Process:* Communication and Documentation; *Client Needs:* Psychosocial Integrity/Sensory/Perceptual Alterations; *Cognitive Ability:* Analysis

Reference: Mohr, W. (2006). *Psychiatric-Mental Health Nursing* (6th ed., p. 647). Philadelphia: Lippincott Williams & Wilkins.

1518. A client who is experiencing paranoid delusions asks a nurse to turn off the television stating, "It controls my thoughts." Which is the most appropriate intervention by the nurse?

1. Refuse the request in order to show control over the client.
2. Comply with the request in order to lessen the client's concerns/fears.
3. Comply with the request to show an understanding of the client's concerns/fears.
4. Refuse the request to avoid supporting the client's delusions.

ANSWER: 4

The most appropriate intervention is to empathize with the client's concerns/fears while making it clear that the nurse does not share the client's delusional thought pattern. This client's delusion does not pose any immediate threat to the nurse's ability to provide a safe, therapeutic setting. The most therapeutic response is one that shows empathy without reinforcing the delusion.

➧ ***Test-taking Tip:*** *Examine options with duplicate information first (options 1 and 4, and then 2 and 3). Eliminate one of each of these to narrow the options.*

Content Area: Mental Health; *Category of Health Alteration:* Cognitive, Schizophrenic, and Psychotic Disorders; *Integrated Process:* Caring; Nursing Process Implementation; *Client Needs:* Psychosocial Integrity/Psychopathology; *Cognitive Ability:* Analysis

Reference: Mohr, W. (2006). *Psychiatric-Mental Health Nursing* (6th ed., p. 650). Philadelphia: Lippincott Williams & Wilkins.

1519. A nurse observes a client with a history of violent command hallucinations mumbling erratically while making threatening gestures directed toward a particular staff member. Which nursing intervention is most appropriate when working with a client with violent command hallucinations?

1. Ask the client to explain the cause of anger.
2. Place the client in seclusion to help de-escalate anger.
3. Inform the client of pending restraint if behavior does not subside.
4. Observe the client for signs of escalating agitation.

ANSWER: 1

When dealing with a client who is hallucinating, the most appropriate intervention is for the nurse to empathize with the client's experience while engaging in therapeutic communication to discuss the root of the client's concern. Asking the client to explain the cause of the anger is client centered and focuses on the behavior. Seclusion is used only as a last resort and in cases of client/milieu safety. Being argumentative by threatening restraint may cause the client to escalate the inappropriate behavior. Observation does nothing to control and/or de-escalate the situation.

➧ ***Test-taking Tip:*** *The key phrase is "most appropriate." Use the process of elimination and focus on the therapeutic management of clients experiencing hallucinations and/or delusions with emphasis on the safety of both the client and those individuals toward whom the violence may be directed.*

Content Area: Mental Health; *Category of Health Alteration:* Cognitive, Schizophrenic, and Psychotic Disorders; *Integrated Process:* Nursing Process Implementation; *Client Needs:* Psychosocial Integrity/Psychopathology; Safe and Effective Care Environment/Safety and Infection Control/Accident and Injury Prevention; *Cognitive Ability:* Analysis

Reference: Varcarolis, E., Carson, V., & Shoemaker, N. (2006). *Foundations of Psychiatric Mental Health Nursing: A Clinical Approach* (5th ed., pp. 397–402, 466). St. Louis, MO: Saunders.

1520. A nurse is reviewing with the family the discharge plan of a client diagnosed with paranoid schizophrenia. A family member asks, "What should I do if the voices come back again?" Which nurse response is most appropriate when advising the family member of what to do during a relapse of paranoid schizophrenia?

1. "Be sure that the client keeps all follow-up appointments."
2. "I will provide you with a list of emergency crisis centers."
3. "Stay with the client and use the distracting techniques we have discussed."
4. "Here is the behavior medicine unit's telephone number: call if there is a problem."

ANSWER: 2

The most appropriate response is for the nurse to provide a list of centers that are prepared to provide immediate crisis intervention for a client experiencing hallucinations. A crisis may occur between appointments and require immediate professional counseling. Distracting the client may only serve to exacerbate the hallucinations. Providing the unit's telephone number does not guarantee immediate crisis intervention.

➧ ***Test-taking Tip:*** *The key phrase is "most appropriate." Use the process of elimination as well as an understanding of the management of a schizophrenic relapse to select the option that is most likely to result in the appropriate, safe management of schizophrenic symptoms.*

Content Area: Mental Health; *Category of Health Alteration:* Cognitive, Schizophrenic, and Psychotic Disorders; *Integrated Process:* Nursing Process Planning; *Client Need:* Psychosocial Integrity/Crisis Intervention; *Cognitive Ability:* Analysis

Reference: Varcarolis, E., Carson, V., & Shoemaker, N. (2006). *Foundations of Psychiatric Mental Health Nursing: A Clinical Approach* (5th ed., pp. 402, 464–466). St. Louis, MO: Saunders.

1521. A nurse is evaluating a client who threatens suicide. The nurse's primary responsibility to the client is to provide a safe, therapeutic environment. Which nursing intervention is most effective in establishing a safe environment for the client?

1. Keep the client involved in structured activities with other clients as directed by the staff.
2. Assign a staff member to stay with the client and provide constant observation.
3. Place the client in a seclusion room designed to minimize stimulation.
4. Remove all potential items that could assist the client in committing suicide.

ANSWER: 2

The most effective nursing intervention to ensure the client is in a safe environment is for the nurse to assign a staff member to constantly observe the client. The client should not be involved in structured activities with others because undivided attention of staff is required in order to reduce or eliminate the risk of suicide. Seclusion should not be considered as an initial intervention since it is the most restrictive of the responses. While removing items that would aid is an act of self-harm, it does not provide the degree of safety that constant one-on-one observation provides.

Test-taking Tip: *The key phrase is "most effective." Use the process of elimination as well as an understanding of the management of a safe and effective milieu, including suicide precautions, to select the option that is most likely to result in the safest environment for this client.*

Content Area: Mental Health; *Category of Health Alteration:* Cognitive, Schizophrenic, and Psychotic Disorders; *Integrated Process:* Nursing Process Planning; *Client Need:* Psychosocial Integrity/Therapeutic Environment; *Cognitive Ability:* Analysis

Reference: Varcarolis, E., Carson, V., & Shoemaker, N. (2006). *Foundations of Psychiatric Mental Health Nursing: A Clinical Approach* (5th ed., pp. 481–482). St. Louis, MO: Saunders.

1522. A nurse attempts to explain to a client who has been experiencing paranoid delusions that laboratory blood work has been ordered. The client begins to shout, "You all just want to drain my blood. Get away from me!" Which nursing response is most therapeutic?

1. "I'll leave and come back later when you are calmer."
2. "What makes you think that I want to drain your blood?"
3. "You know I am not going to hurt you; I am here to help you!"
4. "It must be extremely frightening to think others want to hurt you."

ANSWER: 4

It is most therapeutic for the nurse to empathize with the client's experience while engaging in therapeutic communication to discuss the true root of the client's concern. Leaving avoids the client's concerns. Asking the client to provide a rationale for the fear, being argumentative, or avoiding the client's concerns are not examples of therapeutic communication.

Test-taking Tip: *The key phrase is "most therapeutic." Use the process of elimination and an understanding of therapeutic communication techniques related to the client experiencing delusions to select the option that is likely to result in the greatest positive impact on the client's mental state.*

Content Area: Mental Health; *Category of Health Alteration:* Cognitive, Schizophrenic, and Psychotic Disorders; *Integrated Process:* Communication and Documentation; *Client Needs:* Psychosocial Integrity/Therapeutic Communications; *Cognitive Ability:* Analysis

Reference: Varcarolis, E., Carson, V., & Shoemaker, N. (2006). *Foundations of Psychiatric Mental Health Nursing: A Clinical Approach* (5th ed., pp. 179–193, 412–414). St. Louis, MO: Saunders.

1523. A client experiencing paranoid delusions tells a nurse that "The foreigner who lives next to me wants to kill me." Which nursing response is most therapeutic to assist the client experiencing paranoid delusions?

1. "Do you feel afraid that people are trying to hurt you?"
2. "That's not true. I'm sure your neighbor is a nice person."
3. "What makes you think your neighbor wants to kill you?"
4. "You believe that your foreign neighbor really wants to kill you?"

ANSWER: 1

When communicating with a client with paranoid delusions, the most appropriate response is for the nurse to empathize with the client's experience while engaging in therapeutic communication to discuss the true root of the client's concern. Asking if the client is afraid is client centered and focuses on the paranoia. Disagreeing with the client may make the client more defensive and thus interfere with therapeutic communication. Encouraging discussion only about the delusion is nontherapeutic.

Test-taking Tip: *The key phrase is "most therapeutic." Use the process of elimination and an understanding of therapeutic communication techniques related to the client experiencing delusions to select the option that is likely to result in the greatest positive impact on the client's mental state.*

Content Area: Mental Health; *Category of Health Alteration:* Cognitive, Schizophrenic, and Psychotic Disorders; *Integrated Process:* Nursing Process Implementation; *Client Needs:* Psychosocial Integrity/Sensory/Perceptual Alterations; *Cognitive Ability:* Analysis

Reference: Varcarolis, E., Carson, V., & Shoemaker, N. (2006). *Foundations of Psychiatric Mental Health Nursing: A Clinical Approach* (5th ed., pp. 179–193, 412–414). St. Louis, MO: Saunders.

1524. A client has a history of hallucinations and is at risk to harm self or others. In preparing the client for discharge, a nurse provides instructions regarding interventions directed toward managing hallucinations and anxiety. Which statement indicates that the client has an appropriate understanding of the instructions?

1. "Anxiety is not a typical side effect of my medications."
2. "I should call my therapist when I'm experiencing hallucinations."
3. "I'll learn a lot about my condition by meeting with my support group."
4. "If I eat well and get enough sleep, I will be less likely to hear the voices."

ANSWER: 2

The client should be aware of the importance of discussing hallucinations as they occur with the therapist. There may be an increased risk for impulsive and/or aggressive behavior if a client is experiencing hallucinations, resulting in harm to self or others. Calling the therapist is a specific agreement to seek help and evidences self-responsible commitment and control over one's own behavior. The remaining responses do not provide any specific intervention for the management of hallucinations and/or anxiety.

Test-taking Tip: *Use the process of elimination to select the only option that provides a specific intervention for hallucinations.*

Content Area: Mental Health; *Category of Health Alteration:* Cognitive, Schizophrenic, and Psychotic Disorders; *Integrated Process:* Nursing Process Evaluation; *Client Needs:* Psychosocial Integrity/ Sensory/Perceptual Alterations; Safe and Effective Care Environment/ Safety and Infection Control/Accident and Injury Prevention; *Cognitive Ability:* Analysis

Reference: Varcarolis, E., Carson, V., & Shoemaker, N. (2006). *Foundations of Psychiatric Mental Health Nursing: A Clinical Approach* (5th ed., p. 402). St. Louis, MO: Saunders.

1525. A nurse observes a client who has a history of aggressive behavior toward others swearing and kicking the furniture in the dayroom. Based on the client's behavior, what should be the nurse's immediate priority of care?

1. De-escalate the client's agitation.
2. Provide for a safe, therapeutic milieu.
3. Assess the client's agitation level.
4. Eliminate the source of agitation.

ANSWER: 2

The safety of both the client and staff is a nursing priority. It is important for the nurse to ensure a safe environment for the client as well as for staff and other clients. The remaining responses are client centered and only address the individual client's needs.

Test-taking Tip: *The key phrase is "immediate priority." Use the process of elimination and Maslow's Hierarchy of Needs theory to prioritize the options. Focus on nursing interventions directed toward ensuring client safety.*

Content Area: Mental Health; *Category of Health Alteration:* Cognitive, Schizophrenic, and Psychotic Disorders; *Integrated Process:* Nursing Process Implementation; *Client Need:* Psychosocial Integrity/ Therapeutic Environment; *Cognitive Ability:* Analysis

Reference: Varcarolis, E., Carson, V., & Shoemaker, N. (2006). *Foundations of Psychiatric Mental Health Nursing: A Clinical Approach* (5th ed., pp. 493–500). St. Louis, MO: Saunders.

1526. A nurse is observing a client in a catatonic state. The client is lying in the bed in a fetal position. Which nursing interventions are appropriate in caring for a client in a catatonic state? SELECT ALL THAT APPLY.

1. Assess for safety every 15 minutes.
2. Move the client into the dayroom.
3. Sit quietly beside the client's bed.
4. Encourage client-to-client interaction.
5. Ask occasional open-ended questions.
6. Assign staff to attempt social communication.

ANSWER: 3, 5

A client experiencing catatonic stupor may be immobile and mute; however, the client still requires constant monitoring for safety. While social communication is not possible, therapeutic communication with such a withdrawn client should be maintained since it is believed that the catatonic client is aware of surroundings. Appropriate interventions include the establishment of interpersonal contact and evaluation of safety. The nurse facilitates both safety and communication with the client by sitting in silence and occasionally asking open-ended questions while pausing to provide opportunities for the client to respond. The client should not be left alone or moved into the dayroom since evaluation of safety could not then be assured. The client is not capable of client-to-client interaction. While potentially addressing safety, the nurse is responsible for therapeutic communication and should not assign staff to attempt social communication.

Test-taking Tip: *Use the nursing process and eliminate assessments because the question is asking for interventions. Safety and therapeutic communication are key issues.*

Content Area: Mental Health; *Category of Health Alteration:* Cognitive, Schizophrenic, and Psychotic Disorders; *Integrated Process:* Nursing Process Implementation; *Client Need:* Psychosocial Integrity/ Therapeutic Environment; *Cognitive Ability:* Application

Reference: Varcarolis, E., Carson, V., & Shoemaker, N. (2006). *Foundations of Psychiatric Mental Health Nursing: A Clinical Approach* (5th ed., pp. 414–416). St. Louis, MO: Saunders.

1527. A nurse is assessing a client with a history of aggressive behavior toward others. Which client behavior requires immediate nursing intervention?

1. Refusing to attend a mandatory group session on the unit
2. Stating, "The guy over there needs to sit down and shut up."
3. Petitioning the staff to extend recreation time by 30 minutes
4. Crying while talking on the telephone with family

ANSWER: 2

Making an overtly aggressive statement presents a clear risk to the safety of the other clients as well as to the milieu in general and requires immediate intervention by the nurse. While refusing to attend a mandatory group session requires the nurse's intervention, it does not have the priority of a risk to the safety of others on the unit. Petitioning for the modification of a perceived unfair regulation is a healthy, socially acceptable attempt at change. Crying is an expression of grief not typically of aggression.

➧ ***Test-taking Tip:*** *The key word is "immediate." Note that one option is different from the others.*

Content Area: Mental Health; *Category of Health Alteration:* Cognitive, Schizophrenic, and Psychotic Disorders; *Integrated Process:* Nursing Process Assessment; *Client Needs:* Psychosocial Integrity/Crisis Intervention; Safe and Effective Care Environment/Safety and Infection Control/Accident and Injury Prevention; *Cognitive Ability:* Analysis

Reference: Mohr, W. (2006). *Psychiatric-Mental Health Nursing* (6th ed., pp. 645–650). Philadelphia: Lippincott Williams & Wilkins.

Test 40: **Mental Health: Crisis, Violence, Eating and Sleep Disorders**

1528. A nurse is caring for a client who was violently raped 3 months ago and has a diagnosis of rape-trauma syndrome. Which assessment findings associated with rape-trauma syndrome should a nurse anticipate? SELECT ALL THAT APPLY.

1. Phobias
2. Anorexia
3. Flashbacks
4. Hypertension
5. Sexual promiscuity
6. Migraine headaches

ANSWER: 1, 2, 3, 6

Effects of rape-trauma syndrome begin to occur 2 to 3 weeks after the rape. Symptoms include intrusive thoughts, increased motor activity, increased emotional instability, and fears and phobias. Hypertension may be a result of long-term stress, but it is not recognized as a symptom of rape-trauma syndrome. Fear of sexual encounters rather than excessive sexual activity is a recognized symptom of rape-trauma syndrome.

▶ ***Test-taking Tip:*** *Use the process of elimination to choose the options that represent classic symptoms of rape-trauma syndrome.*

Content Area: Mental Health; *Category of Health Alteration:* Crisis, Violence, Eating, and Sleep Disorders; *Integrated Processes:* Nursing Process Assessment; *Client Need:* Psychosocial Integrity/Mental Health Concepts; *Cognitive Level:* Analysis

Reference: Varcarolis, E., Carson, V., & Shoemaker, N. (2006). *Foundations of Psychiatric Mental Health Nursing: A Clinical Approach* (5th ed., p. 533). St. Louis, MO: Saunders/Elsevier.

1529. A nurse and family members are discussing the treatment goals of a client with a history of drug abuse who is admitted to an acute behavioral medicine unit. The client is experiencing a psychiatric crisis. Which goal should a nurse identify as priority?

1. Successful detoxification of the client
2. Returning client to precrisis level of function
3. Providing the client with effective coping resources
4. Identification of any underlying physical health issues

ANSWER: 2

While the treatment plan may include several goals, the primary goal of crisis intervention is always the return of the client to precrisis level of function. Detoxification and providing effecting coping resources are directed toward treatment of the underlying condition—drug abuse. Identification of an underling health issue is directed toward attaining physical health; it is not a goal of crisis intervention.

▶ ***Test-taking Tip:*** *Use the process of elimination to select the only option directly related to the client's crisis behavior.*

Content Area: Mental Health; *Category of Health Alteration:* Crisis, Violence, Eating, and Sleep Disorders; *Integrated Processes:* Nursing Process Planning; *Client Need:* Psychosocial Integrity/Crisis Intervention; *Cognitive Level:* Application

Reference: Varcarolis, E., Carson, V., & Shoemaker, N. (2006). *Foundations of Psychiatric Mental Health Nursing: A Clinical Approach* (5th ed., p. 459). St. Louis, MO: Saunders/Elsevier.

1530. EBP A nurse is unavoidably late in changing the dressing on a client's leg. The client reacts by becoming verbally aggressive and telling the nurse, "None of you can be trusted. You all just make promises you never intend to keep." The nurse's initial action should be to:

1. alert other staff to the client's apparent escalation.
2. ask the client why he is overreacting to the situation.
3. apologize to the client for being late with the treatment.
4. advise the client that interaction with nursing staff will continue when the client has regained control.

ANSWER: 3

By apologizing for being late with the treatment, the nurse is validating the client's distress and acknowledging his or her role in creating the situation. If the client does not de-escalate, the nurse should then alert the staff. The nurse should first validate the client's feelings and also be careful to use wording that will not alienate the client. The nurse should first validate and then attempt to communicate with the client.

▶ ***Test-taking Tip:*** *Note the key word "initial," and then use the process of elimination and understanding of the nursing role in the de-escalation of an angry client to select the correct option.*

Content Area: Mental Health; *Category of Health Alteration:* Crisis, Violence, Eating, and Sleep Disorders; *Integrated Processes:* Nursing Process Implementation; *Client Need:* Psychosocial Integrity/Crisis Intervention; *Cognitive Level:* Analysis

Reference: Varcarolis, E., Carson, V., & Shoemaker, N. (2006). *Foundations of Psychiatric Mental Health Nursing: A Clinical Approach* (5th ed., p. 495). St. Louis, MO: Saunders/Elsevier.

EBP Reference: National Institute for Clinical Excellence. (2005). *Violence: The Short-Term Management of Disturbed/Violent Behavior in Psychiatric In-Patient Settings and Emergency Departments.* Available at: www.guideline.gov/summary/summary.aspx?doc_id=6570&nbr=004132&string=De-escalation

1531. EBP A young client with a history of drug abuse is admitted to the emergency department after threatening to commit suicide. The client is becoming more agitated as well as physically and verbally abusive to the nursing staff. The priority nursing diagnosis should be:

1. ineffective coping.
2. risk for suicide.
3. risk for self-directed violence.
4. risk for other-directed violence.

ANSWER: 2

While all the options are appropriate for this client, the verbalized threat to commit suicide takes precedence over all other client issues. Although appropriate, the remaining options do not address the client's most serious health issue—threat to commit suicide.

➧ ***Test-taking Tip:*** *Note the key word "priority" in determining the order of severity of the client's physical and psychological issues. By doing so, option 2 should be selected because the client's death is the focal issue.*

Content Area: Mental Health; *Category of Health Alteration:* Crisis, Violence, Eating, and Sleep Disorders; *Integrated Processes:* Nursing Process Analysis; *Client Need:* Psychosocial Integrity/Crisis Intervention; *Cognitive Level:* Application/Analysis

Reference: Varcarolis, E., Carson, V., & Shoemaker, N. (2006). *Foundations of Psychiatric Mental Health Nursing: A Clinical Approach* (5th ed., p. 479). St. Louis, MO: Saunders/Elsevier.

EBP Reference: Substance Abuse and Mental Health Services Administration. (2006). *An Overview of Psychological and Biomedical Issues During Detoxification.* Available at: www.guideline.gov/summary/summary.aspx?doc_id=9117&nbr=004931&string=substance+AND+abuse

1532. A nurse is preparing to document a client's violent episode. Which statements should be included specifically about the violent episode? SELECT ALL THAT APPLY.

1. Client refused to voluntarily enter into seclusion.
2. Client stated, "All of you are just evil people."
3. Client's wife called during escalation cycle.
4. Attempts to identify the cause of client's agitation failed.
5. Five staff members responded to "emergency code."
6. Client asked to leave seclusion room after 30 minutes.

ANSWER: 1, 2, 4, 6

Documentation of a client's violent cycle must include observations of client behavior during the entire cycle, all nursing interventions used and the client's response to the interventions, and how the client was reintegrated into the unit's milieu. The fact that the client received a telephone call during the event does not reflect on the circumstances of the event, and so it does not need to be documented. The number of individuals responding to the emergency need not be documented.

➧ ***Test-taking Tip:*** *Note the key word "specifically." Eliminate options that do not pertain specifically to the violent episode.*

Content Area: Mental Health; *Category of Health Alteration:* Crisis, Violence, Eating, and Sleep Disorders; *Integrated Processes:* Communication and Documentation; *Client Need:* Psychosocial Integrity/Crisis Intervention; *Cognitive Level:* Analysis

Reference: Varcarolis, E., Carson, V., & Shoemaker, N. (2006). *Foundations of Psychiatric Mental Health Nursing: A Clinical Approach* (5th ed., p. 498). St. Louis, MO: Saunders/Elsevier.

1533. To assure that quality care is provided during a client's violent episode, which information should be included in a debriefing session? SELECT ALL THAT APPLY.

1. Client's coping mechanisms post-event
2. The client's history of violent behavior
3. A review of preassault interventions
4. The need for additional/remedial staff training
5. Adherence to instructional policies and procedures
6. Staff feelings regarding the effectiveness of the team

ANSWER: 3, 4, 5, 6

Areas to be included in staff debriefings include team effectiveness and readiness to respond and manage the event, adherence to facility policies and procedures, and staff's ability to respond to the client therapeutically postevent. The client's coping mechanisms and history for violence are not generally pertinent to the postevent debriefing.

➧ ***Test-taking Tip:*** *Apply understanding of appropriate staff management of a violent event. Use the process of elimination to eliminate options that pertain specifically just to the client.*

Content Area: Mental Health; *Category of Health Alteration:* Crisis, Violence, Eating, and Sleep Disorders; *Integrated Processes:* Nursing Process Implementation; *Client Need:* Psychosocial Integrity/Crisis Intervention; *Cognitive Level:* Analysis

Reference: Varcarolis, E., Carson, V., & Shoemaker, N. (2006). *Foundations of Psychiatric Mental Health Nursing: A Clinical Approach* (5th ed., p. 498). St. Louis, MO: Saunders/Elsevier.

1534. EBP Which staff response best indicates an understanding of the risk for client injury regarding the care of a client in restraints?

1. "Can you arrange to order the client's favorite sandwich for his lunch?"
2. "Her feet feel a little cool, but they have a good pulse. I'll get her socks."
3. "I need to make sure the restraints' release mechanisms are working properly."
4. "I'd appreciate it if someone could relieve me for a few minutes and monitor the client."

ANSWER: 4

The client must be constantly monitored when in restraints in order to assess for and prevent any type of client injury. While nutrition, circulation, and properly used restraints are important considerations, the most important action regarding client safety while in restraints is monitoring. Assessing for adequate circulation is important, but it cannot be monitored effectively if the client is not being observed constantly. While the proper working of the restraints is important, it cannot be achieved without appropriate client monitoring.

▶ ***Test-taking Tip:*** *Note the key word "best," and use understanding of continuous monitoring during the use of restraints to select the correct option.*

Content Area: Mental Health; *Category of Health Alteration:* Crisis, Violence, Eating, and Sleep Disorders; *Integrated Processes:* Nursing Process Evaluation; *Client Need:* Safe and Effective Care Environment/Safety and Infection Control/Use of Restraints/Safety Devices; *Cognitive Level:* Analysis

Reference: Varcarolis, E., Carson, V., & Shoemaker, N. (2006). *Foundations of Psychiatric Mental Health Nursing: A Clinical Approach* (5th ed., p. 497). St. Louis, MO: Saunders/Elsevier.

EBP Reference: University of Iowa Gerontological Nursing Interventions Research Center. (2005). *Changing the Practice of Physical Restraint in Acute Care.* Available at: www.guideline.gov/summary/summary.aspx?doc_id=8626&nbr=004806&string=physical+AND+restraint

1535. An older client diagnosed with Alzheimer's disease becomes agitated and insists that he must "go and clean out the barn." Which nursing response is most therapeutic?

1. "What makes you think that the barn needs to be cleaned?"
2. "It's awfully hot today; maybe you should wait until tomorrow."
3. "So you've cleaned a barn. Tell me, did you live on a farm?"
4. "There are no barns around here. Would you like something to eat?"

ANSWER: 3

Rather than attempting to reorient the agitated, cognitively impaired client, asking the client to describe his feelings or memories related to the situation may effectively divert the client's attention to a less problematic focus. While redirecting the client's attention is appropriate, asking the client what makes him think the barn needs to be cleaned may be interpreted as argumentative or challenging and may serve to escalate the client's agitation. Stating there are no barns here and attempting to redirect the client's attention may be viewed as merely putting an obstacle in the client's way.

▶ ***Test-taking Tip:*** *Note the key phrase "most therapeutic," and use understanding of psychopathology of Alzheimer's disease to select the correct option.*

Content Area: Mental Health; *Category of Health Alteration:* Crisis, Violence, Eating, and Sleep Disorders; *Integrated Processes:* Communication and Documentation; *Client Need:* Psychosocial Integrity/Psychopathology; *Cognitive Level:* Analysis

Reference: Varcarolis, E., Carson, V., & Shoemaker, N. (2006). *Foundations of Psychiatric Mental Health Nursing: A Clinical Approach* (5th ed., p. 502). St. Louis, MO: Saunders/Elsevier.

1536. An experienced nurse determines that a new nurse's actions are therapeutic when managing a cognitively impaired client whose agitated behavior is escalating. Which nursing actions should have occurred? SELECT ALL THAT APPLY.

1. Saying, "Mr. Smith, will you look at me, please?"
2. Saying, "You seem upset. How can I help you?"
3. Presenting the client with detailed expectations
4. Telling the client, "Getting so angry will not help you get what you want."
5. Turning off the television in the room to decrease noise
6. Speaking as loud as the client to ensure that the client hears what is being said

ANSWER: 1, 2, 5

Calling the client by name and achieving eye contact may have a calming effect for a cognitively impaired, agitated client. Acknowledging the client's agitation may help the client regain control. Decreasing the stimuli in the area may also have a calming effect on the client. Complex explanations and extensive conversation are likely to be interpreted as more sensory stimuli to the agitated client. The client is not capable of rational thought; telling the client that being angry will not get the client what the client wants may be interpreted as a challenge to the client. Speaking in a loud tone may serve to escalate the client's agitation.

▶ ***Test-taking Tip:*** *Note the key word "therapeutic." Use understanding of the techniques for crisis intervention and managing catastrophic reactions and eliminate options that increase sensory stimuli or can be interpreted as challenging.*

Content Area: Mental Health; *Category of Health Alteration:* Crisis, Violence, Eating, and Sleep Disorders; *Integrated Processes:* Nursing Process Evaluation; *Client Need:* Psychosocial Integrity/Crisis Intervention; *Cognitive Level:* Analysis

Reference: Varcarolis, E., Carson, V., & Shoemaker, N. (2006). *Foundations of Psychiatric Mental Health Nursing: A Clinical Approach* (5th ed., p. 502). St. Louis, MO: Saunders/Elsevier.

1537. A new graduate is working with a cognitively impaired client who has a history of violent behavior. Which statement, made by the new graduate, reflects an immediate need for follow-up by the mentor?

1. "My first concern is the safety of all those on the unit."
2. "I know to turn off the television when he starts pacing the floor."
3. "When he started getting aggressive, I really tried talking to him."
4. "I'm going to try and assign the same staff to work with him each shift."

ANSWER: 3

The mentor should follow-up when the new nurse attempts to talk to the agitated client. Until the client regains control, talking will be interpreted as external stimulation. As the client becomes calmer and more secure, attempts can then be made to redirect the client's attention and behavior. Safety is a major concern and does not require follow-up. Minimizing external stimuli and the use of sound judgment are important in providing a therapeutic milieu for an agitated client and do not require follow-up.

➧ ***Test-taking Tip:*** *Note the key word "immediate," and use understanding of the redirection of agitated clients to select the correct option.*

Content Area: Mental Health; *Category of Health Alteration:* Crisis, Violence, Eating, and Sleep Disorders; *Integrated Processes:* Nursing Process Evaluation; *Client Need:* Safe and Effective Care Environment/ Safety and Infection Control/Accident and Injury Prevention; *Cognitive Level:* Analysis

Reference: Varcarolis, E., Carson, V., & Shoemaker, N. (2006). *Foundations of Psychiatric Mental Health Nursing: A Clinical Approach* (5th ed., p. 502). St. Louis, MO: Saunders/Elsevier.

1538. Which specific client outcome best reflects the primary goal of crisis intervention for a client diagnosed with schizophrenia who is experiencing an alcohol-induced crisis?

1. Client will be successfully detoxified within 20 days.
2. Client will return to former part-time job within 20 days.
3. Client will state two effective coping mechanisms prior to discharge.
4. Client will demonstrate knowledge of proper medication administration prior to discharge.

ANSWER: 2

The primary goal of crisis intervention is to return the client to his or her precrisis level of functioning. Returning to former employment is the most appropriate outcome directed toward that goal. Detoxification is directed toward treatment of the underlying condition, alcohol abuse. The client should be demonstrating the use of effective coping mechanisms, not just stating them. The client's ability to self-administer medication is necessary for treating schizophrenia but is not a goal specific to the crisis situation.

➧ ***Test-taking Tip:*** *Use the process of elimination to select the only option directly related to the client's crisis behavior.*

Content Area: Mental Health; *Category of Health Alteration:* Crisis, Violence, Eating, and Sleep Disorders; *Integrated Processes:* Nursing Process Planning; *Client Need:* Psychosocial Integrity/Crisis Intervention; *Cognitive Level:* Analysis

Reference: Varcarolis, E., Carson, V., & Shoemaker, N. (2006). *Foundations of Psychiatric Mental Health Nursing: A Clinical Approach* (5th ed., p. 459). St. Louis, MO: Saunders/Elsevier.

1539. Staff members have expressed fear of a client who has a history of violent behavior. Which response made by a lead nurse would be most beneficial in addressing the staff's expressed concerns?

1. "Let's not prejudge him. His medication should help him control his behavior."
2. "I will be very attentive to his behavior, monitoring it for any signs of escalation."
3. "It may be hard, but we need to appear calm and nonthreatening but alert to his behavior."
4. "As staff we are all trained to manage violent clients, and we can handle any crisis behavior."

ANSWER: 3

When dealing with potentially violent clients, although it may be very difficult, it is imperative to present a calm, relaxed, nonthreatening demeanor. This option addresses both the staff concerns and offers direction regarding client management. The remaining options fail to address the concerns expressed and a means of controlling the feared behavior.

➧ ***Test-taking Tip:*** *Note the key phrase "most beneficial," and pay attention to the specific focus of the question.*

Content Area: Mental Health; *Category of Health Alteration:* Crisis, Violence, Eating, and Sleep Disorders; *Integrated Processes:* Caring; *Client Need:* Safe and Effective Care Environment/Management of Care/Client Rights; *Cognitive Level:* Analysis

Reference: Varcarolis, E., Carson, V., & Shoemaker, N. (2006). *Foundations of Psychiatric Mental Health Nursing: A Clinical Approach* (5th ed., p. 495). St. Louis, MO: Saunders/Elsevier.

1540. A nurse has suggested that a client newly admitted to the behavioral medicine unit find a suitable place to attempt to gain control over increasing anger. The most therapeutic site the nurse should recommend is:

1. in the client's own private room.
2. an outside sheltered client smoking area.
3. the unit's common TV dayroom.
4. an out-of-the-way corner near the nursing station.

ANSWER: 4

The environment is critical for client de-escalation. A quiet location that is visible to the staff is best. Neither the client's room nor an outside area is visible to the staff. The dayroom is not quiet.

➧ ***Test-taking Tip:*** *Select the only option that is visible to the staff and quiet.*

Content Area: Mental Health; *Category of Health Alteration:* Crisis, Violence, Eating, and Sleep Disorders; *Integrated Processes:* Nursing Process Implementation; *Client Need:* Safe and Effective Care Environment/Safety and Infection Control/Accident and Injury Prevention; *Cognitive Level:* Analysis

Reference: Varcarolis, E., Carson, V., & Shoemaker, N. (2006). *Foundations of Psychiatric Mental Health Nursing: A Clinical Approach* (5th ed., p. 496). St. Louis, MO: Saunders/Elsevier.

1541. EBP A client with a history of aggressive behavior toward staff and peers reports to the nurse that "Everyone is just so touchy; I don't see where I'm being too aggressive." Which nursing action should be included in the therapeutic plan of care to best affect a difference in perceptions?

1. Refamiliarize the client with the rules of the unit.
2. Introduce nonaggressive interpersonal behaviors to the client.
3. Promote a dialog between the staff and client to discuss their perceptions of aggressive behavior.
4. Encourage the staff to show patience to the client since he or she may have poor aggression control.

ANSWER: 3

Research has shown that staff and clients often have different perceptions of aggressive behaviors and how to control or reduce aggression. Thus, promoting a dialog between the client and the staff can clarify the different perceptions. Refamiliarizing the client with unit rules is not an inappropriate option; it may have little impact on the client's aggressive behavior. Providing alternate behaviors is an appropriate option but is not the most therapeutic because the various perceptions need to be addressed first. Suggesting "patience" is not appropriate because the client's aggressive behavior is a risk for injury to the milieu.

➧ ***Test-taking Tip:*** *Note the key word "best" and use the process of elimination. The focus of the question is clarifying misperceptions.*

Content Area: Mental Health; *Category of Health Alteration:* Crisis, Violence, Eating, and Sleep Disorders; *Integrated Processes:* Nursing Process Planning; *Client Need:* Psychosocial Integrity/Therapeutic Environment; *Cognitive Level:* Analysis

Reference: Stuart, G. (2009). *Principles and Practice of Psychiatric Nursing* (9th ed., p. 578). St. Louis, MO: Elsevier/Mosby.

EBP Reference: Sclafani, M., Humphrey, F., Repko, S., Ko, H., Wallen, M., et al. (2008). Reducing patient restraints: A pilot approach using clinical case review. *Perspectives in Psychiatric Care*, 44(1), 32–39.

1542. Which should be a nurse's primary goal of seclusion for a client exhibiting violent behavior?

1. Assist the client in regaining self-control.
2. Assure the safety of the client and others.
3. Regain control over the unit's environment.
4. Provide a consequence for the client's behavior.

ANSWER: 2

The primary goal of seclusion is always safety of the client and others. Regaining self-control and unit control are outcomes of seclusion. Seclusion should never be used as a punishment for behavior.

➧ ***Test-taking Tip:*** *Note the key word "primary." Eliminate options that are outcomes of seclusion.*

Content Area: Mental Health; *Category of Health Alteration:* Crisis, Violence, Eating, and Sleep Disorders; *Integrated Processes:* Nursing Process Planning; *Client Need:* Safe and Effective Care Environment/Safety and Infection Control/Accident and Injury Prevention; *Cognitive Level:* Application

Reference: Varcarolis, E., Carson, V., & Shoemaker, N. (2006). *Foundations of Psychiatric Mental Health Nursing: A Clinical Approach* (5th ed., p. 496). St. Louis, MO: Saunders/Elsevier.

1543. A client is experiencing withdrawal symptoms leading to sleep deprivation. A nurse should recognize that the client is at greatest risk for violent behavior due to:

1. physical withdrawal pain.
2. poor coping mechanisms.
3. a sense of guilt or shame regarding family.
4. anxiety over lack of access to the substance of choice.

ANSWER: 4

A client hospitalized for chemical dependency is at risk for developing violent behavior due to anxiety related to a loss of access to the drug of choice. While inadequately managed physical pain resulting from withdrawal, a sense of guilt or shame regarding family, and the lack of coping skills may result in violent behavior, the primary cause is likely no access to the drug or alcohol.

➧ ***Test-taking Tip:** Note the key word "greatest," and use the process of elimination to determine the primary factor affecting violence in a client who abuses substances.*

Content Area: Mental Health; *Category of Health Alteration:* Crisis, Violence, Eating, and Sleep Disorders; *Integrated Processes:* Nursing Process Assessment; *Client Need:* Psychosocial Integrity/Chemical and Other Dependencies; *Cognitive Level:* Application

Reference: Varcarolis, E., Carson, V., & Shoemaker, N. (2006). *Foundations of Psychiatric Mental Health Nursing: A Clinical Approach* (5th ed., p. 499). St. Louis, MO: Saunders/Elsevier.

1544. A nurse educator is orienting new nursing staff to the behavioral medicine unit when one nurse asks, "How will I know which clients are potentially violent?" Which response by the nurse educator is best?

1. "Just be alert and aware of your client's behavioral clues."
2. "As you plan care, review the client charts to determine who has a history of violence."
3. "Your orientation will include an in-service on violent clients and how to identify them."
4. "A client will usually tell you they are angry about something."

ANSWER: 2

The two most significant predictors of violence are a history of violence and impulsivity. Thus, reviewing the client's chart for this information is best. Suggesting that the staff be alert and aware doesn't effectively address the staff's concerns about identifying potential violent clients. Telling the nurse that the information will be provided during in-service education doesn't answer the nurse's question. The staff needs to be aware of potential violence well before a client verbally expresses the anger.

➧ ***Test-taking Tip:** Note the key word "best." Eliminate any options that do not answer the client's question. Select the option that is most proactive.*

Content Area: Mental Health; *Category of Health Alteration:* Crisis, Violence, Eating, and Sleep Disorders; *Integrated Processes:* Teaching and Learning; *Client Need:* Safe and Effective Care Environment/Management of Care/Information Technology; *Cognitive Level:* Analysis

Reference: Varcarolis, E., Carson, V., & Shoemaker, N. (2006). *Foundations of Psychiatric Mental Health Nursing: A Clinical Approach* (5th ed., p. 500). St. Louis, MO: Saunders/Elsevier.

1545. A nurse is caring for multiple clients on a hospital unit. Which client should the nurse expect to have the greatest risk for violent behavior?

1. A 27-year-old client whose girlfriend recently ended their relationship
2. A 53-year-old client who is preparing for radical facial surgery for cancer
3. An 82-year-old client diagnosed with Alzheimer's disease who has communication deficits
4. A 17-year-old client who suffered various injuries from a fight with a fellow student

ANSWER: 3

Clients with cognitive deficits, such as with Alzheimer's disease, are particularly at risk for acting out aggressively and having violent behavior. The 27-year-old client is at risk due to feelings of rejection, the 53-year-old client is at risk due to feelings of fear, and the 17-year-old client is at risk due to feelings of humiliation and being the focus of physical threats, but these clients are not at the greatest risk from among the options offered.

➧ ***Test-taking Tip:** Note the key word "greatest," and then use understanding of risk factors for violent behavior to choose the correct option.*

Content Area: Mental Health; *Category of Health Alteration:* Crisis, Violence, Eating, and Sleep Disorders; *Integrated Processes:* Nursing Process Assessment; *Client Need:* Psychosocial Integrity/Psychopathology; *Cognitive Level:* Analysis

Reference: Varcarolis, E., Carson, V., & Shoemaker, N. (2006). *Foundations of Psychiatric Mental Health Nursing: A Clinical Approach* (5th ed., p. 501). St. Louis, MO: Saunders/Elsevier.

1546. A nurse manager, concerned about the potential for staff harm on a behavioral health unit, is assessing the unit's milieu. Which milieu situation should be concerning because it is a predictive factor of violence?

1. The unit is currently at less than full client capacity.
2. Several clients have lost smoking privileges.
3. Two clients have a history of spousal abuse.
4. A staff member "is pulled" to work on the unit.

ANSWER: 4

Staff inexperience is a significant environmental predictor of violent behavior of clients. Unit overcrowding, not less than capacity, is also considered an environmental predictor of violence. While revocation of privileges may contribute to the potential for violence, it is a client-oriented factor, not milieu oriented. A history of violent behavior is considered a predictor of potential violence, but it is also a client-oriented factor not a milieu factor.

***Test-taking Tip:** Note the key word "milieu," and use understanding of violence predictors to choose the correct option. Eliminate the two options that relate to the client and not the milieu. Of the two remaining factors, determine which situation is most likely to lead to violence.*

Content Area: Mental Health; *Category of Health Alteration:* Crisis, Violence, Eating, and Sleep Disorders; *Integrated Processes:* Nursing Process Assessment; *Client Need:* Psychosocial Integrity/Therapeutic Environment; *Cognitive Level:* Analysis

Reference: Varcarolis, E., Carson, V., & Shoemaker, N. (2006). *Foundations of Psychiatric Mental Health Nursing: A Clinical Approach* (5th ed., p. 493). St. Louis, MO: Saunders/Elsevier.

1547. In which circumstances should a nurse plan the therapeutic use of seclusion and/or restraints? SELECT ALL THAT APPLY.

1. A client asks to be placed in seclusion.
2. The staff feels the client is likely to harm others.
3. A legally detained client is threatening to "escape."
4. A client expresses the likelihood of self-injury.
5. The staff identifies seclusion as a consequence of a client's behavior.
6. A client's threatening behavior is negatively affecting the therapeutic milieu.

ANSWER: 1, 2, 3, 4

The American Psychiatric Nurses Association has identified the likelihood of harming self or others, escape by an involuntarily detained client, or a client's request to be placed in seclusion or restraints as reasons to therapeutically employ these methods. Neither seclusion nor restraints should ever be used as punishment. While a client's behavior may result in disruption to the milieu, seclusion and restraints are therapeutic only after all alternative interventions have been tried.

***Test-taking Tip:** Look for similarities in options and select the options that can result in self-injury or injury to others.*

Content Area: Mental Health; *Category of Health Alteration:* Crisis, Violence, Eating, and Sleep Disorders; *Integrated Processes:* Nursing Process Planning; *Client Need:* Psychosocial Integrity/Crisis Intervention; *Cognitive Level:* Analysis

Reference: Varcarolis, E., Carson, V., & Shoemaker, N. (2006). *Foundations of Psychiatric Mental Health Nursing: A Clinical Approach* (5th ed., p. 497). St. Louis, MO: Saunders/Elsevier.

1548. During the application of restraints, which action by a team leader will gain the greatest cooperation from a client?

1. Dispassionately explaining why and how the restraints will be applied
2. Showing sympathy by apologizing for the need to restrain the client
3. Affording the client one last opportunity to avoid restraints by "behaving"
4. Offering to remove the restraints as soon as the client can "control the anger"

ANSWER: 1

By providing an explanation of what is to happen and why, the client may resist less or in some instances decide to alter the behavior, especially once an understanding of the intervention is achieved. A dispassionate explanation avoids the nurse's emotions being misinterpreted by the client. The nurse should not view the application of restraints as something to be sorry for; it is in the client's best interest to be assisted in the process of regaining control. To apologize would also give the client the impression that the client is being mistreated. Once the decision is made that restraints are the appropriate intervention, the client is not given an opportunity to negotiate out of their application. The final option will not have much impact on securing the client's cooperation in actually applying the restraints.

***Test-taking Tip:** Note the key word "greatest," and use understanding of the therapeutic use of restraints to choose the correct option.*

Content Area: Mental Health; *Category of Health Alteration:* Crisis, Violence, Eating, and Sleep Disorders; *Integrated Processes:* Nursing Process Implementation; *Client Need:* Safe and Effective Care Environment/Safety and Infection Control/Use of Restraints/Safety Devices; *Cognitive Level:* Analysis

Reference: Varcarolis, E., Carson, V., & Shoemaker, N. (2006). *Foundations of Psychiatric Mental Health Nursing: A Clinical Approach* (5th ed., p. 497). St. Louis, MO: Saunders/Elsevier.

1549. Which assessment observation best indicates to a nurse of a client's readiness to leave involuntary seclusion?

1. The client calmly stating, "I have control over my anger now."
2. Vital signs: P = 82 and regular; R = 16 and regular; BP = 110/64 mm Hg
3. Client observed sitting in seclusion room doorway asking staff for a drink
4. Client history stating, "45 minutes in seclusion resulted in improved control."

ANSWER: 3

The client is showing the ability to tolerate the stimulation provided by being in the doorway and still appropriately asking for needs to be met. The reintegration of a client into the milieu should be done gradually so as to monitor the client's ability to handle increased stimulation. While the client's statement is a positive indicator of regained control, it is not as definitive as observed behavior regarding exposure to increased stimulation. Vital signs may indicate physical calmness, but they are not as definitive as observed behavior regarding exposure to increased stimulation. While past behavior may indicate a pattern, it is not as definitive as observed behavior regarding exposure to increased stimulation.

▶ ***Test-taking Tip:*** *Note the key word "best." Select the option of an observed behavior showing tolerance of increased stimulation.*

Content Area: Mental Health; *Category of Health Alteration:* Crisis, Violence, Eating, and Sleep Disorders; *Integrated Processes:* Nursing Process Evaluation; *Client Need:* Psychosocial Integrity/Behavioral Interventions; *Cognitive Level:* Analysis

Reference: Varcarolis, E., Carson, V., & Shoemaker, N. (2006). *Foundations of Psychiatric Mental Health Nursing: A Clinical Approach* (5th ed., p. 497). St. Louis, MO: Saunders/Elsevier.

1550. A client with poor anger-management skills is visibly upset and while pounding on the desk at the nurses' station shouts, "You're the nurse, so you have to fix this now." The nurse recognizes that the client is a danger to staff and other clients primarily because:

1. if the client is willing to hit the desk, the client is willing to hit someone.
2. the client does not acknowledge his or her role in the problem-solving process.
3. the client has no apparent ability to recognize that he or she is acting inappropriately.
4. the client's main strategy for meeting personal needs and wants is intimidation and anger.

ANSWER: 4

For some, intimidation and anger are the primary strategies for obtaining needs and goals and to achieve feelings of mastery and control. For these clients, angry behavior is a particular risk in the inpatient setting. The remaining options reflect inappropriate assumptions.

▶ ***Test-taking Tip:*** *Note the key word "primarily," and use understanding of the management of an angry client to select the correct option.*

Content Area: Mental Health; *Category of Health Alteration:* Crisis, Violence, Eating, and Sleep Disorders; *Integrated Processes:* Nursing Process Assessment; *Client Need:* Safe and Effective Care Environment/Safety and Infection Control/Accident and Injury Prevention; *Cognitive Level:* Analysis

Reference: Varcarolis, E., Carson, V., & Shoemaker, N. (2006). *Foundations of Psychiatric Mental Health Nursing: A Clinical Approach* (5th ed., p. 499). St. Louis, MO: Saunders/Elsevier.

1551. In planning care for a client who has a cognitive deficit and history of violence following head trauma, the nurse realizes that the primary effect cognitive deficits have in contributing to a client experiencing a catastrophically violent reaction is that:

1. the client has a decreased ability to interpret and tolerate sensory stimuli.
2. the staff has a more difficult time providing appropriate milieu boundaries.
3. the client's ability to process information, including instructions, is limited.
4. the staff's attention is oftentimes diverted to other, more manipulative clients.

ANSWER: 1

Cognitive deficits result in a decreased ability to interpret and tolerate sensory stimuli, which in turn can trigger a catastrophic reaction. The remaining options are not necessarily true of cognitively impaired clients or the staff caring for them.

▶ ***Test-taking Tip:*** *Note that two options pertain to the client and two to the nursing staff. Because the focus should be on the client, eliminate options pertaining to the nursing staff. Of the two remaining options, note that one option describes two problems and the other option only one. Select the more expansive option.*

Content Area: Mental Health; *Category of Health Alteration:* Crisis, Violence, Eating, and Sleep Disorders; *Integrated Processes:* Nursing Process Planning; *Client Need:* Psychosocial Integrity/Sensory/Perceptual Alterations; *Cognitive Level:* Analysis

Reference: Varcarolis, E., Carson, V., & Shoemaker, N. (2006). *Foundations of Psychiatric Mental Health Nursing: A Clinical Approach* (5th ed., pp. 501–502). St. Louis, MO: Saunders/Elsevier.

1552. When debriefing the unit's staff after a client's catastrophic reaction, a nurse stresses the need for the staff to remain calm during the event primarily because:

1. the client's safety is at jeopardy if the staff is feeling threatened.
2. an agitated staff will not be able to manage the situation as effectively.
3. the client will sense the staff's agitation, and aggressive behavior will escalate.
4. an agitated staff response is indicative of a need for additional crisis-control training.

ANSWER: 3

Presence of a second agitated person leads to increased agitation for the client. While an agitated staff member may find it more difficult to keep the client's safety in mind, it is not the primary reason to remain calm. Though an agitated staff member may not be as in control of the situation, it is not the primary reason to remain calm. A staff member's ineffective behavior would require additional training, but it is not the primary reason to remain calm.

▶ ***Test-taking Tip:*** *Note that two options pertain to the client and two to the staff. Eliminate options pertaining to the staff's behavior and focus on the client's response to the behavior.*

Content Area: Mental Health; *Category of Health Alteration:* Crisis, Violence, Eating, and Sleep Disorders; *Integrated Processes:* Teaching and Learning; *Client Need:* Psychosocial Integrity/Stress Management; *Cognitive Level:* Analysis

Reference: Varcarolis, E., Carson, V., & Shoemaker, N. (2006). *Foundations of Psychiatric Mental Health Nursing: A Clinical Approach* (5th ed., p. 502). St. Louis, MO: Saunders/Elsevier.

1553. EBP An indigent client with both emotional and physical diagnoses has just attended a discharge planning session with a nurse. Which client behavior shows the greatest commitment to the client's self-management?

1. Correctly stating the medications prescribed and their administration schedule
2. Asking to stay with a relative until an affordable place to live can be found
3. Researching the names of and calling contact people at local support centers
4. Promising the nurse to keep follow-up appointments at the clinic

ANSWER: 3

Telephoning contacts at support services shows both an understanding of and a willingness to utilize the services. Research has shown that beginning client linkage to services prior to discharge has a positive effect on client outcomes. The remaining options do not show as much commitment to self improvement as does the correct option.

▶ ***Test-taking Tip:*** *Note the key word "greatest," and use the process of elimination to select the only option in which the client's behavior demonstrates an action, not just verbalizing a commitment to self-management.*

Content Area: Mental Health; *Category of Health Alteration:* Crisis, Violence, Eating, and Sleep Disorders; *Integrated Processes:* Nursing Process Evaluation; *Client Need:* Health Promotion and Maintenance/Self-Care; *Cognitive Level:* Analysis

Reference: Stuart, G. (2009). *Principles and Practice of Psychiatric Nursing* (9th ed., p. 578). St. Louis, MO: Elsevier/Mosby.

EBP Reference: Cohen, L. (2006). The importance of staying on therapy. *Psychiatric Times,* 23(4), 15–22.

1554. EBP A father of a teenager diagnosed with an eating disorder states to the nurse, "My wife was always too protective; that's the reason our child has this problem now." The nurse should realize that the father's statement is most likely:

1. a possible indication of the couple's marital discord.
2. a correct interpretation of the result of the protective tendencies.
3. a misconception regarding the cause of the child's eating disorder.
4. an attempt to deflect personal responsibility for his child's eating disorder.

ANSWER: 3

There is no clear agreement regarding the causes of eating disorders. Current research suggests an interaction of biological susceptibility, including genetic markers for both neurobiological vulnerability and personality traits and environmental influences, including family, social, and cultural environments. While there may be marital discord, overprotectiveness or issues related to the father's ineffective coping, no one factor is the likely cause.

▶ ***Test-taking Tip:*** *Note the key word "most." Three options identify a cause, whereas one option is different. Often the option that is different is the correct option.*

Content Area: Mental Health; *Category of Health Alteration:* Crisis, Violence, Eating, and Sleep Disorders; *Integrated Processes:* Nursing Process Analysis; *Client Need:* Psychosocial Integrity/Coping Mechanisms; *Cognitive Level:* Application

Reference: Fortinash, K., & Holoday Worret, P. (2008). *Psychiatric Mental Health Nursing* (4th ed., pp. 391–392). St. Louis, MO: Mosby Elsevier.

EBP Reference: Zucker, M., Losh, M., Bulik, C., LaBar, K., Pevin, J., et al. (2007). Anorexia nervosa and autism spectrum disorders: Guided investigation of social cognitive endophenotypes. *Psychological Bulletin,* 133, 976–1006.

1555. EBP The mother of a teenager diagnosed with anorexia nervosa confides in a nurse that she has always been very protective and is concerned her overprotectiveness is the reason her child developed the eating disorder. The most therapeutic response by the nurse is:

1. "Does your child feel that being overprotected as a child contributed to the problem?"
2. "What makes you feel that your overprotective tendencies caused this problem?"
3. "Don't worry. Your daughter is a teenager, and the cause is more likely the stress of adolescence."
4. "There is no research to confirm that overprotective parenting results in an eating disorder."

ANSWER: 4

Research has shown that overprotective parenting usually exists as a reaction to the disorder not as a causative factor. While asking relevant questions encourages discussion, they in this case do not clarify the misconception. Telling the mother not to worry is a nontherapeutic response.

➧ ***Test-taking Tip:*** *The most therapeutic response is one that addresses the mother's concern.*

Content Area: Mental Health; *Category of Health Alteration:* Crisis, Violence, Eating, and Sleep Disorders; *Integrated Processes:* Communication and Documentation; *Client Need:* Psychosocial Integrity/Psychopathology; *Cognitive Level:* Analysis

Reference: Fortinash, K., & Holoday Worret, P. (2008). *Psychiatric Mental Health Nursing* (4th ed., pp. 391–392). St. Louis, MO: Mosby/Elsevier.

EBP Reference: Zucker, M., Losh, M., Bulik, C., LaBar, K., Pevin, J., et al. (2007). Anorexia nervosa and autism spectrum disorders: Guided investigation of social cognitive endophenotypes. *Psychological Bulletin,* 133, 976–1006.

1556. EBP Which findings should a nurse expect when completing a health history and an assessment for a client diagnosed with anorexia nervosa? SELECT ALL THAT APPLY.

1. Refusal to eat
2. Weighs less than 85% of expected weight for body size and age
3. Age of onset 25 years
4. Intense fear of getting fat despite being underweight
5. Heavy bleeding during menses

ANSWER: 1, 2, 4

Refusal to eat indicates an eating disorder. Criteria for diagnosing anorexia nervosa include weight loss leading to maintaining a body weight less than 85% of that expected and an intense fear of getting fat despite being underweight. The mean age of onset is between 11 to 18 years. While the onset of 25 years is atypical, this is possible. Anorexia can lead to amenorrhea (absence of three consecutive menstrual cycles) rather than heavy bleeding during menses.

➧ ***Test-taking Tip:*** *Read each option carefully. Eliminate options that are opposite those seen with anorexia. Consider that the age of onset can be as young as 8 years old.*

Content Area: Mental Health; *Category of Health Alteration:* Crisis, Violence, Eating, and Sleep Disorders; *Integrated Processes:* Nursing Process Assessment; *Client Need:* Psychosocial Integrity/Psychopathology; *Cognitive Level:* Application

Reference: Fortinash, K., & Holoday Worret, P. (2008). *Psychiatric Mental Health Nursing* (4th ed., pp. 395–396). St. Louis, MO: Mosby/Elsevier.

EBP Reference: American Psychiatric Association. (2006). Treatment of patients with eating disorders (3rd ed.). *American Journal of Psychiatry,* 163(7 Suppl), 4–54. Available at: www.guideline.gov/summary/summary.aspx?doc_id=9318&nbr=004987&string=sudden+AND+cardiac+AND+death+AND+adolescent

1557. A nurse is reviewing the care plan for a client newly diagnosed with anorexia nervosa who is receiving inpatient treatment. According to the client needs, which outcome should a nurse establish as the *most* urgent?

1. Achieves minimum normal weight
2. Resumes normal menstrual cycle
3. Consumes adequate calories for age, height, and metabolic needs
4. Perceives body weight and shape as normal and acceptable

ANSWER: 3

Consuming adequate calories for metabolic needs meets a basic physiological need and is priority. Achieving a minimum normal weight and resuming a normal menstrual cycle are appropriate outcomes but will take time to achieve. The client's perception of body weight and shape as normal is a psychosocial outcome and, while appropriate, is not the most urgent.

➧ ***Test-taking Tip:*** *Use Maslow's Hierarchy of Needs theory to establish a physiological need as the most urgent outcome to be achieved.*

Content Area: Mental Health; *Category of Health Alteration:* Crisis, Violence, Eating, and Sleep Disorders; *Integrated Processes:* Nursing Process Analysis; *Client Need:* Physiological Integrity/Physiological Adaptation/Illness Management; *Cognitive Level:* Application

Reference: Fortinash, K., & Holoday Worret, P. (2008). *Psychiatric Mental Health Nursing* (4th ed., p. 399). St. Louis, MO: Mosby/Elsevier.

1558. EBP A nurse is developing a care plan for a client newly diagnosed with bulimia nervosa who is receiving inpatient treatment. According to the client needs, which outcomes should a nurse establish as the most urgent? Prioritize the outcomes from the most urgent to the least urgent.

______ Demonstrates more effective coping skills to deal with conflicts
______ Ceases binge/purge episodes while in inpatient setting
______ Maintains normal fluid and electrolyte levels
______ Perceives body shape and weight as normal and acceptable
______ Consumes adequate calories for age, height, and metabolic need

ANSWER: 4, 3, 1, 5, 2

According to client needs, physiological needs should be the most urgent. Because the client has been purging, the outcome that the client will maintain normal fluid and electrolyte levels is priority. The next most urgent outcome is the client will consume adequate calories for age, height, and metabolic need. This also is a physiological need. The third priority outcome is the client will cease binge/purge episodes while in inpatient setting. This is a psychosocial outcome but is next because the remaining outcomes cannot be achieved until binging/purging ceases. The fourth priority outcome is demonstrating more effective coping skills to deal with conflicts. The last outcome to be achieved is for the client to perceive body shape and weight as normal and acceptable. According to Maslow's Hierarchy of Needs theory, self-actualization is the highest level of need.

➧ ***Test-taking Tip:*** *Use Maslow's Hierarchy of Needs theory to place items in the correct sequence. Remember that the basic physiological needs are priority, whereas self-actualization is the least urgent need.*

Content Area: Mental Health; *Category of Health Alteration:* Crisis, Violence, Eating, and Sleep Disorders; *Integrated Processes:* Communication and Documentation; *Client Need:* Safe and Effective Care Environment/Management of Care/Establishing Priorities; *Cognitive Level:* Analysis

Reference: Fortinash, K., & Holoday Worret, P. (2008). *Psychiatric Mental Health Nursing* (4th ed., p. 399). St. Louis, MO: Mosby/Elsevier.

EBP Reference: American Psychiatric Association. (2006). Treatment of patients with eating disorders. *American Journal of Psychiatry*, 163(7 Suppl), 4–54.

1559. A 13-year-old client is being discharged from a behavioral health unit with a diagnosis of bulimia nervosa. Which statement should a nurse include when completing the discharge teaching with a parent and the child?

1. "Because the cycle of eating disorder behaviors is life threatening and must be interrupted, continue to monitor your child for at least 1 hour after eating."
2. "The behavior modification program easily changed your child's eating disorder behavior, but you need to continue to offer nourishing foods."
3. "Discourage your child from discussing insights from group and individual therapy because of the potential adverse effects on the entire family."
4. "Continue to prepare separate meals to encourage your child to eat nourishing foods and offer foods that your child desires and will eat."

ANSWER: 1

The cycle of eating disorders must be interrupted because it is life threatening. The client should be monitored for 1 hour or more after meals to discourage the child from purging. Eating disorder behaviors are hard (not easy) to change because gaining weight or stopping purging is terrifying to the client. The child should be encouraged, not discouraged, to share what has been learned in group and individual therapy about the particular psychological issues relating to the eating disorder. The child should be expected to follow family rules, including eating meals prepared for the family. The parent should stop preparing separate meals.

➧ ***Test-taking Tip:*** *Read each option carefully and examine key words and phrases that make an option incorrect, such as "easily changed," "discourage," and "separate meals." Think about the option that should reinforce the child's treatment for bulimia nervosa.*

Content Area: Mental Health; *Category of Health Alteration:* Crisis, Violence, Eating, and Sleep Disorders; *Integrated Processes:* Teaching and Learning; *Client Need:* Physiological Integrity/Physiological Adaptation/Illness Management; *Cognitive Level:* Analysis

Reference: Fortinash, K., & Holoday Worret, P. (2008). *Psychiatric Mental Health Nursing* (4th ed., p. 401). St. Louis, MO: Mosby/Elsevier.

1560. A nurse completing a health history for a client diagnosed with an eating disorder determines that a client is taking 20 laxative products daily and diuretics twice daily and is self-inducing vomiting. Based on this information, which action should the nurse take *next*?

1. Notify the health-care provider.
2. Auscultate the client's apical pulse.
3. Question the client about the consistency and frequency of stools.
4. Ask the client to list the names of the products taken.

ANSWER: 2

By auscultating the client's apical pulse, the nurse can assess the client's heart rate and its regularity to assess whether an irregularity is present. Abuse of laxatives and diuretics and self-induced vomiting can lead to serious electrolyte imbalances that lead to cardiac dysrhythmias. Unless a life-threatening situation exists, a nurse should complete an assessment before notifying the health-care provider of the findings. Questioning the client about his/her stools and obtaining the names of the abused products are important but are not the next action.

➧ ***Test-taking Tip:*** *Think about the effect of laxatives, diuretics, and self-induced vomiting on the client's fluid and electrolyte balance before selecting an option. Use the steps of the nursing process; assessment should be completed before initiating an action unless an initial observation indicates the situation is life-threatening.*

Content Area: Mental Health; *Category of Health Alteration:* Crisis, Violence, Eating, and Sleep Disorders; *Integrated Processes:* Nursing Process Implementation; *Client Need:* Physiological Integrity/Reduction of Risk Potential/Vital Signs; *Cognitive Level:* Analysis

Reference: Fortinash, K., & Holoday Worret, P. (2008). *Psychiatric Mental Health Nursing* (4th ed., p. 406). St. Louis, MO: Mosby/Elsevier.

1561. EBP A nurse is evaluating the attainment of outcomes on the care plan of an adolescent client diagnosed with bulimia nervosa. Based on the diagnosis of bulimia, which behavior indicates that the client is meeting an expected outcome for the disorder?

1. Gains 1 pound after being in treatment for 3 weeks
2. Self-purging decreases in frequency from daily to twice weekly
3. Uses drawing to express feelings about body image and to deal with conflicts
4. Engages staff in conversations that center on food

ANSWER: 3

Using art therapy demonstrates an ability to choose more effective coping skills to deal with conflicts other than preoccupation with food. Because a person diagnosed with bulimia has difficulty naming feelings or finding the words needed for "talk" therapy, art therapy or other expressive therapies allow for greater self-disclosure and exploration of issues. The expected amount of weight gain is 1 pound per week, not 1 pound in 3 weeks. The absence, not just a reduction, of purging is expected. Engaging in conversations about food demonstrates that the client is still preoccupied with food. The expected outcome is absence of preoccupation with food.

➧ ***Test-taking Tip:*** *Think about the issues that clients diagnosed with bulimia nervosa experience and the expected outcomes. Use the process of elimination to eliminate options that demonstrate only progression toward meeting outcomes.*

Content Area: Mental Health; *Category of Health Alteration:* Crisis, Violence, Eating, and Sleep Disorders; *Integrated Processes:* Nursing Process Evaluation; *Client Need:* Physiological Integrity/Physiological Adaptation/Illness Management; *Cognitive Level:* Analysis

Reference: Fortinash, K., & Holoday Worret, P. (2008). *Psychiatric Mental Health Nursing* (4th ed., pp. 400–401). St. Louis, MO: Mosby/Elsevier.

EBP Reference: Finnish Medical Society Duodecim. (2007). Eating disorders among children and adolescents. *EBM Guidelines. Evidence-Based Medicine*. Available at: www.guideline.gov/summary/summary.aspx?doc_id=11035&nbr=005814&string=eating+AND+disorders

---

1562. A nurse is completing a health history for a client diagnosed with narcolepsy. Which finding should a nurse anticipate when completing the assessment?

1. Sudden loss of muscle tone
2. Inability to speak 1 hour before a sleep attack
3. Excessive daytime sleepiness that results in sleep at an inappropriate time
4. Sudden loss of muscle tone after taking a narcotic analgesic

ANSWER: 3

Narcolepsy is a sleep disorder characterized by excessive daytime sleepiness and multiple sleep attacks during the client's normal period of wakefulness, typically taking place at inappropriate times. Cataplexy is the sudden loss of muscle tone and voluntary muscle movement. Approximately 70% of persons with narcolepsy also experience cataplexy. The inability to speak or move just before the onset or upon awakening from a brief sleep attack is sleep paralysis. Persons with narcolepsy may also report sleep paralysis; it occurs just before or after a sleep attack, not 1 hour before an attack. Narcolepsy is not associated with taking a narcotic analgesic medication.

➧ ***Test-taking Tip:*** *Knowledge of narcolepsy (a sleep attack) is needed to answer this question. Use this clue to eliminate options not associated with sleep.*

Content Area: Mental Health; *Category of Health Alteration:* Crisis, Violence, Eating, and Sleep Disorders; *Integrated Processes:* Nursing Process Assessment; *Client Need:* Physiological Integrity/Reduction of Risk Potential/System Specific Assessments; *Cognitive Level:* Application

Reference: Fortinash, K., & Holoday Worret, P. (2008). *Psychiatric Mental Health Nursing* (4th ed., p. 414). St. Louis, MO: Mosby/Elsevier.

1563. Which recommendations should a nurse make when counseling a client who is experiencing insomnia? SELECT ALL THAT APPLY.

1. Eliminate substances such as caffeine and chocolate.
2. Use relaxation skills such as progressive muscle relaxation before bed.
3. Exercise one-half hour each night before bed.
4. Keep a sleep diary, recording when going to bed, number of times awakened, and the number of hours of sleep.
5. If insomnia continues, a referral can be made to a sleep disorder specialist.
6. Consume an alcoholic beverage just before bedtime.

ANSWER: 1, 2, 4, 5

Substances such as caffeine and chocolate are stimulants that can negatively affect restorative sleep. Using relaxation strategies assists the client in managing psychosocial stressors that negatively affect the client's ability to fall asleep. Keeping a sleep diary helps the client to identify patterns of interrupted sleep, possible causes of sleep disturbances, and to identify the amount of sleep attained. A sleep specialist referral may be necessary to identify other physiological causes for insomnia or sleep that is not restorative, such as with sleep apnea. Exercise and alcohol are both stimulants and should be avoided at bedtime.

▶ ***Test-taking Tip:*** *Eliminate any options that include stimulating activities or stimulants because these will impair sleep and should not be recommended activities prior to sleep.*

Content Area: Mental Health; *Category of Health Alteration:* Crisis, Violence, Eating, and Sleep Disorders; *Integrated Processes:* Teaching and Learning; *Client Need:* Health Promotion and Maintenance/Self-Care; *Cognitive Level:* Analysis

Reference: Fortinash, K., & Holoday Worret, P. (2008). *Psychiatric Mental Health Nursing* (4th ed., p. 418). St. Louis, MO: Mosby/Elsevier.

1564. A nurse reads in a 12-year-old client's medical record, "Fracture of left leg from a fall during an episode of somnambulism." Which intervention is most important for the nurse to add to the client's care plan?

1. Restrict visitors to immediate family only
2. Ensure that the bed exit alarm is turned on
3. Instruct the client to turn on the call light when getting out of bed
4. Avoid shadows and whispering when near the client, and monitor for hallucinations

ANSWER: 2

Somnambulism is a sleepwalking disorder in which the individual will participate in complex activities, such as walking, dressing, and toileting, all while in a deep non-REM stage of sleep. A hospitalized client is at risk for a fall or wandering. Turning on a bed exit alarm will alert the staff that the client is getting out of bed. Somnambulism is not associated with visitors. Instructing the client on call light use is useless when sleepwalking because the client is unaware that he or she is sleepwalking. Visual and auditory hallucinations are not associated with sleepwalking.

▶ ***Test-taking Tip:*** *Somnambulism is a sleepwalking disorder. Knowing this information should direct you to the correct option.*

Content Area: Mental Health; *Category of Health Alteration:* Crisis, Violence, Eating, and Sleep Disorders; *Integrated Processes:* Nursing Process Planning; *Client Need:* Safe and Effective Care Environment/Management of Care/Continuity of Care; *Cognitive Level:* Analysis

Reference: Fortinash, K., & Holoday Worret, P. (2008). *Psychiatric Mental Health Nursing* (4th ed., p. 416). St. Louis, MO: Mosby/Elsevier.

1565. A nurse is completing a health history on a client. The client states, "I just can't sleep. I'm only getting a few hours of sleep at night. I just started a new job and I can't do my best without getting enough sleep." The client's history includes a recent breakup with a long-term companion. Which initial statement should be made by the nurse?

1. "Let's try to identify major stressors in your life."
2. "How many hours of sleep do you usually get each night?"
3. "New jobs can be stressful and stress can certainly affect sleep."
4. "Do you think your breakup has something to do with your problem?"

ANSWER: 2

The client should be asked to describe what the client believes to be a healthy sleep pattern in order to assess client expectations and deviation from normal sleep pattern. The other options begin to identify stressors that can affect sleep before fully assessing the extent of the client's sleep problem.

▶ ***Test-taking Tip:*** *Apply the nursing process. A full assessment of the problem should be completed prior to identifying possible causes for intervention.*

Content Area: Mental Health; *Category of Health Alteration:* Crisis, Violence, Eating, and Sleep Disorders; *Integrated Processes:* Nursing Process Assessment; *Client Need:* Physiological Integrity/Basic Care and Comfort/Rest and Sleep; *Cognitive Level:* Analysis

Reference: Varcarolis, E., Carson, V., & Shoemaker, N. (2006). *Foundations of Psychiatric Mental Health Nursing: A Clinical Approach* (5th ed., p. 662). St. Louis, MO: Saunders/Elsevier.

1566. A nurse is overheard responding to a client who reports sleeping only 3 hours at night. Which statement made by the nurse to the client requires the nurse manager to follow up with the nurse?

1. "You sound worried that you may lose your job."
2. "How much sleep do you usually get each night?"
3. "Sleep disorders are common among people who are depressed."
4. "Do you think stress may be interfering with your ability to sleep?"

ANSWER: 3

Telling a client that sleep disorders are common among people who are depressed prematurely informs the client that a sleep disorder has been confirmed or tells that client that he or she is depressed. The statement is inappropriate, and the nurse needs remediation regarding discussing unconfirmed presumptions with clients. The remaining options are not inappropriate since they all seek to gain further information that might be used to assess the client's problem and thus do not require immediate follow-up.

▸ ***Test-taking Tip:*** *Read each option carefully and select a statement in which the nurse is making a medical diagnosis of the client's possible problem.*

Content Area: Mental Health; *Category of Health Alteration:* Crisis, Violence, Eating, and Sleep Disorders; *Integrated Processes:* Nursing Process Assessment; *Client Need:* Psychosocial Integrity/Stress Management; Physiological Integrity/Basic Care and Comfort/Rest and Sleep; *Cognitive Level:* Analysis

Reference: Varcarolis, E., Carson, V., & Shoemaker, N. (2006). *Foundations of Psychiatric Mental Health Nursing: A Clinical Approach* (5th ed., p. 662). St. Louis, MO: Saunders/Elsevier.

1567. Which statement made by an adult client best indicates to a nurse that the client has signs of a sleep disorder?

1. "I realize now that I've never needed more than 5 hours of sleep at night."
2. "Before I had my hyperthyroidism treated with radiation, I was awake for most of the night."
3. "I'm waking up about every 3 hours to go to the bathroom."
4. "I used to sleep 8 hours at night, but now I average about 6 hours and feel tired when I get up."

ANSWER: 4

Sleeping 6 hours indicates a change in the client's sleep pattern and the resulting dysfunction it has created. While the average is 8 hours of sleep at night, the amount of sleep required to feel refreshed varies and some people may need only 5 hours of sleep at night for optimal functioning. Hyperthyroidism can result in hyperactivity, but a statement about its treatment indicates that the problem with sleep has been resolved. Waking up frequently to urinate indicates a problem with elimination that is affecting sleep. The elimination problem should be addressed.

▸ ***Test-taking Tip:*** *Note the key word "best." Use the process of elimination to select an option that indicates a disruption to the normal sleep pattern and the amount of sleep obtained.*

Content Area: Mental Health; *Category of Health Alteration:* Crisis, Violence, Eating, and Sleep Disorders; *Integrated Processes:* Nursing Process Assessment; *Client Need:* Physiological Integrity/Basic Care and Comfort/Rest and Sleep; *Cognitive Level:* Application

Reference: Varcarolis, E., Carson, V., & Shoemaker, N. (2006). *Foundations of Psychiatric Mental Health Nursing: A Clinical Approach* (5th ed., p. 662). St. Louis, MO: Saunders/Elsevier.

Test 41: **Mental Health: End-of-Life Care**

1568. A client with end-stage renal disease has decided to terminate dialysis treatments. The client says to a nurse, "Although I have sought God's guidance in my decision, sometimes I wonder if what I have chosen to do is acceptable to God." The nurse's best response is:

1. "Since you prayed about your decision and feel it is right, your decision to terminate dialysis is probably the right thing to do."
2. "It's good to seek God's guidance when making difficult decisions."
3. "Not knowing about the future and how decisions affect this can be worrisome."
4. "If you are feeling uncertain about your decision to terminate dialysis, you can always go back on dialysis in a few weeks."

ANSWER: 3

The statement in option 3 recognizes the client's feelings. Option 1 denies the client's feelings and provides false reassurance. The statement implies that the client has no cause for worry or concern. Option 2 denies the client's feelings and interjects the nurse's beliefs and values. Option 4 denies the client's feelings and provides incorrect information. With end-stage renal disease, dialysis is performed three times weekly. It is unlikely that the client will live for a few weeks without dialysis.

➧ ***Test-taking Tip:*** *Focus on using therapeutic communication skills and select the option that recognizes the client's feelings.*

Content Area: Mental Health; *Category of Health Alteration:* End-of-Life Care; *Integrated Processes:* Communication and Documentation; *Client Need:* Psychosocial Integrity/End-of-Life Care; *Cognitive Level:* Analysis

Reference: Harkreader, H., Hogan, M., & Thobaben, M. (2007). *Fundamentals of Nursing* (3rd ed., p. 271). St. Louis, MO: Saunders/Elsevier.

1569. An 82-year-old male client, who has just been diagnosed with stage II prostate cancer, informs a nurse of his desire for a DNR order. The nurse's best *initial* action should be to:

1. contact the physician to obtain the order.
2. ask the client to share his feelings related to the new diagnosis.
3. make a referral for the hospital chaplain.
4. ask the client if he knows anyone else who has had prostate cancer.

ANSWER: 2

Asking the client to share his feelings related to the new diagnosis would be the best initial action to determine why the client desires this new DNR order and would encourage communication between the nurse and client. Contacting the physician to obtain the order would be a priority but not the best initial action; the client may be asking for the order as a reaction to fear generated by the new diagnosis. Making a referral for the hospital chaplain also may be helpful if the client desires it, but the nurse should assess the client's feelings first. Asking the client if he knows anyone else who has had prostate cancer may be helpful in the working phase of the relationship when the nurse and client are exploring alternatives together, but it would not be the best initial action.

➧ ***Test-taking Tip:*** *Read the question carefully and choose the best initial action. Apply the nursing process.*

Content Area: Mental Health; *Category of Health Alteration:* End-of-Life Care; *Integrated Processes:* Nursing Process Implementation; *Client Need:* Psychosocial Integrity/End-of-Life Care; *Cognitive Level:* Analysis

Reference: Wilkinson, J., & Van Leuven, K. (2007). *Fundamentals of Nursing: Theory, Concepts & Applications* (Vol. 1, pp. 344–346). Philadelphia: F. A. Davis.

1570. A client says to a nurse, "I wish my family would let me die in peace. I get so angry that my family keeps hovering over me as if I have given up. The doctor told me I have terminal lung cancer and there is no cure!" Which is the best therapeutic response by the nurse?

1. "Your family is hovering over you? I can ask them to leave if you wish."
2. "You are angry because your family thinks that you have given up hope for a cure?"
3. "Have you talked to your family about your feelings?"
4. "You shouldn't feel angry. Your family is just trying to show that they love and care for you."

ANSWER: 2

The nurse is restating what the client says to ensure understanding and to review what the client has said. Restating is a therapeutic communication technique. In option 1, the nurse is repeating what the client has stated as a closed statement and offers a solution. It does not promote a therapeutic interaction. In option 3, the nurse is attempting to assess the client's ability to discuss feelings openly with family members, which is premature. It can also be misconstrued as offering advice, which hinders therapeutic communication. In option 4, the nurse is belittling the client's feelings, which is a hindrance to therapeutic communication.

➧ ***Test-taking Tip:*** *Focus on the option that uses a therapeutic communication technique.*

Content Area: Mental Health; *Category of Health Alteration:* End-of-Life Care; *Integrated Processes:* Communication and Documentation; *Client Need:* Psychosocial Integrity/End-of-Life Care; *Cognitive Level:* Analysis

Reference: Fortinash, K., & Holoday Worret, P. (2008). *Psychiatric Mental Health Nursing* (4th ed., pp. 76–77). St. Louis, MO: Mosby/Elsevier.

1571. A terminally ill, 46-year-old client has an order for morphine sulfate 2 mg to 6 mg intravenously (IV) every 2 hours prn for pain. A nurse administers 2 mg for the first dose, but after 20 minutes the client has no relief and experiences no side effects. What is the nurse's best action?

1. Wait until the 2 hours has elapsed from the time the 2 mg morphine sulfate was administered before giving additional medication, but implement complementary measures for pain control.
2. Call the physician to determine if additional medication can be administered now, since the client had inadequate pain relief.
3. Administer 4 mg of morphine sulfate at the peak effect of the first dose, which would be 20 minutes after the first dose.
4. Repeat the 2 mg of morphine sulfate now and, if not effective, administer the additional 2 mg in 15 minutes.

ANSWER: 3

The client has a range order for morphine sulfate. The total dose is 6 mg in a 2-hour period. Since the client had no relief after 15 minutes and no side effects, 4 mg should be administered to maximize pain control. The peak time for morphine sulfate administered IV is 20 minutes. Complementary measures can be used to distract the client from pain but should not replace analgesic medications for pain control. It is unnecessary to call the physician because the ordered dose is up to 6 mg in 2 hours. The initial dose of 2 mg did not relieve the client's pain; giving an additional 2 mg now and then waiting will only delay when the client can receive the next maximum dose of the medication for adequate pain control.

▶ ***Test-taking Tip:*** *Recognize that the morphine sulfate has been ordered as a range order. Carefully consider the data in the situation.*

Content Area: Mental Health; *Category of Health Alteration:* End-of-Life Care; *Integrated Processes:* Nursing Process Implementation; *Client Need:* Psychosocial Integrity/End-of-Life Care; *Cognitive Level:* Analysis

Reference: Smeltzer, S., Bare, B., Hinkle, J., & Cheever, K. (2008). *Brunner & Suddarth's Textbook of Medical-Surgical Nursing* (11th ed., pp. 280, 464–465). Philadelphia: Lippincott Williams & Wilkins.

1572. EBP The family of a terminally ill client is called to a hospital because the client's death is imminent. Which assessment findings should lead a nurse to conclude that the client's death is near? SELECT ALL THAT APPLY.

1. Cheyne-Stokes respirations
2. Reports seeing persons who have already died
3. States that he or she is dying
4. Extremities feel warm to touch
5. Blood pressure (BP) 80/55 mm Hg
6. Body is held in a rigid, unchanging position

ANSWER: 1, 2, 3, 6

Physical and psychological signs that death is imminent include Cheyne-Stokes respirations, reports of seeing persons who have already died, stating he or she is dying, and a rigid body position. Additional physical signs affect multiple body systems, including musculoskeletal, gastrointestinal (GI), respiratory, cardiovascular, neurological, and renal systems. Extremities will feel cold to the touch, not warm. The systolic BP is below 70 mm Hg and the diastolic BP below 50 mm Hg when death is imminent. A BP of 80/55 mm Hg has a mean arterial pressure of 63, indicating that organs are receiving adequate perfusion.

▶ ***Test-taking Tip:*** *Recall that besides physical signs of imminent death, the client may express feelings of impending death.*

Content Area: Mental Health; *Category of Health Alteration:* End-of-Life Care; *Integrated Processes:* Nursing Process Evaluation; *Client Need:* Psychosocial Integrity/End-of-Life Care; *Cognitive Level:* Application

Reference: Harkreader, H., Hogan, M., & Thobaben, M. (2007). *Fundamentals of Nursing* (3rd ed., p. 1184). St. Louis, MO: Saunders/Elsevier.

EBP Reference: Institute for Clinical Systems Improvement. (2007). *Palliative Care*. Available at: www.guideline.gov/summary/summary.aspx?doc_id=10589&nbr=005531&string=grief

1573. EBP A 65-year-old female client, who has end-stage cardiomyopathy with an ejection fraction of 10%, tells a nurse that she does not want to be resuscitated if she stops breathing. The client currently has a full resuscitation status noted on the medical record. Based on this information, the nurse should *first*:

1. inform the client's health-care provider of the request.
2. ask the client if she wishes to complete a written advance health-care directive.
3. document the client's statements in her medical record.
4. advise the client to discuss her wishes with her surrogate decision maker who will make health-care decisions for her when she is unable to make her own decisions.

ANSWER: 1

A written order instructing the health-care team not to attempt CPR is required. The order must be signed by the health-care provider for it to be valid. The client can complete an advanced health care directive to make her wishes known. This is a directive to the health-care provider indicating the client's wishes requiring resuscitation or other life-sustaining measures; a do not resuscitate (DNR) written order is still required. Health-care professionals can improve the end-of-life decision making for clients by encouraging the use of advance directives. The nurse should document the client's statements and advise the client to discuss her wishes with her surrogate decision maker, but neither of these are the first action.

Test-taking Tip: *The key word is "first."*

Content Area: Mental Health; *Category of Health Alteration:* End-of-Life Care; *Integrated Processes:* Nursing Process Implementation; *Client Need:* Psychosocial Integrity/End-of-Life Care; *Cognitive Level:* Application

Reference: Lewis, S., Heitkemper, M., Dirksen, S., O'Brien, P., & Bucher, L. (2007). *Medical-Surgical Nursing: Assessment and Management of Clinical Problems* (7th ed., pp. 155–156). St. Louis, MO: Mosby.

EBP Reference: Mitty, E., & Ramsey, G. (2008). Advance directives. In E. Capezuti, D. Zwicker, M. Mezey, & T. Fulmer (Eds.), *Evidence-Based Geriatric Nursing Protocols for Best Practice* (3rd ed., pp. 539–563). New York: Springer. Available at: www.guideline.gov/summary/summary.aspx?doc_id=12264&nbr=006348&string=Advance+AND+directives

1574. EBP A client, who has been diagnosed with prostate cancer and received chemotherapy and radiation treatments, is admitted to a hospital for palliative care. A nurse understands that the client:

1. will require minimal nursing care since a cure is no longer a treatment option.
2. is expected to expire within 5 to 7 days.
3. is unable to make decisions independently regarding medical treatment.
4. will receive care that relieves symptoms without hastening or postponing the client's death.

ANSWER: 4

Palliative care is supportive and compassionate care given to clients who opt not to seek curative treatment for a terminal illness. Treatment focuses on symptom control and assisting the client and family through preparation for and through the dying process. Palliative care is often complex since it includes support for clients and their families while controlling symptoms such as pain. There is not a specific timetable involved with the client's life expectancy. Clients are encouraged and often take an active role in planning treatment options in symptom control until progressing to the stage of active dying.

Test-taking Tip: *The issue of the question is what is meant by "palliative care." Information in the stem states the client has cancer and has received treatment. Further care would not be indicated if the cancer were cured. Evaluate each response and choose the option that is more inclusive than the other options.*

Content Area: Mental Health; Fundamentals; *Category of Health Alteration:* End-of-Life Care; *Integrated Processes:* Nursing Process Analysis; *Client Need:* Psychosocial Integrity/End-of-Life Care; *Cognitive Level:* Analysis

Reference: Ignatavicius, D., & Workman, M. (2006). *Medical-Surgical Nursing: Critical Thinking for Collaborative Care* (5th ed., pp. 106–109). St. Louis, MO: Elsevier/Saunders.

EBP References: Qaseem, A., Snow, V., Shekelle, P., Casey, D., Cross, J., et al. (2008). Evidence-based interventions to improve the palliative care of pain, dyspnea, and depression at the end of life: A clinical practice guideline from the American College of Physicians. *Annals of Internal Medicine*, 148(2), 141–146; National Consensus Project for Quality Palliative Care. (2004). *Clinical Practice Guidelines for Quality Palliative Care.* Brooklyn, NY: Author. Available at: www.guideline.gov/summary/summary.aspx?doc_id=5058&nbr=003542&string=grief

1575. A nurse is assessing a 45-year-old client diagnosed with end-stage renal failure who is near death. Which finding suggests that the client has an altered body image?

1. Shows the nurse the internal arteriovenous graft site where the fistula is occluded
2. Begins to cry when the nurse asks about the client's family
3. Tells the nurse that life is no longer worth living
4. Remarks that retaining so much extra fluid is disfiguring and unsightly

ANSWER: 4

Verbalization of negative feelings about the body (disfiguring and unsightly) supports a nursing diagnosis of altered body image. There is no evidence that the client verbalized or displayed negative feelings when showing the nurse an occluded graft site. Crying and stating that life is no longer worth living are signs of grieving.

➧ ***Test-taking Tip:*** *Because altered body image should relate to the client's body, eliminate all options that do not pertain to the client's body. Of the remaining two options, determine which option reflects negative feelings.*

Content Area: Mental Health; *Category of Health Alteration:* End-of-Life Care; *Integrated Processes:* Nursing Process Assessment; *Client Need:* Psychosocial Integrity/Coping Mechanisms; *Cognitive Level:* Application

Reference: Berman, A., Snyder, S., Kozier, B., & Erb, G. (2008). *Kozier & Erb's Fundamentals of Nursing: Concepts, Process, and Practice* (8th ed., pp. 1009, 1084). Upper Saddle River, NJ: Pearson Education.

1576. **EBP** A client with AIDS states to a nurse, "This disease has eaten away my body; I'm nothing but a bag of bones. The sores on my body make my family uncomfortable and reluctant to come near me, even though I am dying." Which interventions should the nurse implement to assist the client to cope with the disturbed body image? SELECT ALL THAT APPLY.

1. Spend extra time with the client
2. Limit self-negation statements
3. Initiate a spiritual care and psychiatric nurse consultant referral
4. Meet with the family to assess their coping and reaction to the change or loss
5. Spend extra time with the client to assist with efforts to enhance appearance
6. Tell the family that they need to spend more time with the client

ANSWER: 1, 2, 3, 4, 5

Frequent contact promotes the client's verbalization of feelings and allows consistent interventions. Self-negating statements can prolong the issue of a disturbed self-image and can interfere with maintaining the highest quality of life possible at the end of life. Collaboration promotes a holistic care plan and can hasten problem solving. Thoughts can influence feelings. Additional information about the family responses can aid in planning interventions for the client and family. The family's reaction could be related to anticipatory grieving and not to the client's appearance or illness. Appearance-enhancing measures can promote the client's sense of control and enhance self-esteem. The family may feel uncomfortable, and telling them to spend more time may increase their discomfort and result in less time with the client.

➧ ***Test-taking Tip:*** *Use the process of elimination to eliminate an option that could increase the client's feelings of a disturbed body image.*

Content Area: Mental Health; *Category of Health Alteration:* End-of-Life Care; *Integrated Processes:* Nursing Process Implementation; *Client Need:* Psychosocial Integrity/Coping Mechanisms; *Cognitive Level:* Application

Reference: Newfield, S., Hinz, M., Tilley, D., Sridaromont, K., & Maramba, P. (2007). *Cox's Clinical Applications of Nursing Diagnosis* (5th ed., pp. 541–548). Philadelphia: F. A. Davis.

EBP Reference: Rumsey, N., Clarke, A., White, P., Wyn-Williams, M., & Garlick, W. (2004). Altered body image: appearance-related concerns of people with visible disfigurement. *Journal of Advanced Nursing,* 48(5), 443–453.

1577. Which nursing direction to a nursing assistant is *inappropriate* when providing care for a dying client with sensory-perceptual alterations?

1. "Ask the client before turning on a bright light, because the client may have a preference for a darkened room."
2. "Be sure to whisper or talk quietly to the client because hearing is the last sense to be lost."
3. "Although touch is diminished, continue to provide comfort to the client with touch, because the pressure of touch can be felt."
4. "Reposition the client slowly, because quick position changes cause dizziness and a sensation of falling for the client."

ANSWER: 2

Hearing is not diminished when a person is dying. Speech should be clear and not whispering. Preferences when dying might include a dark or light room. Light sensitivity may occur, yet shadows may result in confusion or hallucinations. Touch is diminished when dying, but the pressure of touch is felt. A dying person's physiological alterations such as hypotension can cause dizziness and altered sensations.

➧ ***Test-taking Tip:*** *Recall the sensory-perceptual changes and the physiological needs of the dying person. The key word is "inappropriate." Select the option that is incorrect.*

Content Area: Mental Health; *Category of Health Alteration:* End-of-Life Care; *Integrated Processes:* Nursing Process Implementation; *Client Need:* Psychosocial Integrity/Sensory/Perceptual Alterations; *Cognitive Level:* Analysis

Reference: Berman, A., Snyder, S., Kozier, B., & Erb, G. (2008). *Kozier & Erb's Fundamentals of Nursing: Concepts, Process, and Practice* (8th ed., p. 1096). Upper Saddle River, NJ: Pearson Education.

1578. A client who is near death asks a nurse who is sitting nearby to lead a prayer to give him comfort and strength to face the afterlife. The client and the nurse are both of the Baptist faith. Which opening prayer would be most appropriate?

1. "Hail Mary, full of Grace; we beseech you to intercede and provide comfort for Mr. Brown during his last hours on earth and provide him strength as he faces death and eternal life."
2. "O Amida, I take refuge in you, Ocean of Oneness, Eternal Life and Light; I am entrusting my whole heart and mind in your Primal Vow of strength to face the unknown."
3. "Yahweh, ever-present God, and the giver of life, provide comfort to Mr. Brown during his last hours on earth and provide him strength as he faces death and eternal life."
4. "Jesus, you are the light of the world and the giver of strength. Provide comfort to Mr. Brown during his last hours on earth, and provide him strength as he faces death and eternal life."

ANSWER: 4

While prayers may be similar in differing faiths, the addressee of the prayer is different. People of the Baptist faith address their prayer to Jesus. The client's proper name should be included to personalize the prayer. People of the Catholic faith may address their prayer to Mary. People praying a Buddhist prayer may address their prayer to Amida. People of the Jewish faith may address their prayer to God or Yahweh.

➧ ***Test-taking Tip:*** *Note that the prayers are similar but the addressee of the prayer is different. Select the addressee that would be appropriate for a client of the Baptist faith.*

Content Area: Mental Health; *Category of Health Alteration:* End-of-Life Care; *Integrated Processes:* Communication and Documentation; *Client Need:* Psychosocial Integrity/Religious and Spiritual Influences on Health; *Cognitive Level:* Application

Reference: Berman, A., Snyder, S., Kozier, B., & Erb, G. (2008). *Kozier & Erb's Fundamentals of Nursing: Concepts, Process, and Practice* (8th ed., p. 1053). Upper Saddle River, NJ: Pearson Education.

1579. Which action should a nurse plan when caring for four clients of varying religious beliefs who are near death?

1. Repositioning the bed so it is turned toward Mecca for a client of the Jewish faith
2. Calling a priest to anoint the sick and hear the confession of a client of the Methodist faith
3. Arranging for an uninterrupted time for male family members to wash the body of a male client of the Muslim faith who has just died
4. Speaking to the family of a client of the Buddhist faith about cremation within 24 hours to release the soul from any earthly attachment

ANSWER: 3

Persons of the Muslim (Islam) faith believe in special procedures for care of the body after death and a ritual bath with male family members washing male bodies and females washing female bodies. Muslims who are dying also want their body or heads turned toward Mecca. A priest would anoint the sick (formerly Last Rites) for a person of the Catholic faith. Hindus cremate the body within 24 hours to release the soul from any earthly attachment.

➧ ***Test-taking Tip:*** *Focus on both the action and the faith of the client.*

Content Area: Mental Health; *Category of Health Alteration:* End-of-Life Care; *Integrated Processes:* Nursing Process Planning; *Client Need:* Psychosocial Integrity/Religious and Spiritual Influences on Health; *Cognitive Level:* Analysis

References: Berman, A., Snyder, S., Kozier, B., & Erb, G. (2008). *Kozier & Erb's Fundamentals of Nursing: Concepts, Process, and Practice* (8th ed., p. 1048). Upper Saddle River, NJ: Pearson Education; Craven, R., & Hirnle, C. (2009). *Fundamentals of Nursing: Human Health and Function* (6th ed., pp. 1401–1402). Philadelphia: Lippincott Williams & Wilkins.

1580. The parents of a 10-year-old child have just been told that the child has cancer. Which care measure should a nurse identify as a priority for the child and family?

1. Provide support for anticipatory grieving.
2. Provide comfort cares.
3. Teach self-care measures.
4. Allow as much independence as possible.

ANSWER: 1

Anticipatory grieving is psychological and physiological responses to an impending real or imagined loss of a significant person, object, belief, or relationship. Because the child and family will be overwhelmed with the news, this is the priority. Providing comfort cares, teaching, and allowing independence may be pertinent depending on the child's health state, but these are not the priority.

➧ ***Test-taking Tip:*** *The key word is "priority." Use steps of the grieving process to answer this question. The first grief response is shock. Eliminate options 2, 3, and 4, because these do not address interventions during the shock state.*

Content Area: Mental Health; *Category of Health Alteration:* End-of-Life Care; *Integrated Processes:* Caring; *Client Need:* Psychosocial Integrity/Grief and Loss; *Cognitive Level:* Analysis

Reference: Craven, R., & Hirnle, C. (2009). *Fundamentals of Nursing: Human Health and Function* (6th ed., p. 1314). Philadelphia: Lippincott Williams & Wilkins.

1581. An emergency department nurse is present with the family of a client who just died as a result of an automobile accident. Which statements made by the nurse are therapeutic when communicating with the grieving family? SELECT ALL THAT APPLY.

1. "It's all right to grieve."
2. "Tell me how you are feeling."
3. "God had a purpose for everything, and it was your father's life at this time."
4. "Everyone has to die sometime. It was your father's time."
5. "I know how you feel. I lost my dad this time last year."
6. "I will be thinking of and praying for you and your family."

ANSWER: 1, 2, 6

Statements in options 1, 2, and 6 convey nonjudgmental acceptance of grief and offer support and interventions to promote the grieving process. Statements in options 3, 4, and 5 reduce the loss to a common denominator, making one person the same as the next.

▶ ***Test-taking Tip:*** *Focus on therapeutic communication techniques and eliminate options that would be a barrier to communication or grieving.*

Content Area: Mental Health; *Category of Health Alteration:* End-of-Life Care; *Integrated Processes:* Communication and Documentation; *Client Need:* Psychosocial Integrity/Grief and Loss; *Cognitive Level:* Analysis

Reference: Harkreader, H., Hogan, M., & Thobaben, M. (2007). *Fundamentals of Nursing* (3rd ed., p. 1189). St. Louis, MO: Saunders/Elsevier.

1582. A nurse is counseling a mother who has had prolonged grief after the death of her child. Which statement would assist the nurse in assessing whether the mother is experiencing guilt?

1. "Are you especially troubled by a certain memory or thought?"
2. "Tell me about your favorite memories with your child."
3. "Sometimes writing your feelings in a journal helps to deal with guilt feelings."
4. "Are there things you are having trouble doing?"

ANSWER: 1

Asking the mother if she is especially troubled by a certain memory or thought is an assessment-type question that should elicit additional information. Feelings of guilt or regret can delay the normal grieving process. Option 2 is an open-ended statement that supports the mother's expression of positive memories which is an intervention. Option 3 of encouraging journaling is an intervention. Option 4 is a question to assess coping skills.

▶ ***Test-taking Tip:*** *Use the nursing process and eliminate options that do not relate to assessment but rather interventions. Of the two remaining options, determine which would be best.*

Content Area: Mental Health; *Category of Health Alteration:* End-of-Life Care; *Integrated Processes:* Nursing Process Assessment; *Client Need:* Psychosocial Integrity/Grief and Loss; *Cognitive Level:* Application

Reference: Smeltzer, S., Bare, B., Hinkle, J., & Cheever, K. (2008). *Brunner & Suddarth's Textbook of Medical-Surgical Nursing* (11th ed., p. 473). Philadelphia: Lippincott Williams & Wilkins.

1583. A 5-year-old child, involved in a motor vehicle accident in which her mother was killed, tells a nurse that, if she wishes hard enough, she knows her mom will come back from the dead. The nurse understands that the child is:

1. verbalizing perceptions that are characteristic of the child's developmental age.
2. expressing magical thinking.
3. ineffectively coping with the loss of her mother.
4. denying the reality that her mother had died.

ANSWER: 1

Children ages 5 to 6 years perceive death as unnatural, reversible, and avoidable and believe in the power of wishes. Magical thinking is expressed by younger children. The situation as described gives no indication that the child is coping ineffectively or denying the reality of the mother's death.

▶ ***Test-taking Tip:*** *Think about the developmental level of a 5 to 6 year old and his or her experience with death.*

Content Area: Mental Health; *Category of Health Alteration:* End-of-Life Care; *Integrated Processes:* Nursing Process Evaluation; *Client Need:* Psychosocial Integrity/Grief and Loss; *Cognitive Level:* Analysis

Reference: Craven, R., & Hirnle, C. (2009). *Fundamentals of Nursing: Human Health and Function* (6th ed., pp. 1316–1318). Philadelphia: Lippincott Williams & Wilkins.

1584. EBP Which statement by a nurse is best when caring for an adult client who was told an illness is terminal and is offered hospice care?

1. "I know this is not what you wanted to hear."
2. "There is nothing more we can do."
3. "What we are going to focus on now is your pain control and comfort."
4. "Hospice care can assist with symptom control and provide peace at the time of your death."

ANSWER: 3

Focusing on comfort measures is offering the client realistic hope not involving a cure but symptom control. Statements in options 1 and 2 do not offer the client realistic hope. While option 4 offers hope, the focus is on what hospice care can do and not on the immediate needs of the client.

▶ ***Test-taking Tip:*** *Focus on an option that meets the immediate needs of the client.*

Content Area: Mental Health; *Category of Health Alteration:* End-of-Life Care; *Integrated Processes:* Communication and Documentation; *Client Need:* Psychosocial Integrity/Grief and Loss; *Cognitive Level:* Analysis

Reference: Smeltzer, S., Bare, B., Hinkle, J., & Cheever, K. (2008). *Brunner & Suddarth's Textbook of Medical-Surgical Nursing* (11th ed., pp. 462–463). Philadelphia: Lippincott Williams & Wilkins.

EBP Reference: Institute for Clinical Systems Improvement. (2007). *Palliative Care*. Available at: www.guideline.gov/summary/summary.aspx?doc_id=10589&nbr=005531&string=grief

1585. A nurse determines that five clients are in five different stages of grief according to Kübler-Ross's stages. Place the five clients in the order of these stages from the first to the last stage.

______ A 45-year-old client who is terminal with breast cancer says to the nurse, "If only God would let me live until I see my son graduate, then I will be ready to die."

______ A 20-year-old client who was just told that his mother, father, and two younger siblings were killed in an automobile accident says to the nurse, "Check the name again; you must be wrong."

______ A parent, whose child died 6 months previously, says to the nurse, "I have begun to remove items from my baby's room and given them to my sister, who is having a baby."

______ A 75-year-old woman receiving palliative care for throat cancer refuses tube feedings and refuses to look at herself in the mirror.

______ A parent of a brain-injured child says to the nurse, "You keep disturbing my child with your incessant checking; he isn't getting better because you keep trying to wake him."

ANSWER: 3, 1, 5, 4, 2

The five stages of grief, according to Kübler-Ross, are denial, anger, bargaining, depression, and acceptance. The 20-year-old client who was just told that his mother, father, and two younger siblings were killed in an automobile accident is in denial. The parent of a brain-injured child who says to the nurse, "You keep disturbing my child with your incessant checking; he is not get better because you keep trying to wake him" is in the anger phase. The 45-year-old client who is terminal with breast cancer and says to the nurse, "If only God would let me live until I see my son graduate, then I will be ready to die" is bargaining. The 75-year-old woman receiving palliative care for throat cancer who refuses tube feedings and to look at herself in the mirror is exhibiting signs of depression. The parent whose child died 6 months previously and says to the nurse, "I have begun to remove items from my baby's room and given them to my sister, who is having a baby" is displaying signs of acceptance.

▶ ***Test-taking Tip:*** *Recall that the five stages of grief according to Kübler-Ross are denial, anger, bargaining, depression, and acceptance.*

Content Area: Mental Health; *Category of Health Alteration:* End-of-Life Care; *Integrated Processes:* Nursing Process Evaluation; *Client Need:* Psychosocial Integrity/Grief and Loss; *Cognitive Level:* Synthesis

Reference: Smeltzer, S., Bare, B., Hinkle, J., & Cheever, K. (2008). *Brunner & Suddarth's Textbook of Medical-Surgical Nursing* (11th ed., p. 472). Philadelphia: Lippincott Williams & Wilkins.

1586. While a nurse is present, a client tells his family members, "I just can't go on with these chemotherapy treatments anymore. Although I want to be comfortable, I want to go home to die." The wife begins crying and angrily responds, "You are giving up. You got well after being really sick after pneumonia, and you can get over this, too." The son responds, "Dad can get over this if he just tries." The client becomes withdrawn and avoids eye contact with his family. Which nursing diagnosis would be best to add to the client's plan of care?

1. Defensive coping
2. Compromised family coping
3. Anxiety
4. Dysfunctional grieving

ANSWER: 2

Compromised family coping occurs when a supportive person provides insufficient support or encouragement that may be needed by the client to manage adaptive tasks related to the health challenge. The situation does not best describe defensive coping, anxiety, or dysfunctional grieving. Defensive coping is repeated projection of a falsely positive self-evaluation that defends against perceived threats to positive self-regard. Anxiety is a vague uneasy feeling of discomfort or dread accompanied by an autonomic response. Dysfunctional grieving is extended, unsuccessful use of intellectual and emotional responses to work through modifying the self-concept based on the perceptions of the loss.

▶ ***Test-taking Tip:*** *Read the situation carefully and consider the responses of the client and family. The key word is "best."*

Content Area: Mental Health; *Category of Health Alteration:* End-of-Life Care; *Integrated Processes:* Nursing Process Analysis; *Client Need:* Psychosocial Integrity/Family Dynamics; *Cognitive Level:* Analysis

References: Newfield, S., Hinz, M., Tilley, D., Sridaromont, K., & Maramba, P. (2007). *Cox's Clinical Applications of Nursing Diagnosis* (5th ed., pp. 530, 654, 760, 771–772). Philadelphia: F. A. Davis; Potter, P., & Perry, A. (2009). *Fundamentals of Nursing* (7th ed., p. 472). St. Louis, MO: Mosby.

1587. EBP Cardiopulmonary resuscitation is in progress for a client when the client's wife and teenage son arrive. When a nurse intercepts them and tries to move them away from the room the wife cries, "I've got to be with him! He needs us." The son keeps walking toward the room and attempts to enter. Which action is most appropriate?

1. Call for a member of the clergy to be with the wife and son outside the room.
2. Explain that they will be taken into the room by a designated person who will stay with them.
3. Touch the wife and son to console and detain them and explain what is taking place.
4. Ask the code team if they can enter, so the wife can hold her husband's hand and the son can observe.

ANSWER: 2

Research has shown that family member presence during resuscitation have assisted them in dealing with their grief. Recommended procedures include having a designated person (clergy, social worker, or nurse) with them in the room. While being outside the room with a member of the clergy is an option, the room door would be closed to protect the client's privacy. Detaining the wife and son is likely to be met with resistance. Asking the code team is acceptable, but touching the client or the client's bed during defibrillation is harmful to the wife. Code efforts should not be interrupted during the family's presence.

➧ ***Test-taking Tip:*** *Focus on the needs of the family. The key phrase is "most appropriate."*

Content Area: Mental Health; *Category of Health Alteration:* End-of-Life Care; *Integrated Processes:* Nursing Process Implementation; *Client Need:* Psychosocial Integrity/Family Dynamics; *Cognitive Level:* Analysis

Reference: Craven, R., & Hirnle, C. (2009). *Fundamentals of Nursing: Human Health and Function* (6th ed., p. 904). Philadelphia: Lippincott Williams & Wilkins.

EBP Reference: Critchell, C., & Marik, P. (2007). Should family members be present during cardiopulmonary resuscitation? A review of the literature. *American Journal of Hospice and Palliative Medicine,* 24(4), 311–317.

1588. A palliative care nurse visits the wife and an adolescent daughter of a deceased client. Which behaviors exhibited by the daughter should the nurse anticipate may occur due to the adolescent's developmental stage? SELECT ALL THAT APPLY.

1. Personifying the death as a monster who took her dad away
2. Withdrawing into herself
3. Going about her usual activities
4. Trying to take care of her grieving mother
5. Increasing defiance toward her mother
6. Talking on the phone with a friend about the death of her dad

ANSWER: 2, 3, 4, 5, 6

Adolescents may have difficulty tolerating the intense feelings associated with the death of a loved one. They may withdraw into themselves or go about their usual activities in an effort to avoid dealing with the pain of the loss. Some teens act out with aggression or defiance. Others try to take care of their loved ones who are grieving. Adolescents often find it easier to discuss their feelings with their peers rather than adults. Children ages 6 to 9 often personify death in the form of a "boogey man" or monster.

➧ ***Test-taking Tip:*** *Recall that adolescents can have a wide range of responses to the loss of a loved one.*

Content Area: Mental Health; *Category of Health Alteration:* End-of-Life Care; *Integrated Processes:* Nursing Process Assessment; *Client Need:* Psychosocial Integrity/Grief and Loss; *Cognitive Level:* Analysis

Reference: Townsend, M. (2006). *Psychiatric Mental Health Nursing* (5th ed., p. 899). Philadelphia: F. A. Davis.

1589. An 85-year-old spouse of a client, who passed away 2 months ago, states to a clinic nurse, "I am so thankful that my friends and family have been driving me places, because I don't have a driver's license anymore." The nurse interprets the client's statement as:

1. total dependency on others.
2. positive adaptation to the loss.
3. an exaggerated grief response.
4. inhibited grief.

ANSWER: 2

The client is adjusting to changes that have occurred because of the loss. If the client had identified only one person, it could be interpreted as dependence on a particular person. Assistance is provided only for driving, and the client is not totally dependent. An exaggerated grief response would be exhibiting feelings of sadness, helplessness, hopelessness, powerlessness, anger, and guilt as well as somatic complaints that render the individual dysfunctional with daily living. Inhibited grief is absence of grief when ordinarily it would be expected. It may or may not be expected 2 months after the death of a spouse.

➧ ***Test-taking Tip:*** *As each option is read, define the option and eliminate options that do not fit with the woman's statements.*

Content Area: Mental Health; *Category of Health Alteration:* End-of-Life Care; *Integrated Processes:* Nursing Process Analysis; *Client Need:* Psychosocial Integrity/Coping Mechanisms; *Cognitive Level:* Application

Reference: Townsend, M. (2006). *Psychiatric Mental Health Nursing* (5th ed., p. 896). Philadelphia: F. A. Davis.

1590. A nurse is teaching a class to parents who have an adolescent with a terminal illness. Which statement is most appropriate when helping parents with decisions about their child's care?

1. Adolescents should be expected to handle feelings about death in the same way as adults.
2. Adolescents have the right to make all their own decisions related to their health care.
3. The Patient Self-Determination Act of 1990 supports the rights of children 16 years old and older to make their own health-care decisions
4. Adolescents often become angry at their treatment changes, lack of explanations, and threats to their independence.

ANSWER: 4

Adolescents may become angry when changes occur or when they are not involved in decisions. They want to feel independent and be informed of their medical treatment plan. Adolescents handle feelings about death according to their developmental level. Unless the adolescents are emancipated adults, parents are the decision makers related to the health care of children under the age of 18 years. An emancipated minor has the same right as a competent adult to consent to or refuse medical treatment. In some states an unemancipated minor has the right to refuse life-sustaining treatment pursuant to the conditions and procedures of that state.

▶ ***Test-taking Tip:*** *Have an awareness of adolescent developmental stages.*

Content Area: Mental Health; *Category of Health Alteration:* End-of-Life Care; *Integrated Processes:* Teaching and Learning; *Client Need:* Psychosocial Integrity/Coping Mechanisms; *Cognitive Level:* Analysis

Reference: Ball, J., & Bindler, R. (2006). *Child Health Nursing: Partnering with Children and Families* (p. 491). Upper Saddle River, NJ: Pearson/Prentice Hall.

1591. A charge nurse overhears a new nurse talking with a client who is dying. The client states to the nurse, "Today is the day that I know I am going to die." Which statements made by the new nurse indicate that the new nurse is uncomfortable caring for dying clients? SELECT ALL THAT APPLY.

1. "You really don't mean that you want to die. Let's think of something more cheerful."
2. "You think today is the last day of your life?"
3. "I don't think things are really that bad."
4. "Everyone dies sooner or later; what's meant to be will be."
5. "I should go call your family so that they can be near you."

ANSWER: 1, 3, 4, 5

Changing the subject, offering false reassurance, denying what is happening, being fatalistic, blocking the discussion, and avoiding the client are all indicators that the nurse is uncomfortable with dying clients and is impeding the client's attempt to discuss dying and death. Restatement, as in option 2, facilitates therapeutic communication.

▶ ***Test-taking Tip:*** *The key word is "uncomfortable." Select options in which the new nurse changes the subject, offers false reassurance, belittles the client's feelings, blocks therapeutic communication, or avoids the client and eliminate the option that uses therapeutic communication.*

Content Area: Mental Health; *Category of Health Alteration:* End-of-Life Care; *Integrated Processes:* Nursing Process Evaluation; *Client Need:* Psychosocial Integrity/Coping Mechanisms; *Cognitive Level:* Analysis

Reference: Berman, A., Snyder, S., Kozier, B., & Erb, G. (2008). *Kozier & Erb's Fundamentals of Nursing: Concepts, Process, and Practice* (8th ed., p. 1091). Upper Saddle River, NJ: Pearson Education.

1592. An agitated father tearfully tells a crisis counselor, "I hate the man who raped and murdered my son. If he gets off, he will be sorry." What question should the nurse ask *first*?

1. "Do you have enough family or friends nearby to help you cope with your loss?"
2. "Are you thinking of harming yourself or others just like the man who killed your son?"
3. "Are you taking any medications, such as an antidepressant, that may help you through this difficult time?"
4. "How have you been venting your anger?"

ANSWER: 2

A client in crisis may have a distorted concept of reality and may harm self or others. Options 1, 3, and 4, while appropriate to evaluate coping strategies, should not be the nurse's first priority.

▶ ***Test-taking Tip:*** *Use Maslow's Hierarchy of Needs theory of safety before psychosocial interventions to aid in selecting the correct option. Note that options 1, 3, and 4 address interventions for adaptive coping, whereas option 2 is different.*

Content Area: Mental Health; *Category of Health Alteration:* End-of-Life Care; *Integrated Processes:* Communication and Documentation; *Client Need:* Psychosocial Integrity/Crisis Intervention; *Cognitive Level:* Application

Reference: Fortinash, K., & Holoday Worret, P. (2008). *Psychiatric Mental Health Nursing* (4th ed., pp. 456–457). St. Louis, MO: Mosby/Elsevier.

Test 42: **Mental Health: Personality Disorders**

1593. Which behavior should a nurse expect a client diagnosed with paranoid personality disorder to exhibit?

1. Able to trust those who treat the client well
2. Sees the goodwill of others when none exists
3. Acts the opposite of what the client may be thinking or feeling
4. Analyzes the behavior of others to find hidden and threatening meanings

ANSWER: 4

Paranoid personality disorder is characterized by mistrust and suspicion of others such that the behavior of others is analyzed to find hidden and threatening meanings. The person usually feels constant mistrust and suspicion toward others, not able to trust those treating the client well. Rather than seeing the good, a client sees ill will in the actions of others when none exists. Acting the opposite of what the client may be thinking or feeling is descriptive of reaction formation, a defense mechanism often used by persons with an obsessive-compulsive disorder.

Test-taking Tip: *Use the memory cue of the disorders by the clusters:* ***A*** *includes clients whose behavior is odd or eccentric;* ***B*** *includes clients who appear dramatic, emotional, or erratic; and* ***C*** *includes client's who appear anxious and fearful.*

Content Area: Mental Health; *Category of Health Alteration:* Personality and Other Mental Health Disorders; *Integrated Process:* Nursing Process Assessment; *Client Need:* Psychosocial Integrity/Psychopathology; *Cognitive Level:* Analysis

Reference: Videbeck, S. (2006). *Psychiatric Mental Health Nursing* (3rd ed., p. 347). Philadelphia: Lippincott Williams & Wilkins.

1594. **EBP** Individuals with antisocial personality disorder often exhibit poor judgment, emotional distance, aggression, and impulsivity. A nurse understands that besides the limbic system, which other area of the brain is implicated in causing these behaviors? Place an X on the affected area.

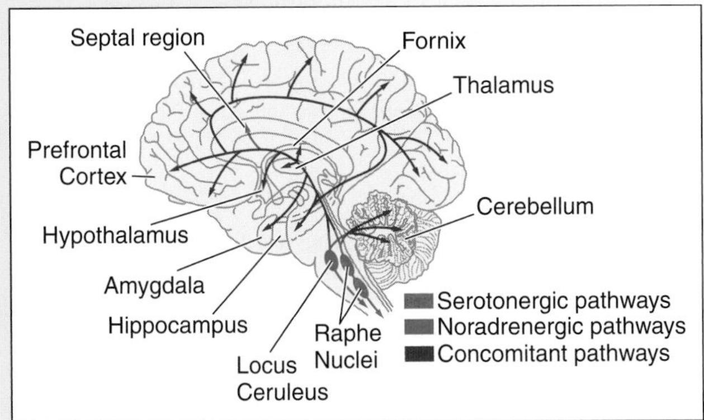

ANSWER:

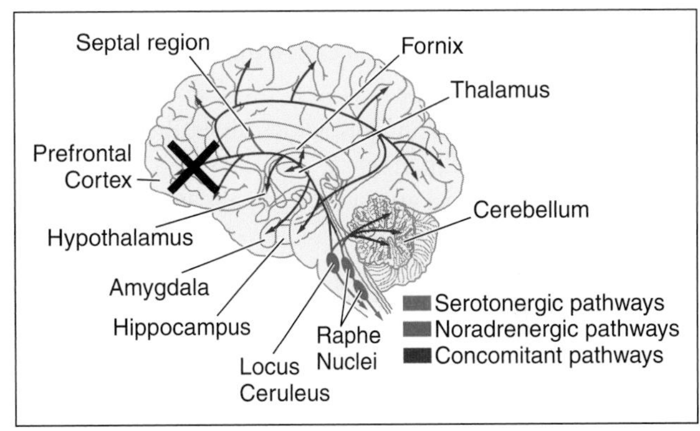

Recent research has implicated failure of control systems in the prefrontal cortex and limbic systems to modulate judgment, emotional distancing, aggression, and impulsivity.

Test-taking Tip: *Study the areas of the brain associated with the behaviors of each individual personality disorder.*

Content Area: Mental Health; *Category of Health Alteration:* Personality and Other Mental Health Disorders; *Integrated Process:* Nursing Process Analysis; *Client Need:* Psychosocial Integrity/Mental Health Concepts; *Cognitive Level:* Analysis

Reference: Boyd, M. (2008). *Psychiatric Nursing Contemporary Practice* (4th ed., p. 463). Philadelphia: Lippincott Williams & Wilkins.

EBP Reference: Siever, L. (2008). Neurobiology of aggression and violence. *American Journal of Psychiatry*, 165, 429–442.

1595. When working with a client with paranoid personality disorder, a nurse should:

1. approach the client in a businesslike manner to work on establishing trust.
2. approach the client first with social conversation to work on developing social relationships.
3. include jokes when conversing with the client to work on reducing the client's serious behavior.
4. arrive 15 minutes after the appointed time to work on eliminating hidden meanings.

ANSWER: 1

Clients with paranoid personality disorder take everything seriously and are attuned to the actions and motivations of others. Social conversation and jokes should be avoided. Punctuality and keeping commitments are necessary.

➧ ***Test-taking Tip:*** *Note that options 2, 3, and 4 are similar and option 1 is different. Often the option that is different is the answer.*

Content Area: Mental Health; *Category of Health Alteration:* Personality and Other Mental Health Disorders; *Integrated Process:* Nursing Process Implementation; *Client Need:* Psychosocial Integrity/Therapeutic Communication; *Cognitive Level:* Application

Reference: Videbeck, S. (2006). *Psychiatric Mental Health Nursing* (3rd ed., p. 347). Philadelphia: Lippincott Williams & Wilkins.

1596. Which behaviors should a nurse expect when working with a client with histrionic personality disorder? SELECT ALL THAT APPLY.

1. Exhibits discomfort in situations in which the client is not the center of attention
2. Shows apathy in conversations until trust is established
3. Lacks close friends or companions other than first-degree relatives
4. Considers relationships to be more intimate than they actually are
5. Harbors recurrent suspicions about the fidelity of their marital partner
6. Uses physical appearance to gain attention

ANSWER: 1, 4, 6

Diagnostic criteria for histrionic personality disorder include discomfort in situations in which the client is not the center of attention, considers relationships to be more intimate than they actually are, and uses physical appearance to gain attention. Individuals display dramatic, colorful, extroverted behavior, and are excitable and emotional. Rather than apathy, the person shows self-dramatization and exaggerated emotional expression. Lacking close friends or companions are behaviors associated with schizoid personality disorder. Harboring suspicions is characteristic of paranoid personality disorder.

➧ ***Test-taking Tip:*** *Use the definition of "histrionic personality disorder" to eliminate incorrect options. This disorder exhibits a pervasive pattern of excessive attention seeking and emotion.*

Content Area: Mental Health; *Category of Health Alteration:* Personality and Other Mental Health Disorders; *Integrated Process:* Nursing Process Assessment; *Client Need:* Psychosocial Integrity/Mental Health Concepts; *Cognitive Level:* Analysis

Reference: Townsend, M. (2006). *Psychiatric Mental Health Nursing, Concepts of Care in Evidence-Based Practice* (5th ed., p. 721). Philadelphia: F. A. Davis.

1597. A nurse is evaluating a client diagnosed with bipolar personality who is currently prescribed lithium (Lithane®) 300 mg tid. The client had a lithium level drawn, and the results are illustrated. The nurse receives an order to add fluoxetine (Prozac®) 20 mg bid and to administer the first dose. Based on the laboratory report findings, the nurse should: SELECT ALL THAT APPLY.

Client Chart

Laboratory Test	4 months ago	2 months ago	Today
Lithium level	1.0 mEq/L	1.2 mEq/L	1.5

1. administer the dose of fluoxetine.
2. question the dose of lithium.
3. question the dose of fluoxetine.
4. notify the physician of the laboratory test results.
5. question the addition of fluoxetine.

ANSWER: 2, 4, 5

The lithium level of 1.5 mEq/L is nearing toxicity (therapeutic range is 0.6–1.2 mEq/L). The physician should be notified, and the dose of lithium and the addition of fluoxetine should be questioned. Fluoxetine will increase the risk of lithium toxicity. Fluoxetine should not be administered. Questioning the dose of fluoxetine is insufficient.

➧ ***Test-taking Tip:*** *Lithium has a very narrow therapeutic range of 0.6 to 1.2 mEq/L and can easily cause toxicity.*

Content Area: Mental Health; *Category of Health Alteration:* Personality and Other Mental Health Disorders; *Integrated Process:* Nursing Process Evaluation; *Client Need:* Physiological Integrity/Reduction of Risk Potential/Laboratory Values; *Cognitive Level:* Analysis

Reference: Skidmore-Roth, L. (2006). *Mosby's Nursing Drug Reference* (pp. 440, 587). St. Louis, MO: Mosby.

1598. EBP When working with a client diagnosed with paranoid personality disorder, a nurse understands that the client most likely:

1. received little affection or approval in childhood.
2. experienced lack of empathy and lack of nurturing during upbringing.
3. experienced an early upbringing characterized by indifference leading to a pattern of discomfort with affection.
4. received recognition for accomplishments in early childhood but not during adolescence.

ANSWER: 1

Individuals with paranoid personality disorder may have been subjected to parental antagonism and harassment. They served as scapegoats for displaced parental aggression and eventually gave up all hope of affection and approval. Lack of an empathetic upbringing and lack of nurturing is associated with schizoid personality disorder. An early upbringing characterized by indifference is associated with schizotypal personality disorder. The client likely received no recognition for accomplishments.

➧ ***Test-taking Tip:*** *Paranoid personality disorder involves mistrust of others and the fear that someone will harm them. This can be a result of lack of affection and lack of recognition of accomplishments in childhood.*

Content Area: Mental Health; *Category of Health Alteration:* Personality and Other Mental Health Disorders; *Integrated Process:* Nursing Process Analysis; *Client Need:* Psychosocial Integrity/Support Systems; *Cognitive Level:* Application

Reference: Townsend, M. (2006). *Psychiatric Mental Health Nursing, Concepts of Care in Evidence-Based Practice* (5th ed., p. 721). Philadelphia: F. A. Davis.

EBP Reference: Westen, D., Shedler, J., & Bradley, R. (2006). A prototype approach to personality disorder diagnosis. *American Journal of Psychiatry*, 163, 846–856.

1599. A 45-year-old male client, with no psychiatric history, is admitted to an emergency department after physically assaulting his wife. The client is frightened by his loss of control. The client tells a nurse he is self-employed, recently expanded his company nationally, and has many well-known friends. The client's wife angrily states, "That's what is important to you; who you know and how it looks!" Despite the business's recent financial loss, the client continues his lavish lifestyle. The nurse determines that the client's behavior is typical of:

1. borderline personality disorder.
2. schizoid personality disorder.
3. narcissistic personality disorder.
4. dependent personality disorder.

ANSWER: 3

Narcissistic personality disorder is characterized by constant seeking of praise and attention, an egocentric attitude, envy, rage, and violence when others are not supportive. A person with borderline personality disorder will engage in self-injury before injuring others. Clients diagnosed with schizoid personality disorder are self-absorbed and exhibit social detachment, and clients diagnosed with dependent personality disorder have low self-esteem and engage in submissive behavior.

➧ ***Test-taking Tip:*** *Read the options before the scenario and then focus on the characteristics of the different personality disorders and the client behaviors. Eliminate options as you read the behaviors.*

Content Area: Mental Health; *Category of Health Alteration:* Personality and Other Mental Health Disorders; *Integrated Process:* Nursing Process Analysis; *Client Need:* Psychosocial Integrity/Psychopathology; *Cognitive Level:* Analysis

Reference: Townsend, M. (2008). *Essentials of Psychiatric Mental Health Nursing* (4th ed., pp. 509–513). Philadelphia: F. A. Davis.

1600. Which should a nurse include as a primary outcome for an individual with schizoid personality disorder?

1. Validates ideas before taking action
2. Able to function independently in the community
3. Cope and control emotions
4. Recognizes limits

ANSWER: 2

An outcome for the individual with schizoid personality disorder focuses on improving functioning within the community. Validating ideas before acting is an outcome for an individual with paranoid personality disorder. Able to cope and control emotions are outcomes for individuals with borderline personality disorder. Recognizes limits is an outcome for individuals with antisocial personality disorder.

➧ ***Test-taking Tip:*** *Use the nursing process and knowledge of schizoid personality disorders to eliminate outcomes that pertain to paranoid, borderline, and antisocial personality disorders.*

Content Area: Mental Health; *Category of Health Alteration:* Personality and Other Mental Health Disorders; *Integrated Process:* Nursing Process Evaluation; *Client Need:* Psychosocial Integrity/Mental Health Concepts; *Cognitive Level:* Application

Reference: Videbeck, S. (2006). *Psychiatric Mental Health Nursing* (3rd ed., p. 347). Philadelphia: Lippincott Williams & Wilkins.

1601. EBP A nurse is caring for a client diagnosed with borderline personality disorder who is self-mutilating. Which actions should be taken by the nurse to prevent further self-mutilation by the client? Prioritize the nurse's actions by placing each step in the correct order.

______ Observe the clients' behavior frequently.
______ Secure a verbal contract with the client that he or she will notify a staff member when the client wishes to self-harm.
______ Care for self-mutilation wounds without giving positive reinforcement by offering sympathy or attention.
______ Encourage client to talk about feelings experienced before the behavior occurred.
______ Teach strategies for appropriate expression of angry feelings.
______ Remove all dangerous objects from the environment.
______ Assign staff on one-to-one basis.

ANSWER: 6, 3, 1, 2, 7, 5, 4

The greatest priority is to care for the client's immediate wounds and allow the client to express feelings. Secure a verbal contract for the individual to notify the staff member if he or she feels like initiating self-harm. Next, ensure the future safety of the client by assigning one-to-one staffing and remove dangerous objects from the environment. Observe closely and frequently. Teach appropriate expression of anger; this is last because the client's behavior needs to de-escalate before teaching will be effective.

▸ ***Test-taking Tip:*** *Use Maslow's Hierarchy of Needs theory; physiological needs are priority, followed by the safety and security needs.*

Content Area: Mental Health; *Category of Health Alteration:* Personality and Other Mental Health Disorders; *Integrated Process:* Nursing Process Planning; *Client Need:* Psychosocial Integrity/Crisis Intervention; *Cognitive Level:* Analysis

Reference: Townsend, M. (2006). *Psychiatric Mental Health Nursing, Concepts of Care in Evidence-Based Practice* (5th ed., p. 721). Philadelphia: F. A. Davis.

EBP Reference: Binks, C., Fenton, M., McCarthy, L., Lee, T., Adams, C., et al. (2006). Psychological therapies for people with borderline personality disorder. *Cochrane Database of Systematic Reviews*, Issue 1, Art. No. CD005652. DOI: 10.1002/14651858.CD005652. Available at: www.cochrane.org/reviews/en/ab005652.html

1602. EBP Which interventions should a nurse plan for a client with avoidant personality disorder? SELECT ALL THAT APPLY.

1. Provide support and reassurance.
2. Explore positive self-aspects.
3. Reframing.
4. De-catastrophizing.
5. Identify negative responses from others.

ANSWER: 1, 2, 3, 4

It is important to provide support and reassurance while helping to explore the positive aspects of self. Reframing is a cognitive behavioral technique where alternative points of view are examined to explain events. De-catastrophizing is a method of learning to assess situations in a realistic manner instead of assuming a catastrophe will happen. Another intervention is exploring positive, not negative, responses from others.

▸ ***Test-taking Tip:*** *Eliminate any option that is similar to the personality disorder.*

Content Area: Mental Health; *Category of Health Alteration:* Personality and Other Mental Health Disorders; *Integrated Process:* Nursing Process Planning; *Client Need:* Psychosocial Integrity/Behavioral Interventions; *Cognitive Level:* Application

Reference: Videbeck, S. (2006). *Psychiatric Mental Health Nursing* (3rd ed., pp. 366, 538, 545). Philadelphia: Lippincott Williams & Wilkins.

EBP Reference: Emmelkamp, P., Benner, A., Kuipers, A., et al. (2006). Comparison of brief dynamic and cognitive-behavioral therapies in avoidant personality disorder. *British Journal of Psychiatry*, 189, 60–64.

1603. EBP Which approach should a nurse use when working with an individual diagnosed with obsessive-compulsive disorder?

1. A rigid autocratic manner
2. Very direct and confrontational
3. Calm and nonconfrontational
4. Direct and hurried

ANSWER: 3

Persons with obsessive-compulsive personality disorder tend to maintain control by carefully and thoroughly following procedures. It is important to adapt a calm and nonconfrontational approach, as any request is likely to result in an increase in the client's anxiety level. A rigid autocratic manner, confrontational approach, and a hurried approach will increase the client's anxiety level.

▸ ***Test-taking Tip:*** *Note that options 1, 2, and 4 are similar and option 3 is different. Often the option that is different is the answer.*

Content Area: Mental Health; *Category of Health Alteration:* Personality and Other Mental Health Disorders; *Integrated Process:* Nursing Process Implementation; *Client Need:* Psychosocial Integrity/Behavioral Interventions; *Cognitive Level:* Analysis

Reference: Boyd, M. (2008). *Psychiatric Nursing Contemporary Practice* (4th ed., p. 474). Philadelphia: Lippincott Williams & Wilkins.

EBP Reference: Torres, A., Prince, M., Bebbington, P., et al. (2006). Obsessive-compulsive disorder: Prevalence, comorbidity, impact, and help-seeking in the British National Psychiatric Morbidity Survey of 2000. *American Journal of Psychiatry*, 163, 1978–1985.

1604. A public health nurse visits a client's home and discovers a multitude of cluttered possessions taking up 75% of the living space, obscuring entrance into the home and access to all rooms except the bathroom. The chairs and table are covered with various objects. The nurse interprets the client's behavior as:

1. inability to focus related to a passive-aggressive personality disorder.
2. inattentiveness to surroundings related to a borderline personality disorder.
3. an attention-seeking behavior related to a histrionic personality disorder.
4. hoarding related to an obsessive-compulsive disorder or obsessive-compulsive personality disorder.

ANSWER: 4
Hoarding behavior is associated with obsessive-compulsive disorder and obsessive-compulsive personality disorder. Options 1, 2, and 3 do not correctly describe the behaviors for the associated disorders.

➧ ***Test-taking Tip:*** *Hoarding is a compulsive behavior done to excess, and this should lead you to associate it with obsessive-compulsive disorder.*

Content Area: Mental Health; *Category of Health Alteration:* Personality and Other Mental Health Disorders; *Integrated Process:* Nursing Process Analysis; *Client Need:* Psychosocial Integrity/Coping Mechanisms; *Cognitive Level:* Analysis

Reference: Townsend, M. (2006). *Psychiatric Mental Health Nursing, Concepts of Care in Evidence-Based Practice* (5th ed., p. 724). Philadelphia: F. A. Davis.

1605. A client on a psychiatric unit is very demanding and belittling of one of the nurses. The client is talking with others and telling them how mean the nurse is to clients. Which nursing diagnosis is most appropriate for the client?

1. Chronic low self-esteem related to use of the defense mechanism splitting
2. Risk for other-directed violence related to negative verbal comments
3. Ineffective coping related to inability to interact with unit personnel
4. Social isolation related to negative behavior

ANSWER: 1
Splitting is a defense mechanism in which the person is unable to integrate and accept both positive and negative feelings and people are considered either all good or all bad. Option 2 is incorrect because the client has not made threats of violence. Option 3 is incorrect because there is no indication that the client has trouble with any other personnel. Option 4 is incorrect because the client is talking with others and is not socially isolated.

➧ ***Test-taking Tip:*** *Consider the current behavior, not what might occur when reviewing the options.*

Content Area: Mental Health; *Category of Health Alteration:* Personality and Other Mental Health Disorders; *Integrated Process:* Nursing Process Analysis; *Client Need:* Psychosocial Integrity/Mental Health Concepts; *Cognitive Level:* Analysis

Reference: Videbeck, S. (2006). *Psychiatric Mental Health Nursing* (3rd ed., p. 362). Philadelphia: Lippincott Williams & Wilkins.

1606. A nurse should anticipate that a client diagnosed with antisocial personality disorder may use the primary ego defense mechanism of:

1. compensation.
2. projection.
3. sublimation.
4. rationalization.

ANSWER: 2
Projection is to attribute a person's thoughts, feelings, or impulses onto another person who does not have these thoughts, feelings or impulses. Coercion and personal profit motivate these individuals, and they attribute these feelings to others. Compensation is a process of counterbalancing weaknesses with strengths. This is a more mature defense mechanism. Sublimation is the channeling of unacceptable impulses, thoughts, and emotions into acceptable ones. Rationalization is putting things into a different, acceptable perspective.

➧ ***Test-taking Tip:*** *Differentiate the more advanced defense mechanisms from the more primitive; individuals with personality disorders are more likely to use the more primitive defense mechanisms.*

Content Area: Mental Health; *Category of Health Alteration:* Personality and Other Mental Health Disorders; *Integrated Process:* Nursing Process Planning; *Client Need:* Psychosocial Integrity/Coping Mechanisms; *Cognitive Level:* Application

Reference: Videbeck, S. (2006). *Psychiatric Mental Health Nursing* (3rd ed., p. 354). Philadelphia: Lippincott Williams & Wilkins.

1607. EBP A physician writes in a client's progress notes, "Will switch medications from the older medications to a newer GABA-ergic anticonvulsant to treat client's instability of mood, transient mood crashes, and inappropriate and intense outbursts of anger." Which medication should a nurse consider when reviewing the physician's new orders?

1. Gabapentin (Neurontin®)
2. Lithium (Lithonate®)
3. Carbamazepine (Tegretol®)
4. Valproic acid (Depakote®)

ANSWER: 1

GABA-ergic (g-aminobutyric acid-ergic) anticonvulsants, such as gabapentin (Neurontin®), appear to act by regulating neural firing in the mesolimbic area. Lithium, carbamazepine, and valproic acid are older medications used to control mood and have a greater number of side effects.

Test-taking Tip: *Be familiar with the use of off-label drugs when psychiatric medications are prescribed. If unsure, correlate the medication classification with the generic name of the medication.*

Content Area: Mental Health; *Category of Health Alteration:* Personality and Other Mental Health Disorders; *Integrated Process:* Communication and Documentation; *Client Need:* Physiological Integrity/Pharmacological and Parenteral Therapies/Expected Actions or Outcomes; *Cognitive Level:* Application

Reference: Boyd, M. (2008). *Psychiatric Nursing Contemporary Practice* (4th ed., p. 449). Philadelphia: Lippincott Williams & Wilkins.

EBP Reference: Silvio, B., Paradiso, E., & Bogetto, F. (2006). Mood stabilizers and novel antipsychotics in the treatment of borderline personality disorder. *Psychiatric Times*, 23(8), 25–33.

1608. A client diagnosed with a borderline personality disorder is prescribed phenelzine (Nardil®) for decreasing impulsivity and self-destructive acts. The client is taught to avoid foods high in tyramine when taking this medication to prevent:

1. cardiac rhythm abnormalities.
2. a hypotensive crisis.
3. a hypertensive crisis.
4. poor absorption of the medication.

ANSWER: 3

The combination of tyramine-containing foods and monoamine oxidase inhibitors (MAOIs) such as phenelzine (Nardil®) can result in a hypertensive crisis. Although the hypertensive crisis state can cause cardiac rhythm abnormalities, this is not the primary reason to avoid foods high in tyramine. Eating foods high in tyramine while taking MAOIs cause hypertension, not hypotension. Foods high in tyramine do not delay absorption of MAOIs.

Test-taking Tip: *Examine options that are opposites first, and eliminate one of these. Then, compare the remaining options with the crisis state to eliminate all but one of these.*

Content Area: Mental Health; *Category of Health Alteration:* Personality and Other Mental Health Disorders; *Integrated Processes:* Teaching and Learning; *Client Need:* Physiological Integrity/Pharmacological and Parenteral Therapies/Adverse Effects/Contraindications/Interactions; *Cognitive Level:* Application

Reference: Pedersen, D. (2008). *Psych Notes* (2nd ed., p. 145). Philadelphia: F. A. Davis.

1609. At 2400 hours, a psychiatrist writes medication orders for a 69-year-old female client admitted to a behavioral health unit. At 0100 hours, a nurse is validating the orders for accurate transcription by pharmacy to the electronic medication administration record (MAR) illustrated. Place an X on the medication order that the nurse should question.

Client A
Medication Administration Record
Date: Today
Allergies: None

Medication	0001–0759	0800–1559	1600–2400
Risperidone (Risperdal®) oral 1 mg bid day 1; 2 mg bid on day 2; 3 mg bid on day 3		0900_____ 2 mg	
Fluoxetine (Prozac®) 10 mg oral daily		0900_____	
Carbamazepine (Tegretol®) 200 mg oral bid		0900_____	2100_____
Docusate sodium (Colace®) 100 mg oral daily		0900_____	

ANSWER:

Medication	0001-0759	0800-1559	1600-2400
Resperidone (Risperdal®) oral **X** 1 mg bid day 1; 2 mg bid on day 2; 3 mg bid on day 3		0900_____ 2 mg	

Risperidone is ordered at the regular adult dose and not an appropriate dose for an older adult. Medications are processed differently in older adults as compared to adults. Metabolism is slowed and adverse reactions can occur quickly in older adults.

▶ ***Test-taking Tip:*** *Be aware of the dosage differences for older adults taking antipsychotic medications.*

Content Area: Mental Health; *Category of Health Alteration:* Personality and Other Mental Health Disorders; *Integrated Process:* Nursing Process Implementation; *Client Need:* Physiological Integrity/Pharmacological and Parenteral Therapies/Expected Actions or Outcomes; *Cognitive Level:* Application

Reference: Deglin, J., & Vallerand, A. (2009). *Davis's Drug Guide for Nurses* (11th ed). Philadelphia: F.A. Davis.

1610. A nurse teaches the communication triad to a client to manage feelings. Which components should the nurse teach? SELECT ALL THAT APPLY.

1. Using an "I" statement to identify the present feeling
2. Using a "you" statement to identify the cause of the feeling
3. Using a "they" statement to examine the effect of the client's feelings on others
4. Making a nonjudgmental statement about an emotional trigger
5. Identifying what would restore comfort to the situation for the client

ANSWER: 1, 4, 5

Using "I" statements, nonjudgmental statements, and a mechanism for restoring comfort are included in the communication triad to manage feelings. Using "you" statements to identify the cause is judgmental. Using "they" statements can also be judgmental and presumptuous.

▶ ***Test-taking Tip:*** *The key word is "triad," so three options are right and two are incorrect.*

Content Area: Mental Health; *Category of Health Alteration:* Personality and Other Mental Health Disorders; *Integrated Process:* Teaching and Learning; *Client Need:* Psychosocial Integrity/Therapeutic Communications; *Cognitive Level:* Application

Reference: Boyd, M. (2008). *Psychiatric Nursing Contemporary Practice* (4th ed., p. 455). Philadelphia: Lippincott Williams & Wilkins.

1611. EBP A nurse understands that milieu therapy can be helpful for a client with antisocial personality disorder because it:

1. sets limits on unacceptable behavior.
2. provides one-on-one interaction and reality orientation with client and nursing personnel.
3. provides a very structured setting that helps the client learn how to behave.
4. simulates a social community where clients can learn to interact with others.

ANSWER: 4

Milieu therapy is helpful because the client can respond adaptively to feedback from peers. The democratic approach with specific rules and regulations, community meetings, and group therapy sessions simulates the societal situation in which the client must live. Limit setting, one-on-one interaction, reality orientation, and a structured setting are all components of milieu therapy, but none is the reason milieu therapy is most helpful for the client.

➧ ***Test-taking Tip:*** *Read each option and select the most global option that would be inclusive of the other options.*

Content Area: Mental Health; *Category of Health Alteration:* Personality and Other Mental Health Disorders; *Integrated Process:* Nursing Process Evaluation; *Client Need:* Psychosocial Integrity/Therapeutic Environment; *Cognitive Level:* Analysis

Reference: Townsend, M. (2006). *Psychiatric Mental Health Nursing, Concepts of Care in Evidence-Based Practice* (5th ed., pp. 187–189, 738). Philadelphia: F. A. Davis.

EBP Reference: Philips, K., Yen, S., & Gunderson, J. (2006). Personality disorders. In R. Hales, & S. Yudofsky (Eds.), *Textbook of Clinical Psychiatry* (5th ed.). Washington, DC: American Psychiatric Publishing.

1612. A nurse is caring for a client who has been diagnosed with psychogenic fugue. In reviewing the client's medical record, which information in the client's history should indicate to the nurse that the diagnosis is correct? SELECT ALL THAT APPLY.

1. The client recently forgot all personal information following an accident.
2. The client left home and assumed a new identity following the loss of a child.
3. The client demonstrates having more than one distinct personality.
4. The client claims to have superhero qualities following a recent suicide attempt.
5. The client resides in a homeless shelter after being physically abused by his or her spouse.

ANSWER: 1, 2

A nurse should identify that the diagnosis of psychogenic fugue is based upon the client's symptoms of assuming a new identity and forgetting previous personal information following a traumatic event or stressor. The other options are not symptoms of or findings associated with psychogenic fugue.

➧ ***Test-taking Tip:*** *Use the process of elimination and review symptoms and diagnosis of dissociative disorders.*

Content Area: Mental Health; *Category of Health Alteration:* Personality and Other Mental Health Disorders; *Integrated Processes:* Nursing Process Analysis; *Client Need:* Psychosocial Integrity/Mental Health Concepts; *Cognitive Level:* Application

Reference: Neeb, K. (2006). *Fundamentals of Mental Health Nursing* (3rd ed., p. 312). Philadelphia: F. A. Davis.

1613. A nurse is treating a client diagnosed with dissociative identity disorder (DID). Which actions should the nurse take when working with this client? SELECT ALL THAT APPLY.

1. Focus on long-term goals.
2. Maintain a calm environment.
3. Use open communication.
4. Observe for signs of suicidal thoughts or behavior.
5. Document changes in the client's behavior.

ANSWER: 2, 3, 4, 5

When working with a client diagnosed with DID, thought to be caused by traumatic events in childhood that trigger a maladaptive response, the nurse should maintain a calm environment, keep open communication, observe for signs of suicide, and document any changes in behavior. The nurse should also focus on short-term goals because this helps to create smaller successes for the client and results in better personality integration.

➧ ***Test-taking Tip:*** *Use the process of elimination and review symptoms and diagnosis of dissociative disorders.*

Content Area: Mental Health; *Category of Health Alteration:* Personality and Other Mental Health Disorders; *Integrated Processes:* Nursing Process Implementation; *Client Need:* Psychosocial Integrity/Mental Health Concepts; *Cognitive Level:* Application

Reference: Neeb, K. (2006). *Fundamentals of Mental Health Nursing* (3rd ed., p. 312). Philadelphia: F. A. Davis.

1614. A nurse is assessing a client who reports that setting and watching fires helps to relieve anxiety. The client reports relieving tension by setting fires, stating, "After I watch something burn, I feel so much better." The nurse is aware that setting fires can be dangerous and believes that the client is suffering from a mental health disorder. Which mental health diagnosis should the nurse expect with regard to this client?

1. Kleptomania
2. Antisocial personality disorder
3. Pyromania
4. Conduct disorder

ANSWER: 3

Pyromania is the most accurate diagnosis to describe the client's behavior. Pyromania is an impulse-control disorder in which a person sets fires to relieve tension. Kleptomania refers to behavior in which a person steals items to relieve tension or to satisfy an uncontrollable urge. Antisocial personality disorder and conduct disorder are not mainly explained through fire-setting behavior; however, some clients diagnosed with these disorders have a history of fire setting.

▶ ***Test-taking Tip:*** *Use the process of elimination and review symptoms of adjustment and impulse control disorders.*

Content Area: Mental Health; *Category of Health Alteration:* Personality and Other Mental Health Disorders; *Integrated Processes:* Nursing Process Assessment; *Client Need:* Psychosocial Integrity/ Mental Health Concepts; *Cognitive Level:* Assessment

References: Townsend, M. (2006). *Psychiatric Mental Health Nursing, Concepts of Care in Evidence-Based Practice* (5th ed., p. 683). Philadelphia: F. A. Davis; American Psychiatric Association. (2000). *Diagnostic and Statistical Manual of Mental Disorders* (Revised 4th ed.). Washington, DC: Author.

1615. An adolescent client diagnosed with conduct disorder is yelling and having temper tantrums in the common area of a psychiatric unit. What is an appropriate nursing intervention for reducing the client's angry outbursts?

1. Instruct the client to stop yelling.
2. Ignore initial yelling and tantrums.
3. Mirror the client's behavior.
4. Use guided walk to move client from common areas.

ANSWER: 2

It is considered an appropriate nursing intervention to ignore initial yelling and tantrums. Lack of feedback often eliminates the behavior. Ignoring the client should be therapeutic and not unintentional. Instructing the client to stop yelling, mirroring the behavior, and using a guided walk may incite the client to become aggressive.

▶ ***Test-taking Tip:*** *Select an option that eliminates positive feedback to the client.*

Content Area: Mental Health; *Category of Health Alteration:* Personality and Other Mental Health Disorders; *Integrated Processes:* Nursing Process Implementation; *Client Need:* Psychosocial Integrity/ Crisis Intervention; *Cognitive Level:* Analysis

Reference: Townsend, M. (2008). *Essentials of Psychiatric Mental Health Nursing* (4th ed., p. 170). Philadelphia: F. A. Davis.

1616. A nurse observes that a client diagnosed with intermittent explosive disorder is becoming aggressive. The client is exhibiting tense posture and clenched fists and has a defiant affect. Which actions should be taken by the nurse to de-escalate the client's aggression? Prioritize the nurse's actions by placing each step in the correct order.

______ Administer medication.
______ Attempt to talk the client down.
______ Provide the use of alternate physical outlets.
______ Apply physical restraints.
______ Call for assistance.

ANSWER: 3, 1, 2, 5, 4

The nurse should begin by attempting to de-escalate the client by talking the client down. The nurse should then provide an appropriate, effective way for the client to release tension by providing alternate physical outlets, such as punching a pillow. If the client continues to be aggressive, medication should be used to calm the client. If the client refuses the medication and aggression escalates to the degree of possible harm, the nurse should remove self and call for assistance. The nurse should not attempt to restrain a client without support. Physical restraint is the last step to take when the client poses harm and is unable to be calmed by talking and/or medication.

▶ ***Test-taking Tip:*** *Visualize steps prior to placing them in the correct order. Focus on using the least restrictive measures first before applying physical restraint.*

Content Area: Mental Health; *Category of Health Alteration:* Personality and Other Mental Health Disorders; *Integrated Processes:* Nursing Process Implementation; *Client Need:* Psychosocial Integrity/ Crisis Intervention; *Cognitive Level:* Analysis

Reference: Townsend, M. (2008). *Essentials of Psychiatric Mental Health Nursing* (4th ed., p. 170). Philadelphia: F. A. Davis.

1617. A client diagnosed with major depressive disorder expresses to a nurse that death would be better than living with depression. The nurse determines that the client is suffering from suicidal ideation and is at risk for committing suicide. Which nursing intervention is priority for the client experiencing suicidal ideation?

1. Talking with the client about reasons to live and instilling positive affirmations
2. Educating the client on medical and psychological treatments for depression
3. Alerting the appropriate authorities and monitoring the client frequently
4. Assessing the surrounding environment for harmful substances or methods to commit suicide

ANSWER: 3

The most appropriate nursing intervention for a client experiencing suicidal ideation is to notify the appropriate authorities of the client's intent to harm. Nurses are obligated under the *Meier v. Ross General Hospital* case to report any suspicion of suicide among clients. Providing positive affirmation, educating the client, and assessing the client's surroundings are other interventions when caring for a client with major depressive disorder, but alerting the appropriate authorities is priority.

➧ ***Test-taking Tip:*** *The key word is "priority," which suggests that other options may be correct, but one option is more important than the other options.*

Content Area: Mental Health; *Category of Health Alteration:* Personality and Other Mental Health Disorders; *Integrated Processes:* Nursing Implementation; *Client Need:* Psychosocial Integrity/Crisis Intervention; *Cognitive Level:* Analysis

Reference: Neeb, K. (2006). *Fundamentals of Mental Health Nursing* (3rd ed., p. 312). Philadelphia: F. A. Davis.

1618. A psychiatric nurse observes a client becoming increasingly agitated and threatening. The nurse is aware of the signs that a crisis situation could occur. What should be the nurse's primary goal while intervening in a crisis?

1. Helping to reconstruct the client's thought process
2. Eliminating and/or resolving present conflicts
3. Encouraging client to talk about feelings that led to the crisis
4. Securing a physician's order for restraints

ANSWER: 2

The nurse's primary goal should be to resolve present conflicts and help the client return to the precrisis state. Helping to alter thought processes would occur during therapeutic intervention. Encouraging the client to talk about feelings is an appropriate intervention but is not the primary goal. The client has shown no harmful behavior that would warrant physical restraint.

➧ ***Test-taking Tip:*** *The key words are "primary goal." Use the process of elimination to eliminate options that are interventions.*

Content Area: Mental Health; *Category of Health Alteration:* Personality and Other Mental Health Disorders; *Integrated Processes:* Nursing Process Implementation; *Client Need:* Psychosocial Integrity/Crisis Intervention; *Cognitive Level:* Application

Reference: Townsend, M. (2008). *Essentials of Psychiatric Mental Health Nursing* (4th ed., p. 167). Philadelphia: F. A. Davis.

1619. A client diagnosed with paraphilia, has been advised to participate in psychoanalytical therapy. The client asks a nurse about what is involved with this type of therapy. Which statement by the nurse accurately describes the focus of psychoanalytical therapy?

1. Psychoanalytical therapy focuses on reducing the level of circulating androgens.
2. Psychoanalytical therapy focuses on aversion techniques.
3. Psychoanalytical therapy focuses on resolving early conflicts.
4. Psychoanalytical therapy focuses on achieving satiation.

ANSWER: 3

Psychoanalytical therapy focuses on resolving unresolved conflicts and trauma from early childhood. The goal is to alleviate anxiety that prevents the client from forming appropriate sexual relationships. Biological treatment focuses on reducing the level of circulating androgens. The goal is to reduce libido by administering antiandrogenic medications that block testosterone synthesis or block androgen receptors. Behavioral therapy focuses on aversion techniques to reduce undesirable behavior. It also focuses on achieving satiation to make the sexual fantasy less arousing or exciting.

➧ ***Test-taking Tip:*** *Use the process of elimination, and review diagnosis and treatment of sexual disorders.*

Content Area: Mental Health; *Category of Health Alteration:* Personality and Other Mental Health Disorders; *Integrated Processes:* Nursing Process Implementation; *Client Need:* Psychosocial Integrity/Mental Health Concepts; *Cognitive Level:* Application

Reference: Townsend, M. (2008). *Essentials of Psychiatric Mental Health Nursing* (4th ed., pp. 448–467). Philadelphia: F. A. Davis.

1620. A nurse is assessing a client who claims to have sexual fantasies that reoccur on a daily basis. Which sexual fantasy described by the client should lead the nurse to consider that the client has paraphilia?

1. Repetitive sexual activity with numerous partners
2. Repetitive sexual activity involving suffering or humiliation
3. Repetitive sexual activity in public places
4. Repetitive sexual activity with members of the same sex

ANSWER: 2

The nurse should be aware that paraphilia involves sexual fantasies or behaviors involving repetitive sexual activity with real or simulated suffering or humiliation. Paraphilias may include a sexual preference for a nonhuman object as well as repetitive sexual activity with nonconsenting partners. Sexual activity with numerous partners, in public places, and with members of the same sex do not meet criteria for paraphilia.

➧ ***Test-taking Tip:*** *Apply knowledge of medical terminology. Select the option that is vastly different from the other options.*

Content Area: Mental Health; *Category of Health Alteration:* Personality and Other Mental Health Disorders; *Integrated Processes:* Nursing Process Implementation; *Client Need:* Psychosocial Integrity/ Mental Health Concepts; *Cognitive Level:* Application

Reference: Townsend, M. (2008). *Essentials of Psychiatric Mental Health Nursing* (4th ed., pp. 448–467). Philadelphia: F. A. Davis.

1621. A nurse is assessing a client who reports symptoms descriptive of hypoactive sexual desire disorder. Which factor, identified by the nurse, is a biological factor that may attribute to hypoactive sexual desire disorder?

1. Past sexual abuse
2. Chronic alcohol use
3. Depression
4. Sexual identity conflicts

ANSWER: 2

The nurse should identify that chronic alcohol use could attribute to hypoactive sexual desire disorder. Other substances that attribute to this disorder are cocaine use and antidepressants. Other options can also attribute to hypoactive sexual desire disorder but are considered psychosocial factors.

▶ ***Test-taking Tip:*** *Note that three options pertain to mental health disorders whereas one option is different. Often the option that is different is the answer.*

Content Area: Mental Health; *Category of Health Alteration:* Personality and Other Mental Health Disorders; *Integrated Processes:* Nursing Process Assessment; *Client Need:* Health Promotion and Maintenance/Lifestyle Choices; *Cognitive Level:* Application

Reference: Townsend, M. (2008). *Essentials of Psychiatric Mental Health Nursing* (4th ed., pp. 448–467). Philadelphia: F. A. Davis.

1622. EBP A client diagnosed with schizophrenia is refusing to take a prescribed psychotropic medication. A nurse attempts to persuade the client to comply with the physician's orders. Under which circumstance could the client be forced to take medication?

1. If the client begins to claim to be God
2. If the client claims to be a terrorist and threatens to kill a nurse
3. If the client threatens to leave the hospital
4. If the client talks about a previous suicide attempt

ANSWER: 2

The client can be forced to take medication if dangerous behavior is exhibited to self or others. The client must also be judged incompetent and the medication must have a reasonable chance of helping the client. Claiming to be God, leaving the hospital, and talking about a previous suicide attempt do not meet the criteria of being a danger to self or others. Discussion of past suicidal behavior does indicate present state of mind.

▶ ***Test-taking Tip:*** *Note that three options pertain to self-harm, whereas one option pertains to harming others. Select the option that is different from the other options.*

Content Area: Mental Health; *Category of Health Alteration:* Personality and Other Mental Health Disorders; *Integrated Processes:* Nursing Process Implementation; *Client Need:* Safe and Effective Care Environment/Safety and Infection Control/Accident and Injury Prevention; *Cognitive Level:* Analysis

Reference: Townsend, M. (2008). *Essentials of Psychiatric Mental Health Nursing* (4th ed., pp. 54–63). Philadelphia: F. A. Davis.

EBP Reference: Gibson, R., & Walcott, G. (2008). Benzodiazepines for catatonia in people with schizophrenia and other serious mental illnesses. *Cochrane Database of Systematic Reviews*, Issue 4, Art. No. CD006570. DOI: 10.1002/14651858.CD006570.pub2. Available at: www.cochrane.org/reviews/en/ab006570.html

---

1623. A client diagnosed with schizoaffective disorder was recently treated for a major depressive episode. Following a 72-hour involuntary commitment, the client is stable and asking to leave the hospital. Which client right should the nurse consider while deciding if the client can be discharged?

1. Right to appropriate service plan
2. Right to least-restrictive treatment
3. Right to freedom from restraint
4. Right to refuse treatment

ANSWER: 2

The nurse should consider the client's right to the least-restrictive environment. If the client is stabilized and no longer displays any suicidal ideation, it is possible to treat the client on an outpatient basis. The right to an appropriate service plan, freedom from restraint, and refuse treatment are important client rights, but they do not directly affect the client's ability to be discharged from involuntary commitment.

▶ ***Test-taking Tip:*** *Use the process of elimination and review ethical and legal issues related to clients with mental health disorders and involuntary commitment.*

Content Area: Mental Health; *Category of Health Alteration:* Personality and Other Mental Health Disorders; *Integrated Processes:* Nursing Process Planning; *Client Need:* Safe and Effective Care Environment/Management of Care/Client Rights; *Cognitive Level:* Analysis

Reference: Townsend, M. (2008). *Essentials of Psychiatric Mental Health Nursing* (4th ed., pp. 54–63). Philadelphia: F. A. Davis.

1624. EBP An adult client diagnosed with obsessive-compulsive personality disorder is being admitted into a psychiatric department after rubbing lesions into both hands and face from excessive washing. The client is refusing to accept any treatment for the wounds or for the mental health diagnosis. What actions should be taken by the nurse? SELECT ALL THAT APPLY.

1. Treat the client's injuries; the client is incompetent.
2. Do not treat the client; the client is competent.
3. Notify the client's physician of the refusal; the client is incompetent.
4. Notify the physician of the refusal; the client is competent.
5. Notify the client's family; the client is incompetent.

ANSWER: 2, 4

The client has the right to refuse treatment. The nurse should withhold treatment and notify the client's physician of the refusal to allow treatment. A diagnosis of obsessive-compulsive disorder does not indicate that the client is incompetent. The nurse could be charged with assault if treatment is administered against the client's will. The nurse cannot disclose confidential health information without the client's consent; the client is competent.

➧ ***Test-taking Tip:*** *First decide whether or not the client is competent, and then review like options and use the process of elimination. Review ethical and legal issues related to clients with mental health disorders.*

Content Area: Mental Health; *Category of Health Alteration:* Personality and Other Mental Health Disorders; *Integrated Processes:* Nursing Process Implementation; *Client Need:* Safe and Effective Care Environment/Management of Care/Client Rights; *Cognitive Level:* Analysis

Reference: Townsend, M. (2008). *Essentials of Psychiatric Mental Health Nursing* (4th ed., pp. 54–63). Philadelphia: F. A. Davis.

EBP Reference: Gava, I., Barbui, C., Aguglia, E., Carlino, D., Churchill, R., et al. (2007). Psychological treatments versus treatment as usual for obsessive compulsive disorder (OCD). *Cochrane Database of Systematic Reviews*, Issue 2, Art. No. CD005333. DOI: 10.1002/14651858.CD005333.pub2. Available at: www.cochrane.org/reviews/en/ab005333.html

---

1625. EBP A nurse in a psychiatric unit cares for clients with unpredictable and often dangerous behaviors. The primary goal of the psychiatric nurse is to keep clients safe. In a psychiatric inpatient unit, which recommended method for managing the safety of multiple clients should the nurse employ?

1. Monitoring client medication
2. Developing trusting relationship with clients
3. Documenting any disturbing client behavior
4. Keeping clients apart as much as possible

ANSWER: 2

Developing a trusting relationship with clients enables the nurse to better predict and prevent dangerous behavior through early intervention. A trusting relationship allows the nurse to use psychological support to reduce risk. Monitoring medication and proper documentation are tasks of a psychiatric nurse, but prove little help on increasing overall unit safety. Keeping clients apart is often not part of the therapeutic process as the goal is to reintegrate clients into society.

➧ ***Test-taking Tip:*** *Use the process of elimination and review techniques for working with clients with mental health diagnoses.*

Content Area: Mental Health; *Category of Health Alteration:* Personality and Other Mental Health Disorders; *Integrated Processes:* Nursing Process Implementation; *Client Need:* Psychosocial Integrity/Therapeutic Communications; *Cognitive Level:* Application

Reference: Townsend, M. (2006). *Psychiatric Mental Health Nursing, Concepts of Care in Evidence-Based Practice* (5th ed., p. 111). Philadelphia: F. A. Davis.

EBP Reference: Bowers, L. (2005). Reasons for admission and their implications for the nature of acute inpatient psychiatric nursing. *Journal of Psychiatric and Mental Health Nursing,* 12, 231–236.

1626. EBP A nurse in an inpatient psychiatric unit is aware of the importance of managing sexual behavior among clients. Which statement is accurate regarding the standard protocol of managing sexual behavior on adult psychiatric inpatient units?

1. Sexual behavior is strictly prohibited.
2. Sexual behavior is governed by least-restrictive legal policies.
3. Sexual behavior can be therapeutic and speed recovery.
4. Sexual behavior is helpful for clients diagnosed with personality disorders.

ANSWER: 2

Due to the legal case *Johnson v. the United States*, clients residing in adult inpatient psychiatric units should be governed by a "least restrictive" policy. This includes developing policies restricting sexual behavior. Therefore, hospitals are restricted from prohibiting sexual behavior. Nevertheless, sexual behavior in inpatient units is not used as a therapeutic tool to speed recovery or to help those diagnosed with personality disorders.

➧ ***Test-taking Tip:*** *Use the process of elimination and review laws governing restrictive policies in inpatient psychiatric units.*

Content Area: Mental Health; *Category of Health Alteration:* Personality and Other Mental Health Disorders; *Integrated Processes:* Nursing Process Implementation; *Client Need:* Health Promotion and Maintenance/Health and Wellness; *Cognitive Level:* Analysis

Reference: Townsend, M. (2006). *Psychiatric Mental Health Nursing, Concepts of Care in Evidence-Based Practice* (5th ed., p. 490). Philadelphia: F. A. Davis.

EBP Reference: Psychiatric Services. (2005). *Managing Sexual Behavior on Adult Acute Care Inpatient Psychiatric Units.* Available at: http://psychservices.psychiatryonline.org

Test 43: **Mental Health: Substance Abuse**

1627. A client says, "I go out just about every weekend and drink pretty heavily with my friends. Does that mean I'm dependent on alcohol?" Which is the best response by the nurse?

1. "Not necessarily. With dependence, you have a strong need to drink and feel uncomfortable if you don't."
2. "You could be dependent. Drinking every week is excessive."
3. "It sounds like you feel guilty about how much you drink."
4. "You're not dependent if you never drink to the point of intoxication."

ANSWER: 1

Dependence involves a compulsive or chronic requirement for a chemical. The need is so strong as to generate physical or psychological distress if left unfilled. Dependency is not defined by frequency, intoxication, or feelings surrounding the drinking behavior.

➧ ***Test-taking Tip:*** *Use the process of elimination. The key word is "dependent." Eliminate any options that do not answer the client's question and then select the most descriptive option.*

Content Area: Mental Health; *Category of Health Alteration:* Substance Abuse; *Integrated Processes:* Communication and Documentation; *Client Need:* Health Promotion and Maintenance/High-Risk Behaviors; *Cognitive Level:* Application

Reference: Townsend, M. (2009). *Psychiatric Mental Health Nursing* (6th ed., p. 442). Philadelphia: F. A. Davis.

1628. A nurse is completing a health history on a client. Which information, obtained during the interview, should indicate to the nurse that the client has a substance dependence problem? SELECT ALL THAT APPLY.

1. Increased concern by family and friends regarding substance use
2. The development of tolerance to increasing amounts of a substance
3. The onset of withdrawal symptoms
4. Continued occupational functioning in spite of increased use
5. Unsuccessful efforts to reduce the amount of substance used
6. Diminished social or recreational activities

ANSWER: 2, 3, 5, 6

The development of tolerance to increasing amounts of a substance, the onset of withdrawal symptoms, unsuccessful efforts to reduce the amount of substance used, and diminished social or recreational activities are all DSM-IV-TR criteria for diagnosis of substance dependence. An increased show of concern by family and friends does not necessarily indicate substance dependence, although this may co-occur in the lives of the client dependent on substances. Increased use would decrease occupational functioning.

➧ ***Test-taking Tip:*** *Use the process of elimination, eliminating option 4 because increased use would decrease occupational functioning and option 1 because the family concerns are not supported by client behaviors of substance use.*

Content Area: Mental Health; *Category of Health Alteration:* Substance Abuse; *Integrated Processes:* Nursing Process Analysis; *Client Need:* Psychosocial Integrity/Chemical and Other Dependencies; *Cognitive Level:* Analysis

Reference: Townsend, M. (2009). *Psychiatric Mental Health Nursing* (6th ed., p. 443). Philadelphia: F. A. Davis.

1629. Four phases have been outlined by Jellinek (1952; Townsend, 2009, p. 447) through which the alcoholic's pattern of drinking progresses. The nurse places a client who is using excessive denial of drinking due to feelings of enormous guilt about drinking in one of the phases. At which phase in the illustration should the nurse place the client? Indicate the area with an X on the illustration.

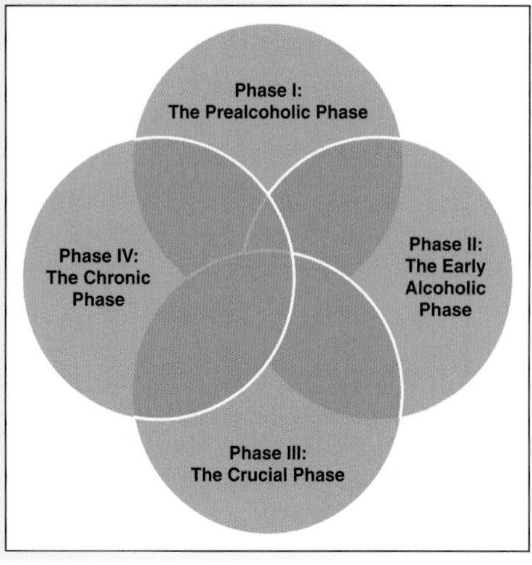

ANSWER:

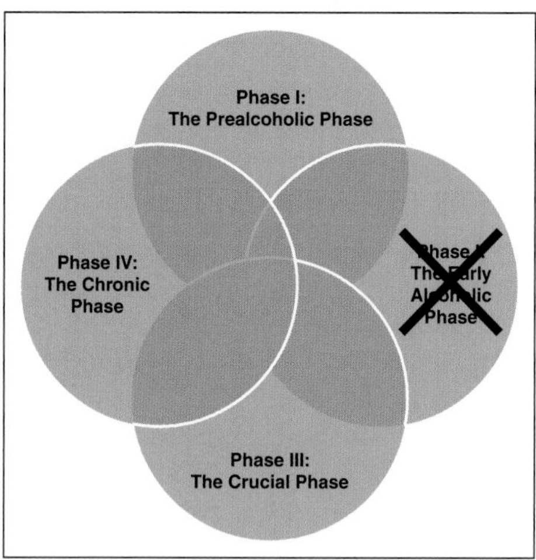

During the early alcoholic phase (phase II) the individual feels guilt and becomes defensive. Excessive use of denial and rationalization become evident. Phase I involves using alcohol to relieve everyday stress. In Phase III control over alcohol is lost, and physiological dependence is evident. Drinking has become the total focus. Phase IV involves emotional and physical disintegration.

▶ ***Test-taking Tip:*** *Think about the progression of substance abuse. Recall that denial occurs early in the alcoholic process. Be familiar with behavioral and functional patterns.*

Content Area: Mental Health; *Category of Health Alteration:* Substance Abuse; *Integrated Processes:* Nursing Process Analysis; *Client Need:* Psychosocial Integrity/Chemical and Other Dependencies; Psychosocial Integrity/Coping Mechanisms; *Cognitive Level:* Analysis

Reference: Townsend, M. (2009). *Psychiatric Mental Health Nursing* (6th ed., p. 447). Philadelphia: F. A. Davis.

1630. A nurse is preparing to lead a group therapy session with a group of clients recovering from alcohol and other substances. Which seating arrangement would be most effective to facilitate group discussion?

1. Clients facing forward with the nurse at the front of the room
2. Clients and nurse seated in a circle around a conference table
3. Clients and nurse seated in chairs arranged in a circle
4. Clients and nurse seated in a circle with new group members observing at the back of the room

ANSWER: 3

The environment should be arranged so that there are no barriers between members. Chairs should be in a circle without tables. All group members, including the leader, should be in the circle. A nurse in the front of the room or a new member observing at the back of the room places members outside of the circle. A conference table is a physical barrier.

▶ ***Test-taking Tip:*** *Focus on the issue: facilitating group discussion. Carefully read each option for possible barriers, then eliminate options that include members outside of the group or that represent a physical barrier.*

Content Area: Mental Health; *Category of Health Alteration:* Substance Abuse; *Integrated Processes:* Nursing Process Planning; *Client Need:* Psychosocial Integrity/Therapeutic Environment; *Cognitive Level:* Application

Reference: Townsend, M. (2009). *Psychiatric Mental Health Nursing* (6th ed., p. 163). Philadelphia: F. A. Davis.

1631. A client receiving treatment for substance dependence has not been attending group therapy. Which is the best response by a nurse to confront this behavior?

1. "Why don't you want to go to group therapy?"
2. "Talking about personal issues with others can be difficult. Try talking to your therapist individually."
3. "You need to attend therapy if you want to get better."
4. "You say you want to get better, but you are not participating in your treatment."

ANSWER: 4

The nurse should address the behavior in a matter-of-fact, nonjudgmental manner by using confrontation with a caring approach. Confrontation interferes with the client's ability to use denial. A caring attitude avoids putting the client on the defensive. A "why" question is a barrier to therapeutic communication and can initiate a defensive response. Other options allow the client to rationalize or blame others or otherwise avoid accepting responsibility for behavior.

➧ ***Test-taking Tip:*** *Use therapeutic communication principles and eliminate options that allow the client to rationalize or blame others or are a barrier to therapeutic communication.*

Content Area: Mental Health; *Category of Health Alteration:* Substance Abuse; *Integrated Processes:* Caring; Communication and Documentation; *Client Need:* Psychosocial Integrity/Chemical and Other Dependencies; Psychosocial Integrity/Therapeutic Communications; *Cognitive Level:* Application

Reference: Townsend, M. (2009). *Psychiatric Mental Health Nursing* (6th ed., pp. 472–473). Philadelphia: F. A. Davis.

1632. A nurse teaches a client that one of the most successful measures for continued recovery for clients with substance abuse disorders is involvement in a 12-step self-help program, such as Alcoholics Anonymous (AA). The nurse informs the client that the major principle associated with the 12-step programs is that:

1. normal substance use can resume with the guidance and support of others.
2. substance abuse disorders can be cured with total abstinence.
3. acceptance of powerlessness over a substance is the first step in recovery.
4. substance abuse is a weakness that can be overcome through the 12 steps.

ANSWER: 3

Admitting powerlessness is the first step in AA recovery. Working the 12 steps and in turn helping others to remain sober are the foundation of 12-step programs. Normal substance use is not possible for the alcoholic/addict. Substance dependence is seen as a disease for which there is no cure. Recovery is a life-long process.

➧ ***Test-taking Tip:*** *Think about the 12-step principles of AA and other self-help groups. Use the process of elimination, eliminating option 1 because substance use should never be resumed. Read the other options carefully.*

Content Area: Mental Health; *Category of Health Alteration:* Substance Abuse; *Integrated Processes:* Teaching and Learning; *Client Need:* Psychosocial Integrity/Chemical and Other Dependencies; Psychosocial Integrity/Religious and Spiritual Influences on Health; *Cognitive Level:* Application

Reference: Townsend, M. (2009). *Psychiatric Mental Health Nursing* (6th ed., p. 479). Philadelphia: F. A. Davis.

1633. Which statement by a client being discharged from inpatient treatment for cocaine abuse would indicate an accurate understanding about the disease process of addiction?

1. "I'm really going to try to stay off the cocaine. I'm not worried about alcohol since I never had any problem with a glass or two of wine with dinner."
2. "Once my cravings go away I won't need to go to Narcotics Anonymous (NA) anymore. I'll be recovered."
3. "I feel so much better after talking to my therapist. I didn't realize I was hurting so much emotionally. I must have been using to deal with my emotional problems."
4. "I didn't realize that staying off drugs meant changing my thoughts and emotions. I thought I could just learn to stop using cocaine. NA will help me make these changes."

ANSWER: 4

An emphasis on the requirement for a total lifestyle change is necessary for preventing relapse. Through NA people learn to change negative attitudes and behaviors into positive ones. Persons addicted to one substance appear to be susceptible to dependency on other substances. There is no cure for addiction. Recovery is a lifelong process. Substance dependence disorders are primary in nature; they are not secondary to other emotional problems.

➧ ***Test-taking Tip:*** *Focus on the concept of total abstinence associated with recovery when answering this question.*

Content Area: Mental Health; *Category of Health Alteration:* Substance Abuse; *Integrated Processes:* Nursing Process Evaluation; *Client Need:* Health Promotion and Maintenance/Principles of Teaching and Learning; Health Promotion and Maintenance/Self-Care; *Cognitive Level:* Analysis

Reference: Kneisl, C., & Trigoboff, E. (2009). *Contemporary Psychiatric-Mental Health Nursing* (2nd ed., p. 355). Upper Saddle River, NJ: Pearson Education.

1634. The spouse of a client who is currently in inpatient treatment for substance abuse makes the following statement: "We've done this so many times. I don't think my spouse is ever going to change. Do you think it's time for me to get a divorce?" Which response by the nurse is most helpful?

1. "I probably would if I were you."
2. "Sounds like you're feeling discouraged in your marriage."
3. "You don't think he's ever going to change?"
4. "I can't tell you that you should get a divorce."

ANSWER: 2

When working with the family, try to help each family member see how he or she is affected by the substance-abusing behavior. Using the technique of validation assists the wife in examining her feelings and facilitates her to further explore how she is being affected. The nurse should refrain from giving a personal opinion. Restatement is a therapeutic technique but is not the best option to encourage facilitation of feelings. A direct answer, while refraining from opinion giving, closes the communication.

Test-taking Tip: *Use the process of elimination when considering all options. Using a therapeutic communication technique that focuses on the client's or spouse's feelings is usually the most therapeutic option.*

Content Area: Mental Health; *Category of Health Alteration:* Substance Abuse; *Integrated Processes:* Caring; Communication and Documentation; *Client Need:* Psychosocial Integrity/Therapeutic Communications; Psychosocial Integrity/Family Dynamics; *Cognitive Level:* Application

Reference: Townsend, M. (2009). *Psychiatric Mental Health Nursing* (6th ed., p. 481). Philadelphia: F. A. Davis.

1635. EBP A nurse working in a medical-surgical nursing unit is caring for a client 3 days post-admission who has a long history of heavy alcohol abuse. For which most acute complications related to alcohol abuse should the nurse initially monitor? SELECT ALL THAT APPLY.

1. Seizures
2. Infections
3. Gastrointestinal bleeding
4. Pancreatitis
5. Delirium tremens

ANSWER: 1, 5

Seizures, delirium tremens, and deregulation of body temperature, pulse, and blood pressure are outcomes in severe alcohol dependence that can lead to fatal consequences. Other medical complications of alcohol withdrawal include infections, hypoglycemia, gastrointestinal (GI) bleeding, undetected trauma, hepatic failure, cardiomyopathy, pancreatitis, and encephalopathy.

Test-taking Tip: *Note the key words "most acute." Use the ABCs (airway, breathing, circulation) to eliminate options that are the least life threatening.*

Content Area: Mental Health; *Category of Health Alteration:* Substance Abuse; *Integrated Processes:* Nursing Process Assess; *Client Need:* Physiological Integrity/Physiological Adaptation/Medical Emergencies; *Cognitive Level:* Application

Reference: Townsend, M. (2009). *Psychiatric Mental Health Nursing* (6th ed., p. 450). Philadelphia: F. A. Davis.

EBP Reference: Substance Abuse and Mental Health Services Administration. (2006). Physical detoxification services for withdrawal from specific substances. In Center for Substance Abuse Treatment (CSAT), *Detoxification and Substance Abuse Treatment* (pp. 41–111). Available at: www.guidelines.gov/summary/summary.aspx?doc_id=9118&nbr=004932

1636. EBP A client tells a nurse, "I usually have a few drinks when I get home from work, but I always limit it to three. I'm not running the risk of becoming addicted, am I?" The nurse's best response is:

1. "As long as you don't have any social problems associated with your use of alcohol, you do not need to be concerned."
2. "If you are concerned, then you might be developing a dependency."
3. "Three drinks a day or a total of seven drinks in a week is considered high-risk drinking for women. You seem concerned that you might be developing an alcohol dependency."
4. "There is no harm in social drinking."

ANSWER: 3

At-risk substance use is defined as the use of any illicit drugs; more than 3 drinks per day or more than 7 drinks per week in women; more than 4 drinks per day or more than 14 drinks per week in men; more than 1 drink per day if over age 65. Alcohol use can have a negative impact on physical health without creating any social problems. Reflecting the client's concern allows for elaboration but does not utilize the opportunity to educate. The client did not describe social drinking behaviors.

Test-taking Tip: *Review the guidelines for safe alcohol use and the use of direct communication when client teaching.*

Content Area: Mental Health; *Category of Health Alteration:* Substance Abuse; *Integrated Processes:* Teaching and Learning; Communication and Documentation; *Client Need:* Health Promotion and Maintenance/High-Risk Behaviors; *Cognitive Level:* Application

Reference: Mohr, W. (2009). *Psychiatric Mental Health Nursing: Evidence-Based Concepts, Skills, and Practices* (7th ed., p. 626). Philadelphia: Lippincott Williams & Wilkins.

EBP Reference: Michigan Quality Improvement Consortium. (2005). *Screening and Management of Substance Use Disorders.* Available at: www.guidelines.gov/summary/summary.aspx?doc_id=8161&nbr=004548

1637. A nurse is preparing to administer thiamine (vitamin B_1) to a client receiving treatment for alcohol dependence. Which statement best describes the rationale for administration of thiamine?

1. Thiamine prevents the neuropathy and confusion associated with chronic alcohol use.
2. Thiamine reduces the risk of withdrawal seizures.
3. Thiamine aids to reverse the malnutrition often associated with alcohol abuse.
4. Thiamine improves peripheral circulation.

ANSWER: 1

Thiamine replacement prevents the neuropathy, confusion, and encephalopathy associated with chronic alcohol use. Anticonvulsants are given to reduce the risk of withdrawal seizures. Although thiamine may aid to reverse the malnutrition, it is not the best rationale for use. Thiamine has no effect on peripheral circulation.

***Test-taking Tip:** Use Maslow's Hierarchy of Needs theory. The key word is "best," indicating that more than one option is correct but one is better than the other. Thiamine reverses malnutrition and also prevents encephalopathy. Decide which is a more acute problem.*

Content Area: Mental Health; *Category of Health Alteration:* Substance Abuse; *Integrated Processes:* Nursing Process Analysis; *Client Need:* Psychosocial Integrity/Chemical and Other Dependencies; Physiological Integrity/Pharmacological and Parenteral Therapies/ Expected Actions or Outcomes; *Cognitive Level:* Application

Reference: Townsend, M. (2009). *Psychiatric Mental Health Nursing* (6th ed., p. 482). Philadelphia: F. A. Davis.

1638. EBP A client admitted to a medical unit 14 hours ago with a diagnosis of gastritis has a health history of moderate alcohol use on a weekly basis. Which symptoms assessed by a nurse suggest that a client may be experiencing alcohol withdrawal? SELECT ALL THAT APPLY:

1. Irritability
2. Polyuria
3. Hypotension
4. Tachycardia
5. Hypervigilance
6. Nausea

ANSWER: 1, 4, 6

Signs and symptoms of alcohol withdrawal may include restlessness, irritability, anxiety, and agitation; anorexia, nausea, and vomiting; tremor, elevated heart rate, and increased blood pressure; insomnia, intense dreaming, nightmares, poor concentration, and impaired memory and judgment; increased sensitivity to sound, light, and tactile sensations; grand mal seizures; and hallucinations and delusions. Hypotension, hypervigilance, and polyuria are not associated with alcohol withdrawal.

***Test-taking Tip:** Think about the signs of alcohol withdrawal, and use the process of elimination.*

Content Area: Mental Health; *Category of Health Alteration:* Substance Abuse; *Integrated Processes:* Nursing Process Assessment; *Client Need:* Physiological Integrity/Physiological Adaptation/Medical Emergencies; Psychosocial Integrity/Chemical and Other Dependencies; *Cognitive Level:* Application

Reference: Townsend, M. (2009). *Psychiatric Mental Health Nursing* (6th ed., p. 450). Philadelphia: F. A. Davis.

EBP Reference: Substance Abuse and Mental Health Services Administration. (2006). Physical detoxification services for withdrawal from specific substances. In Center for Substance Abuse Treatment (CSAT), *Detoxification and Substance Abuse Treatment* (pp. 41–111). Available at: www.guidelines.gov/summary/summary.aspx?doc_id=9118&nbr=004932

1639. A client experiencing severe withdrawal symptoms due to alcohol dependence has an order for chlordiazepoxide (Librium®) 100 mg oral × 1, then 50 mg every 2 hours until symptoms are controlled. The medication is supplied in 50-mg tablets. The nurse administered the initial dose 2 hours ago and is reassessing the client. The client is still agitated and tremulous. The nurse should prepare to administer _____ tablet(s) at this time.

ANSWER: 1

Use a proportion formula. Multiply the extremes and then the means and solve for X.

50 mg : 1 tablet :: 50 mg : X tablets

X = 1.

***Test-taking Tip:** Focus on the information in the question. Use the on-screen calculator if needed. Verify your answer, especially if it seems like an unusual amount.*

Content Area: Mental Health; *Category of Health Alteration:* Substance Abuse; *Integrated Processes:* Nursing Process Implementation; *Client Need:* Physiological Integrity/Pharmacological and Parenteral Therapies/Dosage Calculation; *Cognitive Level:* Analysis

References: Deglin, J., & Vallerand, A. (2007). *Davis's Drug Guide for Nurses* (10th ed., pp. xx–xxii). Philadelphia: F. A. Davis; Townsend, M. (2009). *Psychiatric Mental Health Nursing* (6th ed., p. 481). Philadelphia: F. A. Davis.

1640. A nurse is reviewing information to plan a teaching session on drug abuse prevention and reviews the chart illustrated. Based on the findings presented in the chart, which age group should the nurse target for the substance abuse prevention program to have the greatest impact?

Past Month Illicit Drug Use Among Persons Aged 12 or Older, by Age: 2007

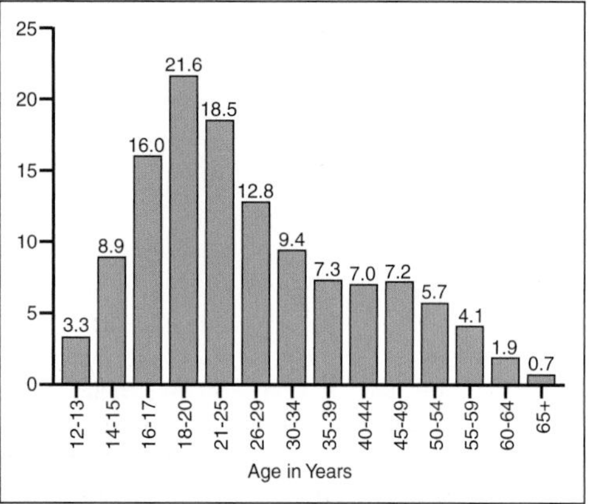

1. 12 to 15 year olds
2. 16 to 25 year olds
3. 18 to 20 year olds
4. 21 to 29 year olds

ANSWER: 1

Primary prevention through health teaching can have a significant impact on preventing youngsters and adolescents from initiating the use of substances through development of self-confidence and self-esteem. Children 12 to 15 years old have a lower rate of use than during the peak years beginning at age 16. Prevention efforts should begin before the rates escalate. The rates of use are highest at the age of 16 until 29 years, with the highest rates of use between 18 and 20 years. Opportunities to prevent drug use are too late at age 16 or older. Rates begin to fall throughout the 20s so targeting this age group is too late.

***Test-taking Tip:** Study the information in the chart and note the key word "prevention."*

Content Area: Mental Health; *Category of Health Alteration:* Substance Abuse; *Integrated Processes:* Nursing Process Planning; *Client Need:* Safe and Effective Care Environment/Management of Care/Information Technology; Psychosocial Integrity/Chemical and Other Dependencies; *Cognitive Level:* Analysis

References: Substance Abuse and Mental Health Services Administration. (2008). *Results from the 2007 National Survey on Drug Use and Health: National Findings.* NSDUH Series H-34, DHHS Publication No. SMA 08-4343. Rockville, MD: Office of Applied Studies. Available at: http://oas.samhsa.gov/nsduh/2k7nsduh/2k7Results.pdf; Varcarolis, E., Carson, V., & Shoemaker, N. (2006). *Foundations of Psychiatric Mental Health Nursing* (5th ed., p. 563). St. Louis, MO: Elsevier.

1641. In the school health center a nurse is caring for a client who is presenting with complaints of generalized fatigue. Which additional finding from the client's history and physical exam should alert the nurse to possible marijuana abuse?

1. Conjunctival infection
2. Flashbacks
3. Gastric disturbances
4. Paranoia

ANSWER: 1

Physical symptoms of cannabis intoxication include conjunctival infection, increased appetite, dry mouth, and tachycardia. Methamphetamine abuse may result in compulsive and aggressive behavior, paranoia, and hallucinations. Flashbacks are contributed to the use of hallucinogens, and gastric disturbances are common in chronic alcohol abuse.

***Test-taking Tip:** Think about the effects of common drugs of abuse.*

Content Area: Mental Health; *Category of Health Alteration:* Substance Abuse; *Integrated Processes:* Nursing Process Analysis; *Client Need:* Psychosocial Integrity/Chemical and Other Dependencies; *Cognitive Level:* Analysis

Reference: Townsend, M. (2009). *Psychiatric Mental Health Nursing* (6th ed., p. 463). Philadelphia: F. A. Davis.

1642. A client states, "I don't see any problem with smoking a little weed. It isn't addictive." A nurse most accurately informs the client:

1. "Marijuana itself is not addictive. The danger is that it often leads to abuse of more illicit drugs."
2. "It is a natural chemical and has many therapeutic uses."
3. "Marijuana has effects similar to alcohol, hallucinogens, and sedatives. All of these substances are addictive."
4. "There do not seem to be any withdrawal symptoms from marijuana; so there is controversy as to whether it is addictive."

ANSWER: 3

Even at moderate doses, cannabis produces effects similar to central nervous system depressants, hallucinogens, and sedative-hypnotics. There is an identified withdrawal syndrome (insomnia and restlessness), so it is considered an addictive substance. Cannabis is believed to have some therapeutic use but still remains a drug with addictive potential.

***Test-taking Tip:** The key words are "most accurately." Select the statement that is most complete. Review the effects of various substances of abuse.*

Content Area: Mental Health; *Category of Health Alteration:* Substance Abuse; *Integrated Processes:* Teaching and Learning; *Client Need:* Health Promotion and Maintenance/Principles of Teaching and Learning; *Cognitive Level:* Application

Reference: Townsend, M. (2009). *Psychiatric Mental Health Nursing* (6th ed., p. 461). Philadelphia: F. A. Davis.

1643. A client who abuses marijuana reports liking the drug for its perceived effects. Which reported experiences should a nurse attribute to marijuana use? SELECT ALL THAT APPLY.

1. Sexual intensity
2. Racing heartbeat
3. Energy
4. Euphoria
5. Appetite suppression
6. Fine muscle coordination

ANSWER: 1, 2, 4

Cannabis use induces tachycardia, euphoria, muscle tremors, and enhancement of sexual experience in both men and women. Central nervous system effects include relaxation, increased appetite (not appetite suppression), and amotivational syndrome, including lethargy (not increased energy) and apathy. Muscle tremors, not fine muscle coordination, are effects of the cannabis.

➧ ***Test-taking Tip:*** *Review the effects of cannabis and use the process of elimination.*

Content Area: Mental Health; *Category of Health Alteration:* Substance Abuse; *Integrated Processes:* Nursing Process Analysis; *Client Need:* Psychosocial Integrity/Chemical and Other Dependencies; *Cognitive Level:* Application

Reference: Townsend, M. (2009). *Psychiatric Mental Health Nursing* (6th ed., pp. 462–463). Philadelphia: F. A. Davis.

1644. A client often avoids talking about his cocaine use by refocusing on other problem areas, such as losing his job and discord within his family. When the client avoids discussing his drug use, the most helpful response by a nurse should be:

1. "It seems like you have multiple problems. Has the cocaine helped you cope with these in the past?"
2. "Can't you see these problems are all related to the cocaine use?"
3. "How do you think these problems will change once you no longer use cocaine?"
4. "You can't do anything about those issues right now. Just focus on getting off cocaine while you are here."

ANSWER: 3

Other problems encountered by the client are often related to drug use. Using a therapeutic communication technique of helping the client see relationships between drug use and other problems helps the client to develop insight into the severity of the substance abuse. Many direct problems will diminish with rehabilitation. Cocaine has likely contributed to other problems, not assisted in coping or resolving them. A closed question may cause defensiveness in a client with little insight. Significant problems should be addressed concurrently in treatment for substance abuse, not avoided.

➧ ***Test-taking Tip:*** *Apply principles of therapeutic communication, as well as knowledge of thought processes commonly associated with substance abuse.*

Content Area: Mental Health; *Category of Health Alteration:* Substance Abuse; *Integrated Processes:* Communication and Documentation; *Client Need:* Psychosocial Integrity/Therapeutic Communications; *Cognitive Level:* Application

Reference: Mohr, W. (2009). *Psychiatric Mental Health Nursing: Evidence-Based Concepts, Skills, and Practices* (7th ed., p. 643). Philadelphia: Lippincott Williams & Wilkins.

1645. A nurse is conducting an admission interview with a client who is under the influence of cocaine. The nurse interprets that which finding is attributable to the client being under the influence of cocaine at the time of the interview?

1. Underreporting the amount of cocaine used on a regular basis
2. Decreased blood pressure and heart rate
3. Hypersensitivity in response to personal questions
4. Lack of attention to the interview process

ANSWER: 3

Cocaine intoxication usually causes changes in sociability, hypervigilance, interpersonal sensitivity, and anxiety. Underreporting is common in all substance abusers and is not specific to cocaine intoxication. Physical effects include tachycardia and either elevated or lowered blood pressure. Hypervigilance and not lack of attention occurs with cocaine intoxication.

➧ ***Test-taking Tip:*** *Note the key phrase "under the influence of cocaine" to rule out the generic response of underreporting the amount used. This response is not specific to cocaine abuse.*

Content Area: Mental Health; *Category of Health Alteration:* Substance Abuse; *Integrated Processes:* Nursing Process Analysis; *Client Need:* Physiological Integrity/Physiological Adaptation/Alterations in Body Systems; *Cognitive Level:* Analysis

Reference: Townsend, M. (2009). *Psychiatric Mental Health Nursing* (6th ed., p. 455). Philadelphia: F. A. Davis.

1646. A client who is addicted to cocaine states, "I don't really need treatment. Things just got a little out of hand, causing some problems. I can handle things on my own. I really need to get back to my business." Which response by the nurse best assists the client to break through denial and get insight into the severity of the addiction?

1. "Tell me about your business."
2. "You don't really need to be here?"
3. "How much cocaine were you using?"
4. "You say you can handle things, but you have found yourself with a lot of problems."

ANSWER: 4

Assist the client to work on accepting the fact that using substances has caused problems in significant life areas. Addressing the business or patterns of cocaine use changes the focus (options 1 and 3). Voicing doubt without presenting reality may cause defensiveness (option 2).

➧ ***Test-taking Tip:*** *Select the option that uses therapeutic communication principles and confrontation.*

Content Area: Mental Health; *Category of Health Alteration:* Substance Abuse; *Integrated Processes:* Communication and Documentation; *Client Need:* Psychosocial Integrity/Therapeutic Communications; *Cognitive Level:* Application

Reference: Townsend, M. (2009). *Psychiatric Mental Health Nursing* (6th ed., pp. 480–481). Philadelphia: F. A. Davis.

1647. EBP A parent expresses concern to a nurse that her son, newly admitted to the mental health unit, may be using methamphetamine. Which physical examination findings by the nurse are consistent with methamphetamine abuse by the client?

1. Hypotension and bradycardia
2. Bruises and scrapes on the extremities
3. Constricted pupils and fatigue
4. Anorexia and recent weight loss

ANSWER: 4

Weight loss is associated with methamphetamine and other stimulant abuse due to their ability to cause a rise in metabolic rate and varying degrees of anorexia. The nurse should expect to find an increase in blood pressure and heart rate, as well as dilated (not constricted) pupils. Bruises and scrapes are often caused by the gait impairment associated with alcohol intoxication. Constricted pupils may indicate opiate abuse. Fatigue can be associated with any drug use.

➧ ***Test-taking Tip:*** *Focus on the issue, effects of stimulant drugs, and then use the process of elimination.*

Content Area: Mental Health; *Category of Health Alteration:* Substance Abuse; *Integrated Processes:* Nursing Process Assessment; *Client Need:* Physiological Integrity/Reduction of Risk Potential/Potential for Alterations in Body Systems; Psychosocial Integrity/Chemical and Other Dependencies; *Cognitive Level:* Analysis

Reference: Townsend, M. (2009). *Psychiatric Mental Health Nursing* (6th ed., p. 455). Philadelphia: F. A. Davis.

EBP Reference: New York State Department of Health. (2005). *Screening and Ongoing Assessment for Substance Use*. Available at: www.guidelines.gov/summary/summary.aspx?doc_id=6848&nbr=004202

1648. A client uses pathological projection to protect against the negative realities resulting from regular methamphetamine use. Which subjective information is the nurse most likely to document when the client uses pathological projection as a coping mechanism?

1. "My dad and I don't get along because he thinks that I'm a failure."
2. "I can't go back to work. I'd be so embarrassed for anyone to find out I've been in treatment."
3. "I'm not giving up alcohol, just the methamphetamine. I never had a problem with alcohol."
4. "Everything will be all right again if I can just stop using drugs."

ANSWER: 1

Projecting involves placing the responsibility for one's behavior somewhere besides the person. When projecting, or blaming, the person is blaming someone or something else for his or her behavior. The client is projecting, or blaming, thoughts that he believes his father has for the client's lack of behavior change. This is negative self-talk and is self-deprecating. Feeling embarrassed displays a fallacy of perfectionism rather than projection. Denial is evidenced in the statement that the client has no problem or intention to alter alcohol use. Believing all problems will be solved if drugs are absent is a fallacy of ignoring.

➧ ***Test-taking Tip:*** *The key word is "projection." Select option 1, noting that it is the only option that does not focus on the client. Review the various defense mechanisms, especially ones commonly used by clients with substance abuse disorders.*

Content Area: Mental Health; *Category of Health Alteration:* Substance Abuse; *Integrated Processes:* Communication and Documentation; *Client Need:* Psychosocial Integrity/Coping Mechanisms; *Cognitive Level:* Analysis

Reference: Mohr, W. (2009). *Psychiatric Mental Health Nursing: Evidence-Based Concepts, Skills, and Practices* (7th ed., p. 644). Philadelphia: Lippincott Williams & Wilkins.

1649. A nurse is interacting with a client who abuses methamphetamine. The client appears not to be willing to give up the drug use, evidenced by statements such as, "I don't plan to quit meth. I can work for days when I'm high." Which is the best response by the nurse to the client's statement?

1. "You'll exhaust yourself doing that."
2. "You can't see the real problem yet because you are in denial."
3. "You think using drugs helps you?"
4. "Good point. You probably do work long hours while you are on meth."

ANSWER: 3

The focus is on current reality and the nurse must be nonjudgmental. Restatement is a neutral response that assists the client in reexamining the thought process. Directive statements do not facilitate the client's thinking and disclosure. Informing the client of denial before he or she indicates readiness does not facilitate the therapeutic relationship. Agreeing with a client's irrational statement reinforces the denial process.

➧ ***Test-taking Tip:*** *Apply principles of therapeutic communication and eliminate options 1, 2, and 4 because these statements use barriers to therapeutic communication.*

Content Area: Mental Health; *Category of Health Alteration:* Substance Abuse; *Integrated Processes:* Communication and Documentation; *Client Need:* Psychosocial Integrity/Therapeutic Communications; *Cognitive Level:* Application

Reference: Townsend, M. (2009). *Psychiatric Mental Health Nursing* (6th ed., pp. 480–481). Philadelphia: F. A. Davis.

1650. A nurse is caring for a client in methamphetamine withdrawal. When caring for this client, the most appropriate action for the nurse should be to:

1. administer sedatives routinely to prevent seizures.
2. allow the client to sleep and eat as desired.
3. administer antipsychotic medications to manage hallucinations.
4. encourage involvement in the treatment milieu.

ANSWER: 2

Treatment of central nervous system (CNS) stimulant withdrawal involves keeping the client in a quiet atmosphere and allowing the client to eat and sleep as much as needed. Sedatives are indicated for withdrawal from CNS depressants. Antipsychotics should be used with caution because of their propensity to lower seizure threshold. Stimulation should be kept to a minimum.

➧ ***Test-taking Tip:*** *Focus on the issue: methamphetamine withdrawal and the expected response.*

Content Area: Mental Health; *Category of Health Alteration:* Substance Abuse; *Integrated Processes:* Nursing Process Implementation; Caring; *Client Need:* Psychosocial Integrity/Therapeutic Environment; *Cognitive Level:* Application

Reference: Townsend, M. (2009). *Psychiatric Mental Health Nursing* (6th ed., p. 482). Philadelphia: F. A. Davis.

1651. A nurse is educating a client on the methadone prescribed for replacement therapy while in an outpatient treatment program for heroin addicts. The client asks how taking a pill is going to help the client stay sober. Which statement is the nurse's best reply?

1. "The methadone will make you high so you won't want heroin anymore."
2. "The methadone will cause you to become very sick if you take heroin at the same time."
3. "The methadone 'replaces' the heroin in your body, so you will not experience withdrawal symptoms and will have fewer cravings for heroin."
4. "The methadone will cause sedation, so you can sleep better, giving you more energy for participating in your treatment."

ANSWER: 3

Methadone is one of the more common medications for opioid detoxification. Methadone is a long-acting agonist that, in effect, displaces heroin (or other abused opioids) and restabilizes the receptor site, thereby reversing opioid withdrawal symptoms. Methadone does not exert the severe high of other abused opiates and has no role in aversion therapy.

➧ ***Test-taking Tip:*** *The key words are "best reply." Focus on the action of methadone.*

Content Area: Mental Health; *Category of Health Alteration:* Substance Abuse; *Integrated Processes:* Teaching and Learning; *Client Need:* Physiological Integrity/Pharmacological and Parenteral Therapies/Expected Actions or Outcomes; *Cognitive Level:* Application

Reference: Mohr, W. (2009). *Psychiatric Mental Health Nursing: Evidence-Based Concepts, Skills, and Practices* (7th ed., p. 632). Philadelphia: Lippincott Williams & Wilkins.

1652. A client is being discharged from treatment for addiction to the prescription anxiolytic, alprazolam (Xanax®) and will be attending an addiction self-help group regularly. Which statement indicates that the client has an accurate understanding of maintaining sobriety according to 12-step self-help principles?

1. "I have learned how to use my nerve pills safely from now on by not overusing them."
2. "I know I can never take sedatives again, but instead I can drink a small glass of wine when I start to feel anxious."
3. "I will have to stay away from situations that I find anxiety-producing."
4. "I cannot take any mood-altering drugs or I run the risk of relapsing."

ANSWER: 4

Alcoholics Anonymous and other 12-step self-help groups promote total abstinence as the only cure. Persons addicted to drugs cannot safely use any mood-altering chemicals. Sobriety involves abstaining from the use of all substances, including anxiety medications and alcohol, in order to maintain optimal wellness. Avoiding anxiety-producing situations is not realistic.

➧ ***Test-taking Tip:** Apply the principles of recovery and sobriety to select the correct response.*

Content Area: Mental Health; *Category of Health Alteration:* Substance Abuse; *Integrated Processes:* Nursing Process Evaluation; *Client Need:* Health Promotion and Maintenance/Principles of Teaching and Learning; *Cognitive Level:* Analysis

Reference: Townsend, M. (2009). *Psychiatric Mental Health Nursing* (6th ed., p. 478). Philadelphia: F. A. Davis.

1653. A mental health nurse explains to a nursing assistant on a mental health unit that opiates have the highest rate of prescription medication abuse and are popular drugs of abuse. Which additional statement should the nurse make to describe the rationale for opiates being abused?

1. Opiates alter the experience of reality and relieve stress.
2. Opiates reduce the feeling of anxiety and induce well-being.
3. Opiates produce feelings of omnipotence and increase awareness.
4. Opiates reduce emotional and physical pain and induce euphoria.

ANSWER: 4

Opioids are popular drugs of abuse because they desensitize an individual to both psychological and physical pain and induce a sense of euphoria. Hallucinogens alter a person's sense of reality. Sedative-hypnotics reduce anxiety but do not produce euphoria. Stimulants produce feelings of omnipotence.

➧ ***Test-taking Tip:** Review the effects of various drugs of abuse and use the process of elimination. Recall that sedative-hypnotics have relaxing effects similar to opiates, but they do not produce euphoria. Select the option that has the greatest effect.*

Content Area: Mental Health; *Category of Health Alteration:* Substance Abuse; *Integrated Processes:* Nursing Process Analysis; *Client Need:* Psychosocial Integrity/Chemical and Other Dependencies; Physiological Integrity/Pharmacological and Parenteral Therapies/Expected Actions or Outcomes; *Cognitive Level:* Application

Reference: Townsend, M. (2009). *Psychiatric Mental Health Nursing* (6th ed., p. 457). Philadelphia: F. A. Davis.

1654. A client is being treated for benzodiazepine abuse. Which interventions should be implemented by a nurse when caring for this client? Rank the interventions in the order that they should be implemented during the client's course of treatment.

______ Review lifestyle changes that will need to be made
______ Take vital signs
______ Administer lorazepam (Ativan®) as ordered
______ Emphasize personal responsibility for abstaining from substance abuse
______ Provide information about the symptoms of withdrawal
______ Encourage oral fluids

ANSWER: 6, 1, 2, 5, 4, 3

Vital signs should be assessed first for impending withdrawal symptoms. Next administer medications to reduce the potentially fatal withdrawal symptoms of the benzodiazepines. Oral fluids are then encouraged to maintain adequate hydration. Education of expected symptoms helps to ease the client's fear of the unknown. Education is accomplished once the client is physically stable and includes information about symptoms of withdrawal and assisting the client to acknowledge personal responsibility for needing to change. Finally, specific changes can be explored to help promote the client's drug-free lifestyle.

➧ ***Test-taking Tip:** Use the nursing process and Maslow's Hierarchy of Needs theory. Recall that assessment and then analysis are priority in the nursing process. Physiological needs are addressed before psychosocial and teaching needs.*

Content Area: Mental Health; *Category of Health Alteration:* Substance Abuse; *Integrated Processes:* Nursing Process Implementation; *Client Need:* Safe and Effective Care Environment/Management of Care/Establishing Priorities; Psychosocial Integrity/Chemical and Other Dependencies; *Cognitive Level:* Analysis

Reference: Isaacs, A. (2005). *Lippincott's Review Series: Mental Health and Psychiatric Nursing* (4th ed., pp. 158–159). Philadelphia: Lippincott Williams & Wilkins.

1655. A nurse is caring for an adolescent diagnosed with attention deficit-hyperactivity disorder who is being placed on a psychostimulant medication. Which stimulant should the nurse expect to be ordered because of its lowest potential for abuse?

1. Amphetamine-dextroamphetamine (Adderall®)
2. Sibutramine (Meridia®)
3. Methylphenidate (Ritalin®)
4. Dextroamphetamine (Dexedrine®)

ANSWER: 3

Methylphenidate produces central nervous system (CNS) stimulation with weak sympathomimetic activity. It is often abused as a last resort among these options because it does not give the user the euphoria they crave. Amphetamine-dextroamphetamine releases norepinephrine and therefore has high abuse potential. Sibutramine raises levels of serotonin, norepinephrine, and dopamine in the body. Dextroamphetamine produces CNS stimulation by releasing norepinephrine. These three medications are more often abused by people who are trying to get a high similar to speed.

Test-taking Tip: *The key words are "lowest potential." Think about the actions of the major prescription stimulants. Consider that methylphenidate has different effects than the medications in the other options.*

Content Area: Mental Health; *Category of Health Alteration:* Substance Abuse; *Integrated Processes:* Nursing Process Analysis; *Client Need:* Psychosocial Integrity/Chemical and Other Dependencies; Physiological Integrity/Pharmacological and Parenteral Therapies/ Expected Actions or Outcomes; *Cognitive Level:* Analysis

References: Richardson, W. (2004). *AD/HD and Stimulant Medication Abuse.* Attention Deficit Disorder Association. Available at: www.add.org/ articles/med_abuse.html; Deglin, J., & Vallerand, A. (2007). *Davis's Drug Guide for Nurses* (10th ed., pp. 779–781). Philadelphia: F. A. Davis.

1656. A nurse is preparing to administer chlordiazepoxide (Librium®) 75 mg orally for a client experiencing severe withdrawal symptoms due to alprazolam (Xanax®) dependency. The medication is supplied in 25-mg capsules. The nurse should prepare to administer _____ capsules of medication to the client.

ANSWER: 3

Use a proportion formula to calculate the dose. Multiply the extremes (outside values) and then the means (inside values) and solve for X.
25 mg : 1 capsule :: 75 mg : X capsule
25X = 75
X = 75/25 = 3.

Test-taking Tip: *Focus on the information in the question and use the on-screen calculator. Verify your answer especially if it seems like an unusual amount.*

Content Area: Mental Health; *Category of Health Alteration:* Substance Abuse; *Integrated Processes:* Nursing Process Implementation; *Client Need:* Psychosocial Integrity/Chemical and Other Dependencies; Physiological Integrity/Pharmacological and Parenteral Therapies/Dosage Calculation; *Cognitive Level:* Analysis

References: Pickar, G. (2007). *Dosage Calculations: A Ratio-Proportion Approach* (2nd ed., pp. 46, 344). Clifton Park, NY: Thomson Delmar Learning; Mohr, W. (2009). *Psychiatric Mental Health Nursing: Evidence-Based Concepts, Skills, and Practices* (7th ed., p. 630). Philadelphia: Lippincott Williams & Wilkins.

1657. EBP A 19-year-old client regularly abuses dextromethorphan (DXM). Which activity, if performed under the influence of dextromethorphan, places the client at highest risk for complications related to DXM abuse?

1. Fishing on the shore of a lake
2. Snow-skiing on spring break
3. Competing in a swim meet
4. Dancing at a night club

ANSWER: 4

When consumed in large quantities, DXM can cause hyperthermia. Hyperthermia is a concern for clients who take DXM while in a hot environment such as exerting themselves at a dance club. Other effects of DXM abuse include hallucinations, loss of motor control, dissociative sensations, confusion, impaired judgment, blurred vision, dizziness, paranoia, excessive sweating, slurred speech, nausea, vomiting, abdominal pain, irregular heartbeat, high blood pressure, headache, and lethargy. Fishing, skiing, and swimming are lower risk activities for inducing complications while taking DXM because of the cooler environments.

Test-taking Tip: *Focus on the actions of the client and the environments. Note that three environments are likely cooler than one environment in the options. Select the option that is different.*

Content Area: Mental Health; *Category of Health Alteration:* Substance Abuse; *Integrated Processes:* Nursing Process Analysis; *Client Need:* Physiological Integrity/Pharmacological and Parenteral Therapies/Adverse Effects/Contradictions/Interactions; *Cognitive Level:* Analysis

Reference: Mohr, W. (2009). *Psychiatric Mental Health Nursing: Evidence-Based Concepts, Skills, and Practices* (7th ed., p. 622). Philadelphia: Lippincott Williams & Wilkins.

EBP Reference: Gavin, M. (2007). Cough and Cold Medicine Abuse. *Kids Health*. Wilmington, DE: The Nemours Foundation. Available at: www.kidshealth.org/parent/system/medicine/cough_cold_medicine_abuse.html

1658. EBP A student participating in college sports is suspected of abusing anabolic steroids and is referred to the college's health service. A nurse completes a health history and assesses the student. Which assessment findings support the suspected abuse? SELECT ALL THAT APPLY.

1. Urinary tract infections
2. Thickening of the hair
3. Edema of the hands or feet
4. Heavy menstruation
5. Acne
6. Aggressiveness

ANSWER: 1, 3, 5, 6

Anabolic steroid abuse is often associated with persons involved with sports and fitness. Certain physiological signs indicating possible steroid abuse include hair loss, acne, dysuria, small testicles, edema of the extremities, and rapid weight gain. Females can develop decreased breast size, acne, virilism, and amenorrhea. Behavioral disturbances such as psychosis or severe aggressiveness can occur. Hair usually thins (not thickens), and females experience cessation of menses (not heavy menstruation).

➧ ***Test-taking Tip:*** *Think about the adverse effects of steroid abuse and use the process of elimination.*

Content Area: Mental Health; *Category of Health Alteration:* Substance Abuse; *Integrated Processes:* Nursing Process Assessment; *Client Need:* Physiological Integrity/Reduction of Risk Potential/Potential for Alterations in Body Systems; Physiological Integrity/Pharmacological and Parenteral Therapies/Adverse Effects/Contraindications/Interactions; *Cognitive Level:* Analysis

Reference: Mohr, W. (2009). *Psychiatric Mental Health Nursing: Evidence-Based Concepts, Skills, and Practices* (7th ed., p. 622). Philadelphia: Lippincott Williams & Wilkins.

EBP Reference: Center for Substance Abuse Treatment. (2006). Anabolic steroids. *Substance Abuse Treatment Advisory*, 5(3), Available at: http://download.ncadi.samhsa.gov/prevline/pdfs/ms991.pdf

1659. EBP A client is seen in a clinic for an annual physical examination. The client asks a nurse if taking the dietary supplement androstenedione, sometimes referred to as "andro," would help to get in shape for football season. Which statement by the nurse is most accurate?

1. "Androstenedione supplements have been proven to be perfectly safe because it is a naturally occurring hormone that is the precursor for testosterone."
2. "Taking androstenedione supplements is similar to taking vitamin supplements. Andro is found in meats, so the tablet forms are safe."
3. "Androstenedione is considered a dietary supplement and therefore is not guaranteed safe by FDA standards."
4. "Benefits of androstenedione have not been proven. In fact, there appear to be more negative effects than benefits."

ANSWER: 4

The nurse has the duty to inform the client of benefits and risks. The available data do not support the use of androstenedione or androstenediol for performance-enhancing effects. In fact, deleterious effects on the lipid profile are suggested by the data. Dietary supplements are not required to have established safety records according to U.S. Food and Drug Administration (FDA) standards. Clients should be encouraged to eat a balanced diet for all needed nutrients and engage in a healthy physical activity program.

➧ ***Test-taking Tip:*** *Review the lack of regulatory standards required for nonpharmaceuticals and dietary supplements. If safety is questionable, remember that client safety should never be compromised.*

Content Area: Mental Health; *Category of Health Alteration:* Substance Abuse; *Integrated Processes:* Teaching and Learning; *Client Need:* Health Promotion and Maintenance/High-Risk Behaviors; Physiological Integrity/Reduction of Risk Potential/Potential for Alterations in Body Systems; *Cognitive Level:* Application

Reference: Mohr, W. (2009). *Psychiatric Mental Health Nursing: Evidence-Based Concepts, Skills, and Practices* (7th ed., p. 622). Philadelphia: Lippincott Williams & Wilkins.

EBP Reference: Mayo Clinic. (2008). *Performance-Enhancing Drugs: Are They a Risk to Your Health?* Mayo Foundation for Medical Education and Research (MFMER). Available at: www.mayoclinic.com/print/performance-enhancing-drugs/HQ01105/METHOD=print

1660. EBP A client has just started taking sustained-release bupropion (Wellbutrin SR®) to aid with smoking cessation. The client has tried to quit smoking with nicotine gum before without success. The client asks the nurse, "How is the Wellbutrin SR® pill any different than the gums or patches that I have tried before?" The best response by the nurse is:

1. "Bupropion is an antidepressant that has shown to be twice as successful as the nicotine patch in helping people quit smoking."
2. "The bupropion pill is more palatable than the gum you tried before, so you should be able to use it longer to abstain from smoking."
3. "The nicotine in bupropion tablets is faster acting than the gums or patches, so it will relieve your cravings more quickly."
4. "You seem skeptical that this will work. How do you feel about giving it a try?"

ANSWER: 1

Bupropion has proven useful in smoking cessation with a 12-month abstinence rate of 35.5% compared to a placebo at 15.6% and the nicotine patch at 16.4%. Palatability of treatment is not a significant factor in smoking abstinence. Bupropion does not contain nicotine. Addressing the client's skepticism may encourage the client to elaborate, but does not address the knowledge deficit that has been indicated.

➧ ***Test-taking Tip:*** *Review the use of antidepressants for obsessive tendencies seen in clients such as those addicted to nicotine or those suffering from eating disorders. When a client indicates a need for information, it is appropriate for the nurse to inform.*

Content Area: Mental Health; *Category of Health Alteration:* Substance Abuse; *Integrated Processes:* Nursing Process Implementation; Teaching and Learning; Communication and Documentation; *Client Need:* Psychosocial Integrity/Chemical and Other Dependencies; Physiological Integrity/Pharmacological and Parenteral Therapies/Expected Actions or Outcomes; *Cognitive Level:* Application

Reference: Townsend, M. (2009). *Psychiatric Mental Health Nursing* (6th ed., p. 482). Philadelphia: F. A. Davis.

EBP Reference: Public Health Service. (2008). *Clinical Practice Guideline: Treating Tobacco Use and Dependence: 2008 Update.* Rockville, MD: U.S. Department of Health and Human Services. Available at: www.ahrq.gov/path/tobacco.htm

---

1661. EBP A client expresses ambivalence about quitting smoking and expresses fears of "getting fat" and "looking like a cow." The client wonders if that is worse than smoking. The most helpful response by the nurse would be:

1. "We could set up a diet for you to start at the same time to prevent you from gaining any weight."
2. "Don't you think it would be much better to be able to breathe easier than to gain a little weight?"
3. "Do you see yourself as overweight?"
4. "It sounds like you are afraid of weight gain. Tell me about both the good and bad things that might happen if you give up smoking."

ANSWER: 4

Fear of weight gain is a barrier for many who want to quit smoking. This is an especially important issue for women and may deter their attempts to stop smoking. Acknowledging fears develops empathy. Exploring fears as well as benefits helps the client in decision making. Cognitive reappraisal helps the client face fears more realistically. Dieting during smoking cessation is not recommended in general and has been shown to increase the likelihood of smoking relapse. Pointing out the health gains of stopping smoking does little to assuage the client's fear of weight gain. Closed-ended questions have limited effectiveness in helping the client discuss fears.

➧ ***Test-taking Tip:*** *Select the therapeutic communication technique that focuses on the client's fears.*

Content Area: Mental Health; *Category of Health Alteration:* Substance Abuse; *Integrated Processes:* Caring; Communication and Documentation; *Client Need:* Health Promotion and Maintenance/High-Risk Behaviors; Psychosocial Integrity/Therapeutic Communications; *Cognitive Level:* Application

Reference: Mohr, W. (2009). *Psychiatric Mental Health Nursing: Evidence-Based Concepts, Skills, and Practices* (7th ed., p. 643). Philadelphia: Lippincott Williams & Wilkins.

EBP Reference: Center for Substance Abuse Treatment. (2006). *Detoxification and Substance Abuse Treatment. Treatment Improvement Protocol (TIP).* Series 45, DHHS Publication No. SMA 06-4131. Rockville, MD: Substance Abuse and Mental Health Services Administration. Available at: http://download.ncadi.samhsa.gov/prevline/pdfs/DTXTIP45(3-30-06).PDF

Test 44: **Mental Health: Pharmacological and Parenteral Therapies**

1662. EBP A client taking sertraline (Zoloft®) for treatment of depression for the past 11 months reports feeling much better and wishes to discontinue the medication. Which is the most appropriate response by a nurse?

1. "The medication will have to be reduced gradually to prevent undesirable symptoms."
2. "It appears that the medication has worked very well. It should be safe to discontinue its use."
3. "You should not stop the medication without talking to your health-care provider first."
4. "You should take this medication indefinitely to prevent recurrence of depressive symptoms."

ANSWER: 1

Sertraline is a selective serotonin reuptake inhibitor (SSRI) antidepressant. Stopping antidepressants abruptly can cause discontinuation/withdrawal symptoms, including dizziness, numbness and tingling, gastrointestinal disturbances (particularly nausea and vomiting), headache, sweating, anxiety, and sleep disturbances. To minimize the risk of discontinuation/withdrawal symptoms, the dose should be reduced gradually over an extended period of time. Antidepressants should not be stopped abruptly. Clients have the right to discontinue medication treatment. Treatment with antidepressants may effectively last for months to several years, but should not be used indefinitely.

▶ ***Test-taking Tip:*** *Use Maslow's Hierarchy of Needs theory, focusing on physiological aspects of SSRI withdrawal. Select an option that should prevent withdrawal.*

Content Area: Mental Health; *Category of Health Alteration:* Pharmacological and Parenteral Therapies; *Integrated Processes:* Communication and Documentation; *Client Need:* Physiological Integrity/Pharmacological and Parenteral Therapies/Medication Administration; *Cognitive Level:* Application

Reference: Townsend, M. (2009). *Psychiatric Mental Health Nursing* (6th ed., p. 314). Philadelphia: F. A. Davis.

EBP Reference: Leydon, G., Rodgers, L., & Kendrick, T. (2007). A qualitative study of patient views on discontinuing long-term selective serotonin reuptake inhibitors. *Family Practice,* 24(6), 570.

1663. A client is to be started on citalopram (Celexa®) for treatment of depression. Which information should be most important for a nurse to include when planning teaching for the client?

1. Activity levels should be increased to include a daily exercise routine.
2. If sexual side effects become unbearable, consult your health-care provider.
3. Avoid processed meats, red wine, and Swiss cheese.
4. Monitor blood pressure regularly, and report any significant changes.

ANSWER: 2

Sexual dysfunction is most commonly associated with the use of serotonin reuptake inhibitors (SSRIs). Weight gain and cardiac effects are associated with the use of tricyclic antidepressants (TCAs). Dietary restriction of foods containing tyramine is necessary for clients taking monoamine oxidase inhibitors (MAOIs).

▶ ***Test-taking Tip:*** *The key word is citalopram; antidepressants ending in "-pram" are members of the SSRI category. Review the common side effects associated with SSRIs.*

Content Area: Mental Health; *Category of Health Alteration:* Pharmacological and Parenteral Therapies; *Integrated Processes:* Nursing Process Planning; Teaching and Learning; *Client Need:* Psychosocial Integrity/Unexpected Body Image Changes; Physiological Integrity/Pharmacological and Parenteral Therapies/Adverse Effects/Contraindications/Interactions; *Cognitive Level:* Analysis

Reference: Townsend, M. (2009). *Psychiatric Mental Health Nursing* (6th ed., p. 313). Philadelphia: F. A. Davis.

1664. EBP A client, who switched to paroxetine (Paxil®) several days ago after taking imipramine (Tofranil®) for several years, presents with tachycardia, hypertension, fever, sweating, and confusion. A nurse notifies the health-care provider, suspecting the client is experiencing:

1. neuroleptic malignant syndrome.
2. discontinuation syndrome.
3. serotonin syndrome.
4. extrapyramidal symptoms.

ANSWER: 3

Tachycardia, hypertension, fever, sweating, and confusion indicate serotonin syndrome, a potentially fatal condition that may occur with concurrent use of other medications that increase serotonin. Neuroleptic malignant syndrome is a rare, potentially fatal condition characterized by hyperpyrexia and severe parkinsonian-like muscle rigidity that can occur with antipsychotics. Discontinuation syndrome may occur with the sudden discontinuation of all antidepressants. Extrapyramidal symptoms (EPS) are associated with the use of antipsychotic medications. Common EPS side effects are involuntary movements, most often affecting the mouth, lips, and tongue, and parkinsonian-like tremors, rigidity, temporary paralysis, and extreme slowness of movement.

▶ ***Test-taking Tip:*** *Remember the action of serotonin reuptake inhibitors, and then relate that action to the potential complications when combining serotonin-elevating medications. If unsure, only one option includes the word serotonin.*

Content Area: Mental Health; *Category of Health Alteration:* Pharmacological and Parenteral Therapies; *Integrated Processes:* Nursing Process Analysis; *Client Need:* Physiological Integrity/Pharmacological and Parenteral Therapies/Adverse Effects/Contraindications/Interactions; *Cognitive Level:* Analysis

Reference: Townsend, M. (2009). *Psychiatric Mental Health Nursing* (6th ed., p. 313). Philadelphia: F. A. Davis.

EBP Reference: Institute for Clinical Systems Improvement. (2008). *Major Depression in Adults in Primary Care.* Available at: www.guideline.gov/summary/summary.aspx?doc_id=12617&nbr=006525&string=psychiatric

1665. A nurse is developing a teaching plan for a client prescribed nortriptyline (Pamelor®). Which self-care aspects should be included to minimize medication side effects and prevent injury? SELECT ALL THAT APPLY.

1. Avoid driving until vision is completely clear to prevent injury.
2. Suck on candy or ice chips to keep your mouth moist.
3. Try running water in the bathroom to stimulate urination.
4. Avoid eating processed meats, cheeses, and wine.
5. Increase fluid and fiber in the diet to prevent constipation.
6. Increase exposure to sunlight to facilitate vitamin D absorption.

ANSWER: 1, 2, 3, 5

Teach the client how to manage the anticholinergic side effects of tricyclic antidepressants (TCAs). Driving is dangerous until vision is clear. Dry mouth can be relieved with hard candy, ice, or water. Running water stimulates urination. Fluid and fiber help relieve constipation. Dietary restrictions are necessary with monoamine oxidase inhibitors (MAOIs), not TCAs. TCAs cause photosensitivity; clients should use sun protection measures.

▶ ***Test-taking Tip:*** *Review the four major anticholinergic side effects of TCAs (blurred vision, urinary retention, dry mouth, and constipation), and then think about nursing actions that should address resolution of those side effects.*

Content Area: Mental Health; *Category of Health Alteration:* Pharmacological and Parenteral Therapies; *Integrated Processes:* Nursing Process Planning; *Client Need:* Health Promotion and Maintenance/Self-Care; Physiological Integrity/Pharmacological and Parenteral Therapies/Medication Administration; *Cognitive Level:* Application

Reference: Townsend, M. (2009). *Psychiatric Mental Health Nursing* (6th ed., pp. 312–313). Philadelphia: F. A. Davis.

1666. A new nurse describes the action of tricyclic antidepressants as relieving symptoms of depression by inhibiting neuronal uptake of the neurotransmitters serotonin and norepinephrine. Based on the illustration, at which labeled site should the new nurse state that inhibition takes place?

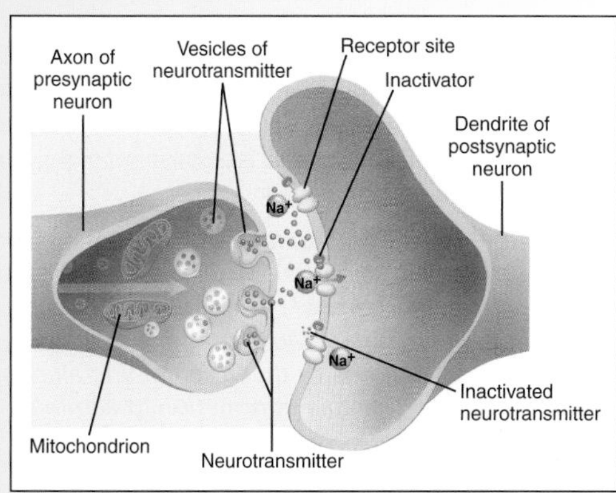

1. Neurotransmitter
2. Receptor site
3. Synapse
4. Dendrites

ANSWER: 2

Neuronal uptake of the neurotransmitters occurs at the receptor sites on the postsynaptic neuron. When the nerve signal reaches the synapse, it causes the release of neurotransmitter from storage vesicles. The synapse is the junction or space between two neurons. The dendrites transmit impulses toward the cell body.

▶ ***Test-taking Tip:*** *Focus on the illustration and the description provided for the action of tricyclic antidepressants to answer this question. Apply knowledge of the normal anatomy and physiology of the neuron and associated terminology.*

Content Area: Mental Health; *Category of Health Alteration:* Pharmacological and Parenteral Therapies; *Integrated Processes:* Nursing Process Analysis; *Client Need:* Physiological Integrity/Pharmacological and Parenteral Therapies/Expected Actions or Outcomes; *Cognitive Level:* Analysis

References: Mohr, W. (2006). *Psychiatric-Mental Health Nursing* (6th ed., p. 290). Philadelphia: Lippincott Williams & Wilkins; Townsend, M. (2008). *Essentials of Psychiatric Mental Health Nursing* (4th ed., p. 36). Philadelphia: F. A. Davis.

1667. Since taking the antidepressant doxepin (Sinequan®), a female client has been reporting a decrease in sexual desire. She says she "just isn't that interested" because she "just doesn't enjoy sex anymore." She and her partner agree that they miss the excitement they used to share. Which is the most helpful response by a nurse?

1. "This often happens when couples are together for a longer period of time. Tell me how you would feel about a referral for counseling."
2. "Try to wait for awhile. This is a temporary effect of your therapy, and as your depression gets better your interest in sexual activity should increase."
3. "Perhaps you could try some alternatives to your normal sexual routines to enhance your sexual relationship."
4. "This may be due to your medication. How would you feel about talking to your doctor about changing to a different type of antidepressant?"

ANSWER: 4

If sexual dysfunction side effects become intolerable, a switch to another antidepressant may be necessary. It is not therapeutic to dismiss the complaint as a normal course for the relationship or boredom within the relationship.

▸ ***Test-taking Tip:*** *Review the side effects of serotonin reuptake inhibitors and use the principles of therapeutic communication to acknowledge the client's concern and provide accurate education.*

Content Area: Mental Health; *Category of Health Alteration:* Pharmacological and Parenteral Therapies; *Integrated Processes:* Caring; Communication and Documentation; *Client Need:* Psychosocial Integrity/Situational Role Changes; Physiological Integrity/Pharmacological and Parenteral Therapies/Adverse Effects/Contraindications/Interactions; *Cognitive Level:* Application

Reference: Townsend, M. (2009). *Psychiatric Mental Health Nursing* (6th ed., p. 313). Philadelphia: F. A. Davis.

1668. Which aspect is most appropriate for a nurse to include in a teaching plan for a client taking amitriptyline (Elavil®)?

1. Establish a calorie-controlled diet plan suitable to the client's preferences.
2. Provide support for concerns of sexual dysfunction.
3. Instruct to discontinue the medication immediately if experiencing a sudden elevation in blood pressure.
4. Encourage to take the medication upon awakening to manage the side effect of insomnia.

ANSWER: 1

Weight gain is often a major concern for clients taking tricyclic antidepressants (TCAs). A calorie-controlled diet plan will assist in avoiding weight gain. Sexual dysfunction is most commonly associated with the use of serotonin reuptake inhibitors (SSRIs) and not TCAs. Sudden hypertension results from food–medication interactions associated with monoamine oxidase inhibitors (MAOIs) and not TCAs. Antidepressants are more likely to cause sedation rather than stimulation and therefore frequently taken at bedtime.

▸ ***Test-taking Tip:*** *Eliminate options that are associated with side effects of SSRIs and MAOIs. Apply knowledge that a side effect of a TCA is sedation to eliminate another option.*

Content Area: Mental Health; *Category of Health Alteration:* Pharmacological and Parenteral Therapies; *Integrated Processes:* Nursing Process Planning; *Client Need:* Physiological Integrity/Pharmacological and Parenteral Therapies/Medication Administration; *Cognitive Level:* Analysis

Reference: Townsend, M. (2009). *Psychiatric Mental Health Nursing* (6th ed., p. 313). Philadelphia: F. A. Davis.

1669. A client taking tranylcypromine (Parnate®) develops a list of possible meal plans. Which meal plans should a nurse determine comprise safe food and beverage selections? SELECT ALL THAT APPLY.

1. Baked chicken, mashed potatoes and gravy, 8 oz 2% milk
2. Grilled salmon, steamed broccoli, 12 oz lemon-lime soda
3. Pepperoni pizza, Caesar salad, 16 oz iced tea
4. Beef burritos with sour cream and guacamole topping, corn chips, 12 oz beer
5. Granola with raisins and almonds, low-fat yogurt, and 8 oz coffee
6. Grilled pork loin, rice, green beans, 12 oz diet clear soda

ANSWER: 1, 2, 6

Tranylcypromine is a monoamine oxidase inhibitor (MAOI), so options should include foods and beverages that contain no tyramine. Baked chicken, mashed potatoes and gravy, 8 oz 2% milk; grilled salmon, steamed broccoli, 12 oz lemon-lime soda; and grilled pork loin, rice, green beans, 12 oz diet clear soda, are menus that include no items containing tyramine. Tyramine is found in pepperoni, sour cream, avocados, beer, raisins, and yogurt.

▸ ***Test-taking Tip:*** *Remember there are only three major MAOIs—isocarboxazid (Marplan®), phenelzine sulfate (Nardil®), and tranylcypromine sulfate (Parnate®)—and foods containing tyramine should be eliminated. Most tyramine-containing foods are processed and aged foods or those containing alcohol, chocolate, and caffeine. Use this information to eliminate options that have tyramine-containing foods.*

Content Area: Mental Health; *Category of Health Alteration:* Pharmacological and Parenteral Therapies; *Integrated Processes:* Nursing Process Evaluation; *Client Need:* Physiological Integrity/Pharmacological and Parenteral Therapies/Adverse Effects/Contraindications/Interactions; *Cognitive Level:* Analysis

Reference: Townsend, M. (2009). *Psychiatric Mental Health Nursing* (6th ed., pp. 310–311). Philadelphia: F. A. Davis.

1670. A nurse is assessing a client for adverse effects of trazodone (Desyrel®). Which assessment finding should the nurse determine is an adverse effect unique to the use of trazodone?

1. Hepatic failure
2. Priapism
3. Weight gain
4. Cardiac dysrhythmias

ANSWER: 2

Prolonged or inappropriate erections are rare but problematic side effects of treatment with trazodone. If left untreated, it can lead to impotence. Hepatic failure is a life-threatening condition reported in the use of nefazodone (Serzone®). Weight gain and cardiac dysrhythmias are associated with many of the tricyclic antidepressants (TCAs).

➧ ***Test-taking Tip:*** *Review side effects of all classes of antidepressants. Note that trazodone is in the class of unique antidepressants, therefore not likely to share side effects in common with the major classifications such as TCAs or serotonin reuptake inhibitors. Use the process of elimination to omit side effects common to the major categories.*

Content Area: Mental Health; *Category of Health Alteration:* Pharmacological and Parenteral Therapies; *Integrated Processes:* Nursing Process Assessment; *Client Need:* Physiological Integrity/Pharmacological and Parenteral Therapies/Adverse Effects/Contraindications/Interactions; *Cognitive Level:* Application

References: Deglin, J., & Vallerand, A. (2009). *Davis's Drug Guide for Nurses* (11th ed., pp. 1200–1201). Philadelphia: F. A. Davis; Townsend, M. (2009). *Psychiatric Mental Health Nursing* (6th ed., p. 314). Philadelphia: F. A. Davis.

1671. After a recreational game of basketball with peers, a client taking lithium for bipolar disorder complains of feeing nauseous and shaky, having blurred vision, and finding it hard to stand. Considering this information, which action should be taken by a nurse?

1. Instruct the client to sit and rest in a cool place.
2. Call the health-care provider (HCP) to request that a stat lithium level be prescribed.
3. Give the client an antiemetic with a large glass of some cool water.
4. Prepare the emergency team for the client's impending cardiac arrest.

ANSWER: 2

The client is showing signs of lithium toxicity, especially apparent after participating in high levels of physical activity. The HCP should be notified for a stat lithium level and corrective action. The therapeutic range for maintenance of bipolar disorder is between 0.6 and 1.2 mEq/L. Signs of toxicity are seen when the serum levels rise above 1.5 mEq/L. Having the client rest or administering an antiemetic will not resolve the serum lithium elevations. A nurse misinterprets the symptoms if preparations are made for impending cardiac arrest.

➧ ***Test-taking Tip:*** *Use the nursing process to perform further assessments before appropriate interventions can be carried out. A health-care provider needs to prescribe a lithium level.*

Content Area: Mental Health; *Category of Health Alteration:* Pharmacological and Parenteral Therapies; *Integrated Processes:* Nursing Process Implementation; *Client Need:* Physiological Integrity/Pharmacological and Parenteral Therapies/Adverse Effects/Contraindications/Interactions; Physiological Integrity/Physiological Adaptation/Medical Emergencies; *Cognitive Level:* Analysis

Reference: Townsend, M. (2009). *Psychiatric Mental Health Nursing* (6th ed., p. 319). Philadelphia: F. A. Davis.

1672. At discharge, a nurse documents that a client taking lithium has an accurate understanding of self-care. On which client statement should the nurse base this judgment?

1. "I know I need to restrict foods high in sugar while I'm taking lithium."
2. "I need to come back and have my blood lithium level checked every 2 weeks."
3. "I should take my lithium on an empty stomach for best absorption."
4. "I need to eat enough foods containing sodium and drink at least 2 to 3 liters of fluid daily."

ANSWER: 4

The client must consume adequate dietary sodium as well as 2,500 to 3,000 mL of fluid per day to prevent dehydration leading to lithium toxicity. Sugary foods should only be avoided if weight gain becomes a problem. Lithium levels should be checked every 1 to 2 months, not every 2 weeks. Lithium often causes stomach upset and can be taken with food for better tolerance.

➧ ***Test-taking Tip:*** *Remember sodium depletion and dehydration will lead to lithium toxicity. Review the properties of lithium, especially its similarities to sodium.*

Content Area: Mental Health; *Category of Health Alteration:* Pharmacological and Parenteral Therapies; *Integrated Processes:* Nursing Process Evaluation; Communication and Documentation; *Client Need:* Physiological Integrity/Pharmacological and Parenteral Therapies/Medication Administration; Health Promotion and Maintenance/Self-Care; *Cognitive Level:* Analysis

Reference: Townsend, M. (2009). *Psychiatric Mental Health Nursing* (6th ed., p. 319). Philadelphia: F. A. Davis.

1673. A mother asks a nurse why the anticonvulsant valproic acid (Depakene®) is being prescribed for her son who is beginning therapy for control of his aggressive behaviors. The nurse's response is based on the fact that anticonvulsants are helpful in reducing manic and impulsive behavior by:

1. enhancing the reuptake of norepinephrine and serotonin in the central nervous system (CNS).
2. blocking the effects of dopamine at the postsynaptic neuron.
3. increasing the levels of gamma-aminobutyric acid (GABA), thereby inhibiting neurotransmission in the CNS.
4. alters sodium channels in neurons decreasing nerve impulse transmission.

ANSWER: 3

Anticonvulsants increase levels of GABA, an inhibitory neurotransmitter in the CNS. Lithium is thought to enhance the reuptake of norepinephrine and serotonin in the CNS. Antipsychotics block the effects of dopamine at the postsynaptic neuron. Another anticonvulsant, such as carbamazepine (Tegretol®), alters sodium channels in neurons, thus decreasing synaptic transmission.

➧ ***Test-taking Tip:*** *Review the role of anticonvulsants in psychiatric treatment. Remember that one effect is sedation; therefore, their use is probable when a calming effect is desired.*

Content Area: Mental Health; *Category of Health Alteration:* Pharmacological and Parenteral Therapies; *Integrated Processes:* Nursing Process Analysis; *Client Need:* Physiological Integrity/Pharmacological and Parenteral Therapies/Expected Actions or Outcomes; *Cognitive Level:* Analysis

Reference: Deglin, J., & Vallerand, A. (2009). *Davis's Drug Guide for Nurses* (11th ed., p. 1212). Philadelphia: F. A. Davis.

1674. A nurse is comparing a client's serum lithium level to a lithium toxicity chart to determine the symptoms of significance for assessment. Place an X on the chart column that depicts signs a client might exhibit if the client's serum lithium level is 3.6 mEq/L.

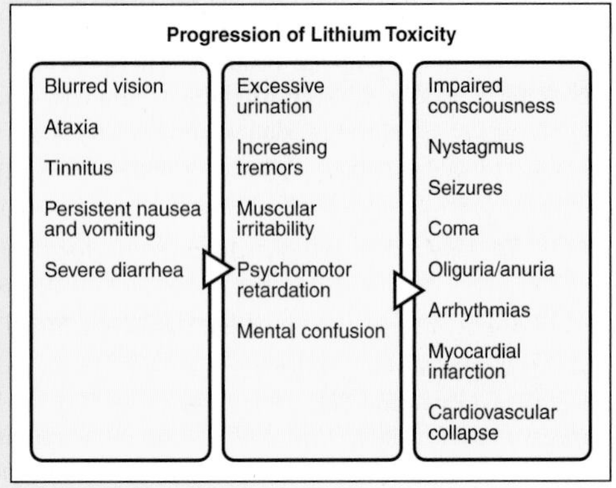

ANSWER:

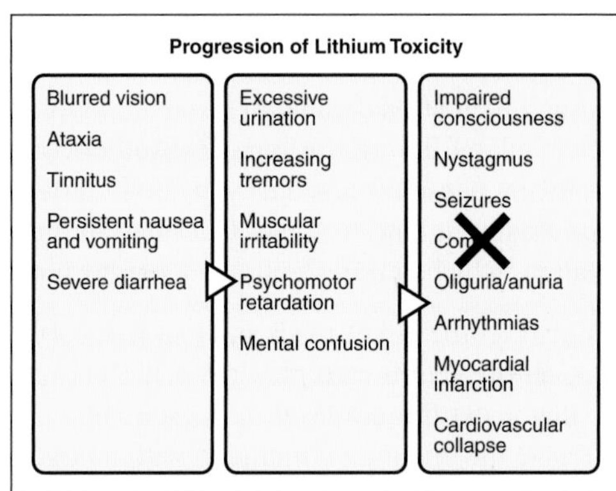

Symptoms of lithium toxicity begin to appear at blood levels greater than 1.5 mEq/L. The third column lists symptoms of lithium levels above 3.5 mEq/L, some of which include impaired consciousness, nystagmus, seizures, and arrhythmias. The first column lists symptoms of lithium levels between 1.5 and 2.0 mEq/L. The middle column lists symptoms of serum levels between 2.0 and 3.5 mEq/L.

➧ ***Test-taking Tip:*** *Review the progression of lithium toxicity. Remember that levels above 3.5 mEq/L are extremely toxic. A method to remember the normal range is to remember that the higher value is double the lower value. It is also similar to serum creatinine, except that serum creatinine is expressed in milligrams per deciliter. A toxic level is also the same as the low normal value for a serum potassium level.*

Content Area: Mental Health; *Category of Health Alteration:* Pharmacological and Parenteral Therapies; *Integrated Processes:* Nursing Process Assessment; *Client Need:* Physiological Integrity/Pharmacological and Parenteral Therapies/Adverse Effects/Contraindications/Interactions; Physiological Integrity/Reduction of Risk Potential/Laboratory Values; *Cognitive Level:* Analysis

Reference: Townsend, M. (2009). *Psychiatric Mental Health Nursing* (6th ed., p. 319). Philadelphia: F. A. Davis.

1675. A nurse is providing instructions to a client. Which substances should a client who is taking alprazolam (Xanax®) be cautioned to avoid? SELECT ALL THAT APPLY.

1. Alcohol
2. Caffeine
3. Antihistamines
4. Narcotics
5. Antidepressants
6. Antioxidants

ANSWER: 1, 3, 4, 5

Alcohol, barbiturates, narcotics, antipsychotics, antidepressants, antihistamines, neuromuscular blocking agents, cimetidine, and disulfiram increase the effects of antianxiety agents. Clients should avoid all agents that depress the central nervous system (CNS), as these medications cause sedation. Caffeine and antioxidants do not depress the CNS or cause additive effects.

▶ ***Test-taking Tip:*** *Use the process of elimination. Consider the desired effect of antianxiety agents. Other medications with similar therapeutic actions would cause undesirable additive effects.*

Content Area: Mental Health; *Category of Health Alteration:* Pharmacological and Parenteral Therapies; *Integrated Processes:* Teaching and Learning; *Client Need:* Health Promotion and Maintenance/ Self-Care; Physiological Integrity/Pharmacological and Parenteral Therapies/ Pharmacological Adverse Effects/Contraindications/Interactions; *Cognitive Level:* Application

Reference: Townsend, M. (2009). *Psychiatric Mental Health Nursing* (6th ed., p. 307). Philadelphia: F. A. Davis.

1676. A hospitalized client is exhibiting occasional anxiety. A nurse notifies a health-care provider to request that a prn anxiolytic medication be prescribed. Which medication, if prescribed, should the nurse question regarding its effectiveness for prn use?

1. Alprazolam (Ativan®)
2. Clonazepam (Klonopin®)
3. Clorazepate (Tranxene®)
4. Buspirone (Buspar®)

ANSWER: 4

Buspirone is not recommended for prn use because of a 10- to 14-day delay in therapeutic onset. Benzodiazepines, such as lorazepam, clonazepam, and clorazepate, have a rapid onset of therapeutic effectiveness.

▶ ***Test-taking Tip:*** *Recognize that all of the options are anxiolytics. Note two medications end in "–am," indicating that they are likely benzodiazepines. Buspirone is the only nonbenzodiazepine. Look for the option that differs from the others.*

Content Area: Mental Health; *Category of Health Alteration:* Pharmacological and Parenteral Therapies; *Integrated Processes:* Nursing Process Analysis; *Client Need:* Physiological Integrity/Pharmacological and Parenteral Therapies/Expected Actions or Outcomes; *Cognitive Level:* Analysis

Reference: Townsend, M. (2009). *Psychiatric Mental Health Nursing* (6th ed., p. 307). Philadelphia: F. A. Davis.

1677. EBP The parent of an adolescent client who is taking chlordiazepoxide (Librium®) for the past 2 months calls a nurse requesting to have the dose increased because of the child's increasing anxiety. The parent states the medication is being administered as directed. Which should be the nurse's best interpretation of this situation?

1. The client may be developing tolerance to chlordiazepoxide and needs the medication dose reevaluated.
2. The client may be skipping doses when not anxious and now needs a double dose of medication when feeling anxious.
3. The client may be becoming resistant to the effects of chlordiazepoxide and should be placed on an alternative medication.
4. The client's anxiety disorder may be hormone-related and larger doses of chlordiazepoxide may be indicated.

ANSWER: 1

Physical and psychological dependence are often associated with the use of benzodiazepines such as chlordiazepoxide. The client is describing tolerance, a sign of dependence. Doses should not be doubled if medication is being skipped. Skipping of the medication reduces the therapeutic effects. Resistance is not the same as dependence; the medication will continue to exert its pharmacological effect with higher doses. Increasing the dosage is not indicated in the development of dependence. Insufficient information is provided in the situation to determine if the client's anxiety is hormone-related.

▶ ***Test-taking Tip:*** *Think about precautions of continued use of benzodiazepines. Remember tolerance and/or withdrawal constitutes drug dependency. Eliminate any options in which there is insufficient information in the situation to make the judgment stated in the option.*

Content Area: Mental Health; *Category of Health Alteration:* Pharmacological and Parenteral Therapies; *Integrated Processes:* Nursing Process Analysis; *Client Need:* Physiological Integrity/Pharmacological and Parenteral Therapies/Adverse Effects/Contraindications/Interactions; *Cognitive Level:* Analysis

Reference: Townsend, M. (2009). *Psychiatric Mental Health Nursing* (6th ed., p. 307). Philadelphia: F. A. Davis.

EBP Reference: Connolly, S., & Bernstein, G. (2007). Work Group on Quality Issues. Practice parameter for the assessment and treatment of children and adolescents with anxiety disorders. *Journal of the American Academy of Child and Adolescent Psychiatry,* 46(2), 267–283. Available at: www.guideline.gov/summary/summary.aspx?doc_id=10549&nbr=005512&string=borderline+AND+personality+AND+disorder

1678. A nurse is reviewing the medications for all assigned clients on an inpatient psychiatric unit. The nurse anticipates assessing for extrapyramidal symptoms (EPS) in clients taking:

1. risperidone (Risperdal®)
2. clozapine (Clozaril®)
3. haloperidol (Haldol®)
4. ziprasidone (Geodon®)

ANSWER: 3

Haloperidol is the only medication listed with a high probability of EPS. Risperidone, clozapine, and ziprasidone are members of the newer generation of antipsychotics with less potential for EPS.

▶ ***Test-taking Tip:*** *Review specific medications included in both the typical and newer, atypical classes of antipsychotics. Recognize one option that does not fit in the same classification as the others and select this option as the answer.*

Content Area: Mental Health; *Category of Health Alteration:* Pharmacological and Parenteral Therapies; *Integrated Processes:* Nursing Process Planning; *Client Need:* Physiological Integrity/Pharmacological and Parenteral Therapies/Adverse Effects/Contraindications/Interactions; *Cognitive Level:* Application

Reference: Townsend, M. (2009). *Psychiatric Mental Health Nursing* (6th ed., pp. 324–325, 511). Philadelphia: F. A. Davis.

1679. A client is being treated with clozapine (Clozaril®). Which findings during a nurse's assessment indicate that the client is experiencing adverse effects of clozapine? SELECT ALL THAT APPLY.

1. Increased restlessness and anxiety
2. Extreme salivation
3. Dehydration
4. Agranulocytosis
5. Blood glucose 192 mg/dL
6. Seizure activity

ANSWER: 2, 4, 5, 6

Clozapine may cause hypersalivation and a significantly higher risk of agranulocytosis (failure of the bone marrow to produce enough neutrophils). Clozapine is also associated with frequent reports of sedation, anticholinergic side effects, hypotension, hyperglycemia, and seizures. Increasing anxiousness or dehydration are not adverse effects of clozapine.

▶ ***Test-taking Tip:*** *Review side effects that are common to all antipsychotics and effects that are medication specific, such as agranulocytosis. Use the process of elimination.*

Content Area: Mental Health; *Category of Health Alteration:* Pharmacological and Parenteral Therapies; *Integrated Processes:* Nursing Process Evaluation; *Client Need:* Physiological Integrity/Pharmacological and Parenteral Therapies/Adverse Effects/Contraindications/Interactions; *Cognitive Level:* Application

Reference: Townsend, M. (2009). *Psychiatric Mental Health Nursing* (6th ed., p. 325). Philadelphia: F. A. Davis.

1680. A client diagnosed with borderline personality disorder (BPD) is taking olanzapine (Zyprexa®). A nurse notes that the medication is effective when observing a reduction in: SELECT ALL THAT APPLY.

1. levels of anxiety.
2. thoughts of paranoia.
3. feelings of depression.
4. expression of hostility.
5. the use of splitting.

ANSWER: 1, 2, 4

Changes measured with olanzapine include a reduction in anxiety, paranoia, anger and hostility, and interpersonal sensitivity. Olanzapine has not shown a significant rate of improvement for depression over time than has placebo. Cognitive restructuring techniques rather than medications are more likely to improve the overuse of the defense mechanism splitting.

▶ ***Test-taking Tip:*** *Review target symptoms of atypical antipsychotics, noting the effects on cognitive improvement and controlled behavioral functioning.*

Content Area: Mental Health; *Category of Health Alteration:* Pharmacological and Parenteral Therapies; *Integrated Processes:* Nursing Process Evaluation; *Client Need:* Physiological Integrity/Pharmacological and Parenteral Therapies/Expected Actions or Outcomes; *Cognitive Level:* Analysis

Reference: Townsend, M. (2008). *Essentials of Psychiatric Mental Health Nursing* (4th ed., p. 521). Philadelphia: F. A. Davis.

1681. A nurse is observing a client on the unit who is being treated with antipsychotics. The client appears unsteady while standing and walking from one location to another and the client's hands are trembling slightly. Based on this information, what is the most appropriate action for the nurse to take?

1. Administer a prn dose of the anticholinergic trihexyphenidyl (Artane®).
2. Approach the client and offer assistance with ambulation back to the client's room for rest.
3. Insist that the client remain seated, using limb restraints if needed for client safety.
4. Call the health-care provider and report indications of early signs of tardive dyskinesia.

ANSWER: 1

Because the client is experiencing extrapyramidal symptoms (EPS) of pseudoparkinsonism, akinesia, and akathesia, the nurse should administer an antiparkinsonian agent to restore the natural balance of acetylcholine and dopamine in the central nervous system. Escorting the client to his or her room or using limb restraints is not the least-restrictive intervention appropriate for this client. The assessment reveals EPS, not tardive dyskinesia.

Test-taking Tip: *The key words are "most appropriate." Note the information in the question regarding the use of antipsychotics. Select the least-restrictive action.*

Content Area: Mental Health; *Category of Health Alteration:* Pharmacological and Parenteral Therapies; *Integrated Processes:* Nursing Process Implementation; *Client Need:* Safe and Effective Care Environment/Management of Care/Establishing Priorities; Physiological Integrity/Physiological Adaptation/Unexpected Response to Therapies; *Cognitive Level:* Application

Reference: Townsend, M. (2009). *Psychiatric Mental Health Nursing* (6th ed., p. 326). Philadelphia: F. A. Davis.

1682. A client in an inpatient psychiatric hospital is experiencing worsening akathesia. A nurse prepares to administer a prn dose of benztropine (Cogentin®). The client's medication record lists benztropine 0.5 mg IM q4h prn. The vial contains 1 mg/mL. In order to provide the correct dose, the nurse should administer _____ mL of the medication.

ANSWER: 0.5 mL

Use a proportion formula to calculate the dosage. Then, multiply the extremes (outside values) and the means (inside values) and solve for X.
1 mg : 1mL :: 0.5 mg : X mL
X = 0.5 mL

Test-taking Tip: *Focus on the information in the question. On the NCLEX-RN® exam, use the on-screen calculator if needed. Verify your answer, especially if it seems like an unusual amount.*

Content Area: Mental Health; *Category of Health Alteration:* Pharmacological and Parenteral Therapies; *Integrated Processes:* Nursing Process Implementation; *Client Need:* Physiological Integrity/Pharmacological and Parenteral Therapies/Dosage Calculation; *Cognitive Level:* Application

Reference: Pickar, G. (2007). *Dosage Calculations: A Ratio-Proportion Approach* (2nd ed., pp. 46, 344). Clifton Park, NY: Thomson Delmar Learning.

1683. A client taking an antipsychotic medication begins to exhibit severe parkinsonian muscle rigidity, a temperature of 105°F (40.6°C), tachycardia, and diaphoresis. Prioritize the steps that a nurse should take to respond to this situation.

______ Notify the health-care provider (HCP) of the symptoms.
______ Withhold all doses of the antipsychotic medication.
______ Assess level of consciousness.
______ Administer bromocriptine (Parlodel®) as prescribed by the HCP stat.
______ Assess degree of muscle rigidity.
______ Take vital signs.

ANSWER: 5, 1, 3, 6, 4, 2

The client is experiencing neuroleptic malignant syndrome (NMS). All neuroleptic medications should be withheld immediately. Further assessment needs to be done before contacting the HCP, beginning with vital signs. Level of consciousness and muscle rigidity will fluctuate in that order of progression. After assessment is completed, the nurse should contact the HCP and report the findings. The HCP should discontinue all neuroleptic medications and prescribe bromocriptine to counteract the effects of NMS. The bromocriptine should then be administered.

Test-taking Tip: *The first action should be to withhold all neuroleptic medications because this is a life-threatening concern. Then, use Maslow's Hierarchy of Needs theory and the nursing process to prioritize the remaining assessments and actions; review the signs of NMS.*

Content Area: Mental Health; *Category of Health Alteration:* Pharmacological and Parenteral Therapies; *Integrated Processes:* Nursing Process Implementation; *Client Need:* Physiological Integrity/Pharmacological and Parenteral Therapies/Adverse Effects/Contraindications/Interactions; Safe and Effective Care Environment/Management of Care/Establishing Priorities; *Cognitive Level:* Analysis

Reference: Townsend, M. (2009). *Psychiatric Mental Health Nursing* (6th ed., p. 326). Philadelphia: F. A. Davis.

1684. A hospitalized adult client is having difficulty falling and staying asleep. A nurse consults standing orders. All medications on the standing orders are included in the table below. Based on the available information presented in the table, which hypnotic medication should a nurse administer to the client to effectively help the client sleep soundly throughout the night?

Medication	Onset (hr)	Peak (hr)	Duration (hr)
Flurazepam (Dalmane®)	0.5	0.5–1	7–8
Temazepam (Restoril®)	0.5	2–3	6–8
Triazolam (Halcion®)	0.5	6–8	10–12
Zolpidem (Ambien®)	Rapid	0.5–2	6–8
Zaleplon (Sonata®)	Rapid	Unknown	3–4
Eszopiclone (Lunesta®)	Rapid	1	6

1. Triazolam (Halcion®)
2. Flurazepam (Dalmane®)
3. Zaleplon (Sonata®)
4. Eszopiclone (Lunesta®)

ANSWER: 1

Triazolam's peak effectiveness is much later than that of the other medications listed in the table and has a slightly longer duration of action. Flurazepam, temazepam, triazolam, zolpidem, zaleplon, and eszopiclone have a rapid to 30-minute onset with moderate variation in duration.

➧ ***Test-taking Tip:*** *Look for information in the chart that stands out as different, such as the peak of triazolam.*

Content Area: Mental Health; *Category of Health Alteration:* Pharmacological and Parenteral Therapies; *Integrated Processes:* Nursing Process Analysis; *Client Need:* Physiological Integrity/ Pharmacological and Parenteral Therapies/Expected Actions or Outcomes; *Cognitive Level:* Application

Reference: Deglin, J., & Vallerand, A. (2009). *Davis's Drug Guide for Nurses* (11th ed., pp. 515, 571, 1202, 1250). Philadelphia: F. A. Davis.

1685. EBP A nurse is working with a family whose 9-year-old child is taking atomoxetine (Strattera®) for attention deficit hyperactivity disorder (ADHD). Which instructions should a nurse include when teaching the parents? SELECT ALL THAT APPLY.

1. Provide ample stimulation for the child as the medication will cause sedation.
2. Administer the child's medication immediately after meals.
3. Administer the medication at least 6 hours before bedtime.
4. Do not skip doses at any time in order to maintain therapeutic levels.
5. Weigh the child weekly to monitor for untoward weight loss.
6. Consult with the health-care provider if the child needs any cold or allergy medication.

ANSWER: 2, 3, 5, 6

The medication should be administered after meals to reduce anorexia. To prevent insomnia, the dose should be administered at least 6 hours before bedtime. Weekly weights are indicated due to potential anorexia and weight loss and the temporary interruption of growth and development. Over-the-counter cold and allergy medications should be avoided because many contain sympathomimetic agents that could compound the effects of the stimulant. Stimuli should be low and the environment kept as quiet as possible. A supervised medication "holiday" should be attempted periodically to determine the effectiveness of the medication and need for continuation.

➧ ***Test-taking Tip:*** *Based on the action, reason the implications for daily use for ADHD and use the process of elimination. Eliminate any options that contain absolute words.*

Content Area: Mental Health; *Category of Health Alteration:* Pharmacological and Parenteral Therapies; *Integrated Processes:* Teaching and Learning; *Client Need:* Health Promotion and Maintenance/Self-Care; Physiological Integrity/Pharmacological and Parenteral Therapies/Medication Administration; *Cognitive Level:* Application

Reference: Townsend, M. (2009). *Psychiatric Mental Health Nursing* (6th ed., pp. 390, 393). Philadelphia: F. A. Davis.

EBP Reference: Institute for Clinical Systems Improvement. (2007). *Diagnosis and Management of Attention Deficit Hyperactivity Disorder in Primary Care for School-Age Children and Adolescents.* Available at: www.guidelines.gov/summary/summary.aspx?doc_id=11080&nbr=005843&string=management+AND+anxiety.

1686. EBP A nurse is performing a health history on a child who is being evaluated for attention deficit hyperactivity disorder (ADHD). Regarding the likelihood of management with psychostimulants, which area is critical to document in the review of systems?

1. Musculoskeletal history
2. Genitourinary history
3. Immunization history
4. Cardiovascular history

ANSWER: 4

Because psychostimulant medications are considered first-line therapy in children with ADHD, a nurse should assess for the presence of cardiovascular conditions because certain cardiovascular conditions would contraindicate the use of psychostimulants. Other absolute contraindications to the use of psychostimulants include psychosis or previous untoward reactions to psychostimulant medications. There are no significant musculoskeletal, genitourinary, or immunologic side effects associated with the use of stimulant medications.

➧ ***Test-taking Tip:*** *Review the side effects of stimulants and think about which body system would be most adversely affected. Use the ABCs (airway, breathing, circulation) to determine a priority body system.*

Content Area: Mental Health; *Category of Health Alteration:* Pharmacological and Parenteral Therapies; *Integrated Processes:* Nursing Process Assessment; Communication and Documentation; *Client Need:* Physiological Integrity/Pharmacological and Parenteral Therapies/Expected Actions or Outcomes; *Cognitive Level:* Analysis

Reference: Townsend, M. (2009). *Psychiatric Mental Health Nursing* (6th ed., pp. 330–331). Philadelphia: F. A. Davis.

EBP Reference: Pliszka, S. (2007). AACAP Work Group on Quality Issues. Practice parameter for the assessment and treatment of children and adolescents with attention-deficit/hyperactivity disorder. *Journal of the American Academy of Child and Adolescent Psychiatry,* 46(7), 894–921. www.guideline.gov/summary/summary.aspx?doc_id=11375&nbr=005912&string=borderline+AND+personality+AND+disorder

1687. A client is taking methylphenidate sustained release tablets (Ritalin SR®) once daily for attention deficit disorder. The medication peaks in 4 to 7 hours and has a duration of 12 hours. At which time should a nurse instruct the client to take the prescribed dose of methylphenidate?

1. At bedtime
2. Six hours before bedtime
3. With the midday meal
4. As soon as the client awakens in the morning

ANSWER: 4

Sustained release forms of methylphenidate may be used for once a day dosage, given in the morning. The 12-hour duration would interfere with nighttime sleep if given anytime after the morning hours.

➧ ***Test-taking Tip:*** *Consider the peak and duration information in the question and calculate when the maximum therapeutic benefit should occur.*

Content Area: Mental Health; *Category of Health Alteration:* Pharmacological and Parenteral Therapies; *Integrated Processes:* Nursing Process Implementation; *Client Need:* Physiological Integrity/Pharmacological and Parenteral Therapies/Medication Administration; *Cognitive Level:* Analysis

References: Deglin, J., & Vallerand, A. (2009). *Davis's Drug Guide for Nurses* (11th ed., p. 978). Philadelphia: F. A. Davis; Townsend, M. (2009). *Psychiatric Mental Health Nursing* (6th ed., p. 392). Philadelphia: F. A. Davis.

1688. A client is prescribed varenicline (Chantix®) for smoking cessation. A nurse concludes that varenicline is being prescribed primarily because it:

1. stimulates the receptors normally stimulated by smoking, producing similar pleasurable effects.
2. blocks receptors in the brain that produce the pleasurable effects of smoking.
3. demonstrates a high degree of attractiveness for a specific receptor.
4. is readily absorbed into the bloodstream for rapid effectiveness.

ANSWER: 2

Varenicline functions as an antagonist. Antagonists cause receptor blockade, thereby resulting in a reduction in transmission and decreased neurotransmitter activity. *Agonists* increase neurotransmitter activity by direct stimulation of specific receptors. *Affinity* is the degree of attractiveness between a medication and a specific receptor. *Absorption* refers to the rate at which the medication enters the bloodstream.

➧ ***Test-taking Tip:*** *Recall that varenicline is antagonistic when selecting the correct option. Apply knowledge of terminology related to pharmacokinetics and pharmacodynamics to delete options that do not relate to antagonism.*

Content Area: Mental Health; *Category of Health Alteration:* Pharmacological and Parenteral Therapies; *Integrated Processes:* Nursing Process Analysis; *Client Need:* Physiological Integrity/Pharmacological and Parenteral Therapies/Expected Actions or Outcomes; *Cognitive Level:* Application

Reference: Townsend, M. (2009). *Psychiatric Mental Health Nursing* (6th ed., p. 304). Philadelphia: F. A. Davis.

1689. A client has been prescribed clonidine (Catapres®) for the unlabeled purpose of easing the discomfort associated with smoking cessation. On which body system should a nurse initially focus the client's physical assessment?

1. Gastrointestinal
2. Musculoskeletal
3. Cardiovascular
4. Neurological

ANSWER: 3

A nurse should focus the initial assessment on the cardiovascular system because the sympathetic activity can cause hypotension and bradycardia. Dry mouth and drowsiness can also be expected with clonidine, so the gastrointestinal system and neurological system should also be assessed but are of less importance than the cardiovascular system. Because there are no anticipated musculoskeletal reactions to clonidine, an assessment of the musculoskeletal system is the least important.

Test-taking Tip: *Remember that clonidine can also be prescribed to treat hypertension. Although there are side effects of clonidine involving other body systems, the cardiovascular system is most acutely affected. Use the ABCs (airway, breathing, circulation) to determine the system that should be priority.*

Content Area: Mental Health; *Category of Health Alteration:* Pharmacological and Parenteral Therapies; *Integrated Processes:* Nursing Process Assessment; *Client Need:* Physiological Integrity/Pharmacological and Parenteral Therapies/Expected Actions or Outcomes; Physiological Integrity/Reduction of Risk Potential/Potential for Alterations in Body Systems; *Cognitive Level:* Application

Reference: Deglin, J., & Vallerand, A. (2009). *Davis's Drug Guide for Nurses* (11th ed., p. 356). Philadelphia: F. A. Davis.

1690. A client is beginning treatment with bupropion (Wellbutrin®) for depression. After meeting with the health-care provider (HCP), the client tells a nurse, "I'm also taking Zyban® to help me stop smoking." Which is the most appropriate action for the nurse to take?

1. Inform the HCP that the client is already taking bupropion, but for smoking cessation.
2. Instruct the client to report any allergic-type reactions after beginning the Zyban®.
3. Provide the client with the telephone number for a smoking cessation support group.
4. Encourage and support the client in following the smoking cessation regimen.

ANSWER: 1

Bupropion is the generic name for both Wellbutrin® and Zyban®. The medication should not be used to treat more than one condition at a time. Additive doses can increase the risk of seizures. Allergic reactions are not likely as the client has already been taking the medication. Encouraging smoking cessation and referring the client to a support group are actions that do not advocate for client safety in this situation.

Test-taking Tip: *Be familiar with both generic and trade names. Recognize that medication duplication is occurring. This can lead to overmedication if not addressed.*

Content Area: Mental Health; *Category of Health Alteration:* Pharmacological and Parenteral Therapies; *Integrated Processes:* Nursing Process Implementation; Caring; *Client Need:* Physiological Integrity/Pharmacological and Parenteral Therapies/Adverse Effects/Contraindications/Interactions; Safe and Effective Care Environment/Management of Care/Advocacy; *Cognitive Level:* Application

Reference: Deglin, J., & Vallerand, A. (2009). *Davis's Drug Guide for Nurses* (11th ed., p. 200). Philadelphia: F. A. Davis.

1691. EBP A severely depressed client tells a nurse, "I don't need these antidepressants, they're too expensive! I'm going to use St. John's wort instead." Which is the most appropriate response by the nurse?

1. "I have some information showing the effective use of St. John's wort. Let's review it."
2. "Although St. John's wort may be less expensive, it has not been shown to improve severe depression."
3. "What would you think about taking the St. John's wort and the antidepressant to maximize the effectiveness?"
4. "That would be a safe alternative, especially if you need to consider your financial resources."

ANSWER: 2

St. John's wort has not been clinically proven to be effective against major depression. It is possibly helpful in mild to moderate depression. St. John's wort should not be taken with other psychoactive medications. Herbal remedies are not subject to FDA approval; therefore, their safety cannot be guaranteed.

Test-taking Tip: *Review the approval process for pharmacological agents, remembering that herbal remedies are not included. Their use should not be encouraged in lieu of clinically effective medications.*

Content Area: Mental Health; *Category of Health Alteration:* Pharmacological and Parenteral Therapies; *Integrated Processes:* Communication and Documentation; *Client Need:* Physiological Integrity/Pharmacological and Parenteral Therapies/Adverse Effects/Contraindications/Interactions; *Cognitive Level:* Application

Reference: Townsend, M. (2009). *Psychiatric Mental Health Nursing* (6th ed., pp. 348, 350). Philadelphia: F. A. Davis.

EBP Reference: Bent, S. (2008). Herbal medicine in the United States: Review of efficacy, safety, and regulation. *Journal of General Internal Medicine,* 23(6), 854–859.

1692. A client seeking treatment for insomnia tells a nurse of researching complementary therapies for promoting sleep. Which herbal remedies should a nurse anticipate that the client may wish to discuss to promote sleep?

1. Feverfew and peppermint
2. Fennel and ginger
3. Echinacea and St. John's wort
4. Chamomile tea and hops

ANSWER: 4

Chamomile tea and hops are believed to relieve insomnia. Feverfew and peppermint are thought to be helpful in treating headaches. Fennel and ginger ease stomachaches, while echinacea and St. John's wort are both used to boost immunity.

➧ ***Test-taking Tip:*** *Knowledge of herbal remedies is necessary to answer this question. Become familiar with common herbal remedies purported to enhance sleep. Because of their affordability and availability, clients may consider their use.*

Content Area: Mental Health; *Category of Health Alteration:* Pharmacological and Parenteral Therapies; *Integrated Processes:* Nursing Process Planning; *Client Need:* Physiological Integrity/Basic Care and Comfort/Nonpharmacological Comfort Interventions; *Cognitive Level:* Application

Reference: Townsend, M. (2009). *Psychiatric Mental Health Nursing* (6th ed., pp. 349–350). Philadelphia: F. A. Davis.

1693. A Native American client is being assessed for emotional distress following a family crisis. In anticipating pharmacological treatment, the nurse understands that a Native American client most likely would:

1. prefer to use herbal remedies and other plant therapies with healing properties.
2. want a well-established relationship with a health-care provider before accepting treatment.
3. attempt to manage emotional problems on his or her own to avoid shame.
4. rely heavily on family for support during treatment for emotional distress.

ANSWER: 1

Native American cultures often use the medicine man or woman and a variety of herbal or other plant and root remedies. Northern European Americans usually value preventive medicine and primary health care, thus already having an established provider. Asian American cultures often see mental illness as shameful and will attempt to manage illness on their own as long as possible. Latino Americans are group oriented, often with the family being the primary social support.

➧ ***Test-taking Tip:*** *Focus on the Native American culture to select the correct option. Eliminate options that pertain to other cultural groups.*

Content Area: Mental Health; *Category of Health Alteration:* Pharmacological and Parenteral Therapies; *Integrated Processes:* Nursing Process Planning; Caring; *Client Need:* Psychosocial Integrity/Cultural Diversity; Physiological Integrity/Basic Care and Comfort/Nonpharmacological Comfort Interventions; *Cognitive Level:* Application

Reference: Townsend, M. (2009). *Psychiatric Mental Health Nursing* (6th ed., pp. 92, 97). Philadelphia: F. A. Davis.

1694. A client, being discharged from treatment for alcoholism, is receiving teaching on taking daily doses of disulfiram (Antabuse®). Which client statement indicates to a nurse that the client correctly understands the safe use of disulfiram?

1. "If I take disulfiram and then drink alcohol, I will become intoxicated much more quickly."
2. "I should take disulfiram at the same time each day to maintain therapeutic effectiveness."
3. "If I do ingest alcohol, I should skip the daily dose of disulfiram to avoid being ill."
4. "I should avoid products such as vanilla extract or certain cough preparations containing alcohol while taking disulfiram."

ANSWER: 4

A client should be aware of alcohol-containing substances such as cough and cold preparations, vanilla extract, aftershave lotion, cologne, mouthwash, nail polish remover, and isopropyl alcohol, which are capable of producing severe adverse symptoms if taking disulfiram. Clients taking disulfiram should totally abstain from alcohol. Ingestion of alcohol will produce severe illness reactions, not intoxication. Disulfiram does not need to be taken at the same time each day. A reaction could occur if alcohol is ingested for up to 2 weeks following the use of disulfiram; thus, just skipping a dose will not prevent the client from becoming ill.

➧ ***Test-taking Tip:*** *Review the purpose of disulfiram and select the option that includes avoiding alcohol-containing products.*

Content Area: Mental Health; *Category of Health Alteration:* Pharmacological and Parenteral Therapies; *Integrated Processes:* Nursing Process Evaluation; *Client Need:* Health Promotion and Maintenance/Self-Care; Physiological Integrity/Pharmacological and Parenteral Therapies/Expected Actions or Outcomes; *Cognitive Level:* Analysis

Reference: Townsend, M. (2009). *Psychiatric Mental Health Nursing* (6th ed., p. 480). Philadelphia: F. A. Davis.

1695. EBP A client who completed inpatient treatment for addiction to heroin is prescribed to take daily doses of methadone during outpatient treatment. The nurse concludes that the primary rationale for the client's outpatient treatment with methadone is to:

1. block the effects of opiates to prevent a "high" if the client uses heroin while in treatment.
2. treat any residual withdrawal symptoms during the outpatient phase of treatment.
3. reduce heroin craving by binding to the brain receptor sites usually occupied by heroin.
4. reduce mania and the potential for self-injury through a legal and safe alternative to heroin use during treatment.

ANSWER: 3

Maintenance treatment with methadone is appropriate for persons with a prolonged history (greater than 1 year) of opioid dependence. Methadone is a long-acting opioid therapeutically used for suppression of withdrawal symptoms during detoxification and maintenance from heroin and other opioids. The goals of treatment are to achieve a stable maintenance dose of opioid agonist and facilitate engagement in a comprehensive program of rehabilitation. Methadone acts as an agonist; an antagonist would block the effect of heroin. Methadone can be used to treat acute withdrawal symptoms, but this question is asking for indications for long-term maintenance therapy. Prescribing methadone for the purpose of legal and safe medication use does not reflect a therapeutic use during concomitant treatment.

▶ ***Test-taking Tip:*** *Read the question carefully. Focus on the use of methadone in outpatient therapy for opioid addiction.*

Content Area: Mental Health; *Category of Health Alteration:* Pharmacological and Parenteral Therapies; *Integrated Processes:* Nursing Process Analysis; *Client Need:* Physiological Integrity/Pharmacological and Parenteral Therapies/Expected Actions or Outcomes; *Cognitive Level:* Application

References: Mohr, W. (2006). *Psychiatric-Mental Health Nursing* (6th ed., p. 632). Philadelphia: Lippincott Williams & Wilkins; Deglin, J., & Vallerand, A. (2009). *Davis's Drug Guide for Nurses* (11th ed., p. 795). Philadelphia: F. A. Davis.

EBP Reference: Work Group on Substance Use Disorders, Kleber, H., Weiss, R., Anton, R., Rounsaville, B., et al. (2006). Treatment of patients with substance use disorders (2nd ed.). *American Journal of Psychiatry,* 163(8 Suppl), 5–82. Available at: www.guidelines.gov/summary/summary.aspx?doc_id=9316&nbr=004985&string=methadone+AND+maintenance+AND+therapy

1696. A client with schizophrenia has a history of nonadherence to the prescribed medication regimen and requires hospitalization for exacerbation of schizophrenic symptoms. Injectable antipsychotic agents are being considered for long-term use to better stabilize the client's symptoms. Which medications, if prescribed by the health-care provider, should the nurse question? SELECT ALL THAT APPLY.

1. Risperidone consta (Risperdal®)
2. Olanzapine (Zyprexa®)
3. Haloperidol decanoate (Haldol®)
4. Fluphenazine decanoate (Prolixin®)
5. Ziprasidone (Geodon®)
6. Aripiprazole (Abilify®)

ANSWER: 2, 5, 6

The nurse should question prescriptions for olanzapine, ziprasidone, and aripiprazole. Olanzapine and ziprasidone injections are indicated for short-term (not long-term) use in acute symptom management. The antipsychotic aripiprazole is not available in injectable form. Risperidone consta, haloperidol decanoate, and fluphenazine decanoate are all sustained release injectable forms of antipsychotic agents. Their duration usually ranges from 2 to 4 weeks, and they are appropriate for long-term use.

▶ ***Test-taking Tip:*** *Note that the three sustained release forms for long-term use have two-word names; thus eliminate these options. Select the options for medications for short-term use or those that are not available for injection.*

Content Area: Mental Health; *Category of Health Alteration:* Pharmacological and Parenteral Therapies; *Integrated Processes:* Nursing Process Implementation; *Client Need:* Physiological Integrity/Pharmacological and Parenteral Therapies/Medication Administration; *Cognitive Level:* Analysis

References: Deglin, J., & Vallerand, A. (2009). *Davis's Drug Guide for Nurses* (11th ed., pp. 111–112, 658–670, 727–729, 1105–1107, 1351–1354, 1614–1616). Philadelphia: F. A. Davis; Mohr, W. (2006). *Psychiatric-Mental Health Nursing* (6th ed., pp. 587–588). Philadelphia: Lippincott Williams & Wilkins.

Chapter Eleven

Reduction of Risk and Physiological Adaptation

Test 45: Altered Fluid and Electrolytes

1697. Which assessment should a nurse perform to obtain the most accurate determination of fluid balance for a child with hydronephrosis?

1. Measuring the client's intake and output
2. Weighing the client
3. Assessing for presence of edema
4. Evaluating serum electrolyte results

ANSWER: 2

Weight is most accurate. Intake and output provides data, but there is additional fluid lost through skin, lungs, and the gastrointestinal tract that cannot be measured. Edema is an indication of fluid retention but is not accurate. Electrolyte levels are not measures of fluid balance, although some are affected by fluid excess or deficit.

Test-taking Tip: *Note the key phrase "most accurate." Think critically about each option, using the process of elimination to rule out incorrect options. Remember that an increase of 1 kg (2.2 lb) is equal to 1,000 mL of fluid.*

Content Area: Child Health; *Category of Health Alteration:* Altered Fluid and Electrolytes; *Integrated Processes:* Nursing Process Assessment; *Client Need:* Physiological Integrity/Reduction of Risk Potential/System Specific Assessments; *Cognitive Level:* Application

Reference: Smeltzer, S., Bare, B., Hinkle, J., & Cheever, K. (2008). *Brunner & Suddarth's Textbook of Medical-Surgical Nursing* (11th ed., p. 304). Philadelphia: Lippincott Williams & Wilkins.

1698. EBP A child is admitted with dehydration following a 24-hour history of vomiting and diarrhea. Oral rehydration therapy is ordered. A nurse should:

1. give 40 to 50 mL/kg of water every 4 hours.
2. give 40 to 50 mL/kg of rehydration solution every 4 hours.
3. give 40 to 50 mL/kg of rehydration solution over 4 hours.
4. give as much rehydration solution as child can tolerate.

ANSWER: 3

Oral rehydration solutions enhance and promote reabsorption of sodium and water. These solutions reduce vomiting, decrease volume loss due to diarrhea, and decrease the duration of illness. Starting with small sips frequently reduces the incidence of further vomiting. Water is not indicated as a fluid to use for rehydration because it lacks the recommended 2 to 3 g/dL of glucose, 45 to 90 mEq/L of sodium, 20 to 25 mEq/L of potassium, and a base solution to equal an osmolality of 200 to 310 mOsm/L.

Test-taking Tip: *Look for key words in the options: "water," "every," "over," and "as much," respectively. Think about what method would be best for rehydration and eliminate options that would not provide for continuous hydration.*

Content Area: Child Health; *Category of Health Alteration:* Altered Fluid and Electrolytes; *Integrated Processes:* Nursing Process Implementation; *Client Need:* Physiological Integrity/Basic Care and Comfort/Nutrition and Oral Hydration; *Cognitive Level:* Application

Reference: Wong, D., Hockenberry, M., Wilson, M., Perry, S., & Lowdermilk, D. (2006). *Maternal Child Nursing Care* (3rd ed., p. 1500). St. Louis, MO: Mosby/Elsevier.

EBP Reference: Bender, B., Ozuah, P., & Crain, E. (2007). Oral rehydration therapy: Is anyone drinking? *Pediatric Emergency Care, 23*(9), 624–626.

1699. EBP A child is admitted to a hospital for observation following an electrical burn. Fluid replacement is ordered. Which indicators should a nurse use to determine adequacy of fluid resuscitation? SELECT ALL THAT APPLY.

1. Capillary refill time (CRT)
2. Sensorium
3. Urine output
4. Blood pressure
5. Skin turgor

ANSWER: 1, 2, 3, 5

The CRT and changes in sensorium, urine output, and skin turgor are all useful in evaluating tissue perfusion. Blood pressure can remain normotensive even with a state of hypovolemia. A child will lose 20% of fluid volume prior to having an impact on blood pressure.

Test-taking Tip: *Remember that a child will lose 20% of fluid volume before the volume loss has an impact on blood pressure.*

Content Area: Child Health; *Category of Health Alteration:* Altered Fluid and Electrolytes; *Integrated Processes:* Nursing Process Assessment; *Client Need:* Physiological Integrity/Physiological Adaptation/Fluid and Electrolyte Imbalances; *Cognitive Level:* Application

Reference: Pillitteri, A. (2007). *Maternal & Child Health Nursing: Care of the Childbearing & Childrearing Family* (5th ed., p. 1672). Philadelphia: Lippincott Williams & Wilkins.

EBP Reference: Csontos, C., Foldi, V., Fischer, T., & Bogar, L. (2007). Factors affecting fluid requirement on the first day after severe burn trauma. *ANZ Journal of Surgery,* 77(9), 745–748.

1700. A nurse is caring for an 8-year-old child following a tonsillectomy. The nurse identifies the nursing diagnosis of *Impaired swallowing related to inflammation and pain.* Which fluids should the nurse plan to administer?

1. Cool water or flavored ice pops
2. Red or brown fluids
3. Colored citrus drinks
4. Ice cream

ANSWER: 1

Cold or frozen fluids can provide comfort while also providing fluid intake. Red and brown fluids should be avoided to distinguish fresh and old blood. Citrus should be avoided, as it can be irritating and is often not tolerated early postoperatively. Milk products coat the throat and may require the child to attempt to clear the throat, which could initiate bleeding.

Test-taking Tip: *Focus on the issue: acceptable fluids after a tonsillectomy.*

Content Area: Child Health; *Category of Health Alteration:* Altered Fluid and Electrolytes; *Integrated Processes:* Nursing Process Planning; *Client Need:* Physiological Integrity/Reduction of Risk Potential/Potential for Complications from Surgical Procedures and Health Alterations; *Cognitive Level:* Application

Reference: Pillitteri, A. (2007). *Maternal & Child Health Nursing: Care of the Childbearing & Childrearing Family* (5th ed., pp. 1248–1250). Philadelphia: Lippincott Williams & Wilkins.

1701. EBP A nurse is asked to provide education to a group of high school students who will be playing sports. Practices begin in early August when the outdoor temperature averages 100 degrees Fahrenheit by noon. Based on this information, which points should the nurse include in the educational session? SELECT ALL THAT APPLY.

1. Gradually increase the amount of activity.
2. Limit activity to 15-minute intervals.
3. Drink fluids before and during practice, even if not thirsty.
4. Wear full gear but remove at breaks.
5. Those with excessive fatigue or headache should rest alone.

ANSWER: 1, 2, 3

Gradually increasing activity allows the body to adjust, especially when there is inactivity prior to starting practices. Limiting activity on hot, humid days allows time to replenish fluids and allows the body to cool down. Drinking fluids during these periods helps to decrease the risk of dehydration. Clothing should be limited to light layers, and gear should be gradually added into the practice for short periods of time. Complaints of headaches, cramps, and excessive fatigue are signs of dehydration. The player should not be left alone and must be encouraged to drink fluids, with attempts made to cool the body down.

Test-taking Tip: *Select options that will prevent dehydration.*

Content Area: Child Health; *Category of Health Alteration:* Altered Fluid and Electrolytes; *Integrated Processes:* Teaching and Learning; *Client Need:* Health Promotion and Maintenance/Health and Wellness; *Cognitive Level:* Application

Reference: Smeltzer, S., Bare, B., Hinkle, J., & Cheever, K. (2008). *Brunner & Suddarth's Textbook of Medical-Surgical Nursing* (11th ed., pp. 2533–2534). Philadelphia: Lippincott Williams & Wilkins.

EBP Reference: Mayo Foundation Medical Education and Research. (2008). *Dehydration and Youth Sports—Curb the Risk.* MayoClinic.com. Available at: www.mayoclinic.com/health/dehydration/SM00037

1702. An adult client presents to a clinic with reports of a significant sore throat that feels like "razor blades when swallowing." The client's throat is reddened with white patches. A rapid strep test is negative. A nurse's discharge teaching includes instructing the client to gargle with saltwater. The nurse explains that the purpose of gargling with saltwater is that:

1. saltwater will take away the pain.
2. saltwater will serve as a cleansing agent.
3. saltwater will reduce inflammation.
4. saltwater will serve as a distraction to the pain.

ANSWER: 3

Osmosis results in movement of fluid from an area of lower solute concentration to higher solute concentration toward equalization. The fluid moves from the inflamed tissue and is mobilized to reduce inflammation. Water alone would be considered a cleansing agent, but this is not the purpose for this client. The pain is relieved because of decreased inflammation.

▶ ***Test-taking Tip:*** *Think about osmosis and the effect it will have on the tissues.*

Content Area: Adult Health; *Category of Health Alteration:* Altered Fluid and Electrolytes; *Integrated Processes:* Nursing Process Implementation; *Client Need:* Physiological Integrity/Basic Care and Comfort/Non-Pharmacological Comfort Interventions; *Cognitive Level:* Application

Reference: Harkreader, H., Hogan, A., & Thobaben, M. (2007). *Fundamentals of Nursing: Caring and Clinical Judgment* (p. 566). St. Louis, MO: Saunders.

1703. A nurse is caring for a client recovering from surgery. Intravenous (IV) therapy is initiated to help maintain normal fluid balance. A physician orders 1,000 mL lactated Ringer's solution to be delivered over 8 hours. In order to infuse the IV fluids over 8 hours, the nurse should set the hourly infusion rate at ____ mL/hr.

ANSWER: 125

1,000 mL divided by 8 hours equals 125 mL/hour.

▶ ***Test-taking Tip:*** *Read the question carefully to determine what is being asked. Remember that to determine the milliliters per hour, divide the volume to be infused by the number of hours over which it should be infused.*

Content Area: Adult Health; *Category of Health Alteration:* Altered Fluid and Electrolytes; *Integrated Processes:* Nursing Process Implementation; *Client Need:* Physiological Integrity/Pharmacological and Parenteral Therapies/Parenteral/Intravenous Therapies; *Cognitive Level:* Application

Reference: Harkreader, H., Hogan, A., & Thobaben, M. (2007). *Fundamentals of Nursing: Caring and Clinical Judgment* (p. 884). St. Louis, MO: Saunders.

1704. A nurse is caring for a client who is comatose and receiving an amount of intravenous (IV) fluid that equals urine output. The client is losing weight. A nurse concludes that the weight loss can best be explained by the fact that:

1. approximately 500 mL of fluid is lost through the gastrointestinal (GI) tract.
2. insensible loss accounts for approximately 400 mL/day.
3. perspiration accounts for greater than 200 mL/day.
4. total fluid loss other than urine can equal 1,000 mL.

ANSWER: 4

Fluid is lost in a variety of ways but most commonly through the urinary system in the form of urine. Additional fluid is lost through perspiration, the GI track, skin, and lungs. This can account for over 1,000 mL/day, which is equal to approximately 1 kg or 2.2 lb. Fluid lost through the GI tract accounts for approximately 100 to 200 mL/day. Insensible fluid loss refers to the fluid lost through the lungs and skin and accounts for approximately 700 to 800 mL/day. Perspiration, under normal conditions, results in the loss of approximately 100 mL/day.

▶ ***Test-taking Tip:*** *Examine each option, noting the amount of fluid lost. Two options excrete too much fluid, and one option excretes too little.*

Content Area: Adult Health; *Category of Health Alteration:* Altered Fluid and Electrolytes; *Integrated Processes:* Nursing Process Analysis; *Client Need:* Physiological Integrity/Physiological Adaptation/Fluid and Electrolyte Imbalances; *Cognitive Level:* Application

Reference: Berman, A., Snyder, S., Kozier, B., & Erb, G. (2008). *Kozier & Erb's Fundamentals of Nursing: Concepts, Process, and Practice* (8th ed., pp. 1429, 1446). Upper Saddle River, NJ: Pearson Education.

1705. A nurse is caring for a client diagnosed with end-stage renal disease (ESRD). The client is 6 feet tall and weighs 180 pounds. The client's total serum protein is 5.8 g/dL. An assessment by the nurse reveals 2+ pitting edema. The nurse determines that this client's edema is most likely the result of:

1. increased capillary hydrostatic pressure.
2. decreased plasma oncotic pressure.
3. increased capillary permeability.
4. decreased serum electrolytes.

ANSWER: 2

A normal serum protein total is 6.0 to 8.0 g/dL. ESRD clients often have low plasma protein from malnutrition and protein restriction. This reduces plasma oncotic pressure and results in fluid remaining in the interstitial space because pressure is not great enough to pull fluid into the capillaries. Although edema can result from increased capillary hydrostatic pressure, decreased plasma oncotic pressure, and increased capillary permeability, the low serum protein suggests reduced oncotic pressure is the most likely cause of the edema. Because the client's kidneys are unable to excrete electrolytes, a higher level of serum electrolytes is present in ESRD.

▶ ***Test-taking Tip:*** *Focus on the client's diagnosis of ESRD and the dietary restrictions that influence fluid shifting between the vascular compartment and the tissues.*

Content Area: Adult Health; *Category of Health Alteration:* Altered Fluid and Electrolytes; *Integrated Processes:* Nursing Process Evaluation; *Client Need:* Physiological Integrity/Physiological Adaptation/Fluid and Electrolyte Imbalances; *Cognitive Level:* Analysis

Reference: Berman, A., Snyder, S., Kozier, B., & Erb, G. (2007). *Kozier & Erb's Fundamentals of Nursing: Concepts, Process, and Practice* (8th ed., p. 136). Upper Saddle River, NJ: Pearson Education.

1706. EBP An 80-year-old client is living in an independent living facility with home health nursing support. The client is diagnosed with pneumonia and started on an oral antibiotic. Which nursing diagnosis would be most appropriate for this client?

1. Risk for imbalanced nutrition
2. Risk for fluid volume deficit
3. Fluid volume deficit
4. Fluid volume excess

ANSWER: 2

The diagnosis of pneumonia may result in fever or increased respiratory rate that increases amount of fluid lost. Additionally, older adults have a decreased sensation of thirst. Nutrition may be affected due to a diagnosis of pneumonia, but fluid volume would be the greatest concern with pneumonia. The client's age and a diagnosis of pneumonia could result in a fluid volume deficit, but there is no information to support that the client is deficient in fluid. There is no information to support an excess fluid volume.

▶ ***Test-taking Tip:*** *The key phrase is "most appropriate." To have an actual nursing diagnosis, rather than a "risk for," information must be present to support the nursing diagnosis.*

Content Area: Adult Health; *Category of Health Alteration:* Altered Fluid and Electrolytes; *Integrated Processes:* Nursing Process Analysis; *Client Need:* Physiological Integrity/Physiological Adaptation/Fluid and Electrolyte Imbalances; *Cognitive Level:* Analysis

Reference: Harkreader, H., Hogan, A., & Thobaben, M. (2007). *Fundamentals of Nursing: Caring and Clinical Judgment* (p. 884). St. Louis, MO: Saunders.

EBP Reference: Mentes, J. (2008). Managing oral hydration. In E. Capezuti, D. Zwicker, M. Mezey, T. Fulmer (Eds.), *Evidence-Based Geriatric Nursing Protocols for Best Practice* (3rd ed., pp. 369–390). New York: Springer Publishing. Available at: www.guideline.gov/summary/summary.aspx?doc_id=12256&nbr=006340&string=Hydration+AND+management

---

1707. A client has a nursing diagnosis of fluid volume deficit. Which vital sign, if decreased, supports this nursing diagnosis?

1. Temperature
2. Respiratory rate
3. Heart rate
4. Blood pressure

ANSWER: 4

Blood pressure is a sensitive measure of changes in blood volume, decreasing in the presence of fluid volume deficit. Temperature and respiratory rate may contribute to volume status, but do not typically change as a result of volume changes. Heart rate may increase as a compensatory mechanism to decreased blood pressure.

▶ ***Test-taking Tip:*** *Think about which vital sign measurement would decrease as a result of fluid volume deficit.*

Content Area: Adult Health; *Category of Health Alteration:* Altered Fluid and Electrolytes; *Integrated Processes:* Nursing Process Evaluation; *Client Need:* Physiological Integrity/Reduction of Risk Potential/Vital Signs; *Cognitive Level:* Analysis

Reference: Berman, A., Snyder, S., Kozier, B., & Erb, G. (2008). *Kozier & Erb's Fundamentals of Nursing: Concepts, Process, and Practice* (8th ed., pp. 1446–1447). Upper Saddle River, NJ: Pearson Education.

1708. A nurse is caring for a client with renal insufficiency. In addition to an ordered fluid restriction, the client needs strict monitoring of intake and output. Which actions should the nurse plan to include when caring for the client? SELECT ALL THAT APPLY.

1. Discussing with the client and family the plan of care and fluid restriction
2. Documenting pureed foods as part of the client's liquid intake
3. Eliminating counting ice chips as intake because this represents such a small amount of intake
4. Providing a collection device for measuring the client's urine output
5. Instructing the family to record any intake they provide to the client on the facility intake record
6. Encouraging the family to bring favorite food items from home for the client to eat

ANSWER: 1, 4

Informing the client and family in the plan of care helps to provide reinforcement for the client and to ensure compliance with the fluid restriction and plan. Measurement and collection devices are necessary and beneficial when strict monitoring is required. Pureed foods are not counted as liquid because they are considered solid in a different form. Ice chips are considered fluid; a 200 mL cup of ice is equal to 100 mL of water. Only health care personnel should document on official agency records. The family should be informed to not provide the client with addition liquid intake. Renal insufficiency will warrant food and fluid restrictions. Bringing favorite food items from home should be discouraged to ensure that the client follows the plan of care for fluid and electrolyte restrictions.

▸ ***Test-taking Tip:*** *Think about the food and fluid restrictions that are likely with renal insufficiency and measures that the nurse can use to ensure that the client adheres to the plan of care.*

Content Area: Adult Health; *Category of Health Alteration:* Altered Fluid and Electrolytes; *Integrated Processes:* Nursing Process Planning; *Client Need:* Physiological Integrity/Basic Care and Comfort/Nutrition and Oral Hydration; *Cognitive Level:* Analysis

Reference: Berman, A., Snyder, S., Kozier, B., & Erb, G. (2008). *Kozier & Erb's Fundamentals of Nursing: Concepts, Process, and Practice* (8th ed., pp. 1447, 1454). Upper Saddle River, NJ: Pearson Education.

1709. A nurse is caring for a client with heart failure who has been placed on a 2,000-mL fluid restriction. The nurse is responsible for establishing a plan for how that restriction should be distributed over a 24-hour period. Which plan, developed by the nurse, is best?

Shift/Time	7–3	3–11	11–7
1.	1,000 mL	1,000 mL	0 mL
2.	900 mL	900 mL	200 mL
3.	1,000 mL	700 mL	300 mL
4.	700 mL	700 mL	600 mL

ANSWER: 3

The general rule is to provide half of the total restriction during the day and the other half between evening and nights, with most fluids offered in the evening. Option 1 is incorrect because fluids should be available during the night. Options 2 and 4 provide for a large amount of fluid intake just before bedtime; this should be avoided because it disrupts sleep.

▸ ***Test-taking Tip:*** *Think about your own fluid intake and when you likely consume the most amount of fluid. Recall that there are usually two meals provided during a 7 a.m.-to 3-p.m. period that would increase fluid intake during this time period.*

Content Area: Adult Health; *Category of Health Alteration:* Altered Fluid and Electrolytes; *Integrated Processes:* Nursing Process Planning; *Client Need:* Physiological Integrity/Basic Care and Comfort/Nutrition and Oral Hydration; *Cognitive Level:* Application

Reference: Berman, A., Snyder, S., Kozier, B., & Erb, G. (2008). *Kozier & Erb's Fundamentals of Nursing: Concepts, Process, and Practice* (8th ed., p. 1454). Upper Saddle River, NJ: Pearson Education.

1710. A 65-year-old client with a history of coronary artery disease is admitted with fluid volume overload. Bumetanide (Bumex®) is administered, and the client's serum potassium level drops to 3.0 mEq/L; intravenous (IV) potassium replacement is ordered. Which factor should a nurse consider when preparing to administer the IV potassium replacement?

1. The potassium concentration should not exceed 20 mEq/L.
2. Ice or warm packs may be needed to reduce vein irritation.
3. The potassium should be administered IV push.
4. The potassium should be added to the IV solution that is infusing.

ANSWER: 2

Potassium can be irritating to the vein, and the client may complain of burning. Strategies to minimize pain and inflammation include ice or warm packs. Although the usual replacement dose is 20 mEq/100 mL with administration of 10 to 20 mEq/hr, concentrations can safely range from 10 to 40 mEq/L. Potassium is never administered as an IV push; it will cause cardiac dysrhythmias. Adding medication to an already-infusing IV solution is unsafe and can result in a faster or slower rate of administration, depending on the volume of solution remaining.

▸ ***Test-taking Tip:*** *Note that options 3 and 4 both address methods of administration. Because both cannot be correct, either one or both are incorrect.*

Content Area: Adult Health; *Category of Health Alteration:* Altered Fluid and Electrolytes; *Integrated Processes:* Nursing Process Planning; *Client Need:* Physiological Integrity/Pharmacological and Parenteral Therapies/Medication Administration; *Cognitive Level:* Application

References: Smeltzer, S., Bare, B., Hinkle, J., & Cheever, K. (2008). *Brunner & Suddarth's Textbook of Medical-Surgical Nursing* (11th ed., p. 323). Philadelphia: Lippincott Williams & Wilkins; Doenges, M., Moorhouse, M., & Murr, A. (2006). *Nursing Care Plans: Guidelines for Individualizing Client Care Across the Life Span* (7th ed., p. 932). Philadelphia: F. A. Davis.

1711. A client is admitted to an emergency department with reports of feeling weak and having "passed out." The outside temperature is 100°F (41.3°C), and the client has been gardening. Physical assessment findings reveal poor skin turgor, dry and dull mucous membranes, heart rate (HR) 120 beats per minute, and blood pressure 92/54 mm Hg. Which nursing diagnosis should the nurse include in the client's plan of care?

1. Impaired oral mucous membrane
2. Fluid volume excess
3. Decreased cardiac output
4. Fluid volume deficit

ANSWER: 4

Signs of dehydration and hypovolemia are evident (weakness, syncope, poor skin turgor, dry and dull mucous membranes, hypotension), suggesting a nursing diagnosis of fluid volume deficit. The client has dry, dull mucous membranes, but impaired oral mucous membrane would not be the most appropriate diagnosis. The client's HR is elevated, indicating that it is compensating for the decreased blood volume. There are no symptoms of decreased cardiac output. The client's mean arterial pressure is 67, suggesting adequate cardiac output for tissue perfusion ([SBP + 2 DBP]/3).

▶ ***Test-taking Tip:*** *Focus on the client's symptoms to establish a nursing diagnosis.*

Content Area: Adult Health; *Category of Health Alteration:* Altered Fluid and Electrolytes; *Integrated Processes:* Nursing Process Analysis; *Client Need:* Physiological Integrity/Physiological Adaptation/Fluid and Electrolyte Imbalances; *Cognitive Level:* Analysis

Reference: Smeltzer, S., Bare, B., Hinkle, J., & Cheever, K. (2008). *Brunner & Suddarth's Textbook of Medical-Surgical Nursing* (11th ed., pp. 312, 316). Philadelphia: Lippincott Williams & Wilkins.

1712. The daughter of an 82-year-old client with Alzheimer's disease contacts a clinic because the client has been unwilling to drink any fluids for over 24 hours. Which instruction by the nurse is most appropriate?

1. Instruct the daughter to bring the client to the emergency department for intravenous fluid replacement.
2. Ask the daughter to bring the client to the clinic for laboratory work.
3. Ask about the presence of other symptoms.
4. Tell the daughter to offer popsicles and then call the clinic again the next day.

ANSWER: 3

Treatment will be dependent upon other symptoms. While the client is at risk for dehydration, admission or diagnostic tests may not be indicated. The nurse should provide education regarding signs and symptoms of dehydration (change in speech, weakness, dry mucous membranes, decreased urine output) and immediate interventions to increase fluid intake. Popsicles, though a source of fluids, would be insufficient to replace fluid needs. Other sources of fluid should also be suggested.

▶ ***Test-taking Tip:*** *The key word is "best." Use the nursing process to determine the best instruction. Additional assessment is needed.*

Content Area: Adult Health; *Category of Health Alteration:* Altered Fluid and Electrolytes; *Integrated Processes:* Nursing Process Implementation; *Client Need:* Physiological Integrity/Physiological Adaptation/Fluid and Electrolyte Imbalances; *Cognitive Level:* Analysis

Reference: Smeltzer, S., Bare, B., Hinkle, J., & Cheever, K. (2008). *Brunner & Suddarth's Textbook of Medical-Surgical Nursing* (11th ed., p. 309). Philadelphia: Lippincott Williams & Wilkins.

1713. A nurse establishes a nursing diagnosis of *Risk for excess fluid volume* for a client diagnosed with heart failure. Which physiological change resulting from heart failure supports this diagnosis?

1. Increased glomerular filtration rate (GFR)
2. Increased antidiuretic hormone (ADH) production
3. Increased sodium excretion
4. Increased cardiac output

ANSWER: 2

ADH is produced in response to changes in intravascular volume. The result is increased water reabsorption. A decrease in GFR (not increase) would put the client at risk for excess fluid volume. Increased sodium excretion usually results in increased fluid output and would not place the client at risk for excess fluid volume. Increased cardiac output usually increases perfusion to the kidney, resulting in increased output, and does not place the client at risk for excess fluid volume.

▶ ***Test-taking Tip:*** *Read each option carefully to determine if it would increase or decrease fluid volume.*

Content Area: Adult Health; *Category of Health Alteration:* Altered Fluid and Electrolytes; *Integrated Processes:* Nursing Process Analysis; *Client Need:* Physiological Integrity/Physiological Adaptation/Illness Management; *Cognitive Level:* Application

Reference: Harkreader, H., Hogan, A., & Thobaben, M. (2007). *Fundamentals of Nursing: Caring and Clinical Judgment* (p. 574). St. Louis, MO: Saunders.

1714. A 1-day-old infant of a mother who is diabetic exhibits jitteriness, apnea, cyanotic episodes, abdominal distention, and a high-pitched cry. Which electrolyte imbalance should a nurse suspect?

1. Early-onset hypocalcemia
2. Late-onset hypocalcemia
3. Hyperglycemia
4. Hypoglycemia

ANSWER: 1

Early-onset hypocalcemia (first 34–48 hours) tends to accompany the hypoglycemia that occurs shortly after birth in an infant of a diabetic mother. Late-onset hypocalcemia occurs 3 to 4 days following birth in infants fed modified cow's milk. Hypoglycemia may occur with newborns of diabetic mothers, but signs would not include abdominal distention and apnea with cyanosis. Hyperglycemia is usually asymptomatic.

➧ ***Test-taking Tip:*** *Focus on the symptoms of abdominal distention, apnea, and cyanosis to select the correct option.*

Content Area: Child Health; *Category of Health Alteration:* Altered Fluid and Electrolytes; *Integrated Processes:* Nursing Process Evaluation; *Client Need:* Physiological Integrity/Physiological Adaptation/Alterations in Body Systems; *Cognitive Level:* Analysis

Reference: Pillitteri, A. (2007). *Maternal & Child Health Nursing: Care of the Childbearing & Childrearing Family* (5th ed., pp. 1532–1533). Philadelphia: Lippincott Williams & Wilkins.

1715. Which electrolyte imbalance should be the priority concern for a nurse when assessing a 10-year-old client diagnosed with acute renal failure?

1. Hypercalcemia
2. Hyperphosphatemia
3. Hyperkalemia
4. Hypernatremia

ANSWER: 3

The normal function of the kidney is to excrete potassium. Acute renal failure in children often results from acute glomerulonephritis with retention of potassium. Hyperkalemia can lead to life-threatening cardiac arrhythmias. Hypercalcemia may result in changes in the neuromuscular system and bradycardia. Hyperphosphatemia may result in the presence of hypocalcemia. Hypernatremia may result in disorientation and lethargy.

➧ ***Test-taking Tip:*** *Use the ABCs (airway, breathing, circulation) to determine which electrolyte imbalance would be the most life-threatening.*

Content Area: Child Health; *Category of Health Alteration:* Altered Fluid and Electrolytes; *Integrated Processes:* Nursing Process Assessment; *Client Need:* Physiological Integrity/Physiological Adaptation/Fluid and Electrolyte Imbalances; *Cognitive Level:* Analysis

Reference: Pillitteri, A. (2007). *Maternal & Child Health Nursing: Care of the Childbearing & Childrearing Family* (5th ed., pp. 1476–1478). Philadelphia: Lippincott Williams & Wilkins.

1716. A client is hypotensive. A nurse closely monitors the client's electrolytes because the nurse knows that renin is released in response to decreased blood flow to the kidneys. Which electrolytes are dependent on the renin angiotensin–aldosterone system and should be closely monitored by the nurse?

1. Sodium, potassium, and chloride
2. Sodium, chloride, and calcium
3. Calcium, phosphate, and magnesium
4. Magnesium, potassium, and sodium

ANSWER: 1

Renin secretion increases plasma levels of angiotensin II, increases serum potassium, and decreases serum sodium. Aldosterone is also released in response to renin. Aldosterone increases sodium reabsorption and potassium excretion, resulting in an increase in chloride. Calcium balance is controlled by the parathyroid hormone, calcitonin, and vitamin D. Phosphorous and magnesium are regulated by the kidneys and influenced by calcium balance, not regulated by the renin–angiotensin system.

➧ ***Test-taking Tip:*** *Focus on the issue of the question: electrolytes dependent on the renin angiotensin–aldosterone system for their regulation.*

Content Area: Adult Health; *Category of Health Alteration:* Altered Fluid and Electrolytes; *Integrated Processes:* Nursing Process Assessment; *Client Need:* Physiological Integrity/Physiological Adaptation/Fluid and Electrolyte Imbalances; *Cognitive Level:* Application

Reference: Berman, A., Snyder, S., Kozier, B., & Erb, G. (2008). *Fundamentals of Nursing: Concepts, Process, and Practice* (8th ed., p. 1431). Upper Saddle River, NJ: Pearson Education.

1717. A nurse is caring for a client admitted with fluid volume overload. The client is receiving diuretic therapy with a loop diuretic. The potassium levels are illustrated in the chart below. On which day should the nurse expect an order for potassium replacement?

Day 1	Day 2	Day 3	Day 4
5.6 mEq/L	4.4 mEq/L	3.5 mEq/L	3.1 mEq/L

1. Day 1
2. Day 2
3. Day 3
4. Day 4

ANSWER: 3

Normal potassium level is 3.5 to 5.0 mEq/L. On day 3, the client is on the low end of normal. Because the client's serum potassium level is decreasing and the client is taking a diuretic, supplementation is needed to prevent a reduction of serum potassium levels below normal. The value on day 1 is high and would not require replacement. The value on day 2 is in the midrange of normal. The value on day 4 is low and would require replacement if replacement were not started on day 3.

➧ ***Test-taking Tip:*** *Recall that a loop diuretic will decrease serum potassium levels. Consider this when selecting an option.*

Content Area: Adult Health; *Category of Health Alteration:* Altered Fluid and Electrolytes; *Integrated Processes:* Nursing Process Implementation; *Client Need:* Physiological Integrity/Pharmacological and Parenteral Therapies/Medication Administration; *Cognitive Level:* Analysis

Reference: Smeltzer, S., Bare, B., Hinkle, J., & Cheever, K. (2008). *Brunner & Suddarth's Textbook of Medical-Surgical Nursing* (11th ed., p. 321). Philadelphia: Lippincott Williams & Wilkins.

1718. A client diagnosed with cardiomyopathy is hyponatremic as a result of fluid volume overload. A fluid restriction of 800 mL/24 hours is ordered by a physician. Which action by the nurse is most appropriate?

1. Provide ice chips and refill the glass every 4 hours.
2. Encourage the client to perform mouth care when feeling thirsty.
3. Offer sugary lozenges for the client to hold in the mouth.
4. Replenish the client's water every 2 hours and have the client take small sips.

ANSWER: 2

Frequent mouth care can help to reduce the sensation of thirst. Ice chips are considered fluid and should be included in the intake volume. A full glass of ice chips is equivalent to 120 mL of fluid. If replaced every 2 hours, ice chips alone would equal 1,440 mL of fluid. Lozenges, especially if high in sugar content, can produce the sensation of thirst. Small frequent sips can quickly add up to high volumes that exceed the client's restriction.

➧ ***Test-taking Tip:*** *The key phrase is "most appropriate." Consider the nurse's action in maintaining the fluid restriction and alleviating the client's thirst.*

Content Area: Adult Health; *Category of Health Alteration:* Altered Fluid and Electrolytes; *Integrated Processes:* Nursing Process Implementation; *Client Need:* Physiological Integrity/Physiological Adaptation/Fluid and Electrolyte Imbalances; *Cognitive Level:* Analysis

References: Smeltzer, S., Bare, B., Hinkle, J., & Cheever, K. (2008). *Brunner & Suddarth's Textbook of Medical-Surgical Nursing* (11th ed., pp. 318–319). Philadelphia: Lippincott Williams & Wilkins; Berman, A., Snyder, S., Kozier, B., & Erb, G. (2008). *Kozier & Erb's Fundamentals of Nursing: Concepts, Process, and Practice* (8th ed., p. 1454). Upper Saddle River, NJ: Pearson Education.

1719. Which assessment findings for a client who is status post-thyroidectomy should direct a nurse to check the client's serum calcium level?

1. Fatigue, decreased cardiac function, and tetany
2. Weakness, tachycardia, and disorientation
3. Muscle cramps, paresthesia, and Trousseau's sign
4. Weakness, edema, and orthostatic hypotension

ANSWER: 3

Muscle cramps, paresthesia, and a positive Trousseau's sign are common manifestations of hypo- or hypercalcemia because of the irritation to the neuromuscular system. Tachycardia is most often associated with abnormal serum magnesium levels. Fatigue is associated with sodium, potassium, and phosphorus imbalances. Hypotension relates most often to volume changes rather than electrolyte imbalances.

➧ ***Test-taking Tip:*** *Focus on calcium's effect on the neuromuscular system to select the correct option.*

Content Area: Adult Health; *Category of Health Alteration:* Altered Fluid and Electrolytes; *Integrated Processes:* Nursing Process Assessment; *Client Need:* Physiological Integrity/Physiological Adaptation/Fluid and Electrolyte Imbalances; *Cognitive Level:* Analysis

Reference: Harkreader, H., Hogan, A., & Thobaben, M. (2007). *Fundamentals of Nursing: Caring and Clinical Judgment* (pp. 570–571). St. Louis, MO: Saunders.

1720. A nurse has gathered assessment data for four assigned clients and is evaluating the data. Which client is most likely experiencing excess fluid volume?

	Client A	Client B	Client C	Client D
Medical Diagnosis	COPD	Renal failure	Heart failure	Postoperative day 1 Abdominal aortic aneurysm (AAA) repair
Physical Exam	Crackles 1+ edema Dyspneic	Crackles No edema No dyspnea	Crackles 1+ edema Dyspnea	Inspiratory crackles 3+ edema Dyspnea cough
Intake/Output	2,250/1,125	2,250/200	2,250/4,250	6,500/1,000
Weight	Up 2 lb	No change	Down 3 lb	Up 10 lb
Laboratory: BUN Hct	 15 mg/dL 46%	 25 mg/dL 40%	 15 mg/dL 32%	 20 mg/dL 32%

1. Client A
2. Client B
3. Client C
4. Client D

ANSWER: 4

Client D is most likely experiencing excess fluid volume. Clients with fluid volume excess may report dyspnea and have crackles. Edema varies from dependent to generalized edema. Common contributing factors to excess fluid volume include chronic kidney disease, heart failure, excessive administration of parenteral fluids, and intake greater than output. Excess fluid volume will most often result in an increased weight and blood urea nitrogen (BUN) and decreased hematocrit because of dilution.

Test-taking Tip: *Carefully review the information about the clients. Recall that weight and intake and output are key findings, so analyze these first for each client.*

Content Area: Adult Health; *Category of Health Alteration:* Altered Fluid and Electrolytes; *Integrated Processes:* Nursing Process Evaluation; *Client Need:* Physiological Integrity/Physiological Adaptation/Fluid and Electrolyte Imbalances; *Cognitive Level:* Synthesis

Reference: Doenges, M., Moorhouse, M., & Murr, A. (2005). *Nursing Care Plans: Guidelines for Individualizing Client Care Across the Life Span* (7th ed., pp. 922–923). Philadelphia: F. A. Davis.

1721. Which assessment findings should prompt a nurse to conclude that interventions have been *ineffective* for a 90-year-old client with hypernatremia?

1. Lethargy and paresthesias
2. Muscle cramps and spasms
3. Restlessness and agitation
4. Decreased body temperature and shivering

ANSWER: 3

Hypernatremia (serum sodium greater than 145 mEq/L) results in water shifting out of cells into the extracellular fluid with resultant dehydration and shrinkage of cells. Dehydration of brain cells results in neurological manifestations such as restlessness, lethargy, agitation, seizures, and even coma. Paresthesias are associated with hyperkalemia. Muscle cramps and spasms are symptoms of hyponatremia. Increased body temperature can be a cause of the hypernatremia; a decrease might suggest improvement.

Test-taking Tip: *Focus on the issue: assessment findings for hypernatremia.*

Content Area: Adult Health; *Category of Health Alteration:* Altered Fluid and Electrolytes; *Integrated Processes:* Nursing Process Evaluation; *Client Need:* Physiological Integrity/Physiological Adaptation/Fluid and Electrolyte Imbalances; *Cognitive Level:* Application

Reference: Smeltzer, S., Bare, B., Hinkle, J., & Cheever, K. (2008). *Brunner & Suddarth's Textbook of Medical-Surgical Nursing* (11th ed., pp. 319–320). Philadelphia: Lippincott Williams & Wilkins.

1722. A nurse is caring for a client with cardiac and renal disease who now has a serum potassium level of 6.0 mEq/L. Which interdependent interventions should the nurse recognize as appropriate for this client? SELECT ALL THAT APPLY.

1. Administer oral sodium polystyrene (Kayexalate®).
2. Administer intravenous (IV) dextrose (D-Glucose®).
3. Administer IV insulin (Humulin®).
4. Administer IV calcium gluconate (Kalcinate®).
5. Administer oral potassium chloride tablets (Klor-Con®).
6. Administer albuterol (Proventil®) inhaler.

ANSWER: 1, 2, 3, 4, 6

Sodium polystyrene is a cation exchange resin that exchanges sodium ions for potassium ions in the intestine. IV glucose and insulin temporarily shift potassium into the cell. Calcium gluconate is administered to stabilize the cardiac cell membrane in the presence of hyperkalemia. Beta-2-adrenergic agonists, such as albuterol, promote cellular reuptake of potassium, possibly via the cyclic guanosine monophosphate (gAMP) receptor cascade. Potassium supplements are contraindicated in clients with hyperkalemia since a further increase in serum potassium concentration in such clients can produce cardiac arrest.

▶ ***Test-taking Tip:*** *Recall that a normal serum potassium level is 3.5 to 5.0 mEq/L. Review treatment of hyperkalemia if having difficulty with this question. Memorization of common laboratory values, such as potassium, is required to answer questions on the NCLEX-RN® examination.*

Content Area: Adult Health; *Category of Health Alteration:* Altered Fluid and Electrolytes; *Integrated Processes:* Nursing Process Planning; *Client Need:* Physiological Integrity/Physiological Adaptation/Fluid and Electrolyte Imbalances; *Cognitive Level:* Analysis

References: Pagana, K., & Pagana, T. (2007). *Mosby's Diagnostic and Laboratory Test Reference* (p. 1153). St. Louis, MO: Mosby/Elsevier; Smeltzer, S., Bare, B., Hinkle, J., & Cheever, K. (2008). *Brunner & Suddarth's Textbook of Medical-Surgical Nursing* (11th ed., pp. 322–324). Philadelphia: Lippincott Williams & Wilkins.

1723. Which recommendation should a nurse teach to a client diagnosed with hypoparathyroidism?

1. Avoid milk and milk products.
2. Avoid carbonated beverages.
3. Ensure a calcium intake of 1,000 to 1,500 mg/day.
4. Perform isometric rather than weight-bearing exercises.

ANSWER: 3

Hypoparathyroidism is decreased function of the parathyroid glands, leading to decreased levels of parathyroid hormone (PTH). In the absence of adequate PTH activity, the ionized calcium concentration in the extracellular fluid falls. The client should be taught to ensure an adequate calcium intake, or supplements may be required. Dairy products are the primary source of calcium and should be increased in the presence of hypoparathyroidism. Carbonated beverages do not impact calcium, but alcohol and caffeinated beverages inhibit calcium absorption. Weight-bearing exercises can decrease the loss of calcium and should be recommended.

▶ ***Test-taking Tip:*** *Apply knowledge that hypoparathyroidism may result in hypocalcemia. Recall that adequate calcium intake is required to prevent hypocalcemia.*

Content Area: Adult Health; *Category of Health Alteration:* Altered Fluid and Electrolytes; *Integrated Processes:* Teaching and Learning; *Client Need:* Physiological Integrity/Physiological Adaptation/Fluid and Electrolyte Imbalances; *Cognitive Level:* Analysis

Reference: Berman, A., Snyder, S., Kozier, B., & Erb, G. (2008). *Kozier & Erb's Fundamentals of Nursing: Concepts, Process, and Practice* (8th ed., p. 1440). Upper Saddle River, NJ: Pearson Education.

1724. **EBP** A nurse is caring for a client who has a magnesium deficiency resulting from alcoholism. Which system should be a nurse's first priority when assessing this client?

1. Cardiovascular system
2. Musculoskeletal system
3. Respiratory system
4. Renal system

ANSWER: 1

Cardiovascular function should be monitored closely because hypomagnesemia can cause life-threatening dysrhythmias, resulting in cardiovascular failure and arrest. Other manifestations of hypomagnesemia include neuromuscular irritability and respiratory difficulties, but assessment of these systems should not be the nurse's first priority.

▶ ***Test-taking Tip:*** *The key phrase is "first priority." Use the ABCs (airway, breathing, circulation) to eliminate options 2 and 4. Of the remaining two options, think about which system is most affected by serum magnesium levels.*

Content Area: Adult Health; *Category of Health Alteration:* Altered Fluid and Electrolytes; *Integrated Processes:* Nursing Process Assessment; *Client Need:* Physiological Integrity/Physiological Adaptation/Fluid and Electrolyte Imbalances; *Cognitive Level:* Application

Reference: Smeltzer, S., Bare, B., Hinkle, J., & Cheever, K. (2008). *Brunner & Suddarth's Textbook of Medical-Surgical Nursing* (11th ed., p. 329). Philadelphia: Lippincott Williams & Wilkins.

EBP Reference: Tong, G., & Rude, R. (2005). Magnesium deficiency in critical illness. *Journal of Intensive Care Medicine,* 20(1), 3–17.

1725. A child with a history of asthma presents to an emergency room and is treated with epinephrine. The child is agitated, sweating profusely while sitting up, and has an oxygen saturation of less than 91% and a respiratory rate of less than 30 breaths per minute. Breath sounds are diminished, and wheezing is absent. Based on this information, which acid-base imbalance should a nurse anticipate?

1. Respiratory acidosis
2. Respiratory alkalosis
3. Metabolic alkalosis
4. Metabolic acidosis

ANSWER: 1

The nurse should anticipate respiratory acidosis. This child is most likely in status asthmaticus with continued respiratory distress despite treatment. Even though the child has a high respiratory rate, there is hypoventilation as a result of bronchoconstriction, which results in carbon dioxide retention. High $Paco_2$ (greater than 42 mm Hg) will result in a lowering of pH or an acidotic state, resulting from primary changes to the respiratory system. Respiratory alkalosis would occur if excess carbon dioxide is blown off with hyperventilation. The client's symptoms are associated with a respiratory and not a metabolic problem; thus, metabolic alkalosis and acidosis are incorrect.

▶ ***Test-taking Tip:*** *Recall that the diminished ventilation will increase the $Paco_2$, which is the respiratory component of acid-base balance. Thus, eliminate options 3 and 4.*

Content Area: Child Health; *Category of Health Alteration:* Altered Fluid and Electrolytes; *Integrated Processes:* Nursing Process Analysis; *Client Need:* Physiological Integrity/Physiological Adaptation/Alterations in Body Systems; *Cognitive Level:* Analysis

Reference: Pillitteri, A. (2007). *Maternal & Child Health Nursing: Care of the Childbearing & Childrearing Family* (5th ed., p. 1417). Philadelphia: Lippincott Williams & Wilkins.

1726. A client has arterial blood gases drawn. The results are pH 7.50, Pco_2 35, HCO_3 30. Which nursing interpretation of the client's acid-base imbalance is correct?

1. Respiratory alkalosis
2. Metabolic alkalosis
3. Respiratory acidosis
4. Metabolic acidosis

ANSWER: 2

A pH of 7.50 indicates alkalosis. A corresponding HCO_3 above the normal range of 20 to 24 mmol/L indicates the primary acid-base imbalance is metabolic alkalosis. A respiratory alkalosis would result in a Pco_2 lower than the normal range of 35 to 45 mm Hg. Respiratory acidosis and metabolic acidosis would result in a pH less than 7.4.

▶ ***Test-taking Tip:*** *Label the pH, the Pco_2 and HCO_3 as either acid or base. Recall that the Pco_2 is the respiratory component and HCO_3 the metabolic component of acid-base balance. The component that matches the pH as acid or base is the system (respiratory or metabolic) initiating the acid-base imbalance.*

Content Area: Adult Health; *Category of Health Alteration:* Altered Fluid and Electrolytes; *Integrated Processes:* Nursing Process Evaluation; *Client Need:* Physiological Integrity/Reduction of Risk Potential/Laboratory Values; *Cognitive Level:* Analysis

References: Berman, A., Snyder, S., Kozier, B., & Erb, G. (2008). *Kozier & Erb's Fundamentals of Nursing: Concepts, Process, and Practice* (8th ed., p. 1444). Upper Saddle River, NJ: Pearson Education; Lewis, S., Heitkemper, M., Dirksen, S., O'Brien, P., & Bucher, L. (2007). *Medical-Surgical Nursing: Assessment and Management of Clinical Problems* (7th ed., pp. 336–337). St. Louis, MO: Mosby.

1727. A nurse is caring for a client diagnosed with respiratory acidosis. Which arterial blood gas findings should indicate to the nurse that the client's kidneys have compensated for the imbalance?

1. pH = 7.43; $Paco_2$ = 60; $Pahco_3$ = 35
2. pH = 7.35; $Paco_2$ = 50; $Pahco_3$ = 30
3. pH = 7.50; $Paco_2$ = 35; $Pahco_3$ = 30
4. pH = 7.44; $Paco_2$ = 45; $Pahco_3$ = 24

ANSWER: 2

Respiratory acidosis results from increased Pco_2. The kidneys respond slowly by retaining $Pahco_3$, which is a base. The normal $Pahco_3$ is 20 to 24 mmol/L. Full compensation occurs when the pH returns to the normal range of 7.35 to 7.45. Option 1 blood gas indicates a metabolic alkalosis with respiratory compensation. A pH of 7.43 is not an acidotic pH, and the body does not overcompensate. Option 3 indicates respiratory alkalosis with the kidneys responding, but the imbalance is not yet compensated. Option 4 is a normal blood gas finding.

▶ ***Test-taking Tip:*** *Compensated means that the pH returns to normal and the system that did not initiate the imbalance will respond in the opposite direction (acid or base) of the imbalance.*

Content Area: Adult Health; *Category of Health Alteration:* Altered Fluid and Electrolytes; *Integrated Processes:* Nursing Process Evaluation; *Client Need:* Physiological Integrity/Physiological Adaptation/Fluid and Electrolyte Imbalances; *Cognitive Level:* Analysis

Reference: Berman, A., Snyder, S., Kozier, B., & Erb, G. (2008). *Kozier & Erb's Fundamentals of Nursing: Concepts, Process, and Practice* (8th ed., p. 1442). Upper Saddle River, NJ: Pearson Education.

1728. A client is admitted with diabetic ketoacidosis (DKA) associated with type 1 diabetes mellitus. The client's blood sugar is 320 mg/dL. The respiratory assessment reveals respiratory rate of 32, with a deep, regular respiratory effort. Which acid-base imbalance is this client most likely experiencing?

1. Respiratory acidosis
2. Respiratory alkalosis
3. Metabolic acidosis
4. Metabolic alkalosis

ANSWER: 3

The elevated blood glucose level is a finding associated with DKA. Kussmaul respirations allow the body to "blow off" excess CO_2 to compensate for the acidotic state and the decreased HCO_3. DKA is a metabolic, not a respiratory, acid-base imbalance. As DKA implies, it is an acidotic, not an alkalotic, imbalance.

➧ ***Test-taking Tip:*** *Recognize that DKA is a metabolic acid-base imbalance and eliminate options that pertain to the respiratory system.*

Content Area: Adult Health; *Category of Health Alteration:* Altered Fluid and Electrolytes; *Integrated Processes:* Nursing Process Evaluation; *Client Need:* Physiological Integrity/Physiological Adaptation/Fluid and Electrolyte Imbalances; *Cognitive Level:* Analysis

References: Harkreader, H., Hogan, A., & Thobaben, M. (2007). *Fundamentals of Nursing: Caring and Clinical Judgment* (p. 572). St. Louis, MO: Saunders; Lewis, S., Heitkemper, M., Dirksen, S., O'Brien, P., & Bucher, L. (2007). *Medical-Surgical Nursing: Assessment and Management of Clinical Problems* (7th ed., pp. 336–337). St. Louis, MO: Mosby.

1729. A nurse is caring for a client suspected of having a pulmonary embolism. The client's arterial blood gas (ABG) results indicate respiratory alkalosis. Which findings support this diagnosis?

1. pH = 7.54; $Paco_2$ = 25; Hco_3 = 24
2. pH = 7.35; $Paco_2$ = 35; Hco_3 = 22
3. pH = 7.50; $Paco_2$ = 40; Hco_3 = 28
4. pH = 7.32; $Paco_2$ = 48; Hco_3 = 24

ANSWER: 1

Because pulmonary emboli interfere with gas exchange, the respiratory center is stimulated to meet oxygenation demands. The tachypnea produces respiratory alkalosis. Thus, the pH is increased above normal of 35 to 45 and the $Paco_2$ is lower than the normal level of 35 to 45 mm Hg. The HCO_3 is normally 22 to 26 mEq/L. The blood gas in option 2 is normal, option 3 represents metabolic alkalosis, and option 4 is indicative of respiratory acidosis.

➧ ***Test-taking Tip:*** *First look at the pH and eliminate the option with a decreased pH because this indicates acidosis. Of the remaining options, look at the $Paco_2$ because it is the respiratory component for arterial blood gases (ABG) analysis. Select the option with the decreased $Paco_2$ because a low $Paco_2$ is present in respiratory alkalosis.*

Content Area: Adult Health; *Category of Health Alteration:* Altered Fluid and Electrolytes; *Integrated Processes:* Nursing Process Assessment; *Client Need:* Physiological Integrity/Physiological Adaptation/Pathophysiology; *Cognitive Level:* Analysis

References: Pagana, K., & Pagana, T. (2007). *Mosby's Diagnostic and Laboratory Test Reference* (pp. 117–125). St. Louis, MO: Mosby/Elsevier; Lewis, S., Heitkemper, M., Dirksen, S., O'Brien, P., & Bucher, L. (2007). *Medical-Surgical Nursing: Assessment and Management of Clinical Problems* (7th ed., pp. 336–337). St. Louis, MO: Mosby.

1730. A nurse assigned to care for multiple clients is reviewing the laboratory reports. Based on the information provided, which clients should the nurse assess first? Prioritize the order in which the nurse should plan to assess the clients.

______ A client diagnosed with renal insufficiency whose serum potassium level is 5.2 mEq/L
______ A client diagnosed with hyperemesis whose serum sodium level is 122 mEq/L
______ A client recovering following head trauma whose serum osmolality is 290 mOsm/kg
______ A client diagnosed with diabetes mellitus whose arterial blood gas results are pH = 7.22; Pco_2 = 35 mm Hg; HCO_3 = 15 mEq/L

ANSWER: 3, 2, 4, 1

The first client to be assessed should be the client diagnosed with diabetes mellitus because the arterial blood gas results indicate metabolic acidosis. A compensatory mechanism will include Kussmaul respirations to eliminate excess acid. Airway assessment is priority, and further assessment is needed to determine the underlying cause for the metabolic acidosis. The client with hyperemesis is experiencing severe hyponatremia with serum sodium below the normal range of 135 to 145 mEq/L and is at risk of seizures. Safety is a second priority. The client diagnosed with renal insufficiency, whose serum potassium level is 5.3 mEq/L, is the third client to be assessed. The serum potassium level is slightly above normal of 3.5 to 5.0 mEq/L. The client recovering following head trauma, whose serum osmolality is 290 mOsm/kg and has a normal serum osmolality level (285–295 mOsm/kg), can be assessed last. This client is the most stable.

Test-taking Tip: Use the ABCs (airway, breathing, circulation) and Maslow's Hierarchy of Needs theory to establish priority.

Content Area: Adult Health; *Category of Health Alteration:* Altered Fluid and Electrolytes; *Integrated Processes:* Nursing Process Assessment; *Client Need:* Safe and Effective Care Environment/Management of Care/Establishing Priorities; *Cognitive Level:* Synthesis

Reference: Lewis, S., Heitkemper, M., Dirksen, S., O'Brien, P., & Bucher, L. (2007). *Medical-Surgical Nursing: Assessment and Management of Clinical Problems* (7th ed., pp. 326–327, 333–335, 1857). St. Louis, MO: Mosby.

1731. EBP A nurse has analyzed the arterial blood gas (ABG) results for a newly admitted client with ethylene glycol toxicity (see table). Which treatment options should the nurse anticipate? SELECT ALL THAT APPLY.

Client's ABG Results	
pH	7.18
$Paco_2$	25 mm Hg
HCO_3	9 mEq/L
Po_2	60%

1. Mechanical hyperventilation of the client
2. Sodium bicarbonate
3. Hemodialysis
4. Intravenous (IV) colloid solution
5. IV potassium replacement
6. Supplemental oxygen

ANSWER: 2, 3, 5, 6

The ABGs reveal partially compensated metabolic acidosis with the pH below the normal of 7.35 to 7.45, the $Paco_2$ below the normal of 35 to 45 mm Hg, and the HCO_3 below the normal of 22 to 26 mEq/L. Ethylene glycol toxicity can produce metabolic acidosis. Half of the total bicarbonate deficit should be replaced during the first few hours of therapy. Hemodialysis is another option for correcting a severe metabolic acidosis associated with ethylene glycol toxicity. Initially, as a compensatory mechanism in metabolic acidosis, potassium would shift out of the vascular compartment and into the cell in exchange for hydrogen ion to reestablish acid-base balance. Until full compensation occurs, potassium replacement is needed. When acid-base balance is achieved, the client should be monitored for hyperkalemia due to shift of potassium back into the vascular compartment. The Po_2 is low, so supplemental oxygen is needed. Mechanical ventilation may be needed to support the client, but not with hyperventilation. The $Paco_2$ is below normal. This occurred because the client would initially hyperventilate as a compensatory mechanism to return the acid-base balance back to normal by increasing the loss of $Paco_2$ through the lungs. At this time, mechanical hyperventilation will increase the loss of carbonic acid and further lower the $Paco_2$ level without correcting the problem. Crystalloids, not colloids, would be used for fluid replacement.

Test-taking Tip: Label the pH, the CO_2, and HCO_3 as either acid or base. Recall that the CO_2 is the respiratory component and HCO_3 the metabolic component of acid-base balance. The component that matches the pH as acid or base is the system (respiratory or metabolic) initiating the acid-base imbalance. The component that is abnormal but does not match the direction of the pH as acid or base is the system that is compensating for the imbalance.

Content Area: Adult Health; *Category of Health Alteration:* Altered Fluid and Electrolytes; *Integrated Processes:* Nursing Process Implementation; *Client Need:* Physiological Integrity/Physiological Adaptation/Fluid and Electrolyte Imbalances; *Cognitive Level:* Analysis

Reference: Lewis, S., Heitkemper, M., Dirksen, S., O'Brien, P., & Bucher, L. (2007). *Medical-Surgical Nursing: Assessment and Management of Clinical Problems* (7th ed., pp. 333–335). St. Louis, MO: Mosby.

EBP References: Naka, T., & Bellomo, R. (2004). Bench-to-bedside review: Treating acid-base abnormalities in the intensive care unit—The role of renal replacement therapy. *Critical Care,* 8(2), 108–114; Levraut, J., & Grimaud, D. (2003). Treatment of metabolic acidosis. *Current Opinion in Critical Care,* 9(4), 260–265; Priestley, M. (2006). Acidosis, metabolic. *E-Medicine*. Available at: www.emedicine.com/PED/topic15.htm

Test 46: **Infectious Disease**

1732. A nurse is caring for a 4-year-old child who is admitted with the diagnosis of chicken pox. Which type of precautions should the nurse plan for this client?

1. Strict airborne isolation with negative airflow
2. Airborne and droplet precautions with positive airflow
3. Contact precautions with negative airflow
4. Droplet precautions with positive airflow

ANSWER: 1

Varicella zoster is transmitted by direct mucous membrane contact, through airborne spread of secretions, and direct lesion contact. In a hospital setting, it is imperative that a negative-airflow room, along with strict droplet and airborne precautions, be used to prevent transmission to vulnerable and susceptible clients. Options 2, 3, and 4 are incorrect because these do not provide sufficient precautions.

▸ ***Test-taking Tip:*** *Note that all options include airflow. First narrow the options by selecting the appropriate type of airflow, positive or negative, and then deciding which would be the most appropriate.*

Content Area: Child Health; *Category of Health Alteration:* Infectious Disease; *Integrated Processes:* Nursing Process Planning; *Client Need:* Physiological Integrity/Physiological Adaptation/Alterations in Body Systems; *Cognitive Level:* Application

References: Hockenberry, M., & Wilson, D. (2007). *Wong's Nursing Care of Infants and Children* (8th ed., pp. 666–667). St. Louis, MO: Mosby/Elsevier; Pillitteri, A. (2007). *Maternal and Child Health Nursing* (5th ed., pp. 1359–1360). Philadelphia: Lippincott Williams & Wilkins.

1733. A medical resident admits a 4-year-old child diagnosed with chicken pox. Which prescribed medication is most important for a nurse to question?

1. Acetaminophen (Tylenol®)
2. Ampicillin (Unasyn®)
3. Acyclovir (Zovirax®)
4. Acetylsalicylic acid (Aspirin®)

ANSWER: 4

Because there is a strong association with the use of acetylsalicylic acid (aspirin) therapy for treating fever in children who have a viral illness and the onset of Reye syndrome, aspirin use is contraindicated for treating fever in children. Acetaminophen can be administered for treating fever. Ampicillin or acyclovir may be appropriate if there is a coinfection.

▸ ***Test-taking Tip:*** *Read the options carefully. Recall that acetylsalicylic acid is aspirin and there is a strong association with Reye syndrome.*

Content Area: Child Health; *Category of Health Alteration:* Infectious Disease; *Integrated Processes:* Nursing Process Implementation; *Client Need:* Physiological Integrity/Pharmacological and Parenteral Therapies/Medication Administration; *Cognitive Level:* Analysis

References: Hockenberry, M., & Wilson, D. (2007). *Wong's Nursing Care of Infants and Children* (8th ed., pp. 666–667). St. Louis, MO: Mosby/Elsevier; Pillitteri, A. (2007). *Maternal and Child Health Nursing* (5th ed., pp. 1359–1360). Philadelphia: Lippincott Williams & Wilkins.

1734. A nurse is caring for a 5-year-old client with the diagnosis of rubeola. Which intervention by the nurse best ensures the comfort of this child?

1. Keeping the lights dim
2. Keeping the skin clean by providing frequent baths
3. Using a warm mist to clear respiratory passages
4. Providing for minimal stimuli

ANSWER: 1

It is common for the client with measles to have photophobia. Keeping the lights dim and covering the windows are extremely important to the client's comfort. Skin should be kept clean and dry. The mist that is used should be cool. "Providing for minimal stimuli" is incorrect, but would be appropriate if "providing diversional activities" was added.

▸ ***Test-taking Tip:*** *This question requires some thought about the specific differences between the different diseases with rashes.*

Content Area: Child Health; *Category of Health Alteration:* Infectious Disease; *Integrated Processes:* Nursing Process Implementation; *Client Need:* Physiological Integrity/Physiological Adaptation/Alterations in Body Systems; *Cognitive Level:* Application

References: Hockenberry, M., & Wilson, D. (2007). *Wong's Nursing Care of Infants and Children* (8th ed., pp. 670–671). St. Louis, MO: Mosby/Elsevier; Pillitteri, A. (2007). *Maternal and Child Health Nursing* (5th ed., pp. 289, 1358–1359). Philadelphia: Lippincott Williams & Wilkins.

1735. A nurse is reviewing serum laboratory results for a 10-year-old child admitted with a diagnosis of chicken pox. Which value should the nurse be most concerned about?

Serum Laboratory Test	Client's Value	Normal Levels
BUN	25 mg/dL	5–25 mg/dL
Creatinine	1.6 mg/dL	0.5–1.5 mg/dL
Na	130 mg/dL	135–145 mEq/L
K	3.4 mg/dL	3.5–5.3 mEq/L
Cl	110 mg/dL	95–105 mEq/L
SGOT	65 unit/L	0–42 unit/L
SGPT	70 unit/L	0–48 unit/L
Amalyse	190 unit/L	less than 200 unit/L

1. Serum glutamic oxaloacetic transaminase (SGOT), because it can indicate compromise of the liver.
2. Potassium, because low potassium can impact cardiac function.
3. No one changed laboratory test value is more important than the other.
4. Creatinine, because it is indicative of decreased renal function.

ANSWER: 1

SGOT is an enzyme released by the liver when it is damaged. Hepatitis is a complication of varicella. There are other laboratory values that are concerning on the chart, but they are not as important as the liver enzymes. Potassium is low and serum creatinine is elevated, but they are not the most concerning. Because the SGOT and serum glutamic pyruvic transaminase (SGPT) are both elevated, these are more concerning than the potassium and creatinine values.

➧ ***Test-taking Tip:*** *Review the chart carefully, and think of the laboratory value alterations that could be indicative of complications from chicken pox.*

Content Area: Child Health; *Category of Health Alteration:* Infectious Disease; *Integrated Processes:* Nursing Process Analysis; *Client Need:* Physiological Integrity Reduction of Risk Potential/Laboratory Values; *Cognitive Level:* Analysis

References: Hockenberry, M., & Wilson, D. (2007). *Wong's Nursing Care of Infants and Children* (8th ed., pp. 666–667). St. Louis, MO: Mosby/Elsevier; Pillitteri, A. (2007). *Maternal and Child Health Nursing* (5th ed., pp. 1359–1360). Philadelphia: Lippincott Williams & Wilkins.

1736. EBP A 2-year-old child, brought to an emergency department by a parent because of a temperature of 103°F (39.4°C), is diagnosed with roseola. Which information should the nurse provide to the parent? SELECT ALL THAT APPLY

1. Expect a rose-pink rash that usually appears once the temperature subsides.
2. Administer aspirin every 3 to 4 hours as needed for an elevated temperature.
3. Use oatmeal baths to reduce the child's itching.
4. Avoid contact with the child's secretions.
5. Remove loose crusts that rub and irritate the skin.
6. Isolate the child from other family members to prevent transmission.

ANSWER: 1, 4

A rose-pink rash appears once the fever drops to normal. It starts usually at the trunk and lasts 1 to 2 days. Transmission is by person-to-person contact through oral secretions and is possible during the febrile and viremic phase of the illness. Aspirin should be avoided with viral illnesses. Acetaminophen (Tylenol®) can be used. The rash does not itch or form scabs. Isolation is unnecessary. Roseola is usually a self-limited illness with no sequelae.

➧ ***Test-taking Tip:*** *Use key words "aspirin," "itching," "removing crusts," and "isolation" to eliminate options.*

Content Area: Child Health; *Category of Health Alteration:* Infectious Disease; *Integrated Processes:* Teaching and Learning; *Client Need:* Physiological Integrity/Physiological Adaptation/Alterations in Body Systems; *Cognitive Level:* Application

Reference: Hockenberry, M., & Wilson, D. (2007). *Wong's Nursing Care of Infants and Children* (8th ed., pp. 668–669). St. Louis, MO: Mosby/Elsevier.

EBP Reference: Zerr, D., Meier, A., Selke, S., Frenkel, L., Huang, M., et al. (2005). A population-based study of primary human herpesvirus 6 infection. *New England Journal of Medicine,* 352(8), 768–776.

1737. A nurse in a clinic is assessing a 5-year-old client who has been exposed to rubeola. Which medication should the nurse anticipate being ordered for this client?

1. Acetaminophen (Tylenol®)
2. Prednisone (Deltasone®)
3. Immunoglobulin intramuscular (BayGam®)
4. Nafcillin

ANSWER: 3

If a person is exposed to the measles, he or she can, within a 6-day window, have a dose of immunoglobulin intramuscular to prevent the disease. Acetaminophen, prednisone, and nafcillin are not used when a child is exposed to rubeola.

Test-taking Tip: *The key word is "exposed." Look at the medications and think about which one would be used to prevent the illness rather than treat it.*

Content Area: Child Health; *Category of Health Alteration:* Infectious Disease; *Integrated Processes:* Nursing Process Analysis; *Client Need:* Physiological Integrity/Pharmacological and Parenteral Therapies/Expected Actions or Outcomes; *Cognitive Level:* Application

References: Hockenberry, M., & Wilson, D. (2007). *Wong's Nursing Care of Infants and Children* (8th ed., pp. 670–671). St. Louis, MO: Mosby/Elsevier; Pillitteri, A. (2007). *Maternal and Child Health Nursing* (5th ed., pp. 289, 1358–1359). Philadelphia: Lippincott Williams & Wilkins.

1738. A nurse is caring for a 3-year-old child with the diagnosis of rubeola. The nurse completes a set of vital signs and a focused assessment at 0800 hours. The child is restless and hard to calm. Upon examination, the child is hot to the touch and is reporting pain. On auscultation of the chest, the child's heart is racing and rales and rhonchi can be heard in the bases of the lung fields. The nurse compares the 0800-hour vital signs to previously obtained vital signs and notes the blood pressure, pulse rate, and temperature to be progressively increasing. What should be the nurse's next priority?

Vital Signs

Time	1600	2000	2400	0400	0800
Pulse	110	115	120	126	130
Respiratory Rate	20	24	26	30	40
Blood Pressure	108/64	110/60	100/60	110/76	120/80
Temperature	100.2°F (37.9°C)		101.6°F (38.7°C)		103.6°F (39.8°C)

1. Double-check the vital signs (VS) in one-half hour.
2. Provide antipyretics to reduce fever.
3. Proceed with the physical assessment and recheck the VS in 1 hour.
4. Have the chart available and contact the primary health-care provider (HCP).

ANSWER: 4

The nurse should contact the primary HCP because the client is presenting with fever and signs and symptoms that are indicative of a respiratory complication secondary to rubeola, with pneumonia being a common complication. The vital signs pattern suggests a potential secondary infection, and another set will not assist the HCP in determining the plan of care. The nurse should administer an antipyretic, but the client would have been receiving this medication already as treatment for fever due to the rubeola viral illness. The nurse should not wait to contact the HCP until after taking vital signs in one-half hour or in 1 hour.

Test-taking Tip: *Consider what is the best option to ensure optimum care and client safety based on the information provided.*

Content Area: Child Health; *Category of Health Alteration:* Infectious Disease; *Integrated Processes:* Nursing Process Evaluation; *Client Need:* Physiological Integrity/Physiological Adaptation/Alterations in Body Systems; *Cognitive Level:* Analysis

References: Hockenberry, M., & Wilson, D. (2007). *Wong's Nursing Care of Infants and Children* (8th ed., pp. 674–675). St. Louis, MO: Mosby/Elsevier; Pillitteri, A. (2007). *Maternal and Child Health Nursing* (5th ed., pp. 289, 1358–1359). Philadelphia: Lippincott Williams & Wilkins.

1739. An 18-year-old client, diagnosed with mumps, is being assessed by a nurse in an emergency department. Which findings should prompt additional assessment by the nurse?

1. Parotid swelling, fever, photophobia
2. Stiff neck, headache, fever
3. Headache, stiff neck, photophobia
4. Vomiting, parotid swelling, photophobia

ANSWER: 3

Headache, stiff neck, and photophobia are associated with aseptic meningitis. Approximately 15% of individuals diagnosed with mumps will develop this complication. Options 1, 2, and 4 all have symptoms that are concerning; it is the combination in option 3 that would require further assessment of the client and communication with primary health-care provider.

▶ ***Test-taking Tip:*** *Think of the physiology of mumps and a neurological complication that is potentially life-threatening.*

Content Area: Child Health; *Category of Health Alteration:* Infectious Disease; *Integrated Processes:* Nursing Process Analysis; *Client Need:* Physiological Integrity/Reduction of Risk Potential/System Specific Assessments; *Cognitive Level:* Application

References: Hockenberry, M., & Wilson, D. (2007). *Wong's Nursing Care of Infants and Children* (8th ed., pp. 672–673). St. Louis, MO: Mosby/Elsevier; Pillitteri, A. (2007). *Maternal and Child Health Nursing* (5th ed., pp. 1364–1365). Philadelphia: Lippincott Williams & Wilkins.

1740. A nurse is assigned to care for a 7-month-old infant. Upon reviewing the history and physical examination, the nurse learns that the infant had been exposed to rubella in utero. For which complications of exposure to rubella in utero should the nurse assess this client?

1. Ophthalmitis, hepatomegaly, blindness
2. Hepatosplenomegaly, delayed hearing loss, hydrocephaly
3. Severe mental retardation, congenital heart defect(s), delayed hearing loss
4. Pneumonia, hydrocephaly, hepatomegaly

ANSWER: 3

Rubella has devastating teratogenic effects on a fetus. These include eye defects, central nervous system effects, congenital heart defects, auditory defects, intrauterine growth retardation, and others. Hepatomegaly is not associated with fetal development in the first trimester.

▶ ***Test-taking Tip:*** *Identify those conditions that would be linked with fetal development in the first trimester. Carefully read options that have similar complications and eliminate those options that have a complication not associated with the first trimester.*

Content Area: Child Health; *Category of Health Alteration:* Infectious Disease; *Integrated Processes:* Nursing Process Assessment; *Client Need:* Physiological Integrity/Physiological Adaptation/Pathophysiology; *Cognitive Level:* Analysis

References: Hockenberry, M., & Wilson, D. (2007). *Wong's Nursing Care of Infants and Children* (8th ed., pp. 674–675). St. Louis, MO: Mosby/Elsevier; Pillitteri, A. (2007). *Maternal and Child Health Nursing* (5th ed., pp. 288, 1357–1358). Philadelphia: Lippincott Williams & Wilkins.

1741. A 17-year-old student is being assessed by a nurse in the high school. The student presents with a sore throat, headache, fever of 101°F (38.3°C), malaise, and abdominal pain. Based on this information, which action should be taken by the nurse?

1. Send the student to a health-care provider (HCP).
2. Provide an antipyretic and have the student remain in the nursing office for an hour.
3. Ask if the student would like to see a HCP for treatment or be sent home.
4. Call a parent and have the student go home with follow-up required.

ANSWER: 4

The student's signs and symptoms are consistent with strep throat. The nurse's responsibility is to provide care for this student and to prevent disease transmission. The parents should make the arrangements for a visit with the HCP. Alhough the student is 17 years old, the student is still under parental guidance and may be under the parent's insurance unless the student is emancipated. Although the antipyretic may decrease the symptoms, these are not administered in a school setting without a HCP prescription.

▶ ***Test-taking Tip:*** *Identify the option that would meet both the needs of the student and those with whom the student would interact.*

Content Area: Child Health; *Category of Health Alteration:* Infectious Disease; *Integrated Processes:* Nursing Process Planning; *Client Need:* Physiological Integrity/Physiological Adaptation/Illness Management; *Cognitive Level:* Analysis

References: Hockenberry, M., & Wilson, D. (2007). *Wong's Nursing Care of Infants and Children* (8th ed., pp. 1320–1321). St. Louis, MO: Mosby/Elsevier; Pillitteri, A. (2007). *Maternal and Child Health Nursing* (5th ed., pp. 290, 364, 789–790, 1366–1370, 1494–1495, 1558–1560, 1601). Philadelphia: Lippincott Williams & Wilkins.

1742. A nurse is preparing to discharge a 10-year-old male client who is hospitalized with the diagnosis of rheumatic fever. The nurse's top priority during the client's discharge teaching should be:

1. providing an avenue for verbalization of feelings regarding illness.
2. providing adequate and appropriate pain medications.
3. ensuring that the client is aware of activity restrictions and the need for adherence.
4. emphasizing the need for long-term prophylactic antibiotic therapy.

ANSWER: 3

Rheumatic fever is a serious illness with many major and minor components. This adolescent is at the developmental age and stage at which it is difficult to ensure compliance with activity level, and the child will want to be very active. Options 1, 2, and 4 are all correct, but option 3 is the priority because nonadherence to activity restrictions can impact cardiac function.

➧ ***Test-taking Tip:*** *Consider the age of the child and the greatest risk upon returning home after being hospitalized.*

Content Area: Child Health; *Category of Health Alteration:* Infectious Disease; *Integrated Processes:* Nursing Process Implementation; *Client Need:* Physiological Integrity/Physiological Adaptation/Illness Management; *Cognitive Level:* Analysis

References: Hockenberry, M., & Wilson, D. (2007). *Wong's Nursing Care of Infants and Children* (8th ed., pp. 1380–1481). St. Louis, MO: Mosby/Elsevier; Pillitteri, A. (2007). *Maternal and Child Health Nursing* (5th ed., pp. 1311–1312). Philadelphia: Lippincott Williams & Wilkins.

1743. A nurse is presenting an educational session for other nurses on erythema and shows the picture illustrated. The nurse should explain that, if observed, the child should see a health-care provider immediately, because this child's erythema pattern is characteristic of:

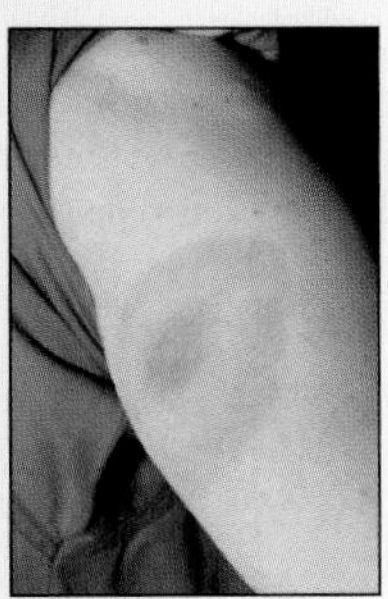

1. a bee sting.
2. a cat scratch.
3. a tick bite.
4. cellulitis.

ANSWER: 3

One of the distinguishing characteristics of Lyme disease is the development of erythema migrans (a bull's-eye-type pattern) 3 to 31 days after a tick bite. The child should be seen and treated immediately to prevent disease development.

➧ ***Test-taking Tip:*** *Focus on the pattern in the illustration. Recall that Lyme disease can present with the distinctive pattern of a bull's-eye.*

Content Area: Child Health; *Category of Health Alteration:* Infectious Disease; *Integrated Processes:* Teaching and Learning; *Client Need:* Physiological Integrity/Physiological Adaptation/Infectious Diseases; *Cognitive Level:* Application

References: Hockenberry, M., & Wilson, D. (2007). *Wong's Nursing Care of Infants and Children* (8th ed., pp. 775–777). St. Louis, MO: Mosby/Elsevier; Pillitteri, A. (2007). *Maternal and Child Health Nursing* (5th ed., pp. 289, 1311, 1360–1361, 1831). Philadelphia: Lippincott Williams & Wilkins.

1744. A college health nurse is providing education to a student athlete who is diagnosed with infectious mononucleosis. The student asks, "Will I be able to play soccer after I rest up for a few weeks?" Which should be the best response by the nurse?

1. "You may not be physically active for 2 to 3 months."
2. "You may be as active as you wish as long as you are not feeling fatigued."
3. "You should not engage in activities in which you may receive a blow to the abdomen."
4. "There are no limitations on activity with this diagnosis."

ANSWER: 3

Hepatosplenomegaly is a potential complication of infectious mononucleosis, which is caused by the Epstein-Barr virus (EBV). Because soccer is a contact sport, injury to the spleen can occur. Persons with acute EBV mononucleosis should be encouraged to rest as much as possible, not return to school until the fever and sore throat are resolved, and should refrain from active physical activity for 3 weeks. It is unnecessary to be physically inactive for 2 to 3 months, yet activity should not be as the client wishes.

➧ ***Test-taking Tip:*** *The key word is "best." Consider the potential complications and the length of the illness when selecting an option.*

Content Area: Child Health; *Category of Health Alteration:* Infectious Disease; *Integrated Processes:* Nursing Process Implementation; *Client Need:* Physiological Integrity/Physiological Adaptation/Alterations in Body Systems; *Cognitive Level:* Analysis

Reference: Hockenberry, M., & Wilson, D. (2007). *Wong's Nursing Care of Infants and Children* (8th ed., pp. 1323–1324). St. Louis, MO: Mosby/Elsevier.

1745. Which instruction by a nurse is best when teaching a parent skin care for a child diagnosed with impetigo?

1. Leave all scabs in place.
2. Remove skin, crusts, and debris by débridement of areas.
3. Avoid bathing the child until all scabs have healed.
4. Wash the crusts daily with soap and water.

ANSWER: 4

Washing the crusts daily with soap and water and not allowing the skin to dry promotes quick healing of the lesions. The scabs may come off with washing. Débridement (removal of undermined skin, crusts, and debris) occurs only after the skin is softened with wet compresses placed over the areas that are to be débrided. The child should be bathed daily.

▶ ***Test-taking Tip:*** *Options 3 and 4 are opposites. Either one or both are incorrect.*

Content Area: Child Health; *Category of Health Alteration:* Infectious Disease; *Integrated Processes:* Teaching and Learning; *Client Need:* Physiological Integrity/Basic Care and Comfort/Nonpharmacological Comfort Interventions; *Cognitive Level:* Application

References: Hockenberry, M., & Wilson, D. (2007). *Wong's Nursing Care of Infants and Children* (8th ed., pp. 767–768). St. Louis, MO: Mosby/Elsevier; Pillitteri, A. (2007). *Maternal and Child Health Nursing* (5th ed. pp. 289, 1368–1370). Philadelphia: Lippincott Williams & Wilkins.

1746. EBP A nurse, working at a local health department, is providing information to a client diagnosed with genital herpes. Which is the priority information that the nurse should provide to the client?

1. Genital herpes simplex virus-2 (HSV-2) is more common in women than men.
2. A herpes simplex virus-1 (HSV-1) genital infection can occur with oral–genital contact or genital contact.
3. After a diagnosis of HSV-2, there is likely to be two to three outbreaks during the first year.
4. Transmission of genital herpes can occur from a partner who does not have a visible sore.

ANSWER: 4

It is imperative to tell the client that transmission can occur from a partner who does not have a visible sore. Information about females being infected more than males and mode of transmission are important, and the client should be informed of these, but these are not the top priority. Typically in the first year after the diagnosis, the client will have four to five outbreaks, not two to three.

▶ ***Test-taking Tip:*** *The key word is "priority." This indicates that more than one option is correct, but one is more important.*

Content Area: Child Health; *Category of Health Alteration:* Infectious Disease; *Integrated Processes:* Nursing Process Implementation; *Client Need:* Safe and Effective Care Environment/Safety and Infection Control/Standard/Transmission-based/Precautions/Surgical Asepsis; *Cognitive Level:* Analysis

Reference: Lewis, S., Heitkemper, M., & Dirksen, S. (2007). *Medical-Surgical Nursing: Assessment and Management of Clinical Problems.* (7th ed., pp. 1496–1497). St. Louis, MO: Mosby/Elsevier.

EBP Reference: Department of Health and Human Services: Centers for Disease Control and Prevention. (2008). *Genital Herpes-CDC Fact Sheet.* Available at: www.cdc.gov/std/Herpes/STDFact-Herpes.htm

---

1747. A school nurse is talking with an adolescent who is concerned about hair loss secondary to tinea capitis. Which should be the nurse's most appropriate response to the adolescent?

1. "You are not the only person who has gone through this. Would you like to talk with someone about this?"
2. "What did your primary health-care provider tell you about your hair growing back?"
3. "You have styled your hair nicely; why is this bothering you?"
4. "Although you lost hair, your hair will grow back in about 6 to 12 months."

ANSWER: 2

Developmentally, adolescence is a time in which peers are very important and personal appearance is of utmost concern. Also important is for the adolescent to be in as much control of any situation as possible and his or her reactions. Asking what information the client already has would allow the nurse to either supplement or clarify the information needed by the student. Telling the student that he or she is not the only person to have experienced this is insensitive. Offering counseling is premature. Asking a why question can block therapeutic communication and initiate defensiveness. Telling the adolescent that the hair will grow back in 6 to 12 months is accurate information, but the client may need further support rather than providing accurate, but challenging information.

▶ ***Test-taking Tip:*** *Identify the most important issues for an adolescent and what responses would continue to allow the adolescent to discuss his or her feelings.*

Content Area: Child Health; *Category of Health Alteration:* Infectious Disease; *Integrated Processes:* Nursing Process Analysis; *Client Need:* Physiological Integrity/Physiological Adaptation/Alterations in Body Systems; *Cognitive Level:* Application

References: Hockenberry, M., & Wilson, D. (2007). *Wong's Nursing Care of Infants and Children* (8th ed., pp. 770–771). St. Louis, MO: Mosby/Elsevier; Pillitteri, A. (2007). *Maternal and Child Health Nursing* (5th ed., pp. 947–950). Philadelphia: Lippincott Williams & Wilkins.

1748. A clinic nurse is assessing a 12-year-old client and observes multiple lesions on the client's face, neck, and arms. Which is the most important question that the nurse should ask?

1. "Do others in your household have similar symptoms?"
2. "When did these lesions occur?"
3. "Do you have an animal at your house?"
4. "Have you been picking at these sores?"

ANSWER: 3

Ringworm is a fungal infection that affects the skin, hair, and nails. Transmission can be human-to-human as well as animal-to-human. Because of the placement of these lesions, they would be consistent with cuddling an animal. While it is important to know if others in the household have similar symptoms, the most important question should focus on the causative agent to establish a diagnosis. The location of the lesions and the adolescent's age should direct the questioning. Unless there is evidence of picking at the sores, the question is irrelevant.

➧ ***Test-taking Tip:*** *Focus on the age of the adolescent and the location of the lesions in selecting the "most important" question.*

Content Area: Child Health; *Category of Health Alteration:* Infectious Disease; *Integrated Processes:* Nursing Process Assessment; *Client Need:* Physiological Integrity/Physiological Adaptation/Alterations in Body Systems; *Cognitive Level:* Analysis

Reference: Hockenberry, M., & Wilson, D. (2007). *Wong's Nursing Care of Infants and Children* (8th ed., p. 770). St. Louis, MO: Mosby/Elsevier.

1749. A clinic nurse is talking with a parent whose 8-year-old child is diagnosed with ringworm. The parent is concerned because the child has developed an extensive, itchy rash. The nurse should instruct the parent to:

1. use topical steroids and antihistamines to treat the reaction.
2. bring the child immediately to the clinic for further assessment by a professional.
3. observe for another 24 hours and call the clinic for further health-care provider instructions.
4. stop all medication immediately.

ANSWER: 1

The extensive, itchy rash is related to the development of a hypersensitivity to the fungal antigen. Topical steroids and antihistamines can and should be used to treat the rash and make the child more comfortable. Because an itchy rash is associated with ringworm, immediate treatment in the clinic is unnecessary. Both topical steroids and antihistamines can be purchased over-the-counter. Observation will not relieve the child's symptoms.

➧ ***Test-taking Tip:*** *Focus on the child's symptoms and measures to relieve the symptoms.*

Content Area: Child Health; *Category of Health Alteration:* Infectious Disease; *Integrated Processes:* Nursing Process Implementation; *Client Need:* Physiological Integrity/Physiological Adaptation/Illness Management; *Cognitive Level:* Application

Reference: Hockenberry, M., & Wilson, D. (2007). *Wong's Nursing Care of Infants and Children* (8th ed., p. 770). St. Louis, MO: Mosby/Elsevier.

1750. A nurse is caring for a 2-year-old child who has undergone a bowel resection with creation of a colostomy placement following a farm accident. During the initial assessment of the client, the nurse observes small threadlike objects on and around the stoma. Based on this information, which critical judgment should be made by the nurse about these objects?

1. These are possible signs of a wound infection.
2. The objects suggest hookworm.
3. The objects suggest pinworms.
4. The objects are fibers left from the surgical procedure.

ANSWER: 3

Enterobiasis, or pinworms, is the most common helminthic infection in the United States. Infection begins when eggs are ingested or inhaled (eggs float in the air). The worms look like tiny pieces of white thread and are about as long as a staple. Threadlike objects are not typical signs of an infection. Although hookworm is a common soil-transmitted helminth infection, hookworm produces an intensely pruritic dermatitis at the entrance site (usually the feet), and as the infection migrates from the pulmonary to the intestinal system, eggs or evidence of the worms would be present in the feces. Suture fibers are not present on the stoma.

➧ ***Test-taking Tip:*** *It is important to think about the fact that a surgical procedure has occurred, but that the child was exposed to a variety of organisms prior to being hospitalized.*

Content Area: Child Health; *Category of Health Alteration:* Infectious Disease; *Integrated Processes:* Nursing Process Analysis; *Client Need:* Physiological Integrity/Physiological Adaptation/Alterations in Body Systems; *Cognitive Level:* Application

References: Hockenberry, M., & Wilson, D. (2007). *Wong's Nursing Care of Infants and Children* (8th ed., pp. 681–682). St. Louis, MO: Mosby/Elsevier; Pillitteri, A. (2007). *Maternal and Child Health Nursing* (5th ed., pp. 1371–1376, 1494, 1499). Philadelphia: Lippincott Williams & Wilkins.

1751. A nurse working in an urgent care setting receives a call from a parent concerned that his or her child may have pinworms. The nurse is providing information about how to obtain a test-tape specimen to accurately make a diagnosis of pinworms. Prioritize the nurse's instruction by placing each statement in the correct order.

____ Place the tongue depressor in a glass jar or in a loose plastic bag.
____ Loop a piece of transparent tape, sticky side out, and place it on the end of a tongue depressor.
____ Repeat the procedure the following day.
____ Bathe the child.
____ Place the tongue depressor firmly against the child's perianal area as soon as the child wakes up in the morning and prior to the child having a bowel movement.

ANSWER: 3, 1, 5, 4, 2

For an accurate diagnosis to be made of pinworms the parents should be given instructions on how to obtain the specimen. The parents should be instructed to loop a piece of transparent tape, sticky side out, and place it on the end of a tongue depressor. As soon as the child wakes up in the morning and prior to the child having a bowel movement or bathing, the end of the tongue depressor is placed against the child's perianal area. The tongue depressor is then placed in a glass jar or loosely in a plastic bag to take to the laboratory. The parent may bathe the child after the specimen is collected. The procedure most likely will need to be repeated again the following day using the same process.

▶ ***Test-taking Tip:*** *Think about the supplies needed to collect the specimen. This should lead you to the first option. Then, review the options and select the last option. Use cues within the options (e.g., following day) to identify the last step in the collection process.*

Content Area: Child Health; *Category of Health Alteration:* Infectious Disease; *Integrated Processes:* Nursing Process Implementation; *Client Need:* Safe and Effective Care Environment/Safety and Infection Control/Standard/Transmission-based/Precautions/Surgical Asepsis; *Cognitive Level:* Analysis

References: Hockenberry, M., & Wilson, D. (2007). *Wong's Nursing Care of Infants and Children* (8th ed., pp. 681–682). St. Louis, MO: Mosby/Elsevier; Pillitteri, A. (2007). *Maternal and Child Health Nursing* (5th ed., pp. 1371–1376, 1494, 1499). Philadelphia: Lippincott Williams & Wilkins.

1752. EBP The mother of a 13-year-old female tells a clinic nurse, "I hope that no one tries to get me to agree to have my daughter get that new vaccine that is supposed to prevent some STDs. My daughter is not and will not be having sex until she is married." What is the nurse's best response?

1. "How do you know that your daughter will not be sexually active prior to marriage?"
2. "It seems that you have some questions about the vaccine Gardasil®. I will make a note for the health-care provider (HCP)."
3. "I believe that you are talking about Gardasil®. Tell me what you have heard about the vaccine."
4. "Here is a pamphlet that talks about the vaccine Gardasil® that is used to prevent some STDs."

ANSWER: 3

Prior to beginning teaching, the nurse should determine what the parent knows about Gardasil®, which is the quadrivalent human papillomavirus (HPV) (types 6, 11, 16, 18) recombinant vaccine. HPV causes genital warts, abnormal Pap tests, and cervical cancer. Because Gardasil® prevents these, it is recommended for females before they become sexually active and routinely given between ages 11 or 12 years. Response 1 is irrelevant and may cause the parent to remove herself from the conversation. Response 2 defers the nurse's responsibility in parent education to the HCP. Response 4 is a passive education method and not beneficial to the needs of this parent at this time.

▶ ***Test-taking Tip:*** *Think about the best method to ensure that the parent has enough information to make an informed decision about refusing the recommended vaccination.*

Content Area: Child Health; *Category of Health Alteration:* Infectious Disease; *Integrated Processes:* Communication and Documentation; *Client Need:* Safe and Effective Care Environment/Management of Care/Informed Consent; *Cognitive Level:* Analysis

EBP References: Department of Health and Human Services: Centers for Disease Control and Prevention. (2007). *Human Papillomavirus Infection.* Available at: www.cdc.gov/std/hpv/default.htm#vaccine; Department of Health and Human Services: Centers for Disease Control and Prevention. (2008). *Human Papillomavirus (HPV) Vaccine Safety.* Available at: www.cdc.gov/vaccinesafety/vaers/gardasil.htm

1753. EBP Multiple clients are being assessed by a nurse working in a clinic for sexually transmitted diseases (STDs). The nurse should specifically assess for signs of cancer when which medical diagnosis is made for a client?

1. Syphilis
2. Chancroid
3. Cytomegalovirus
4. Human papillomavirus

ANSWER: 4

Human papillomavirus causes cervical, vaginal, and penile epithelial changes that can lead to the development of cancer. Clients diagnosed with human papillomavirus infections should be examined regularly for precancerous lesions. Chlamydial infection is also associated with an increased risk of cervical cancer, but syphilis, the chancre of syphilis, and cytomegalovirus have not been associated with an increased risk for cancer in the genital region.

▶ ***Test-taking Tip:*** *Recall that the Centers for Disease Control and Prevention (CDC) recommends administering the HPV vaccine to girls 11 to 12 years of age to prevent the transmission of two strains of HPV.*

Content Area: Adult Health; *Category of Health Alteration:* Infectious Disease; *Integrated Processes:* Nursing Process Assessment; *Client Need:* Physiological Integrity/Physiological Adaptation/Alterations in Body Systems; *Cognitive Level:* Application

Reference: Smeltzer, S., Bare, B., Hinkle, J., & Cheever, K. (2008). *Brunner & Suddarth's Textbook of Medical-Surgical Nursing* (11th ed., pp. 1666, 1977–1978). Philadelphia: Lippincott Williams & Wilkins.

EBP References: New York State Department of Health. (2007). *Human Papillomavirus (HPV)*. Available at: www.guideline.gov/summary/summary.aspx?doc_id=11511&nbr=005964&string=management+AND+women+AND+cervical+AND+intraepithelial+AND+neoplasia; Saslow, D., Castle, P., Cox, J., Davey, D., Einstein, M., et al. (2007). American Cancer Society guideline for human papillomavirus (HPV) vaccine use to prevent cervical cancer and its precursors. *CA: A Cancer Journal for Clinicians,* 57(1), 7–28.

1754. A nurse is planning care for a female client newly diagnosed with herpes simplex virus type 2 (HSV-2, herpes genitalis). In which order should the nurse complete the planned actions? Place the nurse's planned actions in order of priority.

______ Teach abstinence from sexual intercourse during treatment and use of condoms.
______ Determine if the woman is pregnant.
______ Discuss the benefits of joining a support group such as HELP (Herpetics Engaged in Living Productively).
______ Administer an analgesic and suggest a sitz bath.
______ Administer the first dose of acyclovir (Zovirax®).

ANSWER: 4, 1, 5, 2, 3

Knowing whether the woman is pregnant is priority because medications can be teratogenic and there is a substantial risk to a developing fetus. HSV-2 can be contracted by a fetus across the placenta if the mother has a primary infection during pregnancy. It can also be transmitted at birth if the mother has an active herpetic vulvovaginitis at the time of delivery. Administering an analgesic and promoting the woman's comfort is next. Itching, pain, macules, and papules occur initially with HSV-2. The infection can progress to vesicles and ulcers and can involve the labia, cervix, vaginal, and perianal area. The third priority is to administer the first dose of acyclovir. Next, teach abstinence from sexual intercourse during treatment and the use of condoms. Additional teaching should also include other comfort measures, self-care, and STD prevention. The woman is unlikely to be receptive to teaching until some degree of comfort is achieved. Finally, discuss the benefits of joining a support group such as HELP (Herpetics Engaged in Living Productively) because there is no cure for HSV-2 infection.

▶ ***Test-taking Tip:*** *Use the nursing process and Maslow's Hierarchy of Needs theory. Assessment should be completed before interventions.*

Content Area: Adult Health; *Category of Health Alteration:* Infectious Disease; *Integrated Processes:* Nursing Process Planning; *Client Need:* Safe and Effective Care Environment/Management of Care/Establishing Priorities; *Cognitive Level:* Analysis

References: Pillitteri, A. (2007). *Maternal & Child Health Nursing: Care of the Childbearing & Childrearing Family* (5th ed., pp. 289; 790). Philadelphia: Lippincott Williams & Wilkins; Smeltzer, S., Bare, B., Hinkle, J., & Cheever, K. (2008). *Brunner & Suddarth's Textbook of Medical-Surgical Nursing* (11th ed., pp. 1667–1669). Philadelphia: Lippincott Williams & Wilkins.

1755. A client presents at an outpatient clinic with fever, hair loss, joint swelling, and malaise. Findings upon physical assessment include a rash on the trunk, palms, and soles of the feet. Which should be the nurse's *next* action?

1. Ask if the client has had any painless lesions within the last 8 weeks.
2. Determine if the client has had unprotected sexual intercourse with multiple partners.
3. Collect specimens for a fluorescent treponemal antibody absorption test (FTA-ABS).
4. Discuss measures to prevent the spread of sexually transmitted diseases.

ANSWER: 1

Fever, hair loss, joint swelling, malaise, and a rash on the trunk, palms, and soles of the feet are signs of second-stage syphilis. Because these signs occur 2 to 8 weeks after a chancre, the nurse should ask about any painless lesions, which occur in the primary stage of a syphilis infection. A determination of multiple sexual partners is needed in order to notify partners, but syphilis can also be transmitted by other routes, such as oral or anal sex or contact with lesions. Though the nurse may be inclined to conclude the problem is syphilis, further assessment is needed before serological testing. Client education in preventing the spread of syphilis is important, but not the next action.

▶ ***Test-taking Tip:*** *The key phrase is "next action." Note the physical assessment findings. Use the nursing process steps. Additional information should be collected before establishing a nursing diagnosis and planning interventions.*

Content Area: Adult Health; *Category of Health Alteration:* Infectious Disease; *Integrated Processes:* Nursing Process Assessment; *Client Need:* Physiological Integrity/Physiological Adaptation/Alterations in Body Systems; *Cognitive Level:* Analysis

Reference: Smeltzer, S., Bare, B., Hinkle, J., & Cheever, K. (2008). *Brunner & Suddarth's Textbook of Medical-Surgical Nursing* (11th ed., pp. 2505–2507). Philadelphia: Lippincott Williams & Wilkins.

1756. A nurse is assessing a client involved in a motor vehicle accident and notes the lesion illustrated. Rash is also noted on the client's trunk. What precaution should the nurse use to prevent the spread of this infection?

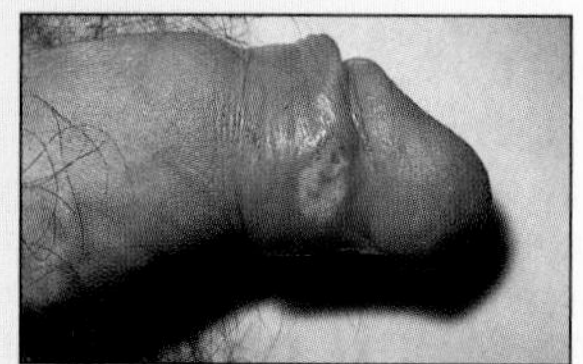

1. Standard precautions should be taken because the lesion appears to be syphilis, which is spread only through sexual contact.
2. Soap and water should be used to wash hands, rather than an alcohol-based hand wash, after contact with the client's skin.
3. A mask, gown, and gloves should be worn by anyone entering the client's room.
4. Gloves should be worn whenever anyone has direct contact with the client's skin.

ANSWER: 4

The lesions of secondary syphilis are highly contagious, and the client's skin should not be touched without wearing gloves. Hand hygiene should be performed when gloves are removed. The microorganisms of syphilis are also present in the client's blood, so standard precautions are also necessary, but they are insufficient when lesions are present. Alcohol-based hand wash is effective in preventing disease transmission. A mask and isolation in a private room is not required. A gown may be needed if clothing is expected to come in contact with skin lesions.

Test-taking Tip: *Use the process of elimination, eliminating options that would take minimal precautions (1 and 2). Considering the two remaining options, think about how syphilis is spread.*

Content Area: Adult Health; *Category of Health Alteration:* Infectious Disease; *Integrated Processes:* Nursing Process Analysis; *Client Need:* Safe and Effective Care Environment/Safety and Infection Control/Handling Hazardous and Infectious Materials; *Cognitive Level:* Application

Reference: Smeltzer, S., Bare, B., Hinkle, J., & Cheever, K. (2008). *Brunner & Suddarth's Textbook of Medical-Surgical Nursing* (11th ed., pp. 2505–2507). Philadelphia: Lippincott Williams & Wilkins.

1757. For which specific signs and symptoms should a nurse assess when a male client is diagnosed with gonorrheal infection? SELECT ALL THAT APPLY

1. Subnormal temperature
2. Purulent urethral discharge
3. Joint pain or stiffness
4. Lesions on the penis
5. Generalized skin rash

ANSWER: 2, 3

Urethral discharge and signs of arthritis, such as joint pain, are associated with an infection caused by *Neisseria gonorrhoeae.* The temperature is elevated, not subnormal. Lesions on the penis and a generalized skin rash are associated with syphilis.

Test-taking Tip: *Focus on a gonorrheal infection, and eliminate options indicative of syphilis.*

Content Area: Adult Health; *Category of Health Alteration:* Infectious Disease; *Integrated Processes:* Nursing Process Assessment; *Client Need:* Physiological Integrity/Physiological Adaptation/Alterations in Body Systems; *Cognitive Level:* Application

References: Lewis, S., Heitkemper, M., Dirksen, S., O'Brien, P., & Bucher, L. (2007). *Medical-Surgical Nursing: Assessment and Management of Clinical Problems* (7th ed., pp. 1367–1368). St. Louis, MO: Mosby/Elsevier; Smeltzer, S., Bare, B., Hinkle, J., & Cheever, K. (2008). *Brunner & Suddarth's Textbook of Medical-Surgical Nursing* (11th ed., p. 2507). Philadelphia: Lippincott Williams & Wilkins.

1758. A female client, who had a past diagnosis of pelvic inflammatory disease (PID) due to a chlamydial infection and gonorrhea, is unable to become pregnant. A health-care provider (HCP) informs a nurse that the PID likely caused the woman's sterility. What is the nurse's best interpretation of the HCP's statement?

1. The infection caused uterine damage such that when fertilization does occur, the fertilized egg does not implant into the uterus.
2. Scarring from the presence of the infection in the fallopian tubes is permanently blocking the tubes.
3. Damage to the cervix from the infection resulted in closure of the cervix such that sperm are blocked from entering the uterus.
4. Ovulation is no longer occurring because the infection damaged the woman's ovaries and less estrogen is being secreted.

ANSWER: 2

Gonorrhea spreads from the vagina into the uterus and then to the tubes and ovaries. Strictures and fallopian tube obstruction can occur. A fertilized egg is unable to pass through a narrowed fallopian tube, thus increasing the chance of an ectopic pregnancy. The blocked fallopian tubes prevent fertilization by not allowing sperm to reach an ovum. While an infection can also cause endometritis and cervicitis, there is less likelihood of generalized uterine damage and cervical obstruction to cause infertility. While ovulation may not occur due to ovarian scarring from the infection, the lack of ovulation is not related to less estrogen production.

➧ ***Test-taking Tip:*** *Think about the spread of the gonorrheal and chlamydial infections within the woman's body. The key word is "best."*

Content Area: Adult Health; *Category of Health Alteration:* Infectious Disease; *Integrated Processes:* Nursing Process Analysis; *Client Need:* Physiological Integrity/Physiological Adaptation/Pathophysiology; *Cognitive Level:* Analysis

Reference: Smeltzer, S., Bare, B., Hinkle, J., & Cheever, K. (2008). *Brunner & Suddarth's Textbook of Medical-Surgical Nursing* (11th ed., p. 1671). Philadelphia: Lippincott Williams & Wilkins.

1759. Which statement made by a client receiving treatment for a sexually transmitted disease indicates a need for teaching?

1. "I should abstain from sexual intercourse while receiving treatment for chlamydia."
2. "I plan to use latex rather than a nonlatex condom because there is less likelihood of the condom breaking."
3. "For the genital warts, I should apply podophyllin resin 10% solution carefully to each wart, and then wash it off in 1 to 4 hours."
4. "There is no cure for genital herpes; I should take the analgesic to control my pain and the antiviral medication to shorten the course of the infection."

ANSWER: 1

Persons treated for chlamydia should abstain from sexual intercourse for 7 days after treatment and until all sexual partners have completed a full course of treatment. All other statements are correct. Nonlatex condoms are more likely to break than latex condoms. Podophyllin is a cytotoxic agent recommended for small external genital warts and should be carefully applied to just the wart, avoiding normal tissue, and washed off in 1 to 4 hours. Genital herpes is caused by the herpesvirus type 2. The virus remains in the body for life. The antiviral medication suppresses viral replication but does not destroy the virus.

➧ ***Test-taking Tip:*** *The key phrase is "need for teaching." Select the option that is an incorrect statement.*

Content Area: Adult Health; *Category of Health Alteration:* Infectious Disease; *Integrated Processes:* Nursing Process Evaluation; *Client Need:* Health Promotion and Maintenance/Principles of Teaching and Learning; *Cognitive Level:* Analysis

References: Lewis, S., Heitkemper, M., Dirksen, S., O'Brien, P., & Bucher, L. (2007). *Medical-Surgical Nursing: Assessment and Management of Clinical Problems* (7th ed., pp. 1371–1377). St. Louis, MO: Mosby/Elsevier; Smeltzer, S., Bare, B., Hinkle, J., & Cheever, K. (2008). *Brunner & Suddarth's Textbook of Medical-Surgical Nursing* (11th ed., pp. 1667–1669). Philadelphia: Lippincott Williams & Wilkins.

1760. An outbreak of hepatitis has occurred at a local factory. Ten factory workers have developed symptoms of the disease within 2 days of each other. The source of the illness is determined to be contaminated cafeteria food. The factory occupational health nurse should notify the Centers for Disease Control and Prevention (CDC) that which type of hepatitis outbreak likely has occurred?

1. Hepatitis A
2. Hepatitis B
3. Hepatitis C
4. Hepatitis D

ANSWER: 1

Foodborne hepatitis A outbreaks are usually due to contamination of food during preparation by an infected food handler. Outbreaks of hepatitis within a group are consistently caused by hepatitis A virus. Hepatitis B and C are transmitted by exposure to blood or body fluids, and therefore neither causes group outbreaks. Hepatitis D virus requires the presence of hepatitis B virus to infect a host.

➧ ***Test-taking Tip:*** *Focus on the different methods of transmission of each type of hepatitis virus. Hepatitis A is the only one that can be transmitted through contaminated food.*

Content Area: Adult Health; *Category of Health Alteration:* Infectious Disease; *Integrated Processes:* Nursing Process Analysis; *Client Need:* Safe and Effective Care Environment/Safety and Infection Control/Reporting of Incident/Event/Irregular Occurrence/Variance; *Cognitive Level:* Application

Reference: Lewis, S., Heitkemper, M., Dirksen, S., O'Brien, P., & Bucher, L. (2007). *Medical-Surgical Nursing: Assessment and Management of Clinical Problems* (7th ed., pp. 1089–1090, 1097). St. Louis, MO: Mosby/Elsevier.

1761. EBP A registered nurse (RN) is caring for a client who is diagnosed with hepatitis A. The client is incontinent of stool. A patient care assistant (PCA) is assisting the RN with the client's care. The RN determines that the PCA understands correct infectious precautions for this client when the PCA is observed:

1. wearing a mask when taking vital signs.
2. wearing a gown and gloves when changing the client's incontinent briefs.
3. wearing gloves when providing perineal care.
4. wearing a gown and gloves when asking the client about food choices for lunch.

ANSWER: 2

Hepatitis A virus is present in the feces for 2 weeks after symptoms appear. The virus can live for several months outside the body; therefore, contact precautions are recommended when caring for clients who are incontinent of stool. There is no need to wear a mask at any time during client care because the virus is not airborne. Wearing gloves when providing perineal care is correct but is not enough protection; gowns should also be worn to protect clothing from contamination and transmission to others. There is no need to wear a gown when talking with the client as long as there is no physical contact.

➧ ***Test-taking Tip:*** *Think about how hepatitis A is transmitted. A memory aid to remember the mode of transmission for hepatitis A would be the letter "A," which is for* ***a****nus. This should enable elimination of options 1 and 4.*

Content Area: Adult Health; *Category of Health Alteration:* Infectious Disease; *Integrated Processes:* Nursing Process Evaluation; *Client Need:* Safe and Effective Care Environment/Management of Care/Supervision; *Cognitive Level:* Application

Reference: Lewis, S., Heitkemper, M., Dirksen, S., O'Brien, P., & Bucher, L. (2007). *Medical-Surgical Nursing: Assessment and Management of Clinical Problems* (7th ed., pp. 1089–1090). St. Louis, MO: Mosby/Elsevier.

EBP Reference: Siegel, J., Rhinehart, E., Jackson, M., & Chiarello, L. (2007). *Guideline for Isolation Precautions: Preventing Transmission of Infectious Agents in the Health Care Setting*. Available at: www.cdc.gov/ncidod/dhqp/pdf/guidelines/Isolation2007.pdf

---

1762. During a home visit to a client who has just been diagnosed with hepatitis A, a nurse is providing education to prevent the spread of the disease to the client's wife and children. Which information should the nurse provide to the family? SELECT ALL THAT APPLY

1. The client should use strict handwashing after bowel movements.
2. Everyone should avoid eating raw foods for the next 2 weeks.
3. Use hot water when washing all the family's laundry together.
4. Clean the common toilet seat with bleach after each use by the client.
5. The client should avoid kissing his children until symptoms disappear.
6. The client should avoid sexual intercourse with his wife until symptoms subside.

ANSWER: 1, 4

Hepatitis A virus is present in the client's feces for 2 weeks after symptoms appear. Careful handwashing after defecation will prevent the spread of the virus. Private toilet facilities are ideal; however, if there is a common family toilet, it should be wiped with bleach after each use by the infected individual. Bleach kills the virus. The virus is not present on raw foods that have been cleansed, in saliva, or in semen, so there is no reason to avoid kissing and intercourse. The client's laundry should be washed separately from the rest of the family in hot soapy water.

➧ ***Test-taking Tip:*** *Think about how hepatitis A is transmitted. A memory aid to remember the mode of transmission for hepatitis A would be the letter "A," which is for* ***a****nus. This should enable elimination of options 2, 5, and 6.*

Content Area: Adult Health; *Category of Health Alteration:* Infectious Disease; *Integrated Processes:* Teaching and Learning; *Client Need:* Safe and Effective Care Environment/Safety and Infection Control/Home Safety; *Cognitive Level:* Analysis

References: Sommers, M., Johnson, S., & Beery, T. (2007). *Diseases and Disorders: A Nursing Therapeutics Manual* (3rd ed., p. 415). Philadelphia: F.A. Davis; Lewis, S., Heitkemper, M., Dirksen, S., O'Brien, P., & Bucher, L. (2007). *Medical-Surgical Nursing: Assessment and Management of Clinical Problems* (7th ed., pp. 1089–1090). St. Louis, MO: Mosby/Elsevier.

1763. EBP A nurse, admitting a client who has a history of ongoing intravenous drug use, reviews the client's serology report. After considering the serology report, which conclusion by the nurse is correct?

Laboratory Test	Patient Values	Normal Values
HBsAg	Positive	Negative
Anti-HBc IgM	Positive	Negative
Aspartate aminotransferase (AST)	200 units/L	8–38 units/L
Alanine aminotransferase (ALT)	150 units/L	10–35 units/L

1. The client has acute hepatitis B and health-care personnel need to be cautioned to emphasize safe injection practices.
2. The client has had hepatitis B in the past and is currently immune.
3. The client has acute hepatitis A, and contact precautions should be initiated.
4. The client is not currently infected with hepatitis, and no extra precautions are required.

ANSWER: 1

The client most likely has contracted hepatitis B. Immunoglobulin M (IgM), an immunoglobulin in the body, is responsible for the primary immune response. Thus, the presence of IgM indicates an acute infection. In this case the positive anti-HBc IgM plus the positive HBsAg (hepatitis B surface antigen) indicates acute infection with hepatitis B. Elevated alanine aminotransferase (ALT) and aspartate aminotransferase (AST) also indicate liver cell injury and acute infection. The primary modes of transmission of the hepatitis B virus are perinatally, percutaneously, and horizontally by mucosal exposure to infectious blood, blood products, or other body fluids. The Centers for Disease Control and Prevention (CDC) has recommended initiation of standard precautions, with an emphasis on safe injection practices for all clients infected with hepatitis B. There is no indication of immunity to hepatitis B in the laboratory report. The laboratory tests for HBsAg and anti-HBc IgM indicate that the client is being tested for hepatitis B, not A. Anti-HBc IgG subtype is indicative of chronic hepatitis infection. A positive anti-HBc IgM and HBsAg indicates acute infection with hepatitis B.

▶ ***Test-taking Tip:*** *The key laboratory values are the positive HBsAg and anti-HBc IgM. Recognizing that these indicate acute infection and are specific for hepatitis B allows elimination of options 2, 3, and 4.*

Content Area: Adult Health; *Category of Health Alteration:* Infectious Disease; *Integrated Processes:* Nursing Process Analysis; *Client Need:* Physiological Integrity/Reduction of Risk Potential/Laboratory Values; *Cognitive Level:* Analysis

Reference: Lewis, S., Heitkemper, M., Dirksen, S., O'Brien, P., & Bucher, L. (2007). *Medical-Surgical Nursing: Assessment and Management of Clinical Problems* (7th ed., pp. 220, 1089, 1093). St. Louis, MO: Mosby/Elsevier.

EBP Reference: Siegel, J., Rhinehart, E., Jackson, M., & Chiarello, L. (2007). Guideline for isolation precautions: Preventing transmission of infectious agents in the health-care setting. Available at: www.cdc.gov/ncidod/dhqp/pdf/guidelines/Isolation2007.pdf

1764. A nurse recognizes the need for additional teaching when a client, newly diagnosed with acute hepatitis C, says:

1. "I know my liver will be enlarged for several more weeks."
2. "Once my jaundice is gone, I will be cured of my hepatitis C."
3. "I understand that my loss of appetite is related to my disease."
4. "I know my liver function will have to be monitored closely in the future."

ANSWER: 2

The disappearance of jaundice does not mean that the client has totally recovered. The majority of hepatitis C infections result in chronic illness. When the client's jaundice begins fading, that is a sign that the convalescent phase of the disease is beginning. Liver enlargement remains for several weeks after the acute phase has ended. The liver inflammation and accumulation of bilirubin cause nausea and anorexia. Hepatitis C carries a high risk of leading to chronic liver disease. The results of liver function tests will be closely monitored.

▶ ***Test-taking Tip:*** *"Need for more teaching" is a false-response item. Select the incorrect statement.*

Content Area: Adult Health; *Category of Health Alteration:* Infectious Disease; *Integrated Processes:* Nursing Process Evaluation; *Client Need:* Physiological Integrity/Physiological Adaptation/Illness Management; *Cognitive Level:* Analysis

Reference: Lewis, S., Heitkemper, M., Dirksen, S., O'Brien, P., & Bucher, L. (2007). *Medical-Surgical Nursing: Assessment and Management of Clinical Problems* (7th ed., pp. 220, 1091–1092). St. Louis, MO: Mosby/Elsevier.

1765. A client diagnosed with hepatitis is reporting pruritus. Which therapy should a nurse suggest to relieve the client's itching?

1. Hot tub baths
2. Rubbing the skin well after showers with a terry cloth bath towel
3. Cool, moist compresses on the affected areas
4. Using an exfoliating brush to scratch affected areas

ANSWER: 3

Cool baths and cool, moist compresses will cause vasoconstriction and thus provide relief. Hot water will increase blood flow to the area and thus increase the itching. Rubbing and scratching affected skin areas increase skin irritation.

▶ ***Test-taking Tip:*** *Focus on the physiological action of heat and cold application. Knowing that heat increases blood flow should allow elimination of option 1.*

Content Area: Adult Health; *Category of Health Alteration:* Infectious Disease; *Integrated Processes:* Nursing Process Implementation; Teaching and Learning; *Client Need:* Physiological Integrity/Basic Care and Comfort/Nonpharmacological Comfort Interventions; *Cognitive Level:* Application

Reference: Craven, R., & Hirnle, C. (2007). *Fundamentals of Nursing, Human Health and Function* (5th ed., p. 1022). Philadelphia: Lippincott, Williams & Wilkins.

1766. A client is seen in a clinic and diagnosed with giardiasis. The client relates a history of just returning on a flight from El Salvador for a medical mission trip, eating food prepared by local residents at a farewell feast, and hiking into the mountains to reach ill residents during the medical mission. The nurse should conclude that the client most likely contracted the infection from:

1. the necessary vaccinations required to travel in El Salvador.
2. close contact with someone who was ill on the return flight from El Salvador.
3. the hike into the mountains and contact with ill residents.
4. eating food and drinking beverages prepared in El Salvador.

ANSWER: 4

Giardiasis, caused from a parasite that attacks the gastrointestinal system, is contracted through ingesting contaminated food and water in areas where sanitation is suspect. Giardiasis is not transmitted through vaccinations, airborne or physical contact, or vectors.

▶ ***Test-taking Tip:*** *Think of the modes of disease transmission. Recall that giardiasis is transmitted through contaminants.*

Content Area: Adult Health; *Category of Health Alteration:* Infectious Disease; *Integrated Processes:* Nursing Process Analysis; *Client Need:* Physiological Integrity/Physiological Adaptation/Alterations in Body Systems; *Cognitive Level:* Analysis

Reference: Lewis, S., Heitkemper, M., Dirksen, S., O'Brien, P., & Bucher, L. (2007). *Medical-Surgical Nursing: Assessment and Management of Clinical Problems* (7th ed., p. 246). St. Louis, MO: Mosby/Elsevier.

1767. Which prescirption by a health-care provider for a client with diarrhea caused by *Escherichia coli* (*E. coli*) 0157:H7 should the nurse question?

1. Lactated Ringer's IV fluids at 125 mL/hr
2. Oral hydration solution (Rehydralyte®) prn
3. Loperamide (Imodium®) 2 mg after each loose stool
4. Bedrest

ANSWER: 3

Loperamide is an antidiarrheal agent that suppresses bowel activity and fluid secretion into the intestinal lumen. Antidiarrheal agents are contraindicated in the treatment of infectious diarrhea because they potentially prolong exposure to the infectious organism. Parenteral fluids and oral solutions containing glucose and electrolytes are used to replace losses. Decreased activity can ease the discomfort of abdominal cramping.

▶ ***Test-taking Tip:*** *Read the orders carefully and focus on the effects of each order. Consider the effects of antidiarrheal agents and how these can prolong exposure to the infectious organism.*

Content Area: Adult Health; *Category of Health Alteration:* Infectious Disease; *Integrated Processes:* Nursing Process Implementation; Communication and Documentation; *Client Need:* Safe and Effective Care Environment/Safety and Infection Control/Error Prevention; *Cognitive Level:* Analysis

References: Lehne, R. (2007). *Pharmacology for Nursing Care* (6th ed., p. 917). St. Louis, MO: Saunders; Monahan, F., Sands, J., Neighbors, M., Marek, J., & Green, C. (2007). *Phipps' Medical-Surgical Nursing: Health and Illness Perspectives* (8th ed., p. 1242). St. Louis, MO: Mosby/Elsevier.

1768. EBP A nurse is assigned to care for four clients. Which client should a nurse closely observe for development of *Clostridium difficile*?

1. Client A, who is 79 years old, takes prednisone for chronic obstructive pulmonary disease and is taking antibiotics for pneumonia.
2. Client B, who is 44 years old, has AIDS.
3. Client C, who is 60 years old, is taking antibiotics after joint replacement surgery.
4. Client D, who is 20 years old, is taking prednisone for Crohn's disease.

ANSWER: 1

The nurse should closely observe client A for the development of a *C. difficile* infection. Development of *C. difficile* is usually preceded by antibiotics that disrupt normal intestinal flora. Older adult clients and those who are immunosuppressed are most at risk. Prednisone is a glucocorticoid that suppresses immune responses. Client A has more risk factors than the clients in options 2, 3, and 4.

▶ ***Test-taking Tip:*** *Read the question carefully. It is asking for the risk factors for development of C. difficile infection. Count the risk factors in each option before making a selection.*

Content Area: Adult Health; *Category of Health Alteration:* Infectious Disease; *Integrated Processes:* Nursing Process Assessment; *Client Need:* Physiological Integrity/Reduction of Risk Potential/Potential for Alterations in Body Systems; *Cognitive Level:* Analysis

Reference: Smeltzer, S., Bare, B., Hinkle, J., & Cheever, K. (2008). *Brunner & Suddarth's Textbook of Medical-Surgical Nursing* (11th ed., p. 2482). Philadelphia: Lippincott Williams & Wilkins.

EBP Reference: Centers for Disease Control and Prevention (CDC). (2008). *Clostridium difficile* Symposium—*Changing Diagnosis, Epidemiology, and Treatment.* Available at: www.cdc.gov/ncidod/dhqp/id_Cdiff.html

1769. EBP A student nurse is caring for a client with a *Clostridium difficile* infection. Which observation made by a registered nurse indicates that the student needs additional information about this disease?

1. Wearing gloves during a physical assessment
2. Entering the room without first putting on a mask
3. Performing frequent hand hygiene with an alcohol-based hand disinfectant
4. Wearing a gown while providing perineal care

ANSWER: 3

According to Centers for Disease Control guidelines, alcohol-based products may not be as effective against C. difficile bacteria as soap and water. Contact isolation is required with this infection; however, wearing a mask in the room is not necessary.

Test-taking Tip: *"Needs more information" is a false-response item. Look for the incorrect statement. Read each option carefully, and consider that C. difficile is a spore-forming microorganism.*

Content Area: Adult Health; *Category of Health Alteration:* Infectious Disease; *Integrated Processes:* Nursing Process Evaluation; *Client Need:* Safe and Effective Care Environment/Management of Care/Supervision; *Cognitive Level:* Analysis

Reference: Smeltzer, S., Bare, B., Hinkle, J., & Cheever, K. (2008). *Brunner & Suddarth's Textbook of Medical-Surgical Nursing* (11th ed., p. 2482). Philadelphia: Lippincott Williams & Wilkins.

EBP Reference: Centers for Disease Control and Prevention (CDC). (2007). *Guideline for Isolation Precautions: Preventing Transmission of Infectious Agents in Healthcare Settings*. Available at: www.cdc.gov/ncidod/dhqp/gl_isolation.html

1770. EBP A client being seen in a walk-in clinic for acute vomiting and diarrhea is diagnosed with a norovirus infection. Which instruction should a nurse include when teaching the client?

1. "Once the symptoms subside, usually in 2 to 3 days, you can return to work and resume usual activities."
2. "The virus continues to be present in the stool for as long as 2 to 3 weeks after you feel better; strict handwashing after using the bathroom and before handling food items is important."
3. "Wash soiled clothing immediately in very hot water to destroy the virus."
4. "Because the virus is also transmitted by respiratory droplets, be sure to wear a mask when in contact with others."

ANSWER: 2

Because the virus is highly contagious and continues to be present in the stool for as long as 2 to 3 weeks, measures must be taken to ensure that the person does not infect others. The Centers for Disease Control and Prevention (CDC) recommends *not* working and avoiding handling or preparing food for others until 2 or 3 days after the person feels better. Washing soiled clothing immediately can reduce the transmission of the virus, but the virus can withstand environmental extremes of heat or cold and are resistant to chemical disinfection. The virus is not transmitted by respiratory droplets, droplets from a violent emesis can be transmitted to water, objects, or surfaces where others can pick up the virus when placing their hands in their mouths. Contact precautions should be used in a health-care setting.

Test-taking Tip: *The client's symptoms are cues to the correct option. Eliminate options that are inconsistent with the client's symptoms.*

Content Area: Adult Health; *Category of Health Alteration:* Infectious Disease; *Integrated Processes:* Teaching and Learning; *Client Need:* Physiological Integrity/Physiological Adaptation/Illness Management; *Cognitive Level:* Analysis

Reference: Smeltzer, S., Bare, B., Hinkle, J., & Cheever, K. (2008). *Brunner & Suddarth's Textbook of Medical-Surgical Nursing* (11th ed., pp. 2501–2502). Philadelphia: Lippincott Williams & Wilkins.

EBP Reference: Centers for Disease Control and Prevention (CDC). (2006). *Norovirus in Healthcare Facilities Fact Sheet.* Available at: www.cdc.gov/ncidod/dhqp/id_norovirusFS.html

1771. A charge nurse on a medical unit is admitting a client diagnosed with meningococcal meningitis. Which room and precautions should the nurse plan for this client?

1. A private room with droplet precautions.
2. A private room with airborne precautions.
3. A semiprivate room with a roommate with a similar diagnosis and standard precautions
4. A semi-private room with a roommate with a similar diagnosis and contact precautions

ANSWER: 2

Meningococcal meningitis is transmitted by contact with pharyngeal secretions and may be airborne. Droplet, standard, or contact precautions alone are insufficient precautions.

▸ ***Test-taking Tip:*** *Recall that meningococcal meningitis is a highly infectious disease. Thus, eliminate options 3 and 4. Of the remaining options, select the option that would provide the most protection.*

Content Area: Adult Health; *Category of Health Alteration:* Infectious Disease; *Integrated Processes:* Nursing Process Planning; *Client Need:* Safe and Effective Care Environment/Management of Care/Concepts of Management; *Cognitive Level:* Analysis

Reference: Smeltzer, S., Bare, B., Hinkle, J., & Cheever, K. (2008). *Brunner & Suddarth's Textbook of Medical-Surgical Nursing* (11th ed., p. 2477). Philadelphia: Lippincott Williams & Wilkins.

1772. EBP A staff nurse has new-onset cough, fever, and a sore throat. The nurse learns of influenza type A exposure from another staff nurse who was diagnosed with influenza 2 days ago. Which recommendation by an occupational health nurse is best?

1. "Immediately make a clinic appointment and request a nasal swab. Oseltamivir (Tamiflu®) can be administered at the onset of symptoms to halt viral replication."
2. "Because you are contagious, you need to use droplet precautions and take sick leave for the next 5 days or so until your symptoms resolve."
3. "Since you had the influenza vaccine, you are not contagious, but you should take sick leave and stay home until you are well."
4. "Go home, take an antipyretic such as acetaminophen (Tylenol®), drink plenty of fluids, and rest. The influenza will likely run its course in 24 to 72 hours."

ANSWER: 1

Influenza type A is highly contagious. Oseltamivir is a new antiviral drug that halts viral proliferation. Because it only halts virus replication, it should be taken at the first signs of illness. Commercial rapid diagnostic tests, collected via nasal swab or other method, are available that can detect influenza viruses within 30 minutes. Although taking sick leave until symptoms abate is correct, having a nasal swab completed is best. The vaccine protects against various known strains of the influenza virus; it does not protect against new mutations of the influenza virus. An antipyretic, fluids, and rest help to alleviate the symptoms, but the individual will be contagious for about 5 days after symptoms appear.

▸ ***Test-taking Tip:*** *The key word is "best," indicating that more than one option could be a correct statement, but one option is better than the other option. Consider that confirming the diagnosis is best.*

Content Area: Adult Health; *Category of Health Alteration:* Infectious Disease; *Integrated Processes:* Nursing Process Implementation; *Client Need:* Physiological Integrity/Physiological Adaptation/Illness Management; *Cognitive Level:* Analysis

Reference: Pillitteri, A. (2007). *Maternal & Child Health Nursing: Care of the Childbearing & Childrearing Family* (5th ed., p. 1257). Philadelphia: Lippincott Williams & Wilkins.

EBP Reference: Fiore, A., Shay, D., Broder, K., Iskander, J., Uyeki, T., et al. (2008). Prevention and control of influenza. Recommendations of the Advisory Committee on Immunization Practices (ACIP). *MMWR*, 57(RR-7), 1–60. Available at: www.guideline.gov/summary/summary.aspx?doc_id=12969&nbr=6678&ss=6&xl=999

1773. EBP Which nursing diagnosis should a nurse add to the plan of care for a client diagnosed with Lyme disease?

1. Imbalanced nutrition: less than body requirements related to diarrhea
2. Disturbed sleep patterns related to hyperalert state
3. Impaired skin integrity related to pruritus
4. Acute pain: joint and muscle related to inflammation

ANSWER: 4

Lyme disease is a spirochetal infection transmitted by the bite of an infected deer tick. Localized erythema occurs at the site of the tick bite 2 to 30 days after exposure and is accompanied by acute viral-like symptoms, including joint and muscle pain. Diarrhea, hyperalertness, and pruritus are not associated with Lyme disease.

▸ ***Test-taking Tip:*** *An understanding of Lyme disease is needed to answer this question. Recall that it is caused by a bite of an infected deer tick.*

Content Area: Adult Health; *Category of Health Alteration:* Infectious Disease; *Integrated Processes:* Nursing Process Analysis; *Client Need:* Physiological Integrity/Physiological Adaptation/Alterations in Body Systems; *Cognitive Level:* Analysis

Reference: Lewis, S., Heitkemper, M., Dirksen, S., O'Brien, P., & Bucher, L. (2007). *Medical-Surgical Nursing: Assessment and Management of Clinical Problems* (7th ed., p. 1714). St. Louis, MO: Mosby/Elsevier.

EBP Reference: Halperin, J., Shapiro, E., Logigian, E., Belman, A., Dotevall, L., et al. (2007). *Practice Parameter: Treatment of Nervous System Lyme Disease (an Evidence-Based Review).* Available at: www.guideline.gov/summary/summary.aspx?doc_id=10858&nbr=005671&string=Lyme+AND+disease

1774. After receiving multiple mosquito bites and experiencing flu-like symptoms, a client consults a nurse at a clinic and asks whether an appointment to see a health-care provider is necessary. Which statement should be the basis for the nurse's response?

1. Antiviral medications can be prescribed to destroy the virus.
2. Clinical signs can be mild flu-like symptoms to fatal encephalitis.
3. If the client has West Nile virus, symptoms will progressively worsen.
4. If the client used insect repellent, the virus would have been destroyed when the mosquito made skin contact.

ANSWER: 2

Clinical signs can be mild flu-like symptoms to fatal encephalitis. The client should be assessed for signs and symptoms of neurological involvement. There is no specific medication to treat an arboviral infection. Cases of West Nile virus can be mild to severe. The insect repellent repels the mosquito and has no effect if the mosquito is infected with the virus.

▶ ***Test-taking Tip:*** *Look for key words in the options, such as "destroy," and eliminate these options.*

Content Area: Adult Health; *Category of Health Alteration:* Infectious Disease; *Integrated Processes:* Caring; *Client Need:* Physiological Integrity/Physiological Adaptation/Illness Management; *Cognitive Level:* Application

References: Smeltzer, S., Bare, B., Hinkle, J., & Cheever, K. (2008). *Brunner & Suddarth's Textbook of Medical-Surgical Nursing* (11th ed., pp. 2274–2275). Philadelphia: Lippincott Williams & Wilkins; Stanhope, M., & Lancaster, J. (2008). *Public Health Nursing: Population-Centered Health Care in the Community* (7th ed., p. 870). St. Louis, MO: Mosby/Elsevier.

1775. EBP A new registered nurse is caring for a client diagnosed with a vancomycin-resistant enterococci (VRE) infection. Which statement to the client indicates the new nurse needs additional orientation when caring for clients diagnosed with a VRE infection?

1. "All hospital personnel should be wearing gown and gloves when they enter your room."
2. "Your visitors should wash their hands well before entering and leaving your room."
3. "You are in a private room because VRE is transmitted via direct or indirect contact."
4. "VRE is a new pathogenic strain of the enterococci microbes normally found in the GI tract."

ANSWER: 1

Gowns are required only if contamination of clothing is likely. Handwashing or hand hygiene is the first line of defense in preventing VRE transmission. A private room is required for infection control. VRE can remain viable on environmental surfaces for weeks, thus room surfaces are disinfected daily and after client discharge. Enterococci genetically mutate and develop antibiotic resistance by producing enzymes that destroy or inactivate the drugs.

▶ ***Test-taking Tip:*** *"Needs further teaching" is a false-response item. Look for the incorrect statement.*

Content Area: Adult Health; *Category of Health Alteration:* Infectious Disease; *Integrated Processes:* Teaching and Learning; *Client Need:* Safe and Effective Care Environment/Safety and Infection Control/Standard/Transmission-based/Precautions/Surgical Asepsis; *Cognitive Level:* Application

Reference: Black, J., & Hokanson Hawks, J. (2009). *Medical-Surgical Nursing: Clinical Management for Positive Outcomes* (8th ed., p. 331). St. Louis, MO: Saunders/Elsevier.

EBP Reference: Siegel, J., Rhinehart, E., Jackson, M., & Chiarellos, L. (2006). *Management of Multidrug-Resistant Organisms in Healthcare Settings, 2006.* Centers for Disease Control and Prevention (CDC). Available at: www.cdc.gov/ncidod/dhqp/pdf/ar/mdroGuideline2006.pdf

1776. A nurse is reviewing the nursing care plan for a client hospitalized with methicillin-resistant *Staphylococcus aureus* (MRSA) infection. Which nursing diagnosis written in the plan should be the nurse's priority?

1. Hyperthermia
2. Social isolation
3. Ineffective coping
4. Risk for deficient fluid volume

ANSWER: 1

Hyperthermia is a physiological need related to the infection and manifested by increased body temperature and increased heart and respiratory rate. Social isolation is a psychosocial need that could be related to the client being placed in MRSA isolation precautions. Ineffective coping is a psychosocial need that could be related to the client's diagnosis and being placed in MRSA isolation precautions. Risk for deficient fluid volume is a potential physiological need related to the loss of fluids from increased metabolic rate, diaphoresis, and decreased oral intake.

➧ *Test-taking Tip: Focus on the key word "priority." According to Maslow's Hierarchy of Needs theory, physiological needs are the priority, followed by safety, then psychosocial needs. Select option 1 because it is the only actual physiological need. Option 4 is a potential physiological need.*

Content Area: Adult Health; *Category of Health Alteration:* Infectious Disease; *Integrated Processes:* Nursing Process Planning; *Client Need:* Physiological Integrity/Physiological Adaptation/Illness Management; *Cognitive Level:* Application

Reference: Lewis, S., Heitkemper, M., Dirksen, S., O'Brien, P., & Bucher, L. (2007). *Medical-Surgical Nursing: Assessment and Management of Clinical Problems* (7th ed., p. 246). St. Louis, MO: Mosby/Elsevier.

1777. EBP An adult client is to receive a booster vaccination for tetanus. Which nursing explanation is correct? "The tetanus vaccination provides:

1. artificial passive immunity through antibodies in the injection that were produced by another."
2. artificial active immunity by injecting a small amount of tetanus antigen, and then your body builds antibodies against tetanus."
3. natural active immunity by exposing you to tetanus in the injection, and then your body builds antibodies against tetanus."
4. natural passive immunity since antibodies were already present, but more were given in the injection to keep you from acquiring tetanus."

ANSWER: 2

The tetanus vaccination provides artificial active immunity by producing antibodies against tetanus. This type of immunity is used to prevent infections or illnesses that have serious consequences, such as tetanus, diphtheria, and polio. Artificial passive immunity is temporary and used if the person is exposed to tetanus. It can also be used for exposure to other serious diseases against which little or no actively acquired immunity exists, such as rabies and poisonous snake bites. Natural active immunity develops when the antigen enters the body without human assistance, and the body responds by actively making antibodies. Antibodies are passed from the mother to the fetus via the placenta or to an infant through breast milk.

➧ *Test-taking Tip: Use the process of elimination. Eliminate options 3 and 4 because they include the word "natural" (entering the body without human assistance). Then eliminate option 1, knowing that passive immunity lasts only days or a few weeks.*

Content Area: Adult Health; *Category of Health Alteration:* Infectious Disease; *Integrated Processes:* Nursing Process Implementation; *Client Need:* Health Promotion and Maintenance/Health and Wellness; *Cognitive Level:* Application

Reference: Ignatavicius, D., & Workman, M. (2006). *Medical-Surgical Nursing: Critical Thinking for Collaborative Care* (5th ed., pp. 372–373). St. Louis, MO: Elsevier/Saunders.

EBP Reference: Kretsinger, K., Broder, K., Cortese, M., Joyce, M., Ortega-Sanchez, I., et al. (2006). Preventing tetanus, diphtheria, and pertussis among adults: Use of tetanus toxoid, reduced diphtheria toxoid and acellular pertussis vaccine. *MMWR*, 55 (No. RR-17). Available at: www.cdc.gov/mmwr/preview/mmwrhtml/rr5517a1.htm

---

1778. EBP An infection control nurse receives confirmation from a hospital laboratory that a client has sputum cultures positive for *Mycobacterium tuberculosis*. According to guidelines issued from the Centers for Disease Control and Prevention (CDC), this is a reportable disease. Which action should be taken by the nurse?

1. Issue a press release to the local news agency.
2. Eliminate health-care workers who have negative tuberculin skin tests from caring for this client.
3. Implement measures to notify the local or state health department of the case.
4. Notify the nearest infectious disease facility and prepare to transfer the client so treatment can be initiated.

ANSWER: 3

The infection control nurse must notify the local or state health department of the case. States mandate which diseases are reportable, and surveillance is managed through local and state health departments. An official report does not involve the local news media. Airborne precautions should already be in place, controlling the risk for transmission of tuberculosis to health-care workers, including those with negative tuberculin tests. Clients diagnosed with respiratory tuberculosis receive treatment in hospitals, clinics, and at home with specific antibiotic and antitubercular medications. Specific tertiary facilities for treatment of clients with tuberculosis are no longer utilized in the United States.

➧ *Test-taking Tip: Read the stem carefully and note that the question calls for a definite requirement to report the disease. Select option 3 because the health departments operate under the guidelines of the CDC.*

Content Area: Adult Health; *Category of Health Alteration:* Infectious Disease; *Integrated Processes:* Nursing Process Analysis; *Client Need:* Safe and Effective Care Environment/Safety and Infection Control/Standard/Transmission-based/Precautions/Surgical Asepsis; *Cognitive Level:* Application

Reference: Craven, R., & Hirnle, C. (2009). *Fundamentals of Nursing: Human Health and Function* (6th ed., pp. 470–472). Philadelphia: Lippincott Williams & Wilkins.

EBP References: Jensen, P., Lambert, L., Iademarco, M., & Ridzon, R. (2005). Guidelines for preventing the transmission of *Mycobacterium tuberculosis* in health-care settings. *MMWR*, 54(17), 1–141; Centers for Disease Control and Prevention. (2009). *Nationally Notifiable Infectious Diseases.* Available at: www.cdc.gov/ncphi/disss/nndss/phs/infdis2009.htm

---

1779. EBP A normally healthy client has a 5-mm skin induration 72 hours after receiving a tuberculin skin test. Which conclusions should the nurse make regarding the test results?

1. This is negative for a normally healthy person.
2. This indicates that active tuberculosis is present and treatment is needed.
3. This is inconclusive, and a chest x-ray is needed to detect active tuberculosis (TB).
4. This is inaccurate because the assessment was done too long after the injection.

ANSWER: 1

An area of induration measuring 15 mm in diameter or greater in a person with no known risk factors for TB and read 48 to 72 hours after injection is a positive TB test. An induration of 5 mm or greater would be a positive result in HIV-infected persons. A positive test indicates exposure to TB. The result is negative for TB rather than inconclusive. Evidence-based practice guidelines indicate that a reading at 72 hours is more accurate than one at 48 hours.

▶ ***Test-taking Tip:*** *Note the key phrase "normally healthy" in both the stem and option 1.*

Content Area: Adult Health; *Category of Health Alteration:* Infectious Disease; *Integrated Processes:* Nursing Process Analysis; *Client Need:* Health Promotion and Maintenance/Health Screening; *Cognitive Level:* Analysis

Reference: Black, J., & Hokanson Hawks, J. (2009). *Medical-Surgical Nursing: Clinical Management for Positive Outcomes* (8th ed., pp. 1605–1606). St. Louis, MO: Saunders/Elsevier.

EBP Reference: Centers for Disease Control and Prevention (CDC). (2007). *Mantoux Tuberculosis Skin Test Facilitator Guide.* Available at: www.cdc.gov/tb/pubs/Mantoux/part2.htm

---

1780. A client who has been sick for several days is being seen in a clinic with a tentative diagnosis of mononucleosis. Which findings should a nurse expect when assessing the client?

1. Weakness, loss of appetite, and extreme constipation
2. Fever, an enlarged spleen, and a rash similar to chickenpox
3. White coating on the throat and depressed lymphocyte levels
4. Extreme fatigue and enlarged lymph nodes in the neck and axilla

ANSWER: 4

During the first 3 days, extreme fatigue, loss of appetite, and chills are present. Then severe reddened sore throat and tonsils with a white coating, high fever, headache, diarrhea, and generalized lymphadenopathy occur. Diarrhea, not constipation, would be present. The spleen enlarges 50% of the time. Occasionally, a rash appears that is similar to measles. Lymphocyte levels would be elevated.

▶ ***Test-taking Tip:*** *Note the key word "expect," and use the process of elimination.*

Content Area: Adult Health; *Category of Health Alteration:* Infectious Disease; *Integrated Processes:* Nursing Process Assessment; *Client Need:* Physiological Integrity/Physiological Adaptation/Alterations in Body Systems; *Cognitive Level:* Application

Reference: Black, J., & Hokanson Hawks, J. (2009). *Medical-Surgical Nursing: Clinical Management for Positive Outcomes* (8th ed., pp. 2030–2031). St. Louis, MO: Saunders/Elsevier.

1781. EBP A nursing student approaches an instructor following a needlestick to the finger from a needle used for an injection with a known HIV-positive client. Which instructor statement is most accurate?

1. Postexposure prophylaxis will need to be started within 1 to 2 hours.
2. HIV antibody testing will need to be done in 6 weeks and then again in 3 months.
3. At the end of the clinical shift, you should make an appointment to see your health-care provider.
4. Flush immediately with water for 10 minutes and cover with a bandage and glove.

ANSWER: 1

Occupational exposure is an urgent medical concern, and medical care should be sought immediately. Prophylactic treatment is started immediately (preferably within 1 to 2 hours) and lasts for 4 weeks. If results of HIV antibody testing returns positive, treatment continues. HIV antibody testing should be completed at baseline, 6 weeks, 3 months, and 6 months after exposure. The exposure site should be washed with soap and water. Flushing with water is required for mucous membrane exposure.

▶ ***Test-taking Tip:*** *Apply disease prevention principles. The only option that will prevent developing the disease is option 1.*

Content Area: Adult Health; *Category of Health Alteration:* Infectious Disease; *Integrated Processes:* Nursing Process Implementation; *Client Need:* Physiological Integrity/Physiological Adaptation/Medical Emergencies; *Cognitive Level:* Analysis

Reference: Black, J., & Hokanson Hawks, J. (2009). *Medical-Surgical Nursing: Clinical Management for Positive Outcomes* (8th ed., p. 2094). St. Louis, MO: Saunders/Elsevier.

EBP Reference: Panlilio, A., Cardo, D., Grohskopf, L., Heneine, W., & Ross, C. (2005). Updated U.S. Public Health Service guidelines for the management of occupational exposures to HIV and recommendations for postexposure prophylaxis. *MMWR*, 54(RR09), 1–17. Available at: www.cdc.gov/mmwr/preview/mmwrhtml/rr5409a1.htm

1782. A client is diagnosed with *Pneumocystis carinii* pneumonia (PCP) secondary to AIDS. Upon assessment for the specific symptoms of PCP, the nurse should expect to find:

1. dyspnea, fever, nonproductive cough, and fatigue.
2. weight loss, night sweats, persistent diarrhea, and hypothermia.
3. dysphagia, yellow-white plaques in the mouth, and sore throat.
4. lung crackles, chest pain, and small, painless purple-blue skin lesions.

ANSWER: 1

PCP is caused by a fungus that produces these symptoms. It is the most common opportunistic infection in HIV/AIDS. Weight loss, night sweats, persistent diarrhea are symptoms of AIDS; hypothermia is not. Dysphagia, yellow-white plaques in the mouth, and sore throat are symptoms of *Candida albicans*. Although PCP could cause lung crackles and chest pain, the skin lesions are found with Kaposi's sarcoma.

➧ ***Test-taking Tip:*** *Focus on the key phrase "specific symptoms of PCP." Look for specific symptoms characteristic of the respiratory system. Eliminate options 2, 3, and 4 because these are not specific to PCP.*

Content Area: Adult Health; *Category of Health Alteration:* Infectious Disease; *Integrated Processes:* Nursing Process Assessment; *Client Need:* Physiological Integrity/Physiological Adaptation/Alterations in Body Systems; *Cognitive Level:* Application

Reference: Black, J., & Hokanson Hawks, J. (2009). *Medical-Surgical Nursing: Clinical Management for Positive Outcomes* (8th ed., pp. 2103, 2106–2107). St. Louis, MO: Saunders/Elsevier.

1783. A client diagnosed with HIV, has a CD4-positive T-lymphocyte count of 160 μL. A nurse evaluates that interventions have been most effective when which outcome is achieved?

1. Soft formed stools daily
2. Skin integrity nonintact
3. Free of opportunistic diseases
4. Current weight maintained or gaining weight

ANSWER: 3

The CD4-positive T-lymphocyte count is low, increasing the client's risk for bacterial, fungal, and viral infections as well as for opportunistic cancers and infections. Interventions have been effective if the client does not develop an infection. Option 1 is an outcome for *altered elimination*. Option 2 is not a desired outcome. Option 4 is an outcome for *altered nutrition: less than body requirements*.

➧ ***Test-taking Tip:*** *Use the knowledge that the client has a depressed immune system. If unsure, focus on the phrase "T-lymphocyte count." Then, after noting the key words "evaluates" and "most effective," select option 3.*

Content Area: Adult Health; *Category of Health Alteration:* Infectious Disease; *Integrated Processes:* Nursing Process Evaluation; *Client Need:* Physiological Integrity/Physiological Adaptation/Illness Management; *Cognitive Level:* Analysis

Reference: Ignatavicius, D., & Workman, M. (2006). *Medical-Surgical Nursing: Critical Thinking for Collaborative Care* (5th ed., pp. 425, 437, 444–445). St. Louis, MO: Elsevier/Saunders.

1784. A nurse is planning care for a client being admitted with newly diagnosed active tuberculosis (TB) secondary to AIDS? Which intervention is most important for the nurse to plan?

1. Monitor for signs of bleeding.
2. Teach strategies for skin care.
3. Institute airborne precautions.
4. Assess CD4 and T-lymphocyte counts.

ANSWER: 3

Active TB can be transmitted by airborne droplet nuclei smaller than 5 microns. The client should be in a private room with negative air pressure and 6 to 12 air exchanges per hour. Persons entering the room should wear a N95 respirator. The client should wear a surgical mask when transported out of the room. The client may be at risk for bleeding due to the effects of antiretroviral therapy, but the situation does not note whether or not the client is receiving treatment. Teaching is important, but not the most important. Although it is important to determine the level of immunodeficiency because the client is at risk for infection, initiating airborne precautions is the most important to prevent transmission of TB.

➧ ***Test-taking Tip:*** *Focus on the client's condition of TB and the key phrase "most important." Select option 3, knowing that TB is transmitted by airborne droplets.*

Content Area: Adult Health; *Category of Health Alteration:* Infectious Disease; *Integrated Processes:* Nursing Process Planning; *Client Need:* Physiological Integrity/Physiological Adaptation/Illness Management; *Cognitive Level:* Application

Reference: Black, J., & Hokanson Hawks, J. (2009). *Medical-Surgical Nursing: Clinical Management for Positive Outcomes* (8th ed., p. 1607). St. Louis, MO: Saunders/Elsevier.

1785. A nurse is teaching a client and the family members about protection measures when the client, diagnosed with AIDS, returns home. Which instruction indicates that the nurse is unclear about the disease transmission?

1. "Disinfect items in your home, using a bleach solution of 1 part bleach to 10 parts of water."
2. "Dispose of contaminated items, except sharps, by placing them in a plastic bag then in the garbage."
3. "Use separate dishes and silverware and wash them with soap and water or place them in the dishwasher."
4. "Wearing gloves, clean body fluid spills with soap and water, and then disinfect the area with bleach solution."

ANSWER: 3

Because sharing eating utensils does not transmit HIV, it is unnecessary to separately wash dishes and silverware used by the client. The client is prone to opportunistic and other infections. This is the required amount for mixing a bleach solution for disinfection. Placing contaminated items in a plastic bag then in the garbage is the correct method for disposing of contaminated articles. Sharps should be placed in a rigid labeled container (such as a tin can), bleach solution added, the lid taped, and then placed in a bag for disposal in the garbage. Cleaning with soap and water and then disinfecting with bleach solution is the correct method for cleaning body fluid spills.

Test-taking Tip: *Note the key word "unclear." Look for the incorrect instruction. Remember that HIV is not transmitted by kissing, hugging, shaking hands, or sharing eating utensils, towels, or bathroom fixtures with an HIV-positive person.*

Content Area: Adult Health; *Category of Health Alteration:* Infectious Disease; *Integrated Processes:* Nursing Process Evaluation; *Client Need:* Safe and Effective Care Environment/Safety and Infection Control/Home Safety; *Cognitive Level:* Application

Reference: Black, J., & Hokanson Hawks, J. (2009). *Medical-Surgical Nursing: Clinical Management for Positive Outcomes* (8th ed., pp. 2093–2095). St. Louis, MO: Saunders/Elsevier.

Test 47: **Medical Emergencies**

1786. A nurse is triaging clients in an emergency department. Which client should be assigned as the highest priority?

1. A 16-year-old client with a severe sunburn injury that is blistering
2. A 55-year-old client experiencing dyspnea, diaphoresis, and chest pain
3. A 40-year-old client with a leg laceration that appears to need stitches
4. A 19-year-old college student who has headaches, diplopia, and a temperature of 102.8°F (39.3°C)

ANSWER: 2

According to the five-level Emergency Severity Index (ESI), clients with chest pain, multiple trauma (unless responsive), child with fever and lethargy, and disruptive psychiatric clients are classified as threatened and are level 2 priority. Level 1 priorities include clients with cardiac arrest, intubated trauma, severe overdose, or SIDS. The clients with a blistering sunburn, leg laceration, and neurological symptoms would be level 3 priorities.

➧ ***Test-taking Tip:*** *Use the ABCs (airway, breathing, circulation) to determine priority. Select the client with a threat to breathing and circulation.*

Content Area: Adult Health; *Category of Health Alteration:* Medical Emergencies; *Integrated Processes:* Nursing Process Implementation; *Client Need:* Safe and Effective Care Environment/Management of Care/Establishing Priorities; *Cognitive Level:* Application

Reference: Lewis, S., Heitkemper, M., Dirksen, S., O'Brien, P., & Bucher, L. (2007). *Medical-Surgical Nursing: Assessment and Management of Clinical Problems* (7th ed., p. 1822). St. Louis, MO: Mosby/Elsevier.

1787. An adult client experiencing diabetic ketoacidosis has been admitted to an emergency department. Which interventions should a nurse initiate immediately? SELECT ALL THAT APPLY.

1. Administer oxygen.
2. Administer D5W with 0.9% NaCl solution after establishing an intravenous (IV) access.
3. Initiate a regular insulin infusion.
4. Determine the time and amount of the last insulin injection.
5. Administer potassium and magnesium to correct electrolyte imbalances.
6. Assess the client's breath for the presence of ketones.

ANSWER: 1, 3, 4

Diabetic ketoacidosis is characterized by hyperglycemia (usually above 300 mg/dL), ketosis, acidosis, and dehydration. Airway management with oxygen administration is necessary. Regular insulin infusion is initiated to lower the client's blood glucose levels. Determining the time and amount of the last insulin injection is needed to ascertain the initial starting dose of the insulin infusion. The initial IV solution is 0.9% NaCl. Once glucose levels approach 250 mg/dL (13.9 mmol/L), 5% dextrose is added. Although electrolyte imbalances occur due to the loss of electrolytes from hyperglycemic diuresis, laboratory assessment of the client's serum values should be completed first. Assessing the breath odor is an assessment not an intervention.

➧ ***Test-taking Tip:*** *Note the key words, "interventions" and "immediately." Eliminate options that are assessments and those that should not be initiated immediately.*

Content Area: Adult Health; *Category of Health Alteration:* Medical Emergencies; *Integrated Processes:* Nursing Process Implementation; *Client Need:* Physiological Integrity/Physiological Adaptation/Medical Emergencies; *Cognitive Level:* Analysis

Reference: Lewis, S., Heitkemper, M., Dirksen, S., O'Brien, P., & Bucher, L. (2007). *Medical-Surgical Nursing: Assessment and Management of Clinical Problems* (7th ed., pp. 1278–1280). St. Louis, MO: Mosby/Elsevier.

1788. Which assessment findings should indicate to a nurse that an adult client experiencing an acute asthma attack warrants urgent medical intervention with an inhaled beta-2 agonist? SELECT ALL THAT APPLY.

1. Respiratory rate (RR) of 32 breaths per minute
2. Pulsus paradoxus
3. Wheezes heard on chest auscultation
4. Client speaking in short sentences to indicate need for oxygen
5. Oxygen saturation 94%
6. Heart rate (HR) 122 beats per minute

ANSWER: 1, 2, 3, 6

The increased RR is the body's attempt to increase oxygen intake. Pulsus paradoxus is a greater than 10 mm Hg drop in systolic blood pressure (BP) or weakening of the pulse during inspiration. It occurs in asthma because of the high negative intrathoracic pressure that increases venous return and right ventricular filling. Consequently, the interventricular septum bulges slightly into the left ventricular outflow tract, decreasing cardiac output and thus BP. Wheezes are expiratory sounds from forced airflow through abnormally collapsed airways with residual air trapping. HR increases to compensate for the decreased oxygenation and pulsus paradoxus. Dyspneic persons speak in words not sentences. An oxygen saturation of 94% correlates with a PaO_2 of 70% (normal PaO_2 is 70%–100%).

➧ ***Test-taking Tip:*** *Select the options that suggest inadequate oxygenation.*

Content Area: Adult Health; *Category of Health Alteration:* Medical Emergencies; *Integrated Processes:* Nursing Process Assessment; *Client Need:* Physiological Integrity/Physiological Adaptation/Medical Emergencies; *Cognitive Level:* Analysis

References: Lewis, S., Heitkemper, M., Dirksen, S., O'Brien, P., & Bucher, L. (2007). *Medical-Surgical Nursing: Assessment and Management of Clinical Problems* (7th ed., pp. 515, 626). St. Louis, MO: Mosby/Elsevier; Merck & Co. (2007). *The Merck Manual's Online Medical Library: The Merck Manual for Medical Professionals.* Whitehouse Station, NJ: Author. Available at: www.merck.com/mmpe/sec07/ch069/ch069a.html

---

1789. An explosion occurred at a nearby factory at 1800 hours. An emergency department charge nurse receives a call from the emergency management systems (EMS) personnel that 35 clients will be transported to the hospital within 10 minutes by ambulance. These clients were triaged at the scene as red and yellow according to the NATO mass casualty categories; others will be coming, and the unit is already short-staffed. Which action should the nurse initiate first?

1. Activate the hospital's emergency response plan.
2. Contact the emergency department nursing director.
3. Notify other emergency nurses of the need for extra help.
4. Call a nearby hospital to determine if 15 clients could be rerouted.

ANSWER: 1

Every health-care facility is required by the Joint Commission to have a plan in place for emergency preparedness. The activation response defines where, how, and when the response should be initiated. Individuals triaged as red have injuries that are life threatening but survivable with minimal intervention. Yellow priority indicates injuries are significant and require medical care, but can wait hours without threat to life. The nursing director would be notified as part of the emergency response plan. The emergency response plan needs to include plans for people and staff management and for coordinated patient care into and out of the facility, including transfers to other facilities. The nurse receiving the call does not call for extra staff or make the determination to reroute clients.

Test-taking Tip: *Consider that emergency response plans are broad and that contacting the director, requesting extra help, and the decision to reroute clients are included in the emergency response plan. Thus, eliminate options 2, 3, and 4.*

Content Area: Adult Health; *Category of Health Alteration:* Medical Emergencies; *Integrated Processes:* Nursing Process Implementation; *Client Need:* Safe and Effective Care Environment/Safety and Infection Control/Emergency Response Plan; Safe and Effective Care Environment/Management of Care/Establishing Priorities; *Cognitive Level:* Application

References: Lewis, S., Heitkemper, M., Dirksen, S., O'Brien, P., & Bucher, L. (2007). *Medical-Surgical Nursing: Assessment and Management of Clinical Problems* (7th ed., p. 1842). St. Louis, MO: Mosby/Elsevier; Smeltzer, S., Bare, B., Hinkle, J., & Cheever, K. (2008). *Brunner & Suddarth's Textbook of Medical-Surgical Nursing* (11th ed., pp. 2560–2562). Philadelphia: Lippincott Williams & Wilkins.

1790. A nurse working in a military hospital's emergency department receives a call that an unknown number of clients have been exposed to a nerve agent during a terrorist attack on a government center. Which medication should the nurse prepare to have readily available in sufficient quantities to treat the clients?

1. Atropine sulfate
2. Labetalol (Trandate®)
3. Dopamine (Intropin®)
4. Phentolamine (Regitine®)

ANSWER: 1

Nerve agents bond with acetylcholinesterase, causing hyperstimulation of the nerve endings. Symptoms are similar to those associated with cholinergic crisis, including bradycardia, copious secretions, and other respiratory, neurological, gastrointestinal, urinary, and visual symptoms. Atropine increases the heart rate and dries secretions. Labetalol is a beta-adrenergic blocking agent that will decrease the heart rate. Dopamine is a vasopressor used to treat cardiac output and increase the blood pressure. Phentolamine is an alpha-adrenergic receptor blocker that will produce hypotension. Phentolamine is administered subcutaneously to treat dopamine extravasation.

Test-taking Tip: *Use the process of elimination, and eliminate medications that will lower the heart rate or blood pressure.*

Content Area: Adult Health; *Category of Health Alteration:* Medical Emergencies; *Integrated Processes:* Nursing Process Planning; *Client Need:* Physiological Integrity/Physiological Adaptation/Medical Emergencies; *Cognitive Level:* Analysis

Reference: Smeltzer, S., Bare, B., Hinkle, J., & Cheever, K. (2008). *Brunner & Suddarth's Textbook of Medical-Surgical Nursing* (11th ed., pp. 2570–2571). Philadelphia: Lippincott Williams & Wilkins.

1791. Five families of clients injured in an apartment fire have arrived at an emergency department to inquire about the health status of their family members. Which is the nurse's best action?

1. Take the families to the triage area so they can be with their loved ones
2. Ask the families to wait in the waiting area until information is available
3. Ensure that there is a designated area for family staffed by available social workers or clergy
4. Direct families to a lounge where a receptionist will be keeping families informed

ANSWER: 3

Families should be in a designated area where social service workers, counselors, therapists, or clergy are available for support. Family members may be feeling intense anxiety, shock, or grief and should be provided with information and updates as soon as possible. Families should not be in the triage or treatment areas to protect the privacy of other clients and to prevent congestion or interference with treatment measures. Support systems would be unavailable in a waiting area or in a lounge.

▶ ***Test-taking Tip:*** *Think about the support families will need in coping with disaster-related injuries or death, and select the option that would provide the families with the most support.*

Content Area: Adult Health; *Category of Health Alteration:* Medical Emergencies; *Integrated Processes:* Nursing Process Implementation; *Client Need:* Psychosocial Integrity/Crisis Intervention; *Cognitive Level:* Application

Reference: Smeltzer, S., Bare, B., Hinkle, J., & Cheever, K. (2008). *Brunner & Suddarth's Textbook of Medical-Surgical Nursing* (11th ed., pp. 2562–2563). Philadelphia: Lippincott Williams & Wilkins.

1792. Which injured client of a mass casualty disaster should a triage nurse in an emergency department establish as the priority client?

1. An unresponsive client with a penetrating head injury.
2. A partially responsive client with a sucking chest wound.
3. A client with a maxilla fracture and facial wounds without airway compromise.
4. A client with third-degree burns over 65% of the body surface area.

ANSWER: 2

A sucking chest wound is a life-threatening but survivable emergency. The client would be triaged as priority 1 (red) according to the NATO triage system. The unresponsive client with a penetrating head injury and the severely burned client have a limited potential for survival, even with definitive care, and would be categorized as a priority 4 level (black). The client with the facial wounds would be classified as priority 2 (yellow) because injuries are significant and require medical care, but can wait hours without threat to life.

▶ ***Test-taking Tip:*** *Use prioritization according to the ABCs (airway, breathing, circulation) and principles of mass casualty disasters. Recall that clients with minimal chance of survival would be the last priority in disaster situations.*

Content Area: Adult Health; *Category of Health Alteration:* Medical Emergencies; *Integrated Processes:* Nursing Process Analysis; *Client Need:* Safe and Effective Care Environment/Management of Care/Establishing Priorities; *Cognitive Level:* Application

Reference: Smeltzer, S., Bare, B., Hinkle, J., & Cheever, K. (2008). *Brunner & Suddarth's Textbook of Medical-Surgical Nursing* (11th ed., p. 2562). Philadelphia: Lippincott Williams & Wilkins.

1793. A health-care provider (HCP) writes orders to transfuse a unit of red blood cells (RBCs) to a client admitted to an emergency department after a disaster. A nurse is completing the compatibility checks between the client's blood type, noted to be blood type B-positive, and the illustrated unit of blood, which had been donated by the client's spouse and obtained from the blood bank. Which clinical judgment by the nurse preparing to administer the unit of blood is correct?

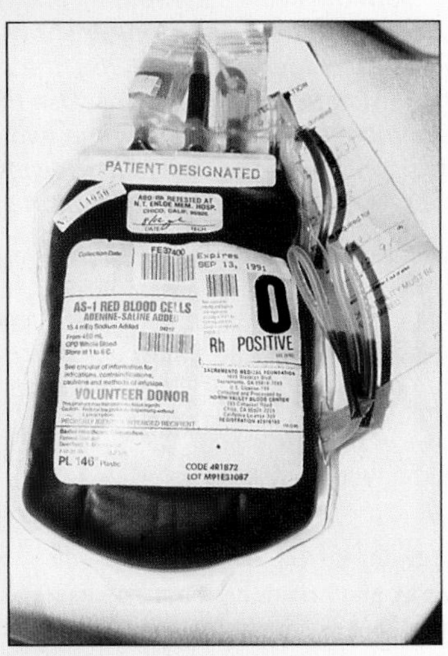

1. The unit of blood is of a different blood type but compatible with the client's blood.
2. The unit of blood is of a different blood type and incompatible with the client's blood.
3. The unit of blood is not the blood component that the HCP prescribed for the client.
4. The unit of blood will cause a hemolytic transfusion reaction and cannot be administered to the client.

ANSWER: 1

Type O blood is compatible for persons with type A, B, or AB blood because it does not have an antigen on the erythrocyte (RBC). A person with type O blood is considered a universal donor. The Rh positive indicates that the Rhesus antigen is present on the cell, whereas Rh negative indicates that the Rh factor is not present. Rh-positive RBCs can only be administered to persons who are Rh positive, whereas Rh-negative RBCs can be administered to persons who are Rh positive or Rh negative. Although the client and spouse have different blood types, the RBCs are compatible. The unit of blood states that it is red blood cells (RBCs). A hemolytic transfusion reaction will occur if there are ABO or Rh incompatibilities.

➧ ***Test-taking Tip:*** *Knowledge of blood administration and blood compatibilities is expected on the NCLEX-RN® exam. Recall that type O blood is the universal donor for RBCs, whereas type AB blood is the universal donor for plasma.*

Content Area: Adult Health; *Category of Health Alteration:* Medical Emergencies; *Integrated Processes:* Nursing Process Evaluation; *Client Need:* Physiological Integrity/Pharmacological and Parenteral Therapies/Blood and Blood Products; *Cognitive Level:* Analysis

Reference: Berman, A., Snyder, S., Kozier, B., & Erb, G. (2008). *Kozier & Erb's Fundamentals of Nursing: Concepts, Process, and Practice* (8th ed., pp. 1472–1473). Upper Saddle River, NJ: Pearson Education.

1794. During resuscitation efforts in an emergency department, the spouse of a trauma victim tells a nurse that her husband has terminal cancer, has completed an advance health care directive (HCD), and does not want cardiopulmonary resuscitation (CPR). What should be the nurse's next action?

1. Contact medical records to see if the client's HCD is on file.
2. In honor of the client's wishes, stop the actions of the resuscitation team.
3. Document the spouse's statement in the client's medical record.
4. Inform the health-care provider (HCP) in charge of the resuscitation team.

ANSWER: 4

A HCP must order whether to withhold or terminate CPR even if it is specified in a client's HCD. Depending on the situation and status of the client, the HCP may want to review the HCD, but this is not the next action because it delays a decision. Even if the client requests no CPR, a HCP's order is required to carry out the request. The spouse's statements should be documented, but this is not the next action.

➧ ***Test-taking Tip:*** *Note the key phrase "next action." Prioritization is required.*

Content Area: Adult Health; *Category of Health Alteration:* Medical Emergencies; *Integrated Processes:* Nursing Process Implementation; *Client Need:* Safe and Effective Care Environment/Management of Care/Advance Directives; *Cognitive Level:* Application

Reference: Lewis, S., Heitkemper, M., Dirksen, S., O'Brien, P., & Bucher, L. (2007). *Medical-Surgical Nursing: Assessment and Management of Clinical Problems* (7th ed., pp. 155–156). St. Louis, MO: Mosby/Elsevier.

1795. An adult client taking warfarin (Coumadin®) for treatment of atrial fibrillation presents to an emergency department complaining of weakness and fatigue. The client's skin is pale and diaphoretic, and the blood pressure is 85/58 mm Hg. When the client is attached to a cardiac monitor, the client's rhythm is atrial flutter with a ventricular rate of 140 beats per minute. A nurse should expect to initiate health-care provider's orders to treat:

1. noncoronary cardiogenic shock.
2. coronary cardiogenic shock.
3. hypovolemic shock.
4. neurogenic shock.

ANSWER: 1

Cardiogenic shock occurs as a result of inadequate supply of oxygen to the heart and tissues due to the heart's inability to contract and pump blood. Noncoronary cardiogenic shock results from conditions that stress the myocardium or result in ineffective myocardial function, such as dysrhythmias. Coronary cardiogenic shock occurs when there is significant damage to the left ventricle such as from an anterior wall myocardial infarction. Though the client is taking warfarin, which can cause bleeding and hypovolemic shock from a decrease in intravascular volume, bleeding is not reported. In neurogenic shock, vasodilatation occurs from a loss of balance between parasympathetic and sympathetic stimulation.

➧ ***Test-taking Tip:*** *Both the client's symptoms and the options suggest shock. Because the cardiac monitor shows a change in rhythm and there is no evidence of bleeding, the shock is likely cardiac in origin. Eliminate options 3 and 4. Use the word "coronary" to eliminate one of the remaining two options. The coronary vessels supply blood to the heart. Because atrial flutter does not involve vessels, eliminate option 2.*

Content Area: Adult Health; *Category of Health Alteration:* Medical Emergencies; *Integrated Processes:* Nursing Process Analysis; *Client Need:* Physiological Integrity/Physiological Adaptation/Medical Emergencies; *Cognitive Level:* Analysis

Reference: Smeltzer, S., Bare, B., Hinkle, J., & Cheever, K. (2008). *Brunner & Suddarth's Textbook of Medical-Surgical Nursing* (11th ed., pp. 366–371). Philadelphia: Lippincott Williams & Wilkins.

1796. A client is admitted to an emergency department with multiple injuries from a motor vehicle accident. A nurse sees that the client's head had been immobilized at the scene. Prioritize the nurse's management of the client during admission to the emergency department.

______ Control hemorrhage.
______ Evaluate for head and neck injuries and other injuries.
______ Splint fractures.
______ Prevent and treat hypovolemic shock.
______ Carry out a more thorough examination.
______ Establish airway patency and ventilation.

ANSWER: 2, 4, 5, 3, 6, 1

The priority is airway and breathing. First establish the airway and maintain ventilation. Next is circulation: control hemorrhage with direct pressure. Third, prevent and treat hypovolemic shock with intravenous fluids and monitor the urine output, all essential components of circulation. Next is disability: assess for head and neck injuries, evaluate for other injuries, and reassess head and neck. Identify deformities and splint fractures, and finally complete the secondary survey, which is a more thorough examination.

➧ ***Test-taking Tip:*** *Use ABCD (airway, breathing, circulation, disability) primary survey method and then complete the secondary survey.*

Content Area: Adult Health; *Category of Health Alteration:* Medical Emergencies; *Integrated Processes:* Nursing Process Implementation; *Client Need:* Safe and Effective Care Environment/Management of Care/Establishing Priorities; *Cognitive Level:* Analysis

References: Lewis, S., Heitkemper, M., Dirksen, S., O'Brien, P., & Bucher, L. (2007). *Medical-Surgical Nursing: Assessment and Management of Clinical Problems* (7th ed., pp. 1823–1826). St. Louis, MO: Mosby/Elsevier; Smeltzer, S., Bare, B., Hinkle, J., & Cheever, K. (2008). *Brunner & Suddarth's Textbook of Medical-Surgical Nursing* (11th ed., pp. 2530–2531). Philadelphia: Lippincott Williams & Wilkins.

1797. EBP A client's wife is allowed to be present during resuscitation efforts for a client in an intensive care unit. Which statement made by a nurse is most correct and appropriate?

1. "You can hold your loved one's hand; sometimes a recovering person remembers that touch."
2. "Another staff member will be with you; I will show you where you can stand near your husband."
3. "Because the resuscitation team needs to work quickly, you need to stay out of their way and not interfere."
4. "If the resuscitation efforts fail, the health-care provider will ask you if you want to terminate resuscitation efforts."

ANSWER: 2

Family members allowed to be present during resuscitation efforts should have a support person with them who is able to answer family member questions and explain expected outcomes of treatment and procedures. Touching the client is unsafe. If a shock is delivered and another person is touching the client or bed, that person will also receive a shock. Telling the wife to stay out of the way and not interfere is insensitive. While the HCP may ask the wife regarding terminating efforts should efforts fail, it is insensitive to present a preconceived idea of failure.

➧ ***Test-taking Tip:*** *Consider the need of family members for support during resuscitation efforts.*

Content Area: Adult Health; *Category of Health Alteration:* Medical Emergencies; *Integrated Processes:* Caring; *Client Need:* Physiological Integrity/Physiological Adaptation/Medical Emergencies; *Cognitive Level:* Analysis

Reference: Smeltzer, S., Bare, B., Hinkle, J., & Cheever, K. (2008). *Brunner & Suddarth's Textbook of Medical-Surgical Nursing* (11th ed., p. 971). Philadelphia: Lippincott Williams & Wilkins.

EBP Reference: American Heart Association. (2005). American Heart Association guidelines for cardiopulmonary resuscitation and emergency cardiovascular care, Part 2: Ethical issues. *Circulation,* 112(Suppl I), IV-6-IV-11. Available at: www.circ.ahajournals.org/cgi/content/full/112/24_suppl/IV-6

1798. EBP Two nurses are performing cardiopulmonary resuscitation (CPR) on an adult client. A nurse performing chest compressions is on the right side of the client, and a nurse performing rescue breathing is on the left side of the client. The nurse performing rescue breathing checks the client's pulse to determine if the nurse's compressions are perfusing. Place an X at the location at which the nurse should check the client's pulse.

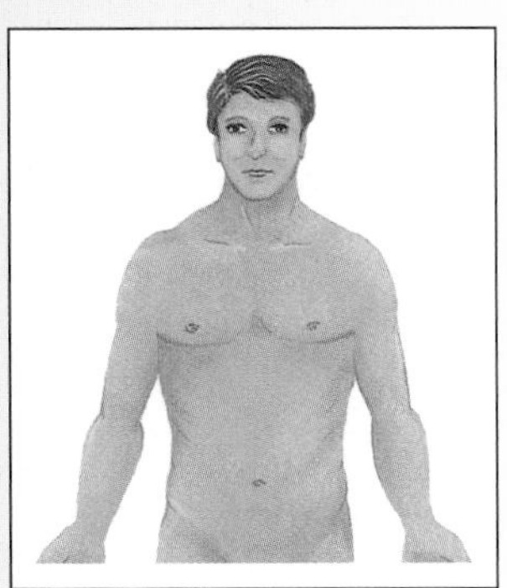

ANSWER:

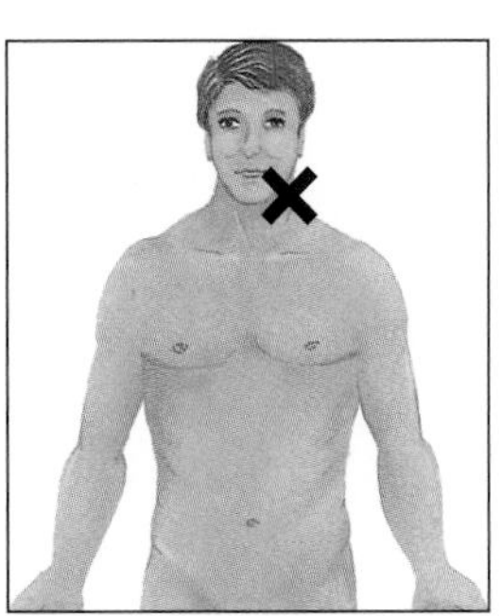

The person performing rescue breathing is on the left, thus the client's left carotid pulse should be checked.

➧ ***Test-taking Tip:*** *Read the scenario carefully to determine where each nurse is located in relation to the client.*

Content Area: Adult Health; *Category of Health Alteration:* Medical Emergencies; *Integrated Processes:* Nursing Process Implementation; *Client Need:* Physiological Integrity/Physiological Adaptation/Medical Emergencies; *Cognitive Level:* Application

Reference: Smeltzer, S., Bare, B., Hinkle, J., & Cheever, K. (2008). *Brunner & Suddarth's Textbook of Medical-Surgical Nursing* (11th ed., pp. 970–971). Philadelphia: Lippincott Williams & Wilkins.

EBP Reference: American Heart Association. (2005). American Heart Association guidelines for cardiopulmonary resuscitation and emergency cardiovascular care. Part 4: Adult health basic life support. *Circulation,* (112), IV-19-IV-34. Available at: www.circ.ahajournals.org/cgi/content/full/112/24_suppl/IV-19

1799. Members of a resuscitation team have arrived at a client's bedside with a defibrillator. A nurse and a nursing assistant are performing cardiopulmonary resuscitation (CPR). What should be the nurse's next action?

1. Stop CPR to apply the conduction pads and analyze the rhythm.
2. Complete a full minute of CPR, then apply the conduction pads and analyze the rhythm.
3. Continue with CPR while the resuscitation team is applying the conduction pads and analyzing the rhythm.
4. Continue with rescue breathing while the resuscitation team is applying the conduction pads.

ANSWER: 4

Rescue breathing should continue until the resuscitation team is ready to analyze the rhythm. The client should not be touched while the rhythm is being interpreted. Rescue breathing can continue; defibrillator pads are placed on the chest or one on the chest and one on the back. Continuing with CPR can delay defibrillation. Every minute that defibrillation is delayed worsens the prognosis. The rhythm cannot be accurately analyzed while CPR is performed.

Test-taking Tip: *Visualize the steps in performing CPR to select the correct option.*

Content Area: Adult Health; *Category of Health Alteration:* Medical Emergencies; *Integrated Processes:* Nursing Process Implementation; *Client Need:* Physiological Integrity/Physiological Adaptation/Medical Emergencies; *Cognitive Level:* Application

Reference: Smeltzer, S., Bare, B., Hinkle, J., & Cheever, K. (2008). *Brunner & Suddarth's Textbook of Medical-Surgical Nursing* (11th ed., pp. 842–843). Philadelphia: Lippincott Williams & Wilkins.

1800. EBP An emergency department nurse is treating a client who presented with hands that are hard, cold, white in appearance, and insensitive to touch. A supervising charge nurse determines that a new nurse is safely able to care for the client when the nurse is noted to: SELECT ALL THAT APPLY

1. massage the client's hands initially to increase circulation.
2. place both of the client's hands in warm water for 30 to 40 minutes.
3. place the client's hands in a dependent position after rewarming to increase circulation.
4. administer an analgesic.
5. wrap the hands tightly after rewarming to retain the heat.
6. encourage active motion of the digits after rewarming.

ANSWER: 2, 4, 6

The findings suggest frostbite. Safe care includes controlled rewarming with warm water immersion and pain control with an analgesic; the rewarming process can be very painful. Active motion promotes maximal restoration of function and helps to prevent contractures. Massage is contraindicated because it increases tissue trauma. Hands should be elevated to prevent edema. Hands are not wrapped; blebs may develop within an hour to a few days. Sterile gauze or cotton is placed between the fingers to prevent maceration.

Test-taking Tip: *Focus on the client's symptoms to select the correct actions.*

Content Area: Adult Health; *Category of Health Alteration:* Medical Emergencies; *Integrated Processes:* Nursing Process Evaluation; *Client Need:* Physiological Integrity/Physiological Adaptation/Medical Emergencies; *Cognitive Level:* Analysis

Reference: Smeltzer, S., Bare, B., Hinkle, J., & Cheever, K. (2008). *Brunner & Suddarth's Textbook of Medical-Surgical Nursing* (11th ed., p. 2539). Philadelphia: Lippincott Williams & Wilkins.

EBP Reference: International Consensus Conference on Cardiopulmonary Resuscitation and Emergency Cardiovascular Care Science with Treatment Recommendations. (2005). First aid. *Circulation*, 112(22 Suppl), III115-25. Available at: www.guideline.gov/summary/summary.aspx? doc_id= 8487&nbr= 004738&string=frostbite.

1801. Five hours after attending a family reunion picnic, three members of a family are admitted to an emergency department with nausea, vomiting, and abdominal cramping. A nurse asks a series of questions as part of the admission assessment. Which should be the nurse's priority question?

1. "How many people were at the reunion?"
2. "What food was served at the reunion?"
3. "Was anyone sick when they came to the reunion?"
4. "What is the relationship of the family members who are sick?"

ANSWER: 2

Nausea, vomiting, and abdominal cramping are classic symptoms of food poisoning with staphylococcal bacteria, which can develop between 30 minutes to 7 hours after ingesting infected food. Knowing how many people were at the reunion may alert the nurse to the potential number of other clients who may develop the same symptoms, but this is not priority. Inquiring about any family member who may have been sick before coming to the reunion might provide information on other sources of the symptoms, as would knowing the relationship of the sick clients.

Test-taking Tip: *Read the situation carefully noting that this is a reunion picnic. Select the only option that relates to food.*

Content Area: Adult Health; *Category of Health Alteration:* Medical Emergencies; *Integrated Processes:* Nursing Process Assessment; *Client Need:* Physiological Integrity/Physiological Adaptation/Medical Emergencies; *Cognitive Level:* Application

Reference: Lewis, S., Heitkemper, M., Dirksen, S., O'Brien, P., & Bucher, L. (2007). *Medical-Surgical Nursing: Assessment and Management of Clinical Problems* (7th ed., pp. 1031–1032). St. Louis, MO: Mosby/Elsevier.

1802. EBP A client is admitted to an emergency department with facial bruises, a broken arm, and rib fractures. The client states she fell down the stairs. During assessment, a nurse notes bruises and lacerations in various stages of healing. Which nursing questions are appropriate? SELECT ALL THAT APPLY.

1. "I noticed you have more bruises. Can you tell me how they happened?"
2. "Has anyone hurt you?"
3. "Have you been falling down a lot lately?"
4. "Have you had any fainting spells or times that you have been weak?"
5. "Are you afraid of anyone at home?"
6. "Why haven't you reported that you have been abused?"

ANSWER: 1, 2, 3, 4, 5

The possibility of abuse should be explored with all women and whenever a person presents with multiples injures in various stages of healing. Questions in options 1, 2, and 5 explore abuse. Neurological alterations, such as transient ischemic attacks, can also result in falls. Questions in options 3 and 4 explore other causes for falling. Asking why the client has not reported abuse is insensitive and presumptuous.

Test-taking Tip: *The key phrase is "various stages of healing." Focus on assessment questions that will help determine the cause of the injuries.*

Content Area: Adult Health; *Category of Health Alteration:* Medical Emergencies; *Integrated Processes:* Communication and Documentation; *Client Need:* Physiological Integrity/Physiological Adaptation/Medical Emergencies; *Cognitive Level:* Application

Reference: Lewis, S., Heitkemper, M., Dirksen, S., O'Brien, P., & Bucher, L. (2007). *Medical-Surgical Nursing: Assessment and Management of Clinical Problems* (7th ed., pp. 2550–2551). St. Louis, MO: Mosby/Elsevier.

EBP Reference: Institute for Clinical Systems Improvement (2006). Domestic violence. Available at: www.guideline.gov/summary/summary.aspx?doc_id=9862&nbr=005286&string=assault

1803. An nurse in an emergency department is admitting an agitated young adult who tried to jump from a bridge after taking a hallucinogenic drug at a party. What should be the nurse's *initial* action?

1. Administer medications to reverse the effects of the hallucinogenic drug.
2. Call the mental health unit to arrange for inpatient treatment.
3. Call security to be present to protect the staff from injury.
4. Stay with the client to protect the client from self-harm until relieved.

ANSWER: 4

Hallucinogenic drugs alter perception; the client should not be left unattended. There are no reversal agents for hallucinogenic drugs. Medications can be administered to decrease agitation. Inpatient treatment may be prescribed, but this is not the initial action. Though agitated, there isn't evidence of violence against others, but the potential exists.

Test-taking Tip: *Note that three options are similar and one is different.*

Content Area: Adult Health; *Category of Health Alteration:* Medical Emergencies; *Integrated Processes:* Nursing Process Implementation; *Client Need:* Physiological Integrity/Physiological Adaptation/Medical Emergencies; *Cognitive Level:* Application

Reference: Ignatavicius, D., & Workman, M. (2006). *Medical-Surgical Nursing: Critical Thinking for Collaborative Care* (5th ed., p. 95). St. Louis, MO: Elsevier/Saunders.

1804. A client has been hospitalized for 48 hours for treatment of symptoms related to chronic obstructive pulmonary disease. Which findings, noted on assessment, should prompt a nurse to implement interventions for alcohol withdrawal? SELECT ALL THAT APPLY.

1. Tremors
2. Reports seeing a bear on the ceiling
3. Inability to recognize familiar objects
4. Disoriented to time and place
5. Decreased blood pressure
6. Bradycardia

ANSWER: 1, 2, 3, 4

Life-threatening alcohol withdrawal is characterized by delirium tremens (tremors and jerky movements), hallucinations, inability to recognize familiar objects or people, disorientation, or global confusion. An increased blood pressure and tachycardia are other findings (not hypotension and bradycardia).

Test-taking Tip: *The key phrase is "alcohol withdrawal." If uncertain, select options related to the neurological system.*

Content Area: Adult Health; *Category of Health Alteration:* Medical Emergencies; *Integrated Processes:* Nursing Process Assessment; *Client Need:* Physiological Integrity/Physiological Adaptation/Medical Emergencies; *Cognitive Level:* Analysis

Reference: Ignatavicius, D., & Workman, M. (2006). *Medical-Surgical Nursing: Critical Thinking for Collaborative Care* (5th ed., pp. 100–101). St. Louis, MO: Elsevier/Saunders.

1805. A young woman presents to an emergency department with palpitations, tachycardia, diaphoresis, chest pain, a feeling of choking, and paresthesias. The woman acknowledges a fear of closed spaces where it is difficult to escape and feelings of "impending doom." Suspecting that the woman is experiencing a panic attack, a nurse should:

1. notify a health-care provider (HCP) to obtain an order for an antianxiety medication.
2. place the client in a treatment room closest to the nurse's station where she can be observed.
3. involve the client in some physical activity to divert her attention from her anxiety.
4. remain with the client and talk her through slow deep-breathing.

ANSWER: 4

To ensure safety, the nurse should stay with the client. Slow deep-breathing may distract the client from focusing on the anxiety. Medication may be needed to control the panic attacks, but client safety is priority. Near a busy nursing station is too stimulating and can increase the state of panic. Physical activity is too stimulating and should be avoided during a panic attack. A calm, controlled environment is needed.

➧ ***Test-taking Tip:*** *The key word is "best," indicating that more than one option is appropriate in a panic situation but one is priority.*

Content Area: Adult Health; *Category of Health Alteration:* Medical Emergencies; *Integrated Processes:* Nursing Process Implementation; *Client Need:* Physiological Integrity/Physiological Adaptation/Medical Emergencies; *Cognitive Level:* Analysis

Reference: Fortinash, K., & Holoday Worret, P. (2008). *Psychiatric Mental Health Nursing* (4th ed., pp. 182–183, 189–190). St. Louis, MO: Mosby/Elsevier.

1806. Four clients present to an emergency department at the same time. Which client should a nurse assess first?

1. An intoxicated 30-year-old who fell and needs stitches for an arm laceration
2. A distraught 45-year-old known cocaine abuser who states he plans to kill himself with the gun he is carrying
3. A 22-year-old who states she was raped but feels guilty because she "may have brought it on herself."
4. An 18-year-old who sustained second-degree hand burns while trying to hide evidence of a methamphetamine lab

ANSWER: 2

The distraught client is at risk for life-threatening harm to himself and others. Depression and suicidal gestures can occur during cocaine withdrawal. Although all other clients need medical attention, none have injuries that are life-threatening.

➧ ***Test-taking Tip:*** *Select the option that poses a life-threatening risk.*

Content Area: Adult Health; *Category of Health Alteration:* Medical Emergencies; *Integrated Processes:* Nursing Process Assessment; *Client Need:* Safe and Effective Care Environment/Management of Care/Establishing Priorities; *Cognitive Level:* Analysis

Reference: Ignatavicius, D., & Workman, M. (2006). *Medical-Surgical Nursing: Critical Thinking for Collaborative Care* (5th ed., p. 95). St. Louis, MO: Elsevier/Saunders.

1807. A multiparous woman in her 42nd week of gestation is experiencing contractions upon her arrival at an emergency department. A nurse determines that the woman is in the second stage of labor. Which nursing action is most important?

1. Transfer the woman to the delivery room.
2. Time the frequency of contractions.
3. Notify a health-care provider (HCP) and prepare for delivery.
4. Check the fetal heart rate.

ANSWER: 3

The nurse should notify a HCP and prepare for delivery. In the second stage of labor, the cervix is fully dilated and 100% effaced, and the infant descends into the birth canal and may crown. Birth may be imminent, and the woman should not be transferred. Timing contractions and checking fetal heart rate are not primary responsibilities at this time. The primary responsibility in the second stage of labor is to support the infant's head and apply slight pressure to control the delivery.

➧ ***Test-taking Tip:*** *Use the nursing process to determine the correct answer option.*

Content Area: Childbearing Families; *Category of Health Alteration:* Medical Emergencies; *Integrated Processes:* Nursing Process Implementation; *Client Need:* Physiological Integrity/Physiological Adaptation/Medical Emergencies; *Cognitive Level:* Analysis

Reference: Pillitteri, A. (2007). *Maternal & Child Health Nursing: Care of the Childbearing & Childrearing Family* (5th ed., pp. 505–506). Philadelphia: Lippincott Williams & Wilkins.

1808. A nurse is admitting a pregnant woman brought in by her friend to an emergency department. Her friend states the woman has been using crystal methamphetamine for the last 3 days and is now "tweaking" (unable to get high anymore). The woman is thrashing about, is agitated, and is becoming violent. Which nursing actions should a nurse plan in the care of the woman? SELECT ALL THAT APPLY.

1. Keep a 7- to 10-foot distance during questioning.
2. Ask nonthreatening questions in a soft tone.
3. Place a fetal monitor on the woman.
4. Keep hands visible where the woman can see them.
5. Call for security.
6. Restrain the woman so she can be examined.

ANSWER: 1, 2, 4

The nurse should keep a safe distance and keep hands visible at all times. Individuals in this state are often paranoid, and that can lead to violence. Individuals in this state often turn violent when they are quiet, indicating that the paranoid thoughts may be taking over the normal thought processes. Do not attempt to touch the woman in any way initially. Placing a fetal monitor or restraining her may cause the woman's behavior to escalate.

▶ ***Test-taking Tip:*** *Think about what interventions could decrease paranoid or violent behaviors.*

Content Area: Childbearing Families; *Category of Health Alteration:* Medical Emergencies; *Integrated Processes:* Nursing Process Planning; *Client Need:* Psychological Integrity/Crisis Interventions; *Cognitive Level:* Analysis

References: Donovan, D., & Wells, E. (2007). "Tweaking 12-Step": The potential role of 12-step self-help group involvement in methamphetamine recovery. *Addiction,* (102 Suppl)1, 121–129; Pillitteri, A. (2007). *Maternal & Child Health Nursing: Care of the Childbearing & Childrearing Family* (5th ed., pp. 480–483). Philadelphia: Lippincott Williams & Wilkins.

1809. A school-aged child is brought to an emergency department by ambulance. The child is minimally responsive, hypotensive, tachycardic, and has a high fever. Orders are written by a health-care provider (HCP). Which order should the nurse initiate *first*?

1. Saline bolus per weight-based protocol
2. Blood cultures times 2
3. Ampicillin (Ampicin®) 25 mg/kg IV q6h
4. Oxygen at 40% FIO_2

ANSWER: 4

The priority is oxygen administration, because hyperthermia increases oxygen demand and the low cardiac output secondary to hypotension decreases the availability of oxygen to tissues. Fluid boluses should then be administered to treat hypotension and increase cardiac output and tissue perfusion. Blood cultures should be drawn prior to the intravenous antibiotics.

▶ ***Test-taking Tip:*** *Use the ABCs (airway, breathing, circulation) and Maslow's Hierarchy of Needs theory to establish priority. Oxygenation is priority; thus select option 4.*

Content Area: Child Health; *Category of Health Alteration:* Medical Emergencies; *Integrated Processes:* Nursing Process Implementation; *Client Need:* Physiological Integrity/Reduction of Risk Potential/Vital Signs; Safe and Effective Care Environment/Management of Care/Establishing Priorities; *Cognitive Level:* Application

Reference: Ball, J., & Bindler, R. (2006). *Clinical Handbook for Pediatric Nursing* (pp. 285–288). Upper Saddle River, NJ: Pearson Education.

1810. A new nurse is caring for an adolescent in the pediatric unit who has injuries secondary to a motor vehicle accident. The nurse has started a blood transfusion. After 30 minutes, the client complains of nausea and a headache. An observing nurse should determine that the new nurse intervened appropriately when the new nurse took which action first?

1. Obtained a set of vital signs
2. Called the primary health-care provider
3. Flushed the infusion tubing with normal saline and restarted the blood
4. Stopped the transfusion

ANSWER: 4

The nurse should immediately stop the transfusion and then take another set of vital signs. The symptoms suggest a transfusion reaction. Obtaining vital signs first will allow additional blood to infuse. Depending on the nurse's findings after data collection, the HCP may be called. If the client is experiencing a transfusion reaction, the line should never be flushed because the client would receive additional blood that is in the tubing.

▶ ***Test-taking Tip:*** *Consider the client's symptoms of nausea and headache. These may or may not suggest a transfusion reaction. Although further assessment is needed, select the option that potentially protects the client from further injury.*

Content Area: Child Health; *Category of Health Alteration:* Medical Emergencies; *Integrated Processes:* Nursing Process Evaluation; *Client Need:* Physiological Integrity/Pharmacological and Parenteral Therapies/Blood and Blood Products; *Cognitive Level:* Analysis

Reference: Ball, J., & Bindler, R. (2008). *Pediatric Nursing: Caring for Children* (4th ed., p. 816). Upper Saddle River, NJ: Prentice Hall.

1811. A nurse is caring for a 2-year-old child who was hit in the head with a softball. The child was stunned after the incident, but had not lost consciousness. On arrival to an emergency department, the toddler is awake and responsive. On exam in one-half hour, the toddler is pale, clammy, and lethargic. Which clinical judgment made by the nurse is correct?

1. This is consistent with the course of a head injury in a pediatric child.
2. The lethargy is most likely due to the toddler being tired and not well hydrated.
3. This is an emergency situation in which a health-care provider needs to be notified immediately.
4. The toddler is arresting; the emergency management system should be activated.

ANSWER: 3

This is an emergency situation. Children are at risk for developing pediatric concussive syndrome. Initially, the injury looks minor, but after minutes or hours the physical status deteriorates drastically. Pale, clammy, and lethargic are not expected signs, nor do they suggest fatigue or poor hydration. A toddler who is arresting would not be breathing or have a pulse.

➧ ***Test-taking Tip:*** *Think about the physiology of a closed head injury with concussion injuries and the fragility of the brain of the infant–toddler.*

Content Area: Child Health; *Category of Health Alteration:* Medical Emergencies; *Integrated Processes:* Nursing Process Analysis; *Client Need:* Physiological Integrity/Physiological Adaptation/Alterations in Body Systems; *Cognitive Level:* Analysis

Reference: Ball, J., & Bindler, R. (2008). *Pediatric Nursing: Caring for Children* (4th ed., p. 1088). Upper Saddle River, NJ: Prentice Hall.

1812. A nurse is working in an emergency department when a 5-year-old child is brought in by ambulance. The child is presenting with shortness of breath, swelling of lips and tongue, is wheezing, and has rhinitis and stridor. The child also has high anxiety and angioedema. The nurse should: SELECT ALL THAT APPLY.

1. put the child in a Trendelenburg's position.
2. administer oxygen.
3. place an intravenous (IV) line.
4. administer epinephrine as prescribed by the health-care provider (HCP).
5. attempt to keep child as calm as possible.
6. administer oral fluids.

ANSWER: 2, 3, 4, 5

The child is most likely presenting with symptoms directly related to anaphylactic shock. Anaphylaxis is a potentially life-threatening systemic reaction to an allergen. Symptoms can occur minutes or up to 2 hours after exposure to the allergen. Interventions are needed to reverse anaphylaxis. Securing the airway and administering oxygen is an initial intervention; the child may require intubation and mechanical ventilation. An IV line is needed for medications that can act quickly. Adrenalin (epinephrine) is an adrenergic (sympathomimetic) agent and cardiac stimulant. Agitation increases oxygen demands. The child should be supine or in the position that is best for optimum ventilation, but not Trendelenburg's position. Legs should be elevated if possible to promote venous return. Fluids may be needed to treat hypotension secondary to vasodilatation and increased vascular permeability but should be delivered by an intravenous route.

➧ ***Test-taking Tip:*** *Use the ABCs (airway, breathing, circulation) to identify interventions that would most quickly reverse anaphylaxis.*

Content Area: Child Health; *Category of Health Alteration:* Medical Emergencies; *Integrated Processes:* Nursing Process Implementation; *Client Need:* Physiologic Integrity/Physiological Adaptation/Medical Emergencies; Physiologic Integrity/Physiological Adaptation/Alterations in Body Systems; *Cognitive Level:* Analysis

Reference: Ball, J., & Bindler, R. (2006). *Clinical Handbook for Pediatric Nursing* (pp. 312–314). Upper Saddle River, NJ: Pearson Education.

1813. Which child, admitted to an emergency department with signs of shock, should a nurse immediately place on latex allergy precautions?

1. A child with spina bifida
2. A child with cardiac anomalies
3. A child with other known allergies
4. A child with a parent who has a latex allergy

ANSWER: 1

An allergy to latex occurs after repeated exposure to latex. Manifestations of reactions to latex can range from redness and blistering to an anaphylactic or systemic option. There is a high prevalence of latex allergy in children with spina bifida, with some sources identifying the prevalence at 80%. This is due to the repeated exposure to latex products during surgeries and numerous catheterizations. Other populations of children most at risk are those who have myelodysplasia and congenital urinary tract anomalies. Only if a child with cardiac anomalies requires frequent surgical procedures would the child be at risk for latex allergy. Though there is a cross-reaction between latex allergy and allergy to a number of foods (banana, kiwi, chestnuts, and avocado), the food allergies should be known before putting a child in latex precautions. There is no evidence supporting the relationship between latex allergy in a parent and subsequently in a child.

➧ ***Test-taking Tip:*** *Focus on the issue: the need for latex allergy precautions.*

Content Area: Child Health; *Category of Health Alteration:* Medical Emergencies; *Integrated Processes:* Nursing Process Implementation; *Client Need:* Physiological Integrity/Reduction of Risk Potential/Potential for Alterations in Body Systems; *Cognitive Level:* Application

Reference: Ball, J., & Bindler, R. (2006). *Clinical Handbook for Pediatric Nursing* (pp. 314–316). Upper Saddle River, NJ: Pearson Education.

1814. EBP A nursing assistant (NA) calls for help after finding an 8-year-old child unresponsive on the floor following a visit with his grandmother in the nursing home. A responding nurse opens the child's airway and attempts rescue breathing while the NA sets up an automated external defibrillator (AED). Which action should the nurse take when observing that the NA has the package of large-sized defibrillator pads opened?

1. Request that the NA hand these to the nurse for application.
2. Ask the NA to open the other package of defibrillator pads.
3. Observe that the NA attaches these correctly to the AED unit.
4. Continue performing CPR until the AED is ready.

ANSWER: 2

The appropriate size defibrillator pads should be used to prevent burning. Depending on the ability of the NA, the nurse might request these to be handed over while the NA continues with rescue breathing until the pads have been applied. The incorrect-sized pads are being selected, so these should not be attached to the AED.

➧ ***Test-taking Tip:*** *Focus on the issue: intervention needed when the adult-sized AED pads are selected for use on a child.*

Content Area: Child Health; *Category of Health Alteration:* Medical Emergencies; *Integrated Processes:* Nursing Process Implementation; *Client Need:* Safe and Effective Care Environment/Safety and Infection Control/Accident or Injury Prevention; *Cognitive Level:* Application

EBP Reference: American Heart Association. (2005). American Heart Association guidelines for cardiopulmonary resuscitation and emergency cardiovascular care: Part 5: Electrical therapies: automated external defibrillators, defibrillation, cardioversion, and pacing. *Circulation,* 112(Suppl I), IV-35-IV-46.

1815. EBP A nurse is performing cardiopulmonary resuscitation (CPR) on a neonate. Which action by the nurse indicates that there is a need for further instruction on performing CPR on a neonate?

1. Performs chest compressions with two thumbs while the fingers encircle the chest
2. Delivers chest compressions on the lower third of the sternum
3. Completes 90 compressions and 30 breaths each minute
4. Lifts the thumbs an inch from the chest between chest compressions

ANSWER: 4

The thumbs should remain on the chest between chest compressions to maintain the correct position. All other actions are correct. Compressions can be performed with two thumbs or with two fingers while a second hand supports the back. Compressions are performed on the lower third of the sternum to a depth of approximately one-third of the anterior-posterior diameter of the chest. A 3:1 ratio of compressions to ventilations, with 90 compressions and 30 breaths to achieve approximately 120 events per minute, is desirable to maximize ventilation at an achievable rate.

➧ ***Test-taking Tip:*** *The phrase "needs further instruction" indicates this is a false-response item. Select the action that is incorrect.*

Content Area: Childbearing Families; *Category of Health Alteration:* Medical Emergencies; *Integrated Processes:* Nursing Process Evaluation; *Client Need:* Physiological Integrity/Physiological Adaptation/Medical Emergencies; *Cognitive Level:* Application

EBP Reference: American Heart Association. (2005). American Heart Association guidelines for cardiopulmonary resuscitation and emergency cardiovascular care: Part 13: Neonatal resuscitation guidelines. *Circulation,* 112(Suppl I), IV-188-IV-195. Available at: www.circ.ahajournals.org/content/vol112/24_suppl/#____AMERICAN_HEART_ASSOCIATION_GUIDELINES_FOR_CARDIOPULMONARY_RESUSCITATION_AND_EMERGENCY_CARDIOVASCULAR_CARE.

1816. A nurse is caring for a child who was pulled from the water after being submersed for 2 minutes. During the day, the child has been alert and oriented and the parents have been staying with the child. At 2200 hours, when beginning an assessment, the nurse has difficulty arousing the child. What should the nurse do *first*?

1. Take a complete set of vital signs and do neurological checks.
2. Call the health-care provider (HCP).
3. Determine if this is the child's normal nighttime behavior.
4. Ask the parent's assistance in rousing the child.

ANSWER: 1

The vital signs and results of the neurological checks are needed to determine the status of the child. A change in neurological status could indicate cerebral edema, which may take up to 12 to 24 hours to develop. Calling the HCP may be an option, but the nursing role is to gather data and then contact the HCP. The child may sleep deeply during the normal time of rest, but for the nurse to assume this could have negative consequences for the child. Asking the parent's assistance in rousing the child may be helpful, but it is more important to complete an independent neurological assessment to determine if the child is developing complications.

➧ ***Test-taking Tip:*** *The key word is "first." Use the steps of the nursing process to determine which nurse action is first. Assessment is the first step of the nursing process.*

Content Area: Child Health; *Category of Health Alteration:* Medical Emergencies; *Integrated Processes:* Nursing Process Implementation; *Client Need:* Physiological Integrity/Reduction of Risk Potential/System Specific Assessments; *Cognitive Level:* Analysis

Reference: Ball, J., & Bindler, R. (2006). *Clinical Handbook for Pediatric Nursing* (pp. 528–529). Upper Saddle River, NJ: Pearson Education.

1817. EBP A nurse working on the pediatric unit takes a call from a parent who is crying. The parent states that her son has just been found with an empty bottle of acetaminophen (Tylenol®). Which should be the nurse's best response?

1. "Let me transfer your call to the emergency department."
2. "Do you have ipecac syrup at home? If so, follow the directions given on the bottle."
3. "Do you have the number for the poison control center?"
4. "How much do you think your child took, and how responsive is he?"

ANSWER: 3

Parents are told to immediately call the local poison control center. The nurse should be ready to provide the number to the parent. The American Academy of Pediatrics no longer recommends that parents keep ipecac in homes. Transferring the call and collecting additional information both waste time and will delay treatment.

▶ ***Test-taking Tip:*** *Identify what is within the scope of nursing practice, and identify the option that best meets the needs of the child in the situation and avoids delay in treatment. Using the process of elimination, discard option 2 because the nurse should not prescribe and options 1 and 4 because these delay treatment.*

Content Area: Child Health; *Category of Health Alteration:* Medical Emergencies; *Integrated Processes:* Communication and Documentation; *Client Need:* Safe and Effective Care Environment/Management of Care/Referrals; *Cognitive Level:* Analysis

Reference: Pillitteri, A. (2007). *Maternal and Child Health Nursing* (5th ed., pp. 1659–1660). Philadelphia: Lippincott Williams & Wilkins.

EBP Reference: Kendrick, D., Coupland, C., Mulvaney, C., Simpson, J., Smith, S., et al. (2007). Home safety education and provision of safety equipment for injury prevention. *Cochrane Database of Systematic Reviews*, Issue 1, Art. No., CD005014. DOI: 10.1002/14651858.CD005014.pub2. Available at: www.mrw.interscience.wiley.com/cochrane/clsysrev/articles/CD005014/frame.html.

1818. A nurse is caring for a 2-year-old toddler who ingested vitamin pills with iron at approximately 0800 hours. The parents brought the child to an emergency department at 1100 hours due to nausea and vomiting, diarrhea, and abdominal pain. The child's vital signs are assessed and documented as illustrated. Based on this information, what should be the nurse's next priority?

Vital Signs

Time	1100	1400	1600	1800	2000
Pulse	130	120	126	118	170
Respiratory Rate	30	28	24	24	40
Blood Pressure	108/58	110/60	100/60	102/56	120/84
Temperature	99.6°F (37.5°C)		99.0°F (37.2°C)		100.6°F (38.1°C)

1. Double-check the vital signs in 1 hour.
2. Obtain the chart and contact the health-care provider (HCP).
3. Recheck the vital signs at the next scheduled time.
4. Ask the parent to try to soothe the child because the child is anxious.

ANSWER: 2

There are 9 hours between the first and last vital sign assessment. Tachycardia and tachypnea are early signs of shock. Between 6 and 12 hours after iron ingestion, there is a potential for hemorrhagic necrosis to occur, with melena and hematemesis occurring by hour 12. If not recognized early, lethargy and coma, cyanosis, and vasomotor collapse result. Rechecking vital signs later (options 1 and 3) will delay interventions to treat impending shock. Although the child may be anxious due to the hospitalization, the extreme change in pulse and respiratory rate, along with the knowledge that the child ingested vitamins with iron, suggest complications, and the HCP should be contacted.

▶ ***Test-taking Tip:*** *Focus on the issue: assessment of a toddler who has ingested iron. Consider the patterns of vital signs in children, early signs of shock, the vulnerability of the child, and the need for accurate and timely assessments when selecting an option.*

Content Area: Child Health; *Category of Health Alteration:* Medical Emergencies; *Integrated Processes:* Nursing Process Analysis; *Client Need:* Physiological Integrity/Physiological Adaptation/Medical Emergencies; *Cognitive Level:* Analysis

References: Pillitteri, A. (2007). *Maternal and Child Health Nursing* (5th ed., pp. 1660–1661). Philadelphia: Lippincott Williams & Wilkins; Ball, J., & Bindler, R. (2006). *Clinical Handbook for Pediatric Nursing* (pp. 154–157). Upper Saddle River, NJ: Pearson Education.

1819. A nurse is auscultating posterior breath sounds in the bases of both lungs of an infant who has undergone a bronchoscopy to remove a foreign body. Which sounds should the nurse anticipate hearing when auscultating the areas illustrated if the lung sounds are normal?

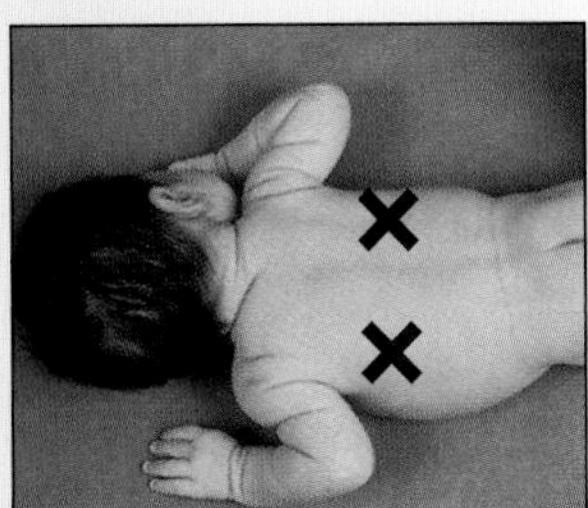

1. Inspiration and expiration (I:E ratio) of equal length
2. Expiration longer than inspiration, with sounds transmitted from the upper airway
3. Inspiration longer than expiration, with sounds transmitted from the upper airway
4. High-pitched sounds with a prolonged inspiration

ANSWER: 3

Vesicular sounds, which have an I:E ratio of 3:1, are heard in the peripheral parts (bases) of an infant's lung fields. Because infants have high body water content and water transmits sound, the upper airway bronchial sounds may also be transmitted. The bronchial sounds can mimic crackles and rhonchi. The I:E ratio of equal length, an I:E ratio of I less than E, and high-pitched sounds are abnormal findings.

➧ ***Test-taking Tip:*** *Consider the findings that would be normal for a young child. Be familiar with normal and abnormal lung sounds for infants and children.*

Content Area: Child Health; *Category of Health Alteration:* Medical Emergencies; *Integrated Processes:* Nursing Process Assessment; *Client Need:* Health Promotion and Maintenance/Techniques of Physical Assessment; *Cognitive Level:* Application

References: Pillitteri, A. (2007). *Maternal and Child Health Nursing* (5th ed., pp. 1004–1005). Philadelphia: Lippincott Williams & Wilkins; Craven, R., & Hirnle, C. (2007). *Fundamentals of Nursing: Human Health and Function* (5th ed., pp. 467–470). Philadelphia: Lippincott Williams & Wilkins.

1820. A nurse is caring for an unresponsive toddler in a pediatric intensive care unit. The child's parent was arrested for alleged child abuse but released on bail. The parent is at the door requesting to visit the child. Which is the most appropriate nursing action?

1. Notify the health-care provider (HCP) to clarify who has access to the child.
2. Allow the parent to enter the room and see the child.
3. Call hospital security.
4. Contact social services.

ANSWER: 3

The nurse's primary responsibility is the safety of the child. If there is not a clear delineation of who should be able to have access to the child, the first thing that must occur is to secure the area by contacting security. The HCP, charge nurse, or social worker may have information about who can access the child, but it is not within their job descriptions to secure the area, thus eliminating options 1 and 4. Without clear orders, the nurse must not allow contact between the parent and child. A report to social services should have already been filed.

➧ ***Test-taking Tip:*** *The key phrase is "most appropriate." Think about the action that would maintain the safety of the child and yet help determine who has access.*

Content Area: Child Health; *Category of Health Alteration:* Medical Emergencies; *Integrated Processes:* Caring; *Client Need:* Safe and Effective Care Environment/Management of Care/Advocacy; *Cognitive Level:* Analysis

Reference: Pillitteri, A. (2007). *Maternal and Child Health Nursing* (5th ed., pp. 1743–1754). Philadelphia: Lippincott Williams & Wilkins.

1821. A nursing assistant (NA) is helping an emergency nurse admit a woman who is the victim of spousal abuse and marital rape. The NA asks the nurse what should be done with the woman's torn and soiled clothing. What is the nurse's best response?

1. "Place items in a plastic bag and avoid blood and body fluid contact."
2. "Place items in separate paper bags and seal them. These may be needed by the police."
3. "Ask the woman what she would like done with her clothing; she may want them discarded."
4. "Fold each article of clothing and leave them with her; she can decide later about disposal."

ANSWER: 2

To preserve the evidence, items are placed in separate paper bags, labeled, and released with appropriate documentation to the requesting police officer. Moisture in a plastic bag will cause mold and mildew and destroy the evidence. Assault is a criminal offense, and evidence should be preserved, so clothing should not be discarded or returned to the woman.

➧ ***Test-taking Tip:*** *Select the option that would preserve the evidence.*

Content Area: Adult Health; *Category of Health Alteration:* Medical Emergencies; *Integrated Processes:* Communication and Documentation; *Client Need:* Physiological Integrity/Physiological Adaptation/Medical Emergencies; *Cognitive Level:* Analysis

Reference: Smeltzer, S., Bare, B., Hinkle, J., & Cheever, K. (2008). *Brunner & Suddarth's Textbook of Medical-Surgical Nursing* (11th ed., pp. 2550–2553). Philadelphia: Lippincott Williams & Wilkins.

Test 48: Nutrition

1822. EBP A clinic nurse is assessing the eating habits of a young adult client to determine the adequacy of daily nutritional intake according to the USDA Food Pyramid for a 2,000-calorie diet. The nurse should determine that the client's nutrient intake is *inadequate* when the client reports eating a total of:

1. 3 cups daily of a variety of fruits, juices, and vegetables.
2. 6 ounces daily of whole grain bread, cereal, and pasta.
3. 5½ ounces of fish or chicken eaten twice weekly each or red meat eaten three times weekly.
4. 3 cups daily of yogurt, cheese, and skim milk products.

ANSWER: 1
For a 2,000-calorie diet, 2½ cups of vegetables and 2 cups of fruits or juices should be eaten every day. Vegetables and fruits are two separate food groups. The amounts of foods in the other food groups are correct for a 2,000-calorie diet.

***Test-taking Tip:** The key word is "inadequate." Think about the foods on the Food Pyramid when selecting an option.*

Content Area: Adult Health; *Category of Health Alteration:* Nutrition; *Integrated Processes:* Nursing Process Evaluation; *Client Need:* Physiological Integrity/Basic Care and Comfort/Nutrition and Oral Hydration; *Cognitive Level:* Analysis

Reference: Harkreader, H., Hogan, M., & Thobaben, M. (2007). *Fundamentals of Nursing* (3rd ed., p. 573). St. Louis, MO: Saunders/ Elsevier.

EBP Reference: U.S. Department of Agriculture. (2005). *MyPyramid.* Available at: www.mypyramid.gov/downloads/MiniPoster.pdf

---

1823. EBP A nurse has developed a client outcome for an overweight client with a body mass index (BMI) of 30 who is attending a health promotion program and weight-loss clinic. Which outcome would be best for the nurse to document in the client's plan of care?

1. Client will lose 2 lb per week for the next 4 weeks.
2. Client will lose 20 lb in 2 weeks.
3. Teach client to increase intake of fruits and vegetables.
4. Inform client to call clinic weekly with weight-loss results.

ANSWER: 1
A correctly stated outcome should be client centered, realistic, and measurable. Teaching and informing the client are interventions, not outcomes.

***Test-taking Tip:** Note the key word "best." Select the outcome that would be most complete.*

Content Area: Adult Health; *Category of Health Alteration:* Nutrition; *Integrated Processes:* Communication and Documentation; *Client Need:* Health Promotion and Maintenance/Health Promotion and Disease Prevention; Physiological Integrity/Basic Care and Comfort/Nutrition and Oral Hydration; *Cognitive Level:* Application

Reference: Lutz, C., & Przytulski, K. (2006). *Nutrition & Diet Therapy: Evidence-Based Applications* (4th ed., p. 28). Philadelphia: F. A. Davis.

EBP Reference: Michigan Quality Improvement Consortium. (2007). *Management of Overweight and Obesity in the Adult.* Available at: www.guideline.gov/summary/summary.aspx?doc_id=10885&nbr=005683&string=obesity

---

1824. EBP A nurse is planning a health fair teaching session on the benefits of including omega-3 fatty acids in the diet. Which food choice recommended by the nurse best provides omega-3 fatty acids?

1. Fish at least twice weekly
2. Leafy green vegetables daily
3. Low-fat mozzarella cheese weekly
4. Cholesterol-free margarine once daily

ANSWER: 1
Fatty fishes—such as mackerel, salmon, bluefish, mullet, sablefish, menhaden, anchovy, herring, lake trout, sardines, and tuna—are recommended foods high in omega-3 fatty acids. All except tuna provide at least 1 gram of omega-3 fatty acids in 100 grams or 3.5 ounces of fish. Leafy green vegetables, low-fat mozzarella cheese, and cholesterol-free margarine do not include omega-3 fatty acids.

***Test-taking Tip:** Note the key phrase "best provides." Use knowledge of foods containing omega-3 fatty acids to answer this question.*

Content Area: Adult Health; *Category of Health Alteration:* Nutrition; *Integrated Processes:* Nursing Process Planning; Teaching and Learning; *Client Need:* Health Promotion and Maintenance/Health Promotion and Disease Prevention; *Cognitive Level:* Application

Reference: Whitney, E., DeBruyne, L., Pinna, K., & Rolfes, S. (2007). *Nutrition for Health and Health Care* (3rd ed., p. 93). Belmont, CA: Thomson Learning.

EBP Reference: Walker K. (2006). Omega-3 fatty acid consumption in the reduction of sudden cardiac death. *American Journal for Nurse Practitioners,* 10 (11/12), 11–14, 15–18, 23–24; Hayes, C. (2005). Relative cardiovascular benefits of n-6 and n-3 fatty acids. *Nutrition and the M.D.,* January, 1–4.

1825. While assessing the dietary intake of a client with gastroesophageal reflux disease (GERD), a nurse should expect the client to report discomfort after consuming which of these foods?

1. Poached salmon, baked potatoes, and apple juice
2. Baked chicken, rice, and milk
3. Hamburger, french fries, and a cola beverage
4. Chef salad, rolls, and sparkling grape juice

ANSWER: 3

Hamburgers and french fries are high-fat foods that decrease the lower esophageal sphincter (LES) pressure, thus allowing gastric contents to reflux back into the esophagus. Cola contains caffeine, which also decreases the LES pressure. The rest of the foods are not high in fat and do not contain caffeine or milk products.

➧ ***Test-taking Tip:*** *Focus on the nutrient content of the foods.*

Content Area: Adult Health; *Category of Health Alteration:* Nutrition; *Integrated Processes:* Nursing Process Assessment; *Client Need:* Physiological Integrity/Basic Care and Comfort/Nutrition and Oral Hydration; *Cognitive Level:* Analysis

References: Lewis, S., Heitkemper, M., Dirksen, S., O'Brien, P., & Bucher, L. (2007). *Medical-Surgical Nursing: Assessment and Management of Clinical Problems* (7th ed., pp. 1004–1005). St. Louis, MO: Mosby/Elsevier; Dudek, S. (2006). Nutrition Essentials for Nursing Practice (5th ed. pp. 193, 494). Philadelphia: Lippincott Williams & Wilkins.

1826. EBP A client is on a low-fat diet for weight reduction and hyperlipidemia. The client asks a nurse to recommend foods high in protein. Which food should the nurse recommend?

1. 1 hard-boiled egg
2. 1 cup of cooked broccoli
3. ½ cup 1% cottage cheese
4. 1 ounce cheddar cheese

ANSWER: 3

A half cup of cottage cheese supplies 16 grams of protein. The grams of protein content of the other foods listed are egg (6), broccoli (4), and cheddar cheese (7).

➧ ***Test-taking Tip:*** *Determine what the question is asking about: high-protein foods. Knowledge of the protein content of foods is necessary to answer this question.*

Content Area: Adult Health; *Category of Health Alteration:* Nutrition; *Integrated Processes:* Nursing Process Implementation; *Client Need:* Physiological Integrity/Basic Care and Comfort/Nutrition and Oral Hydration; *Cognitive Level:* Application

Reference: Whitney, E., DeBruyne, L., Pinna, K., & Rolfes, S. (2007). *Nutrition for Health and Health Care* (3rd ed., pp. A18, A30, A36). Belmont, CA: Thomson Learning.

EBP Reference: Ledikwe, J., Blanck, H., Khan, L., Serdula, M., Seymour, J, et al. (2006). Dietary energy density is associated with energy intake and weight status in U.S. adults. *American Journal of Clinical Nutrition,* 83(6), 1362–1368.

1827. A family notices that their father, who has been diagnosed with cirrhosis, has become increasingly irritable and restless. A health-care practitioner orders a protein-restricted diet. A nurse should explain to the client and family that this dietary change will:

1. help to restore their father's liver function.
2. help reduce the amount of ammonia in their father's blood.
3. give their father's liver a chance to rest, since proteins in the diet make the liver work harder.
4. prevent fluid from leaking into their father's abdomen.

ANSWER: 2

When body protein is deaminated, the resulting ammonia is converted to urea by the liver and excreted by the kidney. Liver damage results due to the increase in serum ammonia, which also causes neurological symptoms. Decreasing protein intake will decrease the amount of ammonia formed in the body. Decreasing the protein will not restore the liver function or rest the liver. Decreasing body protein will not decrease ascites.

➧ ***Test-taking Tip:*** *Focus on the physiology of protein metabolism in the body and the relationship to increased ammonia, which causes hepatic encephalopathy.*

Content Area: Adult Health; *Category of Health Alteration:* Nutrition; *Integrated Processes:* Teaching and Learning; *Client Need:* Physiological Integrity/Basic Care and Comfort/Nutrition and Oral Hydration; Physiological Integrity/Reduction of Risk Potential/Therapeutic Procedures; *Cognitive Level:* Analysis

Reference: Smeltzer, S., Bare, B., Hinkle, J., & Cheever, K. (2008). *Brunner & Suddarth's Textbook of Medical-Surgical Nursing* (11th ed., p. 1307). Philadelphia: Lippincott Williams & Wilkins.

1828. Which low-potassium foods (less than 400 mg of potassium per serving) should a nurse plan to include on a list of acceptable foods for a client experiencing chronic renal failure?

1. Cranberry juice, grapes, fresh string beans, fortified puffed rice cereal
2. Prune juice, dried fruit, tomatoes, and all-bran cereal
3. Milk, cantaloupe, peas, and granola cereal
4. Orange juice, raisins, spinach, and dried beans

ANSWER: 1

Cranberry juice, grapes, fresh string beans, and fortified puffed rice cereal are low-potassium foods. Foods that should be restricted include cantaloupe, tomatoes, prune juice, milk, dried fruit, bananas, and dried beans. Other high-potassium foods include avocados, brussels sprouts, peas, raisins, spinach, winter squash, molasses, all-bran cereal, and nuts. Salt substitutes that contain potassium chloride should also be avoided.

➧ *Test-taking Tip: Identify key high-potassium foods in each option (tomatoes, cantaloupe, and orange juice), and use the process of elimination.*

Content Area: Adult Health; *Category of Health Alteration:* Nutrition; *Integrated Processes:* Nursing Process Planning; *Client Need:* Physiological Integrity/Basic Care and Comfort/Nutrition and Oral Hydration; Physiological Integrity/Physiological Adaptation/Fluid and Electrolyte Imbalances; *Cognitive Level:* Application

Reference: Whitney, E., DeBruyne, L., Pinna, K., & Rolfes, S. (2007). *Nutrition for Health and Health Care* (3rd ed., pp. A10–A14, A18–A19). Belmont, CA: Thomson Learning.

1829. An increase in which specific serum laboratory test should indicate to a nurse that a high-iron diet for a client with early-stage iron-deficiency anemia has been effective?

1. Hemoglobin
2. Folate
3. Ferritin
4. Vitamin B_{12}

ANSWER: 3

Ferritin levels reflect the available iron stores in the body and are specific to iron-deficiency anemia. A level less than 10 ng/mL is diagnostic of iron-deficiency anemia. As the condition improves, ferritin levels rise. In iron deficiency, the body cannot synthesize hemoglobin, but hemoglobin levels drop fairly late in the development of iron-deficiency anemia. Also, other nutrient deficiencies and medical conditions can affect hemoglobin levels. Serum folate is specific to folate-deficiency anemia.

➧ *Test-taking Tip: Note the key words "specific" and "iron-deficiency." Use knowledge of terminology to answer this question (ferritin is an iron-phosphorus-protein complex).*

Content Area: Adult Health; *Category of Health Alteration:* Nutrition; *Integrated Processes:* Nursing Process Evaluation; *Client Need:* Physiological Integrity Reduction of Risk Potential/Laboratory Values; *Cognitive Level:* Analysis

Reference: Whitney, E., DeBruyne, L., Pinna, K., & Rolfes, S. (2007). *Nutrition for Health and Health Care* (3rd ed., pp. E9–E11). Belmont, CA: Thomson Learning.

1830. A nurse teaches a client who is experiencing iron-deficiency anemia to eat foods high in iron and foods that contain vitamin C at the same meal to increase the iron absorption. The nurse evaluates that teaching is effective when which meal is selected by the client?

1. Yogurt and oranges
2. Shrimp and potatoes
3. Lean beef steak and broccoli
4. Chicken and leafy green vegetables

ANSWER: 3

Good sources of iron include lean beef steak, steamed clams, navy beans, enriched cereal, cooked spinach, cooked Swiss chard, beef liver, and black beans. Three ounces of steamed clams have 23.8 mg of iron, compared with cooked beef liver, which has 5.24 mg. Dark green vegetables such as broccoli and bell peppers, citrus fruits, cabbage-type vegetables, cantaloupe, strawberries, lettuce, tomatoes, potatoes, papayas, and mangos are significant sources of vitamin C. Yogurt, shrimp, and chicken contain less iron than do steamed clams.

➧ *Test-taking Tip: Use knowledge of foods high in vitamin C and iron to answer this question.*

Content Area: Adult Health; *Category of Health Alteration:* Nutrition; *Integrated Processes:* Nursing Process Evaluation; *Client Need:* Physiological Integrity/Basic Care and Comfort/Nutrition and Oral Hydration; Physiological Integrity/Physiological Adaptation/Illness Management; *Cognitive Level:* Analysis

Reference: Whitney, E., DeBruyne, L., Pinna, K., & Rolfes, S. (2007). *Nutrition for Health and Health Care* (3rd ed., pp. 210–211, 242). Belmont, CA: Thomson Learning.

1831. A nurse evaluates that a client recognizes foods that are high in calcium when the client selects:

1. 1 cup whole milk, 1 cup spinach, and 3 ounces sardines.
2. 1 cup low-fat yogurt, 1 cup broccoli, and 3 ounces sardines.
3. ½ cup 2% cottage cheese, 1 cup spinach, and 3 ounces frozen tofu.
4. 1 medium baked potato with 1 tbsp fat-free sour cream, 1 cup spinach, and 3 ounces tofu.

ANSWER: 2

One cup of low-fat plain yogurt has 448 mg of calcium, 1 cup of broccoli has 60 mg, and 3 ounces of sardines have 324 mg, for a total of 832 mg of calcium. One cup of whole milk has 300 mg of calcium, 1 cup of spinach has 30 mg calcium, and 3 ounces of sardines have 324 mg, for a total of 654 mg. A half cup of 2% cottage cheese has 78 mg calcium, 1 cup of spinach has 30 mg, and 3 ounces tofu has 310 mg, for a total of 418 mg. A medium baked potato has 38 mg of calcium, 1 tbsp of low-fat sour cream has 20 mg, 1 cup of spinach has 30 mg, and 3 ounces tofu has 310 mg, for a total of 398 mg calcium.

Test-taking Tip: Use the process of elimination, noting that options 1 and 2 both contain sardines and 3 and 4 both contain tofu. Next, look at the dairy content in each option. Eliminate options 3 and 4 because the volume of dairy content is low. Select option 2, knowing that low-fat plain yogurt has more calcium than whole milk.

Content Area: Adult Health; *Category of Health Alteration:* Nutrition; *Integrated Processes:* Nursing Process Evaluation; *Client Need:* Physiological Integrity/Basic Care and Comfort/Nutrition and Oral Hydration; *Cognitive Level:* Analysis

Reference: Whitney, E., DeBruyne, L., Pinna, K., & Rolfes, S. (2007). *Nutrition for Health and Health Care* (3rd ed., pp. 234, A22–A24, A32–A33, A36–A37). Belmont, CA: Thomson Learning.

1832. A client who is recovering from acute diverticulitis is highly motivated to prevent another exacerbation of the disease. A nurse educates the client about the need to increase the amount of dietary fiber in the diet. The nurse evaluates that teaching has been effective when the client makes which menu selection for lunch?

1. A chicken sandwich on whole wheat bread with raw carrots and celery sticks
2. Baked chicken, mashed potatoes, and herbal tea
3. Chicken noodle soup with soda crackers and chocolate pudding
4. Cooked acorn squash, fried chicken, and pasta

ANSWER: 1

Whole wheat bread and raw fruits and vegetables are foods that are high in fiber content.

Test-taking Tip: Recall that cooking food will cause breakdown of the dietary fiber content. Eliminate options 2 and 4.

Content Area: Adult Health; *Category of Health Alteration:* Nutrition; *Integrated Processes:* Nursing Process Evaluation; *Client Need:* Health Promotion and Maintenance/Prevention and Early Detection of Disease/Lifestyle Choices; *Cognitive Level:* Analysis

Reference: Monahan, F., Sands, J., Neighbors, M., Marek, J., & Green, C. (2007). *Phipps' Medical-Surgical Nursing: Health and Illness Perspectives* (8th ed., p. 1239). St. Louis, MO: Mosby/Elsevier.

1833. During preparation for a seminar on healthy living for college students, a nurse outlines content concerning promotion of healthy bowel elimination. The nurse plans to educate the students about the need to consume a minimum of ________ of fiber per day.

1. 5 to 20 grams
2. 20 to 35 grams
3. 35 to 50 grams
4. 50 to 75 grams

ANSWER: 2

The American Dietetic Association recommends an intake of 20 to 35 grams of fiber per day as the minimum daily requirements. The other options are either too low or more than the minimum daily requirement.

Test-taking Tip: The key word is "minimum." Focus on recommended amounts of fiber for a healthy diet.

Content Area: Adult Health; *Category of Health Alteration:* Nutrition; *Integrated Processes:* Nursing Process Planning; Teaching and Learning; *Client Need:* Physiological Integrity/Basic Care and Comfort/Elimination; *Cognitive Level:* Application

Reference: Monahan, F., Sands, J., Neighbors, M., Marek, J., & Green, C. (2007). *Phipps' Medical-Surgical Nursing: Health and Illness Perspectives* (8th ed., p. 1248). St. Louis, MO: Mosby/Elsevier.

1834. EBP A nurse is assessing a malnourished adolescent who has been consuming a vegan diet. For signs of which specific vitamin deficiency should the nurse assess this client?

1. Vitamin A
2. Vitamin B_{12}
3. Vitamin C
4. Vitamin K

ANSWER: 2

Vegans abstain from eating animal products, which provide vitamin B_{12}. Fruits and vegetables that are eaten by vegans contain vitamins A, C, and K, so these are less likely to be deficient.

➧ ***Test-taking Tip:*** *Think about how vitamins A, C, and K are similar and vitamin B_{12} is different.*

Content Area: Child Health; *Category of Health Alteration:* Nutrition; *Integrated Processes:* Nursing Process Assessment; *Client Need:* Physiological Integrity/Basic Care and Comfort/Nutrition and Oral Hydration; *Cognitive Level:* Analysis

Reference: Lutz, C., & Przytulski, K. (2006). *Nutrition & Diet Therapy: Evidence-Based Applications* (4th ed., p. 114). Philadelphia: F. A. Davis.

EBP Reference: U.S. Department of Health and Human Services, U.S. Department of Agriculture. (2005). *Dietary Guidelines for Americans*. Available at: www.guideline.gov/summary/summary.aspx?doc_id= 6417&nbr= 004048&string=Malnutrition

1835. A client who suffered burns of the lower extremities is ordered a high-protein, high-calorie diet. A food diary reveals that the client is not meeting protein or caloric intake goals recommended by the dietician. The client tells a nurse of feeling full quickly when eating meals. Which interventions should the nurse recommend to the client? SELECT ALL THAT APPLY.

1. Include more fresh vegetables in the diet.
2. Eat five to six smaller meals instead of eating three larger sized meals.
3. Include protein bars and whole-milk yogurt as snacks.
4. Drink regular instead of diet sodas.
5. Add protein supplements to cooked cereals.

ANSWER: 2, 3, 5

A client is likely to increase caloric intake by eating more frequent feedings than three traditional meals. Protein bars, whole-milk yogurt, and protein supplements are good sources to add calories and protein to the client's diet. Although fresh vegetables contain needed vitamins, these foods are not good sources of needed calories or protein. Regular soda supplies calories as simple sugars, is not a source of protein, and lacks other nutrients.

➧ ***Test-taking Tip:*** *The issue of the question includes ways to increase protein and calories in the diet. Recall foods that are classified as protein and those high in calories. Evaluate each option and select those that include protein and calories.*

Content Area: Adult Health; *Category of Health Alteration:* Nutrition; *Integrated Processes:* Nursing Process Implementation; *Client Need:* Physiological Integrity/Basic Care and Comfort/Nutrition and Oral Hydration; *Cognitive Level:* Analysis

Reference: Ignatavicius, D., & Workman, M. (2006). *Medical-Surgical Nursing: Critical Thinking for Collaborative Care* (5th ed., pp. 1429, 1645). St. Louis, MO: Elsevier/Saunders.

1836. A client with an ileostomy asks a nurse for nutritional information. The nurse includes all of these points but should emphasize that the most important action is to:

1. identify foods that cause gas and avoid those foods.
2. avoid foods that cause diarrhea.
3. eat a well-balanced diet.
4. drink at least 3,000 mL of fluid per day.

ANSWER: 4

The client with an ileostomy can easily become dehydrated as the stool produced contains large amounts of liquid. The amount of fluid lost depends on whether the client has had previous bowel surgeries with removal of parts of the small bowel.

➧ ***Test-taking Tip:*** *Focus on the anatomy and physiology of the small intestine in relationship to food and fluid absorption.*

Content Area: Adult Health; *Category of Health Alteration:* Nutrition; *Integrated Processes:* Teaching and Learning; *Client Need:* Physiological Integrity/Basic Care and Comfort/Nutrition and Oral Hydration; *Cognitive Level:* Analysis

Reference: Monahan, F., Sands, J., Neighbors, M., Marek, J., & Green, C. (2007). *Phipps' Medical-Surgical Nursing: Health and Illness Perspectives* (8th ed., pp. 1263, 1266). St. Louis, MO: Mosby/Elsevier.

1837. In preparation for discharging a client after a cholecystectomy, a nurse plans to discuss dietary restrictions. Which information is most appropriate for the nurse to include in the discussion?

1. Limiting oral intake to three meals per day; no snacking
2. Drinking fluids between meals, rather than with meals
3. Eating a low-fat diet for the next 4 to 6 weeks
4. Decreasing the amounts of simple sugars in the diet for the next 2 weeks

ANSWER: 3

The client should be instructed to restrict dietary fats for a short period of time until the biliary ducts are able to dilate to accommodate the volume of bile once held by the gallbladder. After that, the client should have no dietary restrictions. There is no reason to limit the oral intake to three meals per day or to drink fluids between meals. Simple sugars are not digested with bile and therefore there is no reason to limit the intake of simple sugars unless the need for weight loss is a concern.

Test-taking Tip: *Focus on the pathophysiology of cholelithiasis and the physiology of the gallbladder. This should allow the elimination of options 1, 2, and 4.*

Content Area: Adult Health; *Category of Health Alteration:* Nutrition; *Integrated Processes:* Nursing Process Implementation; Teaching and Learning; *Client Need:* Physiological Integrity/Physiological Adaptation/Alterations in Body Systems; Physiological Integrity/Basic Care and Comfort/Nutrition and Oral Hydration; *Cognitive Level:* Application

Reference: Smeltzer, S., Bare, B., Hinkle, J., & Cheever, K. (2008). *Brunner & Suddarth's Textbook of Medical-Surgical Nursing* (11th ed., p. 1356). Philadelphia: Lippincott Williams & Wilkins.

1838. EBP A client recovering from an exacerbation of ulcerative colitis is permitted to begin eating solid foods. A nurse recognizes that the client understands the dietary teaching for disease management when the client selects:

1. fried chicken, french fries, and fruit juice.
2. cream of tomato soup, mixed green salad, and whole milk.
3. baked fish, steamed green beans, mashed potatoes with butter, and herbal tea.
4. chili and a glass of wine.

ANSWER: 3

A low-residue diet that is high in calories and protein should be gradually introduced as the client's tolerance for solid food increases. Milk products should be avoided because lactose intolerance is common. Intestinal stimulants such as caffeine, spicy foods, and alcohol should also be avoided.

Test-taking Tip: *Eliminate options 1 and 4 because alcohol, spicy foods, and fried foods are not recommended for any gastrointestinal health deviations. Remember that inflammatory bowel problems cause changes that often promote lactose intolerance. Eliminate option 2 due to high milk content.*

Content Area: Adult Health; *Category of Health Alteration:* Nutrition; *Integrated Processes:* Nursing Process Evaluation; *Client Need:* Physiological Integrity/Basic Care and Comfort/Nutrition and Oral Hydration; *Cognitive Level:* Analysis

Reference: Smeltzer, S., Bare, B., Hinkle, J., & Cheever, K. (2008). *Brunner & Suddarth's Textbook of Medical-Surgical Nursing* (11th ed., p. 1249). Philadelphia: Lippincott Williams & Wilkins.

EBP Reference: Razack, R., & Seidner, D. (2007). Nutrition in inflammatory bowel disease. *Current Opinion in Gastroenterology,* 23(4), 400–405.

1839. EBP A nurse is providing education to a client who is being evaluated for lactose intolerance. The client is scheduled for a breath test for hydrogen excretion. The client is questioning how this test will detect lactose intolerance. The nurse should explain to the client that:

1. undigested lactose causes the breakdown of water molecules in the colon to form oxygen and hydrogen.
2. hydrogen is produced by lactose digestion in the small intestine.
3. undigested lactose produces hydrogen when metabolized by colon bacteria.
4. during the digestive process, lactose is broken down into lactic acid and hydrogen.

ANSWER: 3

Measuring the excretion of hydrogen after lactose ingestion is a sensitive, specific test for lactose intolerance. Undigested lactose produces hydrogen when metabolized by colon bacteria. Lactose does not cause the breakdown of water molecules. Lactose-intolerant individuals are unable to digest lactose.

Test-taking Tip: *Lactose-intolerant individuals are unable to digest lactose; knowing this would enable elimination of options 2 and 4.*

Content Area: Adult Health; *Category of Health Alteration:* Nutrition; *Integrated Processes:* Teaching and Learning; *Client Need:* Health Promotion and Maintenance/Prevention and Detection of Disease/Health Screening; *Cognitive Level:* Application

Reference: Lewis, S., Heitkemper, M., Dirksen, S., O'Brien, P., & Bucher, L. (2007). *Medical-Surgical Nursing: Assessment and Management of Clinical Problems* (7th ed., p. 1079). St. Louis, MO: Mosby/Elsevier.

EBP Reference: Heyman, M. Committee on Nutrition. (2006). Lactose intolerance in infants, children, and adolescents. *Pediatrics,* 118(3), 1279–1286. Available at: www.guideline.gov/summary/summary.aspx?doc_id=9827&nbr=005251&string=hydrogen+AND+breath+AND+test

1840. After completing a wellness seminar at a local manufacturing business, a nurse is answering individual questions. One of the participants tells the nurse his mother has celiac disease and he is afraid he may also have the disease. The nurse agrees that this may be possible when the client states that he experiences diarrhea after eating:

1. eggs.
2. peanut butter.
3. whole wheat bread.
4. spinach and other dark leafy green vegetables.

ANSWER: 3

Celiac disease is an autoimmune disease that results in chronic intestinal inflammation after ingesting gluten. Having a first-degree relative with celiac disease increases the client's risk of developing the disease. Eggs, peanut butter, spinach, and dark leafy green vegetables do not contain gluten.

➧ ***Test-taking Tip:*** *Read the question carefully; it is asking for identification of the nutrient that precipitates bowel inflammation in clients with celiac disease.*

Content Area: Adult Health; *Category of Health Alteration:* Nutrition; *Integrated Processes:* Nursing Process Analysis; *Client Need:* Health Promotion and Maintenance/Health Promotion and Disease Prevention; *Cognitive Level:* Application

Reference: Lewis, S., Heitkemper, M., Dirksen, S., O'Brien, P., & Bucher, L. (2007). *Medical-Surgical Nursing: Assessment and Management of Clinical Problems* (7th ed., p. 1080). St. Louis, MO: Mosby/Elsevier.

1841. A client is hospitalized with a diagnosis of emphysema. Which dietary modifications should a nurse expect to be prescribed for this client, who has no other underlying medical conditions? SELECT ALL THAT APPLY.

1. Mechanical soft
2. Low calorie
3. High protein
4. Restricted potassium
5. Increased calcium

ANSWER: 1, 3

Mechanical soft decreases the chewing effort. Eating, chewing, and digestion increase oxygen demand. Carbohydrate (CHO) metabolism increases CO_2 levels. A high-protein, low-CHO diet is prescribed to provide calories for energy but prevent increased CO_2 levels. A high-calorie diet is prescribed because of the increased energy consumption with eating. Potassium is restricted with renal failure, not emphysema. Calcium is increased with diseases such as tuberculosis or osteoporosis.

➧ ***Test-taking Tip:*** *Recall that there is diminished oxygenation with emphysema and that eating increases oxygen demand and consumption.*

Content Area: Adult Health; *Category of Health Alteration:* Nutrition; *Integrated Processes:* Nursing Process Planning; *Client Need:* Physiological Integrity/Basic Care and Comfort/Nutrition and Oral Hydration; *Cognitive Level:* Analysis

Reference: Craven, R., & Hirnle, C. (2009). *Fundamentals of Nursing: Human Health and Function* (6th ed., p. 972). Philadelphia: Lippincott Williams & Wilkins.

1842. EBP A client receiving chemotherapy is experiencing persistent nausea and occasional vomiting. Based on these symptoms, which interventions should a nurse add to this client's plan of care? SELECT ALL THAT APPLY.

1. Change the client's diet to full liquid.
2. Offer small amounts of food frequently.
3. Administer ondansetron (Zofran®) 1 hour prior to chemotherapy treatments.
4. Encourage liquid consumption throughout the day.
5. Serve a big meal before all chemotherapy treatments.
6. Offer foods that are mild smelling or odorless.

ANSWER: 2, 3, 4, 6

Small meals can be less nauseating than a large, heavy meal. Realistic intake goals are set for the client. Ondansetron is an antiemetic, serotonin receptor antagonist, used to decrease nausea and vomiting caused by chemotherapy. Other medications include metoclopramide (Reglan®) and dexamethasone (Decadron®). Liquids are encouraged to replace fluids lost through emesis. Foods with a strong odor or that are fatty, greasy, or gas forming can increase nausea. A liquid diet does not reduce nausea. A small meal should be served 2 hours prior to chemotherapy.

➧ ***Test-taking Tip:*** *Read each option carefully. The issue of the question is interventions to reduce nausea.*

Content Area: Adult Health; *Category of Health Alteration:* Nutrition; *Integrated Processes:* Nursing Process Analysis; *Client Need:* Physiological Integrity/Basic Care and Comfort/Nutrition and Oral Hydration; *Cognitive Level:* Analysis

Reference: Lewis, S., Heitkemper, M., Dirksen, S., O'Brien, P., & Bucher, L. (2007). *Medical-Surgical Nursing: Assessment and Management of Clinical Problems* (7th ed., pp. 297–298). St. Louis, MO: Mosby/Elsevier.

EBP Reference: American Dietetic Association. (2007). *Oncology Evidence-Based Nutrition Practice Guideline.* Available at: www.guideline.gov/summary/summary.aspx?doc_id=12819&nbr=006621&string=enteral

1843. EBP A nurse is administering an intermittent enteral feeding of 350 mL of formula through a nasogastric tube. To decrease the risk of aspiration, the nurse should:

1. administer the feeding as rapidly as possible.
2. position the client in a supine position for 1 hour after the feeding is complete.
3. confirm tube placement after the feeding has been infused.
4. elevate the client's head to 45 degrees during the feeding.

ANSWER: 4

Positioning the head of the bed at 45 degrees elevation promotes gravity flow of the formula into the stomach and maintains normal functioning of the lower esophageal sphincter. Rapid administration of a bolus feeding reduces lower esophageal sphincter pressure. Tube placement should be confirmed before beginning the feeding. Maintaining the 45-degree elevation of the client's head for 1 hour after the feeding is recommended because it maintains normal functioning of the lower esophageal sphincter.

▶ ***Test-taking Tip:*** *Focus on the anatomy of the stomach and the way in which food passes into the intestines.*

Content Area: Adult Health; *Category of Health Alteration:* Nutrition; *Integrated Processes:* Nursing Process Implementation; *Client Need:* Physiological Integrity/Basic Care and Comfort/Nutrition and Oral Hydration; *Cognitive Level:* Application

Reference: Dudek, S. (2006). *Nutrition Essentials for Nursing Practice* (5th ed., p. 434). Philadelphia: Lippincott Williams & Wilkins.

EBP Reference: American Dietetic Association. (2006). *Critical Illness Evidence-Based Nutrition Practice Guideline.* Available at: www.guideline.gov/summary/summary.aspx?doc_id=12818&nbr=006620&string=enteral+AND+feedings

1844. A mother is concerned about achieving a nutritious intake for her 14-month-old child. Which advice by a nurse would be best?

1. Feed the child before the rest of the family, and then let the child play while the family eats.
2. Because the child's stomach only holds ½ cup, select food from a food group for each meal.
3. Offer 1 to 2 tablespoons of food from each food group with every meal or snack.
4. If on the fourth time of introducing a food, the child still pushes it away, don't retry giving that food; just try other foods.

ANSWER: 3

A 14-month-old child's serving size should be about one-fifth the size of an adult's serving or about a tablespoonful for each year of age. Offering a variety of foods from the food groups will help ensure a nutritious diet and avoid consuming too much or too little food from any one food group. To develop healthy eating habits, the child should eat with the rest of the family and if not hungry should remain at the table. A 1-year-old child's stomach holds about 1 cup. Offering three meals and three nutritious snacks a day increases the likelihood that the toddler will obtain sufficient nourishment. Eight to 15 exposures to a food are needed to effect behavior change.

▶ ***Test-taking Tip:*** *Focus on the issue of achieving a nutritious intake for the toddler, and use the process of elimination.*

Content Area: Child Health; *Category of Health Alteration:* Nutrition; *Integrated Processes:* Teaching and Learning; *Client Need:* Health Promotion and Maintenance/Health and Wellness; *Cognitive Level:* Analysis

References: Harkreader, H., Hogan, M., & Thobaben, M. (2007). *Fundamentals of Nursing* (3rd ed., p. 581). St. Louis, MO: Saunders/Elsevier; Lutz, C., & Przytulski, K. (2006). *Nutrition & Diet Therapy: Evidence-Based Applications* (4th ed., pp. 241–244). Philadelphia: F. A. Davis.

1845. EBP A nurse is caring for a 2-year-old child at risk for iron-deficiency anemia. To prevent iron-deficiency anemia in toddlers, a nurse should recommend: SELECT ALL THAT APPLY.

1. limiting the toddler's milk intake to 24 ounces per day.
2. limiting the toddler's juice intake to 4 to 6 ounces per day.
3. offering iron-rich foods such as beef, lentils, broccoli, and raisins.
4. iron supplementation for 1- to 2-year-old children of parents in a lower economic class.
5. avoiding vegan diets for all toddlers.
6. parental feeding of the toddler to ensure an adequate intake.

ANSWER: 1, 2, 3, 4

To maintain the appetite for iron-enriched cereals, meats, and iron-rich fruits and vegetables, milk should be limited to 24 ounces per day and juice to 4 to 6 ounces per day for children aged 1 to 5 years. Beef, lentils, broccoli, and raisins are some of the iron-rich foods. In a pilot study involving poor and minority populations, prophylactic daily iron supplementation was estimated to reduce the incidence of iron-deficiency anemia by 72%. A toddler can consume a vegan diet and not develop iron-deficiency anemia if the diet is well planned. Toddlers are developing independence and will want to feed themselves. Parental feeding can delay the child's mastering of developmental stages and cause the child to dislike the foods if the parent attempts to force-feed the child.

▶ ***Test-taking Tip:*** *Focus on iron-rich foods, the size of the child's stomach, and child and parental behaviors that could limit the child's intake of iron-rich foods.*

Content Area: Child Health; *Category of Health Alteration:* Nutrition; *Integrated Processes:* Nursing Process Implementation; *Client Need:* Health Promotion and Maintenance/Health and Wellness; *Cognitive Level:* Analysis

Reference: Lutz, C., & Przytulski, K. (2006). *Nutrition & Diet Therapy: Evidence-Based Applications* (4th ed., p. 244). Philadelphia: F. A. Davis.

EBP Reference: U.S. Preventive Services Task Force. (2006). *Screening for Iron Deficiency Anemia—Including Iron Supplementation for Children and Pregnant Women.* Rockville, MD: Agency for Healthcare Research and Quality. Available at: www.guideline.gov/summary/summary.aspx?ss=15&doc_id=9274&nbr=004965&string=Vitamins+and+Minerals

---

1846. A 6-year-old child is being seen in a clinic due to chronic constipation. A health-care provider recommends a high-fiber diet with an increased fluid intake. Which food choices, providing the highest amount of fiber per serving, should a nurse recommend?

1. Whole wheat or rye breads
2. Raw or cooked vegetables
3. Fresh, frozen, or dried fruits
4. Legumes such as baked beans, navy beans, or black-eyed peas

ANSWER: 4

Legumes provide about 8 grams of fiber per serving. Whole wheat or rye breads provide 1 gram of fiber per serving. Raw or cooked vegetables provide 2 to 3 grams of fiber per serving. Fresh, frozen, or dried fruits have about 2 grams of fiber per serving.

➧ ***Test-taking Tip:*** *The key phrase is "highest amount."*

Content Area: Child Health; *Category of Health Alteration:* Nutrition; *Integrated Processes:* Nursing Process Implementation; *Client Need:* Physiological Integrity/Basic Care and Comfort/Nutrition and Oral Hydration; *Cognitive Level:* Analysis

Reference: Whitney, E., DeBruyne, L., Pinna, K., & Rolfes, S. (2007). *Nutrition for Health and Health Care* (3rd ed., p. 77). Belmont, CA: Thomson Learning.

1847. EBP A hospitalized Hispanic child is diagnosed with lactose intolerance and is placed on a lactose-restricted diet. Which dietary supplement should a nurse anticipate being added to the child's diet?

1. Protein
2. Calcium
3. Vitamin B_{12}
4. Beta-carotene

ANSWER: 2

A deficiency of the enzyme lactase results in an inability to digest lactose, the sugar found in dairy products. A lactose-restricted diet, which removes milk and other dairy products from the diet, can result in a calcium, riboflavin, and vitamin D deficiency. Sixty percent or more of Hispanics, Blacks, and Southeast Asians are lactose intolerant. The ability to ingest protein, vitamin B_{12}, and beta-carotene from foods in the meat and bean, grain, vegetable, and fruit food groups is unaffected in persons with lactose intolerance.

➧ ***Test-taking Tip:*** *Recall that lactose is found in milk and other dairy products.*

Content Area: Child Health; *Category of Health Alteration:* Nutrition; *Integrated Processes:* Nursing Process Planning; *Client Need:* Physiological Integrity/Basic Care and Comfort/Nutrition and Oral Hydration; *Cognitive Level:* Analysis

Reference: Whitney, E., DeBruyne, L., Pinna, K., & Rolfes, S. (2007). *Nutrition for Health and Health Care* (3rd ed., p. 252). Belmont, CA: Thomson Learning.

EBP Reference: Greer, F., & Krebs, N. (2006). Optimizing bone health and calcium intakes of infants, children, and adolescents. *Pediatrics,* 117(2), 578–585.

1848. A home health nurse is evaluating a parent's dietary management of a child with celiac disease. Which foods, or food-containing products, should the parents eliminate from their child's diet? SELECT ALL THAT APPLY.

1. Rice
2. Barley
3. Wheat
4. Corn
5. Oats
6. Soybean flour

ANSWER: 2, 3, 5

Celiac disease occurs from an unknown genetic defect. When gluten is ingested, it causes direct destruction of intestinal cells from an autoimmune response. Gluten found in barley, wheat, oats, and rye should be eliminated from the diet. Gluten-containing grains are replaced with rice, corn, soybean flour, or millet.

➧ ***Test-taking Tip:*** *Select the gluten-containing grains in the options.*

Content Area: Child Health; *Category of Health Alteration:* Nutrition; *Integrated Processes:* Nursing Process Evaluation; *Client Need:* Health Promotion and Maintenance/Principles of Teaching and Learning; *Cognitive Level:* Analysis

Reference: Lutz, C., & Przytulski, K. (2006). *Nutrition & Diet Therapy: Evidence-Based Applications* (4th ed., pp. 191–193). Philadelphia: F. A. Davis.

1849. A child is found to be deficient in iron. To increase the child's absorption of iron, which vitamin should a nurse encourage the parents to supplement?

1. Vitamin A
2. Vitamin C
3. Vitamin D
4. Vitamin E

ANSWER: 2

Vitamin C (ascorbic acid) facilitates iron absorption by acting on hydrochloric acid to keep iron in the more absorbable ferrous form. Vitamin A is essential to night vision, the health of epithelial tissue, normal bone growth, and energy regulation. Vitamin D is essential for absorption and use of calcium for bone and tooth growth. Vitamin E is an antioxidant that stimulates the immune system.

➧ ***Test-taking Tip:*** *If unsure, look for similarities and differences; vitamins A, D, E, and K are fat-soluble vitamins, whereas vitamin C is a water-soluble vitamin. An option that is different is likely to be the answer.*

Content Area: Child Health; *Category of Health Alteration:* Nutrition; *Integrated Processes:* Nursing Process Implementation; *Client Need:* Physiological Integrity/Basic Care and Comfort/Nutrition and Oral Hydration; *Cognitive Level:* Application

Reference: Lutz, C., & Przytulski, K. (2006). *Nutrition & Diet Therapy: Evidence-Based Applications* (4th ed., pp. 97–107). Philadelphia: F. A. Davis.

1850. A public health nurse is screening children for nutritional deficiencies. Which illustration depicts a child who is likely experiencing scurvy (vitamin C deficiency)?

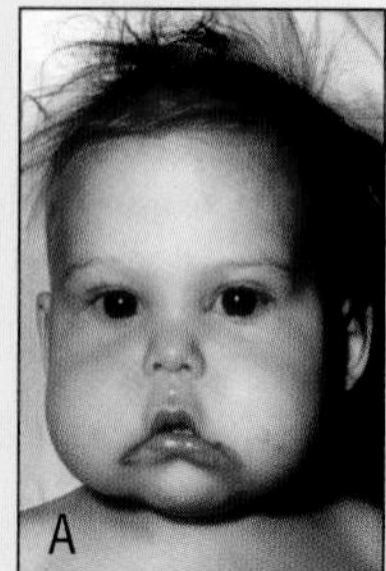

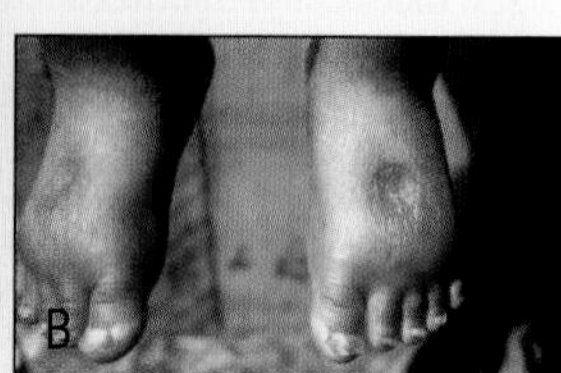

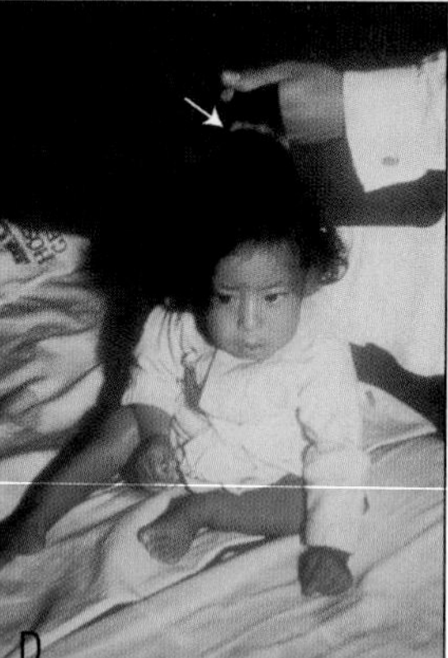

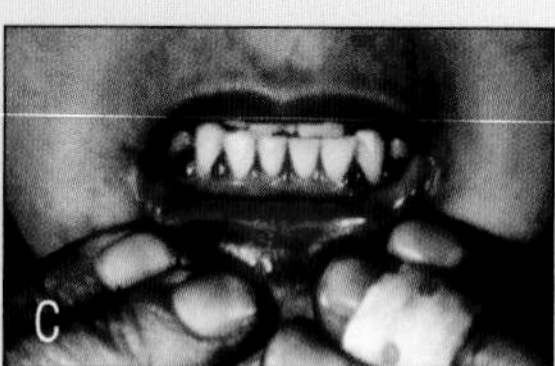

1. Illustration A
2. Illustration B
3. Illustration C
4. Illustration D

ANSWER: 3

The inflamed, spongy, and bleeding gums of the child in illustration C are a clinical manifestation associated with a vitamin C deficiency. The infant presented in illustration A has swollen, red cracks at the corners of the mouth indicative of a vitamin B deficiency. The child with the swollen feet in illustration B is experiencing kwashiorkor due to a severe dietary protein deficiency. The child in illustration D is displaying "flag sign" hair, involving alternating light and dark bands of color along individual hair fibers and thinning hair due to a severe dietary protein deficiency.

➧ ***Test-taking Tip:*** *Recall that vitamin C is essential to tissue growth and repair. Eliminate options 2 and 4 because these do illustrate impaired tissues.*

Content Area: Child Health; *Category of Health Alteration:* Nutrition; *Integrated Processes:* Nursing Process Evaluation; *Client Need:* Physiological Integrity/Basic Care and Comfort/Nutrition and Oral Hydration; *Cognitive Level:* Analysis

Reference: Berman, A., Snyder, S., Kozier, B., & Erb, G. (2008). *Kozier & Erb's Fundamentals of Nursing: Concepts, Process, and Practice* (8th ed., pp. 1256–1257). Upper Saddle River, NJ: Pearson Education.

1851. EBP A nurse is caring for an older adult client who is asking for nutritional information. Good nutrition advice for the older adult should be to:

1. maintain an appropriate weight for height and include nutrient-dense foods.
2. increase vitamin E intake and exercise daily.
3. avoid high-fiber foods and take a multiple-vitamin supplement.
4. become a vegetarian and drink 2 quarts of water per day.

ANSWER: 1

Overall weight control and consumption of foods high in nutrients will promote healthy aging. Supplements, such as vitamin E, are not substitutes for food. Fiber is only part of a healthy diet. A vegan diet does not ensure a nutrient-dense diet.

▶ ***Test-taking Tip:*** *Consider the broad picture of healthy aging before selecting an option.*

Content Area: Adult Health; *Category of Health Alteration:* Nutrition; *Integrated Processes:* Teaching and Learning; *Client Need:* Physiological Integrity/Basic Care and Comfort/Nutrition and Oral Hydration; *Cognitive Level:* Application

Reference: Insel, P., Turner, E., & Ross, D. (2007). *Nutrition* (3rd ed., pp. 702–703). Sudbury, MA: Jones and Bartlett.

EBP Reference: Kuczmarski, M.F., & Weddle, D.O. (2005). Position paper of the American Dietetic Association: Nutrition across the spectrum of aging. *Journal of the American Dietetic Association,* 105, 616–633.

1852. A nurse is counseling a client with cardiac disease who has limited food refrigeration capabilities and prefers using canned vegetables. Which nutrient excess should the nurse caution the client about when eating mainly canned, rather than fresh, vegetables?

1. Potassium
2. Vitamin A
3. Vitamin C
4. Sodium

ANSWER: 4

Canned vegetables, even those low in sodium, have higher sodium levels than fresh or frozen. Potassium and vitamins A and C are not a concern in the processing of canned vegetables.

▶ ***Test-taking Tip:*** *Key words are "excessive" and "canned." Think about how canned vegetables are preserved.*

Content Area: Adult Health; *Category of Health Alteration:* Nutrition; *Integrated Processes:* Teaching and Learning; *Client Need:* Physiological Integrity/Basic Care and Comfort/Nutrition and Oral Hydration; *Cognitive Level:* Application

Reference: Insel, P., Turner, E., & Ross, D. (2007). *Nutrition* (3rd ed., pp. 609–615). Sudbury, MA: Jones and Bartlett.

1853. A clinic nurse is discussing eye health with an older adult. Which nutrients should the nurse encourage the client to consume to protect against vision problems?

1. Minerals
2. Lecithins
3. Antioxidants
4. Amino acids

ANSWER: 3

Oxidative stress plays a role in cataract formation. Antioxidants such as vitamin E and vitamin C may reduce the likelihood of developing cataracts. Minerals generally do not have an antioxidant function. Lecithins are emulsifiers, not antioxidants. Amino acids are building blocks of protein.

▶ ***Test-taking Tip:*** *Think about the nutrient that is most likely to delay cataract formation.*

Content Area: Adult Health; *Category of Health Alteration:* Nutrition; *Integrated Processes:* Nursing Process Implementation; *Client Need:* Physiological Integrity/Basic Care and Comfort/Nutrition and Oral Hydration; *Cognitive Level:* Application

Reference: Insel, P., Turner, E., & Ross, D. (2007). *Nutrition* (3rd ed., p. 715). Sudbury, MA: Jones and Bartlett.

1854. A nurse is caring for an older adult client who has experienced unintended weight loss. Which energy-dense protein foods should the nurse offer to the client when the client requests a snack?

1. Carrot sticks and apple wedges
2. Peanut butter crackers and hard-boiled eggs
3. Whole wheat toast with jelly
4. Yogurt and cottage cheese

ANSWER: 2

Peanut butter and eggs are good sources of complete proteins and are energy and nutrient dense. Fruit and vegetables are not good sources of protein and are generally low in calories per serving. Grain products, such as whole wheat toast, are not good sources of protein and are not energy dense. Yogurt and cottage cheese are not considered energy dense. They are considered good sources of protein.

▶ ***Test-taking Tip:*** *Select the best sources of complete proteins providing the most calories per serving.*

Content Area: Adult Health; *Category of Health Alteration:* Nutrition; *Integrated Processes:* Nursing Process Implementation; *Client Need:* Physiological Integrity/Basic Care and Comfort/Nutrition and Oral Hydration; *Cognitive Level:* Application

Reference: Insel, P., Turner, E., & Ross, D. (2007). *Nutrition* (3rd ed., pp. 711–714). Sudbury, MA: Jones and Bartlett.

1855. A nurse reads in a physician's history and physical note that a hospitalized child has a pica eating disorder. Which conclusions by the nurse are correct? SELECT ALL THAT APPLY.

1. The child consistently eats nonfood substances such as dirt, crayons, and paper.
2. The child regurgitates, chews, and then reswallows previously ingested food.
3. A primary safety concern for the child is the possibility of accidental poisoning.
4. The child's greatest risk is aspiration and therefore should be observed for possible aspiration.
5. Complications can include malabsorption and fecal impaction.
6. Children with a pica disorder are intellectually bright and precocious.

ANSWER: 1, 3, 5

Pica is an eating disorder of young children who persistently eat nonfood substances such as dirt, clay, paint chips, crayons, yarn, or paper. Accidental poisoning from toxic substances in nonfood items is a major concern. Malabsorption, fecal impaction, constipation, and intestinal obstruction are complications associated with eating nonfood substances. The act of regurgitating, chewing, and then reswallowing previously ingested food is a rumination disorder. Regurgitating can increase the risk for aspiration. Aspiration is not the greatest risk associated with a pica disorder. The incidence of a pica disorder increases with children who are cognitively challenged, possibly because of their inability to distinguish edible from inedible substances as early as other children can.

➧ ***Test-taking Tip:*** *Apply knowledge of medical terminology. Pica is the Latin word for magpie (a bird that is an indiscriminate eater).*

Content Area: Child Health; *Category of Health Alteration:* Nutrition; *Integrated Processes:* Nursing Process Analysis; *Client Need:* Physiological Integrity/Basic Care and Comfort/Nutrition and Oral Hydration; *Cognitive Level:* Analysis

Reference: Pillitteri, A. (2007). *Maternal & Child Health Nursing: Care of the Childbearing & Childrearing Family* (5th ed., pp. 1733–1734). Philadelphia: Lippincott Williams & Wilkins.

1856. A clinic nurse is evaluating the effectiveness of parental teaching on interventions for a 10-year-old child diagnosed with an attention deficit hyperactivity disorder (ADHD). Which parental statement indicates that further teaching is needed?

1. "We will restrict our son from eating high-sugar foods, adding sugar to foods, and from foods with red and orange food-coloring additives."
2. "We can use a behavioral contract with our son, who scatters his clothing and belongings throughout the house and then can't find them when needed."
3. "We have developed a chart that lists goals and reward him with a star for progress toward achieving the goals."
4. "Setting limits with our son and increasing his recreational activities may help with his hyperactive behavior."

ANSWER: 1

Studies have consistently found that sugar and food additives do not cause or worsen hyperactive behavior. Behavioral contracts use behavior modification to reinforce positive behaviors and to enhance self-esteem and independence. Using goal charts and rewarding positive behavior with stars is one method to implement behavior modification. Setting limits promotes a safe environment and develops trust, and recreational activities channel excess energy and prevent escalation of disruptive behavior.

➧ ***Test-taking Tip:*** *This is a false-response item. Select the parental statement that is not correct in treating ADHD.*

Content Area: Child Health; *Category of Health Alteration:* Nutrition; *Integrated Processes:* Nursing Process Evaluation; *Client Need:* Psychosocial Integrity/Behavioral Interventions; *Cognitive Level:* Analysis

References: Fortinash, K., & Holoday Worret, P. (2008). *Psychiatric Mental Health Nursing* (4th ed., pp. 384–387). St. Louis, MO: Mosby Elsevier; Whitney, E., DeBruyne, L., Pinna, K., & Rolfes, S. (2007). *Nutrition for Health and Health Care* (3rd ed., p. 307). Belmont, CA: Thomson Learning.

1857. A nurse is caring for a client who does not go outdoors due to agoraphobia and also has an inadequate milk intake. For which vitamin deficiency should a nurse specifically assess when caring for the client?

1. Vitamin B_6
2. Vitamin A
3. Vitamin D
4. Vitamin C

ANSWER: 3

Agoraphobia is a fear of the outdoors, crowds, or uncontrolled social conditions. Milk is a major source of vitamin D, and vitamin D can be synthesized in the body by exposure to sunlight. Vitamin B_6 is primarily found in meat, fish, and poultry and is not synthesized in the body. Vitamins A and C are not synthesized with exposure to sunlight.

➧ ***Test-taking Tip:*** *The key words are "milk" and "sunlight." Focus on the functions and sources of fat-soluble vitamins.*

Content Area: Mental Health; *Category of Health Alteration:* Nutrition; *Integrated Processes:* Nursing Process Assessment; *Client Need:* Physiological Integrity/Basic Care and Comfort/Nutrition and Oral Hydration; *Cognitive Level:* Application

Reference: Insel, P., Turner, E., & Ross, D. (2007). *Nutrition* (3rd ed., pp. 398–405). Sudbury, MA: Jones and Bartlett.

Chapter Twelve

Comprehensive Tests

Comprehensive Exam One

1. A divorced wife of a hospitalized client asks a nurse for a status report on the condition of a hospitalized ex-husband. Which statement by the nurse would be most appropriate?

   1. "He has been comfortable throughout the day. He should be going home tomorrow."
   2. "I'm sorry; I will need to ask for your ex-husband's permission before I can give you any information about his condition."
   3. "You may contact your ex-husband's doctor for an update. Here is the number."
   4. "Because of confidentiality laws, I will need to get your name before I give you any information."

2. EBP When administering which ordered medications should a nurse most definitely plan to wear gloves? SELECT ALL THAT APPLY.

   1. Hydrocortisone (Cortaid®) 0.5% topically to skin lesions
   2. Chlorothiazide (Hydrodiuril®) 250 mg orally
   3. Phytonadione (Aquamephyton®) 10 mg intramuscularly
   4. Insulin aspart (Novolog®) 10 units subcutaneously
   5. Timoptic two drops to right eye daily

3. A client who is being treated for severe depression is receiving information regarding self-help groups. Which statement best demonstrates that the client understands the priority goal for crisis intervention?

   1. "I'm going to attend a self-help group to learn how to best cope with stress."
   2. "Stress causes my depression and I must learn to deal with it effectively."
   3. "I know to take my medication regularly as prescribed by my physician."
   4. "I really think I can learn how to cope so I can get my old life back."

4. EBP A client is admitted to a facility for treatment of alcohol dependence and admits to drinking 12 beers a day for 7 years. Which information, collected during the admission interview, should be *most* significant in planning care during the initial stages of treatment?

   1. High school graduate
   2. Family discord
   3. Tremors in hands
   4. Malnourished

5. EBP A nurse admits a client with assessment findings that include cool, pale extremities; heart rate 110, blood pressure 100/55 mm Hg, restless, and a slight decrease in urine output. Which actions should be taken by the nurse? Prioritize the nurse's actions by placing each intervention in the correct order.

   ___ Administer intravenous (IV) fluids
   ___ Insert urinary catheter
   ___ Provide warm blankets
   ___ Initiate cardiac monitoring

6. EBP After a thorough evaluation, a nurse concludes that the efforts of a client with type 2 diabetes mellitus (DM) to control blood glucose levels have been highly effective over the last 3 months. Which finding supports the nurse's conclusion?

   1. Hemoglobin A_{1c} level of 5%
   2. No incidence of diabetic ketoacidosis (DKA)
   3. No ketones in the urine
   4. Negative oral glucose tolerance test (OGTT)

7. EBP Hydrocortisone (Solu-Cortef®) 2.5 mg/kg IV q 12 hours is ordered for a pediatric client experiencing dyspnea and wheezing from an asthma episode. The child weighs 25 kg. The medication vial contains 100 mg per 2 mL. A nurse should prepare ______ mL of medication for intravenous administration.

8. EBP An operating room nurse is preparing for a client's procedure to begin. How should the nurse ensure that the correct procedure is being done on the correct client?

1. Ask the client to state his or her name
2. Check the medical record for the correct client and date of birth
3. Apply the universal protocol and perform a "time-out"
4. Make sure the operative site is marked

9. EBP Which actions should be taken by a nurse when admitting a client diagnosed with hepatitis C (HCV)?

1. Admits the client to a private room and initiates droplet isolation precautions
2. Admits the client to a semiprivate room and initiates standard precautions
3. Admits the client to a private room and initiates airborne isolation precautions
4. Admits the client to a semiprivate room and initiates contact isolation precautions

10. A nurse has been assigned to care for four newborns. Which newborn should the nurse assess first?

1. Baby A, who is 35 weeks gestation with stable vital signs
2. Baby B, who is large for gestational age (LGA)
3. Baby C, who had an Apgar score of 3 at 1 minute and 5 at 5 minutes
4. Baby D, who was born through meconium-stained fluid

11. EBP A client, diagnosed with severe depression, asks a nurse about taking St. John's wort as an alternative to prescription antidepressants. Which is the best response by the nurse?

1. "Since it is an herbal therapy, it is a safe alternative to antidepressants."
2. "It would take twice the dosage of St. John's wort to equal the effectiveness of a prescription antidepressant."
3. "There isn't enough evidence to support St. John's wort as an effective treatment for depression."
4. "I would suggest you discuss that possibility with your doctor."

12. EBP In the presurgical holding area, a nurse is caring for a client who has a white blood cell count (WBC) of 2.8 K/μL. Which nurse action is *most* important for the nurse to plan prior to initiating an IV?

1. Requesting an order for prophylactic antibiotics
2. Placing the client on respiratory isolation precautions
3. Using antibacterial soap to cleanse the client's arm
4. Performing hand hygiene with alcohol-based rub

13. EBP A nurse is preparing to initiate total parenteral nutrition (TPN) for a client with acute pancreatitis, via a central venous line. The nurse has already properly identified the client and verified the order by comparing the container of TPN solution to the health-care provider's order. Prioritize the remaining steps that the nurse should take in preparing the TPN for administration.

______ Purge the intravenous (IV) tubing with the TPN solution
______ Check patency with saline and then connect the tubing to the client's central line port
______ Assess client's knowledge of TPN and educate as needed
______ Set the infusion pump at the prescribed rate and start the infusion
______ Select the appropriate tubing and filter
______ Place the tubing in a volume control IV pump

14. The mother of a toddler, who is diagnosed with type 1 diabetes mellitus, asks a nurse if her child would benefit from an insulin infusion pump. Which statement should be the basis for the nurse's response?

1. Toddlers are too young to have an insulin pump.
2. Children who have been newly diagnosed with type 1 diabetes mellitus produce insulin in decreasing amounts for about 1 year.
3. The parents must be willing to check blood sugar levels every 3 to 4 hours and adjust insulin, food, and/or physical activity for the child based on the results.
4. A toddler receives only a small amount of insulin in one injection; an insulin pump is not needed until larger amounts of insulin are needed.

15. A nurse assists a physician in placing a central venous catheter for a client while at the client's bedside. The physician is offered a mask and gown but refuses to wear them. During insertion, the nurse notices that the catheter touches the physician's shirt. The nurse speaks up and tells the physician that the catheter is contaminated. The physician disagrees and places the catheter. This is the second time the nurse has had an experience of unsterile technique with the physician. What is the best action to be taken by the nurse?

1. Inform the client that the physician does not use sterile technique
2. Review the institutional policy on reporting physician behaviors
3. Review the standards of care for central venous catheter insertion
4. Ask another nurse to tell the supervisor about the event while discussing it with the physician

16. EBP A client is taking gabapentin (Neurontin®). A nurse evaluates that the medication is effective when noting that the client has:

1. less muscle weakness and decreased spasticity.
2. decreased intensity of chronic pain and decreased frequency of seizures.
3. increased number of white blood cells and increased hemoglobin.
4. improvement in mobility and improvement in cognitive function.

17. A nurse is interpreting a new order written for sertraline (Zoloft®). The dose, written in the chart by a physician, is illegible. What is the best action by the nurse?

1. Call the physician to clarify the order
2. Call the in-house pharmacy for assistance in clarifying the order
3. Consult the medication literature for normal doses and transcribe the order accordingly
4. Obtain a consensus from other nurses on the unit and administer the medication

18. EBP A client, who has undergone several series of chemotherapy treatments for cancer, tells a nurse that he is thinking about foregoing further treatment. The client states he only underwent the last round of therapy to please his family and oncologist. Which is the most appropriate action for the nurse to take?

1. Use therapeutic communication techniques to speak to the client's family about his wishes
2. Listen carefully to the client and encourage him to express his concerns and feelings
3. Ask the client if he has searched the Internet or library for the newest treatment options
4. Notify the primary care provider and request a referral to hospice care

19. EBP A nurse notes the illustrated skin changes on the arm of a client who is 19 days postautologous peripheral blood stem-cell transplantation (PBSCT) for treatment of non-Hodgkin's lymphoma (NHL). A nurse notifies the physician, suspecting that the client is most likely experiencing:

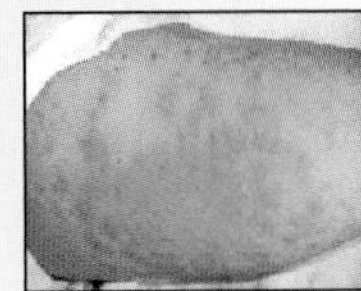

1. herpes zoster.
2. a peripherally inserted central catheter (PICC) line infection.
3. graft-versus-host disease (GVHD).
4. an allergic reaction to a medication.

20. EBP During a clinic visit, a client, who had a transurethral resection of the prostate (TURP) 8 weeks ago, tells a nurse that he no longer ejaculates during sexual intercourse. The client is concerned about this and questions if it is expected after TURP. Which statement should be the basis for the nurse's response?

1. The most common long-term side effect of prostate surgery is retrograde ejaculation.
2. Sexual physical abnormalities are rare after a TURP, and this client may have a psychological problem.
3. Retrograde ejaculation is an early complication of TURP surgery but usually is resolved within 2 weeks.
4. The client is describing an unusual symptom that needs thorough evaluation.

21. A nurse is assessing the lung sounds of a 6-month-old client with bronchiolitis. Place an X over the appropriate area on the illustration where it is most important for the nurse to auscultate for adventitious breath sounds.

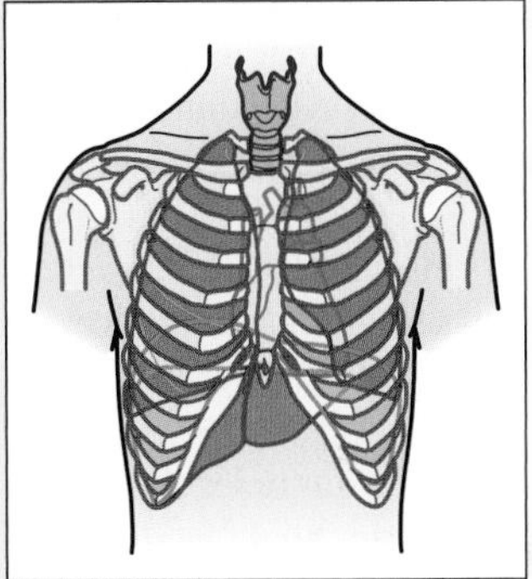

22. A nurse is evaluating a client's understanding of sigmoid colostomy care. The nurse should recognize the need for additional teaching when the client makes which statement?

1. "By utilizing colostomy irrigation I may not need to wear a fecal collecting device at all times."
2. "If I injure the stoma during irrigation, I will know because it will be painful."
3. "I know I need to examine the condition of the skin around the stoma every time I change the appliance."
4. "I know that my stoma should be odor-free if I properly apply and made sure the pouch is sealed."

23. The parent of a 4-year-old boy is concerned about nocturnal enuresis. Which point should the nurse include when educating the parent?

1. Proper handwashing will help prevent nocturnal enuresis.
2. Antipyretics may be administered around the clock.
3. The incidence will increase as the child matures.
4. Bedwetting should not be considered a problem until after the age of 6.

24. A nurse is reviewing the chart of a client admitted for treatment of a pulmonary embolus. Based on the analysis of the chart information, which conclusion by the nurse is correct? SELECT ALL THAT APPLY

Admitting History & Physical	Serum Laboratory Data	Diagnostic Data Results	Medications & Treatments
• Allergies: Latex and sulfonamides • Had been on bedrest at home due to influenza; treated with antibiotics • Severe abdominal cramping and diarrhea • Chest pain on inhalation • Dyspneic • Hemoptysis • Lung sounds: Pleural friction rub	• APTT: 31 seconds • K: 3.2 mEq/L • SCr: 0.7 mg/dL • WBCs: 18.9 K/μL • Stool culture positive for *Clostridium difficile*	• Lung scan: High ventilation-perfusion (V/Q) ratio	• 0.9% NaCl at 100 mL/hr • KCL 10 mEq IV now • Metronidazole (Flagyl®) 500 mg IV q6hr • Initiate heparin intravenous infusion per protocol • Contact isolation precautions • Oxygen 2–4 liters by simple face mask

1. Infection with *Clostridium difficile* is likely from the antibiotics used to treat influenza.
2. Contact isolation precautions are appropriate precautions for preventing an allergic reaction to latex.
3. Potassium chloride (KCL) is ordered to treat the client's low serum potassium level.
4. The metronidazole (Flagyl®) order should be questioned.
5. The heparin infusion order should be questioned.
6. The oxygen order should be questioned.

25. EBP A 4-year-old child has a history of four urinary tract infections over the past year. A physician orders a children's (pediatric) voiding cystourethrogram (CVUG) to determine the cause of the child's urinary tract infections. When preparing the child and parents for the procedure, which statement by the nurse is most accurate?

1. "Your child will need to stay overnight in the hospital to have this test."
2. "You will not be allowed to stay in the room with your child due to the radiation from the test."
3. "A catheter and contrast solution will be inserted into your child's bladder."
4. "Since this procedure is painless, no sedation is necessary during this procedure."

26. EBP Which statement should a nurse make when completing discharge teaching for an 18-year-old client who is hospitalized for treatment of anorexia nervosa?

1. "Now that you have learned to eat again, you are likely to feel hungry often and should give in to the urge to eat."
2. "Expect that you might feel like you are fat and uncomfortable because of your distorted thinking; this is characteristic of an eating disorder."
3. "You should be able to easily gain weight if you ask your parents to prepare the special foods you like to eat."
4. "Isn't it nice to feel that you are in control of your life now? Just continue to follow the meal plan and you will be fine."

27. A nurse is discharging a client following a myocardial infarction (MI) with stent placement and subsequent four-vessel coronary artery bypass graft surgery. The client has a body mass index (BMI) of 30, has a history of hypertension, smokes 1 pack per day (PPD) of cigarettes, and has prescriptions for aspirin, clopidogrel bisulfate (Plavix®), atenolol (Tenormin®), and atorvastatin (Lipitor®). Which discharge instructions are most appropriate? SELECT ALL THAT APPLY.

1. Discontinue the use of your elastic stockings (TEDS®)
2. Use a soft toothbrush and electric razor because you can bleed easily
3. Minimize your alcohol intake
4. Maintain your present weight to promote calorie intake for healing
5. Begin smoking cessation once your incision is completely healed
6. Discontinue the atenolol when your heart rate is less than 60 beats per minute

28. EBP A mother of a school-age child is concerned because her child is overweight and has been eating ice cream due to a dislike for milk. Which nursing action is best?

1. Teach the mother to give her child calcium supplements daily
2. Tell the mother that dairy products will be eaten by the child when the body feels the "need"
3. Teach the mother other options for getting two to three servings of dairy products, such as eating yogurt
4. Tell the mother that she doesn't need to worry about meeting this daily requirement

29. A client weighing 50 kg is diagnosed with a vascular leg ulcer and requires a continuous intravenous infusion of heparin 15 units/kg/hr. In order to administer the correct dose, the nurse should prepare the infusion pump to deliver _______ units of heparin per hour.

30. EBP A nurse is caring for an 85-year-old Native American client with heart failure who has an ejection fraction of 15%. Which nursing action indicates that the nurse needs further instruction on providing culturally competent care because the nurse's action is in conflict with the ethical principle of nonmaleficence?

1. Asking whether the client would like to complete a health-care directive
2. Allowing the client's family to leave tobacco leaves in a dish in the client's room
3. Providing the spouse a chair that folds out into a bed to stay in the client's room
4. Administering morphine sulfate when there are nonverbal and physiological signs of pain

31. At 0700 hours a physician writes medications orders for a newly admitted client:

Clopidogrel bisulfate (Plavix®) 75 mg oral daily
Aspirin 325 mg oral daily
Piperacillin/tazobactam (Zosyn®) 3.37 g IVPB q6h
Potassium chloride (K-Dur®) 40 mEq oral TID

At 0800 a nurse is validating the orders for accurate transcription by the pharmacy onto the client's electronic medication administration record (MAR) prior to administration. Place an X on the medication information that pharmacy has entered incorrectly.

Date: 5/4/09
Scheduled medications

FD: First Dose; LD: Last Dose Medication Order	Medication Name	Dose Frequency (Freq) Route (Rt)	0001–0759	0800–1559	1600–2400
1. FD: 08:00 **5/4/09** LD: OPEN	**PLAVIX**	**75 mg** **Freq: Daily** Rt: oral		08:00 ______	
2. FD: 08:00 **5/4/09** LD: OPEN	**ASA**	**325 mg** **Freq: Daily** Rt: oral		08:00 ______	
3. FD: 08:00 **5/4/09** LD: OPEN	**ZOSYN** Mixed in 100 mL NS	**3.37 g** **Freq: q4HOURS** Rt: IV	02:00 ______	08:00 ______ 14:00 ______	20:00 ______
4. FD: 08:00 **5/4/09** LD: OPEN	**K-Dur**	**40 mEq** **Fq: TID** Rt: oral		08:00 ______ 12:00 ______	17:00 ______

32. A nurse is assisting a 32-year-old new mother who is struggling with breastfeeding her 1-day-old newborn. The mother starts crying and states, "I don't know why I can't get the baby to nurse. Maybe I am not ready to be a mother." Which is the best response by the nurse?

1. "Maybe you should give the baby a bottle."
2. "Of course you are ready to be a mother, you are 32 years old."
3. "Do you know anyone else who has been successful with breastfeeding?"
4. "Tell me about what makes you feel that you are not ready to be a mother."

33. A client, who is not adhering to a physician's advice about dietary modifications and taking lovastatin (Mevacor®) as prescribed, receives additional teaching from a nurse. Based on the results of the client's serum laboratory results at follow-up, which conclusion by the nurse is accurate?

Lipid Profile	Client's Results
Total cholesterol	170 mg/dL
Triglycerides	100 mg/dL
HDL	60 mg/dL
LDL	100 mg/dL

1. The teaching or the medication is ineffective because the LDL level is elevated.
2. The teaching or the medication is ineffective because the total serum cholesterol is elevated.
3. The teaching and the medication are effective because the HDL level and the triglyceride level are within normal limits.
4. The teaching and the medication are effective because the LDL level is within normal limits and the HDL level is elevated.

34. EBP A client who suffered a closed-head injury in an industrial accident remains unresponsive. The client develops hyperthermia. Which interventions should a nurse plan to treat the client's hyperthermia? SELECT ALL THAT APPLY.

1. Administer acetaminophen (Tylenol®) 500 mg rectal suppository
2. Apply covered ice packs to axillary spaces
3. Place the client on a water cooling blanket
4. Administer a tepid bath
5. Administer belladonna and opium (B&O) rectal suppository
6. Administer iced saline through a nasogastric tube (NG) and then apply the NG to suction

35. A nurse, responding to a nursing assistant's call for help, brings the automated external defibrillator (AED) that is available outside a child's room. It appears that the child is not breathing. The nursing assistant (NA) is standing by the child. What should be the nurse's next action?

1. Tell the nursing assistant to open the child's airway and check for breathing
2. Tell the nursing assistant to check the child's pulse
3. Quickly set up the AED and apply the conduction pads
4. Begin cardiopulmonary resuscitation (CPR) and tell the next arriving person to set up the AED

36. EBP A 72-year-old female client is brought to a clinic by her daughter because she has been experiencing fatigue, ataxia, and confusion. The laboratory report indicates that the client has a hemoglobin level of 7.0 g/dL. It is most important for the nurse to collect additional information about the client's:

1. food intake and medication use.
2. exposure to toxic chemicals.
3. ability to care for herself following treatment.
4. daily amount of alcohol consumed and last drink.

37. EBP A nurse instructs a 15-year-old client diagnosed with asthma about using a peak expiratory flow meter. Which *immediate* action should the nurse recommend if the client obtains a reading that falls below 50% of his or her normal personal best reading?

1. Self-administer a nebulizer treatment
2. Use the "as needed" medication for asthma
3. Call the physician
4. Go to the emergency department

38. A parent provides the following food diary to a clinic nurse for a 2-year-old child. Which meal should the nurse address with the parent because the foods are unsafe for a toddler?

Food Diary for a Two-Year-Old

Breakfast	Lunch	Dinner
½ C whole milk ½ C iron-fortified cereal ½ C orange juice	½ C whole milk ½ C vegetables 1 egg ½ C noodles	½ C whole milk 2 oz hot dog slices ¼ C rice ½ C vegetables ¼ C whole cherries
Morning Snack	**Afternoon Snack**	**Evening Snack**
½ C yogurt ½ C fruit	½ C whole milk ½ slice toast 1 Tbs apple butter	½ C whole milk ½ slice buttered toast

1. Breakfast
2. Lunch
3. Dinner
4. Evening snack

39. EBP A psychiatric registered nurse (RN) is caring for clients with multiple mental health diagnoses with the aid of a patient care assistant (PCA). For which client should the RN caution the PCA regarding the client's likelihood of exhibiting aggressive behavior toward other clients and hospital personnel?

1. A client diagnosed with major depressive disorder
2. A client diagnosed with intermittent explosive disorder
3. A client diagnosed with histrionic personality disorder
4. A client diagnosed with oppositional defiant disorder

40. A nurse receives an order to administer a loop diuretic intravenous (IV) push to an adolescent client with hydronephrosis. For which adverse effects should the nurse monitor the client? SELECT ALL THAT APPLY.

1. Ototoxicity
2. Electrolyte abnormalities
3. Orthostatic hypotension
4. Hypertension
5. Hypoglycemia

41. EBP A nurse is teaching clients during a health seminar. In addition to advanced age, which factors associated with the formation of cataracts should the nurse address during the session? SELECT ALL THAT APPLY.

1. Exposure to radiation
2. Chronic exposure to sunlight
3. History of hypertension
4. History of diabetes mellitus
5. Obesity
6. Chronic corticosteroid use

42. A nurse observes the following rhythm on a cardiac monitor. Which should be the most appropriate action by the nurse?

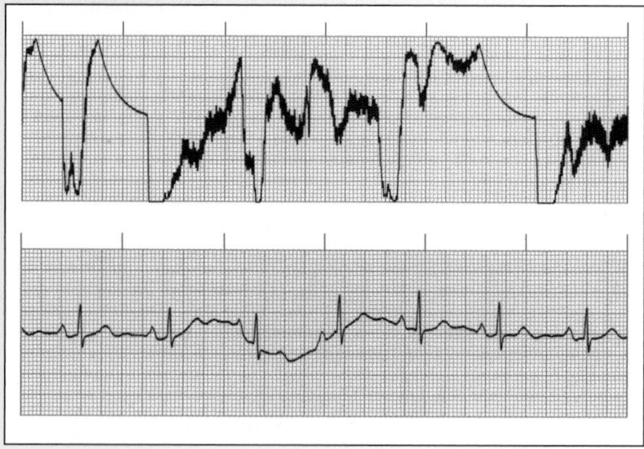

1. Call a code by activating the emergency response system
2. Do nothing because the client is moving; continue to monitor the client
3. Check the client's electrodes, ECG pads, and the electrical outlets in the room
4. Apply the pads for the unit's automated external defibrillator (AED) to interpret the client's rhythm and shock if indicated

43. EBP A 77-year-old client is diagnosed with an abdominal aortic aneurysm measuring 3.5 cm, which was discovered on a routine health physical. The client has a 30 pack-year history of cigarette smoking. Which learning need should a nurse identify as most important for the client?

1. Understand the importance and begin the process of smoking cessation
2. Understand and follow a reduced-sodium and low-saturated fat diet.
3. Follow through with medical supervision so the size of the aneurysm can be monitored at regular intervals
4. Verbalize understanding of preoperative and postoperative care following surgical repair of the aneurysm

44. EBP A client is diagnosed with degenerative joint disease of the left knee, which is to be treated conservatively. A nurse should include which information when planning teaching for the client? SELECT ALL THAT APPLY.

1. Begin a progressive walking program
2. Modify diet for weight reduction
3. Apply cold or heat to the knee joint
4. Obtain a prescription for narcotic analgesics for pain control
5. Avoid prolonged standing, kneeling, squatting, and stair climbing
6. Perform vigorous activities daily, such as rapid flexion and extension of the knee

45. Which signs and symptoms should a nurse expect when assessing a 7-month-old infant diagnosed with pneumonia? SELECT ALL THAT APPLY.

1. Productive cough with white sputum
2. Tachypnea
3. Rhonchi
4. Dullness on percussion
5. Excessive crying
6. Subnormal temperature

46. A nurse is educating a client on the necessary dietary modifications while taking phenelzine sulfate (Nardil®). Of the foods that the client eats frequently, which food should the nurse tell the client is safe to consume while taking phenelzine sulfate?

1. Cheddar cheese
2. Pepperoni
3. Wheat breads
4. Bananas

47. An uninsured client presents to an emergency department. A physician tells the client, "Since you don't have insurance, you will need to go to another hospital." Which statement should a nurse make to the client?

1. "You will need to go to the County Hospital. They will take good care of you there."
2. "I will try to find another doctor who will take care of you."
3. "You have the right to be treated at this hospital. I will talk to the physician."
4. "I will get you something for the pain. I'm sorry, we can't do anything more."

48. EBP A postpartum client tells a nurse that she would like to take ibuprofen (Motrin®) for severe afterpains occurring after breastfeeding her newborn, but she is concerned about the medication passing into her breast milk. The nurse's response to the client should be based on knowing that:

1. naproxen (Naprosyn®) should be the nonsteroidal anti-inflammatory drug (NSAID) of choice for breastfeeding mothers.
2. no medications should be taken when a women is breastfeeding.
3. acetaminophen (Tylenol®) is the only analgesic that should be avoided when breastfeeding.
4. ibuprofen (Motrin®) is poorly transferred into breast milk.

49. A new nurse receives a serum potassium result of 3.1 mEq/L for a client. Which should be the most appropriate action by the new nurse?

1. Document the serum potassium results because this is normal
2. Inform the physician of the test result at the physician's rounds in the morning
3. Consult the charge nurse to receive direction on the next steps
4. Consult the pharmacist to determine the correct amount of potassium to administer

50. EBP Which client behavior should a nurse identify as posing a high-risk for sexual behavior among clients in an inpatient psychiatric unit?

1. Aggression
2. Visual hallucinations
3. Feelings of superiority
4. Independence needs

51. EBP A bedridden client is receiving inpatient hospice care. The client, who has oxygen at 2 liters per nasal cannula, develops respiratory distress including increased respiratory effort and noisy respirations. Which interventions should improve the client's respiratory symptoms? SELECT ALL THAT APPLY.

1. Increase the dosage of morphine sulfate
2. Raise the head of the bed to 60 degrees
3. Administer hyoscyamine (Levsin®)
4. Elevate the client's heels off the bed on pillows
5. Obtain a fan to circulate air within the client's room
6. Administer an expectorant

52. A group of clients is assigned to a team consisting of a registered nurse (RN) and a licensed practical nurse (LPN). Which client should the RN assign to the LPN to provide client care and administer medications?

1. A 14-year-old client with chronic renal failure (CRF) who will need a subcutaneous injection of epoetin (Procrit®)
2. A 6-year-old client with hemophilia A, who has been admitted for a blood transfusion
3. A 12-year-old client who received a stem cell transplant and is to have a bone marrow aspiration
4. A 4-year-old with chemotherapy-induced neutropenia who has an elevated oral temperature

53. A client who had a colon resection for removal of diverticuli also has comorbidities of diabetes and chronic obstructive pulmonary disease (COPD). A team of physicians including a surgeon, hospitalist, endocrinologist, and pulmonologist are involved in the client's care. When a wound infection develops, an infectious disease physician is also consulted. Which plan by the case manager should provide individualized client care?

1. Coordinate communication, plans, and goals from the various physicians
2. Plan a multidisciplinary care conference with all of the physicians present
3. Direct the nurse caring for the client to talk to the physicians on rounds and document their plan of care
4. Recommend to each physician that the hospitalist should be the primary physician

54. A client has the illustrated intravenous (IV) infusion devices operating. Thus far, 700 mL of fluid should have been infused of a 1,000-mL bag of solution. Place an X on the area a nurse should check to confirm that 700 mL of IV fluid has infused.

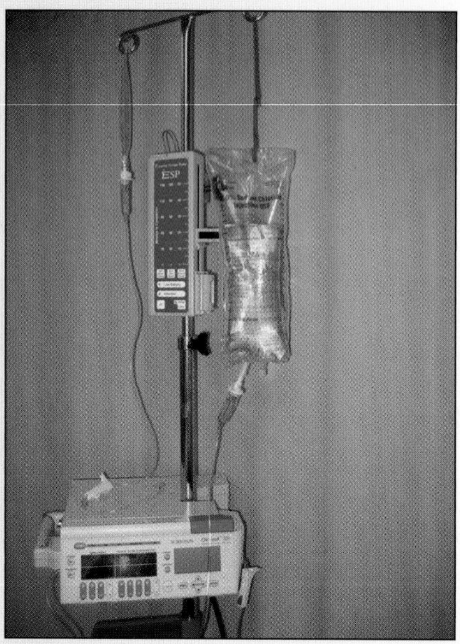

55. EBP A client diagnosed with Parkinson's disease is noted to be at high risk for falls. Which intervention by a nurse would be most effective in fall prevention?

1. Assess the client more frequently than usual
2. Apply restraints to keep the client in bed
3. Ask family members to stay with the client at all times
4. Instruct the nursing assistant to check the client more often

56. A nurse is caring for a toddler who is sitting on the potty chair with a book. When assessing the client, in which stage of Erikson's Stages of Development should a nurse place the toddler?

1. Autonomy versus Shame and Doubt
2. Trust versus Mistrust
3. Initiative versus Guilt
4. Autonomy versus Guilt

57. EBP A nurse identifies the following outcome for a newly delivered full-term infant, "*Area around umbilical cord will remain dry and free of erythema.*" To accomplish this outcome, which intervention should the nurse include in the plan of care?

1. Give the infant sponge baths until the cord falls off
2. Apply a lubricating lotion to the cord twice daily
3. Cover the cord with a transparent dressing to prevent urine contact
4. Move the cord in a circular fashion with each diaper change

58. A mother is devastated and crying after telling a nurse that she was just told that the only chance for her child to live is to have a bone marrow transplant and the only compatible donor is her other child. Which is the most appropriate nursing action to meet the mother's needs at this time?

1. Calling a crisis counselor and making an appointment for the mother
2. Listening quietly while the mother talks and cries
3. Questioning the mother about her fears
4. Describing the process for obtaining the bone marrow for transplant

59. EBP A home-care nurse is visiting the home of a client diagnosed with Alzheimer's disease. Which question by the nurse is most appropriate when attempting to assess the level of depression that the client's husband is experiencing as the primary caregiver?

1. "Do you need some part-time help?"
2. "What do you do in your spare time?"
3. "Do you feel caring for your wife is stressful?"
4. "Caring for your wife must keep you from doing the things you enjoy."

60. A 52-year-old female client tells a nurse that she has not had a menstrual period for 15 months. The client wonders if she still needs to be concerned about an unplanned pregnancy. Which should be the nurse's best response?

1. "As long as a female is having sexual intercourse, pregnancy is possible."
2. "The risk of pregnancy is reduced, but it is still possible."
3. "If you became pregnant at this time in your life, the pregnancy would naturally end in spontaneous abortion."
4. "Since you have not had a menstrual period for so long, it is unlikely that you could become pregnant."

61. When a 4-year-old child arrives on a unit to be admitted for a lymph node biopsy, the child is crying and hugging a teddy bear. Which response by the nurse would be best?

1. "Hello, my name is Chris. Come with me; I am going to show you to your new room."
2. "I see that you are crying. Let's go to the playroom where you can meet other children."
3. "Hi. I know you are feeling scared. I see you brought your special teddy bear. What's your bear's name?"
4. "Can I hold you and your teddy bear, and then take you to the room where you can put teddy to bed?"

62. **EBP** Which statement, made by a nurse caring for an adolescent client reporting "difficulty falling asleep," requires immediate follow-up by a nurse manager?

1. "You sound worried that your loss of sleep has affected your school performance."
2. "How long does it usually take you to fall asleep each night?"
3. "Sleep disorders are common among people who drink too much caffeine."
4. "Are you currently experiencing any unusual stressors in your life?"

63. **EBP** A client is hospitalized with a purulent forearm cut received from a rusty piece of metal. The client has a temperature of 102.8°F (39.3°C) and neck stiffness. The client's last tetanus booster was 6 years ago. Which medications should the nurse anticipate administering?

1. Tetanus and diphtheria toxoid (Td) booster and tetanus immune globulin (TIG)
2. Diazepam (Valium®) and penicillin G (Pfizerpen®)
3. Morphine sulfate and vecuronium (Norcuron®)
4. Fentanyl (Sublimaze®) and metronidazole (Flagyl®)

64. A physician orders 10 mEq of potassium chloride (KCL) intravenously (IV) for an adult client whose serum potassium level prior to surgery is 3.3 mEq/L. Which action should be the nurse's *first* priority?

1. Administering the medication as soon as possible through IV bolus
2. Waiting to start the medication until the client is asleep in surgery
3. Diluting the medication in 100 mL of saline and administer over an hour
4. Applying warm towels to the client's arm to prevent vein irritation during administration

65. **EBP** A client, diagnosed with type 2 diabetes mellitus, is hospitalized during the night with an infected foot ulcer. On admission, a physician writes an order to obtain fingerstick blood glucose levels four times per day before meals and at bedtime, to continue metformin XR (Glucophage®) 500 mg oral daily, and to administer 2 units aspart insulin subcutaneously three times a day, 5 minutes before meals. When reviewing the client's medical record, the on-coming day shift nurse notes that the client has had suboptimal glycemic control with oral hypoglycemic agents. The client's glycosylated hemoglobin level is 10.5%. Which should be the priority action for the on-coming day-shift nurse?

1. Question the physician's order for aspart insulin and metformin XR
2. Review the procedure for glucose monitoring with the client
3. Verify that the morning blood glucose level is greater than 70 mg/dL, and then administer the aspart insulin before breakfast
4. Initiate a consult for the diabetic educator to see the client

66. **EBP** A client, who is considering a Roux-en-y gastric bypass for obesity, asks a nurse to explain how this surgery causes weight loss. Which is the best response by the nurse?

1. "Part of the small bowel is removed so there is less surface for calorie absorption."
2. "The stomach will be bypassed so absorption of calories is decreased."
3. "The part of the stomach which comes into contact with food will be reduced in size, thus decreasing gastric capacity."
4. "Part of the large intestine will be bypassed, thus decreasing the surface area available for nutrient absorption."

67. A registered nurse (RN), with the assistance of a student nurse, is caring for a 24-hour-old infant. The student reports that the newborn's apical pulse is 136 beats per minute. In response to this information, the RN should instruct the student to:

1. monitor the pulse again in 1 hour.
2. place an oximeter on the newborn.
3. document the findings.
4. call the health-care provider immediately to report this information.

68. An elderly client is admitted to the emergency department after a fall. A nurse reviews the client's list of medications to determine if any are psychotropic medications. Which medications, noted in the client's medication list, should the nurse conclude are psychotropic medications that may have contributed to the fall? SELECT ALL THAT APPLY.

1. Alprazolam (Xanax XR®) 1 mg daily
2. Docusate sodium (Colace®) 100 mg daily
3. Hydrochlorothiazide (Hydrodiuril®) 25 mg daily
4. Potassium chloride (Micro K®) 10 mEq twice daily
5. Zolpidem tartrate (Ambien®) 10 mg daily at HS
6. Lisinopril (Zestril®) 10 mg daily

69. EBP A client is transferred from a nursing home to an emergency department with a diagnosis of dehydration secondary to vomiting and emesis from a norovirus infection. Which type of isolation precautions should the nurse initiate?

1. Contact
2. Droplet
3. Airborne
4. Protective

70. EBP A nurse manager's review of clients' medical records indicates that ordered antibiotics are being administered 2 hours prior to incision time. One measure to prevent surgical infection is to ensure that an ordered antibiotic is administered within 1 hour of the incision time. Which action, if taken by the nurse manager, should result in improvement in meeting this objective?

1. Establishment of clear expectations
2. A positive attitude
3. Mandatory staff education
4. Skillful communication

71. A nurse is caring for a client who is receiving intravenous (IV) oxytocin (Pitocin®) for labor induction. The nurse determines that the appropriate dosage of medication is being administered when:

1. 60- to 90-second uterine contractions are occurring every 2 minutes.
2. the client's cervix is 5 cm dilated.
3. three 40- to 60-second uterine contractions are occurring every 10 minutes.
4. the client expresses discomfort when the uterine contractions occur.

72. A nurse is assessing a 76-year-old female client. Which findings require physician consultation? SELECT ALL THAT APPLY.

1. 2+ pitting edema of lower extremities
2. Increased hair thinning
3. Warty growth on the vulva
4. Presence of actinic lentigo
5. Port-wine angioma on the arm
6. 6-mm asymmetric dark lesion on the perineum

73. A nurse is performing an admission assessment on a client with a history of trigeminal neuralgia (tic douloureux). What is the best method for the nurse to assess this client?

1. Ask the client about triggering factors that precipitate pain
2. Gently palpate the face in the areas under the cheekbones, observing for swelling
3. Ask the client to stand, shut both eyes, and alternate hands to touch the nose
4. Count the number of times the client blinks in a minute

74. EBP A 76-year-old client, hospitalized for cancer treatment, has an emergency bowel resection for a bowel obstruction. Four hours postoperatively, the client is experiencing pain. A nurse has the choice of standing postoperative pain orders or standing orders for cancer clients (protocol orders) of which all medications are listed on the client's medication administration record. Which medication should the nurse initially select to treat the client's postoperative pain?

1. Meperidine (Demerol®) 75 mg IM
2. Fentanyl (Duragesic®) transdermal patch 50 mcg/hr
3. Morphine sulfate (Duramorph®) 4 mg IVP q3–4h prn
4. Hydromorphone (Dilaudid®) continuous infusion 15 to 30 mg/hr

75. A nurse is reviewing a serum laboratory report for a client following surgery. Results include WBCs, 18,000 K/μL; SCr, 2.2 mg/dL; K, 3.5 mEq/L; and Hgb, 6.8 mg/dL. Per the physician's orders, the nurse assesses the client, removes the subclavian venous access device, and sends the tip for culture. In which order should the nurse perform the remaining physician's orders? Prioritize the nursing actions.

_____ Administer cephazolin sodium (Ancef®) 1 gram intravenously (IV)
_____ Administer 1 unit packed red blood cells
_____ Prime the blood tubing with 0.9% NaCl
_____ Insert a new intravenous access device
_____ Obtain the blood from blood bank
_____ Verify the client's identification and complete the checks for safe administration of the blood product

Answers

1. ANSWER: 2

The Health Information Portability and Accountability Act (HIPAA) requires nurses to comply with privacy standards, including implementing measures to ensure privacy. No information may be shared with anyone without the client's permission. Telling the divorced spouse about the status of the client is a breach of confidentiality. The physician also is required to follow HIPAA. Obtaining the divorced spouse's name and then providing information is a breach of client confidentiality.

➧ ***Test-taking Tip:*** *This is a positive event question so select an option that "supports" the HIPAA law.*

Content Area: Management of Care; *Category of Health Alteration:* Ethical, Legal, and Safety Issues in Nursing; *Integrated Processes:* Communication and Documentation; *Client Need:* Safe and Effective Care Environment/Management of Care/Informed Consent; *Cognitive Level:* Application

Reference: Jones, R. (2007). *Nursing Leadership and Management: Theories, Processes and Practice* (p. 87). Philadelphia: F. A. Davis.

2. ANSWER: 1, 3, 4, 5

Hydrocortisone can be absorbed through the skin when large amounts are applied. There is the potential for contact with body fluids if skin lesions are exudative. With intramuscular injections, subcutaneous injections, and eye drops, there is the potential for contact with the client's blood and body fluids. The nurse does not need to wear gloves when administering oral medications unless contact with the client's mucous membranes is anticipated. Although there are universal precaution guidelines, research has shown that health-care providers rely on their own judgment of risk rather than on national guidelines. This is a risky behavior and has resulted in injury.

➧ ***Test-taking Tip:*** *Use universal precautions when answering this question.*

Content Area: Fundamentals; *Category of Health Alteration:* Medication Administration; *Integrated Processes:* Nursing Process Implementation; *Client Need:* Safe and Effective Care Environment/ Safety and Infection Control/Standard/Transmission-based/Precautions/ Surgical Asepsis; *Cognitive Level:* Application

Reference: Wilson, B., Shannon, M., Shields, K., & Stang, C. (2008). *Prentice Hall Nurse's Drug Guide 2008* (pp. 306–308, 744–748, 788–790, 1214–1216). Upper Saddle River, NJ: Pearson Education.

EBP Reference: Gammon, J., Morgan-Samuel, H., & Gould, D. (2008). A review of the evidence for suboptimal compliance of healthcare practitioners to standard/universal infection control precautions. *Journal of Clinical Nursing*, 17(2), 157–167.

3. ANSWER: 4

The priority goal for crisis intervention is the client's return to a precrisis level of functioning. Option 1 reflects an outcome of crisis intervention, but it is not the initial goal of crisis intervention. Option 2 reflects an understanding of the role of stress in the development and management of depression, but it is not the initial goal of crisis intervention. Option 3 reflects an understanding of the role medication compliance plays in the prevention of relapse, but it is not the initial goal of crisis intervention.

➧ ***Test-taking Tip:*** *Focus on the information presented in the item's stem while noting the key word "priority." Use your understanding of crisis intervention, focusing on the goal and being able to identify outcomes as well as teaching topics.*

Content Area: Management of Care; *Category of Health Alteration:* Prioritization and Delegation; *Integrated Processes:* Nursing Process Evaluation; *Client Need:* Psychosocial Integrity/Support Systems; *Cognitive Level:* Analysis

Reference: Stuart, G. (2009). *Principles and Practices of Psychiatric Nursing* (9th ed., pp. 282–312). St. Louis, MO: Mosby.

4. ANSWER: 3

A hand tremor is one sign of delirium tremens (DTs). The first priority is protecting the patient's safety during withdrawals. Family discord, nutritional status, and educational level are important information to include in providing appropriate care during the rehabilitation phase of treatment following a safe detoxification from alcohol.

➧ ***Test-taking Tip:*** *Use Maslow's Hierarchy of Needs theory. Physiological problems are the priority. Of the physiological problems, consider which problem is more serious.*

Content Area: Mental Health; *Category of Health Alteration:* Substance Abuse; *Integrated Processes:* Nursing Process Analysis; *Client Need:* Psychosocial Integrity/Chemical and other Dependencies; Physiological Integrity/Reduction of Risk Potential/Potential for Complications from Surgical Procedures and Health Alterations; *Cognitive Level:* Analysis

Reference: Mohr, W. (2009). *Psychiatric Mental Health Nursing: Evidence-Based Concepts, Skills, and Practices* (7th ed., p. 635). Philadelphia: Lippincott Williams & Wilkins.

EBP Reference: Substance Abuse and Mental Health Services Administration. (2006). *Physical Detoxification Services for Withdrawal from Specific Substances.* Available at: www.guidelines.gov/summary/summary.aspx?doc_id=9118&nbr=004932&string=detoxification+AND+substances

5. ANSWER: 3, 4, 1, 2

Shivering increases oxygen demand and warm blankets can be quickly applied. Warm blankets may also promote peripheral vasodilation and make IV catheter insertion easier. Cardiac monitoring should then be initiated. Next, IV fluids should be administered. Finally, insertion of urinary catheter may be indicated for close monitoring of output.

➧ ***Test-taking Tip:*** *Use the ABCs (airway, breathing, circulation) and the nursing process to establish priority. Select an action that decreases oxygen demand as the first action.*

Content Area: Adult Health; *Category of Health Alteration:* Altered Fluid and Electrolytes; *Integrated Processes:* Nursing Process Implementation; *Client Need:* Physiological Integrity/Physiological Adaptation/Fluid and Electrolyte Imbalances; *Cognitive Level:* Analysis

Reference: Smeltzer, S., Bare, B., Hinkle, J., & Cheever, K. (2008). *Brunner & Suddarth's Textbook of Medical-Surgical Nursing* (11th ed.). Philadelphia: Lippincott Williams & Wilkins.

EBP Reference: Wakefield, B., Mentes, J., Holman, J., & Kennith Culp, K. (2008). Risk factors and outcomes associated with hospital admission for dehydration. *Rehabilitation Nursing*, 33(6), 233-242.

6. ANSWER: 1

The client's hemoglobin A_{1c} level supports the nurse's conclusion that the client has been effective in controlling blood glucose levels. Hemoglobin A_{1c} shows the amount of glucose attached to the hemoglobin molecules. This remains attached to the red blood cell (RBC) for the life of the RBC (about 120 days). According to the American Diabetes Association, an ideal hemoglobin A_{1c} is 7% or less for individuals with diabetes. The absence of complications, such as DKA or ketosis, is not the best measure of effective blood glucose control. Type 2 diabetics are more prone to hyperosmolar hyperglycemic syndrome (HHS) because their bodies are able to produce enough insulin to prevent DKA, but not enough to prevent severe hyperglycemia. The OGTT is used to diagnose DM; not for monitoring effective glucose control.

▶ ***Test-taking Tip:*** *The key words are "highly effective" and "3 months." Apply knowledge of the hemoglobin A1c test and normal values to answer this question.*

Content Area: Adult Health; *Category of Health Alteration:* Endocrine Management; *Integrated Processes:* Nursing Process Evaluation; *Client Need:* Physiological Integrity/Physiological Adaptation/Illness Management; *Cognitive Level:* Analysis

Reference: Lewis, S., Heitkemper, M., Dirksen, S., O'Brien, P., & Bucher, L. (2007). *Medical-Surgical Nursing: Assessment and Management of Clinical Problems* (7th ed., pp. 1255, 1258). St. Louis, MO: Mosby.

EBP Reference: American Diabetes Association. (2006). Standards of medical care in diabetes: 2006. *Diabetes Care*, 29(suppl 1), S4–S42.

7. ANSWER: 1.25

First, use a proportion formula to determine the dose, multiply the means (inside values) and extremes (outside values) and solve for X:
2.5 mg : 1 kg :: X mg : 25 kg
X = 62.5 mg
Next: Calculate the amount with the proportion formula:
100 mg : 2 mL :: 62.5 mg : X mL
100X = 125
X = 1.25 mL

▶ ***Test-taking Tip:*** *Focus on the information in the question, noting that first the child's dose should be calculated based on the child's weight and then the amount to administer.*

Content Area: Child Health; *Category of Health Alteration:* Pharmacological and Parenteral Therapies; *Integrated Processes:* Nursing Process Implementation; *Client Need:* Physiological Integrity/ Pharmacological and Parenteral Therapies/Dosage Calculation; *Cognitive Level:* Application

References: Pickar, G. (2007). *Dosage Calculations: A Ratio-Proportion Approach* (2nd ed., pp. 46, 344). Clifton Park, NY: Thomson Delmar Learning; Wilson, B., Shannon, M., Shields, K., & Stang, C. (2008). *Prentice Hall Nurse's Drug Guide 2008* (pp. 744–748). Upper Saddle River, NJ: Pearson Education.

EBP Reference: Kaiser Permanente Care Management Institute. (2006). *Pediatric Asthma: Clinical Practice Guideline.* Available at: www.guideline.gov/summary/summary.aspx?doc_id=10386&nbr=005432&string=atopic+AND+dermatitis

8. ANSWER: 3

The Joint Commission's universal protocol for preventing wrong-site, wrong-procedure, and wrong-person surgery and the Institute for Clinical Systems Improvement safe site protocol includes performing a time-out to verify the correct procedure is being done, on the correct side, and on the correct client. The "time-out" is a verbal confirmation of these measures by the surgical team. Asking the client to state his or her name is not enough information to verify the correct client. A second unique identifier such as birth date or medical record number must also be used. Checking the medical record does not ensure the record is for the client in the room. Marking the operative site will not validate the correct client is present for surgery.

▶ ***Test-taking Tip:*** *Apply knowledge of The Joint Commission's universal protocol. The key words are "correct procedure" on the "correct client." A time-out is needed to do additional checks.*

Content Area: Management of Care; *Category of Health Alteration:* Ethical, Legal, and Safety Issues in Nursing; *Integrated Processes:* Nursing Process Assessment; *Client Need:* Safe and Effective Care Environment/Safety and Infection Control/Error Prevention; *Cognitive Level:* Application

Reference: Wachter, R. (2008). *Understanding Patient Safety* (pp. 58–60). New York: McGraw-Hill.

EBP Reference: Institute for Clinical Systems Improvement. (2009). Health Care Protocol: Perioperative Protocol. Available at: www.icsi.org/perioperative__protocol__36011/perioperative__protocol.html

9. ANSWER: 2

Standard precautions with appropriate needle disposal are the only precautions required. Hepatitis C is transmitted percutaneously through needle sharing and needle stick accidents. It may also be transmitted via blood transfusions. Twenty percent of HCV cases are the result of high-risk sexual behavior. Special isolation precautions and a private room are not required to protect health-care workers from contracting HCV.

▶ ***Test-taking Tip:*** *The focus of this question is the mode of transmission of HCV. Knowing this would allow elimination of options 1, 3, and 4.*

Content Area: Adult Health; *Category of Health Alteration:* Infectious Disease; *Integrated Processes:* Nursing Process Planning; *Client Need:* Safe and Effective Care Environment/Safety and Infection Control/Standard/Transmission-based/Precautions/Surgical Asepsis; *Cognitive Level:* Analysis

References: Berman, A., Snyder, S., Kozier, B., & Erb, G. (2008). *Fundamentals of Nursing: Concepts, Process, and Practice* (8th ed., pp. 688–695). Upper Saddle River, NJ: Pearson Education; Lewis, S., Heitkemper, M., Dirksen, S., O'Brien, P., & Bucher, L. (2007). *Medical-Surgical Nursing: Assessment and Management of Clinical Problems* (7th ed., pp. 1090, 1100). St. Louis, MO: Mosby.

EBP Reference: Siegel, J., Rhinehart, E., Jackson, M., & Chiarello, L. (2007). *Guideline for Isolation Precautions: Preventing Transmission of Infectious Agents in the Health Care Setting.* CDC. Available at: www.cdc.gov/ncidod/dhqp/pdf/guidelines/Isolation2007.pdf

10. ANSWER: 3

An Apgar score below 4 indicates the need for newborn resuscitation. The nurse should assess this infant first to determine if the baby is currently in stable condition. The LGA baby is at increased risk for birth trauma, and the newborn born through meconium-stained fluid is at risk for meconium aspiration. However, neither of these concerns would take priority over the infant with decreased Apgar scores. The preterm infant is at risk for many health concerns but, at present, has stable vital signs. Thus, assessment of this infant could be delayed until the nurse has been assured that the infant with a low Apgar score is currently stable.

▶ ***Test-taking Tip:*** *Prioritize using the ABCs (airway, breathing, circulation). Select the newborn most likely to have concerns in one or all of these areas.*

Content Area: Management of Care; *Category of Health Alteration:* Prioritization and Delegation; *Integrated Processes:* Nursing Process Planning; *Client Need:* Safe and Effective Care Environment/Management of Care/Establishing Priorities; *Cognitive Level:* Analysis

Reference: Davidson, M., London, M., & Ladewig, P. (2008). *Olds' Maternal-Newborn Nursing & Women's Health Across the Lifespan* (8th ed., pp. 670–671, 938, 998). Upper Saddle River, NJ: Prentice Hall Health.

11. ANSWER: 3

For patients with major depression, there is insufficient evidence to recommend hypericum (St. John's wort) as a treatment alternative. Standard therapy may be of greater benefit for moderate to severe depression. The nurse cannot recommend it as a safe alternative nor equate dosages with antidepressant medications. The nurse should provide information to a client's questions rather than simply refer to the physician.

➧ ***Test-taking Tip:*** *Eliminate options that do not provide accurate information in response to the client's question.*

Content Area: Mental Health; *Category of Health Alteration:* Pharmacology and Parenteral Therapies; *Integrated Processes:* Communication and Documentation; Teaching and Learning; *Client Need:* Health Promotion and Maintenance/Principles of Teaching and Learning; Physiological Integrity/Basic Care and Comfort/ Nonpharmacological Comfort Interventions; *Cognitive Level:* Application

Reference: Deglin, J., & Vallerand, A. (2009). *Davis's Drug Guide for Nurses* (11th ed., p. 1316). Philadelphia: F. A. Davis.

EBP Reference: Kaiser Permanente Care Management Institute. (2006). *Depression Clinical Practice Guidelines.* Available at: www.guidelines.gov/summary/summary.aspx?doc_id=9632&nbr=005152&string=antidepressants

12. ANSWER: 4

Since the normal WBC is 3.9 to 11.9 K/μL (3,900 to 11,900 mm^3), the client is at risk for infection. These actions, and using aseptic technique, prevent the introduction of microorganisms. Alcohol-based hand rubs may offer better protection if hands are not visibly soiled. The first line of defense should be preventing the introduction of microorganisms. No data suggest that respiratory isolation is needed. If the client were neutropenic, neutropenic precautions should be used. The insertion site should be cleansed with an alcoholic chlorhexidine solution containing a concentration of chlorhexidine gluconate greater than 0.5%.

➧ ***Test-taking Tip:*** *Knowing the ranges for significant laboratory values will be required when taking the NCLEX-RN® examination. Remember K as a unit of measure represents a thousand (10^3) and μL is equivalent to 1 mm^3.*

Content Area: Adult Health; *Category of Health Alteration:* Perioperative Management; *Integrated Processes:* Nursing Process Planning; *Client Need:* Physiological Integrity/Pharmacological and Parenteral Therapies/Parenteral/Intravenous Therapies; Physiological Integrity/Reduction of Risk Potential/Laboratory Values; *Cognitive Level:* Application

Reference: Ignatavicius, D., & Workman, M. (2006). *Medical-Surgical Nursing: Critical Thinking for Collaborative Care* (5th ed., p. 303). St. Louis, MO: Saunders/Elsevier.

EBP Reference: Marschall, J., Mermel, L., Classen, D., Arias, K., Podgorny, K., et al. (2008). Strategies to prevent central line-associated bloodstream infections in acute care hospitals. *Infection Control and Hospital Epidemiology,* 29(Suppl 1), S22-S30.

13. ANSWER: 3, 5, 1, 6, 2, 4

First, assess client's knowledge of TPN and educate as needed. Client education is essential before new procedures to assist with coping, lessen anxiety, and promote client cooperation. Next, select the appropriate tubing and filter. TPN must be administered through tubing with an in-line filter to prevent contamination. Purging the intravenous (IV) tubing removes the air before the infusion is initiated to protect the client from the risk of air embolus. Next place the tubing in a volume control IV pump. Use of an electronic infusion device prevents fluid overload and insures accurate rate administration. Check patency with saline and then attach the TPN to a central line port. TPN must be administered through a central venous access because it is highly osmotic solution. Finally, set the infusion pump at the prescribed rate and start the infusion.

➧ ***Test-taking Tip:*** *Visualize the steps for administering a medication via IV infusion. The steps are the same, with the exception of using filtered tubing and utilizing a central venous access.*

Content Area: Fundamentals; *Category of Health Alteration:* Safety, Disaster Preparedness, and Infection Control; *Integrated Processes:* Nursing Process Implementation; *Client Need:* Safe and Effective Care Environment/Safety and Infection Control/Safe Use of Equipment; Physiological Integrity/Pharmacological and Parenteral Therapies/Total Parenteral Nutrition; *Cognitive Level:* Application

Reference: Craven, R., & Hirnle, C. (2007). *Fundamentals of Nursing, Human Health and Function* (5th ed., pp. 403, 564, 622, 626, 629). Philadelphia: Lippincott Williams & Wilkins.

EBP Reference: Bishop, L., Dougherty, L., Bodenham, A., Mansi, J., Crowe, P., et al. (2007). *Guidelines on the Insertion and Management of Central Venous Access Devices in Adults.* Available at: www.guideline.gov/summary/summary.aspx?view_id=1&doc_id=11992

14. ANSWER: 3

Insulin pumps are becoming more common in children. Checking the blood sugars, adjusting the insulin, trying to have the child eat the appropriate amounts of food, and getting the activity needed require parental diligence. Toddlers are not too young and are candidates for insulin pumps. Toddlers do produce decreasing amounts of insulin for up to 1 year. It is very difficult to adjust the basal rate for active toddlers when insulin is being produced. It is true that toddlers receive very small amounts of insulin, but that is not an issue affecting whether or not the child can have an insulin pump.

➧ ***Test-taking Tip:*** *Option 1 relates to age, options 2 and 4 relate to insulin production, and option 3 relates to parental responsibility. Focus on the parent's question, whether the child will benefit.*

Content Area: Child Health; *Category of Health Alteration:* Endocrine Management; *Integrated Processes:* Caring; Nursing Process Analysis; *Client Need:* Safe and Effective Care Environment/ Safety and Infection Control/Safe Use of Equipment; *Cognitive Level:* Analysis

Reference: Ball, J., & Bindler, R. (2008). *Pediatric Nursing: Caring for Children* (4th ed., pp. 1226–1227). Upper Saddle River, NJ: Prentice Hall.

15. ANSWER: 2

Nurses have a responsibility to support standards of practice. When standards are not met, they must be reported to the appropriate person or agency. Most institutions have policies for unsafe practices, including those of physicians. The nurse does not have a duty to tell the client of the unsterile technique; however, the nurse should monitor for signs of infection. Reviewing the standards of care will reinforce the need to use sterile technique; however, it will not address the physician's behavior. The nurse should be accountable and take responsibility for reporting unacceptable practice and not ask another to report the event.

➧ ***Test-taking Tip:*** *The key words are "best action." Recognize that the physician's behavior is unsafe and should be reported.*

Content Area: Management of Care; *Category of Health Alteration:* Ethical, Legal, and Safety Issues in Nursing; *Integrated Processes:* Nursing Process Implementation; Caring; *Client Need:* Safe and Effective Care Environment/Management of Care/Legal Rights and Responsibilities; *Cognitive Level:* Analysis

Reference: Wilkinson, J., & Van Leuven, K. (2007). *Fundamentals of Nursing* (pp. 1075–1076). Philadelphia: F. A. Davis.

16. ANSWER: 2

Gabapentin is an adjunct antiepileptic medication used in treating partial or mixed seizures. It also has unlabelled uses in preventing headaches and controlling chronic pain. Side effects of gabapentin include weakness and leukopenia (a reduction of white blood cells). Antiepileptic medications do not decrease spasticity or improve mobility or cognitive function. It has no effect on red blood cells.

➧ *Test-taking Tip: Gabapentin is an antiepileptic medication that can be used for chronic pain control. Eliminate options that do not pertain to these uses.*

Content Area: Adult Health; *Category of Health Alteration:* Pharmacological and Parenteral Therapies; *Integrated Processes:* Nursing Process Evaluation; *Client Need:* Physiological Integrity/ Pharmacological and Parenteral Therapies/Expected Actions or Outcomes; *Cognitive Level:* Analysis

References: Aschenbrenner, D., & Venable, S. (2009). *Drug Therapy in Nursing* (3rd ed., p. 347). Philadelphia: Lippincott Williams & Wilkins; Deglin, J., & Vallerand, A. (2007). *Davis's Drug Guide for Nurses* (10th ed., pp. 561–562). Philadelphia: F. A. Davis.

EBP Reference: Dworkin, R., O'Connor, A., Backonja, M., Farrar, J., Finnerup, N., et al. (2007). Pharmacologic management of neuropathic pain: evidence-based recommendations. *Pain 2007*, 132(3), 237–251. Available at: www.guideline.gov/summary/summary.aspx?doc_id=11724&nbr=006049&string=pain

17. ANSWER: 1

Clarify any order that is not clearly legible with the prescriber. Medication literature will guide in verifying safe dosages, but does not clarify what the client's actual dose should be. The prescribing physician should clarify the order, not the pharmacy or other nursing staff.

➧ *Test-taking Tip: Review the 5 rights of safe medication administration. Never administer any medication if the order is unclear or unsafe.*

Content Area: Mental Health; *Category of Health Alteration:* Pharmacological and Parenteral Therapies; *Integrated Processes:* Communication and Documentation; *Client Need:* Physiological Integrity/Pharmacological and Parenteral Therapies/Medication Administration; *Cognitive Level:* Application

Reference: Deglin, J., & Vallerand, A. (2009). *Davis's Drug Guide for Nurses* (11th ed., pp. 10–11). Philadelphia: F. A. Davis.

18. ANSWER: 2

The nurse should support the client in working through the decision to stop curative treatment by carefully listening to and encouraging the client's expression of feelings and concerns. The client is not asking for assistance to discuss the issue with family members, the primary care provider, or whether other treatment options exist.

➧ *Test-taking Tip: Read the scenario in the stem carefully. Evaluate the options and chose option 2, which focuses on the client and supports him in making treatment decisions.*

Content Area: Mental Health; Fundamentals; *Category of Health Alteration:* End-of-Life Care; *Integrated Processes:* Nursing Process Implementation; Caring; *Client Need:* Psychosocial Integrity/Grief and Loss; *Cognitive Level:* Analysis

Reference: Berman, A., Snyder, S., Kozier, B., & Erb, G. (2008). *Kozier & Erb's Fundamentals of Nursing: Concepts, Process, and Practice* (8th ed., pp. 1094–1095). Upper Saddle River, NJ: Pearson Education.

EBP Reference: Coenen, A., Doorenbos, A., & Wilson, S. (2007). Nursing interventions to promote dignified dying in four countries. *Oncology Nursing Forum*, 34(6), 1151–1156.

19. ANSWER: 3

Acute GVHD may initially appear as a pruritic or painful skin rash. Lesions are red to violet and typically first appear on the palms of the hands, soles of the feet, cheeks, neck, ears, and upper trunk. They can progress to involve the whole body. The median onset is post-transplantation day 19, with a range of 5 to 47 days. Herpes zoster lesions are more commonly noted on the anterior or posterior trunk and face. The vesicles and pustules of herpes zoster are grouped unilaterally, following the pathway of a spinal or cranial nerve (dermatomal distribution); they rupture, weep, and crust, and are very painful. There is no indication that this client had a PICC line. An allergic reaction to a medication is a possibility, but typically the rash appears first on the trunk or back.

➧ *Test-taking Tip: Note the key word, "most likely." Focus on the situation, "19 days postautologous peripheral blood stem-cell transplantation."*

Content Area: Adult Health; *Category of Health Alteration:* Hematological and Oncological Management; *Integrated Processes:* Nursing Process Analysis; *Client Need:* Physiological Integrity/ Reduction of Risk Potential/Potential for Complications of Diagnostic Tests/Treatments/Procedures; *Cognitive Level:* Analysis

References: Ignatavicius, D., & Workman, M. (2006). *Medical-Surgical Nursing: Critical Thinking for Collaborative Care* (5th ed., p. 1598). St. Louis, MO: Saunders/Elsevier; Smeltzer, S., Bare, B., Hinkle, J., & Cheever, K. (2008). *Brunner & Suddarth's Textbook of Medical-Surgical Nursing* (11th ed., p. 1113). Philadelphia: Lippincott Williams & Wilkins.

EBP Reference: Mandanas, R. (2006). Graft versus host disease. *E-Medicine.* Available at: www.emedicine.com/med/topic926.htm

20. ANSWER: 1

Cutting of the prostate during a TURP results in a partial resection of the urinary sphincter mechanism, causing the muscle along the bladder outlet to become weak. As a result, when the individual ejaculates, the sphincter cannot keep the bladder adequately closed. The ejaculate consequently goes backward into the bladder (retrograde ejaculation) rather than forward out of the penis. This occurs to some degree in all types of prostatic surgery. It is not a psychological problem, and it will not resolve within 2 weeks of the surgery.

➧ *Test-taking Tip: Focus on the anatomical alterations that would result in retrograde ejaculation.*

Content Area: Adult Health; *Category of Health Alteration:* Reproductive Management; *Integrated Processes:* Nursing Process Analysis; *Client Need:* Physiological Integrity/Physiological Adaptation/Alterations in Body Systems; *Cognitive Level:* Application

Reference: Lewis, S., Heitkemper, M., Dirksen, S., O'Brien, P., & Bucher, L. (2007). *Medical-Surgical Nursing: Assessment and Management of Clinical Problems* (7th ed., pp. 1421, 1422). St. Louis, MO: Mosby.

EBP Reference: Bird, G., Leveillee, R., & Patel, V. (2006). Prostate hyperplasia, benign. *E-Medicine from WebMD*. Available at: www.emedicine.com/med/TOPIC1919.HTM

21. ANSWER:

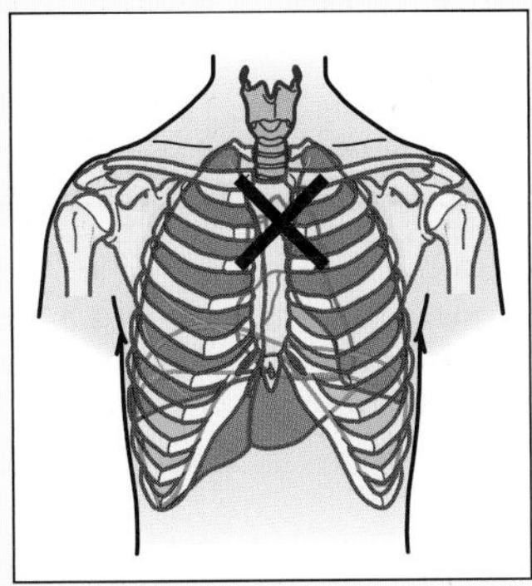

Adventitious breath sounds associated with bronchiolitis are commonly noted over the bronchioles. Placing the stethoscope over the trachea just above the suprasternal notch will allow for the best auscultation.

➧ ***Test-taking Tip:*** *Think about adventitious breath sounds with bronchiolitis. Use medical terminology to determine that auscultation should be over the bronchioles.*

Content Area: Child Health; *Category of Health Alteration:* Respiratory Management; *Integrated Processes:* Nursing Process Assessment; *Client Need:* Health Promotion and Maintenance/Techniques of Physical Assessment; *Cognitive Level:* Application

Reference: Ball, J., & Bindler, R. (2008). *Pediatric Nursing Caring for Children* (4th ed., pp. 700–705). Upper Saddle River, NJ: Pearson Education.

22. ANSWER: 2

The bowel has no sensory nerve endings for pain, so the client would not experience pain if the stoma were injured. By utilizing colostomy irrigations at the same time each day, a client may be able to predict the time of evacuation and thus eliminate the need for wearing a continuous collecting device. The client should be taught to assess peristomal skin with each pouch change, and there should not be apparent odor if a pouch is properly applied and sealed.

➧ ***Test-taking Tip:*** *"The need for additional teaching" indicates a false response item. Look for the incorrect statement.*

Content Area: Adult Health; *Category of Health Alteration:* Gastrointestinal Management; *Integrated Processes:* Nursing Process Evaluation; *Client Need:* Safe and Effective Care Environment/Safety and Infection Control/Safe Use of Equipment; *Cognitive Level:* Application

References: Craven, R., & Hirnle, C. (2007). *Fundamentals of Nursing, Human Health and Function* (5th ed., p. 1147). Philadelphia: Lippincott Williams & Wilkins; Monahan, F., Sands, J., Neighbors, M., Marek, J., & Green, C. (2007). *Phipps' Medical-Surgical Nursing: Health and Illness Perspectives* (8th ed., pp. 1262, 1264–1266). St. Louis, MO: Mosby

23. ANSWER: 4

Nocturnal enuresis, or bedwetting, should not be considered a problem until after age 6 years. Handwashing and the use of antipyretics are unrelated to this condition. The incidence will decline as the child matures.

➧ ***Test-taking Tip:*** *Apply knowledge about developmental milestones to select option 4.*

Content Area: Child Health; *Category of Health Alteration:* Renal and Urinary Management; *Integrated Processes:* Teaching and Learning; *Client Need:* Health Promotion and Maintenance/Growth and Development; *Cognitive Level:* Application

Reference: Berman, A., Snyder, S., Kozier, B., & Erb, G. (2008). *Kozier & Erb's Fundamentals of Nursing: Concepts, Process, and Practice* (8th ed., p. 1288). Upper Saddle River, NJ: Pearson Education.

24. ANSWER: 1, 3, 6

***Clostridium difficile* infection causes mild to severe diarrhea and abdominal cramping and can be associated with antibiotic treatment. Normal serum potassium levels are 3.5 to 5.5 mEq/L. Potassium chloride (KCL) is an appropriate treatment. The oxygen flow should be questioned; at least a flow rate of 5 L per minute is needed to prevent accumulation of expired air in the mask.** A latex allergy requires latex allergy precautions, which include the use of latex-free items. Metronidazole is an antiprotozoal anti-infective medication and is safe to use for clients with latex and sulfonamide allergies. It is used to treat the *Clostridium difficile* infection. While the APTT is within normal range (24 to 33 seconds), the therapeutic range for dosing heparin would be 1.5 to 2.5 times the normal APTT. The heparin infusion order is appropriate for anticoagulant treatment for the pulmonary embolism.

➧ ***Test-taking Tip:*** *Careful analysis of the information in the chart is needed to answer this question. The best strategy is to read the options first and then review the chart. Focus on verifying the appropriateness and/or accuracy of the treatment orders with the information presented.*

Content Area: Management of Care; *Category of Health Alteration:* Ethical, Legal, and Safety Issues in Nursing; *Integrated Processes:* Nursing Process Analysis; *Client Need:* Safe and Effective Care Environment/Safety and Infection Control/Error Prevention; *Cognitive Level:* Analysis

References: Lewis, S., Heitkemper, M., Dirksen, S., O'Brien, P., & Bucher, L. (2007). *Medical-Surgical Nursing: Assessment and Management of Clinical Problems* (7th ed., pp. 641, 1036-1037). St. Louis, MO: Mosby; Monahan, F., Sands, J., Neighbors, M., Marek, J., & Green, C. (2007). *Phipps' Medical-Surgical Nursing: Health and Illness Perspectives* (8th ed., pp. 662–665). St. Louis, MO: Mosby.

25. ANSWER: 3

The nurse should inform the parents that a catheter and contrast solution will be inserted into the child's bladder so that the bladder can be visualized on a fluoroscopic monitor while the bladder is filling to see if any liquid flows backward into one or both ureters, a condition known as vesicoureteral (VU) reflux. The test is performed on an outpatient basis, and a parent is allowed to remain in the room with the child during the procedure if the parent wears a lead apron to prevent exposure of vital organs to radiation. While sedation may not be needed, current studies show that the administration of midazolam (Versed®) eases the child's anxiety and does not affect the results of the test.

➧ ***Test-taking Tip:*** *Use Maslow's Hierarchy of Needs theory. Eliminate any options that do not intervene appropriately with physiological needs. Apply medical terminology to direct you to the correct option. "Cysto-" pertains to bladder. Select the option that includes the word bladder.*

Content Area: Child Health; *Category of Health Alteration:* Renal and Urinary Management; *Integrated Processes:* Teaching and Learning; *Client Need:* Physiological Integrity/Reduction of Risk Potential/Diagnostic Tests; *Cognitive Level:* Application

EBP Reference: Herd, D. (2008). Anxiety in children undergoing VCUG: Sedation or no sedation? *Advances in Urology, 2008*, Article ID 498614. Available at: www.hindawi.com/getarticle.aspx?doi=10.1155/2008/498614

26. ANSWER: 2

Feeling fat and uncomfortable is associated with the distorted thinking that accompanies anorexia nervosa and the client should be prepared and expect that this is characteristic of the disorder. Because of starvation or purging, the client may not feel hungry but should follow the meal plan despite feeling full. Enmeshment should be decreased by not preparing separate or special meals for the client. The client should be expected to follow the meal plan developed. Telling the client that is nice to feel in control of his or her life provides false reassurance. The cycle of eating disorder behaviors is life threatening and must be interrupted.

➧ ***Test-taking Tip:*** *Focus on the option that provides the client insight into the eating disorder and eliminate the other options.*

Content Area: Mental Health; *Category of Health Alteration:* Crisis, Violence, Eating, and Sleep Disorders; *Integrated Processes:* Teaching and Learning; *Client Need:* Psychosocial Integrity/Mental Health Concepts; *Cognitive Level:* Analysis

Reference: Fortinash, K., & Holoday Worret, P. (2008). *Psychiatric Mental Health Nursing* (4th ed., p. 401). St. Louis, MO: Mosby.

EBP Reference: Finnish Medical Society Duodecim. (2007). Eating disorders among children and adolescents. Available at: www.guideline.gov/summary/summary.aspx?doc_id=11035&nbr=005814&string=eating+AND+disorders

27. ANSWER: 2, 3

Both clopidogrel and aspirin prevent platelet aggregation and increase the risk for bleeding. Using bleeding precautions decreases the risk. Alcohol consumption increases caloric intake. A BMI of 30 indicates the client is overweight. Alcohol affects the liver and atorvastatin is metabolized by the liver and can increase liver enzymes. The elastic stockings help to decrease edema in the leg in which the saphenous vein was removed. Edema tends to increase with activity. A healthy diet for weight reduction can be initiated during the healing process. Interventions for smoking cessation should begin immediately, not after healing has occurred. Smoking causes a delay in healing. People who quit smoking after cardiac surgery reduce their risk of death by at least one-third. Atenolol should not be discontinued without a physician's order. Atenolol is used for treating hypertension and decreasing cardiac irritability after a MI and cardiac surgery. For a low heart rate, the client should consult with the physician and not discontinue the atenolol.

➧ ***Test-taking Tip:*** *Focus on the client's risk factors, surgical procedure, and medications ordered to determine appropriate teaching. Eliminate options that increase the potential for complications (options 1, 4, 5, and 6).*

Content Area: Adult Health; *Category of Health Alteration:* Cardiac Management; *Integrated Processes:* Teaching and Learning; *Client Need:* Physiological Integrity/Physiological Adaptation/Illness Management; *Cognitive Level:* Analysis

Reference: Monahan, F., Sands, J., Neighbors, M., Marek, J., & Green, C. (2007). *Phipps' Medical-Surgical Nursing: Health and Illness Perspectives* (8th ed., pp. 746–749, 847–852). St. Louis, MO: Mosby.

28. ANSWER: 3

Teach the mother creative ways to provide calcium in the diet. Calcium is recommended in foods rather than through supplements where absorption is variable. The body may crave certain types of food, but it is essential to develop positive habits in order to eat correctly.

➧ ***Test-taking Tip:*** *The key word is "best." Read each option carefully. Focus on the teaching role of the nurse to select the correct option.*

Content Area: Child Health; *Category of Health Alteration:* Growth and Development; *Integrated Process:* Teaching and Learning; *Client Need:* Health Promotion and Maintenance/Growth and Development; Physiological Integrity/Basic Care and Comfort/Nutrition and Oral Hydration; *Cognitive Level:* Application

Reference: Lutz, C. A., & Przytulski, K. R. (2006). *Nutrition & Diet Therapy: Evidence-Based Applications* (4th ed., p. 242). Philadelphia: F. A. Davis.

EBP Reference: Joanna Briggs Institute. (2007). Effective dietary interventions for managing overweight and obese children. *Best Practice,* 11(1). Available at: www.joannabriggs.edu.au/pdf/BPISEng_11_1.pdf

29. ANSWER: 750

Use a proportion formula to determine the dose. Multiply the means (inside values) and extremes (outside values) and solve for X.
15 units : 1 kg :: X units : 50 kg
X = 15 × 50
X = 750

➧ ***Test-taking Tip:*** *Focus on the information in the question and use the on-screen calculator.*

Content Area: Adult Health; *Category of Health Alteration:* Integument and Other Health Alterations; *Integrated Processes:* Nursing Process Implementation; *Client Need:* Physiological Integrity/Pharmacological and Parenteral Therapies/Dosage Calculation; *Cognitive Level:* Analysis

Reference: Pickar, G. (2007). *Dosage Calculations: A Ratio-Proportion Approach* (2nd ed., pp. 46, 344). Clifton Park, NY: Thomson Delmar Learning.

30. ANSWER: 1

Nonmaleficence is to do no harm. Discussion of advance directives, and issues such as cardiopulmonary resuscitation, are viewed as physically and emotionally harmful to Native American clients. Tobacco is a spiritual aspect of the Native American culture. As long as the tobacco is not burned, it does not cause harm. The family and client have cultural needs for closeness and comfort. Native Americans frequently do not verbalize pain.

➧ ***Test-taking Tip:*** *The key words "needs additional instruction" indicate this is a false-response item. Look for the incorrect answer associated with the Native American culture.*

Content Area: Adult Health; *Category of Health Alteration:* Older Client Needs; *Integrated Processes:* Nursing Process Implementation; *Client Need:* Psychosocial Integrity/Cultural Diversity; Safe and Effective Care Environment/Management of Care/Ethical Practice; *Cognitive Level:* Analysis

Reference: Berman, A., Snyder, S., Kozier, B., & Erb, G. (2008). *Kozier & Erb's Fundamentals of Nursing: Concepts, Process, and Practice* (8th ed., pp. 85, 92, 1194). Upper Saddle River, NJ: Pearson Education.

EBP Reference: Institute for Clinical Systems Improvement. (2008). Assessment and management of acute pain. Available at: www.guideline.gov/summary/summary.aspx?view_id=1&doc_id=12302

31. ANSWER:

3	FD:08:00 **5/4/09** LD: OPEN	**ZOSYN** Mixed in 100 mL NS **Freq: q4HOURS** Rt: IV	**3.37 g**	02:00____	08:00____ 14:00____	20:00____

The medication frequency for piperacillin/tazobactam (Zosyn®) was entered for every 4 hours instead of every 6 hours. Although the times are correct, the frequency is incorrect and could result in a medication error. All other medications were entered correctly.

➧ ***Test-taking Tip:*** *Read the medication orders carefully. Remember, to safely administer medications to clients, all parts of the medication order must be transcribed correctly onto the client's MAR.*

Content Area: Management of Care; *Category of Health Alteration:* Teaching and Learning, Communication, and Cultural Diversity; *Integrated Processes:* Communication and Documentation; *Client Need:* Safe and Effective Care Environment/Management of Care/Information Technology; *Cognitive Level:* Analysis

Reference: Berman, A., Snyder, S., Kozier, B., & Erb, G. (2008). *Kozier & Erb's Fundamentals of Nursing: Concepts, Process, and Practice* (8th ed., pp. 840–843). Upper Saddle River, NJ: Pearson Education.

32. ANSWER: 4

The correct response is to ask an open-ended statement that allows the client and nurse to work together to discuss the mother's issues. Telling the mother to give the baby a bottle does not address the mother's feelings about parenting; it also does not facilitate any communication between nurse and client and may add to the mother's feelings of inadequacy. Telling the mother, "Of course you are ready to be a mother, you are 32 years old," also does not promote any further communication and it gives the message that her feelings are trivial. Asking the mother a yes/no response question can put an end to the conversation quickly and does not address the mother's feelings.

▸ ***Test-taking Tip:*** *Eliminate the obvious incorrect answers. Remember to choose responses that would encourage communication.*

Content Area: Management of Care; *Category of Health Alteration:* Teaching and Learning, Communication, and Cultural Diversity; *Integrated Processes:* Communication and Documentation; *Client Need:* Psychosocial Integrity/Therapeutic Communications; *Cognitive Level:* Application

Reference: Craven, R., & Hirnle, C. (2007). *Fundamentals of Nursing: Human Health and Function* (5th ed., pp. 365–366). Philadelphia: Lippincott Williams & Wilkins.

33. ANSWER: 4

The teaching measures and the medication are effective. HMG-CoA reductase inhibitors (statins) reduce LDL cholesterol and increase HDL cholesterol levels. The normal value of LDL cholesterol is less than 130 mg/dL. The goal is to raise HDL cholesterol to 50 mg/dL or higher with the statin antilipidemics. The LDL cholesterol of 100 mg/dL is normal. The total serum cholesterol of 170 mg/dL is normal (normal is less than 200 mg/dL). The HDL is increased above normal, and the statins do not have an effect on triglycerides.

▸ ***Test-taking Tip:*** *Apply knowledge of the action of HMG-CoA reductase inhibitors (statins). Recall that statins have an effect on the LDL and HDL cholesterol and not triglycerides. Use the process of elimination to eliminate option 3.*

Content Area: Adult Health; *Category of Health Alteration:* Pharmacological and Parenteral Therapies; *Integrated Processes:* Nursing Process Evaluation; *Client Need:* Physiological Integrity/Pharmacological and Parenteral Therapies/Expected Actions or Outcomes; *Cognitive Level:* Analysis

Reference: Lehne, R. (2007). *Pharmacology for Nursing Care* (6th ed., pp. 559–562). St. Louis, MO: Saunders/Elsevier.

34. ANSWER: 1, 2, 3, 4

Interventions to reduce fever in clients with neurological alterations include pharmacologic measures (administration of acetaminophen) and nonpharmacologic measures (ice packs, a water cooling blanket, and a tepid bath), which increase heat loss through conduction. A B&O suppository is used for bladder spasms and does not lower temperature. Iced saline lavage may be used to constrict blood vessels for bleeding esophageal varices. It is not a treatment for hyperthermia.

▸ ***Test-taking Tip:*** *The key words are "hyperthermia" and "appropriate." The prefix "hyper" means excessive; "thermia" refers to temperature. Select option 1 because acetaminophen is known to have an antipyretic effect. Select options 2, 3, and 4 because these interventions will increase heat loss through conduction. Eliminate option 5 because a B&O suppository will not directly lower the temperature. Eliminate option 6 because it is not an appropriate intervention for hyperthermia.*

Content Area: Adult Health; *Category of Health Alteration:* Neurological Management; *Integrated Processes:* Nursing Process Planning; *Client Need:* Physiological Integrity/Reduction of Risk Potential/Vital Signs; *Cognitive Level:* Application

Reference: Berman, A., Snyder, S., Kozier, B., & Erb, G. (2008). *Kozier & Erb's Fundamentals of Nursing: Concepts, Process, and Practice* (8th ed., p. 531). Upper Saddle River, NJ: Pearson Education.

EBP Reference: Thompson, H., Kirkness, C., Mitchell, P., & Webb, D. (2007). Fever management practices of neuroscience nurses: national and regional perspectives. *Journal of Neuroscience Nursing*, 39(3), 151–162.

35. ANSWER: 1

The child's airway should be opened, and this is something that the NA should be able to manage because CPR certification is a requirement of employment in a health-care setting. The initial shock of seeing an unresponsive child for the first time can immobilize a person, but directions from another will assist the NA to act accordingly. The pulse is checked after opening the airway and checking for breathing. If defibrillation is required, every minute that defibrillation is delayed worsens the child's prognosis. The nurse can be setting up the AED while telling the NA to assess ABCs, and the NA should be able to begin CPR if needed.

▸ ***Test-taking Tip:*** *Note that the nurse's initial assessment of the situation is that the child is not breathing.*

Content Area: Child Health; *Category of Health Alteration:* Medical Emergencies; *Integrated Processes:* Nursing Process Implementation; *Client Need:* Physiological Integrity/Physiological Adaptation/Medical Emergencies; *Cognitive Level:* Application

Reference: Pillitteri, A. (2007). *Maternal & Child Health Nursing: Care of the Childbearing & Childrearing Family* (5th ed., pp. 1316–1317). Philadelphia: Lippincott Williams & Wilkins.

36. ANSWER: 1

Fatigue, ataxia, confusion, and a hemoglobin level of 7.0 g/dL suggests an anemia. The majority of anemias in older adults are due to nutritional deficiencies and medication use for chronic conditions. Exposure to chemical toxins is less common than nutritional deficiencies as a cause of anemia in older adults. The symptoms of ataxia and confusion can occur because of inadequate tissue oxygenation from the low hemoglobin. The symptoms are likely to resolve with blood replacement. Although alcohol consumption can cause ataxia and confusion and falls could cause bleeding, the situation does not indicate that the client has bruising or has been bleeding.

▸ ***Test-taking Tip:*** *Think about the major causes of anemia in the elderly prior to answering the question.*

Content Area: Adult Health; *Category of Health Alteration:* Hematological and Oncological Management; *Integrated Processes:* Nursing Process Assessment; *Client Need:* Physiological Integrity/Physiological Adaptation/Alterations in Body Systems; *Cognitive Level:* Analysis

Reference: Smeltzer, S., Bare, B., Hinkle, J., & Cheever, K. (2008). *Brunner & Suddarth's Textbook of Medical-Surgical Nursing* (11th ed., p. 1047). Philadelphia: Lippincott Williams & Wilkins.

EBP Reference: Killip, S. (2007). Iron deficiency anemia. *American Family Physician*, 75(5), 619–621, 671–678, 756.

37. ANSWER: 2

The appropriate first action to take when the peak flow rate is less than 50% of the personal best is to immediately take the "as needed" medication for asthma, which should be a short-acting bronchodilator. Severe airway narrowing may be occurring. Preparing for a nebulizer treatment will delay intervention. If the peak expiratory flow rate does not return immediately and stays in the yellow range (50% to 79% of personal best), then the physician should be notified or the child should go to the emergency department.

Test-taking Tip: Recognize that the child is in respiratory distress and immediate intervention is needed.

Content Area: Child Health; *Category of Health Alteration:* Respiratory Management; *Integrated Processes:* Teaching and Learning; *Client Need:* Physiological Integrity/Physiological Adaptation/Illness Management; *Cognitive Level:* Application

Reference: Hockenberry, M., & Wilson, D. (2007). *Wong's Nursing Care of Infants and Children* (8th ed., p. 1359). St. Louis, MO: Mosby.

EBP Reference: National Asthma Education and Prevention Program. (2007). *Expert panel report 3: Guidelines for the diagnosis and management of asthma.* Bethesda, Maryland: National Heart, Lung, and Blood Institute. Available at: www.guideline.gov/summary/summary.aspx?doc_id=11678&nbr=006027&string=asthma

38. ANSWER: 3

Infants and young children should not have hot dogs or cherries because these pose a choking risk. Hot dogs expand in the child's airway, and the fibrous skins of both hot dogs and cherries make sufficient chewing of these difficult. The other meals contain safe foods that don't pose a risk for choking. Eggs are introduced when the child is 1 year of age, but the child should be monitored for an egg allergy. Between 2 to 3½ cups of whole milk daily is sufficient to meet the nutrient needs of the 1-year-old. The overall food diary shows a balanced diet for the child's age.

Test-taking Tip: The key words are "most concerning." Think ABCs (airway, breathing, circulation). Examine each meal to determine if any food could compromise the airway of a 2-year-old.

Content Area: Child Health; *Category of Health Alteration:* Nutrition; *Integrated Processes:* Nursing Process Analysis; *Client Need:* Physiological Integrity/Reduction of Risk Potential/Potential for Alterations in Body Systems; *Cognitive Level:* Analysis

Reference: Whitney, E., DeBruyne, L., Pinna, K., & Rolfes, S. (2007). *Nutrition for Health and Health Care* (3rd ed., p. 287). Belmont, CA: Thomson Learning.

39. ANSWER: 2

A client diagnosed with intermittent explosive disorder is most likely to exhibit aggressive behavior. Intermittent explosive disorder is characterized by a history of aggressive behavior to others and destruction of property. Major depressive disorder and histrionic personality disorder are not characterized by aggressive behavior. Oppositional defiant disorder is more typically diagnosed in adolescents and is not typically characterized by aggression.

Test-taking Tip: Use the process of elimination, focusing on the key words "aggressive behavior."

Content Area: Management of Care; *Category of Health Alteration:* Prioritization and Delegation; *Integrated Processes:* Nursing Process Analysis; *Client Need:* Safe and Effective Care Environment/Safety and Infection Control/Injury Prevention; *Cognitive Level:* Analysis

Reference: Stuart, G. (2009). *Principles and Practices of Psychiatric Nursing* (9th ed.). St. Louis, MO: Mosby.

EBP Reference: Hazlett, E., Speiser, L., Goodman, M., Roy, M., Carrizal, M., Wynn, J. K., et al. (2007). Exaggerated affect-modulated startle during unpleasant stimuli in borderline personality disorder. *Biological Psychiatry*, 62(3), 250–255.

40. ANSWER: 1, 2, 3

Ototoxicity, electrolyte abnormalities, and orthostatic hypotension are common side effects of loop diuretic therapy. Diuretics are used for treatment of hypertension and would therefore be unlikely to cause hypertension. Hyperglycemia, not hypoglycemia, and glycosuria are side effects of loop diuretics.

Test-taking Tip: Note that options 3 and 4 are opposites, so one of these is likely to be incorrect.

Content Area: Child Health; *Category of Health Alteration:* Renal and Urinary Management; *Integrated Processes:* Nursing Process Implementation; *Client Need:* Physiological Integrity/Pharmacological and Parenteral Therapies/Adverse Effects/Contradictions; *Cognitive Level:* Application

Reference: Lewis, S., Heitkemper, M., Dirkson, S., O'Brien, P., & Bucher, L. (2007). *Medical-Surgical Nursing: Assessment and Management of Clinical Problems* (7th ed., p. 773). St. Louis, MO: Mosby.

41. ANSWER: 1, 2, 4, 6

Cataracts form under conditions that promote water loss and increase density of the lens. Exposure to toxic agents such as radiation, ultraviolet light from the sun, elevated glucose levels that occur with diabetes mellitus, and corticosteroid use damage the lens. The cumulative effects of aging also lead to cataract formation. Hypertension and obesity are not associated with cataract formation.

Test-taking Tip: Recall the pathophysiology involved with cataract formation. Consider each option and select the options that pose a risk to toxic agents.

Content Area: Adult Health; *Category of Health Alteration:* Integumentary Management and Other Health Alterations; *Integrated Processes:* Nursing Process Analysis; *Client Need:* Physiological Integrity/Reduction of Risk Potential/Potential for Alterations in Body Systems; *Cognitive Level:* Analysis

Reference: Ignatavicius, D., & Workman, M. (2006). *Medical-Surgical Nursing: Critical Thinking for Collaborative Care* (5th ed., pp. 1092–1093). St. Louis, MO: Saunders/Elsevier.

EBP Reference: American Academy of Ophthalmology. (2006). Cataract in the adult eye. Preferred practice pattern. In: *American Academy of Ophthalmology (AAO).* San Francisco: Author. Available at: www.guideline.gov/summary/summary.aspx?doc_id=10173&nbr5357

42. ANSWER: 3

Loose leads can cause artifact, which is a distortion of the ECG baseline and waveforms caused by factors other than the heart's electrical activity, such as client movement or loose leads. The electrodes should be removed and securely replaced in areas less affected by movement. The dark, wider tracing suggests electrical interference in addition to loose leads; the electrical plugs should be checked for loose connections. The nurse should first assess the client to determine if a code should be initiated. The artifact indicates the leads are loose. Accurate rhythm interpretation is difficult if artifact is present. Applying an AED is premature. The nurse should first assess the client.

Test-taking Tip: Always check the client first. Read each option carefully to determine if it is an appropriate intervention for the monitor rhythm illustrated. Even though you may not initially recognize the rhythm, the information provided in the options may assist in interpreting the rhythm.

Content Area: Adult Health; *Category of Health Alteration:* Cardiac Management; *Integrated Processes:* Nursing Process Implementation; *Client Need:* Physiological Integrity/Physiological Adaptation/Hemodynamics; *Cognitive Level:* Analysis

Reference: Lewis, S., Heitkemper, M., Dirksen, S., O'Brien, P., & Bucher, L. (2007). *Medical-Surgical Nursing: Assessment and Management of Clinical Problems* (7th ed., pp. 844–846). St. Louis, MO: Mosby.

43. ANSWER: 3

With a 3.5 cm aneurysm, continued medical supervision is indicated, including frequent computerized tomography (CT) exams to monitor the size of the aneurysm and risk for rupture. Smoking cessation and following a diet that lowers the risk of arteriosclerosis are indicated, but not the priority. Asymptomatic abdominal aortic aneurysms less than 6 cm in older adults are usually managed nonsurgically.

Test-taking Tip: *The age of the client and size of the aneurysm are cues in the stem to the correct option. The words "most important" are key words that indicate the need to prioritize. Note that option 2 addresses surgical management and option 3 addresses medical management; thus one of these options must be incorrect.*

Content Area: Adult Health; *Category of Health Alteration:* Vascular Management; *Integrated Processes:* Teaching and Learning; *Client Need:* Physiological Integrity/Physiological Adaptation/Illness Management; *Cognitive Level:* Application

Reference: Ignatavicius, D., & Workman, M. (2006). *Medical-Surgical Nursing: Critical Thinking for Collaborative Care* (5th ed., p. 807). St. Louis, MO: Saunders/Elsevier.

EBP Reference: Cosford, P., & Leng, G. (2007). Screening for abdominal aortic aneurysm. *Cochrane Database of Systematic Reviews* 2007, *2*, Article no. CD002945. Available at: www.cochrane.org/reviews/en/ab002945.html

44. ANSWER: 1, 2, 3, 5

Progressive walking strengthens bone and muscles and helps reduce obesity. Walking should be for a duration that is well tolerated initially and then walking is gradually increased to a duration of 30–60 minutes 5 to 7 days per week. Weight reduction decreases stress on the joints. Cold will reduce swelling and inflammation; heat increases circulation to the area and increases comfort. Avoiding prolonged standing, kneeling, squatting, and stair climbing will protect the knee joint. First-line medications include acetaminophen (Tylenol®) or, if not effective, a nonsteroidal anti-inflammatory drug (NSAID). Vigorous activities that produce prolonged pain and inflammation should be avoided because these stress the joint.

Test-taking Tip: *Focus on initial measures to protect the knee joint, reduce pain, and increase activity tolerance.*

Content Area: Adult Health; *Category of Health Alteration:* Musculoskeletal Management; *Integrated Processes:* Nursing Process Planning; *Client Need:* Physiological Integrity/Physiological Adaptation/Illness Management; *Cognitive Level:* Application

Reference: Smeltzer, S., Bare, B., Hinkle, J., & Cheever, K. (2008). *Brunner & Suddarth's Textbook of Medical-Surgical Nursing* (11th ed., pp. 1914–1917). Philadelphia: Lippincott Williams & Wilkins.

EBP Reference: American Academy of Orthopaedic Surgeons (AAOS). (2008). Treatment of osteoarthritis of the knee (non-arthroplasty). Rosemont (IL): AAOS. Available at: www.guideline.gov/summary/summary.aspx?doc_id=14279&nbr=7155

45. ANSWER: 1, 2, 3, 4

Coughing is due to the excessive sputum production with pneumonia. The blocked airways increases respiratory effort (tachypnea) and mucus in the airways causes scattered rhonchi throughout the lung fields. Consolidation causes dullness on percussion. Excessive crying is not usually noted; children are lethargic and listless. Children with pneumonia usually have high fever (not subnormal temperature) and are warm to the touch.

Test-taking Tip: *Focus on the condition and eliminate options opposite of those expected.*

Content Area: Child Health; *Category of Health Alteration:* Respiratory Management; *Integrated Processes:* Nursing Process Assessment; *Client Need:* Physiological Integrity/Reduction of Risk Potential/System Specific Assessments; *Cognitive Level:* Application

Reference: Ball, J., & Bindler, R. (2008). *Pediatric Nursing Caring for Children* (4th ed., pp. 705–706). Upper Saddle River, NJ: Pearson Education.

46. ANSWER: 3

Foods high in tyramine should be avoided when taking monoamine oxidase inhibitors (MAOIs). Wheat bread is allowed because it is low in tyramine. Cheddar cheese, pepperoni, and bananas all contain moderate to high levels of tyramine and should be avoided during MAOI therapy.

Test-taking Tip: *Review that phenelzine sulfate (Nardil®) is an MAOI. Remember which medications are MAOIs and that those who take MAOIs need to avoid ingestion of tyramine. Review tyramine-containing foods and use the process of elimination.*

Content Area: Mental Health; *Category of Health Alteration:* Pharmacology and Parenteral Therapies; *Integrated Processes:* Teaching and Learning; *Client Need:* Health Promotion and Maintenance/Self-Care; Physiological Integrity/Pharmacological and Parenteral Therapies/Adverse Effects/Contraindications/Interactions; *Cognitive Level:* Application

Reference: Townsend, M. (2009). *Psychiatric Mental Health Nursing* (6th ed., p. 311). Philadelphia: F. A. Davis.

47. ANSWER: 3

The Emergency Medical Treatment and Active Labor Act (EMTALA) ensures public access to emergency services regardless of ability to pay. Sending the client to another hospital violates the client's rights as does sending the client home. The physician is required to see the client even if the client is uninsured.

Test-taking Tip: *Note that three options deny care, whereas one is different. Often the option that is different is correct.*

Content Area: Management of Care; *Category of Health Alteration:* Ethical, Legal, and Safety Issues in Nursing; *Integrated Processes:* Caring; *Client Need:* Safe and Effective Care Environment/Management of Care/Client Rights; *Cognitive Level:* Analysis

Reference: Wilkinson, J., & Van Leuven, K. (2007). *Fundamentals of Nursing* (p. 1072). Philadelphia: F.A. Davis.

48. ANSWER: 4

Of the nonsteroidal anti-inflammatory drugs (NSAIDs), ibuprofen is the preferred choice because it has poor transfer into milk and has been well-studied in children. Long half-life NSAIDs, such as naproxen, can accumulate in the infant's system with prolonged use. Breastfeeding mothers do not need to avoid all medications. The transfer of medications into breast milk depends on a concentration gradient that allows passive diffusion of nonionized, non-protein–bound drugs. The infant's medication exposure can be limited by prescribing medications to the breastfeeding mother that are poorly absorbed orally, by avoiding breastfeeding during times of peak maternal serum drug concentration, and by prescribing topical therapy when possible. Acetaminophen can be used safely in breastfeeding women.

▸ *Test-taking Tip: Eliminate option 2 as this option is too extreme to be true. Select the option that has poor transfer in breast milk.*

Content Area: Childbearing Families; *Category of Health Alteration:* Postpartum Management; *Integrated Processes:* Nursing Process Implementation; *Client Need:* Physiological Integrity/Pharmacological and Parenteral Therapies/Expected Actions or Outcomes; *Cognitive Level:* Analysis

Reference: Davidson, M., London, M., & Ladewig, P. (2008). *Olds' Maternal-Newborn Nursing & Women's Health Across the Lifespan* (8th ed., pp. 1080–1081, 1159). Upper Saddle River, NJ: Prentice Hall Health.

EBP References: Werler, M., Mitchell, A., Hernandez-Diaz, S., & Honein, M. (2005). Use of over-the-counter medications during pregnancy. *Am J Obstet Gynecol*, 193(3 Pt 1), 771–777; Wilbeck, J., Schorn, M., & Daley, L. (2008). Pharmacologic management of acute pain in breastfeeding women. *Journal of Emergency Nursing*, 34(4), 340–344.

49. ANSWER: 3

The serum potassium level is low. When the nurse lacks the knowledge to solve a problem, it is appropriate to consult with a person who has more experience, such as the charge nurse or mentor. Waiting until the next morning to inform the physician could result in a delay of necessary client treatment and is inappropriate. The pharmacist may be consulted to learn about potassium supplements, but cannot prescribe potassium for the nurse to administer.

▸ *Test-taking Tip: Eliminate options that would delay client treatment or relate to performing an action that is outside of the professional's role.*

Content Area: Management of Care; *Category of Health Alteration:* Leadership and Management; *Integrated Processes:* Nursing Process Analysis; *Client Need:* Safe and Effective Care Environment/ Management of Care/Collaboration with Interdisciplinary Team; *Cognitive Level:* Application

Reference: Harkreader, H., Hogan, M., & Thobaben, M. (2007). *Fundamentals of Nursing* (3rd ed., pp. 195, 208). St. Louis, MO: Saunders/Elsevier.

50. ANSWER: 1

A nurse should identify that certain client behaviors indicate a higher risk for sexual behavior. Aggression is a behavior associated with the potential for increased sexual behavior. Auditory hallucinations and not visual hallucinations and perception of inferiority, not superiority, are other indicators. Deep dependency needs, and not independence needs, identify another indicator of potential for increased sexual behavior.

▸ *Test-taking Tip: Carefully read the options for behaviors that are opposite those expected for a client with high-risk for sexual behavior with other clients.*

Content Area: Mental Health; *Category of Health Alteration:* Personality and Other Mental Health Disorders; *Integrated Processes:* Nursing Process Assessment; *Client Need:* Psychosocial Integrity/Mental Health Concepts; *Cognitive Level:* Application

EBP Reference: Waddell, A., Ross, L., Ladd, L., & Seeman, M. (2006). Safe minds–perceptions of safety in a rehabilitation clinic for serious persistent mental illness. *International Journal of Psychosocial Rehabilitation*, 11(1), 4–10.

51. ANSWER: 1, 2, 3, 5

Dyspnea in hospice clients is treated with morphine sulfate to decrease venous return and ease the effort of breathing. Raising the head of the bed improves lung expansion. Levsin® is an anticholinergic medication that will dry respiratory secretions. The flow of circulating air from the fan often diminishes the sense of effort the client feels in trying to breathe. Elevation of the heels will prevent skin breakdown on the heels but does not affect breathing. An expectorant will thin secretions and may increase coughing.

▸ *Test-taking Tip: Read the scenario in the stem carefully. Evaluate each option as to easing respiratory effort or decreasing respiratory secretions.*

Content Area: Mental Health; Fundamentals; *Category of Health Alteration:* End-of-Life Care; *Integrated Processes:* Nursing Process Intervention; *Client Need:* Physiological Integrity/Basic Care and Comfort/ Nonpharmacological Comfort Interventions; *Cognitive Level:* Analysis

Reference: Ignatavicius, D., & Workman, M. (2006). *Medical-Surgical Nursing: Critical Thinking for Collaborative Care* (5th ed., pp. 111–112). St. Louis, MO: Saunders/Elsevier.

EBP Reference: Wee, B., & Hillier, R. (2008). Interventions for noisy breathing in patients near to death. *Cochrane Database of Systematic Reviews 2008*, *1*, Article no. CD005177. Available at: www.mrw.interscience.wiley.com/cochrane/clsysrev/articles/CD005177/frame.html

52. ANSWER: 1

The client with CRF is the most stable. Subcutaneous administration of epoetin is within the LPN scope of practice. The other clients require skills that are more complex, sterile technique, or judgments about the client's care.

▸ *Test-taking Tip: Think about the LPN scope of practice. Eliminate options that require complex skills, assessments, or if the client's condition may be unstable.*

Content Area: Management of Care; *Category of Health Alteration:* Prioritization and Delegation; *Integrated Processes:* Nursing Process Planning; *Client Need:* Safe and Effective Care Environment/ Management of Care/Delegation; *Cognitive Level:* Application

References: Berman, A., Snyder, S., Kozier, B., & Erb, G. (2008). *Kozier & Erb's Fundamentals of Nursing: Concepts, Process, and Practice* (8th ed., pp. 518–520). Upper Saddle River, NJ: Pearson Education; Weiss, D., & Tappen, R. (2007). *Essentials of Nursing Leadership and Management* (4th ed., pp. 123–137). Philadelphia: F. A. Davis Company.

53. ANSWER: 1

Coordination of care is a primary function of case managers. Overseeing services and resources to avoid duplication and breakdowns in quality are important to the role of the case manager. Planning a conference with all physicians may be difficult due to scheduling constraints. The conference also excludes the client and family, which would be inappropriate. A case manager should not delegate coordination of care to the nurse caring for the client. It would be inappropriate for the nurse to recommend one physician be the primary physician.

▸ *Test-taking Tip: The key words include case manager. The issue of the question is coordinating care from a variety of physicians and disciplines, which is part of the correct answer.*

Content Area: Management of Care; *Category of Health Alteration:* Leadership and Management; *Integrated Processes:* Nursing Process Planning; *Client Need:* Safe and Effective Care Environment/ Management of Care/Case Management; *Cognitive Level:* Analysis

Reference: Whitehead, D., Weiss, S., & Tappen, R. (2007). *Essentials of Nursing Leadership and Management* (p. 147). Philadelphia: F.A. Davis.

54. ANSWER:

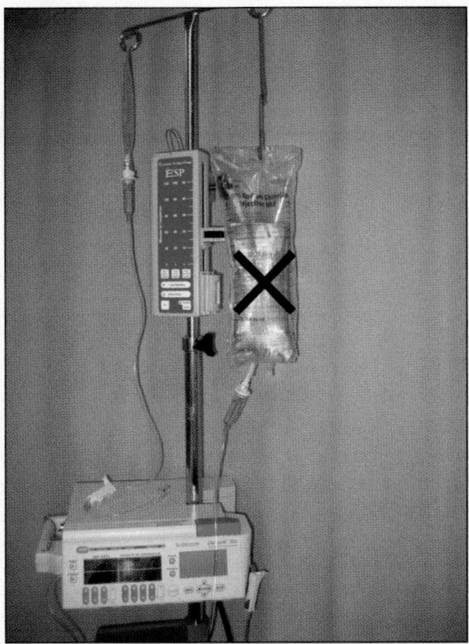

To ensure proper IV infusion pump function, the nurse should confirm that the infusion rate is consistent with changes in the volume of fluid remaining in the IV bag. In this illustration, the infusion rate must be incorrect or the IV infusion pump must be malfunctioning because only approximately 200 mL of solution has infused. The X should not be placed on the pump itself because the pump may read that 700 mL has infused whereas the bag may show only 200 mL has infused.

➧ ***Test-taking Tip:*** *The key word is "confirm." The only sure method to confirm the volume infused is to check the IV solution bag that is infusing and not the pump.*

Content Area: Management of Care; *Category of Health Alteration:* Ethical, Legal, and Safety Issues in Nursing; *Integrated Processes:* Nursing Process Implementation; *Client Need:* Safe and Effective Care Environment/Safety and Infection Control/Safe Use of Equipment; *Cognitive Level:* Application

Reference: Jones, R. (2007). *Nursing Leadership and Management: Theories, Processes and Practice* (p. 76). Philadelphia: F.A. Davis.

55. ANSWER: 1

Assessing the client more frequently is the most effective intervention of the options provided. Restraints should only be applied if the client demonstrates noncompliance and a physician order is obtained for the restraints. Family members may not be able to prevent a fall. Instructing the nursing assistant to check the client more frequently may be helpful; however the delegation lacks specific time frequency.

➧ ***Test-taking Tip:*** *Pay attention to the key word of this question, "most effective." Apply knowledge of fall prevention interventions. It is important that the nurse provide care and interventions for clients unless specified in the question that the nurse is delegating to another staff member. Therefore, the best option is for the nurse to assess the client rather than having a family member or a nursing assistant monitor the client. The nursing process can also be used to answer this question. Assessment is the first step in the nursing process.*

Content Area: Management of Care; *Category of Health Alteration:* Ethical, Legal, and Safety Issues in Nursing; *Integrated Processes:* Nursing Process Implementation; *Client Need:* Safe and Effective Care Environment/Safety and Infection Control/Accident and Injury Prevention; *Cognitive Level:* Application

Reference: Harkreader, H., Hogan, M., & Thobaben, M. (2007). *Fundamentals of Nursing* (3rd ed., pp. 555–556). St. Louis, MO: Saunders/Elsevier.

EBP Reference: Best Practice Committee of the Health Care Association of New Jersey. (2006). Fall management guidelines. Available at: www.guideline.gov/summary/summary.aspx?doc_id=9743&nbr=005216&string=fall+AND+prevention

56. ANSWER: 1

The toddler stage of development based on Erikson's developmental theory is Autonomy versus Shame and Doubt. Trust versus Mistrust is the stage for an infant. Initiative versus Guilt is the stage for a preschooler. Autonomy versus Guilt is not a stage.

➧ ***Test-taking Tip:*** *Apply knowledge of Erikson's Stages of Development. Examine options that have some of the same terms and use the process of elimination to eliminate one or both of these.*

Content Area: Child Health; *Category of Health Alteration:* Growth and Development; *Integrated Processes:* Nursing Process Assessment; *Client Need:* Health Promotion and Maintenance/Developmental Stages and Transitions; *Cognitive Level:* Analysis

Reference: Pillitteri, A. (2007). *Maternal & Child Health Nursing: Care of the Childbearing & Childrearing Family* (5th ed., pp. 814–815). Philadelphia: Lippincott Williams & Wilkins.

57. ANSWER: 1

Until the umbilical cord falls off, it should be kept dry. Therefore the infant should be given sponge baths rather than immersed in a tub of water. The use of lotions near the cord should be discouraged because this can decrease drying and predispose the area to infection. The cord should be uncovered to promote drying and the diaper placed such that urine does not come in contact with the cord. The cord should not be moved as manipulation can cause infection to develop.

➧ ***Test-taking Tip:*** *Focus on the action that would best promote drying of the cord and eliminate options that increase cord moistness or injury.*

Content Area: Childbearing Families; *Category of Health Alteration:* Neonatal and High-Risk Neonatal Management; *Integrated Processes:* Nursing Process Implementation; *Client Need:* Health Promotion and Maintenance/Antepartum/Intrapartum/Postpartum and Newborn Care; *Cognitive Level:* Application

Reference: Pillitteri, A. (2007). *Maternal & Child Health Nursing: Care of the Childbearing & Childrearing Family* (5th ed., p. 712). Philadelphia: Lippincott Williams & Wilkins.

EBP Reference: National Collaborating Centre for Primary Care. (2006). Postnatal care. Routine postnatal care of women and their babies. Available at: www.guideline.gov/summary/summary.aspx?doc_id=9630&nbr=005150&string=newborn+AND+umbilical+AND+care

58. ANSWER: 2

Because the mother just received devastating news, the nurse's presence acknowledges the mother's feelings and is needed for support as the mother begins to cope with the news. A crisis counselor may be helpful, but what is needed at this time is the nurse's presence. Questioning the mother about her fears is a barrier to therapeutic communication. While information is helpful in coping, the timing is inappropriate. What is needed at this time is listening and caring.

➧ ***Test-taking Tip:*** *Focus on selecting the option that best demonstrates caring.*

Content Area: Child Health; *Category of Health Alteration:* Hematological and Oncological Management; *Integrated Processes:* Caring; *Client Need:* Psychosocial Integrity/Crisis Intervention; *Cognitive Level:* Analysis

References: Ball, J., & Bindler, R. (2008). *Pediatric Nursing: Caring for Children* (4th ed., pp. 870–871). Upper Saddle River, NJ: Pearson Education; Berman, A., Snyder, S., Kozier, B., & Erb, G. (2008). *Kozier & Erb's Fundamentals of Nursing: Concepts, Process, and Practice* (8th ed., pp. 469–471). Upper Saddle River, NJ: Pearson Education.

59. ANSWER: 2

The nurse should use an open-ended questioning technique that provides the client's husband with an opportunity to share any information deemed appropriate. The answers would then provide the nurse with the chance to ask questions that are more specific to areas of concern. Closed-ended questions require only a yes or no answer and limit discussion. The nurse should not presume that the client is experiencing stress since doing so may cause him to become defensive.

➧ ***Test-taking Tip:*** *Key words are "most appropriate." Use the process of elimination and focus on therapeutic communication techniques as well as the needs of caregivers.*

Content Area: Mental Health; *Category of Health Alteration:* Cognitive, Schizophrenic, and Psychotic Disorders; *Integrated Process:* Nursing Process Assessment; *Client Needs:* Psychosocial Integrity/ Mental Health Concepts; Communication and Documentation; *Cognitive Ability:* Analysis

Reference: Mohr, W. (2006). *Psychiatric-Mental Health Nursing* (6th ed., pp. 65–76, 755). Philadelphia: Lippincott Williams & Wilkins.

EBP Reference: Family Caregiver Alliance. (2006). Caregiver assessment: principles, guidelines and strategies for change. Report from a national consensus development conference. Volume I. San Francisco: Author. Available at: www.guideline.gov/summary/summary.aspx?doc_id=9670&nbr=005179&string=alzheimer's+AND+disease

60. ANSWER: 4

Menopause is the physiological cessation of menses associated with declining ovarian function. It is usually considered complete after 1 year of amenorrhea. Once menopause is complete, reproductive function ends. The other statements are incorrect.

➧ ***Test-taking Tip:*** *Recall the relationship between menopause and reproduction. Once a female is menopausal, pregnancy is not physiologically possible.*

Content Area: Adult Health; *Category of Health Alteration:* Reproductive Management; *Integrated Processes:* Nursing Process Implementation; Teaching and Learning; *Client Need:* Health Promotion and Maintenance/Health and Wellness; *Cognitive Level:* Application

References: Lewis, S., Heitkemper, M., Dirksen, S., O'Brien, P., & Bucher, L. (2007). *Medical-Surgical Nursing: Assessment and Management of Clinical Problems* (7th ed., p. 1390). St. Louis, MO: Mosby; Smeltzer, S., Bare, B., Hinkle, J., & Cheever, K. (2008). *Brunner & Suddarth's Textbook of Medical-Surgical Nursing* (11th ed., p. 1633). Philadelphia: Lippincott Williams & Wilkins.

61. ANSWER: 3

Stating that the child is likely afraid and making reference to the stuffed animal acknowledges the child's feelings as well as focuses on a familiar object of security. The nurse's introduction and directions to the child does not acknowledge the child's feelings and is an attempt to control the child. Diverting the child by taking them to the playroom will not alleviate fear and anxiety. Asking the child a question that allows for a yes-no response is a close-ended question and, because of the child's fear and anxiety, will likely get a "no" response.

➧ ***Test-taking Tip:*** *Select an option that will decrease fear and anxiety for the child.*

Content Area: Child Health; *Category of Health Alteration:* Hematological and Oncological Management; *Integrated Processes:* Communication and Documentation; *Client Need:* Psychosocial Integrity/Therapeutic Communications; *Cognitive Level:* Analysis

References: Ball, J., & Bindler, R. (2008). *Pediatric Nursing: Caring for Children* (4th ed., p. 421). Upper Saddle River, NJ: Pearson Education; Berman, A., Snyder, S., Kozier, B., & Erb, G. (2008). *Kozier & Erb's Fundamentals of Nursing: Concepts, Process, and Practice* (8th ed., pp. 469–471). Upper Saddle River, NJ: Pearson Education.

62. ANSWER: 3

Telling the client that sleep disorders are associated with caffeine intake prematurely informs the client that a sleep disorder has been confirmed and/or makes assumptions about the client's caffeine intake. This statement is inappropriate and the nurse needs to be remediated regarding discussing unconfirmed presumptions with a client. The remaining options either respond to the client's concern or further assesses a sleep problem, are not inappropriate, and thus do not require immediate follow-up.

➧ ***Test-taking Tip:*** *Note the key words "requires immediate follow-up." This is a false-response option. Select the statement that should not be made by the nurse. Eliminate options that respond to the client's concern or further assess a sleep problem.*

Content Area: Mental Health; *Category of Health Alteration:* Crisis, Violence, Eating, and Sleep Disorders; *Integrated Processes:* Nursing Process Evaluation; *Client Need:* Physiological Integrity/Basic Care and Comfort/Rest and Sleep; *Cognitive Level:* Analysis

Reference: Varcarolis, E., Carson, V., & Shoemaker, N. (2006). *Foundations of Psychiatric Mental Health Nursing: A Clinical Approach* (5th ed., p. 662). St. Louis, MO: Saunders/Elsevier.

EBP Reference: American Psychiatric Association (2006). Practice guideline for the psychiatric evaluation of adults. Available at: www.guideline.gov/summary/summary.aspx?doc_id=9317&nbr=004986&string=Mental+AND+disorders

63. ANSWER: 1

Both Td and TIG are initially administered in different sites to neutralize circulating toxins. Diazepam is used for skeletal muscle relaxation to control spasms (which the client is not exhibiting), and penicillin is used to inhibit further growth of *Clostridium tetani.* Morphine sulfate, a narcotic analgesic, is used for pain control, which is appropriate, but vecuronium is a neuromuscular blocking agent for treating severe cases of muscle spasm, which the client is not exhibiting. Fentanyl, a sedative and narcotic analgesic, is for severe pain control and is not indicated at this time. Metronidazole, an anti-infective, antiprotozoal agent, is an alternative to penicillin G and would be appropriate.

➧ ***Test-taking Tip:*** *For the option to be the answer, both the medications must be appropriate for treating the client at this time. Avoid reading into the question.*

Content Area: Adult Health; *Category of Health Alteration:* Infectious Disease; *Integrated Processes:* Nursing Process Planning; *Client Need:* Physiological Integrity/Pharmacological and Parenteral Therapies/Expected Actions or Outcomes; *Cognitive Level:* Analysis

Reference: Lewis, S., Heitkemper, M., Dirksen, S., O'Brien, P., & Bucher, L. (2007). *Medical-Surgical Nursing: Assessment and Management of Clinical Problems* (7th ed., pp. 1588–1589). St. Louis, MO: Mosby.

EBP Reference: CDC. (2009). Recommended adult immunization schedule—United States, 2009. *MMWR Weekly*, 57(53), Q1–Q4. Available at: www.cdc.gov/mmwr/PDF/wk/mm5753-Immunization.pdf

64. ANSWER: 3

Potassium chloride must be diluted prior to administration as a preventative measure since concentrated doses or rapid infusion can cause hyperkalemia, cardiac arrhythmias, or arrest. Administration of concentrated potassium chloride can cause cardiac arrhythmias or arrest. A low serum potassium level increases the client's risk of dysrhythmias during anesthesia administration. The client's serum potassium level should be within the normal range prior to surgery. Hot packing may provide comfort since the medication is irritating to the veins, but this is not most important.

Test-taking Tip: *Waiting to administer delays the benefits of the medication. Administering the medication through the IV is unsafe. Diluting the medication is more important than hot packing.*

Content Area: Adult Health; *Client Need:* Physiological Integrity/Pharmacological and Parenteral; *Integrated Processes:* Nursing Process Planning; *Client Need:* Physiological Integrity/ Pharmacological and Parenteral Therapies/Medication Administration; *Cognitive Level:* Application

Reference: Wilson, B., Shannon, M., Shields, K., Stang, C. (2008). *Prentice Hall Nurse's Drug Guide 2008* (pp. 1243–1245). Upper Saddle River, NJ: Pearson Education.

65. ANSWER: 3

Most people with type 2 diabetes eventually need to start taking insulin to achieve optimal control of blood glucose and prevent complications such as retinopathy, nephropathy, neuropathy, and cardiovascular disease. Research has shown that, with the addition of insulin, glycosylated hemoglobin levels decrease to near-normal levels. Questioning the order is unnecessary. The order is correct. The procedure for glucose monitoring may need to be taught or reviewed with the client, but this is not priority. The nurse should initiate a consult because the client has already developed a complication (foot ulcer), but this is not priority.

Test-taking Tip: *Note the key word "priority." Read the situation carefully, noting that the nurse is an on-coming day-shift nurse. Determine which action must be first. Use the nursing process to determine the priority.*

Content Area: Adult Health; *Category of Health Alteration:* Endocrine Management; *Integrated Processes:* Nursing Process Implementation; *Client Need:* Physiological Integrity/Pharmacological and Parenteral Therapies/Medication Administration; *Cognitive Level:* Analysis

Reference: Lewis, S., Heitkemper, M., Dirksen, S., O'Brien, P., & Bucher, L. (2007). *Medical-Surgical Nursing: Assessment and Management of Clinical Problems* (7th ed., pp. 1268–1273). St. Louis, MO: Mosby.

EBP References: Kvapil, M., Swatko, A., Hilberg, C., & Shestakova, M. (2006). Biphasic insulin aspart 30 plus metformin: an effective combination in type 2 diabetes. *Diabetes, Obesity, and Metabolism,* 8, 39–48; Holman, R., Thornem, K., Farmer, A., Davies, M., Keenan, J., Sanjoy, P., et al. (2007). Addition of biphasic, prandial, or basal insulin to oral therapy in type 2 diabetes. *New England Journal of Medicine,* 357(17), 1716–1730. Available at: content.nejm.org/cgi/content/full/NEJMoa075392

66. ANSWER: 3

A Roux-en-y gastric bypass reduces the size of the upper part of the stomach to approximately 20 mL to 30 mL. None of the small bowel is removed in this surgery. The stomach and large bowel are not bypassed.

Test-taking Tip: *Eliminate options that do not address "gastric." Of the remaining two options, visualize the procedure to select the best option.*

Content Area: Adult Health; *Category of Health Alteration:* Gastrointestinal Management; *Integrated Processes:* Teaching and Learning; *Client Need:* Physiological Integrity/Reduction of Risk Potential/Potential for Complications from Surgical Procedures and Health Alterations; *Cognitive Level:* Application

Reference: Smeltzer, S., Bare, B., Hinkle, J., & Cheever, K. (2008). *Brunner and Suddarth's Textbook of Medical-Surgical Nursing* (11th ed., pp. 1218–1219). Philadelphia: Lippincott Williams & Wilkins.

EBP Reference: Institute for Clinical Systems Improvement. (2006). Prevention and management of obesity (mature adolescents and adults). Available at: www.guideline.gov/summary/summary.aspx?doc_id=10226&nbr=005389&string=gastric+AND+bypass

67. ANSWER: 3

The expected range for the newborn's apical pulse is 100 to 160 beats per minute (bpm). While crying, the newborn's heart rate may increase up to 180 bpm and drop as low as 90 bpm when the infant is sleeping. Because this assessment finding is within the normal range, the student should document the findings without further action. There is no need to recheck the pulse in 1 hour, to apply an oximeter, or to notify the health-care provider.

Test-taking Tip: *The question is asking for the normal heart rate parameters for a newborn. Knowledge of the expected range is required to answer this question.*

Content Area: Childbearing Families; *Category of Health Alteration:* Neonatal and High-Risk Neonatal Management; *Integrated Processes:* Nursing Process Implementation; *Client Need:* Physiological Integrity/ Reduction of Risk Potential/Vital Signs; *Cognitive Level:* Application

Reference: Pillitteri, A. (2007). *Maternal & Child Health Nursing: Care of the Childbearing & Childrearing Family* (5th ed., p. 683). Philadelphia: Lippincott Williams & Wilkins.

68. ANSWER: 1, 5

A psychotropic medication is any medication that affects the mind, emotion, or behavior. Research has shown that psychotropic medications are associated with the risk of falls in older adult clients. Alprazolam, a benzodiazepine, prescribed to control anxiety, and zolpidem tartrate, a hypnotic, prescribed for short-term insomnia, are both considered psychotropic medications. Docusate sodium is a stool softener. Hydrochlorothiazide is a diuretic. Potassium chloride is a potassium supplement. Lisinopril is an angiotensin-converting enzyme (ACE) inhibitor that blocks the conversion of angiotensin I to the vasoconstrictor angiotensin II. It is used to treat hypertension.

Test-taking Tip: *Determine the category of each medication and whether it is psychotropic. Eliminate options in which the medication classification is known to be other than psychotropic.*

Content Area: Adult Health; *Category of Health Alteration:* Neurological Management; *Integrated Processes:* Nursing Process Evaluation; *Client Need:* Physiological Integrity/Pharmacological and Parenteral Therapies/Adverse Effects/Contradictions/Interactions; *Cognitive Level:* Application

Reference: Wilson, B., Shannon, M., Shields, K., & Stang, C. (2008). *Prentice Hall Nurse's Drug Guide 2008* (pp. 46–48, 741–743, 890–891, 1243–1245, 1619–1620). Upper Saddle River, NJ: Pearson Education.

69. ANSWER: 1

Noroviruses are present in the stool and vomit of infected persons and can be found from the day they start to feel ill to as long as 2 weeks after they feel better. Contact precautions should be used. Modes of transmission include touching surfaces or objects contaminated with norovirus and then placing the hand in the mouth, eating food or drinking liquids that are contaminated with norovirus, and having direct contact with another person who is infected and showing symptoms. Masks should be worn if cleaning heavily soiled areas. Norovirus is not spread by droplets. The high-efficiency particulate (HEPA) masks and negative air-flow room of airborne precautions are unnecessary. Those coming in contact with the client need self-protection measures.

➧ ***Test-taking Tip:*** *Recall that the virus is present in stool and emesis.*

Content Area: Adult Health; *Category of Health Alteration:* Infectious Disease; *Integrated Processes:* Nursing Process Implementation; *Client Need:* Physiological Integrity/Physiological Adaptation/Alterations in Body Systems; *Cognitive Level:* Application

Reference: Smeltzer, S., Bare, B., Hinkle, J., & Cheever, K. (2008). *Brunner & Suddarth's Textbook of Medical-Surgical Nursing* (11th ed., pp. 2501–2502). Philadelphia: Lippincott Williams & Wilkins.

EBP Reference: Centers for Disease Control and Prevention (CDC). (2006). *Norovirus in healthcare facilities fact sheet.* Available at: www.cdc.gov/ncidod/dhqp/id_norovirusFS.html

70. ANSWER: 3

Learning takes place in all encounters. Staff education is important in establishing expectations and ensuring consistency in timing of antibiotic administration. Although the manager may have established clear expectations, if the staff is not appropriately informed, they will not be prepared to meet the defined expectations. A positive attitude from management may be helpful, but does not replace staff education. It is important to provide skillful communication; however, staff education ensures that all staff receives the same communication.

➧ ***Test-taking Tip:*** *The key word is "action." Eliminate options that are passive.*

Content Area: Management of Care; *Category of Health Alteration:* Leadership and Management; *Integrated Processes:* Teaching and Learning; *Client Need:* Safe and Effective Care Environment/ Management of Care/Performance Improvement (Quality Improvement); *Cognitive Level:* Application

Reference: Catalano, J. (2006). *Nursing Now! Today's Issues, Tomorrow's Trends* (4th ed., p. 252). Philadelphia: F.A. Davis.

EBP Reference: Medicare Quality Improvement Community. (2006). *Surgical Care Improvement Project (SCIP).* Harrisburg, PA: Author. Available at: medqic.org/dcs/ContentServer?cid=1122904930422&pagename=Medqic%2FContent%2FParentShellTemplate&parentName=Topic&siteVersion=null&c=MQParents

71. ANSWER: 3

The goal of IV oxytocin administration for labor induction is to achieve a contraction pattern of three 40- to 60-second uterine contractions over a 10 minute period. Cervical dilation and reports of client discomfort are not part of the criteria that determines if the induction goal has been achieved. Contractions lasting 60 to 90 seconds and occurring every 2 minutes is a contraction pattern that exceeds the criteria limits.

➧ ***Test-taking Tip:*** *Recall that oxytocin causes the uterus to contract. Eliminate options that do not address the process of uterine contractions.*

Content Area: Childbearing Families; *Category of Health Alteration:* Pharmacological and Parenteral Therapies; *Integrated Processes:* Nursing Process Evaluation; *Client Need:* Physiological Integrity/ Pharmacological and Parenteral Therapies/Expected Actions or Outcomes; *Cognitive Level:* Application

Reference: Davidson, M., London, M., & Ladewig, P. (2008). *Olds' Maternal-Newborn Nursing & Women's Health Across the Lifespan* (8th ed., p. 521). Upper Saddle River, NJ: Prentice Hall Health.

72. ANSWER: 1, 3, 6

Pitting edema can be a sign of fluid volume overload from cardiac, renal, endocrine, medication-related, or another problem. The warty growth on the vulva could be a sign of human papillomavirus (HPV) infection. The 6-mm asymmetric dark lesion is a hallmark sign for cancer. Increased hair thinning and actinic lentigo (sun freckles or age spots) are normal findings in the older adult population. Port-wine angioma is a benign vascular tumor that involves the skin and the subcutaneous tissues that are present at birth, usually persisting indefinitely.

➧ ***Test-taking Tip:*** *Eliminate normal age-related changes and any options that can occur at birth that are considered normal findings.*

Content Area: Adult Health; *Category of Health Alteration:* Infectious Disease; *Integrated Processes:* Nursing Process Assessment; *Client Need:* Safe and Effective Care Environment/Management of Care/Consultation; *Cognitive Level:* Analysis

Reference: Smeltzer, S., Bare, B., Hinkle, J., & Cheever, K. (2008). *Brunner & Suddarth's Textbook of Medical-Surgical Nursing* (11th ed., pp. 233, 1666, 1978). Philadelphia: Lippincott Williams & Wilkins.

73. ANSWER: 1

The nurse should ask the client about the pain and its triggers before proceeding to an examination because clients are often fearful of initiating an episode of the facial pain. Pain associated with trigeminal neuralgia is very severe and occurs in spasms. Palpating the face may trigger a pain episode that would prevent additional data gathering about the client's symptoms. Testing for cerebella function is not indicated. The trigeminal nerve functions in the blink reflex, but counting the blinks is not a useful assessment.

➧ ***Test-taking Tip:*** *Focus on the key words "trigeminal neuralgia" and "initial." A neuralgia is a painful nerve condition (suffix "-algia" indicates pain). Consider that the nurse must be careful in performing any assessment that would initiate a pain episode. Select option 1 because it addresses the pain, client concern, and does not risk initiating pain. Eliminate option 2 because it does not address the pain issue. Eliminate options 3 and 4 because they are not related to the issue of the question.*

Content Area: Adult Health; *Category of Health Alteration:* Neurological Management; *Integrated Processes:* Nursing Process Assessment; *Client Need:* Health Promotion and Maintenance/ Techniques of Physical Assessment; *Cognitive Level:* Analysis

Reference: Ignatavicius, D., & Workman, M. (2006). *Medical-Surgical Nursing: Critical Thinking for Collaborative Care* (5th ed., pp. 1023–1024). St. Louis, MO: Saunders/Elsevier.

74. ANSWER: 3

Morphine sulfate is recommended for severe, acute pain. It alters the client's perception and response to painful stimuli while producing generalized CNS depression. Meperidine has been reported to cause delirium in the elderly; older adults are at increased risk for meperidine toxicity. Fentanyl is recommended for moderate to severe chronic pain requiring continuous opioid analgesic therapy. Hydromorphone will take additional time to prepare; although it is a good option to obtain the medication for later dosing. Starting at the lowest dose (15 mg/hr) is recommended for older adult clients.

➧ ***Test-taking Tip:*** *Knowledge of analgesics for older adults is necessary to answer this question. If unsure, use the process of elimination, eliminating options 2 and 4 because of the longer time of onset and the client is in acute pain.*

Content Area: Fundamentals; *Category of Health Alteration:* Medication Administration; *Integrated Processes:* Nursing Process Evaluation; *Client Need:* Physiological Integrity/Pharmacological and Parenteral Therapies/Pharmacological Pain Management; *Cognitive Level:* Application

Reference: Wilson, B., Shannon, M., Shields, K., & Stang, C. (2008). *Prentice Hall Nurse's Drug Guide 2008* (pp. 631–632, 748–750, 942–945, 1023–1025). Upper Saddle River, NJ: Pearson Education.

EBP References: Manworren, R. (2006). Pain Control. A call to action to protect range orders. A consensus statement supports this important nursing responsibility. *American Journal of Nursing,* 106(7), 65–68; Institute for Clinical Systems Improvement. (2008). Assessment and management of acute pain. Available at: www.guideline.gov/summary/summary.aspx?view_id=1&doc_id=12302

75. ANSWER: 2, 6, 4, 1, 3, 5

First insert an intravenous access device and then start the Ancef®. It will take about 20 minutes to infuse the Ancef®. Because blood would need to be returned to the blood bank if out for more than 30 minutes, the IV should be started before obtaining the blood. Next, obtain the blood from the blood bank. Prime the blood tubing with 0.9% NaCl infusion while waiting for the blood (the blood tubing would not be used for administering Ancef®). Complete the identification and blood administration checks to ensure it is the correct blood product for this client, and then start the blood infusion. The blood should infuse between 2 and 4 hours.

Test-taking Tip: *When establishing priorities, determine the amount of time each action will take. Remember blood must be started within 30 minutes of retrieving it from the blood bank and medications administration with the blood is contraindicated.*

Content Area: Adult Health; *Category of Health Alteration:* Perioperative Management; *Integrated Processes:* Nursing Process Implementation; *Client Need:* Safe and Effective Care Environment/Management of Care/Continuity of Care; Safe and Effective Care Environment/Management of Care/Establishing Priorities; *Cognitive Level:* Analysis

Reference: Berman, A., Snyder, S., Kozier, B., & Erb, G. (2008). *Kozier & Erb's Fundamentals of Nursing: Concepts, Process, and Practice* (8th ed., pp. 217–218). Upper Saddle River, NJ: Pearson Education.

Comprehensive Exam Two

1. EBP A nurse is preparing to administer medications to an adult client. Which medication order is most accurate and should be the safest for the nurse to administer?

   1. Heparin sodium 5,000 U. subq bid
   2. Digoxin (Lanoxin®) .25 mg oral daily
   3. Levofloxacin (Levaquin®) 500 mg daily
   4. Timolol 0.5% 2 drops right eye bid

2. EBP A 2-month-old infant is brought to a clinic for evaluation of pyloric stenosis. Which findings is a clinic nurse most likely to observe?

   1. Vomiting, diarrhea, weight loss, and lethargy
   2. Nonbilious vomiting, weight loss, hunger after vomiting, and lethargy
   3. Bilious vomiting, vomiting related to feeding position, weight loss, and diarrhea
   4. Vomiting, diarrhea, severe pain, and lethargy

3. Two patient care assistants (PCAs) are helping a client with left-sided weakness to get up from a chair and return to bed. Based on the illustration provided, which action by a nurse observing this transfer is *best*?

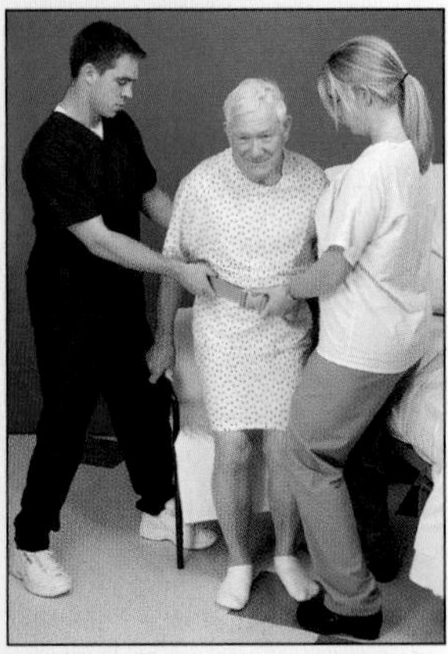

   1. Intervene because the chair is incorrectly placed for transferring the client back to bed
   2. Compliment the female PCA because she is supporting the client's weak side
   3. Compliment the male PCA because he is using a wide base of support
   4. Praise the client for using his hand for support on the chair to help prevent a fall

4. A nurse is caring for a client receiving a fluid challenge for treatment of prerenal failure caused by severe hypotension. The nurse evaluates that the fluid challenge has been most effective for treating the prerenal failure when which observation is noted?

   1. Blood pressure 140/72 mm Hg
   2. Increased cardiac output
   3. Urine output 70 mL per hour
   4. Heart rate 120 beats per minute (bpm)

5. A nurse, working in a junior high school, is approached by a seventh-grade female. The student is concerned about her best friend who had a sexual encounter with a popular eighth-grade boy. Now her friend thinks that she is pregnant. Prioritize the manner in which the nurse should best approach this situation.

   ______ Ask the student the name of her friend and approach her friend in a private setting to discuss the situation
   ______ Contact the parents of the student and ask to set up an appointment with them
   ______ Make a referral to a primary health-care provider
   ______ Ask the student her friend's name and tell her that you would like to meet with them together.

6. Two nurses are having a conflict about whose turn it is to float to a unit outside of their home unit. Which statement by one of the nurses indicates negotiation toward conflict resolution?

   1. "It's not my turn to float, so you should go. I will take my turn next time."
   2. "I'm willing to float today if you could come in 15 minutes early for me tomorrow."
   3. "If you don't float today, I will end up floating 2 days in a row, and that's not fair."
   4. "We all float too much so neither of us should float. Let's talk with our nurse manager."

7. For an adult who experienced a seizure, which notation is a nurse most likely to document in the client's medical record about the postictal period?

   1. Whether the client experienced an "aura"
   2. What the client was doing immediately preceding the seizure
   3. What the condition of the client was immediately following the seizure
   4. Where tonic-clonic activity started and how long the client was unresponsive

8. A community nurse is teaching a group of mothers with children between the ages of 1 and 4 years. Which nurse's statement should best inform the mothers about measures to prevent the most common cause of death in children in this age group?

1. "Ensure that your children receive the annual influenza vaccine to prevent pneumonia."
2. "Apply sunscreen whenever you take your children outdoors to prevent skin cancer."
3. "Place medications and knives in locked cabinets to prevent unintentional injury."
4. "Avoid physical punishment of children to prevent unintentional homicide."

9. A mother, who is holding her newly delivered, full-term newborn, questions a nurse about the intermittent pauses she sees in her baby's breathing. Which statement should be the basis for the nurse's response to the client?

1. This type of breathing will typically cause changes in skin color, and the mother should be prepared for this development.
2. Initial newborn respirations should be regular in rate, periodic pauses warrant further investigation.
3. Periodic breathing is expected as the newborn transitions to life outside the uterus.
4. Pauses in the respiratory rate are a symptom of decreased surfactant production in the term newborn.

10. A client reports continued but improving insomnia, anorexia, and crying spells following the death of the client's spouse 1 month ago. Which is the most appropriate nursing diagnosis that a nurse should establish for the client?

1. Impaired adjustment
2. Ineffective coping
3. Dysfunctional grieving
4. Family processes interrupted

11. In the process of preparing a Native American Navajo female for an esophagogastroduodenoscopy (EGD) procedure, a nurse sits down, faces the client directly, and uses a picture diagram during an education session. Later that day, the client requests that the nurse, who had given preprocedure instructions, not be allowed to provide postprocedure care. The nurse evaluates that the client was likely uncomfortable with the first nurse's teaching because:

1. Native American females do not make health-care decisions and do not feel comfortable receiving medical information.
2. Native Americans form a personal friendship with their health-care providers and are uncomfortable with strangers providing health-care information.
3. Native Americans consider direct eye contact disrespectful.
4. Native Americans consider pictures of body parts inappropriate.

12. EBP A hospitalized client, experiencing chronic abdominal pain, is receiving the maximum recommended dose of fentanyl (Duragesic®) by transdermal patch and intravenous morphine sulfate for breakthrough pain. The client continues to rate the pain at a level of 8 on a scale of 0 to 10. The client agrees to include progressive relaxation techniques through guided imagery as an intervention to lessen pain. Which should be the best method for the nurse to evaluate the effectiveness of progressive relaxation in controlling the client's pain?

1. Monitor the client's blood pressure and pulse rate and compare to previous readings
2. Ask the client to describe and rate the pain
3. Ask the client's significant other to describe any changes in the client's behavior
4. Monitor the client's facial expression

13. EBP Immediately after the delivery of a client's placenta, a health-care provider orders an intravenous infusion of oxytocin (Pitocin®) at 20 milliunits/minute. A nurse should evaluate that the medication was effective when which assessment information is collected?

1. Systolic blood pressure is above 100 mm Hg
2. Lochia flow is small
3. Mother reports no afterpains
4. Uterine fundus is firm

14. EBP A nurse is reviewing the serum laboratory report of a 7-year-old child who has been rehydrated following acute vomiting and diarrhea. Which laboratory value change should the nurse expect with successful rehydration?

1. Hemoglobin was 9.5 mg/dL; now 12.5 mg/dL
2. Hematocrit was 32%; now 37%
3. Blood urea nitrogen (BUN) was 28 mg/dL; now 16 mg/dL
4. Serum creatinine (SCr) was 1.2 mg/dL; now 0.9 mg/dL

15. A nurse is caring for a client following a left tibial osteotomy with bone graft from the left hip and cast application to the left lower leg. Which assessment finding should be a priority and requires the nurse to intervene immediately?

1. Has not voided for 6 hours
2. Numbness and tingling of the left toes
3. Left hip dressing saturated with serosanguineous drainage
4. Experiencing nausea

16. Which intervention should a nurse implement when caring for a client immediately after a transurethral resection of the prostrate (TURP)?

1. Monitor the abdominal dressings for blood or urine drainage
2. Alert the surgeon if blood clots are noted in the urinary drainage bag
3. Encourage sitting at the side of the bed as soon as possible
4. Monitor the urinary catheter to assure it remains patent

17. Two nurses are approaching a client to begin cardiopulmonary resuscitation (CPR). One nurse goes to the right side of the client's head to check the client's airway. In which location should the other nurse be positioned?

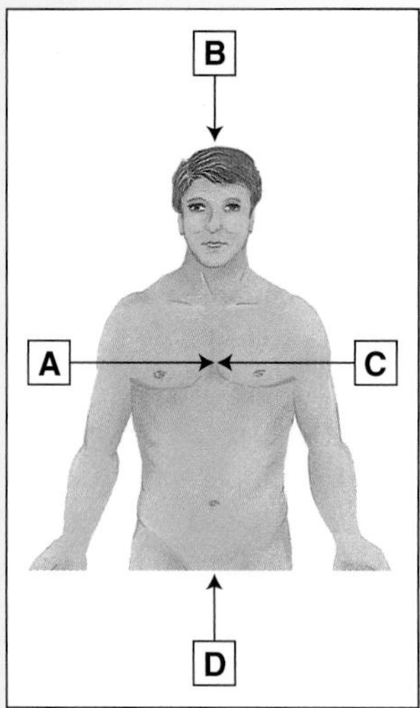

1. Location A
2. Location B
3. Location C
4. Location D

18. EBP A nurse plans to include the family in the treatment of a client who abuses substances. What should be the nurse's primary rationale for including family members?

1. Helping the family learn ways to protect the client from additional harm
2. Assisting the family in reducing temptations for the client to drink or use substances
3. Reducing distress in the relationship to lessen the risk for relapse
4. Encouraging the family to confront the client about the harm caused by substance abuse

19. EBP When a powdered chemotherapy medication spills on a hard surface in a clinical area, which required safety practices should a nurse use to clean the spill?

1. Wear protective gown, gloves, goggles, and head covering and use double-bag clean-up pads with open waste disposal bags
2. Wear protective gown, gloves, face shield, and foot coverings and use single-bag clean-up pads with an open waste disposal bag
3. Wear protective gown, gloves, face shield, and head covering and use single-bag clean-up pads with an open waste disposal bag
4. Wear protective gown, gloves, goggles and a respirator mask and use double-bag clean-up pads with open waste disposal bags

20. A client is being admitted to a medical unit with a diagnosis of acute rejection following a liver transplant. Multiple intravenous (IV) medications have been ordered. A charge nurse should plan to assign the client to which nurse?

1. An intensive care (ICU) registered nurse (RN) who floated to the medical unit for the day.
2. A licensed practice nurse (LPN) who has worked on the medical unit for 5 years.
3. A newly licensed RN on the medical unit who needs experience with IV medications.
4. A RN who has worked on the medical unit for 10 years and is working a double shift.

21. An adult client with a viral upper respiratory infection has an order for guaifenesin (Robitussin®) 400 mg orally every 4 hours. Which client statement should indicate to a nurse that the client needs additional teaching about the medication?

1. Take the medication with food
2. Increase fluid intake to 3000 mL/day
3. Take acetaminophen if experiencing the side effect of a headache
4. Chew sugarless gum to help alleviate the discomfort caused by a nonproductive cough

22. EBP A nurse is teaching a woman who is 8 weeks pregnant and had a Roux-en-Y gastric bypass surgical procedure 19 months ago. The woman's body mass index (BMI) is now 30.3%, down from 39.5%. Which nutritional deficits associated with gastric bypass should the nurse address with this client? SELECT ALL THAT APPLY.

1. Iron deficiency
2. Vitamin B_{12} deficiency
3. Vitamin C deficiency
4. Vitamin A deficiency
5. Calcium deficiency
6. Protein deficiency

23. Which illustration should a nurse choose when educating the parents of a child diagnosed with asthma about the best way to deliver medication via a metered dose inhaler? Place an X on the illustration that the nurse should select.

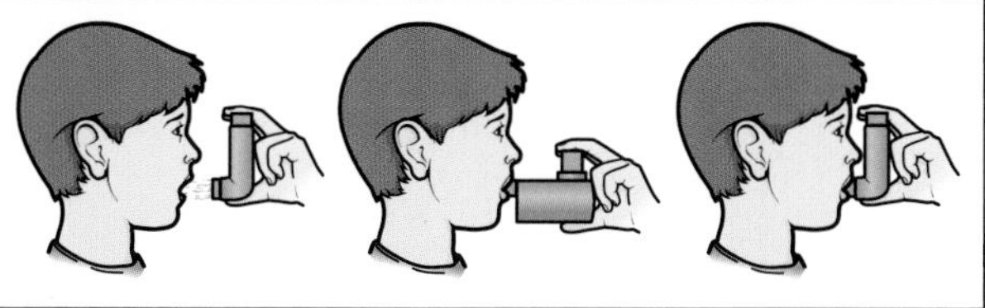

24. EBP A client, who had a femoral popliteal bypass graft surgery 2 days earlier, requests nicotine patches because he does not want to begin smoking again. The nurse provides the client with positive encouragement for beginning smoking cessation with nicotine replacement therapy (NRT). Which statement should be the basis for the nurse's support?

1. NRT eliminates withdrawal symptoms.
2. NRT delivered intradermally is superior to other forms such as chewing gum.
3. NRT gradually allows the client to decrease the number of cigarettes smoked.
4. NRT increases the long-term success rate of the client remaining smoke free.

25. A nurse is assessing a client for possible scabies. Identify the circle with an X where the nurse would most frequently locate the grey-brown burrows of the scabies parasite.

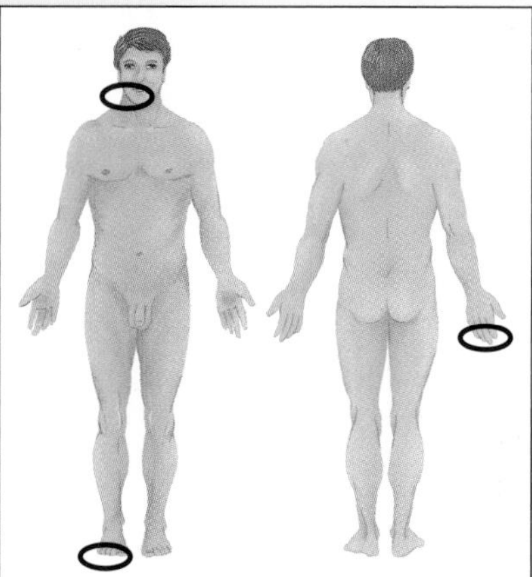

26. The parents of a toddler with cerebral palsy express concern about the child's weight. A nurse advises the parents about nutrition. On a subsequent home visit, which observation by the nurse indicates further teaching is needed?

1. Gives small frequent feedings
2. Provides solid foods
3. Gives the child utensils with large, padded handles
4. Includes a high-calorie supplement

27. EBP Which action should a nurse perform *first* when receiving a client in the operating room?

1. Assess the client's level of anxiety
2. Confirm that the operative consent is signed
3. Verify the correct operative site with the client
4. Check the client's name band and ask the client's name

28. EBP In making a decision for the first clinic appointment following hospital discharge for a postpartum mother and her baby, which most important information should a nurse consider?

1. The standard of care that a clinic visit should be 2 days following hospitalization
2. Relevant factors from the prenatal, intrapartum, and postnatal period
3. How long the mother and baby were in the hospital
4. The age of the mother and ability to care for her newborn

29. EBP A nurse, retrieving a medication from a hospitalized client's medication box, finds four ordered medications with the labels illustrated below. The nurse should complete a variance report after finding which medication in the client's medication box?

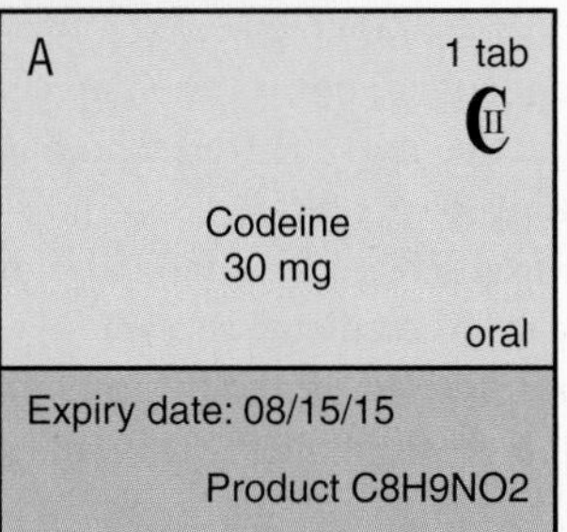

A
1 tab
CII
Codeine
30 mg
oral
Expiry date: 08/15/15
Product C8H9NO2

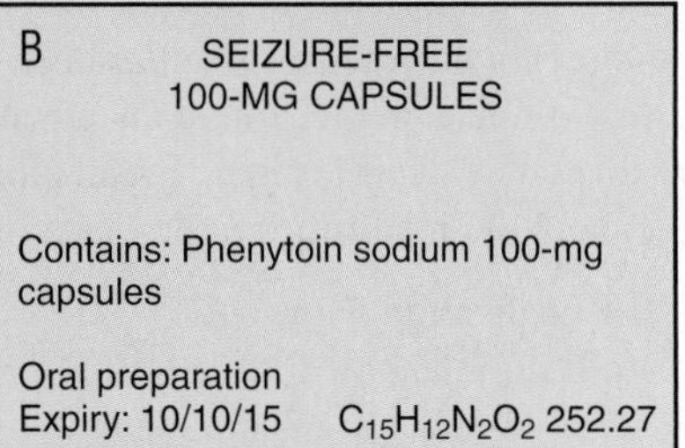

B
SEIZURE-FREE
100-MG CAPSULES
Contains: Phenytoin sodium 100-mg capsules
Oral preparation
Expiry: 10/10/15 $C_{15}H_{12}N_2O_2$ 252.27

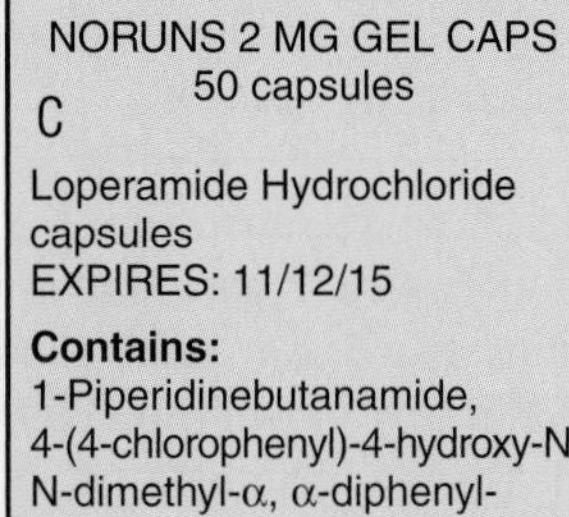

NORUNS 2 MG GEL CAPS
50 capsules
C
Loperamide Hydrochloride capsules
EXPIRES: 11/12/15
Contains:
1-Piperidinebutanamide,
4-(4-chlorophenyl)-4-hydroxy-N,
N-dimethyl-α, α-diphenyl-

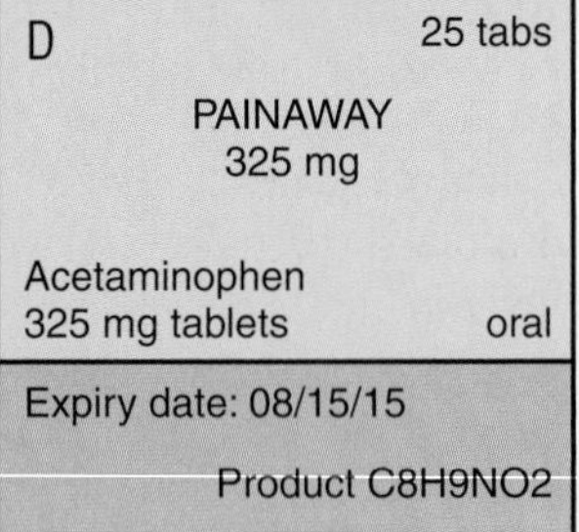

D
25 tabs
PAINAWAY
325 mg
Acetaminophen
325 mg tablets
oral
Expiry date: 08/15/15
Product C8H9NO2

1. A
2. B
3. C
4. D

30. EBP A bridging strategy is designed to assure that a homeless client with a history of violent behavior will experience positive outcomes upon discharge. Which statement made by the client best shows the need for *further* understanding regarding the importance of a bridging strategy?

1. "I want to thank you for giving me places to go for help."
2. "I want to get better and because I know these places can help me I have contacted one of them."
3. "I will keep the list of outpatient services' telephone numbers where I won't lose it."
4. "I'll go to these places when I can no longer get the things I need to be healthy and safe."

31. A nurse is caring for a client who has been transferred from the coronary care unit following a myocardial infarction (MI). The client frequently calls the nurse to check on the ECG monitor rhythm. When the cardiac rehabilitation therapist arrives to transport the client for cardiac rehabilitation exercises, the client questions if he or she is ready for activity so soon after an MI. Which behavioral response should the nurse determine that the client is exhibiting?

1. Depression
2. Denial
3. Anger
4. Dependency

32. EBP A child is admitted to a hospital in hyperglycemic crisis. Which initial intravenous (IV) fluid order should a nurse expect for this child?

1. 0.9% sodium chloride at a rate of 10 to 20 mL/kg per hour for the first hour
2. D5W with 20 mEq potassium chloride at a rate of 50 mL/kg over a 4-hour period
3. D10W and 0.45% sodium chloride at a rate of 5 to 10 mL/kg for the first 4 hours
4. Ringer's lactate solution at a rate of 10 to 20 mL/kg per hour for the first hour

33. EBP A nurse in the Post-Anesthesia Care Unit (PACU) is caring for a client who received general anesthesia. Which interventions should the nurse implement when caring for this client? SELECT ALL THAT APPLY.

1. Teach the client how to use an incentive spirometer
2. Move the client into a lateral position to protect the airway
3. Administer morphine sulfate intravenously (IV) for pain control
4. Protect IV lines to prevent dislodgement during emergence delirium
5. Repeat orientation explanations until the amnesiac anesthesia wears off

34. EBP A client presents with oral mucositis after receiving radiation therapy for pharyngeal cancer. Which signs and symptoms should a nurse expect to find upon assessment of this client?

1. Gingivitis, plaque, and halitosis
2. Candidiasis, inflammation, and cheilitis
3. Oral erythema, pain, and dysguesia
4. Oral ulceration, caries, and leukoplakia

35. EBP A nurse is caring for a client who is to receive a unit of packed red blood cells (PRBCs). Which safety measure should the nurse implement when administering the blood transfusion?

1. Monitor vital signs every 15 minutes during the transfusion to detect complications early
2. Administer the unit of PRBCs slowly over 5 hours to prevent a transfusion reaction
3. Stop the transfusion if a reaction occurs and administer 0.9% NaCl at the IV catheter hub to keep the intravenous (IV) site patent
4. Deliver the PRBCs through an infusion pump with standard tubing to ensure a consistent rate

36. A new nurse is caring for a 78-year-old client diagnosed with dementia, who experienced a stroke 3 weeks ago. A nurse manager recognizes the need for further education regarding appropriate delegation of the client care when the new nurse states:

1. "I've watched the nursing aide and I believe the nurse aide can feed the client safely."
2. "I'll have the nursing aide reinforce with the client that swearing at staff is unacceptable."
3. "The client's skin needs checked; the nurse aide (NA) can do that when showering the client."
4. "The client needs new slippers; the NA can show the client's family the old slippers when they visit today."

37. A client, diagnosed with depression and fibromyalgia, is started on a tricyclic antidepressant. About which common side effect should a nurse inform the client while taking a tricyclic antidepressant?

1. Agranulocytosis
2. Unintentional tremor
3. Dry mouth
4. Diarrhea

38. Which action should a nurse take when caring for a client with thrombocytopenia?

1. Teach the client to use dental floss after teeth brushing to prevent dental caries
2. Treat an elevated temperature of 102°F (39°C) or greater with two 325-mg aspirin tablets
3. Prevent injury by maintaining the client on strict bedrest
4. Assess for signs of blurred vision, headache, or mental status changes

39. EBP When a nurse removes a syringe after giving an intravenous (IV) push medication through a heparin lock port on a central line, the lock port adheres to the syringe and is removed from the central line catheter hub. The nurse notes that the clamp on the central line catheter is still open and suspects that air may have entered the central line catheter. Which immediate actions should be taken by the nurse? SELECT ALL THAT APPLY.

1. Notify the health-care provider
2. Close the clamp on the central line catheter
3. Turn the client onto the right side with the feet higher than the head
4. Attach a 10-mL syringe to the catheter, open the clamp, and aspirate until blood returns
5. Flush the line with 0.9% NaCl and then heparin if ordered

40. EBP A nurse completes the measurements for the electrocardiogram (ECG) monitor rhythm strips for four different clients. Following analysis of the ECG rhythms, the nurse determines that one of the clients requires an immediate intervention. Which measurement findings warrant immediate intervention?

1. PRI = 0.20 sec.; QRS = 0.10 sec.; QT = 0.38 sec.; ventricular rate = 102 beats per minute (bpm)
2. P waves fibrillatory; PR unmeasureable; QRS = .08 sec.; QT unmeasureable; ventricular rate = 90 bpm
3. PRI inconsistent; more Ps than QRSs and no correlation between Ps and QRSs; QRS = .14 sec; atrial rate = 60 bpm; ventricular rate = 30 bpm
4. PRI = 0.24 sec.; QRS = .10 sec.; QT = .44 sec.; ventricular rate = 58 bpm

41. A nurse is assessing the mental status of a client diagnosed with bipolar disorder. Which client behavior is the nurse most likely to assess during a manic episode?

1. Social withdrawal
2. Somatic-type delusions
3. Flight of ideas
4. Trembling or shaking

42. A nurse, assisting a physician during the placement of a central venous catheter, observes that the catheter tip touches a hair that has fallen from the client's head into the sterile field. Which is the most appropriate action by the nurse?

1. Do nothing because the hair that fell in the sterile field is from the client's head
2. Immediately inform the physician of the break in sterile technique and obtain replacement supplies
3. Inform the physician that the catheter tip touched a hair and let the physician decide what action should be taken
4. Obtain an antiseptic solution for the physician to cleanse the catheter tip so that the catheter is free of microorganisms before insertion

43. A client returns to a clinic for a follow-up visit and is diagnosed as positive for human immunodeficiency virus (HIV). The client expresses fear related to lack of finances, fear of social avoidance, and hopelessness. Which action by the nurse should provide the most client support?

1. Referral to a physician infectious disease specialist
2. Referral to a community-based HIV clinic
3. Referral to the local public health department
4. Recommendation to disclose the diagnosis to family

44. A nurse assesses a 30-year-old client 30 minutes after a vaginal delivery and obtains the following information.

B/P: 120/80 mm Hg
Pulse: 70 beats per minute
Respirations: 20 breaths per minute
Fundus: boggy
Lochia: large rubra
Perineum: bruised and swollen
Pain: Perineal pain; 6 out of 10 on numeric scale

In response to the information, which intervention should the nurse initiate *first*?

1. Apply ice to the perineum
2. Massage the fundus until it is firm
3. Give the client pain medication
4. Provide perineal care

45. A nurse is teaching a 6-year-old child, diagnosed with precocious puberty, about physiological changes that are taking place. Which statement should be helpful in facilitating a positive body image for this child?

1. "You may want to dress like a teenager now that you are going through puberty."
2. "All children will go through these changes when they become adults."
3. "The changes in your body are normal but occurring at an earlier age. Your friends will experience the same changes eventually."
4. "You are going to look older than your chronological age. Remember to always tell others your real age so they don't ask you to do things that you are not ready to do."

46. A hospice nurse is caring for a 4-year-old client diagnosed with a terminal, congenital heart defect who is dying. In meeting the psychosocial needs of the client and family, the nurse employs a variety of techniques. Which nursing action demonstrates uncaring behaviors?

1. Minimally touching the client and conversing, in a soft voice, as if the client is alert
2. Allowing the client and family privacy to express feelings and comfort one another
3. Encouraging the family to talk with and reassure the child who is dying
4. Encouraging the client and family to verbalize feelings of sadness, loss, and forgiveness

47. EBP A nurse is caring for a client receiving negative-pressure wound therapy (vacuum-assisted closure) for a large, sacral pressure sore wound. For which problem, associated with negative pressure wound therapy, should the nurse plan to monitor the client?

1. Saturated dressings
2. Drainage of fluids
3. Air leaks
4. Air bubbles

48. EBP A health-care provider (HCP) writes the following orders for a client admitted in sickle cell crisis: "oxygen 2L/NC, one unit MS 4 mg IV now, one unit packed red blood cells, and hydroxyurea (Hydrea®) 250 mg oral daily." In response to these orders, what action should a nurse take?

1. Initiate all orders as prescribed
2. Call the HCP to clarify the MS order
3. Prepare 4 mg MS for administration after initiating the oxygen
4. Verify with another nurse that MS should be morphine sulfate based on this client's condition

49. A nurse is developing the plan of care for a client hospitalized with an acute case of pneumonia. No orders have been written, so the nurse contacts a physician. Which intervention should the nurse ensure that the physician includes in the client's plan of care?

1. Avoiding antipyretics because of liver toxicity
2. Including antiviral medication, such as amantadine (Symmetrel®)
3. Increasing intravenous (IV) and oral fluid intake
4. Obtaining a physical therapy consult for increasing activity

50. A clinic nurse is assessing a 9-year-old boy whose blood pressure is 112/72 mm Hg. Based on the findings, which nursing action is most appropriate?

1. Begin counseling including a low-sodium diet, weight control, and exercise
2. Refer the child for a workup for hypertension
3. Discuss with the physician the need for antihypertensive therapy
4. Document the child's blood pressure findings only

51. Which initial behavior demonstrates to a nurse on a mental health unit that a client is beginning to assume responsibility for the management of his or her anger?

1. The client develops a plan on how to react when feeling stressed
2. The client identifies stressors that have led to violent outbursts in the past
3. The client states plans to start a regular exercise program to help "work off the anger"
4. The client apologizes to all those friends and family he/she has directed his/her anger toward

52. After attempting other interventions, a nurse on a mental health unit decides to place a client, who is exhibiting dangerous and physically abusive behavior, in seclusion. Which statement should a nurse consider when placing the client in seclusion?

1. A standing order may be used to place a client in seclusion.
2. A client should be removed from seclusion as soon as possible.
3. It is illegal to seclude a client on a mental health unit.
4. Clients in seclusion should be monitored every 2 hours.

53. When using an otoscope to view the tympanic membrane of a 12-month-old infant brought to the well-baby clinic, a nurse should: SELECT ALL THAT APPLY.

1. select the smallest otoscope tip that will allow for visualization.
2. pull the pinna down and back to properly align the ear canal.
3. note the color of the tympanic membrane.
4. rest the otoscope on the nondominant hand.
5. pull the pinna up and back to properly align the ear canal.
6. rest the otoscope on the child's head.

54. A nurse is caring for a young client scheduled for cystectomy with urinary diversion for treatment of bladder cancer. The client states to a nurse, "With all the smokers around, why couldn't one of them get bladder cancer instead of me? I've never smoked in my life!" Which is the best response by the nurse?

1. "It seems unfair that you developed cancer?"
2. "Smoking isn't the only cause of bladder cancer."
3. "With your upcoming surgery, I can understand why you are afraid."
4. "You're angry and I know you really don't mean to wish this on someone else."

55. EBP A home-care nurse visits a client who lives alone and is independent with self-care. The client is receiving palliative care for a progressive cancer. Which nursing intervention best ensures that the client is receiving adequate pain control?

1. Teaching to keep a pain diary and contacting the nurse if breakthrough pain medication is needed more than 3 times in 24 hours.
2. Instructing to include ample fluids and high-fiber foods to prevent constipation associated with narcotic analgesics.
3. Assisting to recognize anxiety and employing relaxation techniques as soon as possible.
4. Scheduling opioid medications at bedtime to ensure being able to sleep through the night.

56. A nurse is calculating a 24-hour carbohydrate intake for a client with type 1 diabetes mellitus. Based on the client's food intake record and considering that one carbohydrate choice (CHO) equals 15 grams of carbohydrate, the nurse should calculate that the client consumed ______ grams of carbohydrate in the last 24 hours.

24-Hour Food Intake

Breakfast	Lunch	Dinner
1 C whole milk (1 CHO) ½ C cooked oatmeal (1 CHO) 1 C apple juice (1 CHO) 1 slice bacon	1 C whole milk (1 CHO) Carrot sticks 3 oz tuna 2 slices bread (2 CHO)	1 C whole milk (1 CHO) 3 oz beef patty ½ C corn (1 CHO) ⅓ C pasta 1 C orange juice (2 CHO)
	Afternoon Snack	**Evening Snack**
	1 slice toast (1 CHO) 1 Tbsp apple butter	1 small banana (1 CHO)

57. EBP A client, diagnosed with a personality disorder, is hospitalized on a medical unit. A psychiatrist orders mirtazapine (Remeron®) to be continued. Prior to administering a dose of mirtazapine, a nurse reviews the results of the client's serum laboratory test. Based on the report, which action should the nurse take?

Serum Lab Test	Client's Value	Normal Values
Cholesterol	240 mg/dL	0–200 mg/dL
Triglycerides	300 mg/dL	30–150 mg/dL
HDL	28 mg/dL	35 mg/dL or greater
LDL	160 mg/dL	Less than 130 mg/dL
Albumin	4.9 g/dL	3.4–4.7 U/L
AST/SGOT	52 U/L	8–45 U/L
ALT/SGPT	48 U/L	0.2–1.3 mg/dL
Total bilirubin	1.6 mg/dL	38–126 mU/mL
Alkaline phosphatase	128 mU/mL	

1. Administer the prescribed mirtazapine
2. Consult with the psychiatrist regarding increasing the dose of mirtazapine
3. Consult with the psychiatrist regarding decreasing the dose of mirtazapine
4. Consult with the general practitioner regarding the mirtazapine and whether additional serum laboratory tests should be drawn to assess for another comorbid condition

58. A nurse is preparing to administer ondansetron (Anzemet®) 12.5 mg intravenously (IV) to a client with postoperative nausea. The medication is supplied in 20 mg per 1-mL vials. The nurse should prepare to administer________ mL of medication.

59. EBP A 70-year-old male client, diagnosed with diabetes mellitus, arrives at a clinic to receive an influenza vaccination. The client informs the nurse of his health history, states he received an influenza vaccination last year, and denies having any allergies. What is the nurse's best action?

1. Administer the vaccination as requested with live, attenuated influenza vaccine (LAIV)
2. Administer the vaccination as requested with trivalent inactivated influenza vaccine (TIV)
3. Inform the client that he is not a candidate for the vaccination because of the severity of his heart disease
4. Inform the client that the influenza vaccination is good for 5 years and vaccination is not necessary at this time

60. EBP A client, diagnosed with benign prostatic hyperplasia (BPH), is given a prescription for tamsulosin (Flomax®). The client is questioning the need for this medication. Which explanation by a nurse about this medication is correct?

1. Reduces the size of the prostate gland and thus relieve the obstructive BPH symptoms
2. Decreases the inflammation caused by the prostatic enlargement
3. Relaxes the smooth muscle in the prostate and thus facilitate urinary flow
4. Decreases the specific gravity of the urine and therefore decreases the risk of urinary tract infection

61. EBP While in labor, a first-time mother informs a nurse that she wants to breastfeed her infant but is concerned about her ability to successfully breastfeed. Based on this information, which intervention should the nurse plan to implement immediately after the delivery to promote successful breastfeeding?

1. Allowing the mother to rest for 1 to 2 hours after the delivery before attempting to breastfeed
2. Providing privacy by allowing the mother and infant to be alone during the first feeding
3. Placing the infant skin-to-skin with the mother
4. Giving the newborn a bottle of formula to stimulate bowel peristalsis before breastfeeding

62. An orthopedic nurse is caring for a client who is being discharged to home following the repair of a fractured leg. Which orthopedic device is being used in the illustration and which nursing intervention is required to maintain this device?

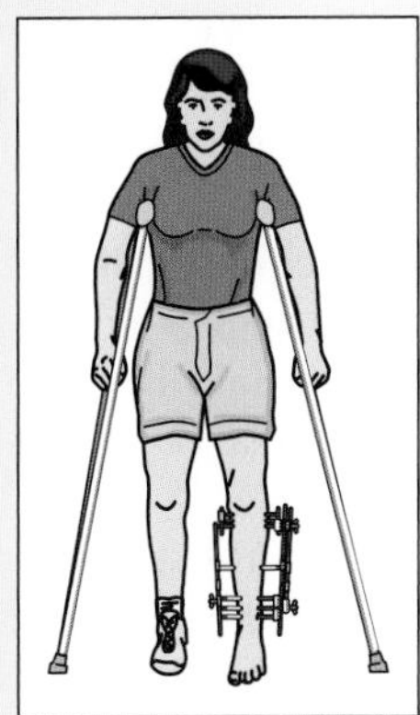

1. Internal fixation device, which requires pin care with hydrogen peroxide and saline on a daily basis
2. Buck's traction, which should be removed when the client retires to bed to sleep at night
3. Brace cast, which involves monitoring the client to remain non-weight bearing on the affected extremity
4. External fixation device, which requires daily inspection of the surrounding skin for redness

63. EBP A nurse receives an order to administer glycopyrrolate (Robinul®) intravenously through a central line access to a client 30 minutes prior to surgery. After explaining the procedure to the client, the nurse gathers supplies, performs hand hygiene, and applies gloves. Which steps should the nurse take to administer the medication through an existing single lumen peripherally inserted central venous catheter (PICC) that has 0.9% NaCl infusing at 30 mL per hour? Prioritize the nurse's actions by placing each step in the correct order.

______ Cleanse injection port with antiseptic swab and allow the port to dry

______ Occlude IV line and gently pull back syringe plunger to check for a blood return

______ Select injection port of IV tubing closest to client

______ Release tubing and inject medication within recommended time

______ Remove syringe, and recheck fluid infusion rate

______ Assess IV insertion site for signs of infiltration or phlebitis

______ Connect a 10-mL syringe with the medication to the injection port

64. A nurse manager is observing a new nurse who is applying topical triamcinolone (Kenalog®) 0.025% cream to a toddler's skin areas affected by dermatitis. Which action in the nurse's procedure should be corrected by the nurse manager?

1. Inspects skin for signs of infection, including increased pain, erythema, and purulent exudate
2. Performs hand hygiene and then dons exam gloves to apply the cream
3. Spreads cream over the toddler's buttock and affected areas and applies a disposable diaper
4. Asks the mother to hold the toddler while applying cream to affected areas on the back

65. A child, diagnosed with acute nonlymphoid leukemia is admitted to a hospital with a fever and neutropenia. To avoid the complications associated with neutropenia, which nursing interventions should a nurse include in the child's plan of care?

1. Placing the child in a private room, restricting ill visitors, and using strict handwashing techniques
2. Encouraging a well-balanced diet, including iron-rich foods, and helping the child avoid overexertion
3. Offering a moist, bland, soft diet, using toothettes rather than a toothbrush, and providing frequent saline mouthwashes
4. Avoiding rectal temperatures, avoiding injections, and applying direct pressure for 5 to 10 minutes after venipuncture

66. EBP A female client, who was abused and sexually assaulted for the second time by her estranged husband, is receiving treatment in an emergency department. The client is distraught and states, "The police can't keep him away, and I am afraid I might get pregnant." Which interventions should the nurse plan in treating this client? SELECT ALL THAT APPLY.

1. Obtain specimens of vaginal secretions
2. Administer a douche, if ordered
3. Administer emergency contraception if results of the pregnancy test are negative
4. Ask the woman about making arrangements at a woman's shelter
5. Keep the room door open when out of the room so the woman does not feel alone
6. Notify security to prevent the estranged husband from having access to the woman

67. EBP A client, with the diagnosis of congestive heart failure (CHF), contacts a clinic nurse and states, "I don't know why my ankles are so fat." What is the most appropriate initial response by the clinic nurse?

1. "Tell me about your activity level."
2. "What have you eaten in the last 24 hours?"
3. "Have you weighed yourself today?"
4. "How different are they from yesterday?"

68. A registered nurse (RN) and a licensed practical nurse (LPN) are preparing for the delivery of a small-for-gestational-age (SGA) newborn. Which action by the LPN indicates to the RN that the LPN needs additional orientation about the probable complications associated with an SGA infant?

1. Gathers equipment for newborn resuscitation
2. Discusses delayed cord clamping with the client's spouse
3. Places the radiant warmer close to the client's delivery bed
4. Prepares equipment needed for glucose monitoring

69. EBP A client, diagnosed with bipolar disorder, is in an acute manic state. The nursing staff is unable to verbally deescalate the situation and a physician orders a stat dose of aripiprazole (Abilify®) intramuscularly. Which client behavior indicates that the medication has been effective?

1. Client is sedated
2. Client's excitability is reduced
3. Client's psychotic symptoms are reduced
4. Client's mood swings are equalized

70. EBP A parish nurse is monitoring blood pressures at a blood pressure–screening clinic. A client, who just finished smoking a cigarette, asks the nurse for a blood pressure check. Which is the nurse's best action?

1. Ask the client to have the blood pressure taken on another day
2. Immediately take the client's blood pressure
3. Ask the client to return in 30 minutes and upon return take the client's blood pressure
4. Ask the client if the client knows that smoking leads to heart disease and cancer

71. A nurse, working in a college health center, receives a call from a first-year student who has had flu-like symptoms with neck stiffness for the past 4 hours. Which is the initial question the nurse should ask the student?

1. "Have you been able to drink anything?"
2. "Do you have a fever?"
3. "What do you mean 'flu-like symptoms'?"
4. "Do you have a rash anywhere on your body?"

72. EBP A client, who has worn contacts for over 15 years, asks a nurse about a surgical procedure to correct vision. The client asks about laser in-situ keratomileusis (LASIK) surgery. The nurse explains that this procedure corrects refraction errors by:

1. enhancing the outflow of aqueous humor.
2. reshaping the cornea.
3. flattening of the retina.
4. decreasing density of the lens.

73. A nurse is caring for a client with severe lymphedema in the right lower extremity. A sequential compression device is ordered at a specific pressure for 2 hours twice daily. The nurse is initiating the device. Prioritize the nurse's actions to safely provide this treatment.

_____ Assess and document baseline color, temperature, and presence of peripheral pulses in the lower extremities

_____ Explain the purpose, expected outcome and procedure to the client

_____ Mark the skin and measure the lower extremity with lymphedema as recommended by the manufacturer of the sequential compression device

_____ Monitor the client for pain and toleration during the treatment

_____ Measure the lower extremity with lymphedema again, reassess the circulation in the lower extremities, and document.

_____ Apply a stocking over the leg and then the sequential compression sleeve, connect, set the control unit at the prescribed pressure, and turn on the unit

74. Nurse A is documenting administration of morphine sulfate in a client's electronic medical record (EMR). The nurse is called away to talk with a physician and quickly leaves the computer. Seeing a free computer, Nurse B selects a different client for documentation. Nurse B is also called away. Nurse A returns to the computer and completes documentation on Nurse B's client's record. Which nursing actions should have prevented this incorrect medical record entry? SELECT ALL THAT APPLY.

1. Log out of the system before leaving the computer
2. Check that the correct client is selected before beginning documentation
3. Tell Nurse B to make sure to select the right client before documenting
4. Ask another nurse to complete the documentation
5. Always log in when accessing a record
6. Always use the assigned user ID and created password when documenting in an EMR

75. Immediately following surgery, a surgical nurse is caring for a client who has normal lung function and is receiving 40% oxygen by mask. The client's oxygen saturation (SpO_2) reading is 90%. Which action should the nurse implement based on this reading?

1. Decrease the oxygen level to 30%
2. Increase the oxygen level to 50%
3. Leave the oxygen level at 40%
4. Place the client on room air

Answers

1. ANSWER: 4

Timolol, the generic name of a medication, is ordered correctly with the correct concentration. The dose of the medication, the route, and the frequency are clearly identifiable. In some facilities, only generic names are permitted. The U is an unacceptable abbreviation noted on The Joint Commission's Do Not Use List. The .25 mg lacks a leading zero and is also an unacceptable abbreviation. The route for administering levofloxacin is missing.

Test-taking Tip: *Read each option carefully to determine if essential parts of the medication order are noted and whether acceptable abbreviations are being used. Eliminate options where missing components are noted within the option.*

Content Area: Fundamentals; *Category of Health Alteration:* Medication Administration; *Integrated Processes:* Communication and Documentation; *Client Need:* Physiological Integrity/ Pharmacological and Parenteral Therapies/Medication Administration; *Cognitive Level:* Analysis

Reference: Berman, A., Snyder, S., Kozier, B., & Erb, G. (2008). *Kozier & Erb's Fundamentals of Nursing: Concepts, Process, and Practice* (8th ed., p. 840). Upper Saddle River, NJ: Pearson Education.

EBP Reference: The Joint Commission. (2005). Patient Safety Do Not Use List. Available at: www.jointcommission.org/NR/rdonlyres/ 2329F8F5-6EC5-4E21-B932-54B2B7D53F00/0/06_dnu_list.pdf

2. ANSWER: 2

Nonbilious vomiting, weight loss, hunger after vomiting, and lethargy are characteristic of pyloric stenosis. Diarrhea is not characteristic of pyloric stenosis. In pyloric stenosis, vomiting is unrelated to feeding position, and diarrhea is also not a symptom of pyloric stenosis. Vomiting, diarrhea, severe pain, and lethargy are signs and symptoms of intussusception.

Test-taking Tip: *Examine options with duplicate information first. Note that all options except option 2 include diarrhea. Often, the option that is different is the answer.*

Content Area: Child Health; *Category of Health Alteration:* Gastrointestinal Management; *Integrated Processes:* Nursing Process Assessment; *Client Need:* Physiological Integrity/Physiological Adaptation/ Alterations in Body Systems; *Cognitive Level:* Application

Reference: Kyle, T. (2008). *Essentials of Pediatric Nursing* (pp. 687–689). Philadelphia: Lippincott Williams & Wilkins.

EBP Reference: Cincinnati Children's Hospital Medical Center. (2007). Evidence-based clinical practice guideline for hypertrophic pyloric stenosis. Available at: www.guideline.gov/summary/summary.aspx? view_id=1&doc_id=12095

3. ANSWER: 1

To transfer a client with left-sided weakness back to bed, the client's strong side (not the weak side) should be toward the bed. Though the female PCA is supporting the client's weak side, the male PCA is using a wide base of support, and the client is using the strong side to push from the chair, complimenting and praising are not the best actions to protect the client from injury.

Test-taking Tip: *Select the option that uses ergonomic principles in transferring a client safely. Note three options are similar (complimentary) and one is different.*

Content Area: Fundamentals; *Client Need:* Safe and Effective Care Environment/Safety and Infection Control; *Integrated Processes:* Nursing Process Implementation; *Client Need:* Safe and Effective Care Environment/Safety and Infection Control/Ergonomic Principles; *Cognitive Level:* Analysis

References: Berman, A., Snyder, S., Kozier, B., & Erb, G. (2008). *Kozier & Erb's Fundamentals of Nursing: Concepts, Process, and Practice* (8th ed., pp. 1142–1144). Upper Saddle River, NJ: Pearson Education; Monahan, F., Sands, J., Neighbors, M., Marek, J., & Green, C. (2007). *Phipps' Medical-Surgical Nursing: Health and Illness Perspectives* (8th ed., pp. 1433–1434). St. Louis, MO: Mosby.

4. ANSWER: 3

A clinical finding in prerenal failure is a decreased urine output. A urine output of greater than 30 mL per hour indicates the fluid challenge is effective. Although improvement is noted in the blood pressure, the focus of the question is on treating the prerenal failure and not the blood pressure. Although improvement is noted in the cardiac output, the focus of the question is on treating the prerenal failure and not the cardiac output. Tachycardia is a manifestation of prerenal failure. If treatment is effective, the client's heart rate should be 60 to 100 bpm.

Test-taking Tip: *Focus on the key words "for treating the prerenal failure." Eliminate options 1, 2, and 4 because they do not evaluate kidney function.*

Content Area: Adult Health; *Category of Health Alteration:* Renal and Urinary Management; *Integrated Processes:* Nursing Process Evaluation; *Client Need:* Physiological Integrity/Reduction of Risk Potential/Therapeutic Procedures; *Cognitive Level:* Analysis

Reference: Ignatavicius, D., & Workman, M. (2006). *Medical-Surgical Nursing: Critical Thinking for Collaborative Care* (5th ed., p. 1732). St. Louis, MO: Saunders/Elsevier.

5. ANSWER: 2, 3, 4, 1

The best approach should be to see if the student could get the friend to visit the nurse with her. This would be the least threatening to the student and would not cause conflicts between the friends. If the friend is unwilling to visit the nurse with the student, then the nurse should approach the student. Because the student is a minor, the parents need to be apprised of the situation. Because of privacy laws and rights of minors, it would be best if the girl is ready to talk with the parents while the nurse is present. The girl will need to see a primary care provider. A referral can be made by the nurse if the parents do not currently have one.

Test-taking Tip: *Approach this situation in relation to privacy laws, trust issues, ethical practice, and parental rights and responsibilities.*

Content Area: Management of Care; Child Health; *Category of Health Alteration:* Prioritization and Delegation; *Integrated Processes:* Nursing Process Implementation; *Client Need:* Safe and Effective Care Environment/Management of Care/Legal Rights and Responsibilities; *Cognitive Level:* Analysis

References: Hockenberry, M., & Wilson, D. (2007). *Wong's Nursing Care of Infants and Children* (8th ed., pp. 838–839, 859–862). St. Louis, MO: Mosby; Ball, J., & Binder, R. (2006). *Clinical Handbook for Pediatric Nursing* (pp. 285–288). Upper Saddle River, NJ: Pearson Education.

6. ANSWER: 2

Generating possible solutions is an important step in conflict resolution. Emotional involvement usually clouds the issue making it more difficult to resolve. Response such as "not my turn," "that's not fair," "all float too much," do not offer steps toward resolution.

Test-taking Tip: *Focus on the option that demonstrates conflict resolution first and then negotiation.*

Content Area: Management of Care; *Category of Health Alteration:* Leadership and Management; *Integrated Processes:* Nursing Process Analysis; *Client Need:* Safe and Effective Care Environment/Management of Care/Concepts of Management; *Cognitive Level:* Application

Reference: Wilkinson, J., & Van Leuven, K. (2007). *Fundamentals of Nursing* (p. 966). Philadelphia: F. A. Davis.

7. ANSWER: 3

The word 'postictal' period is the time following a seizure. If an aura is present, it appears before the onset of the seizure. The prefix "post' indicates that it follows, or comes after, therefore the word "preceding" in this answer selection is clearly false. Tonic-clonic activity and loss of consciousness occur during a grand-mal seizure.

➧ ***Test-Taking Tip:*** *Notice prefixes and suffixes for clues.*

Content Area: Adult Health; *Category of Health Alteration:* Neurological and Musculoskeletal Management; *Integrated Processes:* Communication and Documentation; *Client Need:* Safe and Effective Care Environment/Management of Care/Continuity of Care; *Cognitive Level:* Application

Reference: *Taber's Cyclopedic Medical Dictionary*. (2007). Philadelphia: F. A. Davis.

8. ANSWER: 3

Over the last decade, unintentional injury has been the leading cause of death in children ages 1 to 4 years. Pneumonia, cancer, and homicide are other causes of death related to this age group, but these are not the leading causes.

➧ ***Test-taking Tip:*** *The key words are "most common." Focus on the age group and the causes.*

Content Area: Fundamentals; *Category of Health Alteration:* Safety, Disaster Preparedness, and Infection Control; *Integrated Processes:* Communication and Documentation; *Client Need:* Safe and Effective Care Environment/Safety and Infection Control/Accident and Injury Prevention; *Cognitive Level:* Application

Reference: Ball, J., & Binder, R. (2006). *Clinical Handbook for Pediatric Nursing* (pp. 16–17). Upper Saddle River, NJ: Pearson Education.

9. ANSWER: 3

Periodic pauses of up to 15 seconds in newborn respirations are expected during early newborn life. Rapid eye movement sleep, gross motor activity, sucking, and crying will increase the frequency of the pauses. Periodic breathing is rarely associated with changes in skin color. At 35 weeks gestation, surfactant production is adequate to maintain good respiratory gas exchange in the majority of newborn infants. Healthy term newborns are not lacking in surfactant.

➧ ***Test-taking Tip:*** *Eliminate option 4 because lack of surfactant production is not a concern in full-term newborns.*

Content Area: Childbearing Families; *Category of Health Alteration:* Neonatal and High-Risk Neonatal Management; *Integrated Processes:* Nursing Process Analysis; *Client Need:* Health Promotion and Maintenance/Developmental Stages and Transitions; *Cognitive Level:* Application

Reference: Davidson, M., London, M., & Ladewig, P. (2008). *Olds' Maternal-Newborn Nursing & Women's Health Across the Lifespan* (8th ed., pp. 793, 798). Upper Saddle River, NJ: Prentice Hall Health.

10. ANSWER: 4

The most appropriate nursing diagnosis is *Family processes, interrupted*. This response is the only diagnosis that supports uncomplicated grief. Grief is an emotional state following the death of a loved one that affects a client's physical and emotional well-being with impairment of functioning lasting for days, weeks, or months. Impaired adjustment, ineffective coping, and dysfunctional grieving support a maladaptive grief response. Impaired adjustment is the inability to modify behavior in a manner consistent with a change in health status. Ineffective coping is the inability to form a valid appraisal of the stressors, inadequate choices of practical response, and/or inability to use available resources. Dysfunctional grieving is the risk for extended, unsuccessful use of intellectual and emotional responses by which individuals, families, communities attempt to work through the process of modifying self-concept based upon the perception of loss.

➧ ***Test-taking Tip:*** *Use the process of elimination. The key words in the stem are "improving" and "1 month ago."*

Content Area: Mental Health; *Category of Health Alteration:* Anxiety and Mood Disorders; *Integrated Processes:* Nursing Process Analysis; *Client Need:* Psychosocial Integrity/Grief and Loss; *Cognitive Level:* Analysis.

Reference: Pedersen, D. (2008). *Psych Notes* (2nd ed., p. 167). Philadelphia: F. A. Davis.

11. ANSWER: 3

Native Americans often avoid direct eye contact and consider it disrespectful or aggressive. Decision making is mutual in Native American Navajo families and they will accept care from Western health-care practitioners. Looking at pictures of body parts for education is unacceptable.

➧ ***Test-taking Tip:*** *Read the question carefully and focus on the first nurse's actions during the instruction session.*

Content Area: Management of Care; *Category of Health Alteration:* Teaching and Learning, Communication, and Cultural Diversity; *Integrated Processes:* Communication and Documentation; *Client Need:* Psychosocial Integrity/Cultural Diversity; *Cognitive Level:* Analysis

References: Lewis, S., Heitkemper, M., Dirksen, S., O'Brien, P., & Bucher, L. (2007). *Medical-Surgical Nursing: Assessment and Management of Clinical Problems* (7th ed., p. 31). St. Louis, MO: Mosby; Harkreader, H., Hogan, M., & Thobaben, M. (2007). *Fundamentals of Nursing* (3rd ed., pp. 56–57). St. Louis, MO: Saunders/Elsevier.

12. ANSWER: 2

The single most important indicator of pain and its intensity is the client's report of pain; whether treatment includes medication, nonpharmacological interventions, or both. Clients with chronic pain are less likely to have physiological changes because the autonomic nervous system adapts to the pain. Asking the client's significant other's opinion and assessing client facial expression are not as reliable as asking the client about pain.

➧ ***Test-taking Tip:*** *Read the scenario in the stem carefully. Determine that the question is asking the best method to evaluate pain. Consider the options and the option that focuses directly on the client's individual pain experience.*

Content Area: Fundamentals; *Category of Health Alteration:* Basic Care and Comfort; *Integrated Processes:* Nursing Process Evaluation; *Client Need:* Physiological Integrity/Basic Care and Comfort/Nonpharmacological Comfort Interventions; *Cognitive Level:* Analysis

Reference: Berman, A., Snyder, S., Kozier, B., & Erb, G. (2008). *Kozier & Erb's Fundamentals of Nursing: Concepts, Process, and Practice* (8th ed., pp. 1198, 1202). Upper Saddle River, NJ: Pearson Education.

EBP Reference: Institute for Clinical Systems Improvement. (2008). Assessment and management of acute pain. Available at: www.guideline.gov/summary/summary.aspx?view_id=1&doc_id=12302

13. ANSWER: 4

Prevention of postpartum hemorrhage (PPH) involves the routine administration of oxytocin immediately following delivery of the placenta to promote uterine contraction and vasoconstriction, thus preventing the uterus from becoming atonic. A firm fundus would indicate that the oxytocin was effective. A side effect of oxytocin is mild transient hypertension. Thus a systolic blood pressure above 100 mm Hg would be expected. The purpose of the oxytocin is to contract the uterus. In response, the lochia flow should be moderate to small unless the client had experienced a perineal laceration. If the oxytocin causes continuous uterine contraction, the client will not experience afterpains. However, if the uterus contracts and relaxes, as sometimes happens with multigravidas, the client may feel afterpains when the oxytocin is infusing.

▶ ***Test-taking Tip:*** *Recall the action of oxytocin is to contract the uterus. Select the option that best describes that action.*

Content Area: Childbearing Families; *Category of Health Alteration:* Pharmacological and Parenteral Therapies; *Integrated Processes:* Nursing Process Evaluation; *Client Need:* Physiological Integrity/Pharmacological and Parenteral Therapies/Expected Actions or Outcomes; *Cognitive Level:* Application

Reference: Davidson, M., London, M., & Ladewig, P. (2008). *Olds' Maternal-Newborn Nursing & Women's Health Across the Lifespan* (8th ed., pp. 1080–1081, 1160–1161). Upper Saddle River, NJ: Prentice Hall Health.

EBP Reference: Briggs, G., & Wan, S. (2006). Drug therapy during labor and delivery: Part 2. *American Journal of Health-System Pharmacy*, 63(12), 1131–1139.

14. ANSWER: 3

The BUN has normalized. A normal BUN for a child is 4 to 17 mg/dL. The hemoglobin, hematocrit, BUN, and creatinine elevate with acute diarrhea and normalize with rehydration. The hemoglobin and hematocrit should be elevated with hemoconcentration and then normalize with rehydration. Normal hemoglobin is 11.5 to 15.5 g/dL, and hematocrit is 35 to 45%. A normal SCr is 0.3 to 0.7 mg/dL. The SCr is still elevated.

▶ ***Test-taking Tip:*** *Even if normal values for a 7-year-old child are unknown, look at the laboratory value changes and consider that changes that should occur with hemoconcentration and then rehydration.*

Content Area: Child Health; *Category of Health Alteration:* Gastrointestinal Management; *Integrated Processes:* Nursing Process Evaluation; *Client Need:* Physiological Integrity/Reduction of Risk Potential/Laboratory Values; *Cognitive Level:* Analysis

Reference: Hockenberry, M., & Wilson, D. (2007). *Wong's Nursing Care of Infants and Children* (8th ed., pp. 1182, 1867–1869). St. Louis, MO: Mosby.

EBP Reference: Levine, A. (2008). Pediatrics: Gastroenteritis. *E-Medicine from WebMD*. Available at: www.emedicine.com/emerg/TOPIC380.HTM

15. ANSWER: 2

Numbness and tingling suggest circulatory impairment from compartment syndrome. Inability to void, dressing saturation, and nausea also should be addressed; but are not the priority.

▶ ***Test-taking Tip:*** *Use the ABCs—airway, breathing, and circulation—to establish priority.*

Content Area: Adult Health; *Category of Health Alteration:* Musculoskeletal Management; *Integrated Processes:* Nursing Process Analysis; *Client Need:* Physiological Integrity/Physiological Adaptation/Illness Management; *Cognitive Level:* Analysis

Reference: Lewis, S., Heitkemper, M., Dirksen, S., O'Brien, P., & Bucher, L. (2007). *Medical-Surgical Nursing: Assessment and Management of Clinical Problems* (7th ed., pp. 1643–1648). St. Louis, MO: Mosby.

16. ANSWER: 4

During the first 24 to 48 hours after prostatectomy, it is critical that the patency of the catheter be assessed and maintained. The risk of blood clots forming and obstructing the flow of urine is greatest during this time period. Parts of the gland are removed through a scope inserted into the urethra. Therefore, an abdominal incision is not required. Blood clots are expected after prostate surgery for the first 24 to 36 hours, and thus there is no need to notify the surgeon of this development. Activities that increase abdominal pressure such as sitting should be avoided as they predispose the client to increased bleeding.

▶ ***Test-taking Tip:*** *The key phrase is "immediately after a TURP." Recall that bleeding is a major concern in the early postoperative period. Select the option that decreases bleeding or the complications of bleeding.*

Content Area: Adult Health; *Category of Health Alteration:* Reproductive Management; *Integrated Processes:* Nursing Process Implementation; *Client Need:* Physiological Integrity/Physiological Adaptation/Illness Management; *Cognitive Level:* Application

References: Lewis, S., Heitkemper, M., Dirksen, S., O'Brien, P., & Bucher, L. (2007). *Medical-Surgical Nursing: Assessment and Management of Clinical Problems* (7th ed., p. 1421). St. Louis, MO: Mosby; Smeltzer, S., Bare, B., Hinkle, J., & Cheever, K. (2008). *Brunner & Suddarth's Textbook of Medical-Surgical Nursing* (11th ed., p. 1761). Philadelphia: Lippincott Williams & Wilkins.

17. ANSWER: 3

If the person performing rescue breathing is on the right side of the client, then the person performing compressions should be on the left side of the client. A person doing rescue breathing with a bag-mask resuscitator might stand at the head of the bed. In this case the person doing compressions could be on either side of the bed. Position D is only assumed for abdominal thrusts on an unresponsive choking victim.

▶ ***Test-taking Tip:*** *Read the scenario carefully and visualize the position of the rescue breather.*

Content Area: Adult Health; *Category of Health Alteration:* Medical Emergencies; *Integrated Processes:* Nursing Process Implementation; *Client Need:* Physiological Integrity/Physiological Adaptation/Medical Emergencies; *Cognitive Level:* Application

Reference: Smeltzer, S., Bare, B., Hinkle, J., & Cheever, K. (2008). *Brunner & Suddarth's Textbook of Medical-Surgical Nursing* (11th ed., pp. 970–971). Philadelphia: Lippincott Williams & Wilkins.

18. ANSWER: 3

Studies show that reducing relationship distress lessens the risk of relapse. One of the goals of therapy includes helping families become aware of their own needs and providing genuine, enduring healing for family members; working to shift power to the parental figures in a family and to improve communication; helping the family make interpersonal, intrapersonal, and environmental changes affecting the person using alcohol or drugs; and keeping substance abuse from moving from one generation to another (i.e., prevention). Families are not responsible for the consequences of the client's actions or reducing the client's temptation to use (options 1, 2, and 4).

▶ ***Test-taking Tip:*** *Note that option 3 focuses on the family's needs whereas the other options focus on the client's needs.*

Content Area: Mental Health; *Category of Health Alteration:* Substance Abuse; *Integrated Processes:* Nursing Process Planning; Caring; *Client Need:* Psychosocial Integrity/Chemical and Other Dependencies; Health Promotion and Maintenance/Self-Care; *Cognitive Level:* Analysis

Reference: Mohr, W. (2009). *Psychiatric Mental Health Nursing: Evidence-Based Concepts, Skills, and Practices* (7th ed., p. 646). Philadelphia: Lippincott Williams & Wilkins.

EBP References: Substance Abuse and Mental Health Service Administration's National Registry of Evidence-Based Programs and Practices. (2006). Available at: www.nrepp.samhsa.gov/programfulldetails.asp?PROGRAM_ID=70; Center for Substance Abuse Treatment. (2006). Substance abuse: clinical issues in intensive outpatient treatment. Available at: www.guideline.gov/summary/summary.aspx?doc_id=12196&nbr=006293&string=%22substance+abuse%22+and+%22family+therapy%22

19. ANSWER: 4

Wearing protective gown, gloves, goggles, and a respirator mask and using double-bag clean-up pads with open waste disposal bags provides adequate protection for cleaning up powder chemotherapy spills. If the spill involves liquid chemotherapy drugs, the nurse would need protective gown, gloves, and goggles only, but would still double-bag the spilled waste.

▸ ***Test-taking Tip:*** *Note the key word "safety practices" and focus on the issues of the medication spill. Examine options with duplicate words first. If unsure, eliminate options using a single-bag and focus on options using a double-bag.*

Content Area: Adult Health; *Category of Health Alteration:* Hematological and Oncological Management; *Integrated Processes:* Nursing Process Implementation; *Client Need:* Safe and Effective Care Environment/Safety and Infection Control/Handling Hazardous and Infectious Materials; *Cognitive Level:* Application

Reference: Black, J., & Hokanson Hawks, J. (2009). *Medical-Surgical Nursing: Clinical Management for Positive Outcomes* (8th ed., p. 284). St. Louis, MO: Saunders/Elsevier.

EBP Reference: Connor, T., & McDiarmid, M. (2009). Preventing Occupational Exposures to Antineoplastic Drugs in Health Care Settings. Available at: www.intl-caonline.amcancersoc.org/cgi/reprint/56/6/354

20. ANSWER: 1

The RN from ICU would have the most experience in monitoring the client and preparing IV medications for administration. The LPN would be unable to prepare and administer the IV medications that will be required. The newly licensed RN would not have the experience needed to prepare the IV medications. The nurse's inexperience will likely prolong the time before the client receives the ordered medications. Fatigue increases the risk for errors.

▸ ***Test-taking Tip:*** *Use the process of elimination, focusing on the key phrase "multiple IV medications" and determine which nurse is best experienced to handle multiple medications.*

Content Area: Management of Care; *Category of Health Alteration:* Prioritization and Delegation; *Integrated Processes:* Nursing Process Planning; *Client Need:* Safe and Effective Care Environment/Management of Care/Continuity of Care; *Cognitive Level:* Application

References: Ignatavicius, D., & Workman, M. (2006). *Medical-Surgical Nursing: Critical Thinking for Collaborative Care* (5th ed., p. 276). St. Louis, MO: Saunders/Elsevier; Berman, A., Snyder, S., Kozier, B., & Erb, G. (2008). *Kozier & Erb's Fundamentals of Nursing: Concepts, Process, and Practice* (8th ed., p. 518). Upper Saddle River, NJ: Pearson Education.

21. ANSWER: 1

Guaifenesin (Robitussin®) aids in expectoration by reducing adhesiveness and surface tension of secretions. It should be taken with a full glass of water. Increasing fluids helps to liquefy secretions. Side effects include headache, which can be relieved with acetaminophen. Sugarless gum or hard candy will help alleviate the discomfort caused by a nonproductive cough.

▸ ***Test-taking Tip:*** *Recall that guaifenesin is an expectorant. The key words are "needs additional teaching." Select the option that is incorrect.*

Content Area: Adult Health; *Category of Health Alteration:* Pharmacological and Parenteral Therapies; *Integrated Processes:* Nursing Process Evaluation; *Client Need:* Health Promotion and Maintenance/Principles of Teaching and Learning; *Cognitive Level:* Analysis

Reference: Deglin, J., & Vallerand, A. (2009). *Davis's Drug Guide for Nurses* (11th ed., pp. 610–611). Philadelphia: F. A. Davis.

22. ANSWER: 1, 2, 4, 5, 6

Reduced intake can result in nutritional deficits. Those most likely to occur after gastric bypass surgery include iron (from malabsorption), vitamin B_{12} (from reduced intrinsic factor production secondary to parietal cell loss and malabsorption), and vitamin A (from bypassed duodenum where these are primarily absorbed), and calcium and protein (from reduce intake). Vitamin C deficiency has not been associated with Roux-en-Y gastric bypass.

▸ ***Test-taking Tip:*** *Consider which nutrients are absorbed in the stomach and which have the highest potential to be malabsorbed after Roux-en-Y gastric bypass.*

Content Area: Childbearing Families; *Category of Health Alteration:* Prenatal and Antepartal Management; *Integrated Processes:* Nursing Process Analysis; *Client Need:* Physiological Integrity/Basic Care and Comfort/Nutrition and Oral Hydration; *Cognitive Level:* Analysis

EBP Reference: Poitou, B., Ciangura, C., Coupaye, M., Czernichow, S., Bouillot, J., & Basdevant, A. (2007). Nutritional deficiency after gastric bypass: Diagnosis, prevention and treatment. *Diabetes Metabolism*, 33(1), 13–24.

23. ANSWER:

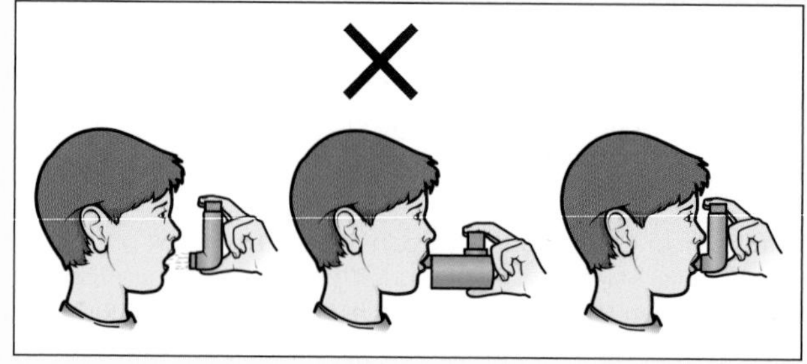

Using a spacer for pediatric clients facilitates the best absorption of aerosolized medication. Children often have trouble coordinating their inspiration with the dispensing of the medication. Holding the inhaler two or three fingers away from the mouth and depressing the canister is ineffective in children. They often have difficulty coordinating inspiratory efforts with discharge of the metered dose inhaler (MDI), and the desired medication is lost in the air. In illustration C, wrapping the lips around the spacer to obtain a tight seal before depressing the canister are appropriate forms and can be used with older clients and adults, but is not the best method of delivery for clients of this age. Medication is often concentrated in the buccal cavity and is absorbed, but is less effective.

▶ ***Test-taking Tip:*** *Focus on the age of the child and select the option that is best for this client's age. Review medications administration with a metered dose inhaler if you had difficulty answering this question.*

Content Area: Child Health; *Category of Health Alteration:* Respiratory Management; *Integrated Processes:* Nursing Process Implementation; *Client Need:* Physiological Integrity/Pharmacological and Parenteral Therapies/Medication Administration; *Cognitive Level:* Analysis

Reference: Karch, A. (2008). *Focus on Nursing Pharmacology* (4th ed., p. 910). Philadelphia: Lippincott Williams & Wilkins.

24. ANSWER: 4

A review of studies of nicotine replacement therapy (NRT) for smoking cessation found that nicotine replacement therapy helped persons quit smoking and almost doubled long-term success rates. NRT reduces, but does not eliminate, withdrawal symptoms. There is no evidence of one form of NRT being superior to others. Smoking cigarettes while using NRT, even if reduced, increases the risk of serious adverse effects, especially cardiovascular effects.

▶ ***Test-taking Tip:*** *The issue of the question is NRT. Use the process of elimination to select the statement that demonstrates the best outcome for smoking cessation.*

Content Area: Adult Health; *Category of Health Alteration:* Vascular Management; *Integrated Processes:* Nursing Process Implementation; *Client Need:* Health Promotion and Maintenance/Health Promotion and Disease Prevention; Physiological Integrity/Pharmacological and Parenteral Therapies/Expected Actions or Outcomes; *Cognitive Level:* Application

Reference: Lewis, S., Heitkemper, M., Dirksen, S., O'Brien, P., & Bucher, L. (2007). *Medical-Surgical Nursing: Assessment and Management of Clinical Problems* (7th ed., pp. 170–174). St. Louis, MO: Mosby.

EBP References: Department of Health and Human Services. (2008). Treating tobacco use and dependence: Available at: www.guideline.gov/summary/summary.aspx?doc_id=12520&nbr=006444&string=tobacco+AND+cessation; Stead, L., Perera, R., Bullen, C., Mant, D., & Lancaster, T. (2008). Nicotine replacement therapy for smoking cessation. *Cochrane Database of Systematic Reviews 2008, 1*, Article no. CD000146. Available at: www.cochrane.org/reviews/en/ab000146.html

25. ANSWER:

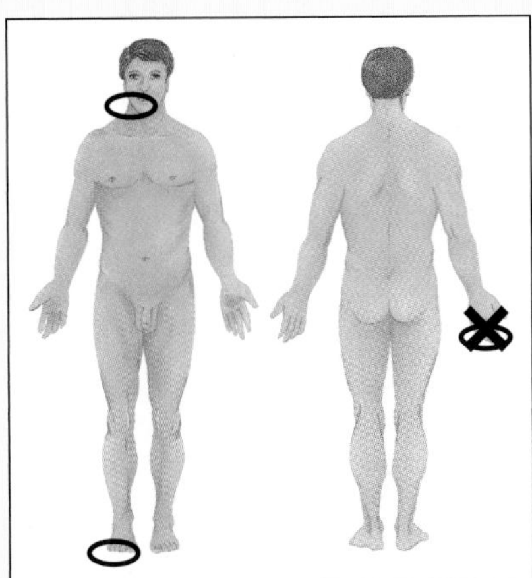

Scabies lesions tend to be concentrated in the web spaces of the fingers.

▶ ***Test-taking Tip:*** *Focus on the key word "most frequently locate" and "scabies parasite." Recall that the papules appear most frequently in finer webs, axillae, wrist folds, umbilicus, groin and genitals.*

Content Area: Adult Health; *Category of Health Alteration:* Integumentary Management and Other Health Alterations; *Integrated Processes:* Nursing Process Assessment; *Client Need:* Physiological Integrity/Physiological Adaptation/Alterations in Body Systems; *Cognitive Level:* Application

Reference: Monahan, F., Sands, J., Neighbors, M., Marek, J., & Green, C. (2007). *Phipps' Medical-Surgical Nursing: Health and Illness Perspectives* (8th ed., p. 1874). St. Louis, MO: Mosby.

26. ANSWER: 2

Soft foods and not solid should be provided because they require less work of mastication. Small, frequent feedings, high-calorie supplements, and utensils with large padded handles help the child to get adequate calories and engage in self-feeding when possible.

▶ ***Test-taking Tip:*** *Select an option that would increase energy expenditure.*

Content Area: Child Health; *Category of Health Alteration:* Neurological and Musculoskeletal Management; *Integrated Processes:* Nursing Process Evaluation; *Client Need:* Physiological Integrity/Basic Care and Comfort/Nutrition and Oral Hydration; *Cognitive Level:* Application

Reference: Ball, J., & Bindler, R. (2008). *Pediatric Nursing: Caring for Children* (4th ed., p. 508). Upper Saddle River, NJ: Pearson Education.

27. ANSWER: 4

To protect the client from unintentional harm, the client's identity should be confirmed first. Though the client's level of anxiety is important, ensuring client safety is first. Before checking a client's medical record, the nurse should determine if the client is the correct client for the operative procedure. Before verifying the correct operative site, the nurse must have admitted the correct client.

▶ ***Test-taking Tip:*** *Use Maslow's Hierarchy of Needs theory to eliminate options.*

Content Area: Adult Health; *Category of Health Alteration:* Perioperative Management; *Integrated Processes:* Nursing Process Implementation; *Client Need:* Safe and Effective Care Environment/Safety and Infection Control/Error Prevention; *Cognitive Level:* Application

Reference: Ignatavicius, D., & Workman, M. (2006). *Medical-Surgical Nursing: Critical Thinking for Collaborative Care* (5th ed., p. 318). St. Louis, MO: Saunders/Elsevier.

EBP Reference: The Joint Commission. (2009). Universal Protocol. Available at: www.jointcommission.org/NR/rdonlyres/AEA17A06-BB67-4C4E-B0FC-DD195FE6BF2A/0/UP_HAP_20080616.pdf

28. ANSWER: 2

Relevant factors from the prenatal, intrapartum, and postnatal period influence the decision for the first clinic appointment after hospitalization. The timing of the follow-up clinic visit is individualized to the needs of the mother and infant. The newborn should have a health maintenance visit 2 to 4 weeks after birth and the woman 4 to 6 weeks postpartum. Many times babies and mothers are to return to the clinic in 2 days, but this may not always be the case and is not a required standard of care. When a mother is young, she may come to the clinic in 2 days; however, many young mothers are very mature. The criteria for a clinic visit cannot be based on age alone.

▶ ***Test-taking Tip:*** *Use the nursing process, considering the need for individualizing care.*

Content Area: Child Health; *Category of Health Alteration:* Growth and Development; *Integrated Processes:* Nursing Process Analysis; *Client Need:* Safe and Effective Care Environment/Management of Care/Collaboration with Interdisciplinary Team; *Cognitive Level:* Application

Reference: Pillitteri, A. (2007). *Maternal & Child Health Nursing: Care of the Childbearing & Childrearing Family* (5th ed., p. 650). Philadelphia: Lippincott Williams & Wilkins.

EBP Reference: National Collaborating Centre for Primary Care. (2006). *Postnatal care. routine postnatal care of women and their babies.* Available at: www.guideline.gov/summary/summary.aspx?ss=15&doc_id=9630&nbr=5150.

29. ANSWER: 1

The ℭ on the label indicates that codeine is a controlled substance. The categorization of schedule I to V indicates the potential for abuse. Schedule I controlled substances have the highest potential for abuse and are not acceptable for medical use (such as heroin). Schedule II medications have a high potential for abuse. Controlled substances must be signed out from a locked drawer or box at the time of administration. Because the other medications have been ordered and they are not controlled substances, they should be in the client's medication box.

▶ ***Test-taking Tip:*** *Note the focus of the question, finding medications in a client's medication box and needing to complete a variance report. Apply knowledge of reading medication labels to answer this question.*

Content Area: Fundamentals; *Category of Health Alteration:* Medication Administration; *Integrated Processes:* Nursing Process Analysis; *Client Need:* Safe and Effective Care Environment/Safety and Infection Control/Reporting of Incident/Event/Irregular Occurrence/Variance; *Cognitive Level:* Application

Reference: Craven, R., & Hirnle, C. (2007). *Fundamentals of Nursing: Human Health and Function* (5th ed., pp. 589–593). Philadelphia: Lippincott Williams & Wilkins.

EBP Reference: Food and Drug Administration (ND). *Controlled Substances Act: Part C—Registration of Manufacturers, Distributors, and Dispensers of Controlled Substances.* Available at: www.fda.gov/RegulatoryInformation/Legislation/ucm148726.htm#cntlsbc

30. ANSWER: 4

The statement about accessing the services when the client can no longer get the things needed to be healthy and safe shows a lack of understanding regarding the need to access these services before breakdown of the plan of care occurs. Thanking the staff for information about places for help provides some indication of an understanding of the importance of outpatient services. Acknowledging that a service has been contacted and keeping a list of outpatient services' telephone numbers available shows an understanding of the importance of a bridging strategy.

▶ ***Test-taking Tip:*** *The key words are "need for further understanding." This is a false-response question. Select the option that demonstrates that the client would utilize a service only as a last resort.*

Content Area: Mental Health; *Category of Health Alteration:* Crisis, Violence, Eating, and Sleep Disorders; *Integrated Processes:* Teaching and Learning; *Client Need:* Health Promotion and Maintenance/Self-Care; *Cognitive Level:* Analysis

Reference: Stuart, G. (2009). *Principles and Practice of Psychiatric Nursing* (9th ed., p. 578). St. Louis, MO: Mosby.

EBP Reference: Cohen, L. (2006). The importance of staying on therapy. *Psychiatric Times,* 23(4), 15–22.

31. ANSWER: 4

Dependency is a state of reliance on another and can be a behavioral response to acute coronary syndrome. Depression is usually manifested by symptoms of withdrawal, crying, or apathy. These behaviors are not noted in the situation. Denial is a defense mechanism that allows minimization of a threat. It may be manifested by minimizing the severity of the medical condition or ignoring activity restrictions, or avoids discussing illness or its significance. Anger is often manifested by antagonistic behaviors that may be directed at family, staff, or medical regimen.

▶ ***Test-taking Tip:*** *Focusing on the client's behaviors of "frequently calling" and "questions" will direct you to option 4.*

Content Area: Adult Health; *Category of Health Alteration:* Cardiac Management; *Integrated Processes:* Nursing Process Evaluation; *Client Need:* Psychosocial Integrity/Coping Mechanisms; *Cognitive Level:* Analysis

Reference: Lewis, S., Heitkemper, M., Dirksen, S., O'Brien, P., & Bucher, L. (2007). *Medical-Surgical Nursing: Assessment and Management of Clinical Problems* (7th ed., p. 814). St. Louis, MO: Mosby.

32. ANSWER: 1

Initial fluid therapy is directed toward expansion of the intravascular and extravascular volume and restoration of renal profusion. Therefore, an isotonic solution of 0.9% sodium chloride is needed for the first hour. The usual rate is 10 to 20 mL/kg. This fluid is then continued at 1.5 times the 24-hour maintenance rate, or replaced with 0.45% sodium chloride at the same rate. Potassium is not added to the IV fluids until renal function is assured and then 20 to 40 mEq potassium is added. D5W, D10W, and Ringer's lactate are not isotonic solutions.

▶ ***Test-taking Tip:*** *Focus on eliminating the solutions with glucose because the child is already hyperglycemic. Of the remaining options, focus on whether or not potassium should be administered in the early phases of hyperglycemic crisis.*

Content Area: Child Health; *Category of Health Alteration:* Endocrine Management; *Integrated Processes:* Nursing Process Planning; *Client Need:* Physiological Integrity/Pharmacological and Parenteral Therapies/Parenteral/Intravenous Therapies; *Cognitive Level:* Analysis

References: Ball, J., & Bindler, R. (2006). *Child Health Nursing: Partnering with Children & Families* (pp. 1263–1285). Upper Saddle River, NJ: Pearson Education; Hockenberry, M., & Wilson, D. (2007). *Wong's Nursing Care of Infants and Children* (8th ed., pp. 1705–1711). St. Louis, MO: Mosby.

EBP Reference: Wolfsdorf, J., Glaser, N., & Sperling, M. (2006). Diabetic ketoacidosis in infants, children, and adolescents: a consensus statement from the American Diabetes Association. *Diabetes Care,* 29(5), 1150.

33. ANSWER: 2, 3, 4, 5

Unless contraindicated, the side-lying position will prevent aspiration of secretions. Turning also will mobilize secretions. Analgesics are administered IV in the PACU for a rapid onset in controlling pain. Some clients emerge from anesthesia in an agitated state for a short period of time. This is termed emergence delirium. Amnesiac anesthesia causes a loss of memory. Repeat explanations such as "Mr. Brown, surgery is over; you are in the recovery room." The client would not be alert enough to be able to comprehend using the incentive spirometer and would not be ready to sit up to use it.

➧ ***Test-taking Tip:*** *Visualize a client recovering from anesthesia and use the ABCs (airway, breathing, circulation) and Maslow's Hierarchy of Needs theory to assist in identifying appropriate interventions.*

Content Area: Adult Health; *Category of Health Alteration:* Perioperative Management; *Integrated Processes:* Nursing Process Implementation; *Client Need:* Physiological Integrity/Reduction of Risk Potential/Potential for Complications from Surgical Procedures and Health Alterations; *Cognitive Level:* Application

Reference: Lewis, S., Heitkemper, M., Dirksen, S., O'Brien, P., & Bucher, L. (2007). *Medical-Surgical Nursing: Assessment and Management of Clinical Problems* (7th ed., pp. 361–371, 381). St. Louis, MO: Mosby.

EBP Reference: Institute for Clinical Systems Improvement. (2008). Assessment and management of acute pain. Available at: www.guidelines.gov/summary/summary.aspx?doc_id=12302&nbr=6371

34. ANSWER: 3

Oral erythema, inflammation, ulceration, pain, and dysguesia (taste changes) commonly occur with oral mucositis. Gingivitis, plaque, halitosis (bad breath), candidiasis, cheilitis (lip inflammation), caries (dental cavities), and leukoplakia (white oral lesions) are not signs or symptoms of mucositis.

➧ ***Test-taking Tip:*** *Note the keywords "oral mucositis" and focus on conditions associated with the mouth. Options 1, 2, and 4 are not associated with mucositis and can be eliminated.*

Content Area: Adult Health; *Category of Health Alteration:* Hematological and Oncological Management; *Integrated Processes:* Nursing Process Assessment; *Client Need:* Physiological Integrity/Reduction of Risk Potential/Potential for Complications of Diagnostic Tests/Treatments/Procedures; *Cognitive Level:* Analysis

Reference: Langhorne, M., Fulton, J., & Otto, S. (2007). *Oncology Nursing* (5th ed., p. 505). St. Louis, MO: Mosby.

EBP Reference: Keefe, D., Schubert, M., Elting, L., Sonis, S., Epstein, J., et al. (2007). Updated clinical practice guidelines for the prevention and treatment of mucositis. *Cancer,* 109(5), 820–831. Available at: www.guidelines.gov/summary/summary.aspx?doc_id=12094&nbr=006223&string=mucositis

35. ANSWER: 3

If the client experiences symptoms of a transfusion reaction, the transfusion should be stopped immediately. The line should be kept open for emergency medications, but saline should not be administered through the existing blood tubing because the client will receive the blood remaining in the tubing. Vital signs are assessed before the transfusion begins, 15 minutes after it is started, and then hourly until the transfusion is completed. Upon completion, the vital signs are taken and then repeated an hour later. PRBCs should infuse in 4 hours or less to avoid the risk of septicemia. Special tubing with a filter is used to administer blood.

➧ ***Test-taking Tip:*** *Carefully read each of the options. Apply knowledge of blood administration to answer this question.*

Content Area: Adult Health; *Category of Health Alteration:* Hematological and Oncological Management; *Integrated Processes:* Nursing Process Implementation; *Client Need:* Safe and Effective Care Environment/Safety and Infection Control/Injury Prevention; Physiological Integrity/Pharmacological and Parenteral Therapies/Blood and Blood Products; *Cognitive Level:* Application

Reference: Ignatavicius, D., & Workman, M. (2006). *Medical-Surgical Nursing: Critical Thinking for Collaborative Care* (5th ed., pp. 913–915). St. Louis, MO: Saunders/Elsevier.

EBP Reference: Finnish Medical Society Duodecim. (2008). Blood transfusion: indications and administration. In: *EBM Guidelines. Evidence-Based Medicine.* Helsinki, Finland: Wiley Interscience. John Wiley & Sons. Available at: http://www.guidelines.gov/summary/summary.aspx?doc_id=12787&nbr=006589&string=Blood+AND+transfusion

36. ANSWER: 3

The scope of practice for ancillary staff does not include the management of client care. Assessing the client's skin is not a responsibility that the RN can delegate to the ancillary staff. Feeding, reinforcement, and securing supplies are activities that may be assumed by ancillary staff as deemed appropriate by the RN.

➧ ***Test-taking Tip:*** *The key phrase "needs further education" indicates this is a false-response item. Select the option that indicates incorrect delegation, which includes assessment, planning, evaluation, or teaching; these are responsibilities that the RN cannot delegate.*

Content Area: Management of Care; *Category of Health Alteration:* Prioritization and Delegation; *Integrated Processes:* Nursing Process Planning; *Client Need:* Safe and Effective Care Environment/Management of Care/Delegation; *Cognitive Level:* Application.

References: Berman, A., Snyder, S., Kozier, B., & Erb, G. (2008). *Kozier & Erb's Fundamentals of Nursing: Concepts, Process, and Practice* (8th ed., pp. 518–520). Upper Saddle River, NJ: Pearson Education; Potter, P., & Perry, A. (2009). *Fundamentals of Nursing* (7th ed., pp. 287, 309–311). St. Louis, MO: Mosby.

37. ANSWER: 3

Tricyclic antidepressants block acetylcholine receptors, which cause anticholinergic effects, including dry mouth, blurred vision, constipation, and urinary retention. Agranulocytosis is a rare and serious side effect of traditional antipsychotic medications that can be fatal. Unintentional tremor and diarrhea are common side effects with selective serotonin reuptake inhibitors (SSRIs), a different class of antidepressant medication.

➧ ***Test-taking Tip:*** *The key word is "common." Use the process of elimination and review side effects related to tricyclic antidepressants.*

Content Area: Mental Health; *Category of Health Alteration:* Anxiety and Mood Disorders; *Integrated Processes:* Teaching and Learning; *Client Need:* Safe and Effective Care Environment/Management of Care/Ethical Practice; *Cognitive Level:* Analysis

Reference: Varcarolis, E., Carson, V., & Shoemaker, N. (2006). *Foundations of Psychiatric Mental Health Nursing* (5th ed., pp. 343, 348). St. Louis, MO: Saunders/Elsevier.

38. ANSWER: 4

Bleeding can occur with low platelet levels (usually less than 50,000/mm^3 or 50 K/μL). Blurred vision, headache, or mental status changes can be signs of intracranial bleeding. Because the client is prone to bleeding, dental flossing and aspirin are contraindicated. A client should be ambulated with assistance.

➧ ***Test-taking Tip:*** *Apply knowledge of bleeding precautions to select the correct answer. If uncertain, select the option that uses the first step of the nursing process.*

Content Area: Adult Health; *Category of Health Alteration:* Hematological and Oncological Management; *Integrated Processes:* Nursing Process Implementation; *Client Need:* Physiological Integrity/Reduction of Risk Potential/System Specific Assessments; *Cognitive Level:* Application

Reference: Smeltzer, S., Bare, B., Hinkle, J., & Cheever, K. (2008). *Brunner & Suddarth's Textbook of Medical-Surgical Nursing* (11th ed., pp. 1076, 1087). Philadelphia: Lippincott Williams & Wilkins.

39. ANSWER: 1, 2, 4, 5

The health-care provider should be notified; an echocardiogram may be ordered, and the client should be assessed by a physician. The clamp should be closed to prevent additional air from entering the line. Attaching a syringe and aspirating until blood returns may prevent air in the line from entering the central circulation. The line should be flushed with 0.9% NaCl and then heparin, if ordered, to maintain patency of the central line and prevent it from clotting. The client should be placed the client on the left side, not the right side, with the feet higher than the head. This position traps air in the right atrium, which can then be removed directly by intracardiac aspiration if necessary.

➧ ***Test-taking Tip:*** *Visualize each option, recalling that the goals are to prevent air from entering the central circulation or to trap the air in the right atrium. Remember that air rises so the client should be positioned on the left side.*

Content Area: Fundamentals; *Category of Health Alteration:* Medication Administration; *Integrated Processes:* Nursing Process Implementation; *Client Need:* Physiological Integrity/Pharmacological and Parenteral Therapies/Central Venous Access Devices; *Cognitive Level:* Application

References: Craven, R., & Hirnle, C. (2007). *Fundamentals of Nursing: Human Health and Function* (5th ed., pp. 624, 626–627). Philadelphia: Lippincott Williams & Wilkins; Ingram, P. (2006). The safe removal of central venous catheters. *Nursing Standard*, 20(49), 42–46.

EBP Reference: Bishop L., Dougherty L., Bodenham, A., Mansi, J., Crowe, P., et al. (2007). Guidelines on the insertion and management of central venous access devices in adults. *International Journal of Laboratory Hematology*, 29(4), 261–278. Available at: www.guideline.gov/summary/summary.aspx?view_id=1&doc_id=11992

40. ANSWER: 3

Complete heart block is a life-threatening dysrhythmia because, if untreated, it results in reduced cardiac output and subsequent ischemia. The atrial rate is usually sinus, 60 to 100 bpm. If the AV node initiates an impulse, the ventricular rate is 40 to 60 bpm; if the His Purkinje system initiates an impulse, it is 20 to 40 bpm. The QRS is widened if the impulse is initiated below the bundle of His. The PRI is variable and there is no relationship between the P waves and the QRS complexes. Option 1 is sinus tachycardia. A normal PRI = 0.12 to 0.20 secs; QRS = 0.06 to 0.10 secs; QT is rate dependent; and ventricular rate is 60 to 100 bpm. A rate greater than 100 bpm is tachycardia. Option 2 is atrial fibrillation, and option 4 is sinus bradycardia with a first-degree AV block (PRI is greater than 0.20 secs).

➧ ***Test-taking Tip:*** *Read each option carefully. If unsure of normal waveform measurements, eliminate options 1 and 4 because these have waveforms that are measurable. Of options 2 and 3, note that option 3 has more abnormal waveforms than option 2.*

Content Area: Adult Health; *Category of Health Alteration:* Cardiac Management; *Integrated Processes:* Nursing Process Analysis; *Client Need:* Physiological Integrity/Physiological Adaptation/Medical Emergencies; *Cognitive Level:* Analysis

Reference: Lewis, S., Heitkemper, M., Dirksen, S., O'Brien, P., & Bucher, L. (2007). *Medical-Surgical Nursing: Assessment and Management of Clinical Problems* (7th ed., pp. 847–854). St. Louis, MO: Mosby.

EBP Reference: Institute for Clinical Systems Improvement. (2008). Diagnosis and treatment of chest pain and acute coronary syndrome. Available at: http://www.guidelines.gov/summary/summary.aspx?doc_id=13480&nbr=6889

41. ANSWER: 3

A client experiencing a manic episode may speak whatever comes to mind and rapidly change topics (flight of ideas). Social withdrawal is a symptom of a major depressive episode. Somatic-type delusions is associated with a major depressive episode with psychosis. Trembling or shaking is more likely to be observed in a client with panic disorder.

➧ ***Test-taking Tip:*** *"Mental status" and "manic episode" are the key words in the stem. Use the process of elimination and review symptoms of manic episodes.*

Content Area: Mental Health; *Category of Health Alteration:* Anxiety and Mood Disorders; *Integrated Processes:* Nursing Process Assessment; *Client Need:* Psychosocial Integrity/Mental Health Concepts; *Cognitive Level:* Analysis

Reference: Townsend, M. (2008). *Essentials of Psychiatric Mental Health Nursing* (4th ed., p. 356). Philadelphia: F. A. Davis.

42. ANSWER: 2

Contaminated supplies should never be used for a sterile procedure. A person who sees a sterile object become contaminated must correct or report the situation. The hair in the sterile field contaminates the sterile field. The hair is not sterile. The nurse has an ethical and legal responsibility to protect the client from injury. Thus, allowing the physician to decide is a breach of duty to the client. An antiseptic agent is one that inhibits the growth of some microorganisms, but does not render an object sterile.

➧ ***Test-taking Tip:*** *Implement principles of sterile technique when answering this question.*

Content Area: Adult Health; *Category of Health Alteration:* Safety, Disaster Preparedness, and Infection Control; *Integrated Processes:* Nursing Process Implementation; *Client Need:* Safe and Effective Care Environment/Safety and Infection Control/Surgical Asepsis; Safe and Effective Care Environment/Management of Care/Legal Rights and Responsibilities; *Cognitive Level:* Application

Reference: Berman, A., Snyder, S., Kozier, B., & Erb, G. (2008). *Kozier & Erb's Fundamentals of Nursing: Concepts, Process, and Practice* (8th ed., pp. 687–688). Upper Saddle River, NJ: Pearson Education.

43. ANSWER: 2

A specialty clinic with experience in management of clients with newly diagnosed HIV will provide the most support for the type of concerns expressed by the client. Referral to the physician may not address the psychosocial needs of the client, nor will disclosure to the family. The local public health department may be able to provide resources; however, it is likely the specialty clinic is better prepared to deal with the holistic needs of the client.

➧ ***Test-taking Tip:*** *Key word is "most client support." Focus on what each option can provide in fulfilling client needs according to Maslow's Hierarchy of Needs theory, including the need for love and belonging.*

Content Area: Management of Care; *Category of Health Alteration:* Leadership and Management; *Integrated Processes:* Nursing Process Implementation; *Client Need:* Safe and Effective Care Environment/Management of Care/Referrals; *Cognitive Level:* Application

Reference: Harkreader, H., Hogan, M., & Thobaben, M. (2007). *Fundamentals of Nursing* (3rd ed., pp. 1146–1149). St. Louis, MO: Saunders/Elsevier.

44. **ANSWER: 2**

If the nurse detects a soft, boggy uterine fundus, it should be massaged immediately until it is firm. Postpartum hemorrhage is a leading cause of maternal morbidity and mortality in the United States and uterine atony is the most common cause of postpartum hemorrhage. Since postpartum hemorrhage can be life-threatening, the nurse should make prevention of this problem a priority. Providing pain control with ice and medication are also important and should be addressed after the fundus is firm. Providing perineal care would be the lowest priority.

➧ ***Test-taking Tip:*** *Apply Maslow's Hierarchy of Needs theory and address the potentially life-threatening concern first.*

Content Area: Childbearing Families; *Category of Health Alteration:* Postpartum Management; *Integrated Processes:* Nursing Process Implementation; *Client Need:* Safe and Effective Care Environment/ Management of Care/Establishing Priorities; *Cognitive Level:* Analysis

References: Davidson, M., London, M., & Ladewig, P. (2008). *Olds' Maternal-Newborn Nursing & Women's Health Across the Lifespan* (8th ed., p. 1164). Upper Saddle River, NJ: Prentice Hall Health; Wong, D., Hockenberry, M., Wilson, D., Perry, S., & Lowdermilk, D. (2006). *Maternal Child Nursing Care* (3rd ed., p. 659). Philadelphia: Lippincott Williams & Wilkins.

45. **ANSWER: 3**

Reassuring the child that pubertal changes are normal, and that the child's friends will eventually develop the same characteristics, should be helpful in facilitating a positive body image. The other statements only reinforce to the child that there are differences.

➧ ***Test-taking Tip:*** *Focus on the issue: positive body image development. Use the process of elimination to eliminate options 1 and 2 because these do not focus on the child's body changes. Eliminate option 4 because the focus is on looking older and not the body changes.*

Content Area: Child Health; *Category of Health Alteration:* Endocrine Management; *Integrated Processes:* Communication and Documentation; *Client Need:* Psychosocial Integrity/Support Systems; *Cognitive Level:* Application

References: Ball, J., & Bindler, R. (2006). *Child Health Nursing: Partnering with Children & Families* (pp. 1248–1250). Upper Saddle River, NJ: Pearson Education; Hockenberry, M., & Wilson, D. (2007). *Wong's Nursing Care of Infants and Children* (8th ed., p. 722). St. Louis, MO: Mosby; McCance, K., & Huether, S. (2006). *Pathophysiology: The Biologic Basis for Disease in Adults and Children* (5th ed., p. 725). St. Louis, MO: Mosby.

46. **ANSWER: 1**

When a client is near death, they may seem to be withdrawn from the physical environment, maintaining the ability to hear while not able to respond. The nurse should touch the client gently (not minimally) and converse as if the client is alert, using a soft voice. Allowing for privacy and encouraging talking, reassuring, and verbalizing feelings are important elements of saying goodbye.

➧ ***Test-taking Tip:*** *The key word in the stem is "uncaring." This is a false-response question so the answer is the action that the nurse should not do when caring for the client and family.*

Content Area: Child Health; *Category of Health Alteration:* Cardiovascular Management; *Integrated Processes:* Caring; *Client Need:* Psychosocial Integrity/End-of-Life Care; *Cognitive Level:* Application

Reference: Lewis, S., Heitkemper, M., Dirkson, S., O'Brien, P., & Bucher, L. (2007). *Medical-Surgical Nursing: Assessment and Management of Clinical Problems* (7th ed., p. 160). St. Louis, MO: Mosby.

47. **ANSWER: 3**

Maintaining an airtight seal is often a problem during negative-pressure wound therapy. The negative pressure removes drainage of fluid and prevents saturation of dressings. Air bubbles are not a problem with the negative-pressure wound therapy.

➧ ***Test-taking Tip:*** *Focus on the key words of "negative-pressure wound therapy." Use association to select an option that would suggest inadequate pressure.*

Content Area: Adult Health; *Category of Health Alteration:* Integument & Other Health Problems; *Integrated Processes:* Nursing Process Planning; *Client Need:* Safe and Effective Care Environment/ Safety and Infection Control/Safe Use of Equipment; *Cognitive Level:* Analysis

Reference: Lewis, S., Heitkemper, M., Dirksen, S., O'Brien, P., & Bucher, L. (2007). *Medical-Surgical Nursing: Assessment and Management of Clinical Problems* (7th ed., p. 205). St. Louis, MO: Mosby.

EBP Reference: Ubbink, D., Westerbos, S., Evans, D., Land, L., & Vermeulen, H. (2008). Topical negative pressure for treating chronic wounds. *Cochrane Database of Systematic Reviews, 3*. Available at: www.cochrane.org/reviews/en/ab001898.html

48. **ANSWER: 2**

The abbreviation MS is on the "do not use" list of abbreviations by The Joint Commission (formerly the Joint Commission on Accreditation of Healthcare Organizations [JCAHO]). It could be interpreted as morphine sulfate or magnesium sulfate. Initiating all orders, preparing and administering MS, or verifying the abbreviations MS with another nurse are unsafe actions.

➧ ***Test-taking Tip:*** *Carefully read each prescribed order, noting that all would be appropriate for a client in sickle cell crisis except MS. MS could be either morphine sulfate (which is appropriate) or magnesium sulfate (which would be inappropriate).*

Content Area: Adult Health; *Category of Health Alteration:* Hematological and Oncological Management; *Integrated Processes:* Nursing Process Analysis; *Client Need:* Physiological Integrity/ Pharmacological and Parenteral Therapies/Medication Administration; *Cognitive Level:* Analysis

Reference: Smeltzer, S., Bare, B., Hinkle, J., & Cheever, K. (2008). *Brunner & Suddarth's Textbook of Medical-Surgical Nursing* (11th ed., pp. 1056–1057). Philadelphia: Lippincott Williams & Wilkins.

EBP Reference: The Joint Commission. (2005). *Official "do not use" list.* Available at: www.jointcommission.org/NR/rdonlyres/2329F8F5-6EC5-4E21-B932-54B2B7D53F00/0/06_dnu_list.pdf

49. **ANSWER: 3**

The plan of care for a client with pneumonia should provide both curative and supportive measures, including increased fluid intake. Antipyretics, analgesics, and oxygen therapy are also included in the therapeutic regimen. The client should get lots of rest with restricted activity levels, especially in the acute phase of the illness. The situation does not state whether or not the source of the infection is viral or bacterial.

➧ ***Test-taking Tip:*** *Do not assume information if it is not given. In this case, the stem does not explicitly say that the infection is viral or bacterial, so the pharmacological therapy option should be eliminated.*

Content Area: Adult Health; *Category of Health Alteration:* Respiratory Management; *Integrated Processes:* Nursing Process Evaluation; *Client Need:* Safe and Effective Care Environment/ Management of Care/Collaboration with Interdisciplinary Team; *Cognitive Level:* Analysis

References: Lewis, S., Heitkemper, M., Dirksen, S., O'Brien, P., & Bucher, L. (2007). *Medical-Surgical Nursing: Assessment and Management of Clinical Problems* (7th ed., pp. 566–567). St. Louis, MO: Mosby; Doenges, M., Moorhouse, M., & Murr, A. (2006). *Nursing Care Plans: Guidelines for Individualizing Client Care Across the Life Span.* (7th ed., pp. 128–140). Philadelphia: F. A. Davis.

50. ANSWER: 4

The systolic blood pressure of 112 is at 25% of the client's age and the diastolic of 72 is at 10%. No intervention is necessary. The client should be rescreened periodically as per the guidelines set by age.

Test-taking Tip: Note that options 1, 2, and 3 are related to treating for hypertension, whereas option 4 is the only option that considers the blood pressure reading a normal finding.

Content Area: Child Health; *Category of Health Alteration:* Cardiovascular Management; *Integrated Processes:* Nursing Process Implementation; *Client Need:* Physiological Integrity/Reduction of Risk Potential/Vital Signs; *Cognitive Level:* Application

Reference: Hockenberry, M., & Wilson, D. (2007). *Wong's Nursing Care of Infants and Children* (8th ed., Appendix). St. Louis, MO: Mosby.

51. ANSWER: 2

The client must first identify the stressors before being able to act on controlling the anger they create in him or her. The stressors must first be identified before a plan or coping skills can be addressed.

Test-taking Tip: Note the key words "initial." Focus on the use of the nursing process. An assessment should be completed prior to planning.

Content Area: Mental Health; *Category of Health Alteration:* Crisis, Violence, Eating, and Sleep Disorders; *Integrated Processes:* Nursing Process Evaluation; *Client Need:* Psychosocial Integrity/Behavioral Interventions; *Cognitive Level:* Analysis

Reference: Varcarolis, E., Carson, V., & Shoemaker, N. (2006). *Foundations of Psychiatric Mental Health Nursing: A Clinical Approach* (5th ed., p. 498). St. Louis, MO: Saunders/Elsevier.

52. ANSWER: 2

Every alternative intervention should be attempted to remove a client from seclusion as soon as possible, such as negotiating or diversion. Negative psychological effects of seclusion should be minimized by reducing the time in seclusion. Standing orders may never be used for seclusion or restraints. Clients demonstrating harm to themselves or others may legally be restrained or secluded. Clients in seclusion are at risk of death due to their uncontrollable behavior. Minimum monitoring must be every 15 minutes.

Test-taking Tip: Focus on what the question is asking. You are asked to find which answer is "true" or "correct" regarding a client in seclusion.

Content Area: Management of Care; *Category of Health Alteration:* Ethical, Legal, and Safety Issues in Nursing; *Integrated Processes:* Nursing Process Analysis; *Client Need:* Safe and Effective Care Environment/Safety and Infection Control/Use of Restraints/Safety Devices; *Cognitive Level:* Analysis

Reference: Department of Health and Human Services, Centers for Medicare & Medicaid Services. (2006). *Medicare and Medicaid programs; Hospital conditions of participation: patients' rights; final rule.* DHHS Publication 42 CFR Part 482. Baltimore, MD. Author. Available at: www.cms.hhs.gov/CertificationandCompliance/Downloads/PatientsRights.pdf

53. ANSWER: 1, 2, 3, 4

Otoscope tips are available in different sizes, and using the smallest tip decreases the chance for injury. Pulling the pinna down and back properly aligns the ear canal for children under 2 years old. Noting the color of the tympanic membrane is important in an ear assessment. Pulling the pinna up and back should be done for children 2 years and older and adults. Resting the otoscope on a hand rather than the child's head allows the otoscope to move with the child's movement so the tympanic membrane will not be injured.

Test-taking Tip: Note the child's age. First review options that are similar (2 and 5; 4 and 6), eliminate one of each of these, and then review the other options. Assessing the ear of a child up to 2 years of age is a different procedure from that of an adult.

Content Area: Child Health; *Category of Health Alteration:* Integumentary Management and Other Health Alterations; *Integrated Processes:* Nursing Process Assessment; *Client Need:* Health Promotion and Maintenance/Techniques of Physical Assessment; *Cognitive Level:* Application

Reference: Pillitteri, A. (2007). *Maternal & Child Health Nursing: Care of the Childbearing & Childrearing Family* (5th ed., pp. 1000–1001). Philadelphia: Lippincott Williams & Wilkins.

54. ANSWER: 1

The client is in the "why me" stage of acceptance. Clarifying encourages communication and allows the client to express feelings and move toward acceptance. Telling the client that smoking is not the only cause of bladder cancer ignores the client's feelings and blocks communication. Telling a client his or her feelings are understood belittles the client's feelings and blocks communication. Telling the client that he or she is angry and doesn't mean to wish cancer on another is making a conclusion without sufficient data. This is also a judgmental response, which blocks therapeutic communication.

Test-taking Tip: Note the key word "best." Eliminate responses that do not address the client's concerns and promote therapeutic communication.

Content Area: Adult Health; *Category of Health Alteration:* Renal and Urinary Management; *Integrated Processes:* Communication and Documentation; Caring; *Client Need:* Psychosocial Integrity/Therapeutic Communications; *Cognitive Level:* Analysis

Reference: Berman, A., Snyder, S., Kozier, B., & Erb, G. (2008). *Kozier & Erb's Fundamentals of Nursing: Concepts, Process, and Practice* (8th ed., pp. 469–473). Upper Saddle River, NJ: Pearson Education.

55. ANSWER: 1

For able clients, maintaining a pain diary is an effective way to monitor pain control. The client needs to know how to determine when pain is no longer adequately controlled and the action to take. Dietary practices to avoid constipation and using relaxation techniques are appropriate interventions but do not ensure pain control. Opioid medications for palliative pain control should be administered around the clock.

Test-taking Tip: Read the scenario in the stem carefully. The words "best ensures" identifies the need to select the option that is the priority intervention for pain control. Eliminate an option that incorrectly describes the use of opioid medications for pain control.

Content Area: Mental Health; Fundamentals; *Category of Health Alteration:* End-of-Life Care; *Integrated Processes:* Nursing Process Intervention; *Client Need:* Physiological Integrity/Pharmacological and Parenteral Therapies/Pharmacological Pain Management; *Cognitive Level:* Analysis

Reference: Smeltzer, S., Bare, B., Hinkle, J., & Cheever, K. (2008). *Brunner & Suddarth's Textbook of Medical-Surgical Nursing* (11th ed., pp. 464–465). Philadelphia: Lippincott Williams & Wilkins.

EBP Reference: Aubin, M., Vezina, L., Parent, R., Fillion, L., Allard, P., et al. (2006). Impact of an educational program on pain management in patients with cancer living at home. *Oncology Nursing Forum,* 33(6), 1183–1188.

56. ANSWER: 180

To determine the 24-hour grams of carbohydrate intake, add the CHO choices (12 total CHO choices). Multiply the 12 CHO choices and the 15 grams of carbohydrate per choice to obtain the total of 180 grams of carbohydrates.

➧ **Test-taking Tip:** *Read the question carefully. The question is asking for grams of carbohydrates and not carbohydrate choices. This question requires a calculation.*

Content Area: Adult Health; *Category of Health Alteration:* Nutrition; *Integrated Processes:* Nursing Process Evaluation; *Client Need:* Physiological Integrity/Basic Care and Comfort/Nutrition and Oral Hydration; *Cognitive Level:* Analysis

Reference: Whitney, E., DeBruyne, L., Pinna, K., & Rolfes, S. (2007). *Nutrition for Health and Health Care* (3rd ed., p. 523). Belmont, CA: Thomson Learning.

57. ANSWER: 3

The client's serum lipid level and liver function tests are elevated. A reduced dose is warranted with hepatic impairment because mirtazapine is metabolized in the liver. The dose should not be administered without first consulting with the psychiatrist. An increased dose will cause toxic effects because the current dose cannot be metabolized when the liver is impaired. The psychiatrist ordering the medication should be consulted and has the expertise in psychiatric conditions, whereas a general practitioner does not.

➧ **Test-taking Tip:** *Focus on the two options that are opposite first and eliminate one of these. Then, examine the other options.*

Content Area: Mental Health; *Category of Health Alteration:* Personality and Other Mental Health Disorders; *Integrated Processes:* Nursing Process Evaluation; *Client Need:* Physiological Integrity/Pharmacological and Parenteral Therapies/Adverse Effects/Contraindications/Interactions; *Cognitive Level:* Analysis

Reference: Wilson, B., Shannon, M., Shields, K., & Stang, C. (2008). *Prentice Hall Nurse's Drug Guide 2008* (pp. 1007–1008). Upper Saddle River, NJ: Pearson Education.

EBP Reference: Bienenfeld, D. (2008). Personality disorders. *E-Medicine from WebMD.* Available at: www.emedicine.com/med/TOPIC3472.HTM#Medication

58. ANSWER: 0.625

Use the formula for calculating medication dosages. 0.625 mL is the usual dose for ondansetron (Anzemet®) for treating postoperative nausea.
Ratio-Proportion Formula:
20 mg : 1 mL :: 12.5 mg : X mL
Multiply the outside and inside values and solve for X.
20 X = 12.5
X = 0.625

➧ **Test-taking Tip:** *Focus on the information in the question and use the on-screen calculator. Verify your response, especially if it seems like an unusual amount.*

Content Area: Adult Health; *Category of Health Alteration:* Perioperative Management; *Integrated Processes:* Nursing Process Implementation; *Client Need:* Physiological Integrity/Pharmacological and Parenteral Therapies/Dosage Calculation; *Cognitive Level:* Analysis

Reference: Pickar, G. (2007). *Dosage Calculations: A Ratio-Proportion Approach* (2nd ed., pp. 46, 344). Clifton Park, NY: Thomson Delmar Learning.

59. ANSWER: 2

Vaccination with TIV is recommended for persons who are at increased risk for severe complications from influenza, such as those with a chronic illness. TIV should not be administered to persons known to have anaphylactic hypersensitivity to eggs or to other components of the influenza vaccine. LAIV is used in vaccinating healthy, nonpregnant persons aged 5 to 49 years. The influenza vaccine is repeated annually because it is developed from representative influenza viruses anticipated to circulate in the United States during that year's influenza season.

➧ **Test-taking Tip:** *Read each option carefully. Eliminate options that include administering live, attenuated vaccines because these are only administered to healthy individuals.*

Content Area: Adult Health; *Category of Health Alteration:* Cardiac Management; *Integrated Processes:* Nursing Process Implementation; *Client Need:* Health Promotion and Maintenance/Health Promotion and Disease Prevention; Physiological Integrity/Pharmacological and Parenteral Therapies/Medication Administration; *Cognitive Level:* Analysis

EBP Reference: Fiore, A., Shay, D., Broder, K., Iskander, J., Uyeki, T., et al. (2008). Prevention and control of influenza. Recommendations of the Advisory Committee on Immunization Practices (ACIP) 2008, *MMWR Recommendations and Reports*, 57(RR07);1–60. Available at: www.cdc.gov/mmwr/preview/mmwrhtml/rr5707a1.htm

60. ANSWER: 3

Flomax® is a alpha-adrenergic receptor blocker, which relaxes the smooth muscle in the prostate. This ultimately facilitates urinary flow through the urethra. Alpha-adrenergic blockers are recommended as first-line medical therapy for clients with bothersome symptoms. Tamsulosin does not actually decrease the size of the prostate, and it does not have anti-inflammatory actions. Specific gravity of the urine will not be altered by tamsulosin.

➧ **Test-taking Tip:** *Eliminate option 4 because decreasing specific gravity would not be a treatment for BPH. Note the similarities in options 1, 2, and 4 (reduce, decrease, and decrease, respectively) and that option 3 is different.*

Content Area: Adult Health; *Category of Health Alteration:* Reproductive Management; *Integrated Processes:* Teaching and Learning; *Client Need:* Physiological Integrity/Pharmacological and Parenteral Therapies/Expected Actions or Outcomes; *Cognitive Level:* Application

Reference: Lewis, S., Heitkemper, M., Dirksen, S., O'Brien, P., & Bucher, L. (2007). *Medical-Surgical Nursing: Assessment and Management of Clinical Problems* (7th ed., p. 1417). St. Louis, MO: Mosby.

EBP Reference: Finnish Medical Society Duodecim. (2008). Benign prostatic hyperplasia. In: *EBM Guidelines. Evidence-Based Medicine.* Helsinki, Finland. Available at: www.guidelines.gov/summary/summary.aspx?doc_id=13191&nbr=006739&string=prostatic+AND+hypertrophy

61. ANSWER: 3

Skin-to-skin contact after birth leads to an eightfold increase in spontaneous nursing and may be a critical component in breastfeeding success. For the first hour after birth, the infant is usually active, alert, and ready to breastfeed. Thirty minutes after birth, newborn activity begins to decrease, and the newborn enters a period of deep sleep. Allowing the mother to rest for 1 to 2 hours immediately after delivery would bypass the initial period of newborn activity. Most women appreciate having an experienced nurse with them for a first feeding to offer support and advice. Leaving the mother and infant alone during the first feeding does not help to promote successful breastfeeding. Supplemental bottle-feedings for the breastfeeding infant are not recommended for normal, healthy newborns as they may lead to nipple confusion and decrease infant stimulation of the mother's breast.

▶ ***Test-taking Tip:*** *Read each option carefully. Select an option that will also promote infant bonding.*

Content Area: Childbearing Families; *Category of Health Alteration:* Neonatal and High-Risk Neonatal Management; *Integrated Processes:* Nursing Process Planning; *Client Need:* Physiological Integrity/Basic Care and Comfort/Nutrition and Oral Hydration; *Cognitive Level:* Application

References: Davidson, M., London, M., & Ladewig, P. (2008). *Olds' Maternal-Newborn Nursing & Women's Health Across the Lifespan.* (8th ed., pp. 813, 904, 913). Upper Saddle River, NJ: Prentice Hall Health; Pillitteri, A. (2007). *Maternal & Child Health Nursing: Care of the Childbearing & Childrearing Family* (5th ed., p. 730). Philadelphia: Lippincott Williams & Wilkins.

EBP Reference: Moore E.R., Anderson G.C., & Bergman N. (2007). Early skin-to-skin contact for mothers and their healthy newborn infants. *Cochrane Database of Systematic Reviews 2007*, 3, Article no. CD003519. Available at: www.cochrane.org/reviews/en/ab003519.html

62. ANSWER: 4

The diagram shows an external fixation device that is placed percutaneously after the fracture has been reduced. A potential complication, pin-tract infection, necessitates daily inspection of the skin at the pin sites for redness and drainage. An internal fixation involves the use of metal pins, screws, rods, or plates to immobilize the fracture, which are internal and inserted during open surgery. Buck's traction is applied to the skin and immobilizes the lower extremity after a hip fracture. A brace cast is a patellar weight-bearing cast used with midshaft or distal fracture of the femur.

▶ ***Test-taking Tip:*** *Study the diagram carefully. Evaluate each option and compare the description to the diagram. Use the process of elimination to rule out incorrect options.*

Content Area: Fundamentals; *Category of Health Alteration:* Basic Care and Comfort; *Integrated Processes:* Nursing Process Analysis; *Client Need:* Physiological Integrity/Basic Care and Comfort/Mobility/Immobility; *Cognitive Level:* Analysis

Reference: Ignatavicius, D., & Workman, M. (2006). *Medical-Surgical Nursing: Critical Thinking for Collaborative Care* (5th ed., p. 1202). St. Louis, MO: Saunders/Elsevier.

63. ANSWER: 3, 5, 2, 6, 7, 1, 4

The nurse should first assess the IV insertion site for signs of infiltration or phlebitis. Then the nurse should select the port closest to the client and cleanse the port and allow it to dry. The nurse should use a 10-mL syringe for administering medications through a central venous access because too much pressure is exerted with smaller syringes, which can damage the catheter. After connecting the syringe, the nurse occludes the IV line, pulls back the plunger to check for a blood return, releases the tubing, and injects the medication. The nurse removes the syringe and rechecks the infusion rate. This is the correct procedure for administering an intravenous medication through an existing IV line.

▶ ***Test-taking Tip:*** *Use visualization to focus on the data in the question and then visualize the remaining steps of the procedure. Prioritizing is placing items in the correct sequence.*

Content Area: Management of Care; *Category of Health Alteration:* Prioritization and Delegation; *Integrated Processes:* Nursing Process Implementation; *Client Need:* Physiological Integrity/Pharmacological and Parenteral Therapies/Central Venous Access Devices; *Cognitive Level:* Application

Reference: Potter, P., & Perry, A. (2009). *Fundamentals of Nursing* (7th ed., p. 760). St. Louis, MO: Mosby.

EBP Reference: Bishop, L., Dougherty, L., Bodenham, A., Mansi, J., Crowe, P., et al., (2007). Guidelines on the insertion and management of central venous access devices in adults. *International Journal of Laboratory Hematology*, 29(4), 261–278. Available at: www.guideline.gov/summary/summary.aspx?view_id=1&doc_id=11992.

64. ANSWER: 3

Triamcinolone is a corticosteroid. Covering the area with an occlusive dressing can result in systemic absorption. The medication should be withheld if signs of infections are present. Creams should be applied to skin surfaces with gloved fingers. The gloves do not need to be sterile. The mother can help to ensure that the cream is applied to all affected areas.

▶ ***Test-taking Tip:*** *Think about the process for applying topical creams and ointments as well as the action of the medication to select the correct option.*

Content Area: Fundamentals; *Category of Health Alteration:* Medication Administration; *Integrated Processes:* Nursing Process Evaluation; *Client Need:* Physiological Integrity/Pharmacological and Parenteral Therapies/Medication Administration; *Cognitive Level:* Application

Reference: Craven, R., & Hirnle, C. (2007). *Fundamentals of Nursing: Human Health and Function* (5th ed., p. 570). Philadelphia: Lippincott Williams & Wilkins.

65. ANSWER: 1

Induction with myelosuppressant therapy lowers the neutrophil count. Children with leukemia most often die of infection. A well-balanced diet, iron-rich foods, and avoiding overexertion are appropriate for treating anemia. A soft diet, using toothettes, and providing frequent saline mouthwash are used to treat stomatitis. Avoiding rectal temperatures and injections, and applying direct, prolonged pressure are more appropriate for preventing hemorrhage.

▶ ***Test-taking Tip:*** *Neutropenia increases the client's risk for infection. Select an option that decreases this risk.*

Content Area: Child Health; *Category of Health Alteration:* Hematological and Oncological Management; *Integrated Processes:* Nursing Process Implementation; *Client Need:* Safe and Effective Care Environment/Safety and Infection Control/Standard Precautions/Transmission-based Precautions/Surgical Asepsis; *Cognitive Level:* Analysis

Reference: Pillitteri, A. (2007). *Maternal & Child Health Nursing: Care of the Childbearing & Childrearing Family* (5th ed., p. 1696). Philadelphia: Lippincott Williams & Wilkins.

66. ANSWER: 1, 2, 3, 4

Multiple specimens should be collected to examine for sperm, semen, and sexually transmitted diseases (STDs). A douche may then be ordered to cleanse the vagina. Emergency contraception is an oral contraceptive medication containing levonorgestrel and ethinyl estradiol and can prevent unwanted pregnancy if taken no later than 72 hours after intercourse. A woman's shelter can help maintain the woman's safety and provide support. The woman should never be left alone in the room. If available in the community, a volunteer from the Rape Victim Companion Program should be called. Notifying security is premature. There is no indication that the estranged husband is trying to access the woman.

Test-taking Tip: Focus on the goals of treating a client of sexual assault: sympathetic support, reducing emotional trauma, gathering evidence, and managing problems.

Content Area: Adult Health; *Category of Health Alteration:* Medical Emergencies; *Integrated Processes:* Nursing Process Planning; *Client Need:* Physiological Integrity/Physiological Adaptation/Medical Emergencies; *Cognitive Level:* Analysis

Reference: Smeltzer, S., Bare, B., Hinkle, J., & Cheever, K. (2008). *Brunner & Suddarth's Textbook of Medical-Surgical Nursing* (11th ed., pp. 2551–2552). Philadelphia: Lippincott Williams & Wilkins.

EBP Reference: Polis, C., Schaffer, K., Blanchard, K., Glasier, A., Harper, C., & Grimes, D. (2007). Advance provision of emergency contraception for pregnancy prevention (full review). *Cochrane Database of Systematic Reviews* 2007, 2, Article no. CD005497. Available at: www.cochrane.org/reviews/en/ab005497.html.

67. ANSWER: 3

Weight is a critical indicator of fluid loss or gain. Clients with CHF are taught to monitor weight daily at the same time using the same scale. Asking about activity level, foods eaten, and whether the client's ankles are different in appearance from the previous day are additional appropriate assessments and will direct necessary client education, but asking about the client's weight is the most appropriate question.

Test-taking Tip: The key word is "initial." Remember that 1 kg (2.2 pounds) is equivalent to 1,000 mL of fluid gain.

Content Area: Adult Health; *Category of Health Alteration:* Altered Fluid and Electrolytes; *Integrated Processes:* Nursing Process Assessment; *Client Need:* Physiological Integrity/Physiological Adaptation/Fluid and Electrolyte Imbalances; *Cognitive Level:* Analysis

Reference: Harkreader, H., Hogan, A., & Thobaben, M. (2007). *Fundamentals of Nursing: Caring and Clinical Judgment* (p. 884). St. Louis, MO: Saunders/Elsevier.

EBP Reference: Michigan Quality Improvement Consortium. (2009). Adults with systolic heart failure. Available at: www.guidelines.gov/summary/summary.aspx?doc_id=13822&nbr=7051

68. ANSWER: 2

The RN should be educating the client and her spouse. Delayed cord clamping is avoided in SGA babies because it increases the amount of blood shifted from the placenta to the infant and may produce polycythemia. Polycythemia is a complication already common in SGA babies because increased red blood cells are a physiological response to in utero chronic hypoxia stress. Polycythemia may contribute to hypoglycemia and hyperbilirubinemia. The other actions are within the LPN scope of practice. Birth asphyxia is a common problem for SGA infants because they have underdeveloped chest muscles and because they are at risk for meconium aspiration due to anoxia during labor. Therefore, many SGA infants require resuscitation at birth. Diminished subcutaneous fat, depletion of brown fat in utero, and a large surface area decrease the ability of SGA babies to conserve heat. A controlled environment is needed to maintain body temperature. Hypoglycemia is the most common metabolic complication of SGA babies due to poor hepatic glycogen stores and inadequate enzymes to activate gluconeogenesis.

Test-taking Tip: Recall the physiological complications of SGA babies. Think about the effects of delayed cord clamping. Consider the scope of practice for the RN and LPN.

Content Area: Childbearing Families; *Category of Health Alteration:* Neonatal and High-Risk Neonatal Management; *Integrated Processes:* Nursing Process Evaluation; *Client Need:* Safe and Effective Care Environment/Management of Care/Supervision; *Cognitive Level:* Analysis

References: Davidson, M., London, M., & Ladewig, P. (2008). *Olds' Maternal-Newborn Nursing & Women's Health Across the Lifespan* (8th ed., pp. 669, 932). Upper Saddle River, NJ: Prentice Hall Health; Pillitteri, A. (2007). *Maternal & Child Health Nursing: Care of the Childbearing & Childrearing Family* (5th ed., p. 758). Philadelphia: Lippincott Williams & Wilkins.

69. ANSWER: 2

The desired outcome of aripiprazole is a reduction in excitable or paranoid behavior. It does not cause sedation or reduce psychotic symptoms or mood swings.

Test-taking Tip: Note that no information is presented in the question suggesting the client has psychotic symptoms, thus eliminate any options pertaining to psychotic symptoms. Review the multiple uses of antipsychotics to select the correct option.

Content Area: Mental Health; *Category of Health Alteration:* Pharmacological and Parenteral Therapies; *Integrated Processes:* Nursing Process Evaluation; *Client Need:* Physiological Integrity/Pharmacological and Parenteral Therapies/Expected Actions or Outcomes; *Cognitive Level:* Analysis

Reference: Deglin, J., & Vallerand, A. (2009). *Davis's Drug Guide for Nurses* (11th ed., pp. 191–192). Philadelphia: F. A. Davis.

EBP Reference: McClellan, J., Kowatch, R., & Findling, R. (2007). Work Group on Quality Issues. Practice parameter for the assessment and treatment of children and adolescents with bipolar disorder. *Journal of the American Academy of Child and Adolescent Psychiatry*, 46(1), 107–125. Available at: www.guideline.gov/summary/summary.aspx?doc_id=10548&nbr=005511&string=bipolar+AND+disorder

70. ANSWER: 3

The nurse should ask the client to return after 30 minutes when the effects of smoking are no longer affecting the blood pressure reading. The nurse does not need to delay the blood pressure reading more than 30 minutes when the effects of nicotine have worn off. Rather than telling the client the ills of smoking, it would be more effective to determine the client's understanding and concerns about smoking.

Test-taking Tip: Read the scenario in the stem carefully. Consider the short-term effects of smoking on blood pressure. Evaluate each response and select option 3, which focuses on obtaining an accurate blood pressure reading on the client.

Content Area: Fundamentals; *Category of Health Alteration:* Basic Care and Comfort; *Integrated Processes:* Nursing Process Planning; *Client Need:* Physiological Integrity/Reduction of Risk Potential/Vital Signs; *Cognitive Level:* Analysis

EBP Reference: Springhouse. (2007). *Best Practices: Evidence-based Nursing Procedures* (2nd ed., p. 28). Philadelphia: Lippincott Williams & Wilkins.

71. ANSWER: 4

People living in close quarters, such as college students, are at a greater risk than the general population for meningococcal meningitis, a life-threatening illness. Meningococcal meningitis presents as flu-like symptoms that last a short period of time, with the subsequent development of a petechial rash. Nuchal rigidity is a significant sign of meningeal irritation. The condition becomes critical in 12 to 48 hours after onset, thus asking if the client has a rash is priority. Asking about liquid intake, a fever, or to explain the symptoms are appropriate, but not the most important question.

Test-taking Tip: The key words are "college student" and "flu-like symptoms."

Content Area: Adult Health; *Category of Health Alteration:* Infectious Disease; *Integrated Processes:* Nursing Process Assessment; *Client Need:* Physiological Integrity/Reduction of Risk/Potential for Alterations in Body Systems; *Cognitive Level:* Application

References: Black, J., & Hokanson Hawks, J. (2009). *Medical-Surgical Nursing: Clinical Management for Positive Outcomes* (8th ed., pp. 1834–1836). St. Louis, MO: Saunders/Elsevier; Ball, J., & Bindler, R. (2006). *Clinical Handbook for Pediatric Nursing* (pp. 334–335). Upper Saddle River, NJ: Pearson Education.

72. ANSWER: 2

LASIK surgery reshapes the cornea to correct the shape of the cornea in clients with refraction errors from myopia, hyperopia, and astigmatism. LASIK surgery does not include the retina, lens, or the flow tract of aqueous humor.

➧ ***Test-taking Tip:*** *The issue of the question is to define what area of the eye is involved with LASIK surgery. Recall the prefix "kerato-" refers to cornea and select option 2.*

Content Area: Adult Health; *Category of Health Alteration:* Integumentary Management and Other Health Alterations; *Integrated Processes:* Teaching and Learning; *Client Need:* Physiological Integrity/Reduction of Risk Potential/Potential for Complications from Surgical Procedures and Health Alterations; *Cognitive Level:* Application

Reference: Ignatavicius, D., & Workman, M. (2006). *Medical-Surgical Nursing: Critical Thinking for Collaborative Care* (5th ed., pp. 1103–1105). St. Louis, MO: Saunders/Elsevier.

EBP Reference: American Academy of Ophthalmology Refractive Management/Intervention Panel. (2007). Refractive errors & refractive surgery. Available at: www.guideline.gov/summary/summary.aspx?doc_id=11754&nbr006058&string=refractive+and+errors.

73. ANSWER: 2, 1, 3, 5, 6, 4

The nurse would first explain the treatment and procedure to the client. A baseline assessment is done before the treatment. Mark the skin and make initial measurements according to manufacturer recommendations. Apply a stocking to protect the skin and complete the application of the device. Monitor the client during the treatment including pain. Reassess the extremity including assessment and measurement and compare to pretreatment status.

➧ ***Test-taking Tip:*** *Focus on the data in the question and then proceed with listing in the steps in completing the treatment. Prioritizing is placing the actions in the correct sequence.*

Content Area: Adult Health; *Category of Health Alteration:* Vascular Management; *Integrated Processes:* Nursing Process Implementation; *Client Need:* Safe and Effective Care Environment/Safety and Infection Control/Safe Use of Equipment; Physiological Integrity/Reduction of Risk Potential/Therapeutic Procedures; *Cognitive Level:* Analysis

Reference: Berman, A., Snyder, S., Kozier, B., & Erb, G. (2008). *Kozier & Erb's Fundamentals of Nursing: Concepts, Process, and Practice* (8th ed., pp. 1417–1418). Upper Saddle River, NJ: Pearson Education.

74. ANSWER: 1, 2, 5, 6

Nurses should always log in with their personal user ID and password before documenting on a medical record and always log out before leaving the computer. Never use another person's computer access. Always make sure the correct client is selected. Nurse B did select the correct client, however, did not log out. A nurse should never have another nurse complete incomplete documentation.

➧ ***Test-taking Tip:*** *Read each option carefully and think about actions that would prevent inappropriate documentation in an EMR. Apply knowledge of using information technology for accurate documentation.*

Content Area: Management of Care; *Category of Health Alteration:* Ethical, Legal, and Safety Issues in Nursing; *Integrated Processes:* Communication and Documentation; *Client Need:* Safe and Effective Care Environment/Management of Care/Information Technology; *Cognitive Level:* Application

Reference: Harkreader, H., Hogan, M., & Thobaben, M. (2007). *Fundamentals of Nursing* (3rd ed., p. 251). St. Louis, MO: Saunders/Elsevier.

75. ANSWER: 2

The oxygen saturation level, 90%, is below a normal level of greater than 95% for a client with normal lung function. Decreasing the oxygen level to a lower level, leaving the client at the same oxygen level, or removing the oxygen may expose the client to tissue hypoxia and inhibit the normal healing process after surgery.

➧ ***Test-taking Tip:*** *Remember the normal oxygen saturation (SpO_2) is greater than 95%. Use this knowledge to eliminate options.*

Content Area: Adult Health; *Category of Health Alteration:* Perioperative Management; *Integrated Processes:* Nursing Process Analysis; *Client Need:* Physiological Integrity/Reduction of Risk Potential/Therapeutic Procedures; *Cognitive Level:* Analysis

Reference: Lewis, S., Heitkemper, M., Dirksen, S., O'Brien, P., & Bucher, L. (2007). *Medical-Surgical Nursing: Assessment and Management of Clinical Problems* (7th ed., pp. 514–515). St. Louis, MO: Mosby.

Illustration Credits

CHAPTER 2

Unnumbered Figure 2-1: Wilkinson, J. & Van Leuven, K. (2007). Fundamentals of Nursing: Theory, Concepts & Applications (Vol. 1). Philadelphia: F. A. Davis.

Test 2

Unnumbered Figures T2-1, T2-2, T2-3: Williams, L. & Hopper, P. (2007). Understanding Medical-Surgical Nursing (3rd ed.). Philadelphia: F. A. Davis.

Unnumbered Figures T2-4, T2-5: Wilkinson, J. & Van Leuven, K. (2007). Fundamentals of Nursing: Thinking & Doing (Vol. 2). Philadelphia: F. A. Davis.

Test 5

Unnumbered Figures T5-1, T5-2: Dillon, P. (2007). Nursing Health Assessment (2nd ed.). Philadelphia: F. A. Davis.

Test 6

Unnumbered Figure T6-1: Wilkinson, J. & Van Leuven, K. (2007). Fundamentals of Nursing: Theory, Concepts & Applications (Vol. 2). Philadelphia: F. A. Davis.

Unnumbered Figures T6-2, T6-3: Nugent, P. & Vitale, B. (2004). Fundamentals Success: A Course Review Applying Critical Thinking to Test Taking (p. 348). Philadelphia: F. A. Davis.

Unnumbered Figure T6-5: Wilkinson, J. & Van Leuven, K. (2007). Fundamentals of Nursing: Theory, Concepts & Applications (Vol. 1). Philadelphia: F. A. Davis.

Test 7

Unnumbered Figures T7-1, T7-2, T7-3: Wilkinson, J. & Van Leuven, K. (2007). Fundamentals of Nursing: Theory, Concepts & Applications (Vol. 2). Philadelphia: F. A. Davis.

Unnumbered Figure T7-4: Wilkinson, J. & Van Leuven, K. (2007). Fundamentals of Nursing: Thinking & Doing (Vol. 2). Philadelphia: F. A. Davis.

Unnumbered Figures T7-5, T7-6: Wilkinson, J. & Van Leuven, K. (2007). Fundamentals of Nursing: Thinking & Doing (Vol. 2). Philadelphia: F. A. Davis.

Test 8

Unnumbered Figures T8-1, T8-2: Dillon, P. (2007). Nursing Health Assessment: A Critical Thinking, Case Studies Approach (2nd ed.). Philadelphia: F. A. Davis.

Unnumbered Figures T8-3, T8-4, T8-5, T8-6: Dillon, P. (2007). Nursing Health Assessment: A Critical Thinking, Case Studies Approach (2nd ed., p. 75-76). Philadelphia: F. A. Davis.

Test 9

Unnumbered Figures T9-1, T9-2, T9-3: Dillon, P. (2007). Nursing Health Assessment: A Critical Thinking, Case Studies Approach (2nd ed.). Philadelphia: F. A. Davis.

Unnumbered Figures T9-5, T9-6: Dillon, P. (2007). Nursing Health Assessment: Clinical Pocket Guide (2nd ed.). Philadelphia: F. A. Davis.

Test 11

Unnumbered Figure T11-1: Ward, S. & Hisley, S. (2009). Maternal-Newborn Nursing: Optimizing Outcomes for Mothers, Children and Newborns. Philadelphia: F. A. Davis.

Test 12

Unnumbered Figures T12-1, T12-2: Dillon, P. (2007). Nursing Health Assessment: Clinical Pocket Guide (2nd ed.). Philadelphia: F. A. Davis.

Test 13

Unnumbered Figures T13-1, T13-2: Dillon, P. (2007). Nursing Health Assessment: Clinical Pocket Guide (2nd ed.). Philadelphia: F. A. Davis.

Test 14

Unnumbered Figures T14-1, T14-2, T14-3, T14-4, T14-5: Dillon, P. (2007). Nursing Health Assessment: Clinical Pocket Guide (2nd ed.). Philadelphia: F. A. Davis.

Test 15

Unnumbered Figures T15-1, T15-2: Myers, E. (2003). RN Notes: Nurses Clinical Pocket Guide (2nd ed.). Philadelphia: F.A. Davis.

Unnumbered Figure T15-3: Jones, S. (2005). ECG Notes: Interpretation and Management Guide. Philadelphia: F. A. Davis.

Test 16

Unnumbered Figures T16-6, T16-7, T16-10: Williams, L. & Hopper, P. (2007). Understanding Medical-Surgical Nursing (3rd ed.). Philadelphia: F. A. Davis.

Unnumbered Figures T16-8, T16-9: Dillon, P. (2007). Nursing Health Assessment: A Critical Thinking, Case Studies Approach (2nd ed.) Philadelphia: F. A. Davis.

Test 17

Unnumbered Figures T17-1, T17-2: Scanlon, V. & Sanders, T. (2007). Essentials of Anatomy & Physiology (5th ed.). Philadelphia: F. A. Davis.

Test 18

Unnumbered Figure T18-1: Scanlon, V. & Sanders, T. (2007). Essentials of Anatomy & Physiology (5th ed.). Philadelphia: F. A. Davis.

Unnumbered Figures T18-2, T18-3: Dillon, P. (2007). Nursing Health Assessment: A Critical Thinking, Case Studies Approach (2nd ed.). Philadelphia: F. A. Davis.

Test 19

Unnumbered Figures T19-1, T19-2: Dillon, P. (2007). Nursing Health Assessment: A Critical Thinking, Case Studies Approach (2nd ed.). Philadelphia: F. A. Davis.

Test 20

Unnumbered Figures T20-1, T20-2, T20-3, T20-4, T20-5, T20-6: Williams, L. & Hopper, P. (2007). Understanding Medical-Surgical Nursing (3rd ed.). Philadelphia: F. A. Davis.

Test 22

Unnumbered Figures T22-1, T22-2, T22-3: Williams, L. & Hopper, P. (2007). Understanding Medical-Surgical Nursing (3rd ed.). Philadelphia: F. A. Davis.

Test 23

Unnumbered Figures T23-1, T23-2: Williams, L. & Hopper, P. (2007). Understanding Medical-Surgical Nursing (3rd ed.). Philadelphia: F. A. Davis.

Test 24

Unnumbered Test 24-1: Dillon, P. (2007). Nursing Health Assessment: A Critical Thinking, Case Studies Approach (2nd ed.). Philadelphia: F. A. Davis.

Test 25

Unnumbered Test 25-1: Wilkinson, J. & Van Leuven, K. (2007). Fundamentals of Nursing: Theory, Concepts & Applications (Vol. 1). Philadelphia: F. A. Davis.

Test 26

Unnumbered Figure T26-1: Dillon, P. (2007). Nursing Health Assessment: A Critical Thinking, Case Studies Approach (2nd ed.). Philadelphia: F. A. Davis.

Test 27

Unnumbered Figures T27-1, T27-2, T27-3, T27-4, T27-5: Dillon, P. (2007). Nursing Health Assessment: A Critical Thinking, Case Studies Approach (2nd ed.). Philadelphia: F. A. Davis.

Unnumbered Figures T27-6, T27-7, T27-8: Phillips, L. (2005). Manual of IV Therapeutics (4th ed.). Philadelphia: F. A. Davis.

Unnumbered Figure T27-9: Williams, L. & Hopper, P. (2007). Understanding Medical-Surgical Nursing (3rd ed.). Philadelphia: F. A. Davis.

Unnumbered Figures T27-10, T27-11, T27-12, T27-13: Dillon, P. (2007). Nursing Health Assessment: A Critical Thinking, Case Studies Approach (2nd ed.). Philadelphia: F. A. Davis.

Test 28

Unnumbered Figures T28-1, T28-2, T28-3, T28-4, T28-5: Dillon, P. (2007). Nursing Health Assessment: A Critical Thinking, Case Studies Approach (2nd ed.). Philadelphia: F. A. Davis.

Test 29

Unnumbered Figures T29-1, T29-2, T29-3, T29-4: Scanlon, V. & Sanders, T. (2007). Essentials of Anatomy & Physiology (5th ed.). Philadelphia: F. A. Davis.

Test 30

Unnumbered Figure T30-1: Gylys, B. A. & Masters, R. M. (2004). Medical Terminology Specialties: A Medical Specialties Approach with Patient Records. Philadelphia: F. A. Davis.

Test 31

Unnumbered Figures T31-1, T31-2: Scanlon, V. & Sanders, T. (2007). Essentials of Anatomy & Physiology (5th ed.). Philadelphia: F. A. Davis.

Test 32

Unnumbered Figures T32-1, T32-2: Wilkinson, J. & Van Leuven, K. (2007). Fundamentals of Nursing: Theory, Concepts & Applications (Vol. 2). Philadelphia: F. A. Davis.

Test 33

Unnumbered Figures T33-1, T33-2: Dillon, P. (2007). Nursing Health Assessment: A Critical Thinking, Case Studies Approach (2nd ed.). Philadelphia: F. A. Davis.

Test 34

Unnumbered Figures T34-1, T34-2: Scanlon, V. C. & Sanders, T. (2007). Essentials of Anatomy and Physiology (5th ed.). Philadelphia: F. A. Davis.

Test 37

Used with permission from Pfizer, Inc.

Test 42

Unnumbered Figures T41, T42: Townsend, M. T. (2005). Psychiatric Mental Health Nursing (4th ed.). Philadelphia: F. A. Davis.

Test 43

Unnumbered Figure T43-3: Substance Abuse and Mental Health Services Administration. (2008). Results from the 2007 National Survey on Drug Use and Health: National Findings (Office of Applied Studies, NSDUH Series H-34, DHHS Publication No. SMA 08-4343). Rockville, MD. http://oas.samhsa.gov/nsduh/2k7nsduh/2k7Results.pdf

Test 44

Unnumbered Figure T46-1: Townsend, M. T. (2008). Essentials of Psychiatric Mental Health Nursing (4th ed.). Philadelphia: F. A. Davis.

Test 46

Unnumbered Figure T46-1: Center for Disease Control.

Unnumbered Figure T46-2: Williams, L. & Hopper, P. (2007). Understanding Medical-Surgical Nursing (3rd ed.). Philadelphia: F. A. Davis.

Test 47

Unnumbered Figure T47-1: Phillips, L. (2005). Manual of IV Therapeutics (4th ed., p. 588). Philadelphia: F. A. Davis.

Unnumbered Figures T47-2, T47-3: Scanlon, V. & Sanders, T. (2007). Essentials of Anatomy & Physiology (5th ed., p. 13). Philadelphia: F. A. Davis.

Unnumbered Figure T47-4: Dillon, P. (2007). Nursing Health Assessment: A Critical Thinking, Case Studies Approach (2nd ed., p. 866). Philadelphia: F. A. Davis.

Test 48

Unnumbered Figures T48-1, T48-2, T48-3, T48-4: Center for Disease Control.

Index

Note: Page numbers followed by t refer to tables; page numbers followed by b refer to boxes.

B

C

D

E

F

N

O

P

Q

R

S

X

Z